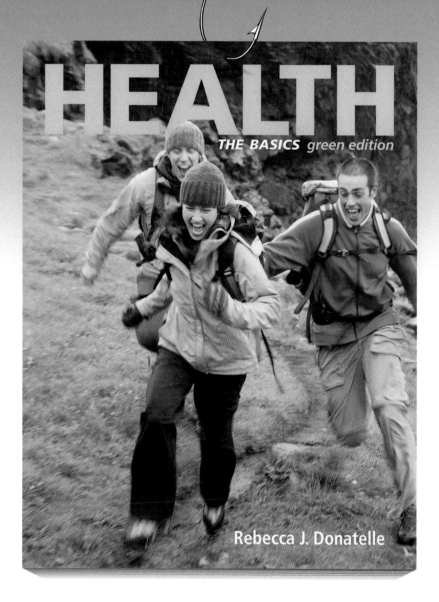

Hook students with exciting new content

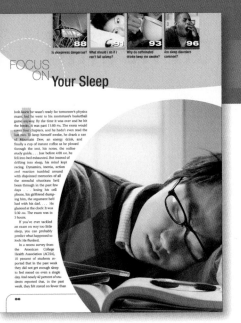

NEW! Four mini **Focus On** chapters address subjects that relate to many aspects of one's health and wellness, but that aren't generally given sufficient coverage in personal health texts.

The "Focus On" chapters cover:

Your Sleep

Your Body Image

Your Risk for Diabetes

Your Spiritual Health

Assess Yourself

Are You Sleeping Well?

myhealthlab

Read each statement below, then circle True of False according to whether or not it applies to you in the current school term.

1. I sometimes doze off in my morning classes. — True False
2. I sometimes doze off in my last class of the day. — True False
3. I go through most of the day feeling tired. — True False
4. I feel drowsy when I'm a passenger in a bus or car. — True False
5. I often fall asleep while reading or studying. — True False
6. I often fall asleep at the computer or watching TV. — True False
7. It usually takes me a long time to fall asleep. — True False
8. My roommate tells me I snore. — True False
9. I wake up frequently throughout the night. — True False
10. I have fallen asleep while driving. — True False

If you answer true more than once, you may be sleep-deprived. Try the strategies in this chapter for getting more or better quality sleep, but if you still experience sleepiness, see your healthcare provider.

Get your students hooked into their own health with mini Focus On chapters and newly designed Assess Yourself and Your Plan for Change boxes.

Assess Yourself self-assessments have been designed individually so that each is unique, fun, and appealing. They encourage students to evaluate their behaviors and health risks, and to pursue their own behavior change projects.

Your Plan for Change now accompanies the self-assessments in each chapter, offering practical, targeted, time-based lists of suggestions for behavior change.

YOUR PLAN FOR CHANGE

This chapter gave you the opportunity to learn why sleep is so important for your health and your academic success, and to compare your typical sleep patterns with the recommendations of experts. Below are some steps you can take to improve your sleep tonight, and by the end of the semester.

Today, you can:

○ Evaluate your behaviors and identify things you're doing that get in the way of a good night's sleep. Develop a plan. What can you do differently starting today?

○ Write a list of personal Dos and Don'ts. For instance: *Do* turn off your cell phone after 11:00 PM. *Don't* drink anything with caffeine after 3:00 PM.

Within the next 2 weeks, you can:

○ Keep a sleep diary, noting not only how many hours of sleep you get each night, but also how you feel and how you function the next day.
○ Arrange your room to promote restful sleep. Remember the "cave": Keep it quiet, cool, and dark, and replace any uncomfortable bedding.

○ Visit your campus health center and ask for more information about getting a good night's sleep.

By the end of the semester, you can:

○ Establish a regular sleep schedule. Get in the habit of going to bed and waking up at the same time, even on weekends.
○ Create a ritual, such as stretching, meditation, light reading, or listening to music, that you follow each night to help your body ease from the activity of the day into restful sleep.
○ If you are still having difficulty sleeping and feel you may have a sleep disorder or an underlying health problem disrupting your sleep, contact your health care provider.

An overhauled art program presents concepts and facts creatively, with a goal of drawing the student into the subject matter. The art uses compelling graphics and photographs to convey health information quickly and clearly, promoting better understanding of the topic while enlivening the study experience.

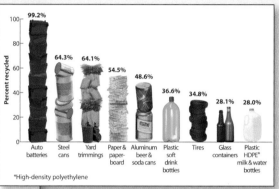

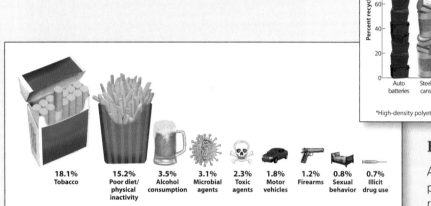

18.1% Tobacco | 15.2% Poor diet/ physical inactivity | 3.5% Alcohol consumption | 3.1% Microbial agents | 2.3% Toxic agents | 1.8% Motor vehicles | 1.2% Firearms | 0.8% Sexual behavior | 0.7% Illicit drug use

How Much Do We Recycle?

Although experts believe that up to 90 percent of our trash is recyclable, our recycling rates for most types of trash fall far short of this goal.

Leading Causes of Preventable Death in the United States

Chronic diseases, unintentional injuries, and intentional injuries are all leading causes of death that are closely linked to these modifiable risk factors and health behaviors.

College Students' Patterns of Alcohol Use

A study by the Harvard School of Public Health found that 44.4 percent of students were binge drinkers, and, of those, 22.8 percent were frequent bingers (people who binge drink three times or more in a 2-week period).

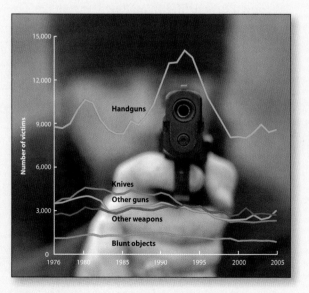

Homicide in the United States by Weapon Type, 1976–2005

Like the homicide rate generally, gun-involved incidents increased sharply in the late 1980s and early 1990s before falling to a low in 1999.

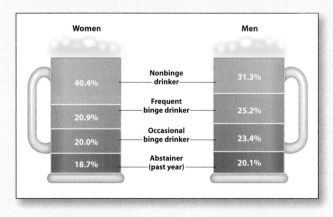

Women | Men
Nonbinge drinker — 40.4% | 31.3%
Frequent binge drinker — 20.9% | 25.2%
Occasional binge drinker — 20.0% | 23.4%
Abstainer (past year) — 18.7% | 20.1%

Get your students **hooked on the environment** with the new Green Edition

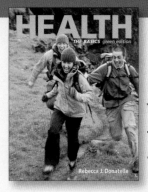

HEALTH
THE BASICS green edition
Rebecca J. Donatelle

What Makes Us Green

The Green Edition is written, produced, and manufactured according to a Green Edition Standard.

- **Printing on recycled paper using soy ink** helps preserve our forest and petroleum resources.

- **Printing this book in the United States** helps to lower the usage of carbon-emitting ship fuel and ensures that strict environmental regulations are applied to its manufacture.

- **Pearson eText** eliminates printing and shipping altogether, and gives students access to the text wherever they have access to the Internet. Pearson eText provides the full text, formatted just as it is in the print edition, with the added benefits of an annotation tool, a zoom feature, and hyperlinks.

- **The Instructor Resource DVD is packaged in a new FSC-certified Eco Pak** that contains no plastic. It has been reduced from five CD-ROMS to one DVD, and now includes transparency masters as PDF files, eliminating the printed acetates entirely.

Green Guide Topics

- Our Planet Needs You!
- Bedding Down in Green
- Old Phones Given New Life
- Greening Your Wedding
- Diaper Dilemma: Cloth or Disposable?
- Clear the Air!
- Bottled Water Boom: Who Pays the Price?
- Toward Sustainable Seafood
- Go Green against Cancer
- Be Eco-Clean and Allergen Free
- Green Goodbyes
- Sustainability on Campus
- Environmental Mindfulness
- Perils of Medical Waste
- Sustainable Supplements

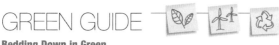

GREEN GUIDE

Bedding Down in Green

We may not lie awake thinking about our bed's impact on the environment, but we can still make healthier and environmentally sound choices through the bedding products we buy. To begin with, ecofriendly choices for most textile products—including sheets and blankets—have become widely available. Organic cotton and bamboo are both gaining popularity, and they offer comfortable advantages.

During the production of conventional cotton, or nonorganic cotton, synthetic pesticides and other environmentally harmful chemicals are used. Conversely, organic cotton reduces global pesticide use and is grown using organic farming techniques, such as crop rotation and biological pest control. These techniques are aimed at producing crops without exhausting the soil or polluting the environment.

After harvest, there are other aspects of nonorganic cotton production that can be environmentally harmful. The conventional cotton industry uses a large number of chemicals including bleach, and petroleum-based dyes. Organic cotton products are typically processed without bleach and use natural dyes.

Bamboo is another useful fiber that has environmental benefits. The use of bamboo fiber in textiles offers a soft fabric from a rapidly renewable resource. Bamboo is actually a type of grass that can grow extremely fast, up to several feet per day! Further, bamboo does not require replanting and helps offset greenhouse gases by absorbing CO_2 from the atmosphere. This plant is naturally resistant to pests and infection, so no pesticides are used in its cultivation, and its natural antibacterial and antifungal properties are an added bonus of using bamboo bedding.

For most people, a mattress is an extremely important purchase: The bed you choose can affect the quality of your rest and can impact your overall health for years. Your choice of mattress can impact the planet's health, too. Synthetic materials used in conventional mattresses, such as polyurethane foam, can emit volatile organic compounds that have been associated with poor respiratory function. Moreover, conventional mattresses are often treated with synthetic chemicals (e.g., formaldehyde, fire retardants, and stain repellants) that are known to "off-gas," affecting indoor air quality and potentially causing future negative health consequences.

More healthful and environmentally responsible mattress materials include organic cotton, wool, and natural latex. Some ecofriendly mattresses combine organic cotton with wool, a natural fire retardant. Wool is also nonabsorbent and, consequently, is less hospitable to microorganisms than more absorbent materials, meaning no antimicrobial chemicals are necessary on wool products.

Similarly, natural latex mattresses and pillows can offer a comfortable night's sleep without the company of mold or bacteria. Natural latex products, derived from the resin of the rubber tree, are hypoallergenic, mold- and mildew-resistant, and breathable. They are also biodegradable and are produced from a renewable resource—rubber trees are not killed or damaged by the process of tapping them for their resin, so they can continue producing resin and contributing to counterbalancing greenhouse gases for years.

With ecofriendly beds and bedding, you can sleep easily knowing that your choices are healthier for you and for the environment, both inside and outside your home.

NEW! Green Guides

What does the environment have to do with personal health? Your students will find out when they read these engaging features! Concrete, informative, and practical, they get students thinking about ways to be both healthy and environmentally responsible.

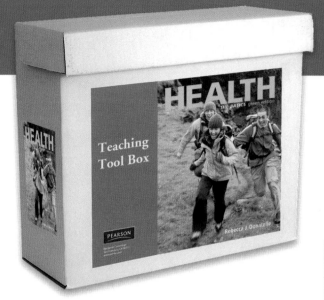

Teaching Tool Box

No matter what your teaching style, the Teaching Tool Box has the resources you need!

978-0-321-66718-2 | 0-321-66718-2

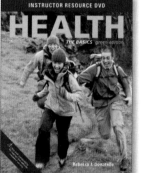

Instructor Resource and Support Manual

Easier to use than a typical instructor's manual, this key guide provides a step-by-step visual walkthrough of all the resources available to you for preparing your lectures. Also included are tips and strategies for new instructors, sample syllabi, and suggestions for integrating MyHealthLab® into your classroom activities and homework assignments.

Instructor Resource DVD

The Instructor Resource DVD includes 30 new *ABC News* Lecture Launcher videos, clicker questions, Quiz Show questions, PowerPoint® lecture outlines, all illustrations and tables from the text, selected photos, and Transparency Masters, as well as Microsoft® Word files for the Instructor Resource and Support Manual and the Test Bank. The DVD also holds the Computerized Test Bank, which includes all the questions from the printed test bank in a format that allows instructors to incorporate these questions into their exams.

Also in the Teaching Tool Box:

- Course-at-a-Glance Quick Reference Guide
- Instructor Access Kit for MyHealthLab
- Printed Test Bank
- *Live Right! Beating Stress in College and Beyond*
- *Eat Right! Healthy Eating in College and Beyond*
- *Behavior Change Log Book and Wellness Journal*
- Take Charge Self-Assessment Worksheets

Great Ideas! Active Ways to Teach Health & Wellness

A resource filled with ideas submitted by other health instructors, this revised manual provides 17 new ideas for classroom activities related to specific health and wellness topics.

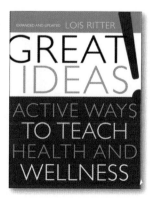

Make **teaching and learning** online easy

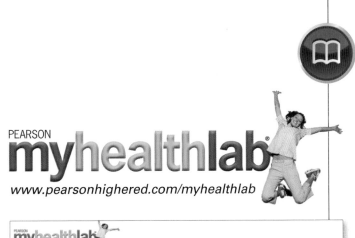

PEARSON
myhealthlab®

www.pearsonhighered.com/myhealthlab

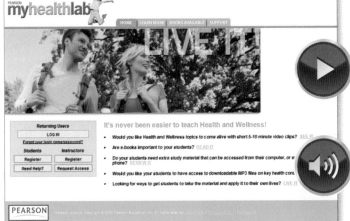

Newly organized by learning areas, and a snap to navigate, MyHealthLab makes it easier than ever to learn about personal health and wellness.

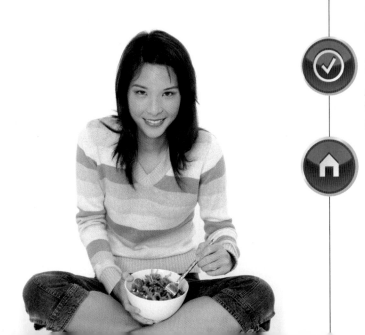

Read It

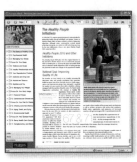

In addition to chapter objectives that direct student learning, this section of MyHealthLab contains the new Pearson eText, a full-featured electronic book. Pearson eText is laid out just like the book, so it is easy and engaging for your students to read, but it also allows them to create notes, highlight text in different colors, create book marks, zoom, click hyperlinked words and phrases to view definitions, and view an animation or visit a website as they read the text. Also available in this section are chapter-specific RSS feeds.

See It

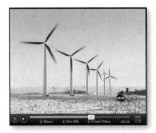

Students can't help but learn when they watch the more than 40 *ABC News* videos, each 5-10 minutes long, about important health topics.

Hear It

MP3 files explain the big picture concepts for each chapter and new audio case studies encourage students to think about real-life health choices.

Do It

Activities related directly to the book's Green Guides encourage students to work on becoming more environmentally healthy, while critical thinking questions, case studies, and weblinks provide further opportunities for student learning.

Review It

An online glossary, flashcards that speak to cell phones, and four types of study quizzes for each chapter mean your students will always be ready come exam time.

Live It

This brand NEW electronic toolkit helps jumpstart your students' behavior change project. More than 30 assessments from the book plus worksheets help your students target the health behaviors they wish to change. The site guides students through planning for change, creating a behavior change contract, journaling and logging their behaviors as they implement change, and preparing a reflection piece to aid in behavior change evaluation.

Outstanding media tools
help you teach and students learn

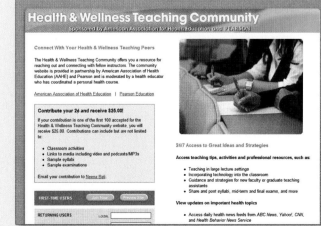

Robust teaching and learning resources keep 'em hooked

For Instructors

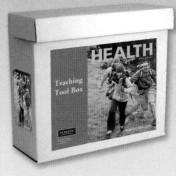

Teaching Tool Box

978-0-321-66718-2
0-321-66718-2

Save hours of valuable planning time with one comprehensive course planning kit. Gathered in one handy box are a wealth of supplements and resources that reinforce key learning from the text and suit virtually any teaching style. The Teaching Tool Box provides all the prepping and lecture tools an instructor needs:

- The Course-at-a-Glance Quick Reference Guide to quickly find resources

- An Instructor Resource DVD including PowerPoint® Lecture Outlines, PRS Clicker Questions, Quiz Show questions, *ABC News* Video Clips, and Transparency Masters to engage students in the classroom

- A MyHealthLab access kit so you can get online quickly

- The Instructor Resource and Support Manual to easily find visual assets

- *Great Ideas! Active Ways to Teach Health and Wellness*

- Printed and Computerized Test Banks

- *Take Charge of Your Health! Worksheets**

- *Behavior Change Log Book and Wellness Journal**

- *Eat Right! Healthy Eating in College and Beyond!**

- *Live Right! Beating Stress in College and Beyond!**

*Student supplements now included for your reference

MyHealthLab®

www.pearsonhighered.com/myhealthlab

WebCT

www.pearsonhighered.com/elearning

BlackBoard

www.pearsonhighered.com/elearning

Companion Website

www.pearsonhighered.com/donatelle

For Students

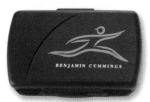

Digital 5-Step Pedometer

978-0-321-51803-3 • 0-321-51803-9

Help students take strides to better health with this pedometer, a first step toward overall health and wellness. This pedometer measures steps, distance (miles), activity time, and calories, and provides a time clock. Available for only $8.50 when packaged with any text.

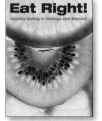

Eat Right! Healthy Eating in College and Beyond

978-0-8053-8288-4 • 0-8053-8288-7

Practical guidelines, tips, shopper's guides, and recipes make this fun booklet the student's best resource for turning healthy eating principles into blueprints for action.

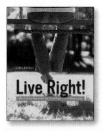

Live Right! Beating Stress in College and Beyond

978-0-321-49149-7 • 0-321-49149-1

College is stressful, but this fun and practical booklet can help. It's filled with useful tips for coping with the stress of classes, relationships, finances and more both during college and throughout life.

Behavior Change Log Book and Wellness Journal

978-0-8053-7844-3 • 0-8053-7844-8

This assessment tool helps students track daily exercise and nutritional intake and create a long-term nutritional and fitness prescription plan.

Take Charge of Your Health! Worksheets

978-0-321-49942-4 • 0-321-49942-5

A total of 50 self-assessment exercises are available as a gummed pad and can be packaged with the text at no additional charge.

Companion Website

www.pearsonhighered.com/donatelle

BEHAVIOR CHANGE CONTRACT

Complete the Assess Yourself questionnaire. After reviewing your results and considering the various factors that influence your decisions, choose a health behavior that you would like to change, starting this quarter or semester. Sign the contract at the bottom to affirm your commitment to making a healthy change and ask a friend to witness it.

My behavior change will be:

_____

My long-term goal for this behavior change is:

_____

These are three obstacles to change (things that I am currently doing or situations that contribute to this behavior or make it harder to change):

1. _____

2. _____

3. _____

The strategies I will use to overcome these obstacles are:

1. _____

2. _____

3. _____

Resources I will use to help me change this behavior include:

a friend/partner/relative: _____

a school-based resource: _____

a community-based resource: _____

a book or reputable website: _____

In order to make my goal more attainable, I have devised these short-term goals:

_____	_____	_____
short-term goal	target date	reward
_____	_____	_____
short-term goal	target date	reward
_____	_____	_____
short-term goal	target date	reward

When I make the long-term behavior change described above, my reward will be:

_____   target date: _____

I intend to make the behavior change described above. I will use the strategies and rewards to achieve the goals that will contribute to a healthy behavior change.

Signed: _____   Witness: _____

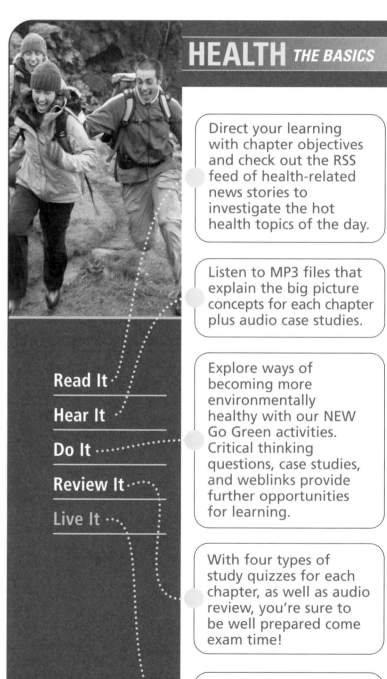

There's more in store!

All of the tools described below are available to you on your companion website at www.pearsonhighered.com/donatelle.

HEALTH *THE BASICS*

Read It
Hear It
Do It
Review It
Live It

Direct your learning with chapter objectives and check out the RSS feed of health-related news stories to investigate the hot health topics of the day.

Listen to MP3 files that explain the big picture concepts for each chapter plus audio case studies.

Explore ways of becoming more environmentally healthy with our NEW Go Green activities. Critical thinking questions, case studies, and weblinks provide further opportunities for learning.

With four types of study quizzes for each chapter, as well as audio review, you're sure to be well prepared come exam time!

Work to improve your health with all of the Behavior Change resources (for more information, flip to the other side).

Become a healthier you!

Access this Behavior Change Contract, and all of the tools you need to change behaviors for the better, at www.pearsonhighered.com/donatelle.

HEALTH *THE BASICS*

Live It

Read It
Hear It
Do It
Review It
Live It

Assess Yourself

Access electronic versions of the self-assessments from your book, along with a host of additional assessments.

Plan Change

Here are all the tools you need to successfully plan for change and fill out a behavior change contract.

Implement Change

Track and log your progress with the tools provided here.

Evaluate Change

How did you do? Here you'll be able to reflect on your journey.

In addition to these healthy behavior change tools, turn to the flip side to see the other valuable resources available online!

BEHAVIOR CHANGE CONTRACT

Complete the Assess Yourself questionnaire. After reviewing your results and considering the various factors that influence your decisions, choose a health behavior that you would like to change, starting this quarter or semester. Sign the contract at the bottom to affirm your commitment to making a healthy change and ask a friend to witness it.

My behavior change will be:

_____

My long-term goal for this behavior change is:

_____

These are three obstacles to change (things that I am currently doing or situations that contribute to this behavior or make it harder to change):

1. _____
2. _____
3. _____

The strategies I will use to overcome these obstacles are:

1. _____
2. _____
3. _____

Resources I will use to help me change this behavior include:

a friend/partner/relative: _____

a school-based resource: _____

a community-based resource: _____

a book or reputable website: _____

In order to make my goal more attainable, I have devised these short-term goals:

short-term goal	target date	reward
short-term goal	target date	reward
short-term goal	target date	reward

When I make the long-term behavior change described above, my reward will be:

_____ target date: _____

I intend to make the behavior change described above. I will use the strategies and rewards to achieve the goals that will contribute to a healthy behavior change.

Signed: _____   Witness: _____

HEALTH
THE BASICS green edition

REBECCA J. DONATELLE
Oregon State University

Benjamin Cummings

Boston   Columbus   Indianapolis   New York   San Francisco   Upper Saddle River
Amsterdam   Cape Town   Dubai   London   Madrid   Milan   Munich   Paris   Montréal   Toronto
Delhi   Mexico City   São Paulo   Sydney   Hong Kong   Seoul   Singapore   Taipei   Tokyo

Senior Acquisitions Editor: Sandra Lindelof
Project Editor: Kari Hopperstead
Development Manager: Barbara Yien
Development Editor: Cheryl Cechvala
Art Development Manager: Laura Southworth
Art Development Editor: Kari Hopperstead
Editorial Assistant: Brianna Paulson
Associate Media Producer: Molly Crowther
Project Editor, Supplements: Katie Cook
Managing Editor: Deborah Cogan
Production Supervisor: Beth Masse

Production Management and Composition: Progressive
    Publishing Alternatives
Senior Photo Editor: Donna Kalal
Interior Designer: Hespenheide Design
Cover Designer: Studio A
Illustrator: Precision Graphics
Photo Researcher: Kristin Piljay
Manufacturing Buyer: Jeff Sargent
Senior Marketing Manager: Neena Bali
Cover Photo Credit: Steve Casimiro

Library of Congress Cataloging-in-Publication Data

Donatelle, Rebecca J., 1950–
   Health : the basics / Rebecca J. Donatelle. — Green ed.
     p. cm.
   Includes index.
   ISBN-13: 978-0-321-62640-0
   ISBN-10: 0-321-62640-0
  1. Health—Textbooks. I. Title.
   RA776.D663 2010
   613—dc22

               2009045020

Planet Friendly Publishing
GREEN EDITION
✔ Made in the United States
✔ Printed on Recycled Paper
   Text: 10%   Cover: 10%
   Learn more: www.greenedition.org

At Pearson Education we're committed to producing books in an earth-friendly manner and to helping our customers make greener choices.

Manufacturing books in the United States ensures compliance with strict environmental laws and eliminates the need for international freight shipping, a major contributor to global air pollution.

And printing on recycled paper helps minimize our consumption of trees, water and fossil fuels. The text of *Health: The Basics*, Green Edition was printed on paper made with 10% post-consumer waste, and the cover was printed on paper made with 10% post-consumer waste. According to Environmental Defense's Paper Calculator, by using this innovative paper instead of conventional papers, we achieved the following environmental benefits:

Trees Saved: 131 • Air Emissions Eliminated: 21,722 pounds
Water Saved: 51,715 gallons • Solid Waste Eliminated: 5,751 pounds

Benjamin Cummings
is an imprint of

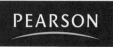

www.pearsonhighered.com

ISBN 10: 0-321-62640-0; ISBN 13: 978-0-321-62640-0 (Student edition)
ISBN 10: 0-321-66727-1; ISBN 13: 978-0-321-66727-4 (Professional copy)
ISBN 10: 0-321-67785-4; ISBN 13: 978-0-321-67785-3 (Books a la carte edition)

1 2 3 4 5 6 7 8 9 10—CRK—11 12 10 09

Manufactured in the United States of America.

Brief Contents

Contents

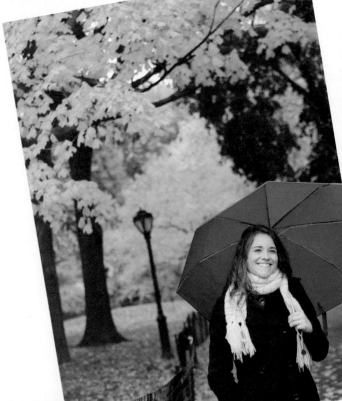

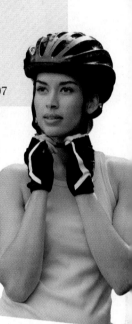

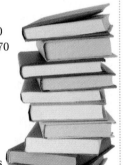

Part Two: Creating Healthy and Caring Relationships

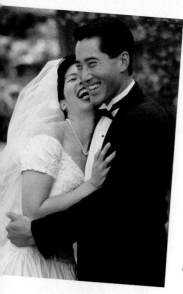

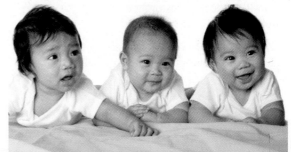

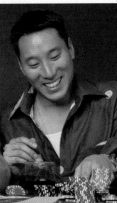

10 Managing Your Weight 288

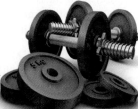

FOCUS ON: Your Body Image 314

11 Personal Fitness 326

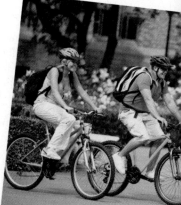

Part Five: Preventing and Fighting Disease

12 Cardiovascular Disease and Cancer   352

FOCUS ON: Your Risk for Diabetes   386

13 Infectious and Noninfectious Conditions   397

Part Six: Facing Life's Challenges

14 Aging, Death, and Dying 432

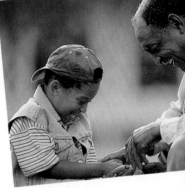

15 Environmental Health 453

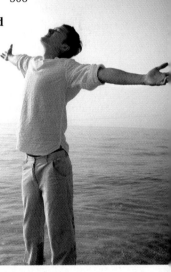

Feature Boxes

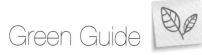
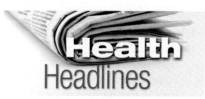

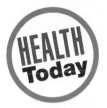
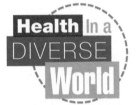
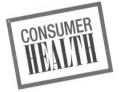
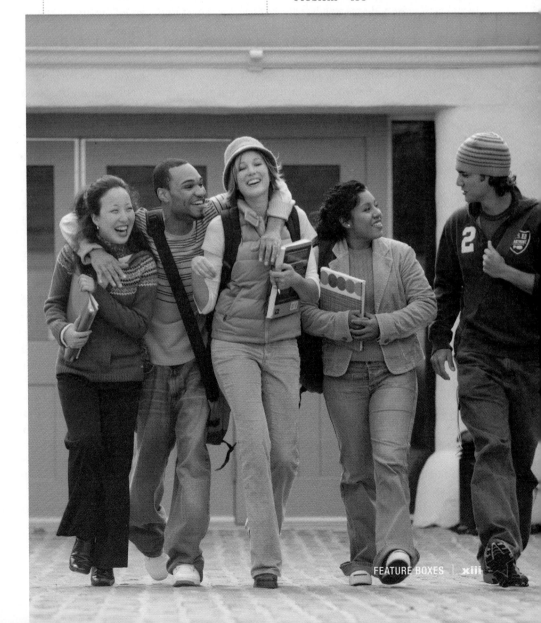

Preface

In today's world, health is headline news. The issues may seem so big, so far-reaching, that you may wonder if there is anything you can do to make a difference; to ensure a life that is healthy and long and a planet that is preserved for future generations. You're not alone! Getting healthy and staying healthy is a challenge for many, but it is not impossible. No matter how old you are, no matter how many health challenges you face, you can make positive changes for a healthier future, you can help others maintain health, and you can become an agent for healthy change in your community.

My goal in writing *Health: The Basics*, Green Edition, is to empower students to identify their health risks, create plans for change, and make healthy lifestyle changes part of their daily routines. This book provides the most scientifically valid information available to help students be smarter in their health decision making, more involved in their personal health, and more active as an advocate for healthy changes in their community. As many of today's health concerns know no geographical boundaries, my aim is to challenge students to think globally as they consider health risks and seek creative solutions to health problems.

Exciting revisions have been made to the art and design of the book in this new edition, with the purpose of capturing students' interest and engaging them in the subject matter. The book is designed to help students quickly grasp the information presented and understand its relevance to their own lives, both now and in the future. In addition, four Focus On chapters have been added to delve into areas of health that are of practical importance to college students but are not always given sufficient coverage in a personal health text: sleep, body image, diabetes risk, and spiritual health.

With this latest edition of *Health: The Basics*, I have endeavored to acknowledge and emphasize the connections between personal health, social health, and environmental health by creating a Green Edition. Global and local environmental health issues are integrated throughout the text, and Green Guide features in the text and accompanying activities on the website encourage students to consider environmental responsibility while improving their health. The creation of the Green Edition involved evaluating the environmental impact of the book itself and developing ways to produce and deliver a more sustainable book and supplements package.

I am gratified by the overwhelming success that *Health: The Basics* has enjoyed through its many revisions and changes. I hope that this edition's rich foundation of scientifically valid information, its wealth of technological tools and resources, and its thought-provoking features will continue to stimulate students to share my enthusiasm for health and to actively engage in health promotion and disease prevention.

New to This Edition

Health: The Basics, Green Edition maintains many features that the text has become known for, while incorporating several major revisions and exciting new features. The most noteworthy changes to the text as a whole include the following:

- **The Green Edition** contains an increased focus on environmental awareness throughout and is manufactured using a green edition standard that includes using recycled paper and soy inks, and printing in the United States to minimize fuel required for transportation and to ensure strict environmental and labor regulation. The Green Edition also has a supplement package that has been modified for greenness through reduction in packaging and a focus on paperless delivery of content.
- **New Green Guide** features encourage students to think about the impact the environment has on their health and to explore ways of reducing their own impact on the environment in order to improve their health and the health of the local and global community.
- **Four new Focus On mini-chapters** address subjects that relate to many aspects of one's health and wellness, but that aren't generally covered sufficiently in personal health texts: Your Sleep, Your Body Image, Your Risk for Diabetes, and Your Spiritual Health.
- **A completely overhauled art program** presents concepts and facts creatively, with a goal of drawing the student into the subject matter. There is more art than ever before, and it uses compelling graphics and photographs to convey health information quickly and clearly, promoting better understanding of the topic while enlivening the study experience.
- **A new, innovative design** "hooks" students into the material through its bold, eye-catching features, including a pulled statistic feature.
- **New Gender & Health boxes** highlight key gender differences in health status, as well as focus on health concerns specific to either men or women.
- **Skills for Behavior Change** features have been revised to present practical checklists of behavior changes students can incorporate into their lives. The book contains more of these helpful boxes than ever.
- **Assess Yourself self-assessments** have been designed individually so that each is unique, fun, and appealing. They encourage students to evaluate their behaviors and health risks, and to pursue their own behavior change projects. The assessments are all available as electronic assignments through MyHealthLab.
- **New Your Plan for Change** sections now accompany the self-assessments in each chapter, offering targeted suggestions

for steps students can take right away, within the next 2 weeks, and by the end of the semester to change their behaviors.

- **MyHealthLab and the Companion Website** have been reorganized by learning areas and now incorporate the new Live It! behavior-change module.
- **An extensively revised media package** includes the reorganized and expanded MyHealthLab and Companion Website; a new Live It! behavior-change module; Pearson eText; an Instructor Resource DVD that contains PowerPoint® lecture slides, 30 new *ABC News* videos, new clicker questions, transparency masters, and the full test bank; as well as a new Health & Wellness Teaching Community site.

Chapter-by-Chapter Revisions

The Green Edition has been updated line by line to provide students with the most current information and references for further exploration. Portions of chapters have been reorganized to improve the flow of topics, while figures, tables, feature boxes, and photos have all been added, improved on, and updated. The following is a chapter-by-chapter listing of some of the most noteworthy changes, updates, and additions.

Chapter 1: The Basics of Healthy Change Revised introduction focuses on the scope and impact of health, the variety of student experience, and the importance of behavior change. New feature boxes discuss health disparities, gender differences in health, and environmental health. Focus on healthy behavior change includes an expanded discussion of the Transtheoretical Model. New table provides statistics on some of the *Healthy People 2010* objectives. New figures illustrate public health achievements of the twentieth century, the wellness continuum, the dimensions of health, leading causes of preventable death, and a sample Behavior Change Contract.

Chapter 2: Psychosocial Health New section and figure describe Maslow's hierarchy of needs. Other new figures illustrate the components of psychosocial health and mental health concerns of college students. New sections cover posttraumatic stress disorder and personality disorders. New table presents information on medications commonly prescribed to treat mental illnesses. New feature boxes explore adult attention deficit/hyperactivity disorder (ADHD) and self-injury.

Chapter 3: Managing Your Stress New sections cover stress and digestive problems, Type C and Type D personalities, downshifting, and procrastination. Revised section on personal sources of stress includes discussion of relationships and living environments. New feature boxes discuss stress-related hair loss and weight gain, positive psychology approaches to stress reduction, and money management. New figures illustrate the physical symptoms of stress, diaphragmatic breathing, and progressive muscle relaxation. A revised self-assessment includes the student stress scale and new stressful "scenarios."

Focus On: Your Sleep ALL NEW Focus On chapter covers the important functions of sleep, mechanics of sleep, sleep needs, ways to improve sleep habits, and sleep disorders. Includes new figures of the sleep cycle, impact of sleep duration, and a sleep diary. New feature boxes include tips for dealing with jet lag, green bedding, and gender differences in sleep disorders. New self-assessment looks at personal sleep habits.

Chapter 4: Preventing Violence and Injury Chapter now begins with a revised section on violence on U.S. campuses. New feature boxes cover gun violence, intimate partner violence against men, donating cell phones to battered women shelters, social networking safety, and noise-induced hearing loss. New figures detail crime rates in the United States and homicide by weapon type. New sections discuss the impact of violence in the media, elder abuse, emotionally abusive relationships, and rape on campus. New section on unintentional injuries covers driving and cycling safety.

Chapter 5: Healthy Relationships and Sexuality A new self-assessment looks at communication skills. New feature boxes cover gender differences in communication, listening skills, green weddings, and tips for ending a relationship. New sections discuss self-esteem as an aspect of communication skills, nonverbal communication, unmet expectations, menstrual problems, and responsible sexual behavior. New tables present parenting styles and types of sexual dysfunction. New figures show the structure of families in the United States, marital status of U.S. adults, healthy versus unhealthy relationship characteristics, and differences in men's and women's communication styles.

Chapter 6: Your Reproductive Choices Revised table shows latest information on effectiveness, sexually transmitted infection (STI) protection, frequency of use, and cost of contraceptive methods. Reorganized text consistently presents the advantages and disadvantages of each contraceptive method. A new section covers choosing a method of contraception. New figures show how to use a female condom, types of contraception used by college students, when women have abortions (in weeks), and changes in a woman's body during pregnancy. New feature boxes cover pregnancy preparation steps for both mothers and fathers, and cloth versus disposable diapers.

Chapter 7: Addiction and Drug Abuse New sections added on compulsive spending, exercise addiction, and technology addiction. A new table provides an overview of the uses and effects of different drugs of abuse. Reorganized coverage of drug dynamics and different classes of drugs includes new sections on how drugs affect the brain, over-the-counter (OTC) drug abuse, prescription drug abuse, and reasons students do and do not use drugs. New sections discuss misuse and abuse of amphetamine-like ADHD drugs, caffeine as a stimulant recreational drug, benzodiazepines and barbiturates, steroid use in U.S. society, treatment and recovery from drug addiction, and harm reduction strategies in public health. New figures illustrate the action of drugs in the brain, reasons college students use drugs, nonmedical use of ADHD drugs, and caffeine content of various products. New feature boxes cover buying medications online and drug abuse among women.

Chapter 8: Alcohol and Tobacco New sections cover the definition of a standard drink, fetal alcohol spectrum disorders, alcohol and prescription drug abuse, reasons college students smoke, nicotine addiction, and the financial benefit of quitting smoking. New figures illustrate college students' patterns of alcohol use, alcohol-related problems among college students, standard drink equivalencies, approximate blood alcohol concentration and accompanying effects, effects of alcohol on the body, smoking trends among college students, and health effects of smoking. In addition to the self-assessment on alcohol use, there is a new self-assessment covering nicotine addiction. New feature boxes discuss women and alcohol use, alcohol and ethnic differences, tips for cutting down on drinking, smoking among women, environmental tobacco policies, and tips for quitting smoking.

Chapter 9: Nutrition and You Expanded water coverage includes discussion of hyponatremia and recommended water consumption amounts. Reorganized discussion of carbohydrates includes new sections on glycemic index and glycemic load. Revised illustrated tables present water-soluble vitamins, fat-soluble vitamins, major minerals, and trace minerals separately. A new self-assessment helps you track and evaluate your food intake. New and revised figures illustrate trends in per capita nutrient consumption, the digestive process, complementary plant proteins, sustainable seafood, interpreting a food label, and MyPyramid. New feature boxes look at global nutrition, environmental impact of bottled water, increasing fiber intake, reducing fat consumption, environmental threats to seafood, health benefits of soy products, making sense of nutrition hype, women's nutrition needs, eating on a budget, and reducing the risk of foodborne illness.

Chapter 10: Managing Your Weight New sections added on youth and body mass index (BMI), as well as general factors contributing to overweight and obesity. Revised coverage of metabolic rates includes discussion of the thermic effect of food, yo-yo dieting, and adaptive thermogenesis. New tables present percent body fat recommendations and analysis of popular diet books. New and revised figures show obesity trends over the past 20 years, health consequences of overweight, BMI, different methods of assessing body composition, and portion comparisons. New feature boxes discuss globesity and sitting behavior.

Focus On: Your Body Image ALL NEW Focus On chapter covers the nature of body image and factors that impact it, body image disorders, explanation of eating disorders and risk factors relating to them, tips for dealing with eating disorders in yourself or in friends, and exercise disorders. New figures depict the body image continuum, the eating issues continuum, health effects of anorexia nervosa, health effects of bulimia nervosa, and the female athlete triad. New feature box offers tips for developing a positive body image. New self-assessment evaluates possible disordered eating.

Chapter 11: Personal Fitness New feature boxes discuss gender differences in exercise, performance-enhancing drugs, evaluating fitness products and services, and active transportation.

Discussion of strength-training expanded to cover variation, reversibility, exercise selection and order, sets and repetitions, and rest periods. New and revised figures illustrate components of physical fitness, health benefits of exercise, and calories burned by different activities. New illustrated tables present forms of resistance training and different exercise equipment.

Chapter 12: Cardiovascular Disease and Cancer New sections discuss peripheral artery disease, cardiometabolic risks, metabolic syndrome, inflammation and C-reactive protein, homocysteine, and stress as a cancer risk factor. New feature boxes cover the warning signs of a stroke, heart healthy "super foods," green actions that can lower cancer risk, breast self-examination, and testicular self-examination. Table of cholesterol levels updated with recommendations from the American Heart Association (AHA); table of cancer screening guidelines updated with the latest from the American Cancer Society. New and revised figures illustrate the prevalence of cardiovascular disease (CVD) in U.S. adults, deaths from CVD, atherosclerosis, metastasis, and breast self-examination. In addition to the self-assessment on cancer risk, there is a new self-assessment covering CVD risk.

Focus On: Your Risk for Diabetes ALL NEW Focus On chapter discusses the different types of diabetes and their prevalence and causes, symptoms and potential complications, treatment and management, and ways to prevent developing pre-diabetes. New figures depict the prevalence of diabetes among U.S. adults, biology of diabetes, complications of diabetes, and blood glucose level tests. New feature box offers tips for reducing diabetes risk. A new self-assessment evaluates personal diabetes risk.

Chapter 13: Infectious and Noninfectious Conditions New discussions cover the inflammatory response, methicillin-resistant staphylococcus aureus, multidrug resistant and extensively drug resistant tuberculosis, tickborne bacterial diseases, and H1N1. Reorganized sections on sexually transmitted diseases consistently present symptoms, complications, diagnosis, and treatment. New figures illustrate the body's defenses, a continuum of risk for sexual behaviors, and the methods of human immunodeficiency virus (HIV) transmission among U.S. men and women. New photos of herpes, human papillomavirus (HPV), gonorrhea, and pubic lice reinforce the reality of infectious disease threats to college students. New feature boxes cover tips for reducing risk of infectious disease, vaccine safety, avoiding flu viruses, practicing safer sex, STI complications in women, the HPV vaccine, HIV/AIDS in women, and using green cleaners to combat allergens.

Chapter 14: Aging, Death, and Dying New text discussions include the aging of the baby boomer generation, effects of aging on the senses, importance of exercise throughout the life span, the *Five Wishes* living will, and palliative care. A new table presents exercise recommendations for adults over age 65 from the American College of Sport Medicine (ACSM) and the AHA. A new figure illustrates the normal effects of aging on the body. New feature boxes discuss osteoporosis, living with grief, and green burial options.

Chapter 15: Environmental Health New sections discuss factors contributing to population growth, different growth rates in different nations, zero population growth, particle pollution, carbon footprint, the Air Quality Index (AQI), and lead as an indoor air pollutant. New tables list U.S. cities with the cleanest and dirtiest air and ten of the most "eco-enlightened" college campuses. New and revised figures illustrate world liquid fuels consumption, the AQI, trash composition, recycling rates, and noise levels. New feature boxes cover tips for environmentally responsible consumerism, ways to eliminate mold in the home, and sustainability on campus.

Focus On: Your Spiritual Health ALL NEW Focus On chapter discusses the nature of spirituality and its distinction from religion, the potential benefits of focusing on spiritual health, and ways to enhance spiritual health. New figures depict the facets of spirituality and the elements of mindfulness. New feature boxes look at cultivating spirituality through service and practicing environmental mindfulness. New self-assessment evaluates spiritual IQ.

Chapter 16: Savvy Health Care Consumerism New sections cover patient rights, prescription and OTC drugs, and the debate over health care reform and national health care. New figures illustrate the OTC medicine label, health care spending in different nations, and health care funds sources and expenditures. A new table looks at common OTC drugs. New feature boxes discuss the placebo effect, evaluating online health information, and the environmental effects of medical waste.

Chapter 17: Complementary and Alternative Medicine New text discussion compares complementary and alternative medicine (CAM) with conventional medicine. A new illustrated table presents common herbal remedies, while another new table shows other common dietary supplements. New figures illustrate the ten most popular forms of CAM in the United States, diseases and conditions for which CAM is most often used, and the four domains of CAM. New feature boxes consider sustainable supplements and CAM and self-care. A new self-assessment looks at how savvy students are regarding CAM consumerism.

Text Features and Learning Aids

Health: The Basics includes the following special features, all of which have been revised and improved upon for this edition:

● **Chapter objectives** summarize the main competencies students will gain from each chapter and alert students to the key concepts.
● **Chapter opener questions** capture students' attention and engage them in what they will be learning. Questions are repeated and answered in photo legends within the chapter.

● **What Do You Think?** critical thinking questions appear throughout the text, encouraging students to pause and reflect on material they have read.
● **Assess Yourself** boxes help students evaluate their health behaviors. The Your Plan for Change section within each box (new to this edition) provides students with targeted suggestions for ways to implement change.
● **Skills for Behavior Change** boxes focus on practical strategies that students can use to improve health or reduce their risks from negative health behaviors.
● **Health Headlines** boxes highlight new discoveries and research, as well as interesting trends in the health field.
● **Health Today** boxes focus attention on specific health and wellness issues that relate to today's college students.
● **Health in a Diverse World** boxes expand discussion of health topics to diverse groups within the United States and around the world.
● **Gender & Health** boxes (new to this edition) help students understand unique aspects of health for both genders.
● **Consumer Health** boxes promote critical-thinking skills and informed consumerism of health-related products.
● **Green Guides** (new to this edition) offer information on how health topics relate to environmental concerns and suggest ways for students to be both healthy and environmentally friendly.
● **A running glossary** in the margins defines terms where students first encounter them, emphasizing and supporting understanding of material.
● The sections at the ends of chapters focus on student application: **Summary** wraps up chapter content, **Pop Quiz** multiple choice questions and **Think about It!** discussion questions encourage students to evaluate and apply new information, **Accessing Your Health on the Internet** and **References** sections offer more opportunities to explore areas of interest.
● **Behavior Change Contracts** for students to fill out are included at the front of the book.

Supplementary Materials

Available with *Health: The Basics*, Green Edition, is a comprehensive set of ancillary materials designed to enhance learning and to facilitate teaching.

Student Supplements

● **MyHealthLab** (www.pearsonhighered.com/myhealthlab). MyHealthLab is newly organized by learning areas. *Read It* houses the new Pearson eText, with which users can create notes, highlight text in different colors, create bookmarks, zoom, click hyperlinked words for definitions, and change page view. Pearson eText also links to associated media files. *See It* includes more than 60 *ABC News* videos on important health topics and the key concepts of each chapter presented in PowerPoint® lecture outline form. *Hear It* contains MP3 files of the big-picture concepts for the text and audio case studies. *Do It* contains activities related to the Green

Guides, critical thinking questions, case studies, and weblinks. *Review It* contains four types of study quizzes for each chapter. *Live It* is a new electronic tool kit designed to help jumpstart students' behavior-change projects with assessments and resources to plan change; students can fill out a Behavior Change Contract, journal and log behaviors, and prepare a reflection piece.

- **Companion Website** (www.pearsonhighered.com/donatelle). This website is organized by learning areas. Students can study chapter objectives (Read It), listen to MP3 clips of main concepts and case studies (Hear It), learn hands-on with selected Green Guide activities plus critical thinking questions (Do It), take practice quizzes (Review It), and access a brand new electronic behavior-change tool kit (Live It).
- *Take Charge of Your Health!* **Worksheets.** This pad of 50 self-assessment activities allows students to further explore their health behaviors.
- *Behavior Change Log Book and Wellness Journal.* This assessment tool helps students track daily exercise and nutritional intake and create a long-term nutrition and fitness prescription plan. It includes Behavior Change Contracts and topics for journal-based activities.
- *Eat Right! Healthy Eating in College and Beyond.* This booklet provides students with practical nutrition guidelines, shopper's guides, and recipes.
- *Live Right! Beating Stress in College and Beyond.* This booklet gives students useful tips for coping with stressful life challenges both during college and for the rest of their lives.
- **Digital 5-Step Pedometer.** Take strides to better health with this pedometer, which measures steps, distance (miles), activity time, and calories, and provides a time clock.
- **MyDietAnalysis** (www.mydietanalysis.com). Powered by ESHA Research, Inc., MyDietAnalysis features a database of nearly 20,000 foods and multiple reports. It allows students to track their diet and activity using up to three profiles, and to generate and submit reports electronically.

Instructor Supplements

A full resource package accompanies *Health: The Basics* to assist the instructor with classroom preparation and presentation.

- **MyHealthLab** (www.pearsonhighered.com/myhealthlab). This tool provides a one-stop spot for accessing a wealth of preloaded content and makes paper-free assigning and grading easier than ever. Instructors can electronically assign the self-assessments to students, who can complete them anonymously and still have their work reflected in the gradebook. Reports on cumulative class responses allow instructors to better target certain issues in lectures. MyHealthLab contains the Pearson eText, which allows for instructor annotation to be shared with the class; includes over 60 *ABC News* videos; and provides robust electronic behavior-change tools.
- *ABC News* **Health and Wellness Lecture Launcher Videos.** Thirty brand-new videos, each 5 to 10 minutes long, help instructors stimulate critical discussion in the class-room. Videos are provided already linked within PowerPoint® lectures and are available separately in large-screen format with optional closed captioning on the Instructor Resource DVD and through MyHealthLab.
- **Instructor Resource DVD.** The Instructor Resource DVD includes 30 new *ABC News* Lecture Launcher videos, clicker questions, Quiz Show questions, PowerPoint® lecture outlines, all illustrations and tables from the text, selected photos, Transparency Masters, as well as Microsoft Word® files for the Instructor Resource and Support Manual and the Test Bank. The DVD also holds the Computerized Test Bank.
- **Teaching Tool Box.** This kit offers all the tools necessary to guide an instructor through the course: Instructor Resource and Support Manual; Test Bank; Instructor Resource DVD with *ABC News* Lecture Launcher videos and Computerized Test Bank; Course-at-a-Glance grid; MyHealthLab Instructor Access Kit; *Great Ideas! Active Ways to Teach Health and Wellness*; *Behavior Change Logbook and Wellness Journal*; *Eat Right!*, *Live Right!*; and *Take Charge of Your Health* worksheets.
- **Course-at-a-Glance Quick Reference Guide.** This supplement is a road map to the Teaching Tool Box. It breaks down all the available resources by chapter and page number. The side for instructors lists assets for use in preparing lectures or while in class. The student side outlines resources to aid in homework or in-class activities. Now printed in a smaller trim size and in a recyclable format.
- **Instructor Resource and Support Manual.** This teaching tool provides chapter summaries and outlines, and a step-by-step visual walkthrough of all the resources available to instructors. It includes information on available PowerPoint® lectures with the accompanying figures and art, integrated *ABC News* Lecture Launcher video discussion questions, tips and strategies for managing large classrooms, ideas for in-class activities, and suggestions for integrating MyHealthLab and MyDietAnalysis into your classroom activities and homework assignments.
- **Test Bank.** The Test Bank is organized around Bloom's Taxonomy, or the Higher Order of Learning, to help instructors create exams that encourage students to think analytically and critically.
- *Great Ideas! Active Ways to Teach Health & Wellness.* This manual provides ideas for classroom activities related to specific health and wellness topics, as well as suggestions for activities that can be adapted to various topics and class sizes.
- *Clickers in the Classroom.* This handbook provides detailed guidance in enhancing lectures using clicker (Classroom Response Systems) technology.
- **Course Management.** In addition to MyHealthLab, WebCT and Blackboard are available. Contact your Benjamin Cummings sales representative for details.
- **Community Website** (www.pearsonhighered.com/healthcommunity). The new Health & Wellness Teaching Community website, sponsored by American Association for Health Education (AAHE) and Pearson, serves instructors by offering teaching tips and ideas, and has a forum for peers to talk to one another about health-related issues.

Acknowledgments

It is hard for me to believe that *Health: The Basics* is in its ninth edition! Since its inception, the health textbook market has undergone remarkable changes. While the text remains the foundation of information, the ability to communicate with students through the Internet and other media provides textbook authors and publishers entirely new and exciting ways of teaching and sharing information. Each step along the way in planning, developing, and marketing a high-quality textbook and supplemental materials requires a tremendous amount of work from many dedicated professionals, and I cannot help but think how fortunate I have been to work with the gifted publishing professionals at Benjamin Cummings. Through time constraints, decision making, and computer meltdowns, this group handled every detail, every obstacle with patience, professionalism, and painstaking attention to detail. From this author's perspective, the personnel personify key aspects of what it takes to be successful in the publishing world: (1) drive and motivation; (2) commitment to excellence; (3) a vibrant, youthful, and enthusiastic approach; and (4) personalities that motivate an author to continually strive to produce market-leading texts.

In particular, credit goes to Ms. Kari Hopperstead, Project Editor *par excellance!* Over nine editions of this text, I have worked with several excellent editors, each of whom represented the best qualities to be found in publishing today. Without a doubt, Kari is among the absolute finest! Under her leadership and guidance this text has been able to develop, become more refined, more cutting edge, and even more accessible to students. She has wonderful instincts about student interests and needs; goes above and beyond the call of duty to see that her books are of high quality; and has a creative, youthful flare in her editorial capacity that is unique. She is truly a gem in the editorial field and a huge asset for me as an author.

Further praise and thanks go to the highly skilled and hardworking, creative, and charismatic Senior Acquisitions Editor Sandra Lindelof, without whose efforts the book could never even get off the ground. In addition, I would like to acknowledge the wonderful contributions of Development Editor Cheryl Cechvala. As a relative newcomer to the book's team, she did a terrific job suggesting organizational change, doing comparative reviews, and merging content and updates with new information and ideas. Overall, she brought a fresh perspective to the work that helped us do the kind of thorough revision that was necessary. This was a huge and complicated task, and Cheryl did an exemplary job.

Although these three women were key contributors to the finished work, there were many other people who worked on this revision of *Health: The Basics*. In particular, I would like to thank Production Supervisor Beth Masse who skillfully navigated production pitfalls and kept the book moving along with grace and good humor. Thanks also to Linda Kern, Crystal Clifton, and the many hardworking staff at Progressive Publishing Alternatives who put everything together to make a polished finished product. Development Editor Laura Bonazzoli played a critical role in crafting the new Focus On mini-chapters, while Holly Smith and the talented artists at Precision Graphics deserve many thanks for making our innovative new art program a reality. Gary Hespenheide and his staff at Hespenheide Design worked wonders in giving the book an exciting and fresh new look, and designer Jana Anderson's cover is a thing of beauty. Project Editor Katie Cook gets major kudos for overseeing the print supplements package, and Molly Crowther, Associate Media Producer, put together our most innovative and comprehensive media supplements package yet. Additional thanks go to the rest of the team at Benjamin Cummings, especially Production Coordinator Philip Minitte, Editorial Assistant Brianna Paulson, Production Supervisor Dorothy Cox, Managing Editor Deborah Cogan, and Development Manager Barbara Yien.

The editorial and production teams are critical to a book's success, but I would be remiss without thanking another key group who ultimately help determine a book's success: the textbook representative and sales group and their leader, Senior Marketing Manager Neena Bali. Neena does a superb job of making sure that *Health: The Basics* gets into instructors' hands and that adopters receive the service they deserve. In keeping with my overall experiences with Benjamin Cummings, the marketing and sales staff are among the best of the best. I am very lucky to have them working with me on this project and want to extend a special thanks to all of them!

Contributors to the Green Edition

Many colleagues, students, and staff members have provided the feedback, reviews, extra time, assistance, and encouragement that have helped me meet the rigorous demands of publishing this book over the years. Whether acting as reviewers, generating new ideas, providing expert commentary, or revising chapters, each of these professionals has added his or her skills to our collective endeavor.

I would like to thank specific contributors to chapters in this edition: As always, I would like to give particular thanks to Dr. Patricia Ketcham (Oregon State University) who has helped with the *Health: The Basics* series since its beginnings. As Associate Director of Health Promotion in Student Health Services on campus, Dr. Ketcham provides a unique perspective on the challenges facing today's students. She contributed to Chapter 6, Your Reproductive Choices; Chapter 7, Addiction and Drug Abuse; Chapter 8, Alcohol and Tobacco; and Chapter 16, Savvy Health Care Consumerism. Dr. Peggy Pederson (Western Oregon State University) completed major revisions of Chapter 2, Psychosocial Health; and Chapter 5, Healthy Relationships and Sexuality. As an associate professor in health promotion and health education, Dr. Pederson provided both her expertise in this area and an engaging writing style that greatly enhanced the quality and presentation of updates to this chapter. Dr. Amy Eyler (St. Louis University) applied her significant expertise and a wealth of teaching and research knowledge to updating Chapter 11, Personal Fitness. Dr. Karen Elliot, assistant professor in the health promotion and health behavior program at Oregon State University, contributed to the revision of Chapter 14, Aging, Death, and Dying, and Chapter 17, Complementary and Alternative Medicine, and provided major updates to the STI and HIV/AIDS sections of Chapter 13.

Thanks also to the talented people who contributed to the supplement package: Daniel Czech (Georgia Southern University), Karen Elliot (Oregon State University), John Kowalczyk (University of Minnesota at Duluth), Bridget Melton (Georgia Southern University), Karen Nein, Teresa Snow (Georgia Institute of Technology), Caile Spear (Boise State University), Natalie Stickney (Georgia Perimeter College),

David Wassmer (Harrisburg Area Community College), Scott Wolf (Southwestern Illinois College), and Lana Zinger (Queensborough Community College).

Reviewers for the Green Edition

With each new edition of *Health: The Basics*, we have built on the combined expertise of many colleagues throughout the country who are dedicated to the education and behavioral changes of students. We thank the many reviewers of the past eight editions of *Health: The Basics* who have made such valuable contributions. For the Green Edition, reviewers who have helped us continue this tradition of excellence include Elizabeth Barrington (San Diego Mesa College), Kimberly Bayer (Sierra College), Carol Biddington (California University of Pennsylvania), Daniel Czech (Georgia Southern University), Carrie Edwards (Cerritos College), James W. Forkum (Sierra College), Guoyuan Huang (University of Southern Indiana), Mary E. Iten (University of Nebraska at Kearney), Cathy Kennedy (Colorado State University), La Tonya D. Lewis (Elizabeth City State University), Kirstin Maanum (New Mexico State University), Tanya J. Morgan (West Chester University of Pennsylvania), Andrea S. Salis (Queensborough Community College), Ann Sebren (Arizona State University), Karen Vail-Smith (East Carolina University), and Brandi Weaver (University of Tennessee at Martin).

Many thanks to all!
Rebecca J. Donatelle, PhD

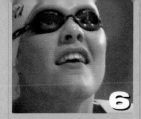

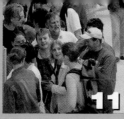

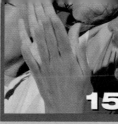

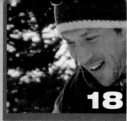

6

11

15

18

What is meant by "quality of life"?

Why should I be concerned about health conditions in other places?

How do my friends and family influence my health?

What can I do to change an unhealthy habit?

The Basics of Healthy Change

1

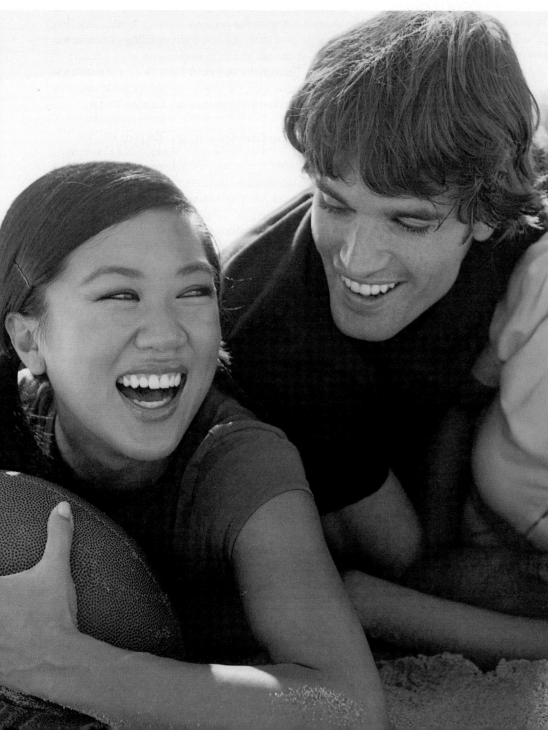

Objectives

✱ Discuss health in terms of its dimensions and historical, current, and future perspectives.

✱ Explain the importance of a healthy lifestyle in preventing premature disease and promoting wellness.

✱ Discuss the health status of Americans and the significance of *Healthy People 2010* and *2020* and other national initiatives to promote health.

✱ Understand the importance of a global perspective on health, and recognize how gender, racial, and cultural backgrounds influence disparities in health status, research, and risk.

✱ Examine your role in protecting global health through adoption of a green lifestyle.

✱ Evaluate sources of health information, particularly the Internet, to determine reliability.

✱ Focus on current risk behaviors, and realize how they can impact your current and future health.

✱ Learn how to apply behavior-change techniques to your own lifestyle.

1

Do you have health on your mind? Do you try to eat nutritious foods and exercise regularly? Do you avoid tobacco and alcohol use? Or do you prefer not to think about your health? Maybe you feel you have plenty of time to worry about it later in life, or maybe you just don't know where to begin. The health habits of college students, be they 19 or 39, vary widely. While many of you engage in less-than-healthy behaviors, many of you also take the opposite track and do your best to improve and maintain good health.

But what does it mean to be in good health? More importantly, do you think that you are healthy? If you feel fine and have no problems conducting your life from day to day, does that mean you enjoy optimal health?

You might be surprised to learn that *health* is much more complex than just the absence of disease. Optimal health habits can lead to a robust and thriving life, while marginal habits can lead to poor health later in life even though you may feel okay now. In addition to the physical health that helps ensure a sound body, your social, intellectual, emotional, environmental, and spiritual health all play a role in maintaining your well-being, and poor health in any of these areas can have negative impacts not just today, but next month, next year, and 20 years from now. Your health is affected by your environment, genetics, and, importantly, your lifestyle, and the choices you make every day help sustain, improve, or destroy it.

health The ever-changing process of achieving individual potential in the physical, social, emotional, mental, spiritual, and environmental dimensions.

wellness The achievement of the highest level of health possible in each of several dimensions.

The good news is that adopting healthy behaviors, while not necessarily easy, does not have to be painful, and achieving behavior change can be a fun and rewarding process. The purpose of this book is to explore the various areas of your life that affect your short- and long-term health. As you learn more about the health effects of specific behaviors, you are encouraged to consider how your actions today will affect you tomorrow, and you will learn how your behaviors also affect the health of the people around you, as well as the health of the planet. In the face of conflicting media messages and pressure from your peers, you have the power to make decisions that lead to better health for yourself, for others, and for the planet.

Putting Your Health in Perspective

Although we use the term **health** almost unconsciously, few people understand the broad scope of the word. For some, health simply means the antithesis of sickness. To others, it means being in good physical shape and able to resist illness. Still others use terms such as **wellness,** or *well-being,* to include a wide array of factors that lead to positive health status. Why do all of these variations exist?

In part, the differences in perception are due to an increasingly enlightened way of viewing health that has taken shape over time. As our understanding of illness has improved, so has our ability to understand what it means to be healthy. Although our current understanding of health has evolved over centuries, we face many challenges in ensuring that everyone has equal opportunities for achieving it.

Health: Yesterday and Today

Prior to the 1800s, if you weren't sick, you were regarded as lucky. When childhood diseases such as diphtheria and deadly epidemics such as bubonic plague, influenza, and cholera killed millions of people, survivors were believed to be of hearty, healthy stock. Not until the late 1800s did researchers recognize that entire populations were victims of environmental factors (such as microorganisms found in contaminated water, air, and human waste) over which they had little control. Public health officials moved swiftly to clean water supplies and enact other policies to help populations at greatest risk. As a result, *health* became synonymous with *good hygiene.*

The twentieth century brought dramatic changes in life expectancy, with continued improvements in sanitation and the development of vaccinations and antibiotics that stopped the spread of many infectious diseases.

Today, scientists recognize that health is much more than the absence of disease. It includes the physical, social, and mental elements of life, as well as environmental, spiritual, emotional, and intellectual dimensions. To be truly healthy, a person must be capable of functioning at an optimal level in each of these areas, as well as interacting with others and the greater environment in a productive and healthy manner. Poor health and unhealthy habits involve and impact all areas of your life, from your relationships to your environment to your academic success (see Figure 1.1). Rather than simply looking at how long we live, or the number of disease-free years we enjoy, public health researchers know that the quality of those years is also

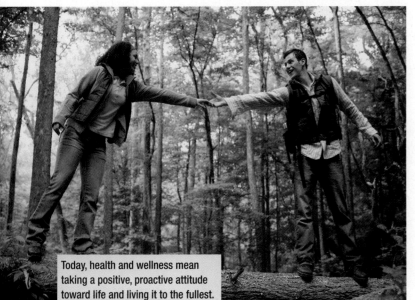

Today, health and wellness mean taking a positive, proactive attitude toward life and living it to the fullest.

vital. Today, *quality of life* is considered as important as years of life. It's not just how long we live, but also how *well* we live.

Improvements to health have not occurred just at the personal level. Over the past 100 years, numerous policies, individual actions, and public services have advanced our health status on a large scale (see **Figure 1.2**). Current **morbidity,** or illness rates, indicate that people are less likely to contract common infectious diseases that devastated previous generations. Today, most childhood diseases are preventable or curable because of improvements in education, socioeconomic conditions, medical technology, vaccinations, and other public health measures. For these reasons, people are now living longer than at any other time in our history. According to **mortality** statistics, the average life expectancy at birth in the United States has risen to 77.8 years (compare this to the average 47-year life expectancy of an individual born in the early 1900s).[1] Although the average life expectancy of Americans as a whole has increased over the past century, our average life expectancy at birth lags behind 49 other countries. Japan and other nations leading the pack have life expectancies of 82 years and higher.[2]

Will this trend continue? A recent study projects that today's newborns will be the first generation to have a lower life expectancy than that of their parents.[3] Largely attributable

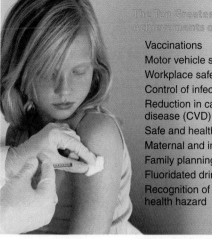

FIGURE 1.2 **The Ten Greatest Public Health Achievements of the Twentieth Century**

Vaccinations
Motor vehicle safety
Workplace safety
Control of infectious diseases
Reduction in cardiovascular disease (CVD) and stroke deaths
Safe and healthy foods
Maternal and infant care
Family planning
Fluoridated drinking water
Recognition of tobacco as a health hazard

Source: Adapted from Centers for Disease Control and Prevention, "Ten Great Public Health Achievements—United States, 1900–1999," *Morbidity and Mortality Weekly Report* 48, no. 12 (April 1999): 241–43.

to the consequences of obesity, researchers report that life expectancy could decline by as much as 5 years over the next few decades.[4] It is also important to note that life expectancy predictions are just an average of the total population and that there continue to be large disparities in life expectancy across different groups according to such factors as gender, race, and income. For example, a baby girl born in the United States in 2005 could expect to live 80.4 years, 5.2 years longer than her male counterpart, whose life expectancy is 75.2 years.[5] (See the **Gender & Health** box on page 4 for more on the differences between men's and women's health status.) According to the same report, the life expectancy for a white girl born in 2005 was 80.8 years, but only 76.3 years for a black girl born the same year; for a white boy born in 2005, life expectancy was 75.7 years versus 69.5 for a black boy born the same year.

morbidity The relative incidence of disease.

mortality The proportion of deaths to population.

The Evolution toward Wellness

René Dubos, a twentieth-century biologist and philosopher, aptly summarized the thinking of his contemporaries by defining health as "a quality of life,

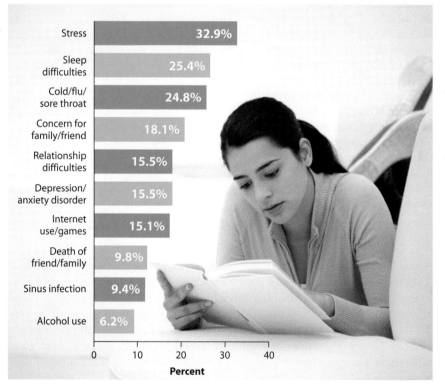

Stress	32.9%
Sleep difficulties	25.4%
Cold/flu/sore throat	24.8%
Concern for family/friend	18.1%
Relationship difficulties	15.5%
Depression/anxiety disorder	15.5%
Internet use/games	15.1%
Death of friend/family	9.8%
Sinus infection	9.4%
Alcohol use	6.2%

0   10   20   30   40
Percent

FIGURE 1.1 **Top Ten Reported Impediments to Academic Performance—Past 12 Months** Your personal health and wellness can affect your academic success. In a recent National College Health Association survey, students indicated specific health problems that prevented them from performing at their best.

Source: Data are from American College Health Association. *American College Health Association—National College Health Assessment (ACHA-NCHA) Web Summary.* 2008. Available at www.acha-ncha.org.

Health: His and Hers

You don't have to be a health expert to know that there are physiological differences between men and women. Though much of the male and female anatomy is identical, researchers are discovering that the same diseases and treatments can affect men and women very differently. Many illnesses—for example, osteoporosis, multiple sclerosis, diabetes, and Alzheimer's disease—are much more common in women, even though rates for these diseases seem to be increasing in men. Why do these differences exist? Is it simply a matter of lifestyle? Clearly it is much more complicated than that. Consider the following:

✳ The size, structure, and function of the brain differ in women and men, particularly in areas that affect mood and behavior and in areas used to perform tasks. Reaction time is slower in women, but accuracy is higher.

✳ Bone mass in women peaks when they are in their twenties; in men, it increases gradually until age 30. At menopause, women lose bone at an accelerated rate, and 80 percent of osteoporosis cases are women.

✳ Women's cardiovascular systems are different in size, shape, and nervous system impulses; women have faster heart rates.

✳ Women's immune systems are stronger than men's, but women are more prone to autoimmune diseases (disorders in which the body attacks its own tissues, such as multiple sclerosis, lupus, and rheumatoid arthritis). Men and women experience pain in different ways and may react to pain medications differently.

Differences do not stop there, according to a report by the Society for Women's Health Research:

✳ When consuming the same amount of alcohol, women have a higher blood alcohol content than men, even allowing for size differences.

✳ Women who smoke are 20 to 70 percent more likely to develop lung cancer than men who smoke the same number of cigarettes.

✳ Women are more likely than men to suffer a second heart attack within 1 year of their first heart attack.

✳ The same drug can cause different reactions and different side effects in women and men—even common drugs such as antihistamines and antibiotics.

✳ Women are two times more likely than men to contract a sexually transmitted infection and are ten times more likely to contract HIV when having unprotected intercourse.

✳ Depression is two to three times more common in women than in men, and women are more likely than men to attempt suicide; however, men are more likely to succeed at suicide.

Surprisingly, although countless disparities in health have long been recognized, researchers largely ignored the unique aspects of women's health until the 1990s, when the National Institutes of Health (NIH) funded a highly publicized 15-year, $625 million study. Known as the Women's Health Initiative (WHI), this study was designed to focus research on the uniqueness of women when it came to drug trials, development of surgical instruments, and other health issues, rather than assuming that women were just like the men who had been studied. This research and the follow-up studies are providing invaluable information about women's health risks and potential strategies for prevention, intervention, and treatment.

Sources: National Heart, Lung and Blood Institute, "News from the Women's Health Initiative: Reducing Total Fat Intake May Have Small Effect on Risk of Breast Cancer, No Effect on Risk of Colorectal Cancer, Heart Disease, or Stroke," NIH News, February 7, 2006, www.nhlbi.nih.gov/new/press/06-02-07.htm; Society for Women's Health Research, "Sex Differences in Cardio/Cerebrovascular Diseases," 2007, www.womenshealthresearch.org/site/PageServer?pagename=hs_facts_cardio; Society for Women's Health Research, "Top Five Women's Health Stories of 2006," 2006, www.womenshealthresearch.org/site/News2?page=NewsArticle&id=6319.

involving social, emotional, mental, spiritual, and biological fitness on the part of the individual, which results from adaptations to the environment."[6] The concept of adaptability, or the ability to successfully cope with life's ups and downs, became a key element of the overall health definition. Eventually the term *wellness* became popular. It included the previously mentioned elements and also implied that there were levels of health within each category. To achieve *high-level wellness,* a person must move progressively higher on a continuum of positive health indicators (see **Figure 1.3**). Those who fail to achieve these levels may move to the illness side of the continuum. Today, the terms *health* and *wellness* are often used interchangeably to mean the dynamic, ever-changing process of trying to achieve one's potential in each

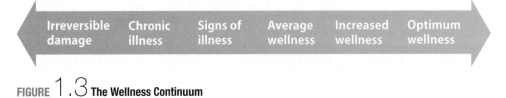

| Irreversible damage | Chronic illness | Signs of illness | Average wellness | Increased wellness | Optimum wellness |

FIGURE 1.3 **The Wellness Continuum**

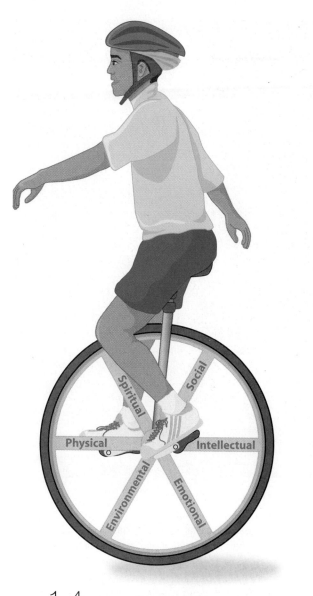

FIGURE 1.4 **The Dimensions of Health**
When all the dimensions are in balance and well developed, they can support your active and thriving lifestyle.

successes and mistakes and making responsible decisions that take into consideration all aspects of a situation.
● *Environmental health* refers to an appreciation of the external environment and the role individuals play to preserve, protect, and improve environmental conditions.
● *Emotional health* refers to the ability to express emotions when they are appropriate, controlling them when they are not, and avoiding expressing them inappropriately. Self-esteem, self-confidence, self-efficacy, trust, love, and many other emotional reactions and responses are all part of emotional health.
● *Spiritual health* involves subscribing to a way of life or a belief in a supreme being based on a particular religious doctrine or feeling of unity with a greater force and a guiding sense of meaning or value in all life. True spiritual health typically goes well beyond an organized religion and includes many more aspects of living a balanced, introspective, and meaningful life.

Although typically not considered a dimension in most wellness continuums, **mental health** is an important concept. Often confused with emotional, social, spiritual, or intellectual health, it is a broader concept that encompasses all of these dimensions. According to the U.S. surgeon general, this umbrella term refers to the "successful performance of mental function,

mental health The thinking part of psychosocial health; includes your values, attitudes, and beliefs.

resulting in productive activities, fulfilling relationships with others, and the ability to adapt to change and cope with adversity. From early childhood until late life, mental health is the springboard of thinking and communication skills, learning, emotional growth, resilience, and self-esteem."[7]
Many people believe that the best way to achieve wellness is to adopt a *holistic* approach, which emphasizes the integration of and balance among mind, body, and spirit. Achieving wellness means attaining the optimal level of wellness for a person's unique limitations and strengths. A physically disabled person may function at his or her optimal level of performance; enjoy satisfying interpersonal relationships; maintain emotional, spiritual, and intellectual health; and have a strong interest in environmental concerns. In contrast, a person who spends hours lifting weights to perfect the size and shape of each muscle but pays little attention to nutrition may look healthy but not have a good balance in all areas of health. Although we often consider physical attractiveness and other external trappings in measuring overall health, these are only two indicators of wellness and indicate little about the other dimensions.

How healthy are you? Complete the **Assess Yourself** at the end of the chapter to gain perspective on your own level of wellness in each dimension.

of several interrelated dimensions, which typically include the following (and are presented in **Figure 1.4**):

● *Physical health* includes characteristics such as body size and shape, sensory acuity and responsiveness, susceptibility to disease and disorders, body functioning, physical fitness, and recuperative abilities. Newer definitions of *physical health* also include our ability to perform normal *activities of daily living (ADLs)*, or those tasks that are necessary to normal existence in today's society.
● *Social health* refers to the ability to have satisfying interpersonal relationships, including interactions with others, adaptation to social situations, and appropriate daily behaviors in society.
● *Intellectual health* refers to the ability to think clearly, reason objectively, analyze critically, and use brain power effectively to meet life's challenges. It means learning from

what do you think?
Based on the wellness dimensions discussed, what are your key strengths in each dimension? ● What are your key deficiencies? ● What one or two things can you do to enhance your strong areas? ● To improve your weaknesses?

The *Healthy People* Initiatives

In 1990, the U.S. surgeon general proposed a national plan for promoting health among individuals and groups. Known as *Healthy People 2000,* the plan outlined a series of long-term objectives. Although many communities worked toward achieving these goals, as a nation we still had a long way to go by the new millennium, when a new plan, *Healthy People 2010,* came into effect.

Healthy People 2010 and Other Initiatives

The *Healthy People 2010* plan took the original initiative to the next level. *Healthy People 2010* is a nationwide program with two broad goals: (1) increase life span and quality of life and (2) eliminate health disparities. Each of these goals has the potential to make real changes in the population's health.

National Goal: Improving Quality of Life

For decades, we have looked at our steadily increasing life expectancy rates and proudly proclaimed that Americans' health has never been better. Recently, however, health organizations and international groups have attempted to quantify the number of years a person lives with a disability or illness, compared with the number of healthy years. The World Health Organization summarizes this concept as **healthy life expectancy.** Simply stated, *healthy life expectancy* refers to the number of years a newborn can expect to live in full health, based on current rates of illness and mortality and also on the quality of their lives. For example, if we could delay the onset of diabetes so that a person didn't develop the disease until he or she was 60 years old, rather than developing it at 30, there would be a dramatic increase in this individual's healthy life expectancy.

healthy life expectancy The number of years a newborn can expect to live in full health, based on current rates of illness and mortality

This new focus on *quality of life* has become increasingly important. By the year 2030, the number of older Americans is expected to reach 71 million, or roughly 20 percent of the U.S. population.[8] Will those Americans continue to be productive or suffer from largely avoidable, disabling chronic diseases? Will the numbers of persons in America disabled by mental illnesses, such as depression and anxiety disorders, or by substance abuse lead to nonproductive and destructive years of life for many? Will people be able to fully realize their dreams for happiness, education, healthy lifestyle, homes, families, and so on,

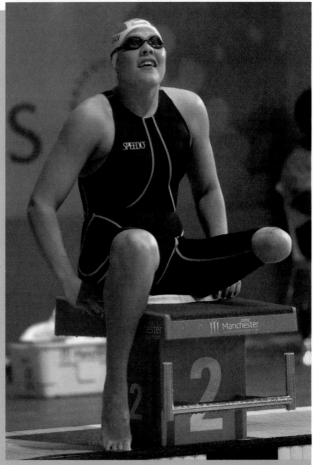

What is meant by "quality of life"?

Health-related quality of life refers to a person's or group's perceived physical and mental health over time. Just because a person has an illness or disability doesn't mean his or her quality of life is necessarily low. The South African swimmer Natalie du Toit lost her leg in a motorcycle accident at the age of 14, but that hasn't prevented her from achieving her goals and a high quality of life. In 2008 she swam in Beijing, the first amputee to qualify for and compete in the Olympic Games.

or will large numbers of them report low quality of life? Concerns over health-related quality of life prompt health professionals to call for policies, programs, and services that emphasize health status, opportunity, and promotion of func-

67 & 71 are the *healthy* life expectancies of men and women, respectively, in the U.S. Note that the average total life expectancies of men and women in the U.S. are 75 and 80, respectively, demonstrating that many people live their last years with significant health problems that affect their quality of life.

tional capacity at all ages and stages of life. A mentally and physically healthy population that can look forward to quality years of life is an important international health priority.

Healthy People 2010 also includes 28 focus areas, each representing a public health priority such as nutrition, tobacco use, substance abuse, access to quality health services, and common health conditions (for example, heart disease and diabetes). Under these focus areas is a list of leading health indicators (LHIs) that spell out specific health issues. For each focus area, the plan presents objectives for the nation to achieve during this decade. For instance, nutrition data show that only 42 percent of Americans aged 20 and older are at

their healthy weight; the *Healthy People 2010* goal is to raise that number to 60 percent. In the focus area of physical activity and fitness, 40 percent of Americans aged 18 and older do not engage in any leisure-time physical activity. The objective is to reduce this number to 20 percent.[9] Table 1.1 lists some of the objectives included in *Healthy People 2010*.

TABLE
1.1

A Sampling of *Healthy People 2010* Objectives

Objective	Baseline Statistic	Target 2010 Goal	Latest Statistic	Progress
Increase the proportion of persons with health insurance	83%	100%	83%*	No change
Increase the proportion of persons who use protective measures that may reduce the risk of skin cancer (e.g., sunscreen of SPF 15 or higher, sun-protective clothing, avoiding artificial sources of UV light)	59%	85%	71%‡	Moved toward target
Increase the proportion of adults with diabetes whose condition has been diagnosed	64%	78%	71%§	Moved toward target
Reduce the number of persons exposed to harmful air pollutants	137,019	0	115,149§	Moved toward target
Improve the nation's air quality by increasing the proportionate use of cleaner alternative fuels	0.8%	8%	2.4%†	Moved toward target
Reduce deaths caused by motor vehicle crashes	14.7 per 100,000 persons	8 per 100,000 persons	14.4 per 100,000 persons†	Moved toward target
Increase percentage of people using safety belts in motor vehicles	69%	92%	82%‡	Moved toward target
Reduce the annual rate of rape or attempted rape	0.9 per 1,000 persons	0.8 per 1,000 persons	0.6 per 1,000 persons*	Exceeded target
Increase the proportion of adults who are at a healthy weight	42%	60%	32%†	Moved away from target
Reduce the proportion of adults who are obese	23%	15%	33%†	Moved away from target
Increase the proportion of persons aged 2 years and older who consume at least three daily servings of vegetables	4%	50%	4%§	No change
Increase the proportion of adults who engage regularly, preferably daily, in moderate physical activity for at least 30 minutes per day	32%	50%	31%*	Moved away from target
Reduce deaths from HIV infection	5.3 deaths per 100,000 persons	0.7 deaths per 100,000 persons	4.0 deaths per 100,000 persons†	Moved toward target
Decrease the rate of binge drinking among college students	39%	20%	41%*	Moved away from target
Reduce proportion of adults who smoke cigarettes	24%	12%	20%*	Moved toward target
Increase the proportion of women smokers who stop smoking during their first trimester of pregnancy	14%	30%	11%‡	Moved away from target
Increase smoke-free and tobacco-free environments in schools, including all school facilities, property, vehicles, and school events	37%	100%	64%†	Moved toward target

*Latest data are from 2007.
†Latest data are from 2006.
‡Latest data are from 2005.
§Latest data are from 2004.

Sources: DATA2010 . . . *The Healthy People* 2010 Database, Centers for Disease Control and Prevention, http://wonder.cdc.gov/data2010/index.htm, updated September 2009; U.S. Department of Health and Human Services, *Healthy People 2010,* 2d ed., with *Understanding and Improving Health and Objectives for Improving Health,* 2 vols. (Washington, DC: U.S. Government Printing Office, November 2000), available at www.health.gov/healthypeople.

As 2010 arrives, health professionals have been taking input and planning for a whole new set of national objectives. Known as *Healthy People 2020*, these objectives are expected to have an even greater emphasis on diverse health needs and healthy disparities among selected populations and should be available soon. This increased focus on disparities is particularly important as we consider the increasingly diverse population in the United States. According to the 2000 U.S. Census, approximately 30 percent of the population currently belongs to a racial or ethnic minority group. It is projected that by the year 2060, non-Hispanic whites will make up less than 50 percent of the U.S. population.[10]

National Goal: Improving Health and Reducing Disparities

Are we making progress? From all indicators, national priorities are shifting, and health professionals and public and private organizations are beginning to work together to help people make better health decisions. For example, cities across the United States are passing legislation that bans *trans* fats from restaurant food items, and a majority of major cities have now gone "smoke-free." More and more states and cities are adopting green policies and programs in an effort to do their part in reducing global warming. Colleges and universities are ramping up their efforts to reduce waste, use less energy, and create more sustainable living environments on campus. These landmark actions and others are designed to improve life span, quality of life, and the state of our environment. On the flip side, there are still disparities in health care. Some populations are at a distinct disadvantage when it comes to getting and staying healthy. For example, if you are a college student without health insurance and are on a limited budget, you may put off visiting the doctor or not go at all. If you have a serious illness, this delay can lower your chance of successful treatment. Factors such as language barriers can also negatively impact an individual's health. Studies have shown that people whose primary language is not English or who cannot read prescription labels or follow written medical instructions have significant barriers to overall health.[11]

Recognizing the changing demographics of the U.S. population and the vast differences in health status based on racial or ethnic background, *Healthy People 2010* included strong language about the importance of reducing **health disparities.**[12] See the **Health in a Diverse World** box for examples of groups that often experience health disparities.

health disparities Differences in the incidence, prevalence, mortality, and burden of diseases and other health conditions among specific population groups.

health promotion Combined educational, organizational, policy, financial, and environmental supports to help people reduce negative health behaviors and promote positive change.

risk behaviors Actions that increase susceptibility to negative health outcomes.

sex The biological and physiological aspects that make an individual male or female.

gender The socially accepted roles and attributes of being male or female.

A New Focus on Health Promotion

The objectives of *Healthy People 2010* and *2020* and other programs are to promote health and to prevent premature disability through social, environmental, policy-related, and community-based programming. In addition, a new emphasis on assisting individuals in their pursuit of specific behavior changes is emerging. Although *change* seems to be a persistent buzzword at all levels of society today, making changes without knowledge, a plan, and appropriate resources is not easy. The term **health promotion** describes the educational, organizational, procedural, environmental, social, and financial supports that help individuals and groups reduce negative health behaviors and promote positive change. Health promotion programs identify healthy people who are engaging in **risk behaviors,** motivate them to change their actions, and provide support to increase chances of success. Effective stop-smoking programs, for instance, don't simply say, "Just do it." Instead, they provide information about possible consequences to smokers and the people they expose to secondhand smoke

46.3 million
Americans do not have health insurance.

(educational support); encourage smokers to participate in smoking cessation classes and allow employees time off to attend or set up buddy systems to help them (organizational support); establish policies governing smokers' behaviors and supporting their decisions to change, such as banning smoking in the workplace and removing cigarettes from vending machines (environmental support); and provide monetary incentives to motivate people to participate (financial support).

Health promotion programs also encourage people with sound health habits to maintain them. By attempting to modify behaviors, increase skills, change attitudes, increase knowledge, influence values, and improve health decision making, health promotion goes well beyond the simple information campaign. By basing services in communities, organizations, schools, and other places where most people spend their time, health promotion programs increase the likelihood of long-term success on the road to health and wellness.

Whether we use the term *health* or *wellness,* we are talking about a person's overall responses to the challenges of living. Occasional dips into the ice cream bucket and other deviations from optimal behavior should not be viewed as major failures. Actually, the ability to recognize that each of us is an imperfect being attempting to adapt in an imperfect world signals individual well-being.

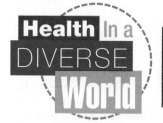

Health In a DIVERSE World

The Challenge of Health Disparities

Among the factors that can affect an individual's ability to attain optimal health are the following:

✳ **Race and ethnicity.** Research indicates dramatic health disparities among people of certain racial and ethnic backgrounds. Socioeconomic differences, stigma based on "minority status," poor access to health care, cultural barriers and beliefs, discrimination, and limited education and employment opportunities can all impact health status. Some groups are also genetically predisposed to certain diseases; for example, sickle cell disease is most common among people of African ancestry, Tay-Sachs disease afflicts people of Eastern European heritage and French Canadians, and multiple sclerosis disproportionately afflicts Caucasians.

Although genes are clearly important to discussions of chronic disease susceptibility, there is considerable debate about the actual role of race and ethnicity in disparity research. One view approaches race as a biologically meaningful category and indicates that racial disparities in health reflect inherited susceptibility to disease. A second view treats race as a proxy for class and views socioeconomic status as the real culprit behind racial disparities. There are other views that combine various theories on why such disparities exist.

✳ **Inadequate health insurance.** A large and growing number of people are *uninsured* or *underinsured.* Those without adequate insurance coverage may face high copayments, high deductibles, or limited care in their area. In the past two decades, numerous health professionals, health-related groups, politicians, and government leaders have sought to address the looming crisis in health care in the United States. The complexity of the topic, the large numbers of special-interest groups that would be affected by any major changes, and concerns over economic and personal impacts of change have made significant progress difficult.

✳ **Sex and gender.** There are numerous instances of tremendous health disparities by **sex** and **gender,** not the least of which is the vast difference in life expectancy between men and women. At all ages and stages of life, men and women experience major differences in rates of disease and disability.

✳ **Lifestyle behaviors.** Persistent poverty may make it difficult to buy healthy food, get enough rest and exercise, cope with stress, and seek preventive medicine. Obesity, smoking, and lack of exercise are examples of health problems related directly to behavioral and cultural patterns we adopt from our families.

✳ **Geographic location/transportation access.** Whether you live in an urban or rural area and have access to public transportation or your own vehicle can have a huge impact on what you choose to eat and your ability to visit the doctor or dentist. Older people, people with disabilities, and people who lack the financial means to travel for preventive tests such as mammograms are clearly at a health disadvantage. In addition, persons who live in rural areas or small communities might not have ready access to high-tech diagnostic and treatment centers or may have difficulty getting referrals to specialists when facing chronic diseases.

✳ **Sexual orientation.** The 5 to 10 percent of Americans who identify themselves as gay, lesbian, bisexual, or transgender experience high levels of health disparities. These individuals may lack social support, are often denied health benefits due to unrecognized marital status, and face unusually high stress levels and stigmatization by other groups. They are also more likely to engage in risky behaviors such as smoking, unprotected sex, and drug and alcohol abuse and report higher levels of depression and suicide in adolescence.

✳ **Disability.** Today, over 50 million Americans, or 1 in 5 people, are living with at least one disability, and most Americans will experience a disability at

Many people in the United States experience several impediments to receiving proper health care, such as geographic isolation, poverty, and lack of health insurance, One of the ways public health officials attempt to address this problem is to organize Remote Area Medical (RAM) clinics. At a clinic like this, rural families, most with little or no insurance, wait in line for hours to receive free health care from hundreds of professional doctors, nurses, dentists, and other health workers.

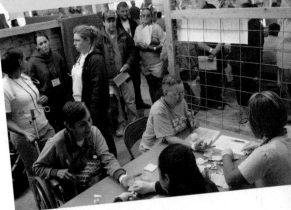

some time in their lives. Although some are easy to recognize, such as a person using a wheelchair, others, such as autism or learning disabilities, are harder to detect. Regardless of the type of disability, problems with major life activities are often present. Disproportionate numbers of disabled individuals lack access to health care services, social support, and community resources that would enhance their quality of life.

Sources: National Institutes of Health, *National Institutes of Health (NIH) Strategic Research Plan and Budget to Reduce and Ultimately Eliminate Health Disparities: Volume 1, Fiscal Years 2002–2006* (Bethesda, MD: National Institutes of Health, May 12, 2006); Centers for Disease Control and Prevention, "People with Disabilities Can Lead Long, Healthy Lives," www.cdc.gov/ Features/Disabilities. Updated October 6, 2008; Centers for Disease Control and Prevention, "Uninsured Americans: Newly Released Health Insurance Statistics," www.cdc.gov/Features/ Uninsured. Updated April 9, 2009; Centers for Disease Control and Prevention, "Lesbian, Gay, Bisexual and Transgender Health," www.cdc.gov/ Features/LGBT. Updated August 7, 2008.

We must also remember to be tolerant of others. Rather than be warriors against pleasure in our zeal to change the health behaviors of others, we need to be supportive, non-judgmental, and helpful to people trying to achieve their own health goals. Ultimately, we all have to find our own best way to make change happen.

Health Status Report: How Are We Doing?

Table 1.2 summarizes the leading causes of death in the United States. Note that adolescents and young adults aged 15 to 24 are most likely to die from unintentional injuries, followed by homicide and suicide. Alcohol is a leading factor in many of these deaths. Unintentional injuries are also the major killer in the next age group, aged 25 to 44, followed by malignant neoplasms (cancer) and heart disease. In 2005, for the first time in U.S. history, cancer replaced cardiovascular disease as the number one cause of death for all persons under the age of 85.[13] When all age groups are included, cardiovascular disease remains the number one cause of death in the United States and worldwide.

In the United States, chronic diseases account for seven of the ten leading causes of death and are linked to preventable lifestyle behaviors such as tobacco use, poor nutrition, and lack of physical activity, all of which can lead to obesity, alcohol use, car crashes, risky sexual behavior, and drug use.[14] Currently, more than half of Americans suffer from one or more chronic diseases at a cost to our economy of over $1 trillion.[15] Many of these diseases are the result of preventable risk behaviors, and with earlier diagnosis and increased attention to reducing risks, billions of dollars could be saved each year. The modifiable behavioral risk factors in Figure 1.5 are the leading causes of preventable disease and death in the United States. By conserva-

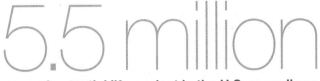

years of potential life are lost in the U.S. annually as a direct result of cigarette smoking.

tive estimates, these preventable risk behaviors affect quality of life for nearly 100 million Americans and account for 70 percent of total medical expenditures.[16] Primary and secondary

TABLE 1.2	Leading Causes of Death in the United States by Age (Years), 2006		
All Ages		**Aged 15–24**	
Diseases of the heart	629,191	Unintentional injuries	15,859
Malignant neoplasms (cancer)	560,102	Homicide	5,596
Cerebrovascular diseases	137,265	Suicide	4,097
Chronic lower respiratory diseases	124,614	Malignant neoplasms	1,643
Unintentional injuries	117,748	Diseases of the heart	1,021
Under 1 Year		**Aged 25–44**	
Congenital anomalies	5,827	Unintentional injuries	30,949
Short gestation or low birth weight	4,841	Malignant neoplasms	17,604
Sudden infant death syndrome	2,145	Diseases of the heart	14,873
Newborn affected by maternal complications	1,694	Suicide	11,240
Unintentional injuries	1,119	Homicide	7,525
Aged 1–4		**Aged 45–64**	
Unintentional injuries	1,591	Malignant neoplasms	151,654
Congenital anomalies	501	Diseases of the heart	101,588
Malignant neoplasms	372	Unintentional injuries	29,505
Homicide	350	Diabetes mellitus	17,012
Diseases of the heart	160	Cerebrovascular diseases	16,779
Aged 5–14		**Aged 65+**	
Unintentional injuries	2,228	Diseases of the heart	510,934
Malignant neoplasms	916	Malignant neoplasms	387,828
Homicide	387	Cerebrovascular diseases	117,284
Congenital anomalies	330	Chronic lower respiratory diseases	107,058
Diseases of the heart	242	Alzheimer's disease	72,135

Source: M. Heron, "Deaths: Preliminary Data for 2006," in *National Vital Statistics Reports* 56, no. 16 (Hyattsville, MD: National Center for Health Statistics, 2008).

FIGURE 1.5 Leading Causes of Preventable Death in the United States

Sources: Data are from A. Mokdad et al., "Actual Causes of Death in the United States, 2000," *Journal of the American Medical Association* 291, no. 10 (2004): 1238–45; A. Mokdad et al., "Actual Causes of Death in the United States, 2000—Correction," *Journal of the American Medical Association* 293, no. 3 (2005).

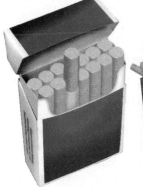 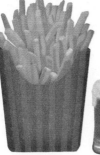 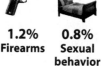 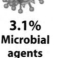

18.1%	15.2%	3.5%	3.1%	2.3%	1.8%	1.2%	0.8%	0.7%
Tobacco	Poor diet/ physical inactivity	Alcohol consumption	Microbial agents	Toxic agents	Motor vehicles	Firearms	Sexual behavior	Illicit drug use

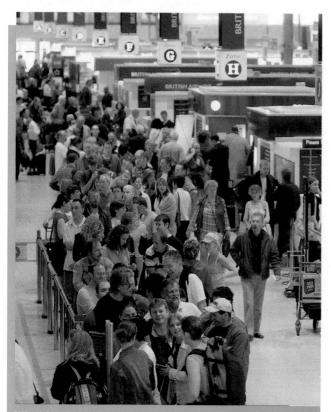

Why should I be concerned about health conditions in other places?

With the rise of global travel, commerce, and communication, we are living in an increasingly global society in which everyone's health and wellness is becoming interdependent. The health status of one nation—the environmental pollutants it produces, the diseases it harbors, even the eating habits it promotes—can impact the health of people in surrounding nations and around the world. For example, infectious disease can spread much more quickly now than in the past. The deadly flu pandemic of 1918 took over 1 year to travel around the globe, whereas people today could transmit illness globally in a matter of weeks.

preventions offer our best hope for reducing the **incidence** and **prevalence** of disease and disability.

Health educators in our schools and communities offer an effective delivery mechanism for prevention and intervention programs. **Certified Health Education Specialists (CHESs)** make up a trained cadre of public health educators with special credentials and competencies in developing prevention programs that offer scientifically and behaviorally sound methods to help individuals and communities increase the likelihood of success in achieving optimal health. These specialists have the skills and experience to greatly enhance the nation's health. A major shift in focus from treatment to prevention is necessary to achieve our national goals.

incidence The number of new cases.
prevalence The number of existing cases.
Certified Health Education Specialist (CHES) Academically trained health educator who has passed a national competency examination for prevention and intervention programming.

what do you think?

Think about your own health right now. On a scale from 1 to 10, with 1 being the lowest and 10 the highest, how would you rate your fitness level? ● Your ability to form and maintain healthy relationships? ● Your ability to cope with daily stressors?

Global Health Issues

Everyone's health is profoundly affected by economic, social, behavioral, scientific, and technological factors. The world economy has become increasingly interconnected and globalized; every day, millions of people move across national borders, leading to many new challenges for health around the world. Current concern over pandemic flu, resistant tuberculosis, and methicillin-resistant *Staphylococcus aureus* (MRSA) as well as the impact of global warming on health status provides a grim reminder for the need for a proactive international response to disease prevention. Health risks are not limited to

GREEN GUIDE

Our Planet Needs You!

The health of our environment has always been important, but today scientists agree that global environmental conditions pose dire threats to all living things. While debate rages over the causes and potential consequences of our environmental health concerns, it's becoming increasingly clear that the nonsustainable practices of an elite cluster of nations—including the United States—are primarily responsible for the severity of the problems we now face. Indeed, according to the Center for Environment and Population, the United States alone is responsible for 25 percent of the world's energy consumption—this in spite of the United States being home to only 5 percent of the global population.

Some of the greatest environmental challenges facing us are

✴ Climate change brought about by greenhouse gas emissions from the burning of fossil fuels in our homes; our factories; our businesses; and, perhaps most devastatingly, our cars, buses, trucks, and airplanes.

✴ Over-reliance on fossil fuels and other nonrenewable energy sources, resulting in pollution and resource depletion.
✴ Exploitation of natural resources and the endangerment of species and habitats resulting from unsustainable fishing, logging, and mining practices; urban expansion; and excess water usage.
✴ Pollution of our land, water, food supply, and air by fossil-fuel emissions, medical waste, electronic waste, toxic wastes, and nonbiodegradable trash.
✴ Deforestation and desertification driven by overpopulation, poverty, nonsustainable farming techniques, and ever-increasing demands for wood and paper products.

As more and more people become aware of these major threats to our environmental health, there has been an increasing recognition of the need to adopt environmentally responsible, or "green," practices in our homes and communities. While the next decade will undoubtedly bring about rapid changes in the cars we drive, the types of energy we develop, and the way

we preserve our natural resources, the real impetus for positive change should start right here, right now, with the actions of individual Americans each and every day.

Throughout this text, we will provide useful suggestions for environmentally responsible changes that you can make as you explore different areas of your own personal health. These include ideas on how to select healthy foods that are produced sustainably, ways to reduce your environmental impact during your leisure time, and tips for locating green health care products. As a start, this text itself is a green product, utilizing recycled paper and environmentally friendly inks at no additional cost to you.

As with all behavior changes, small and incremental changes often reap huge rewards over time. If each of us makes the commitment today and initiates these behaviors for the rest of the term and beyond, it will help move us in the right direction. We hope to challenge you to be the change agent you want others to be.

---

disease—contaminants of food, air, and water supplies; climate change; and chemical toxins are modern health threats to the global community (see the **Green Guide** above).

Likewise, health disparities are not just a national concern. They exist in every nation around the globe. Those nations that lack adequate resources such as food, water, and shelter; have weak economies; or have ongoing political unrest are especially likely to experience extreme health disparities. In developed nations, the leading causes of death are ischemic heart disease, stroke, and chronic obstructive respiratory diseases. In developing nations, leading causes of death are HIV/AIDS, lower-respiratory infections, heart disease, and diarrheal diseases, which are largely a result of a lack of clean water.

what do you think?

What implications do developments in global health have for people living in the United States today? ● What international programs, policies, or services might help control the world's health problems in the next decade? ● Are there actions that individuals can take to help?

Changing Your Health Behaviors

People engage in unhealthy behaviors even when they know these behaviors are risky. In fact, a recent study of the Behavioral Risk Factor Surveillance System (BRFSS) data indicates that only 3 percent of the population adheres to the top four health recommendations.[17] This means that many of us still smoke, avoid exercise, and consume *trans* fats, even though we are bombarded with public health messages that tell us to do otherwise. While we may make resolutions every January 1 to lose weight, stop smoking, exercise more, eat better, and find more friends, usually by January 5 we've given up on these seemingly simple tasks. However, every individual has the potential to adopt healthier habits. The key is to do so one step at a time.

Major factors that influence behavior and behavior-change decisions can be divided into three general categories: predisposing, enabling, and reinforcing.

- **Predisposing factors.** Our life experiences, knowledge, cultural and ethnic heritage, and current beliefs and values are all *predisposing factors* that influence behavior. Factors that may predispose us to certain health conditions include age, sex, race, income, family background, educational background, and access to health care. For example, if your parents smoked, you are 90 percent more likely to start smoking than someone whose parents didn't. If your peers smoke, you are 80 percent more likely to smoke than someone whose friends don't.
- **Enabling factors.** Skills and abilities; physical, emotional, and mental capabilities; community and government priorities and commitment to health; and safe and convenient resources and facilities that make health decisions easy or difficult are *enabling factors.* Positive enablers encourage you to carry through on your intentions to change. Negative enablers work against your intentions to change. For example, if you would like to join a fitness center but discover that the closest one is 4 miles away, closes at 9:00 p.m., and the membership fee is $500, those negative enablers may convince you to stay home. By contrast, if your school's fitness center is two blocks away, stays open until midnight, and offers a special student membership, those positive enablers will probably convince you to join. Identifying positive and negative enabling factors and devising alternative plans when the negative factors outweigh the positive are part of planning for behavior change.

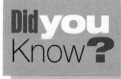

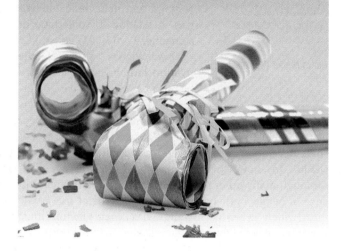

- **Reinforcing factors.** *Reinforcing factors* include the presence or absence of support, encouragement, or discouragement that significant people in your life bring to a situation; employer actions and policies; health provider costs and access; community resources; and access to health education. For example, if you decide to stop smoking and your family and friends continue smoking in your presence, you may be tempted to start smoking again. In other words, your smoking behavior is reinforced. If, however, you are overweight, you lose a few pounds, and all your friends tell you how terrific you look, your positive behavior is reinforced, and you will likely continue your weight-loss plan.

The manner in which you reward or punish yourself in the process of change also plays a role. Accepting small failures and concentrating on your successes can foster further achievements. Berating yourself because you binged on potato chips or haven't found time to use that fitness club membership may create an internal environment in which failure becomes almost inevitable. Telling yourself that you're worth the extra effort and giving yourself a pat on the back for small accomplishments are often overlooked factors in positive behavior change.

Beliefs and Attitudes

We often assume that when rational people realize their behaviors put them at risk, they will change those behaviors and reduce that risk. But this is not necessarily true. Consider the number of health professionals who smoke, consume junk food, and act in other unhealthy ways. They surely know better, but their "knowing" is disconnected from their "doing." Why is this so? Two strong influences on behavior are beliefs and attitudes.

Skills for Behavior Change

How Many of These Healthy Behaviors Do *You* Practice?

* Get a good night's sleep (minimum of 7 hours)
* Maintain healthy eating habits and manage your weight
* Participate in physical recreational activities
* Practice safer sex
* Limit your intake of alcohol and avoid tobacco products
* Schedule regular self-exams and medical checkups

Several other actions may not add years to your life, but they can add significant life to your years:

* Control real and imaginary stressors
* Maintain meaningful relationships with family and friends
* Make time for yourself and be kind to others
* Participate in at least one fun activity each day
* Respect the environment and the people in it
* Consider alternatives when making decisions; view mistakes as learning experiences
* Value each day and make the best of opportunities
* Understand the health care system and use it wisely

A **belief** is an appraisal of the relationship between some object, action, or idea (for example, smoking) and some attribute of that object, action, or idea (for example, "smoking is expensive, dirty, and causes cancer"—or, "smoking is sociable and relaxing"). An **attitude** is a relatively stable set of beliefs, feelings, and behavioral tendencies in relation to something or someone.

Psychologists studying the relationship between beliefs and health behaviors have determined that although beliefs may subtly influence behavior, they may not actually cause people to behave differently. In 1966, psychologist I. Rosenstock developed a classic theory, the **Health Belief Model (HBM),** to show when beliefs affect behavior change.[18] Although many other models attempt to explain the influence of beliefs on behaviors, the HBM remains one of the most widely accepted. It holds that several factors must support a belief before change is likely:

- **Perceived seriousness of the health problem.** How severe would the medical and social consequences be if the health problem was to develop or be left untreated? The more serious the perceived effects, the more likely that action will be taken.
- **Perceived susceptibility to the health problem.** What is the likelihood of developing the health problem? People who perceive themselves at high risk are more likely to take preventive action.

- **Cues to action.** A person who is reminded or alerted about a potential health problem is more likely to take action. For example, having your doctor tell you that your blood sugar levels indicate a pre-diabetic state may be the cue that pushes you to lose weight and exercise.

People follow the Health Belief Model many times every day. Take, for example, smokers. Older smokers are likely to know other smokers who have developed serious heart or lung problems. They are thus more likely to perceive tobacco as a threat to their health than are teenagers who have just begun smoking. The greater the perceived threat of health problems caused by smoking, the greater the chance a person will quit.

However, many chronic smokers know the risks yet continue to smoke. Why do they miss these cues to action? According to Rosenstock, some people do not believe they will be affected by a severe problem—they act as though they are immune to it—and are unlikely to change their behavior. They also may feel that the immediate pleasure outweighs the long-range cost.

Our attitudes tend to reflect our emotional responses to situations and follow from our beliefs. The more consistent your attitude is toward an action and the more you are influenced by others to take that action, the more likely you are to be motivated to change the behavior and to ultimately succeed in doing so. The key is being able to recognize potential barriers that you may face as you try modifying your behaviors. Figure 1.6 lists some of the common barriers people encounter when trying to make behavior change and some suggested ways to overcome them.

belief Appraisal of the relationship between some object, action, or idea and some attribute of that object, action, or idea.

attitude Relatively stable set of beliefs, feelings, and behavioral tendencies in relation to something or someone.

Health Belief Model (HBM) Model for explaining how beliefs may influence health behaviors.

If you think... then	try this strategy...
"I don't have enough time"	Chart your hourly activities for 1 day. What are your highest priorities? What can you eliminate? Plan to make some time for a healthy change next week.
"I'm too stressed"	Assess your major stressors right now. List those you can control and those you can change or avoid. Then identify two things you enjoy that can help you reduce stress now.
"I worry about what others may think"	Ask yourself how much others influence your decisions about drinking, sex, eating habits, etc. What is most important to you? What actions can you take to act in line with these values?
"I don't think I can do it"	Just because you haven't before doesn't mean you can't now. To develop some confidence, take baby steps and break tasks into small pieces.
"It's a habit I can't break"	Habits are difficult to break but not impossible. What triggers your behavior? List ways you can avoid these triggers. Ask for support from friends and family.

FIGURE 1.6 **Common Barriers to Behavior Change**
There are several types of obstacles that can make it difficult to succeed in making a behavior change. Each strategy shown can help overcome these obstacles.

Source: From D. L. Watson and R. G. Tharp, *Self-Directed Behavior: Self-Modification for Personal Adjustment.* 9th ed. © 2007 Reprinted with permission of Wadsworth Publishing, a division of Cengage Learning.

Self-Efficacy

Self-efficacy—an individual's belief that he or she is capable of achieving certain goals or of performing at a level that may influence events in life—is one of the most important factors that influence our health status. People who have it are more likely to take action to improve their health, stick to their plan of action, and experiment with other options for making improvements. In general, people who exhibit high self-efficacy are confident that they can succeed, and they approach challenges with a positive attitude. Prior success in academics, athletics, or social interactions will lead to expectations of success in the future. Self-efficacious people are more likely to feel a sense of personal control over situations. People who approach challenges, such as changing an unhealthy behavior, with confidence (that "I can do it" mentality) may be more motivated to change and achieve a greater level of success.

On the other hand, someone with low self-efficacy or with self-doubts about what they can and cannot do may give up easily or never even try to change a behavior. These people tend to shy away from difficult challenges. They may have failed before, and when the going gets tough, they are more likely to give up or revert to old patterns of behavior.

External versus Internal Locus of Control

The conviction that you have the power and ability to change is a powerful motivator. Individuals who feel that they have limited control over their lives often find it more difficult to initiate positive changes.[19] If they believe that someone or something else controls a situation or that they dare not act in a particular way because of peer repercussions, they may become easily frustrated and give up. People with these characteristics have an *external* **locus of control.** In contrast, people who have a stronger *internal* locus of control believe they have power over their own actions. They are more driven by their own thoughts and are more likely to state their opinions and be true to their own beliefs.

Having an internal or external locus of control can vary according to circumstance. For instance, someone who finds out that diabetes runs in their family may resign himself to one day facing the disease, instead of taking an active role in modifying his lifestyle to minimize his risk of developing diabetes. On this front, he would be demonstrating an external locus of control. However, the same individual might exhibit an internal locus of control when being pressured by friends to smoke. He knows that he does not want to smoke and does not want to risk the potential consequences of the habit, so he takes charge and resists the pressure. In general, developing and maintaining an internal locus of control can help you take charge of your health behaviors.

what do you think?

In general, do you have an internal or an external locus of control? ● Can you describe a situation where you demonstrated an internal locus of control? ● Can you think of some good friends who you'd describe as more internally controlled? Externally controlled? How have you seen these demonstrated?

Significant Others as Change Agents

Many of us are highly influenced by the approval or disapproval (real or imagined) of close friends, loved ones, and the social and cultural groups to which we belong. Such influences can support healthy behavior, or they can interfere with even the best intentions.

Your Family From the time of your birth, your parents and other family members have given you strong cues about which actions are and are not socially acceptable. Brushing your teeth, bathing, and chewing food with your mouth closed are behaviors that your family probably instilled in you long ago. Your family and local culture influenced your food choices, your religious beliefs, your political beliefs, and many of your other values and actions. If you deviated from your family's norms, a family member probably let you know fairly quickly. Strong and positive family units provide care, trust, and protection; are dedicated to the healthful development of all family members; and work to reduce problems.

self-efficacy Belief in one's ability to perform a task successfully.
locus of control The "location," *external* (outside oneself) or *internal* (within oneself), an individual perceives as the source and underlying cause of events in his or her life.

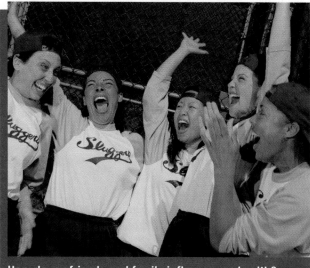

How do my friends and family influence my health?

The people in your life can play a huge role—both positive and negative—in the health choices you make. The behaviors of those around you can predispose you to certain health habits, at the same time enabling and reinforcing them. Seeking out the support and encouragement of friends who have similar goals and interests will strengthen your commitment to develop and maintain positive health behaviors.

When the loving family unit does not exist or when it does not provide for basic human needs, it becomes difficult for a child to learn positive health behaviors. Often, healthy behaviors get their start in healthy homes; unhealthy homes breed unhealthy habits. Healthy families provide the foundation for a clear and necessary understanding of what is right and wrong, what is positive and negative. Without this fundamental grounding, many young people have great difficulties.

Social Bonds and the Influence of Others Just as your family influences your actions during your childhood, your friends and significant others influence your behaviors as you grow older. Most of us desire to fit the "norm" and avoid hassles in our daily interactions with others. If you deviate from the actions expected in your hometown or among your friends, you may suffer ostracism, strange looks, and other negative social consequences. Understanding the subtle and not-so-subtle ways in which other people influence our actions is an important step toward changing our behaviors.

Transtheoretical Model of Health Behavior Change (Stages of Change model) Model of behavior change that identifies six distinct stages people go through in altering behavior patterns.

The influence of others serves as a powerful *social support* for positive change. If friends offer encouragement (subjective norms), for example, by becoming "workout buddies," you are more likely to remain motivated to change your behavior. However, if you believe your friends will think you are a "nerd" for going to the gym, you may quickly lose your motivation. The importance of cultivating and maintaining close *social bonds* with others is an important part of overall health. Finding friends who share your personal values can greatly affect your behaviors. The key people in our lives play a powerful role in our motivation to change for the better—or for the worse.

Motivation and Readiness to Change

On any given morning, many of us get out of bed and resolve to change a given behavior that day. Whether it be losing weight, drinking less, exercising more, being nicer to others, managing time better, or some other change, we start out with enthusiasm and high expectations. However, a vast majority of people return to their old behavior. Wanting to change is a prerequisite of the change process, but there is much more to the process than motivation. *Motivation* must be combined with common sense, commitment, and a realistic

understanding of how best to move from point A to point B. *Readiness* is the state of being that precedes behavior change, and those who are ready are likely to make the actual effort. People who are ready to change possess the attitudes, knowledge, skills, and internal and external resources that make change possible.[20]

Why do so many good intentions fail? According to Dr. James Prochaska of the University of Rhode Island and Dr. Carlos DiClemente of the University of Maryland, it's because we are going about things in the wrong way; fewer than 20 percent of us are really prepared to take action. After considerable research, they have concluded that behavior changes usually do not succeed if they start with the change itself. Instead, we must go through a series of stages to adequately prepare ourselves for that eventual change.[21] According to Prochaska and DiClemente's **Transtheoretical Model of Health Behavior Change** (also called the **Stages of Change model**), our chances of keeping those New Year's resolutions will be greatly enhanced if we have proper reinforcement and help during each of the following stages.

1. Precontemplation. People in the precontemplation stage have no current intention of changing. They may have tried to change a behavior before and given up, or they may be in denial and unaware of any problem. Sometimes a few frank yet kind words from friends may be enough to make precontemplators take a closer look at themselves. Recommending readings or making tactful suggestions can be useful in helping precontemplators consider making a change.

2. Contemplation. In this phase, people recognize that they have a problem and begin to contemplate the need to change. Acknowledgment usually results from increased awareness, often due to feedback from family and friends or access to information. Despite this acknowledgment, people can languish in this stage for years, realizing that they have a problem but lacking the time or energy to make the change.

Often, contemplators need a little push to get them started. This may come in the form of someone helping them set up a change plan (for example, an exercise routine), buying a helpful gift (such as a low-fat cookbook), sharing articles about a particular problem, or inviting them to go hear a speaker on a related topic. See the **Consumer Health** box on page 19 for tips on using the Internet to gather valuable health information.

3. Preparation. Most people at this point are close to taking action. They've thought about what they might do and may even have come up with a plan. Rather than thinking about why they can't begin, they have started to focus on what they can do.

There are some standard guidelines to follow when you are preparing for change. Set realistic goals (large and small), take small steps toward change, change only a couple of things at once, reward small milestones, and seek support from friends. Identify factors that have enabled or obstructed success in the past, and modify them where possible. Complete a Behavior Change Contract to help you commit to making these changes.

4. Action. In this stage, people begin to follow their action plans. Those who have prepared for change, thought about alternatives, engaged social support, and made a plan of action are more ready for action than those who have given it little thought. Unfortunately, too many people start behavior change here rather than going through the first three stages. Without a plan, without enlisting the help of others, or without a realistic goal, failure is likely.

Publicly stating the desire to change helps ensure success. Encourage friends who are making a change to share their plans with you. Offer to help, and try to remove potential obstacles from the person's intended action plan. Social support and the buddy system can motivate even the most reluctant person.

5. Maintenance. Maintenance requires vigilance, attention to detail, and long-term commitment. Many people reach a goal, only to relax and slip back into the undesired behavior. In this stage, it is important to be aware of the potential for relapses and to develop strategies for dealing with such challenges. Common causes of relapse include overconfidence, daily temptations, stress or emotional distractions, and self-deprecation.

During maintenance, continue taking the same actions that led to success in the first place. Find fun and creative ways to maintain positive behaviors. This is where a willing and caring support group can be vital. Knowing where on your campus to turn for help when you don't have a close support network is also helpful.

6. Termination. By this point, the behavior is so ingrained that the current level of vigilance may be unnecessary. The new behavior has become an essential part of daily living. Do you know someone who has made a major behavior change that has now become an essential part of that person's life?

Choosing a Behavior-Change Technique

Once you have analyzed all the factors that influence your behaviors, consider what actions you can take to change the negative ones. Behavior-change techniques include shaping, visualization, modeling, controlling the situation, reinforcement, and changing self-talk. The options don't stop here, but these are the most common strategies.

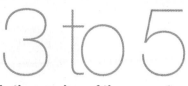

is the number of times most people will attempt to change an unhealthy behavior before succeeding.

Shaping

Regardless of how motivated you are, some behaviors are almost impossible to change immediately. To reach your goal, you may need to take a number of individual steps, each designed to change one small piece of the larger behavior. This process is known as **shaping.**

For example, suppose that you have not exercised for a while. You decide that you want to get into shape, and your goal is to jog 3 miles every other day. But you realize that you'd face a near-death experience if you tried to run even a few blocks in your current condition. So you decide to build up to your desired fitness level gradually. During week 1, you will walk for 1 hour every other day at a slow, relaxed pace. During week 2, you will walk for the same amount of time but speed up your pace and cover slightly more ground. During week 3, you will speed up even more and try to go even farther. You will continue taking such steps until you reach your goal.

Whatever the desired behavior change, all shaping involves the following actions:

- Start slowly, and try not to cause undue stress during the early stages of the program.
- Keep the steps small and achievable.
- Be flexible. If the original plan proves uncomfortable or you deviate from it, don't give up! Start again, and move forward.
- Don't skip steps or move to the next step until you have mastered the previous one.
- Reward yourself for meeting regular, previously-set goals.

Remember, behaviors don't develop overnight, so they won't change overnight.

Visualization

Mental practice can transform unhealthy behaviors into healthy ones. Athletes and others use a technique known as **imagined rehearsal** to reach their goals. By visualizing their planned action ahead of time, they are better prepared when they put themselves to the test.

For example, suppose you want to ask someone out on a date. Imagine the setting (walking together to class). Then practice in your mind and out loud exactly what you want to say. Mentally anticipate different responses ("Oh, I'd love to, but I'm busy that evening. . . .") and what you will say in reaction ("How about if I call you sometime this week?"). Careful mental and verbal rehearsal—you could even try out your scenario on a friend—will greatly improve the likelihood of success.

shaping Using a series of small steps to gradually achieve a particular goal.

imagined rehearsal Practicing, through mental imagery, to become better able to perform an event in actuality.

Modeling

Modeling, or learning behaviors by watching others perform them, is one of the most effective strategies for changing behavior. For example, suppose that you have trouble talking to people you don't know very well. One of the easiest ways to improve your communication skills is to select friends whose social skills you envy. Observe them. Do they talk more or listen more? How do people respond to them? Why are they such good communicators? If you observe behaviors you admire and isolate their components, you can model the steps of your behavior-change technique on a proven success.

Controlling the Situation

Sometimes, the right setting or the right group of people will positively influence your behaviors. Many situations and occasions trigger certain actions. For example, in libraries, houses of worship, and museums, most people talk softly. Few people laugh at funerals. The term **situational inducement** refers to an attempt to influence a behavior by using occasions and social settings to control it.

For example, you may be more apt to stop smoking if you work in a smoke-free office, a positive situational inducement. But working in a smoke-filled bar, a negative situational inducement, may tempt you to resume. By carefully considering which settings will help and which will hurt your effort to change, and by deciding to seek the first and avoid the second, you will improve your chances for change.

modeling Learning specific behaviors by watching others perform them.
situational inducement Attempt to influence a behavior through situations and occasions that are structured to exert control over that behavior.
positive reinforcement Presenting something positive following a behavior that is being reinforced.
self-talk The customary manner of thinking and talking to yourself, which can impact your self-image.

Reinforcement

Another way to promote positive behavior change is to reward yourself for it. This is called **positive reinforcement.** Each of us is motivated by different reinforcers.

Most positive reinforcers can be classified into five categories: consumable, activity, manipulative, possessional, and social.

- *Consumable reinforcers* are delicious edibles, such as candy, cookies, or gourmet meals.
- *Activity reinforcers* are opportunities to do something enjoyable, such as watching TV or going on vacation.
- *Manipulative reinforcers* are incentives, such as getting a lower rent in exchange for mowing the lawn or the promise of a better grade for doing an extra-credit project.
- *Possessional reinforcers* are tangible rewards, such as a new TV or a sports car.
- *Social reinforcers* are signs of appreciation, approval, or love, such as loving looks, affectionate hugs, and praise.

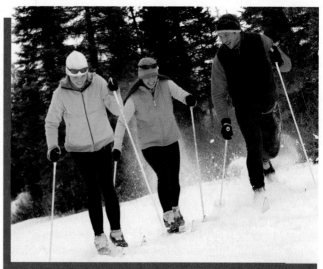

What can I do to change an unhealthy habit?

Many people find it easiest to change an unhealthy habit by making small incremental changes, working toward a goal, and rewarding themselves along the way. The people in your life can help you change by modeling healthy behaviors, supporting your efforts to change, and offering reinforcement.

When choosing reinforcers, determine what would motivate you to act in a particular way. Research has shown that people can be motivated to change their behaviors, such as not smoking during pregnancy or abstaining from cocaine, if they set up a token economy system whereby they earn tokens or points that can be exchanged for meaningful rewards, such as money.[22] The difficulty often lies in determining which incentive will be most effective. Your reinforcers may initially come from others (extrinsic rewards), but as you see positive changes in yourself, you will begin to reward and reinforce yourself (intrinsic rewards). Although reinforcers should immediately follow a behavior, beware of overkill. If you reward yourself with a movie every time you go jogging, this reinforcer will soon lose its power. It would be better to give yourself this reward after, say, a full week of adhering to your jogging program.

what do you think?

What type of reinforcers would most likely get you to change a behavior? Money? Praise or recognition from someone in particular? ● Why would you find this reinforcer motivating? ● Can you think of some healthy options for reinforcing your own behavior changes?

Changing Self-Talk

Self-talk, the way you think and talk to yourself, can also play a role in modifying health-related behaviors. Self-talk can reflect your feelings of self-efficacy, discussed earlier in this chapter. When we don't feel self-efficacious, it's tempting to engage in negative self-talk, which can sabotage our

Surfing for the Latest in Health

The Internet can be a wonderful resource for rapid answers: 72 percent of college students obtain health information from the Web. However, the Web can also be a source of much *misinformation*. If you're not careful, you could end up feeling frazzled, confused, and—worst of all—misinformed. To ensure that the sites you visit are reliable and trustworthy, follow these tips:

✳ Look for websites sponsored by an official government agency, a university or college, or a hospital/medical center. These typically offer accurate, up-to-date information about a wide range of health topics. Government sites are easily identified by their *.gov* extensions (for example, the National Institute of Mental Health's website is www.nimh.nih.gov); college and university sites typically have *.edu* extensions (e.g., Johns Hopkins University's website is www.jhu.edu). Hospitals often have a *.org* extension (e.g., the Mayo Clinic's

website is www.mayoclinic.org). Major philanthropic foundations, such as the Robert Wood Johnson Foundation, the Legacy Foundation, the Kellogg Foundation, and others, often provide information about selected health topics. In addition, national nonprofit organizations, such as the American Heart Association and the American Cancer Society, are often good, authoritative sources of information. Foundations and nonprofits usually have URLs ending with a .org extension.
✳ Search for well-established, professionally peer-reviewed journals such as the *New England Journal of Medicine* (http://content.nejm.org) or the *Journal of the American Medical Association (JAMA;* http://jama.ama-assn.org). Although some of these sites require a fee for access, you can often locate concise abstracts and information, such as a weekly table of contents, that can help you conduct a search. Other times, you can pay a basic fee

for a certain number of hours of unlimited searching. Your college may have Internet access to these journals that they make available to students for no cost.
✳ Consult the Centers for Disease Control and Prevention (www.cdc.gov) for consumer news, updates, and alerts.
✳ For a global perspective on health issues, visit the World Health Organization (www.who.int/en).
✳ There are many government- and education-based sites that are independently sponsored and reliable. The following is just a sample. We'll provide more in each chapter as we cover specific topics:

1. Aetna Intelihealth: www.intelihealth.com
2. FamilyDoctor.org http://familydoctor.org
3. MedlinePlus: www.nlm.nih.gov/medlineplus
4. Go Ask Alice!: www.goaskalice.columbia.edu

5. WebMD health: http://my.webmd.com

✳ The nonprofit health care accrediting organization URAC (www.urac.org) has devised over 50 criteria that health sites must satisfy to display its seal. Look for the "URAC Accredited Health Web Site" seal on websites you visit. In addition to policing the accuracy of health claims, URAC evaluates health information and provides a forum for reporting misinformation, privacy violations, and other complaints.
✳ And, finally, don't believe everything you read. Cross-check information against reliable sources to see whether facts and figures are consistent. Be especially wary of websites that try to sell you something. Just because a source claims to be a physician or an expert does not mean that this is true. When in doubt, check with your own health care provider, health education professor, or state health division website.

---

best intentions. Here are some strategies for changing self-talk.

Rational-Emotive Therapy
Rational-emotive therapy, a form of cognitive therapy or self-directed behavior change, is based on the premise that there is a close connection between what people say to themselves and how they feel. According to psychologist Albert Ellis, most emotional problems and related behaviors stem from irrational statements that people make to themselves when events in their lives are different from what they would like them to be.[23]

For example, suppose that after doing poorly on a test, you say to yourself, "I can't believe I flunked that easy exam. I'm so stupid." By changing this irrational, "catastrophic" self-talk into rational, positive statements about what is

really going on, you increase the likelihood that you will make a positive behavior change. Positive self-talk might be phrased as follows: "I really didn't study enough for that exam, and I'm not surprised I didn't do well. I'm certainly not stupid. I just need to prepare better for the next test." Such self-talk will help you to recover quickly and take positive steps to correct the situation.

Blocking/Thought Stopping
By purposefully blocking or stopping negative thoughts, a person can concentrate on taking positive steps toward behavior change. For example, suppose you are preoccupied with your ex-partner, who has recently deserted you for someone else. You consciously stop thinking about the situation and force yourself to think about something more pleasant (perhaps dinner tomorrow with your best friend). By refusing to dwell on negative images

and forcing yourself to focus elsewhere, you can avoid wasting energy, time, and emotional resources and move on to positive change.

Planning Behavior Change

Before you begin the process of behavior change, take stock of the factors that have made you maintain the current behavior. Assessing the causes of your existing behaviors will help you determine where you need to make changes.

Self-Assessment: Antecedents and Consequences

Behaviors, thoughts, and feelings always occur in a context, that is, in a situation. Situations can be divided into two components: the events that come before and those that come after. *Antecedents* are the setting events for a behavior; they stimulate a person to act in certain ways. Antecedents can be physical events, thoughts, emotions, or the actions of other people. *Consequences*—the results of behavior—affect whether a person will repeat that action. Consequences also can consist of physical events, thoughts, emotions, or the actions of other people.

Suppose you are shy and must give a speech in front of a large class. The antecedents include walking into the class, feeling frightened, wondering whether you are capable of doing a good job, and being unable to remember a word of your speech. If the consequences are negative—if your classmates laugh or you get a low grade—your terror about speaking in public will be reinforced, and you will continue to dread this kind of event. In contrast, if you receive positive feedback from the class or instructor, you may actually learn to like speaking in public.

Learning to recognize the antecedents of a behavior and acting to modify them is one method of changing behavior. A diary noting your undesirable behaviors and identifying the settings in which they occur can be a useful tool.

Self-Assessment: Analyzing Personal Behavior

Successful behavior change requires determining what you want to change. All too often we berate ourselves by using generalities: "I'm lousy to my friends; I need to be a better person." Determining the specific behavior you would like to modify—in contrast to the general problem—will allow you to set clear goals. What are you doing that makes you a lousy friend? Are you gossiping or lying about your friends? Have you been a taker rather than a giver? Or are you really a good friend most of the time?

Let's say the problem is gossiping. You can analyze this behavior by examining the following components.

- **Frequency.** How often do you gossip—all the time or only once in a while?
- **Duration.** How long have you been doing this?
- **Seriousness.** Is your gossiping just idle chatter, or are you really trying to injure other people? What are the consequences for you? For your friends? For your relationships?
- **Basis for problem behavior.** Is your gossip based on facts, perceptions of facts, or deliberate embellishment of the truth?
- **Antecedents.** What kinds of situations trigger your gossiping? Do some settings or people bring it out in you more than others do? What triggers your feelings of dislike or irritation toward your friends? Why are you talking behind their backs?

Once you assess your actions and determine what motivates you, consider what you can do to change your behavior.

Setting Realistic Goals

Changing behavior is not easy, but sometimes we make it even harder by setting unrealistic and unattainable goals. To start making positive changes, ask yourself these questions:

1. **What do I want?** What is your ultimate goal—to lose weight? Exercise more? Reduce stress? Have a lasting relationship? Whatever it is, you need a clear picture of the target outcome.

2. **Which change is the greatest priority at this time?** Often people decide to change several things all at once. Suppose that you are gaining unwanted weight. Rather than saying, "I need to eat less, start jogging, and really get in shape," be specific about the current behavior you need to change. Are you eating too many sweets? Too many high-fat foods? Perhaps a realistic goal would be to try to eat less fat during dinner every day. Choose the behavior that constitutes your greatest problem, and tackle that first. You can always work on something else later. Take small steps, experiment with alternatives, and find the best way to meet your goals.

3. **Why is this important to me?** Think through why you want to change. Are you doing it because of your health? To look better? To win someone else's approval? Usually, doing something because it's right for you rather than to win others' approval is a sound strategy. If you are changing for someone else, what happens when that other person isn't around?

4. **What are the potential positive outcomes?** What do you hope to accomplish?

5. **What health-promoting programs and services can help me get started?** Nearly all campuses offer helpful resources. You might buy a self-help book at the campus bookstore, speak to a counselor, or enroll in an aerobics class at the local fitness center.

6. **Are there family or friends whose help I can enlist?** Social support is one of your most powerful allies. Getting a friend to exercise with you, asking your partner to help you stop smoking by quitting at the same time you do, and making a commitment with a friend to never let each other drive if you've been drinking alcohol—these are all examples of how people can help each other make positive changes.

Decision Making: Choices for Change

Now it is time to make a decision that will lead to positive health outcomes. Try anticipating what might occur in a given setting and think through all possible safe alternatives.

For example, suppose you know you will likely be offered a drink at parties. What response would be okay in your social group? If someone is flirting with you and the situation takes on a distinct sexual overtone, how can you prevent the situation from turning unpleasant for you? Advance preparation will help you stick to your behavior plan.

Fill out the Behavior Change Contract at the beginning of this book to help you set a goal, anticipate obstacles, and create strategies to overcome those obstacles. **Figure 1.7** shows an example of a completed contract. Remember that things typically don't "just happen." Making a commitment by completing a contract helps you stay alert to potential problems, to be aware of your alternatives, to maintain a good sense of your values, and to stick to your beliefs under pressure.

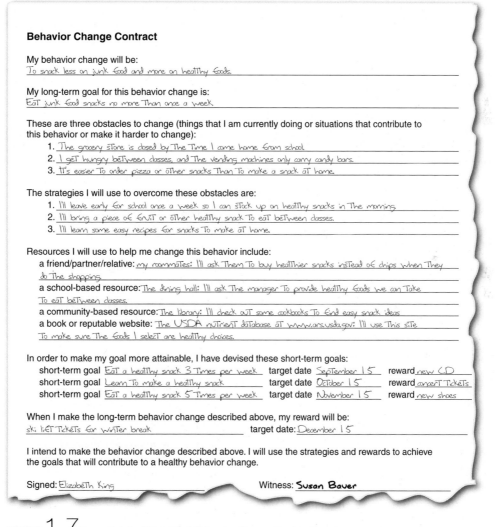

Behavior Change Contract

My behavior change will be:
To snack less on junk food and more on healthy foods.

My long-term goal for this behavior change is:
Eat junk food snacks no more than once a week

These are three obstacles to change (things that I am currently doing or situations that contribute to this behavior or make it harder to change):
1. The grocery store is closed by the time I come home from school
2. I get hungry between classes, and the vending machines only carry candy bars.
3. It's easier to order pizza or other snacks than to make a snack at home.

The strategies I will use to overcome these obstacles are:
1. I'll leave early for school once a week so I can stock up on healthy snacks in the morning.
2. I'll bring a piece of fruit or other healthy snack to eat between classes.
3. I'll learn some easy recipes for snacks to make at home.

Resources I will use to help me change this behavior include:
a friend/partner/relative: my roommates: I'll ask them to buy healthier snacks instead of chips when they do the shopping.
a school-based resource: The dining hall: I'll ask the manager to provide healthy foods we can take to eat between classes.
a community-based resource: The library: I'll check out some cookbooks to find easy snack ideas
a book or reputable website: The USDA nutrient database at www.ars.usda.gov: I'll use this site to make sure the foods I select are healthy choices.

In order to make my goal more attainable, I have devised these short-term goals:
short-term goal Eat a healthy snack 3 times per week   target date September 15   reward new CD
short-term goal Learn to make a healthy snack   target date October 15   reward concert tickets
short-term goal Eat a healthy snack 5 times per week   target date November 15   reward new shoes

When I make the long-term behavior change described above, my reward will be:
ski lift tickets for winter break   target date: December 15

I intend to make the behavior change described above. I will use the strategies and rewards to achieve the goals that will contribute to a healthy behavior change.

Signed: Elizabeth King   Witness: Susan Bauer

FIGURE 1.7 Example of a Completed Behavior Change Contract

Assess Yourself

How Healthy Are You?

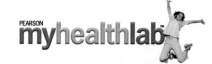

Although we all recognize the importance of being healthy, it can be a challenge to sort out which behaviors are most likely to cause problems or which ones pose the greatest risk. *Before* you decide where to start, it is important to look at your current health status.

By completing the following assessment, you will have a clearer picture of health areas in which you excel and those that could use some work. Taking this assessment will also help you to reflect on components of health that you may not have thought about.

Answer each question, then total your score for each section and fill it in on the Personal Checklist at the end of the assessment for a general sense of your health profile. Think about the behaviors that influenced your score in each category. Would you like to change any of them? Choose the area that you'd like to improve, then complete the Behavior Change Contract at the front of your book. Use the contract to

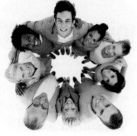

Fill out this assessment online at www.pearsonhighered.com/myhealthlab or www.pearsonhighered.com/donatelle.

think through and implement a behavior change over the course of this class.

Each of the categories in this questionnaire is an important aspect of the total dimensions of health, but this is not a substitute for the advice of a qualified health care provider. Consider scheduling a thorough physical examination by a licensed physician or setting up an appointment with a mental health counselor at your school if you need help making a behavior change.

For each of the following, indicate how often you think the statements describe you.

1 Physical Health

	Never	Rarely	Some of the Time	Usually or Always
1. I am happy with my body size and weight.	1	2	3	4
2. I engage in vigorous exercises such as brisk walking, jogging, swimming, or running for at least 30 minutes per day, three to four times per week.	1	2	3	4
3. I get at least 7 to 8 hours of sleep each night.	1	2	3	4
4. My immune system is strong, and my body heals itself quickly when I get sick or injured.	1	2	3	4
5. I listen to my body; when there is something wrong, I try to make adjustments to heal it or seek professional advice.	1	2	3	4

Total score for this section: _____

2 Social Health

	Never	Rarely	Some of the Time	Usually or Always
1. I am open, honest, and get along well with others.	1	2	3	4
2. I participate in a wide variety of social activities and enjoy being with people who are different from me.	1	2	3	4
3. I try to be a "better person" and decrease behaviors that have caused problems in my interactions with others.	1	2	3	4
4. I am open and accessible to a loving and responsible relationship.	1	2	3	4
5. I try to see the good in my friends and do whatever I can to support them and help them feel good about themselves.	1	2	3	4

Total score for this section: _____

3 Emotional Health

	Never	Rarely	Some of the Time	Usually or Always
1. I find it easy to laugh, cry, and show emotions like love, fear, and anger, and try to express these in positive, constructive ways.	1	2	3	4
2. I avoid using alcohol or other drugs as a means of helping me forget my problems.	1	2	3	4
3. I recognize when I am stressed and take steps to relax through exercise, quiet time, or other calming activities.	1	2	3	4
4. I try not to be too critical or judgmental of others and try to understand differences or quirks that I note in others.	1	2	3	4
5. I am flexible and adapt or adjust to change in a positive way.	1	2	3	4

Total score for this section: _____

4 Environmental Health

	Never	Rarely	Some of the Time	Usually or Always
1. I buy recycled paper and purchase biodegradable detergents and cleaning agents, or make my own cleaning products, whenever possible.	1	2	3	4
2. I recycle paper, plastic, and metals; purchase refillable containers when possible; and try to minimize the amount of paper and plastics that I use.	1	2	3	4
3. I try to wear my clothes for longer periods between washing to reduce water consumption and the amount of detergents in our water sources.	1	2	3	4
4. I vote for proenvironment candidates in elections.	1	2	3	4
5. I minimize the amount of time that I run the faucet when I brush my teeth, shave, or shower.	1	2	3	4

Total score for this section: _____

5 Spiritual Health

	Never	Rarely	Some of the Time	Usually or Always
1. I take time alone to think about what's important in life—who I am, what I value, where I fit in, and where I'm going.	1	2	3	4
2. I have faith in a greater power, be it a supreme being, nature, or the connectedness of all living things.	1	2	3	4
3. I engage in acts of caring and goodwill without expecting something in return.	1	2	3	4
4. I sympathize/empathize with those who are suffering and try to help them through difficult times.	1	2	3	4
5. I go for the gusto and experience life to the fullest.	1	2	3	4

Total score for this section: _____

6 Intellectual Health

	Never	Rarely	Some of the Time	Usually or Always
1. I carefully consider my options and possible consequences as I make choices in life.	1	2	3	4
2. I learn from my mistakes and try to act differently the next time.	1	2	3	4
3. I have at least one hobby, learning activity, or personal growth activity that I make time for each week, something that improves me as a person.	1	2	3	4
4. I manage my time well rather than let time manage me.	1	2	3	4
5. My friends and family trust my judgment.	1	2	3	4

Total score for this section: _____

Although each of these six aspects of health is important, there are some factors that don't readily fit in one category. As college students, you face some unique risks that others may not have. For this reason, we have added a section to this self-assessment that focuses on personal health promotion and disease prevention. Answer these questions and add your results to the Personal Checklist in the following section.

7 Personal Health Promotion/ Disease Prevention

	Never	Rarely	Some of the Time	Usually or Always
1. If I were to be sexually active, I would use protection such as latex condoms, dental dams, and other means of reducing my risk of sexually transmitted infections.	1	2	3	4
2. I can have a good time at parties or during happy hours without binge drinking.	1	2	3	4
3. I have eaten too much in the last month and have forced myself to vomit to avoid gaining weight.	4	3	2	1
4. If I were to get a tattoo or piercing, I would go to a reputable person who follows strict standards of sterilization and precautions against bloodborne disease transmission.	1	2	3	4
5. I engage in extreme sports and find that I enjoy the highs that come with risking bodily harm through physical performance.	4	3	2	1

Total score for this section: _____

Personal Checklist

Now, total your scores for each section on the next page and compare them to what would be considered optimal scores. Are you surprised by your scores in any areas? Which areas do you need to work on?

	Ideal Score	Your Score
Physical health	20	_____
Social health	20	_____
Emotional health	20	_____
Environmental health	20	_____
Spiritual health	20	_____
Intellectual health	20	_____
Personal health promotion/ disease prevention	20	_____

What Your Scores in Each Category Mean

Scores of 15–20:

Outstanding! Your answers show that you are aware of the importance of these behaviors in your overall health. More important, you are putting your knowledge to work by

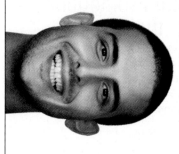

practicing good health habits that should reduce your overall risks. Although you received a very high score on this part of the test, you may want to consider areas where your scores could be improved.

Scores of 10–14:

Your health risks are showing! Find information about the risks you are facing and why it is important to change these behaviors. Perhaps you need help in deciding how to make the changes you desire. Assistance is available from this book, your professor, and student health services at your school.

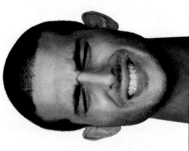

Scores below 10:

You may be taking unnecessary risks with your health. Perhaps you are not aware of the risks and what to do about them. Identify each risk area and make a mental note as you read the associated chapter in the book. Whenever possible, seek additional resources, either on your campus or through your

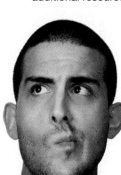

local community health resources, and make a serious commitment to behavior change. If any area is causing you to be less than functional in your class work or personal life, seek professional help. In this book you will find the information you need to help you improve your scores and your health. Remember that these scores are only indicators, not diagnostic tools.

YOUR PLAN FOR **CHANGE**

The **Assess yourself** activity gave you the chance to look at the status of your health in several dimensions. Now that you have considered these results, you can take steps toward changing certain behaviors that may be detrimental to your health.

Today, you can:

○ Evaluate your behavior and identify patterns and specific things you are doing.

○ Select one pattern of behavior that you want to change.

○ Fill out the Behavior Change Contract at the front of your book. Be sure to include your long- and short-term goals for change, the rewards you'll give yourself for reaching these goals, the potential obstacles along the way, and the strategies for overcoming these obsta-

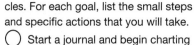

cles. For each goal, list the small steps and specific actions that you will take.

○ Start a journal and begin charting your progress toward your behavior change goal.

○ Tell a friend or family member about your behavior change goal, and ask them to support you along the way.

Within the next 2 weeks, you can:

○ Review your journal entries and consider how successful you have been in following your plan. What helped you be successful? What

made change more difficult? What will you do differently next week?

○ Revise your plan as needed: Are the short-term goals attainable? Are the rewards satisfying?

○ Practice safer sex.

○ Maintain healthy eating habits and manage your weight.

○ Control real and imaginary stressors.

○ Maintain meaningful relationships with family and friends.

By the end of the semester, you can:

○ Schedule a regular self-exam.

○ Understand the health care system.

○ Value each day and make the best of opportunities.

Summary

✳ Health encompasses the entire dynamic process of fulfilling one's potential in the physical, social, emotional, spiritual, intellectual, and environmental dimensions of life. Wellness means achieving the highest level of health possible in several dimensions.

✳ Although the average American life span has increased over the past century, we also need to increase the quality of life. Programs such as *Healthy People 2010* have established national objectives for achieving longer life and quality of life for all Americans through health promotion and disease prevention.

✳ Health disparities contribute to increased disease risks. Factors such as gender, race, and socioeconomic status continue to play a major role in health status and care. Women have longer lives but have more medical problems than do men. To close the gender gap in health care, researchers have begun to include more women in medical research and training.

✳ For the U.S. population as a whole, the leading causes of death are heart disease, cancer, and stroke. In the 15- to 24-year-old age group, the leading causes are unintentional injuries, homicide, and suicide. Many of the risks associated with cancer, heart disease, and stroke can be reduced through lifestyle changes. Many of the risks associated with accidents, homicide, and suicide can be reduced through preventive measures, particularly reductions in the use of alcohol and other drugs.

✳ Several factors contribute to a person's health status, and a number of them are within our control. Beliefs and attitudes, self-efficacy, locus of control, intentions to change, support from significant others, and readiness to change are factors over which individuals have some degree of control. Access to health care, genetic predisposition, health policies that support positive choices, and other factors are all potential reinforcing, predisposing, and enabling factors that may influence health decisions.

✳ Behavior-change techniques, such as shaping, visualization, modeling, controlling the situation, reinforcement, changing self-talk, and problem solving help people succeed in making behavior changes.

✳ Decision making has several key components. Each person must explore his or her own problems, the reasons for change, and the expected outcomes. The next step is to plan a course of action best suited to individual needs and fill out a Behavior Change Contract.

Pop Quiz

1. Our ability to perform everyday tasks, such as walking up the stairs or tying your shoes, is an example of
   a. improved quality of life.
   b. physical health.
   c. health promotion.
   d. activities of daily living.

2. Janice describes herself as confident and trusting, and she displays both high self-esteem and high self-efficacy. The dimension of health this relates to is the
   a. social dimension.
   b. emotional dimension.
   c. spiritual dimension.
   d. intellectual dimension.

3. What statistic is used to describe the number of new cases of AIDS in a given year?
   a. morbidity
   b. mortality
   c. incidence
   d. prevalence

4. Because Craig's parents smoked, he is 90 percent more likely to start smoking than someone whose parents didn't. This is an example of what factor influencing behavior change?
   a. circumstantial factor
   b. enabling factor
   c. reinforcing factor
   d. predisposing factor

5. Which of the following is likely to be a reinforcing factor in your efforts at healthy behavior change?
   a. Your friend tells you how great it is that you're sticking to your exercise plan and offers to take you to the movies if you keep it up.
   b. Your parents buy you a gym membership as it's too cold for you to exercise outdoors.
   c. Your parents tell you not to worry about a few extra pounds, because you're "big boned."
   d. Your friends agree not to allow you to "bum" cigarettes when you're at a party.

6. Suppose you want to lose 20 pounds. To reach your goal, you take small steps. You start by joining a support group and counting calories. After 2 weeks, you begin an exercise program and gradually build up to your desired fitness level. What behavior change strategy are you using?
   a. shaping
   b. visualization
   c. modeling
   d. reinforcement

7. After Kirk and Tammy pay their bills, they reward themselves by watching TV together. The type of positive reinforcement that motivates them to pay their bills is
   a. activity reinforcer.
   b. consumable reinforcer.
   c. manipulative reinforcer.
   d. possessional reinforcer.

8. The setting events for a behavior that cue or stimulate a person to act in certain ways are called
   a. antecedents.
   b. frequency of events.
   c. consequences.
   d. cues to action.

9. What strategy for change is advised for an individual in the preparation stage of change?
   a. seeking out recommended readings
   b. finding creative ways to maintain positive behaviors
   c. setting realistic goals
   d. publicly stating the desire for change

10. Spiritual health is
    a. exclusive to religiosity.
    b. optional for achieving wellness.
    c. related to one's purpose in life.
    d. finding fulfilling relationships.

Answers to these questions can be found on page A-1.

Think about It!

1. How are the terms *health* and *wellness* similar? What, if any, are important distinctions between these terms? What is health promotion? Disease prevention?

2. How healthy is the U.S. population today? Are we doing better or worse in terms of health status than we have done previously? What factors influence today's disparities in health?

3. What are some of the major differences in the way men and women are treated in the health care system? Why do you think these differences exist? How do race, sexual orientation, religion, marital status, and age affect how people are treated in the health care system?

4. What is the Health Belief Model? How may this model be working when a young woman decides to

smoke her first cigarette? Her last cigarette?

5. Explain the predisposing, reinforcing, and enabling factors that might influence a young mother who is dependent on welfare as she decides whether to sell drugs to support her children.

6. Using the Stages of Change model, discuss what you might do (in stages) to help a friend stop smoking. Why is it important that a person be ready to change before trying to change?

Accessing Your Health on the Internet

The following websites explore further topics and issues related to personal health. For links to the websites below, visit the Companion Website for *Health: The Basics*, Green Edition at www.pearsonhighered.com/donatelle.

1. *CDC Wonder.* Clearinghouse for comprehensive information from the Centers for Disease Control and Prevention (CDC), including special reports, guidelines, and access to national health data. http://wonder.cdc.gov

2. *MayoClinic.com.* Reputable resource for specific information about health topics, diseases, and treatment options provided by the staff of the Mayo Clinic. Easy to navigate and consumer friendly. www.mayoclinic.com

3. *National Center for Health Statistics.* Outstanding place to start for information about health status in the United States. Links to key documents such as *Health, United States* (published yearly); national survey information; and information on mortality by age, race, gender, geographic location, and other important data. Includes comprehensive information provided by the CDC, as well as easy links to at least ten of the major health resources currently

being used for policy and decision making about health in the United States. www.cdc.gov/nchs

4. *National Health Information Center.* Excellent resource for consumer information about health. www.health.gov/nhic

5. *World Health Organization.* Excellent resource for global health information. Provides information on the current state of health around the world, such as illness and disease statistics, trends, and illness outbreak alerts. www.who.int/en

References

1. National Center for Health Statistics, *Health, United States, 2008, with Chartbook on Trends in the Health of Americans* (Hyattsville, MD: National Center for Health Statistics, 2009).

2. Central Intelligence Agency, "Rank Order: Life Expectancy at Birth," in *The World Fact Book* (Washington, DC: CIA, 2009); National Center for Health Statistics, *Health, United States, 2007*; R. Dubos, *So Human an Animal* (New York: Scribners, 1968), 15.

3. S. J. Olshansky et al., "A Potential Decline in Life Expectancy in the United States in the 21st Century," *New England Journal of Medicine* 352, no. 11 (March 17, 2005): 1138–45.

4. Ibid.

5. U.S. Department of Health and Human Services, Health Resources and Services Administration, *Women's Health USA 2008* (Rockville, Maryland: U.S. Department of Health and Human Services, 2008).

6. R. Dubos, *So Human an Animal*, 15.

7. K. Braithwaite, "Mending Our Broken Mental Health Systems," *American Journal of Public Health* 96, no. 10 (2006): 1724.

8. Centers for Disease Control and Prevention and the Merck Company Foundation, *The State of Aging and Health in America 2007* (Whitehouse Station, NJ: The Merck Company Foundation, 2007).

9. National Center for Health Statistics, "About *Healthy People 2010*," www.cdc.gov/nchs.

10. Centers for Disease Control and Prevention, Office of Minority Health and Health Disparities, "Racial and Ethnic Populations," 2009, www.cdc.gov/omhd/Populations/populations.htm.

11. G. F. Kominski et al., *Language Barriers Pose a Risk for California HMO Enrollees* (Los Angeles: UCLA Center for Health Policy Research, May 2006); G. Glores,

"Language Barriers in Health Care in the United States," *New England Journal of Medicine* 355, no. 3 (2006): 229–331.

12. National Institutes of Health, *National Institutes of Health (NIH) Strategic Research Plan and Budget to Reduce and Ultimately Eliminate Health Disparities: Volume 1, Fiscal Years 2002–2006* (Bethesda, MD: National Institutes of Health, May 12, 2006).

13. A. Jemal et al., "Cancer Statistics," *A Cancer Journal for Clinicians* 55 (January/February 2005): 10–30; E. Ward, News Conference: American Cancer Society, ACS (January 19, 2005).

14. Centers for Disease Control and Prevention, "Chronic Disease Prevention and Health Promotion," www.cdc.gov/nccdphp. Updated April 8, 2009.

15. R. DeVol et al., *An Unhealthy America: The Economic Burden of Chronic Disease—Charting a New Course to Save Lives and Increase Productivity and Economic Growth* (Santa Monica, CA: The Milken Institute, 2007).

16. Centers for Disease Control and Prevention, *The Burden of Chronic Diseases and Their Risk Factors: National and State Perspectives, 2004* (Atlanta: U.S. Department of Health and Human Services, 2004).

17. M. Reeves and A. Rafferty, "Healthy Lifestyle Characteristics Among Adults in the United States," *Archives of Internal Medicine* 165, no. 8 (2005): 854–57.

18. I. Rosenstock, "Historical Origins of the Health Belief Model," *Health Education Monographs* 2, no. 4 (1974): 328–35.

19. J. M. Twenge, Z. Liqing, and C. Im, "It's Beyond My Control: A Cross-Temporal Meta-Analysis of Increasing Externality in Locus of Control, 1960–2002," *Personality and Social Psychology Review* 8 (2004): 308–20.

20. M. Hesse, "The Readiness Ruler as a Measure of Readiness to Change Polydrug Use in Drug Abusers," *Journal of Harm Reduction* 3, no. 3 (2006): 1477–81; M. Cismaru, "Using Protection Motivation Theory to Increase the Persuasiveness of Public Service Communications," The Saskatchewan Institute of Public Policy, Public Policy Series paper no. 40 (February 2006); A. Fallon et al., "Health Care Provider Advice for African American Adults Not Meeting Health Behavior Recommendations," *Preventing Chronic Disease* 3, no. 2 (2006): A45; M. R. Chacko et al., "New Sexual Partners and Readiness to Seek Screening for Chlamydia and Gonorrhea: Predictors among Minority Young Women," *Sexually Transmitted Infections* 82 (2006): 75–79.

21. J. O. Prochaska and C. C. DiClemente, "Stages and Processes of Self-Change of Smoking: Toward an Integrative Model of Change," *Journal of Consulting and Clinical Psychology* 51 (1983): 390–95.

22. R. J. Donatelle et al., "Using Incentives and the 5A's in Clinical Practice to Motivate Pregnant Smokers to Quit: The Maternal Intervention to Stop Smoking (MISS) Trial" (forthcoming); S. Higgins et al., "The Effects of Monetary Value of Voucher-Based Incentives on Abstinence in Cocaine Users," *Addiction* 102, no. 2 (2007): 271–81.

23. A. Ellis and M. Benard, *Clinical Application of Rational Emotive Therapy* (New York: Plenum, 1985).

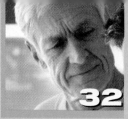

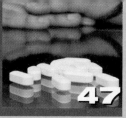

32 How do others influence my psychosocial health?

36 Is laughter really the best medicine?

40 What are the symptoms of depression?

47 What should I do if someone I know is suicidal?

2 Psychosocial Health

Objectives

✱ Define each of the four components of psychosocial health, and identify the basic traits shared by psychosocially healthy people.

✱ Learn what factors affect your psychosocial health; discuss the positive steps you can take to enhance your psychosocial health.

✱ Identify common psychosocial problems, such as anxiety disorders and depression, and explain their causes and treatments.

✱ Explain the methods of different types of mental health professionals, and examine how they can play a role in preventing specific types of psychosocial health problems.

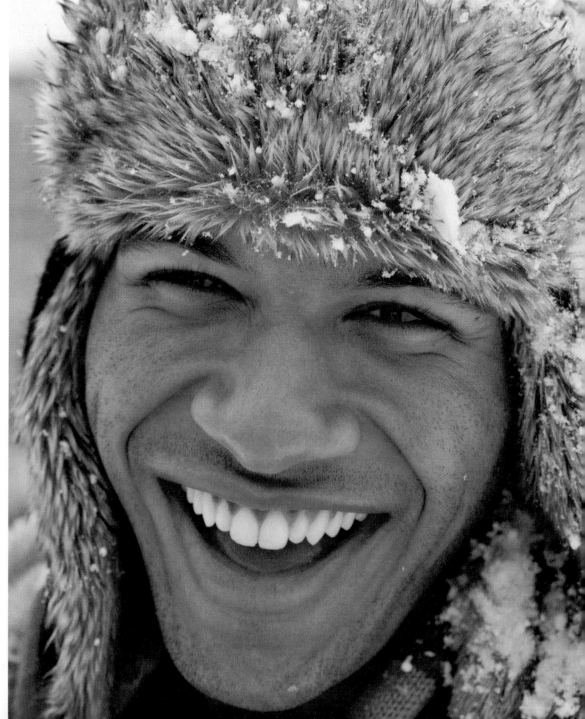

Although the vast majority of college students describe their college years as among the best of their lives, many find the pressure of grades, financial concerns, relationship problems, and the struggle to understand who they are to be extraordinarily difficult. Steven Hyman, provost of Harvard University and former director of the National Institutes of Mental Health, sounded this alarm about student mental health: "The mental state of many students is so precarious that it is interfering with the core mission of the university."[1] Psychological distress caused by relationship issues, family issues, academic competition, and college life adjustment is rampant on college campuses today. Experts believe that the anxiety-prone campus environment is a major contributor to poor health decisions such as high alcohol consumption and, in turn, to health problems that ultimately affect academic success and success in life.

Fortunately, even though we often face seemingly insurmountable pressures, human beings possess a resiliency that enables us to cope, adapt, and thrive, regardless of life's challenges. How we feel and think about ourselves, those around us, and our environment can tell us a lot about our psychosocial health and whether we are healthy emotionally, spiritually, and mentally. Increasingly, health professionals recognize that having a solid social network, being emotionally and mentally healthy, and developing spiritual capacity don't just add years to life—they put life into years.

What Is Psychosocial Health?

Psychosocial health encompasses the mental, emotional, social, and spiritual dimensions of what it means to be healthy (Figure 2.1). It is the result of a complex interaction between a person's history and his or her thoughts about and interpretations of the past and what it means to the present. Psychosocially healthy people are emotionally, mentally, socially, intellectually, and spiritually resilient. They respond to challenges and frustrations in appropriate ways most of the time, despite occasional slips (Figure 2.2). When they do slip, they recognize it and take action to rectify the situation. Once they are informed about the resources that are available to help them get through tough situations, they use them. Most authorities identify several basic characteristics shared by psychosocially healthy people.[2]

● **They feel good about themselves.** They typically are not overwhelmed by fear, love, anger, jealousy, guilt, or worry. They know who they are, have a realistic sense of their capabilities, and respect themselves even though they realize they aren't perfect.
● **They feel comfortable with other people.** They enjoy satisfying and lasting personal relationships and do not take advantage of others or allow others to take advantage of them. They recognize that there are others whose needs are greater than their own. They can give love, consider others'

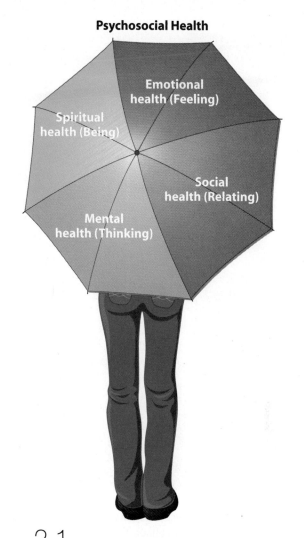

Psychosocial Health

Emotional health (Feeling)
Spiritual health (Being)
Social health (Relating)
Mental health (Thinking)

FIGURE 2.1 **Psychosocial Health**
Psychosocial health is a complex interaction of mental, emotional, social, and spiritual health. Possessing strength and resiliency in these dimensions can maintain your overall well-being and help you weather the storms of life.

interests, take time to help others, respect personal differences, and feel responsible for their fellow human beings.
● **They control tension and anxiety.** They recognize the underlying causes and symptoms of stress in their lives and consciously avoid irrational thoughts, hostility, excessive excuse making, and blaming others for their problems. They use resources and learn skills to control reactions to stressful situations.

psychosocial health The mental, emotional, social, and spiritual dimensions of health.

● **They meet the demands of life.** They try to solve problems as they arise, accept responsibility, and plan ahead. They set realistic goals, think for themselves, and make independent decisions. Acknowledging that change is inevitable, they welcome new experiences.
● **They curb hate and guilt.** They acknowledge and combat tendencies to respond with anger, thoughtlessness, selfishness, vengeful acts, or feelings of inadequacy. They do not try

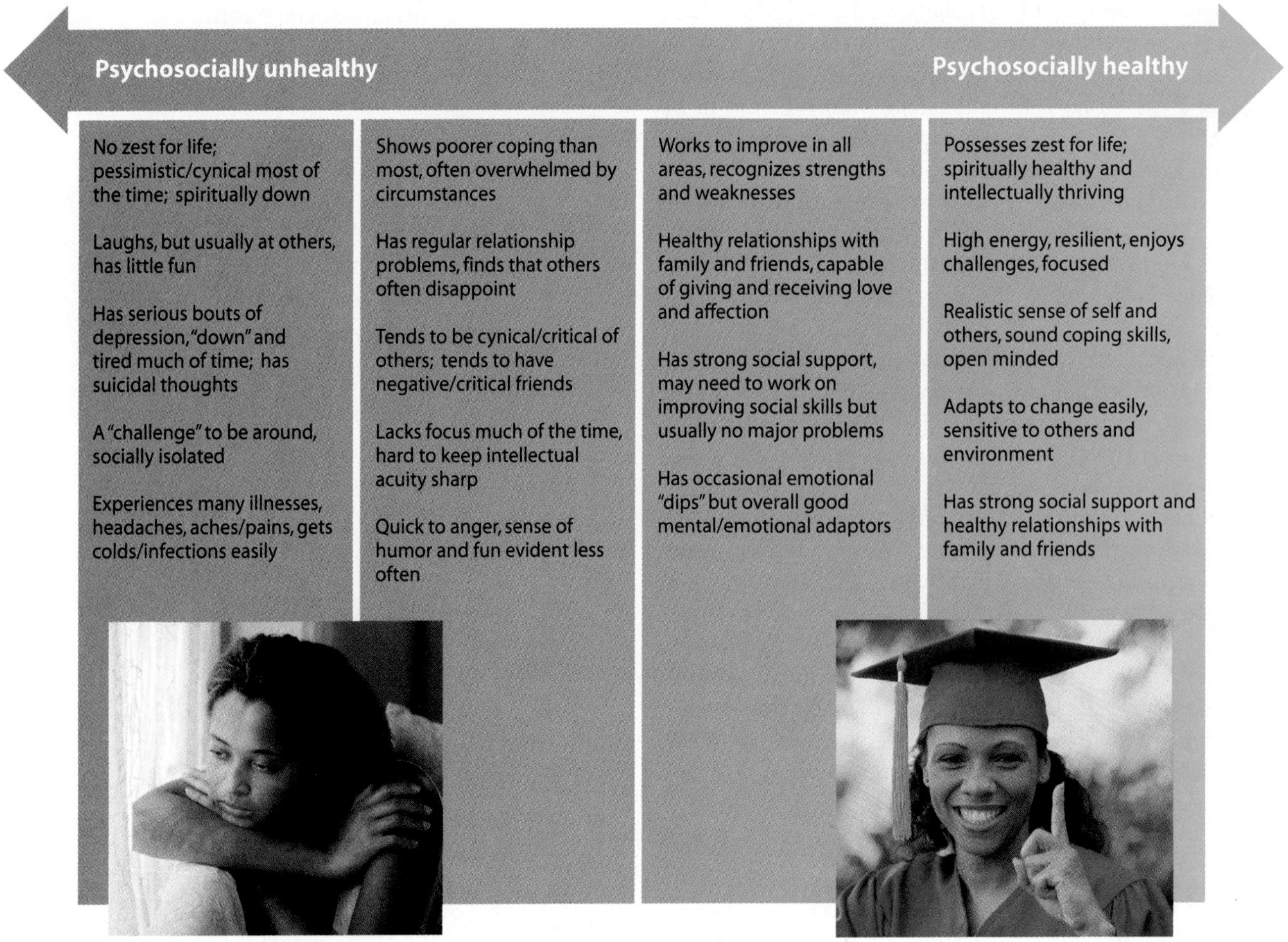

No zest for life; pessimistic/cynical most of the time; spiritually down	Shows poorer coping than most, often overwhelmed by circumstances	Works to improve in all areas, recognizes strengths and weaknesses	Possesses zest for life; spiritually healthy and intellectually thriving
Laughs, but usually at others, has little fun	Has regular relationship problems, finds that others often disappoint	Healthy relationships with family and friends, capable of giving and receiving love and affection	High energy, resilient, enjoys challenges, focused
Has serious bouts of depression, "down" and tired much of time; has suicidal thoughts	Tends to be cynical/critical of others; tends to have negative/critical friends	Has strong social support, may need to work on improving social skills but usually no major problems	Realistic sense of self and others, sound coping skills, open minded
A "challenge" to be around, socially isolated	Lacks focus much of the time, hard to keep intellectual acuity sharp	Has occasional emotional "dips" but overall good mental/emotional adaptors	Adapts to change easily, sensitive to others and environment
Experiences many illnesses, headaches, aches/pains, gets colds/infections easily	Quick to anger, sense of humor and fun evident less often		Has strong social support and healthy relationships with family and friends

FIGURE 2.2 **Characteristics of Psychosocially Healthy and Unhealthy People**
Where do you fall on this continuum?

to knock others aside to get ahead but rather reach out to help others—even people they don't particularly like.

● **They maintain a positive outlook.** They approach each day with a presumption that things will go well. They look to the future with enthusiasm rather than dread. Reminders of good experiences brighten their day. Fun and making time for themselves are integral parts of their lives.

● **They value diversity.** They do not feel threatened by people of a different race, gender, religion, sexual orientation, ethnicity, or political party. They are nonjudgmental and do not force their beliefs and values on others.

● **They appreciate and respect nature.** They take the time to enjoy their surroundings, are conscious of their place in the universe, and act responsibly to preserve their environment.

● **They enrich the lives of others.** They "tune in," and rather than being narcissistic and self-serving, they often think of others' needs and try to help whenever possible.

Psychologists have long argued that before we can achieve any of the above characteristics of psychologically and socially healthy people, we must have certain basic needs met in our lives. In the 1960s, human theorist Abraham Maslow developed a *hierarchy of needs* to describe this idea (Figure 2.3):

At the bottom of his hierarchy are basic *survival needs,* such as food, sleep, and water; at the next level are *security needs,* such as shelter and safety; at the third level—*social needs*—is a sense of belonging and affection; at the fourth level are *esteem needs,* self-respect and respect for others; and at the top are needs for *self-actualization* and self-transcendence.

According to Maslow's theory, a person's needs must be met at each of these levels before that person can ever truly be healthy. Failure to meet one of the lower levels of needs will interfere with a person's ability to address the upper-level ones. For example, someone who is homeless or worried about threats from violence will be unable to focus on fulfilling social, esteem, or actualization needs. Maslow believed that people are more likely to behave badly if they are frustrated by a lack of need fulfillment.[3]

what do you think?

Which psychosocial qualities do you value most in your friends? ● What area do you think is your greatest psychosocial strength? Your greatest weakness? ● Do you agree with Maslow's assessment that people behave badly socially when their needs are not being met? Can you think of an example?

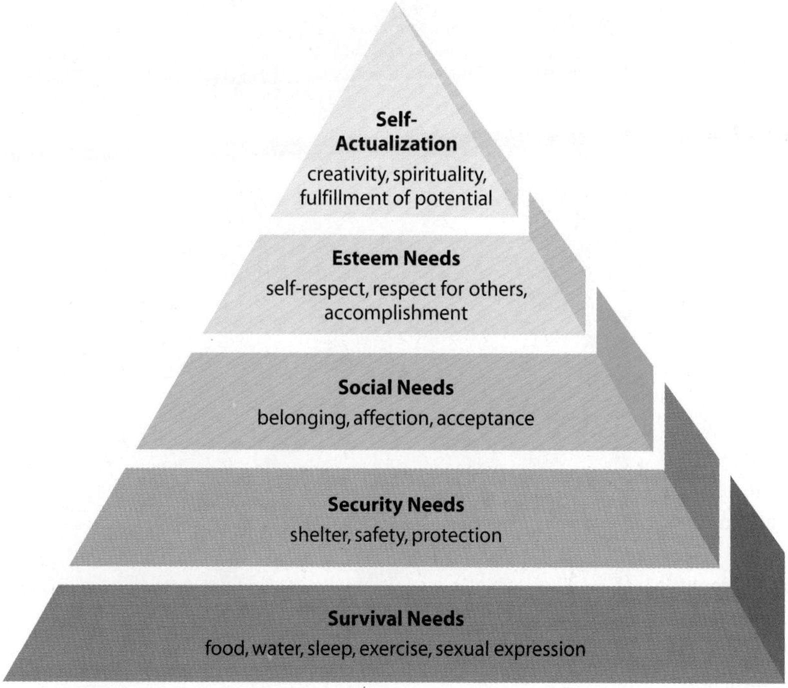

FIGURE 2.3 **Maslow's Hierarchy of Needs**

Attaining psychosocial health and wellness involves many complex processes. This chapter will help you understand not only what it means to be psychosocially well, but also why we may run into problems in our psychosocial health. Learning how to assess your own health and take action to help yourself are important aspects of psychosocial health.

Mental Health: The Thinking You

The term **mental health** is often used to describe the "thinking" or "rational" part of psychosocial health. It is defined as the successful performance of mental function and results in productive activities, fulfilling relationships, and the ability to cope with life's challenges. Mental health plays a role in the way we think, communicate, express emotion, and feel about ourselves. A mentally healthy person has the intellectual ability to sort through information, messages, and life events, to attach meaning, and to respond appropriately.

A mentally healthy person is likely to respond to life's challenges constructively. For example, suppose you spend your spring break with friends on the beaches of Mexico, knowing that you have a major term paper due on the first day back from vacation. The night before the paper is due, you quickly throw it together. Rather than falling off the deep end and blaming the instructor if you get a D on the paper, as a mentally healthy student you would accept responsibility for the choices you made, learn from mistakes, and plan differently next time.

When mentally healthy individuals realize that they are getting into trouble with classes, relationships, and life in general, they know when they are still okay and when they are starting to slide. Knowing when to seek help, talk to a trusted friend, or take time out for rest and regrouping are all part of healthy adapting and coping.

Emotional Health: The Feeling You

The term **emotional health** is often used interchangeably with *mental health.* Although the two are closely intertwined, emotional health more accurately refers to the feeling, or subjective, side of psychosocial health that includes emotional reactions to life. **Emotions** are intensified feelings or complex patterns of feelings that we experience on a regular basis. Love, hate, frustration, anxiety, and joy are only a few of the many emotions we feel.

Emotionally healthy people usually respond appropriately to upsetting events. Rather than respond in an extreme fashion or behave inconsistently or offensively, they are able to express their feelings, communicate with others, and show emotions in appropriate ways. Have you ever seen someone react with extreme anger by shouting or punching a wall? Ex-lovers who become jealous of new relationships and who then damage cars or property are classic examples of people exhibiting unhealthy and dangerous emotional reactions. Such violent responses and emotional volatility have become a problem of epidemic proportions in the United States (see Chapter 4).

Emotional health also affects *social health.* People who feel hostile, withdrawn, or moody may become socially isolated.[4] Because they are not much fun to be around, their friends may avoid them at the very time they are most in need of emotional support. For students, a more immediate concern is the impact of emotional trauma on academic performance. Have you ever tried to study for an exam after a fight with a close friend or family member? Emotional turmoil may seriously affect your ability to think, reason, and act rationally. Many otherwise rational, mentally healthy people do ridiculous things when they are going through a major emotional upset. Mental functioning and emotional responses are intricately connected.

mental health The thinking part of psychosocial health; includes your values, attitudes, and beliefs.
emotional health The feeling part of psychosocial health; includes your emotional reactions to life.
emotions Intensified feelings or complex patterns of feelings we constantly experience.
social health Aspect of psychosocial health that includes interactions with others, ability to use social supports, and ability to adapt to various situations.

Social Health: Interactions with Others

Social health, an important part of the broader concept of psychosocial health, includes your interactions with others on an individual and group basis, your ability to use social resources and support in times of need, and your ability to adapt to a variety of social situations. Socially healthy individuals have a wide range of interactions with family, friends, and acquaintances and are able to have a healthy interaction with an intimate partner. Typically, socially healthy individuals are able to listen, express themselves, form healthy attachments, act in socially acceptable and responsible ways, and find the best fit for themselves in society. Numerous studies have documented the importance of positive relationships with family members, friends, and one's significant other in overall well-being and healthy longevity.[5]

Social bonds reflect the level of closeness and attachment that we develop with individuals. They provide intimacy, feelings of belonging, opportunities for giving and receiving nurturance, reassurance of one's worth, assistance and guidance, and advice. Social bonds take multiple forms, the most common of which are social support and community engagements.

social bonds Degree and nature of interpersonal contacts.
social support Network of people and services with whom you share ties and from whom you get support.
spiritual health The aspect of psychosocial health that relates to having a sense of meaning and purpose to one's life, as well as a feeling of connection with others and with nature.

The concept of **social support** is more complex than many people realize. In general, it refers to the networks of people and services with whom and which we interact and share social connections. These ties can provide *tangible support,* such as babysitting services or money to help pay the bills, or *intangible support,* such as encouraging you to share intimate thoughts. Sometimes, support can be felt as perceiving that someone would be there for us in a crisis. Generally, the closer and the higher the quality of the social bond, the more likely a person is to ask for and receive social support. For example, if your car broke down on a dark country road in the middle of the night, whom could you call for help and know that they would do everything possible to get there? Common descriptions of strong social support include the following:[6]

- Being cared for and loved, with shared intimacy
- Being esteemed and valued; having a sense of self-worth
- Sharing companionship, communication, and mutual obligations with others; having a sense of belonging
- Having "informational" support—access to information, advice, community services, and guidance from others

Social health also reflects the way we react to others. In its most extreme forms, a lack of social health may be represented by aggressive acts of prejudice toward other individuals or groups.

Spiritual Health: An Inner Quest for Well-Being

Although mental health and emotional health are key factors in overall psychosocial functioning, it is possible to be mentally and emotionally healthy and still not achieve optimal well-being. What is missing? For many people, the difficult-to-describe element that gives meaning to life is the spiritual dimension.

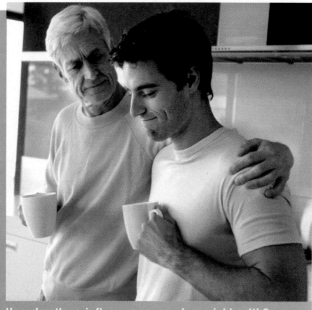

How do others influence my psychosocial health?

Support from family and friends is a vital component of your social health. Your general sense of well-being can be strongly affected by the positive or negative nature of your social bonds.

According to the National Center for Complementary and Alternative Medicine, *Spirituality* is broader than religion and is defined as an individual's sense of purpose and meaning in life; it goes beyond material values.[7] Spirituality may be practiced in many ways, including religion; however, religion does not have to be part of a spiritual person's life. **Spiritual health** refers to the sense of belonging to something greater than the purely physical or personal dimensions of existence. For some, this unifying force is nature; for others, it is a feeling of connection to other people; for still others, the unifying force is a god or other higher power.

On a day-to-day basis, many of us focus on acquiring material possessions and satisfying basic needs. But there comes a point when we discover that material possessions do not automatically bring happiness or a sense of self-worth. As we develop into spiritually healthy beings, we recognize our identity as unique individuals and gain a better appreciation of our strengths and shortcomings and our place in the universe.

Focus On: Your Spiritual Health beginning on page 474 will help you explore your spiritual health in more detail and to better understand the role spirituality plays in your overall psychosocial health.

Factors Influencing Psychosocial Health

Most of our mental, emotional, and social reactions to life are a direct outcome of our experiences and social and cultural expectations. Our psychosocial health is based, in part, on how we perceive life experiences.

Build Your Self-Esteem

＊ Pay attention to your own needs and wants. Listen to what your body, mind, and heart are telling you.

＊ Take good care of yourself. Eat healthy foods, get plenty of sleep, exercise, and plan fun activities for yourself.

＊ Take time to do things you enjoy. Make a list of things that make you happy and do something from that list every day.

＊ Do something that you have been putting off, such as cleaning out your closet or paying a bill that you've been ignoring, to give yourself sense of accomplishment.

＊ Give yourself rewards. Acknowledge that you are a great person by rewarding yourself occasionally.

＊ Spend time with people who make you feel good about yourself. Avoid people who treat you badly or make you feel bad about yourself.

＊ Display or keep close by items that you like and that remind you of your achievements, your friends, or special times.

＊ Take advantage of any opportunity to learn something new—you'll feel better about yourself and be more productive.

＊ Do something nice for another person. There is no greater way to feel better about yourself than to help someone in need.

The Family

Families have a significant influence on psychosocial development. Children raised in healthy, nurturing, happy families are more likely to become well-adjusted, productive adults. Children raised in **dysfunctional families,** in which there is violence; negative behavior; distrust; anger; dietary deprivation; drug abuse; parental discord; or sexual, physical, or emotional abuse, may have a harder time adapting to life and run an increased risk of psychosocial problems. In dysfunctional families, love, security, and unconditional trust are so lacking that children often become confused and psychologically bruised. Yet, not all people raised in dysfunctional families become psychosocially unhealthy, and not all children from healthy environments become well adjusted. Obviously, more factors are involved in our "process of becoming" than just our family.

The Macro Environment

Although isolated negative events may do little damage to psychosocial health, persistent stressors, uncertainties, and threats can cause significant problems. Drugs, neighborhood crime and threats to safety, injury, school failure,

unemployment, financial problems, natural disasters, and a host of other bad things can happen to good people. But it is believed that certain protective factors, such as having a positive role model in the midst of chaos, or certain positive personality traits can help children from even the worst environments remain healthy and well adjusted. They are often more resilient in the face of adversity and are more likely to have the resources to cope more effectively.

Another important influence is access to health services and programs designed to enhance psychosocial health. Attending a support group or seeing a trained therapist is often a crucial first step in prevention and intervention efforts. Memberships in church groups, athletics, or other socially bonding situations can also help a person feel connected and supported. Individuals from poor socioeconomic environments who cannot afford professional help and who don't have community and social networks of support, often find it difficult to secure help in improving their psychosocial health.

Self-Efficacy and Self-Esteem

During our formative years, successes and failures in school, athletics, friendships, intimate relationships, our jobs, and every other aspect of life subtly shape our beliefs about our own personal worth and abilities. These beliefs are internal influences on our psychosocial health.

Self-efficacy describes a person's belief about whether he or she can successfully engage in and execute a specific behavior. **Self-esteem** refers to one's sense of self-respect or self-worth. It can be defined as one's evaluation of oneself and one's personal worth as an individual. People with a high sense of self-efficacy and self-esteem tend to express a positive outlook on life. People with low self-esteem may demean themselves and doubt their ability to succeed.

Our self-esteem is a result of the relationships we have with our parents and family during our formative years; with our friends as we grow older; with our significant others as we form intimate relationships; and with our teachers, coworkers, and others throughout our lives. How can you build up your self-esteem? The **Skills for Behavior Change** box on this page suggests small things you can do every day that can significantly impact the way you feel about yourself.

dysfunctional families Families in which there is violence; physical, emotional, or sexual abuse; parental discord; or other negative family interactions.

self-efficacy Belief in one's own ability to perform a task successfully.

self-esteem Sense of self-respect or self-worth.

learned helplessness Pattern of responding to situations by giving up because of repeated failure in the past.

Learned Helplessness versus Learned Optimism

Psychologist Martin Seligman has proposed that people who continually experience failure may develop a pattern of responding known as **learned helplessness,** in which they give up and fail to take any action to help themselves. Seligman

what do you think?

What impact has your family had on your psychosocial health?
● Are you primarily an optimist or a pessimist? Why do you think you have this outlook? ● Do you ever struggle with low self-esteem or feelings of helplessness?

ascribes this response in part to society's tendency toward victimology, blaming one's problems on other people and circumstances.[8] Although viewing ourselves as victims may make us feel better temporarily, it does not address the underlying causes of a problem. Ultimately, it can erode self-efficacy and foster learned helplessness by making us feel that we cannot do anything to improve the situation.

Today, many people have developed self-help programs that utilize elements of Seligman's principle of **learned optimism.** Foundational to these self-help programs is the thought that just as we learn to be helpless, so can we teach ourselves to be optimistic. By changing our self-talk, examining our reactions and the way we assess what happens to us in life, and blocking negative thoughts, we can "unlearn" negative thought processes that have become habitual. Some programs practice "positive affirmations" with clients, teaching them the sometimes difficult task of learning to write and/or verbalize positive things about themselves. Often we are our own worst critics, and taking praise from others and learning to be kinder to ourselves are difficult.

learned optimism Teaching oneself to think positively.

Personality

Your personality is the unique mix of characteristics that distinguish you from others. Heredity, environment, culture, and experience influence how each person develops. Personality determines how we react to the challenges of life, interpret our feelings, and resolve conflicts.

Most of the recent schools of psychosocial theory promote the idea that we have the power not only to understand our behavior, but also to change it and thus mold our own personalities. Although much has been written about the importance of a healthy personality, there is little consensus on what that concept really means. In general, people who possess the following traits often appear to be psychosocially healthy:[9]

● **Extroversion,** the ability to adapt to a social situation and demonstrate assertiveness as well as power or interpersonal involvement
● **Agreeableness,** the ability to conform, be likable, and demonstrate friendly compliance as well as love
● **Openness to experience,** the willingness to demonstrate curiosity and independence (also referred to as inquiring intellect)
● **Emotional stability,** the ability to maintain social control
● **Conscientiousness,** the qualities of being dependable and demonstrating self-control, discipline, and a need to achieve
● **Resiliency,** the ability to adapt to change and stressful events in healthy and flexible ways

Life Span and Maturity

Our temperaments change as we move through life, as illustrated by the extreme emotions that many young teens experience. Most of us learn to control our emotions as we advance toward adulthood.

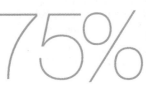

75% of the general U.S. population is estimated to be extroverted, as measured by the Myers–Briggs Type Indicator personality test.

The college years mark a critical transition period for young adults as they move away from families and establish themselves as independent adults. The transition to independence will be easier for those who have successfully accomplished earlier developmental tasks, such as learning how to solve problems, make and evaluate decisions, define and adhere to personal values, and establish both casual and intimate relationships. People who have not fulfilled these earlier tasks may find their lives interrupted by recurrent "crises" left over from earlier stages. For example, if they did not learn to trust others in childhood, they may have difficulty establishing intimate relationships as adults.

Strategies to Enhance Psychosocial Health

As we have seen, psychosocial health involves four dimensions. Attaining self-fulfillment is a lifelong, conscious process that involves enhancing each of these components. Strategies include building self-efficacy and self-esteem, understanding and controlling emotions, maintaining support networks, and learning to solve problems and make decisions. In addition to the advice in this chapter, see Chapter 3 for tips on effective

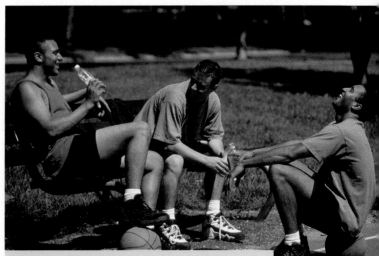

Fostering a solid support group can be as simple as spending time playing a team sport, like basketball, with friends.

stress reduction, relaxation techniques, and other tools for enhancing psychosocial health. Below are a few healthy steps you can start acting on today:

- **Find a support group.** A support group of peers who share your values can make you feel good about yourself and encourage you to take an honest look at your actions and choices. Keeping in contact with old friends and important family members can provide a foundation of unconditional love that will help you through life's transitions.
- **Complete required tasks.** A good way to boost your sense of self-efficacy is to learn new skills and develop a history of success. Most college campuses provide study groups and learning centers that can help you manage time, develop study skills, and prepare for tests.
- **Form realistic expectations.** If you expect perfect grades, a steady stream of Saturday-night dates, and the perfect job, you may be setting yourself up for failure. Assess your current resources and the direction in which you are heading. Set small, incremental goals that you can actually meet.
- **Make time for you.** Taking time to enjoy yourself is another way to boost your self-esteem and psychosocial health. View a new activity as something to look forward to and an opportunity to have fun. Anticipate and focus on the fun things you have to look forward to each day.
- **Maintain physical health through exercise.** Regular exercise fosters a sense of well-being. A growing body of research supports the role of exercise in improved mental health.
- **Examine problems and seek help when necessary.** Knowing when to seek help from friends, support groups, family, or professionals is another important factor in boosting self-esteem. Sometimes you can handle life's problems alone; at other times, you need assistance.
- **Get adequate sleep.** Getting enough sleep on a daily basis is a key factor in physical and psychosocial health. Not only do our bodies need to rest to conserve energy for our daily activities, but we also need to restore supplies of many of the neurotransmitters that we use up during our waking hours. For more information on the importance of sleep, see **Focus On: Your Sleep** beginning on page 86.

The Mind–Body Connection

Can negative emotions make us physically ill? Can positive emotions and happiness help us stay well? Researchers are exploring the interaction between emotions and health, especially in conditions of uncontrolled, persistent stress. In fact, the National Institutes of Health's National Center for Complementary and Alternative Medicine (NCCAM) and other organizations are investing more and more dollars in large research projects designed to explore the link between mind and body.

At the core of the mind–body connection is the study of **psychoneuroimmunology (PNI),** or how the brain and behavior affect the body's immune system. The science of PNI focuses on the relationship between emotions, psychosocial factors, the central nervous system, the immune system, and disease and illness.

Happiness and Health

One area of study that appears to be particularly promising in enhancing physical health is *happiness*—defined as a kind of placeholder for several positive states in which individuals actively embrace the world around them.[10] In examining the characteristics of happy people, scientists have found that this emotion can have a profound impact on the body. Happiness, or related mental states like hopefulness, optimism, and contentment, appears to reduce the risk or limit the severity of cardiovascular disease, pulmonary disease, diabetes, hypertension, colds, and other infections. Laughter can promote increases in heart and respiration rates and can reduce levels of stress hormones in much the same way as light exercise. For this reason, it has been promoted as a possible risk reducer for people with hypertension and other forms of cardiovascular disease.[11]

Subjective well-being refers to that uplifting feeling of inner peace or an overall "feel-good" state, which includes happiness. Subjective well-being is defined by three central components: satisfaction with present life, relative presence of positive emotions, and relative absence of negative emotions.[12] You do not have to be happy all the time to achieve overall subjective well-being. Everyone experiences disappointments, unhappiness, and times when life seems unfair. However, people with high subjective well-being are typically resilient, are able to look on the positive side and get back on track fairly quickly, and are less likely to fall into despair over setbacks.

Scientists suggest that some people may be biologically predisposed to happiness. Psychologist Richard Davidson proposes that happiness may, in part, be related to actual differences in brain physiology—that *neurotransmitters*, the chemicals that transfer messages between neurons, may function more efficiently in happy people.[13] Other psychologists suggest that

> **psychoneuroimmunology (PNI)** The science that examines the relationship between the brain and behavior and how this affects the body's immune system.
> **subjective well-being** An uplifting feeling of inner peace.

Calming your mind may help heal your body.

we can develop happiness by practicing positive psychological actions.[14]

Whereas positive emotions appear to benefit physical health, evidence is accumulating that negative emotions can impair it. Studies of widowed and divorced people reveal below-normal immune-system functioning and higher rates of illness and death than among married people. Other studies have shown unusually high rates of cancer among depressed people.[15] Some researchers suggest that people who are divorced, widowed, or depressed are more likely to drink and smoke, use drugs, eat and sleep poorly, and be sedentary—all of which may affect the immune system. In fact, the immune system changes measured in studies of the mind–body connection are relatively small. The health consequences of such minute changes are difficult to gauge, and researchers continue to seek the answer to this question.[16]

Does Laughter Enhance Health?

Do you remember the last time you laughed so hard that you cried? Remember how relaxed you felt afterward? Scientists are just beginning to understand the role of humor in our lives and health. For example, researchers have found that stressed-out people with a strong sense of humor become less depressed and anxious than those whose sense of humor is less well developed. Couples who reminisce and laugh about positive shared experiences have more stable, lasting relationships, while students who use humor as a coping mechanism report that it predisposes them to a positive mood.[17]

Learning to laugh puts more joy into everyday experiences and increases the likelihood that fun-loving people will keep company with us. Psychologist Barbara Fredrickson argues that positive emotions such as joy, interest, and contentment serve valuable life functions.[18] Joy is associated with playfulness and creativity. Interest encourages us to explore our world, which enhances knowledge and cognitive ability. Contentment allows us to savor and integrate experiences, an important step in achieving mindfulness and insight. By building our physical, social, and mental resources, these positive feelings empower us to cope effectively with life's challenges. Subsequent research has demonstrated that although the actual emotions may be transient, their effects can be permanent and provide lifelong enrichment.[19]

Using Positive Psychology to Enhance Happiness

If happiness is good for your health, how does one "get happy"? In his book *The Geography of Bliss*, author Eric Weiner reports on an explosion in happiness writings, research, and public interest. He defines happiness as "the mirror image of depression. . . . It is a stable disposition to feel good in the same way that depression is a stable disposition to feel sad or melancholy."[20] The emerging discipline of *positive psychology* focuses on helping us achieve the happiness we desire, find meaning in life, build our character strengths, and in general approach life from a more "positivistic" perspective.[21] Though this body of research is still in its early stages, several key aspects have emerged. You can implement the following strategies to enhance happiness and employ a more positive outlook on life:[22]

- **Develop gratitude.** Gratitude is a sense of thankfulness and appreciation for the good things in your life as well as for life's lessons. In one study, Seligman required individuals to write down three positive occurrences that happened each day for 1 week, then write an answer to the question, "Why did this good thing happen?" Try this yourself for 1 week.
- **Use capitalization.** Capitalization refers to the process by which we focus on the good things that happen to us and share those things with others. Research in this area indicates that telling others about a positive experience increases the positive emotion associated with the event and prolongs the good feelings.
- **Know when to say when.** Researchers have found that people who are always trying to do their absolute best and are not meeting their own high expectations may be more prone to depression, frustration, anxiety, and other problems. Find a level of achievement that you will be satisfied with, make sure it is realistic, and stick to it.
- **Grow a signature strength.** Traits such as wisdom, courage, humanity, hope, vitality, curiosity, and love are all considered virtues one should work hard to develop. These

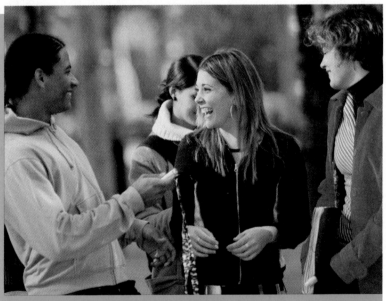

Is laughter really the best medicine?

Research is inconclusive regarding whether the act of laughing actually improves your health, but we've all experienced the sense of well-being that a good laugh can bring. Whether or not it increases blood flow, boosts immune response, lowers blood sugar levels, or facilitates better sleep, there is no doubting that sharing laughter and fun with others can strengthen social ties and bring joy to your everyday life.

strengths are believed to be among the most important to one's overall health.

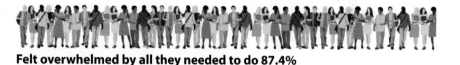

When Psychosocial Health Deteriorates

U.S. adults suffer from a diagnosable mental disorder in any given year.

Sometimes circumstances overwhelm us to such a degree that we need outside assistance to help us get back on track toward healthful living. Abusive relationships, stress, anxiety, loneliness, financial upheavals, and other traumatic events can sap our spirits, causing us to turn inward or to act in ways that are outside what might be considered normal. Chemical imbalances, drug interactions, trauma, neurological disruptions, and other physical problems also may contribute to these behaviors. **Mental illnesses** are disorders that disrupt thinking, feeling, moods, and behaviors and cause a varying degree of impaired functioning in daily life. They are believed to be caused by life events in some cases and by biochemical or brain dysfunction in others.[23] As with physical disease, mental illnesses can range from mild to severe and exact a heavy toll on the quality of life, both for people with the illnesses and for those who come in contact with them.

Mental disorders are common in the United States and worldwide. An estimated 26.2 percent of Americans aged 18 and older—about 1 in 4 adults—suffer from a diagnosable mental disorder in a given year. This translates to 57.7 million people. Out of these, about 6 percent, or 1 in 17, suffer from a serious mental illness requiring close monitoring, residential care in many instances, and medication. Mental disorders are the leading cause of disability in the United States and Canada for people aged 15 to 44. Nearly half (45 percent) of those with any mental disorder meet criteria for two or more disorders at the same time.[24] In the United States, mental disorders are diagnosed based on the American Psychiatric Association's *Diagnostic and Statistical Manual of Mental Disorders,* Fourth Edition, Text Revision *(DSM-IV-TR).*

Mental Health Threats to College Students

Today's students face increasing threats from difficulties in relationships, anxiety, depression, sexual assaults, pressures to take drugs, and a swirling morass of social and environmental problems. The pressures to succeed in an increasingly fast-paced and depersonalized environ-

ment often result in significant mental health problems for students. According to a recent American College Health Association survey of students from across the United States, 18.2 percent had been diagnosed with depression at some time in their lives.[25] Figure 2.4 shows more results from this survey. The **Health Headlines** box on page 38 highlights one growing mental health concern among young adults, attention deficit/hyperactivity disorder.

mental illnesses Disorders that disrupt thinking, feeling, moods, and behaviors and that impair daily functioning.

Although there are many types of mental illness, we will focus here on those most likely to be experienced by large numbers of college students. For information about other disorders, consult the websites at the end of this chapter, or ask your instructor for local resources.

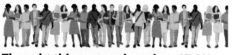

Felt overwhelmed by all they needed to do 87.4%

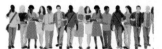

Thought things were hopeless 47.0%

Had difficulty functioning because of depression 30.6%

Seriously considered suicide 6.4%

Intentionally injured themselves 5.5%

Attempted suicide 1.3%

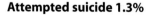

= 2%

FIGURE 2.4 **Mental Health Concerns of American College Students, Past 12 Months**
Source: Data are from American College Health Association (ACHA), *ACHA-National College Health Assessment II, Reference Group Data Report, Fall 2008.* (Baltimore: ACHA, 2009).

Health Headlines

WHEN ADULTS HAVE ADHD

Attention deficit/hyperactivity disorder (ADHD) is a common neurobehavioral disorder that affects 5 to 8 percent of school-aged children. In as many as 60 percent of cases, symptoms persist into adulthood. In any given year, 4.1 percent of adults are identified as having ADHD.

People with ADHD are hyperactive or distracted most of the time. Even when they try to concentrate, they find it hard to pay attention. They have a hard time organizing things, listening to instructions, remembering details, and controlling their behavior. As a result, people with ADHD often have problems getting along with other people at home, at school, or at work. ADHD may run in families.

ADULT ADHD MYTHS AND FACTS

MYTH: ADHD is just a lack of willpower. Persons with ADHD focus well on things that interest them; they could focus on any other tasks if they really wanted to.
FACT: ADHD looks very much like a willpower problem, but it isn't. It's essentially a chemical problem in the management systems of the brain.
MYTH: Everybody has the symptoms of ADHD, and anyone with adequate intelligence can overcome these difficulties.
FACT: ADHD affects persons of all levels of intelligence. And although everyone sometimes is prone to distraction or impulsivity, only those with chronic impairments from ADHD symptoms warrant an ADHD diagnosis.
MYTH: Someone can't have ADHD and also have depression, anxiety, or other psychiatric problems.

FACT: A person with ADHD is six times more likely to have another psychiatric or learning disorder than most other people. ADHD usually overlaps with other disorders.
MYTH: Unless you have been diagnosed with ADHD as a child, you can't have it as an adult.
FACT: Many adults struggle all their lives with unrecognized ADHD impairments. They haven't received help because they assumed that their chronic difficulties, like depression or anxiety, were caused by other impairments that did not respond to usual treatment.

EFFECTS OF ADULT ADHD

Left untreated, ADHD can disrupt everything from your career to your relationships and financial stability. Although most of us sometimes have challenges in these areas, the persistent chaos and disorganization of ADHD can make managing the problems worse and worse. Some key areas of disruption might include the following:

✳ **Health.** Impulsivity and trouble with organization can lead to problems with health, such as compulsive eating, alcohol and drug abuse, or forgetting medication for a chronic condition.
✳ **Work and finances.** Difficulty concentrating, completing tasks, listening, and relating to others can lead to trouble at work. Managing finances also may be a concern. You may find yourself struggling to pay your bills, losing paperwork, missing deadlines, or spending impulsively, resulting in debt.
✳ **Relationships.** You might wonder why loved ones constantly nag you to tidy up, get organized, and take care of business. Or if your loved one has ADHD, you might be hurt that your loved one doesn't seem to listen to you, blurts out hurtful things, and leaves you with the bulk of organizing and planning.

GET EDUCATED ABOUT ADHD

If you suspect you or someone close to you has ADHD, learn as much as you can about adult ADHD and treatment options. Children and Adults with

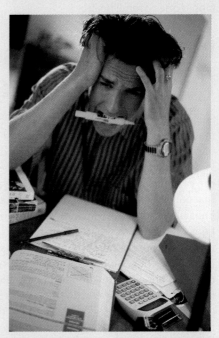

Disorder and chaos can be headaches for us all, but ADHD sufferers may find them insurmountable obstacles.

Attention-Deficit Hyperactivity Disorder (CHADD) is a good source of information and support (www.chadd.org). Adult ADHD can be a challenge to diagnose, as there is no simple test for it. Many symptoms of ADHD overlap with other conditions, and ADHD often occurs concurrently with other conditions, such as depression or anxiety disorders. To ensure that you have the best treatment plan, secure a diagnosis and treatment plan from a qualified professional with experience in ADHD.

Sources: Centers for Disease Control and Prevention, "Attention-Deficit Hyperactivity Disorder," www.cdc.gov/ncbddd/adhd, accessed March 8, 2009; National Institute of Mental Health, "The Numbers Count," www.nimh.nih.gov/health/publications/the-numbers-count-mental-disorders-in-america/index.shtml, 2008; H. R. Searight, J. M. Burke, and F. Rottnek, "Adult ADHD: Evaluation and Treatment in Family Medicine," *American Family Physician* 62, no. 9 (2000): 2091–92; J. Saisan, J. Jaffe, T. de Benedictis, M. Smith, and R. O. Segal, "Adult ADD/ADHD: Signs, Symptoms, Effects, and Getting Help," Helpguide.org, updated March 2009, www.helpguide.org/mental/adhd_add_adult_symptoms.htm; T. Brown, *Attention Deficit Disorder: The Unfocused Mind in Children and Adults* (New Haven, CT: Yale University Press, 2005).

Mood Disorders

Chronic mood disorders are disorders that affect how you feel, such as persistent sadness or feelings of euphoria. They include depression, dysthymia, bipolar disorder, and seasonal affective disorder. In any given year, approximately 10 percent of Americans aged 18 or older—or 20.9 million people—suffer from a mood disorder.[26]

Depressive disorders are the most common mood disorders. The president of the American Psychological Association once remarked, "Depression has been called the common cold of psychological disturbances, which underscores its prevalence, but trivializes its impact."[27] Each year, depression affects approximately 14.8 million American adults, or about 7 percent of the U.S. population, and it is the leading cause of disability in the United States for people aged 15 to 44.[28] These numbers may reflect just the tip of the iceberg when it comes to determining how many people suffer from depression. Many more are misdiagnosed or underdiagnosed, are not receiving treatment, or are not treated with the right combinations of therapy.[29] Some people experience one bout of depression and never have problems again, but others suffer recurrences throughout their lives. Stressful life events are often catalysts for these recurrences.

Depressive Disorders

Sometimes life throws us down the proverbial stairs. We experience loss, pain, disappointment, and frustration, and we can be left feeling beaten and bruised. How do we know whether those emotions are really signs of a **major depressive disorder**? It's important to note that true depressive disorders are not the same as having a bad day or feeling down after a negative experience. It also isn't something that can be willed or wished away, or just a matter of learning to "grow a thicker skin." True depressive disorders are characterized by a combination of symptoms that interfere with work, study, sleep, eating, relationships, and enjoyment of life. Symptoms can last for weeks, months, or years and vary in intensity.[30]

Sadness and despair are the main symptoms of depression. Other common signs include the following:

- Loss of motivation or interest in pleasurable activities
- Preoccupation with failures and inadequacies; concern over what others are thinking
- Difficulty concentrating; indecisiveness; memory lapses
- Loss of sex drive or interest in close interactions with others
- Fatigue and loss of energy; slow reactions
- Sleeping too much or too little; insomnia
- Feeling agitated, worthless, or hopeless
- Withdrawal from friends and family
- Diminished or increased appetite
- Significant weight loss or weight gain
- Recurring thoughts that life isn't worth living; thoughts of death or suicide

30 years old is the median age of onset for mood disorders.

Although most people only think of major depression when they think of depression, many people suffer from **dysthymic disorder,** a less severe syndrome of chronic, mild depression. Dysthymia can be harder to recognize than major depression. Dysthymic individuals may appear to function okay, but they may lack energy or may fatigue easily; be short-tempered, overly pessimistic, and ornery; or just not quite feel up to par without having any really overt symptoms. People with dysthymia may cycle into major depression over time. For a diagnosis, symptoms must persist for at least 2 years in adults (1 year in children). This disorder affects approximately 1.5 percent of the U.S. population aged 18 and older in a given year, or about 3.3 million American adults.[31]

Another type of depressive mood disorder is **bipolar disorder,** also called *manic depression*. People with bipolar disorder often have severe mood swings, ranging from extreme highs (mania) to extreme lows (depression). Sometimes these swings are dramatic and rapid; other times they are slow and gradual. When in the manic phase, people may be overactive, talkative, and have tons of energy; in the depressed phase, they may experience some or all of the typical major depressive symptoms.

Although the exact cause of bipolar disorder is unknown, biological, genetic, and environmental factors, such as drug abuse and stressful or psychologically traumatic events, seem to be involved in triggering episodes of the illness. Once diagnosed, persons with bipolar disorder have several counseling and pharmaceutical options, and most will be able to live a healthy, functional life while being treated.

An estimated 6 percent of Americans suffer from another form of depression called **seasonal affective disorder (SAD),** and an additional 14 percent experience a milder form of the illness known as the *winter blues*. SAD strikes during the winter months and is associated with reduced exposure to sunlight. People with SAD suffer from irritability, apathy, carbohydrate craving and weight gain, increased sleep time, and general sadness. Several factors are implicated in SAD development, including disruption in the body's natural circadian rhythms and changes in levels of the hormone melatonin and the brain chemical serotonin.[32]

The most beneficial treatment for SAD is light therapy, in which patients are exposed to lamps that simulate sunlight. Eighty percent of patients experience relief from their symptoms within 4 days. Other treatments for SAD include diet change (eating more complex carbohydrates), increased

chronic mood disorder Experience of persistent emotional states, such as sadness, despair, and hopelessness.
major depressive disorder Severe depression that entails chronic mood disorder, physical effects such as sleep disturbance and exhaustion, and mental effects such as the inability to concentrate.
dysthymic disorder A less severe type of depression than major depressive disorder that is milder, chronic, harder to recognize, and often characterized by fatigue, pessimism, or a short temper.
bipolar disorder Form of mood disorder characterized by alternating mania and depression.
seasonal affective disorder (SAD) A type of depression that occurs in the winter months, when sunlight levels are low.

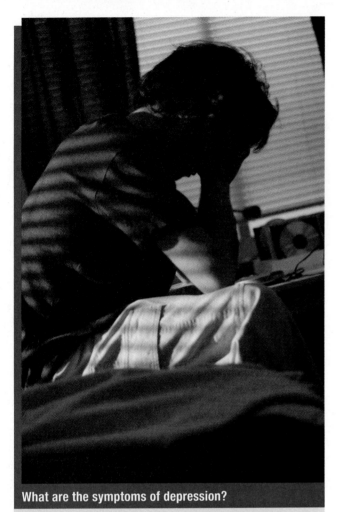

What are the symptoms of depression?

There is more to depression than simply feeling blue. When a person is clinically depressed, he finds it difficult to function, sometimes struggling just to get out of bed in the morning or to follow a conversation.

exercise, stress-management techniques, sleep restriction (limiting the number of hours slept in a 24-hour period), psychotherapy, and prescription medications.

Causes of Depressive Disorders Depressive disorders are caused by the interaction between biology, learned behavioral responses, cognitive factors, environment, and situational triggers and stressors. The biology of mood disorders is related to individual levels of brain chemicals called *neurotransmitters*. Some types of depression, such as bipolar disorder, appear to have a genetic component and to run in families. People who have low self-esteem, who consistently view themselves and the world with pessimism, or who are readily overwhelmed by stress are prone to depression. Depression can also be triggered by a serious loss, difficult relationships, financial problems, and pressure to get good grades or succeed in athletics. In recent years, researchers have shown that changes in the body's physical

health can be accompanied by mental changes, particularly depression. Stroke, heart attack, cancer, Parkinson's disease, problems with chronic pain, type 2 diabetes, certain medications, alcohol, hormonal disorders, and a wide range of afflictions can cause you to become depressed, frustrated, and angry. When this happens, recovery is often more difficult. A person who feels exhausted and defeated may lack the will to fight illness and do what is necessary to optimize recovery.

Depression in College Students Mental health problems, particularly depression, have gained increased recognition as major obstacles to success and healthy adjustment on campuses throughout the country. Students who have weak communication skills; who find that college isn't what they expected; or who find that people they've known seem different, causing them to lose their "lifeboats" in a sea of strangers, often have difficulties. Stressors such as anxiety over relationships, pressure to get good grades and win social acceptance, abuse of alcohol and other drugs, poor diet, and lack of sleep can create a toxic cocktail that can overwhelm even the most resilient students.

The National College Health Assessment found that over a 6-year period, from 2002 to 2008, the number of students who reported "having been diagnosed with depression" increased from 11 percent to 15 percent. Predictably, stress and depression are among students' top five impediments to academic success.[33] See the **Health Today** box on page 41 for information on another, often related, psychological disorder of growing concern among young people—self-mutilation.

International students are particularly vulnerable to depression and other mental health concerns. Being far from home without the security of family and friends can exacerbate problems and make coping difficult. Most campuses have counseling centers, cultural centers, and other services available; however, many students do not use them because of persistent stigma about going to a counselor.

Depression in Women Women are almost twice as likely as men to experience depression. Hormonal changes related to the menstrual cycle, pregnancy, miscarriage, postpartum period, premenopause, and menopause may be factors in this increased rate.[34] Additionally, women face various stressors in their lives related to multiple responsibilities—work, child-rearing, single parenthood, household work, and caring for older parents—at rates that are higher than those of men. New research indicates that women have more difficulties obtaining restorative sleep, which may contribute to these problems.[35]

Researchers have observed gender differences in coping strategies (responses to certain events or stimuli) and have proposed that some women's strategies make them more vulnerable to depression. Presented with a list of things people do when depressed, college students were asked to indicate how likely they were to engage in each behavior. Men were

HEALTH Today

Cutting through the Pain

When some people are unable to deal with the pain, pressure, and stress they experience in everyday life, they may resort to self-injury in order to cope. *Self-injury,* also termed *self-mutilation, self-harm,* or *nonsuicidal self-injury* (NSSI), is the act of deliberately harming one's body in an attempt to cope with overwhelming negative emotions. Self-injury is a coping mechanism; it is not an attempt at suicide.

The most common method of self-harm is cutting (with razors, glass, knives, or other sharp objects). Other methods include burning, bruising, excessive nail biting, breaking bones, pulling out hair, and embedding sharp objects under the skin. Seventy-five percent of those who harm themselves do so in more than one way.

Researchers estimate that between 2 and 8 million Americans have engaged in self-harm at some point in their lives and the prevalence of NSSI in college students is reported between 17 and 38 percent. Many people who inflict self-harm suffer from larger mental health conditions and have experienced sexual, physical, or emotional abuse as children or adults. Self-harm is also commonly associated with mental illnesses such as borderline personality disorder, depression, anxiety disorders, substance abuse disorders, post-traumatic stress disorder, and eating disorders.

Signs of self-injury include multiple scars, current cuts and abrasions, and implausible explanations for wounds and ongoing injuries. A self-injurer may attempt to conceal scars and injuries by wearing long sleeves and pants. Other symptoms can include difficulty handling anger, social withdrawal, sensitivity to rejection, or body alienation. If you or someone you know is engaging in self-injury, seek professional help. Treatment is challenging; not only must the self-injurious behavior be stopped, but the sufferer must learn to recognize and manage the feelings that triggered the behavior.

Recovering cutters use some of the following steps in their treatment:

1. Start by being aware of feelings and situations that trigger your urge to cut.

2. Identify a plan of what you can do instead of cutting when you feel the urge.

3. Create a list of alternatives, including:
* Things that might distract you
* Things that might soothe and calm you
* Things that might help you express the pain and deep emotion
* Things that might help release physical tension and distress
* Things that might help you feel supported and connected
* Things that might substitute for the cutting sensation

For more information, try these resources: American Self-Harm Information Clearinghouse, www.selfinjury.org; S. A. F. E. Alternatives, www.selfinjury.com; and Self-Injury Support, www.sisupport.org.

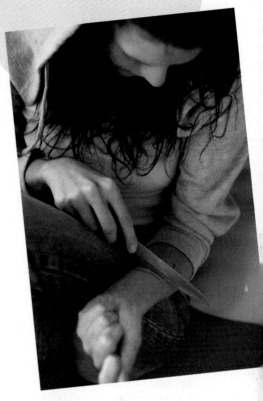

Previously, self-injury was thought to be more common in females, but recent research indicates that rates are generally the same for men and women.

Sources: J. Bennett, "Why She Cuts," *Newsweek* Web Exclusive, December 29, 2008, www.newsweek.com/id/177135; M. J. Prinstein, "Introduction to the Special Section on Suicide and Nonsuicidal Self-Injury: A Review of Unique Challenges and Important Directions for Self-Injury Science," *Journal of Consulting and Clinical Psychology* 76, no. 1 (2008): 1–8; Mayo Clinic Staff, "Self-Injury/Cutting," August 2, 2008, www.mayoclinic.com.

---

more likely to assert, "I avoid thinking of reasons why I am depressed," "I do something physical," or "I play sports." Women were more likely to answer, "I try to determine why I am depressed," "I talk to other people about my feelings," and "I cry to relieve the tension." In other words, the men tried to distract themselves from a depressed mood, whereas the women focused on it. If focusing obsessively on negative feelings intensifies these feelings, women who do this may predispose themselves to depression. This hypothesis has not been directly tested recently, but some early supporting evidence suggested its validity.[36]

Depression in Men Six million men in the United States are currently in treatment for depression, and countless others suffering from the disorder are untreated. Depression in men is often masked by alcohol or drug abuse or by the socially acceptable habit of working excessively long hours. Typically, depressed men present not as hopeless and helpless, but as irritable, angry, and discouraged, often personifying a "tough guy" image. Men are less likely to admit they are depressed, and doctors are less likely to suspect it, based on what men report during doctor's visits.[37]

Depression can also affect men's physical health differently from women's. Although depression is associated with an increased risk of coronary heart disease in both men and women, it is also associated with a higher risk of death by heart disease in men.[38] Men are also more likely to act on suicidal feelings than women, and they are usually more successful at suicide as well; suicide rates among depressed men are four times those of women.[39] Encouragement and support from families and friends may help men recognize symptoms and seek treatment.

what do you think?

Why do you think that women experience more depression than men? ● Do you think men and women cope with depression differently? In what ways? ● Who is most likely to seek counseling for depression on campus? Why?

Depression in Older Adults
Many adults in their middle and older years are emotionally stable and lead active and satisfying lives. However, when depression does occur, it is often undiagnosed or untreated, particularly in people in lower income groups or those who do not have access to community resources and supports or medications. Older adults may be less likely to discuss feelings of sadness, loss, helplessness, or other symptoms, or they may attribute their own depression to aging. Those who have insurance may take multiple medications, many of which may result in depression symptoms and may increase their risks for related problems.

Depression in Children
Today, depression in children is an increasingly reported phenomenon, with shocking cases of suicide and other outcomes in children as young as 4 and 5 years old. Depressed children may pretend to be sick, refuse to go to school, sleep incessantly, engage in self-mutilation, get into trouble with drugs or alcohol, and attempt suicide. Parents of children who are depressed may find it difficult to find therapists trained in working with depressed children or physicians skilled in determining which adult antidepressants may be best for children.

Treating Mood Disorders

The best treatment for mood disorders involves determining the person's type and degree of depression and its possible causes. Both psychotherapeutic and pharmacological modes of treatment are recommended for clinical (severe and prolonged) depression. Drugs often relieve the symptoms of depression, such as loss of sleep or appetite, and psychotherapy can be equally helpful by improving the ability to function.

Psychotherapeutic Treatment In some cases, psychotherapy alone may be the most successful treatment. The two most common psychotherapeutic treatments for depression are cognitive therapy and interpersonal therapy.

Cognitive therapy helps a patient look at life rationally and correct habitually pessimistic thought patterns. It focuses on the present rather than analyzing a patient's past. To pull a person out of depression, cognitive therapists usually need 6 to 18 months of weekly sessions that include reasoning and behavioral exercises.

Interpersonal therapy, sometimes combined with cognitive therapy, also addresses the present but focuses on correcting chronic relationship problems. Interpersonal therapists focus on patients' relationships with their families and other people.

Pharmacological Treatment Antidepressant drugs offer several options for treating depressive disorders. The most common antidepressants are the selective serotonin reuptake inhibitors (SSRIs), but in the past few years new drugs with different methods of action have also become available. Table 2.1 on page 43 lists some of the common psychiatric medications prescribed to treat depression as well as those commonly prescribed to treat the other mental disorders discussed later in this chapter.

The potency, dosage, and side effects of each drug vary greatly. Antidepressants should be prescribed only after a thorough psychological and physiological examination. In 2004, the U.S. Food and Drug Administration asked the makers of antidepressant drugs to add a warning to the labels advising that patients taking these drugs be monitored for "worsening depression or the emergence of suicidality." Recent reports of suicidal tendencies among some youth taking antidepressants have stirred controversy over the use of these drugs in certain populations.[40]

If your doctor suggests an antidepressant, ask these questions first:

● What biological indicators are you using to determine whether I really need this drug?
● What is the action of this drug? When will I start to feel the benefits? What are the side effects of using this drug? What happens if I stop taking it?
● What is your rationale for selecting this antidepressant over others?

TABLE 2.1 Types of Medications Used to Treat Various Mental Illnesses

Antidepressants	**Used to treat depression, panic disorders, anxiety disorders**	
Selective serotonin reuptake inhibitors (SSRIs)	*Examples:* fluoxetine (Prozac), paroxetine (Paxil, Seroxat), escitalopram (Lexapro, Esipram), citalopram (Celexa), and sertraline (Zoloft)	The current standard drug treatment for depression; also frequently prescribed for anxiety disorders
Noradrenergic and specific serotonergic antidepressants (NaSSAs)	*Examples:* mirtazapine (Avanza, Zispin, Remeron)	Reportedly have fewer sexual dysfunction side effects than SSRIs
Serotonin-norepinephrine reuptake inhibitors (SNRIs)	*Examples:* venlafaxine (Effexor), duloxetine (Cymbalta)	Also sometimes prescribed for ADHD
Norepinephrine-dopamine reuptake inhibitors (NDRIs)	*Examples:* bupropion (Wellbutrin, Zyban)	Also used in smoking cessation; fewer weight gain or sexual dysfunction side effects than SSRIs
Tricyclic antidepressants (TCAs)	*Examples:* imipramine, amitriptyline, nortriptyline, and desipramine	Negative side effects; usually used as a 2nd or 3rd line of treatment when other medications prove ineffective
Monoamine oxidase inhibitors (MAOIs)	*Examples:* phenelzine (Nardil), tranylcypromine (Parnate), and isocarboxazid (Marplan)	Dangerous interactions with many other drugs and substances in food; generally no longer prescribed
Anxiolytics (antianxiety drugs)	**Used to treat anxiety disorders including OCD, GAD, panic disorders, phobias, PTSD**	
Benzodiazepines	*Examples:* lorazepam (Ativan), clonazepam (Klonopin), alprazolam (Xanax), diazepam (Valium)	Short-term relief, sometimes taken on an as-needed basis; dangerous interactions with alcohol; possible to develop tolerance or dependence
Serotonin 1A agonists	*Examples:* buspirone (BuSpar)	Longer-term relief; must be taken for at least 2 weeks to achieve antianxiety effects
Mood stabilizers	**Used to treat bipolar disorder, schizophrenia**	
Lithium	*Examples:* lithium carbonate	Drug most commonly used to treat bipolar disorder; blood levels must be closely monitored to determine proper dosage and avoid toxic effects
Anticonvulsants	*Examples:* valproic acid (Depakene), divalproex sodium (Depakote), sodium valproate (Depacon)	Used more frequently for acute mania than for long-term maintenance of bipolar disorder
Antipsychotics (neuroleptics)	**Used to treat schizophrenia, mania, bipolar disorder**	
Atypical antipsychotics	*Examples:* clozapine (Clozaril), risperidone (Risperdal)	First line of treatment for schizophrenia; fewer adverse effects than earlier antipsychotics
First-generation antipsychotics	*Examples:* haloperidol (Haldol), chlorpromazine (Thorazine)	Earliest forms of antipsychotics; unpleasant side effects such as tremor and muscle stiffness
Stimulants	**Used to treat ADHD, narcolepsy**	
Methylphenidate	*Brand names:* Ritalin, Metadate, Concerta	Can lead to tolerance and dependence; frequently abused for both performance enhancement and recreational use
Amphetamines	*Examples:* amphetamine (Adderall), dextroamphetamine (Dexedrine, Dextrostat), pemoline (Cylert)	Can lead to tolerance and dependence; frequently abused for both performance enhancement and recreational use

- How long can I be on this medication without significant risk to my health?
- How will you follow up or monitor the levels of this drug in my body? How often will I need to be checked?

You may not feel the therapeutic effects of antidepressants for several weeks, so patience is important. Also, you should not stop taking medication all at once, but rather gradually, and always under your doctor's supervision. In addition, be careful when taking antidepressant medications to avoid alcohol or illicit drug consumption, as the interactions between these drugs can be life threatening.

Anxiety Disorders

Anxiety disorders include generalized anxiety disorder, panic disorders, obsessive-compulsive disorder, and phobic disorders. They are characterized by persistent feelings of threat and worry. Consider John Madden, former head coach of the Oakland Raiders and a true "man's man," who outfitted his own bus and, for many years, drove every weekend across the country to serve as commentator on NFL football games. What was the reason behind this exhausting driving schedule? Madden is terrified of getting on a plane.

Anxiety disorders are the number-one mental health problem in the United States, affecting over 40 million people aged 18 to 54 each year, or about 18 percent of all adults.[41] Anxiety is also a leading mental health problem among adolescents, affecting 13 million youngsters aged 9 to 17. Costs associated with an overly anxious populace are growing rapidly; conservative estimates cite nearly $50 billion a year spent in doctors' bills and workplace losses in America. These numbers don't begin to address the human costs incurred when a person is too fearful to leave the house or talk to anyone outside the immediate family.

anxiety disorders Disorders characterized by persistent feelings of threat and worry in coping with everyday problems.
generalized anxiety disorder (GAD) A constant sense of worry that may cause restlessness, difficulty in concentrating, tension, and other symptoms.
panic attack Severe anxiety reaction in which a particular situation, often for unknown reasons, causes terror.

Generalized Anxiety Disorder

One common form of anxiety disorder, **generalized anxiety disorder (GAD),** is severe enough to significantly interfere with daily life. Generally, the person with GAD is a consummate worrier who develops a debilitating level of anxiety. Often multiple sources of worry exist, and it is hard to pinpoint the root cause of the anxiety. To be diagnosed with GAD, one must exhibit at least three of the following symptoms for more days than not during a 6-month period: restlessness or feeling keyed up or on edge; being easily fatigued; difficulty concentrating or mind going blank; irritability; muscle tension; and sleep disturbances.[42] Often GAD runs in

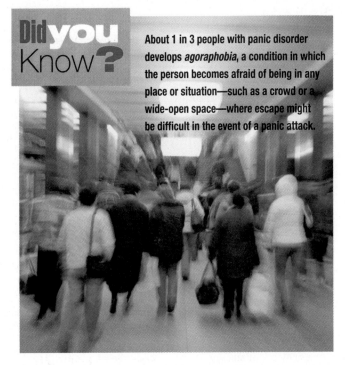

families and is readily treatable with benzodiazepines such as Librium, Valium, and Xanax, which calm the person for short periods. Individual therapy can be a more effective long-term treatment.

Panic Disorders

Panic disorders are characterized by the occurrence of **panic attacks,** a form of acute anxiety reaction that brings on an intense physical reaction. You may dismiss the feelings as the jitters from too much stress, or the reaction may be so severe that you fear you will have a heart attack and die. Approximately 6 million Americans aged 18 and older experience panic attacks each year, usually in early adulthood. Panic attacks and disorders are increasing in incidence, particularly among young women. Although highly treatable, panic attacks may become debilitating and destructive, particularly if they happen often and cause the person to avoid going out in public or interacting with others.

A panic attack typically starts abruptly, peaks within 10 minutes, lasts about 30 minutes, and leaves the person tired and drained.[43] Symptoms include increased respiration, chills, hot flashes, shortness of breath, stomach cramps, chest pain, difficulty swallowing, and a sense of doom or impending death.

Although researchers aren't sure what causes panic attacks, heredity, stress, and certain biochemical factors may play a role. Your chances of having a panic attack increase if you have a close family member who has them. Some researchers believe that people who suffer panic attacks are experiencing an overreactive fight-or-flight physical response (see Chapter 3).

Phobic Disorders

Phobias, or phobic disorders, involve a persistent and irrational fear of a specific object, activity, or situation, often out of proportion to the circumstances. Phobias result in a compelling desire to avoid the source of the fear. About 13 percent of Americans suffer from phobias, such as fear of spiders, snakes, public speaking, and so on.

Social phobias are perhaps the most common. A **social phobia** is an anxiety disorder characterized by the persistent fear and avoidance of social situations. Essentially, the person dreads these situations for fear of being humiliated, embarrassed, or simply looked at. These disorders vary in scope. Some cause difficulty only in specific situations, such as getting up in front of the class to give a report. In more extreme cases, a person avoids all contact with others.

Obsessive-Compulsive Disorder

People who feel compelled to perform rituals over and over again; are fearful of dirt or contamination; have an unnatural concern about order, symmetry, and exactness; or have persistent intrusive thoughts that they can't shake may be suffering from **obsessive-compulsive disorder (OCD).** Approximately 2 million Americans aged 18 or over have OCD.[44] Not to be confused with being a perfectionist, a person with OCD often knows the behaviors are irrational and senseless yet is powerless to stop them. According to the *DSM-IV-TR*, to be diagnosed as OCD, the obsessions must consume more than 1 hour per day and interfere with normal social and/or life activities. Although the exact cause is unknown, genetics, biological abnormalities, learned behaviors, and environmental factors have all been considered. OCD usually begins in adolescence or early adulthood, and the median age of onset is 19.

As with other anxiety-based disorders, medication and cognitive behavioral therapy are often the keys to treatment. Some individuals are given antidepressants, antianxiety drugs, or other drug combinations, which often prevent future attacks. Cognitive therapy can help sufferers recognize and avoid triggers or deal with triggers through meditation, deep breathing, and other relaxation techniques.

Post-Traumatic Stress Disorder

According to the American Psychiatric Association, one-third to one-half of individuals exposed to a traumatic life event will develop some form of psychopathology. In severe cases, an individual may develop **post-traumatic stress disorder (PTSD).** PTSD generally develops within the first hours or days after a traumatic event, but occasionally symptoms do not begin until months or years later.

Often PTSD affects soldiers returning home from war, particularly those who saw friends killed or mangled or who experienced terrible wounds. Responses from a survey given to a sample of service personnel deployed to Iraq indicated that 90 percent had been shot at and a high percentage reported knowing someone who was injured or had been killed, or had killed an enemy combatant. Almost 50 percent had handled dead bodies. This study of armed services members found that one in eight reported symptoms of PTSD.[45] Unfortunately, less than half of those with problems sought help, fearing stigma and damage to their careers. Many of these soldiers continue to suffer from these experiences for decades afterward. Other traumatic events that can cause PTSD include rape or other physical attacks, severe accidents, witnessing a murder or death, being caught in a natural disaster, or terrorist attacks.

Symptoms of PTSD include the following:

- Dissociation, or perceived detachment of the mind from the emotional state or even the body. The person may have a sense of the world as a dreamlike or unreal place and have little memory of the events—a form of dissociative amnesia.
- Acute anxiety or nervousness, in which the person is hyperaroused; may cry easily or experience mood swings; and experience flashbacks, nightmares, and recurrent thoughts or visual images. Some people may sense vague uneasiness or feel like the traumatic event is happening again and again. Others may experience intense physiological reactions, such as shaking or nausea, when something reminds them of the event. In some cases, they may have difficulty returning to areas that remind them of the trauma.

> **phobia** A deep and persistent fear of a specific object, activity, or situation that results in a compelling desire to avoid the source of the fear.
> **social phobia** A phobia characterized by fear and avoidance of social situations.
> **obsessive-compulsive disorder (OCD)** A form of anxiety disorder characterized by recurrent, unwanted thoughts and repetitive behaviors.
> **post-traumatic stress disorder (PTSD)** A collection of symptoms that may occur as a delayed response to a serious trauma.

As our knowledge about this disorder grows, therapies designed to help trauma victims recover are becoming increasingly effective. Schools, communities, and workplaces now routinely bring in crisis experts immediately after a traumatic event to help survivors talk through their feelings and gain support from others. New generations of antianxiety drugs can help individuals who have difficulties. Sleep aids and other options are available to ease short-term symptoms.

Sources of Anxiety Disorders

Because anxiety disorders vary in complexity and degree, scientists have yet to find clear reasons why one person develops them and another doesn't. The following factors are often cited as possible causes.[46]

- **Biology.** Some scientists trace the origin of anxiety to the brain and brain functioning. Using sophisticated positron emission tomography scans (PET scans), scientists can analyze areas of the brain that react during anxiety-producing events. Families appear to display similar brain and physiological reactivity, indicating that we may inherit our tendencies toward anxiety disorders.

● **Environment.** Anxiety can be a learned response. Although genetic tendencies may exist, experiencing a repeated pattern of reacting to certain situations programs the brain to respond in a certain way. For example, if your mother or father screamed whenever a large spider crept into view or if other anxiety-raising events occurred frequently, you might be predisposed to react with anxiety to similar events later in your life. Interestingly, animals also experience such anxieties—perhaps from being around their edgy owners.

● **Social and cultural roles.** Cultural and social roles also may be a factor in risks for anxiety. Because men and women are taught to assume different roles in society (for example, man as protector, woman as victim), women may find it more acceptable to scream, shake, pass out, and otherwise express extreme anxiety. Men, by contrast, may have learned to suppress such anxieties rather than act on them.

Personality Disorders

According to the *DSM-IV-TR,* **personality disorders** are "enduring patterns of inner experience and behavior that deviate markedly from the expectation of the individual's culture and are pervasive and inflexible."[47] Researchers at the National Institutes of Mental Health have found that about 9 percent of adults in the United States have some form of personality disorder as defined by the *DSM-IV-TR.*[48] People who live, work, or are in relationships with individuals suffering from personality disorders often find them to be very challenging and destructive interactions.

Common types of personality disorders include *paranoid personality disorders,* which involve pervasive, unfounded suspicion and mistrust of other people, irrational jealousy, and secretiveness. Persons with this illness have delusions of being persecuted by everyone, from their family members and loved ones to the government. *Narcissistic personality disorders* involve an exaggerated sense of self-importance and self-absorption. Persons with narcissistic personalities are fascinated with themselves and are preoccupied with fantasies of how wonderful they are.[49] Typically they are overly needy and demanding and believe that they are "entitled" to nothing but the best. Most are so self-absorbed that they don't have time to be supportive of anyone else.

personality disorders A class of mental disorders that is characterized by inflexible patterns of thought and beliefs that lead to socially distressing behavior.

schizophrenia A mental illness with biological origins that is characterized by irrational behavior, severe alterations of the senses (hallucinations), and often an inability to function in society.

Borderline personality disorder (BPD) is characterized by impulsiveness and engaging in risky behaviors such as gambling sprees, unsafe sex, use of illicit drugs, and risky driving.[50] Seventy to 80 percent of persons diagnosed with BPD self-mutilate or self-harm.[51] Sufferers have trouble stabilizing their moods and can experience erratic mood swings. Other characteristics of this mental illness include reality distortion and the tendency to see things in only "black and white" terms.

Schizophrenia

Perhaps the most frightening of all psychological disorders is **schizophrenia,** which affects about 1 percent of the U.S. population. Schizophrenia is characterized by alterations of the senses (including auditory and visual hallucinations); the inability to sort out incoming stimuli and make appropriate responses; an altered sense of self; and radical changes in emotions, movements, and behaviors. Typical symptoms of schizophrenia include fluctuating courses of such things as delusional behavior, hallucinations, incoherent and rambling speech, inability to think logically, erratic movement and odd gesturing, and difficulty with normal activities of daily living.[52] The net effect is that such individuals are often regarded by an unknowing society as being "odd;" as such, they have difficulties in social interactions and may withdraw. Contrary to popular belief, schizophrenia is not the same as split personality or multiple personality disorder.

For decades, scientists believed that schizophrenia was an environmentally provoked form of madness. They blamed abnormal family interactions or early childhood traumas. Since the mid-1980s, however, when magnetic resonance imaging (MRI) and positron-emission tomography (PET)

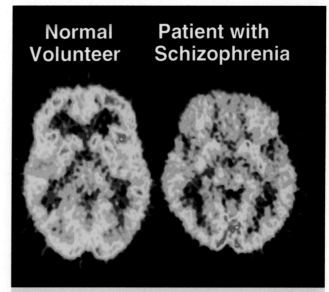

These brain images reveal significant differences between normal brain activity and that of a person with schizophrenia. Yellow and red identify areas of greatest activity, and blue signifies reduced activity.

allowed us to study brain function more closely, scientists have recognized that schizophrenia is a biological disease of the brain. The brain damage occurs early in life, possibly as early as the second trimester of fetal development. Fetal exposure to toxic substances, infections, or medications have all been studied as possible risks. In addition, possible hereditary links are being explored. Symptoms usually appear in men in their late teens and twenties and in women in their late twenties and early thirties.[53]

Even though environmental theories of the causes of schizophrenia have been discarded in favor of biological ones, a stigma remains attached to the disease. Families of people with schizophrenia frequently experience anger and guilt. They often need information, family counseling, and advice on how to meet the schizophrenic person's needs for shelter, medical care, vocational training, and social interaction.

At present, schizophrenia is treatable but not curable. Treatments usually include some combination of hospitalization, medication, and supportive psychotherapy. Supportive psychotherapy, as opposed to psychoanalysis, can help the patient acquire skills for living in society. With proper medication, public understanding, support of loved ones, and access to therapy, many schizophrenics lead normal lives. In the absence of these forms of assistance and treatment, they may have great difficulty.

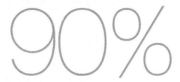

90% of people who kill themselves have a diagnosable mental disorder, most commonly a depressive disorder or a substance abuse disorder.

choose not to go to college but who are searching for direction in careers, relationships, and other life goals are also at risk. Specific risk factors include a family history of suicide, previous suicide attempts, excessive drug and alcohol use, prolonged depression, financial difficulties, serious illness in oneself or a loved one, and loss of a loved one through death or rejection. Societal pressures often serve as a catalyst.

Recent studies indicate that suicide is the eighth leading cause of death for men and the sixteenth leading cause of death for women. Whether they are more likely to attempt suicide or are more often successful in their attempts, nearly four times as many men die by suicide than women. Overall, firearms, suffocation, and poison are by far the most common methods of suicide. However, men are almost twice as likely as women to commit suicide with firearms, while women are almost three times as likely as men to commit suicide by poisoning.[56]

Warning Signs of Suicide

In most cases, suicide does not occur unpredictably. In fact, 75 to 80 percent of people who commit suicide give a warning of their intentions, though they are not always recognized as such by the people around them. Anyone who expresses a desire to kill himself or herself or who has made an attempt is at risk. Common signs that a person may be contemplating suicide include the following:[57]

Suicide: Giving Up on Life

Each year there are over 32,000 reported suicides in the United States.[54] Experts estimate that there may actually be closer to 100,000 cases; the discrepancy is due to the difficulty in determining the causes of many suspicious deaths. More lives are lost to suicide than to any other single cause except cancer and cardiovascular disease. It is the third leading cause of death for 15- to 24-year-olds and the fourth leading cause of death for 10- to 14-year-olds.[55]

College students are more likely than the general population to attempt suicide; it is the second leading cause of death on college campuses (accidents are the first). The pressures, joys, disappointments, challenges, and changes of the college environment are believed to be partially responsible for the emotional turmoil that can lead a young person to contemplate suicide. However, young adults who

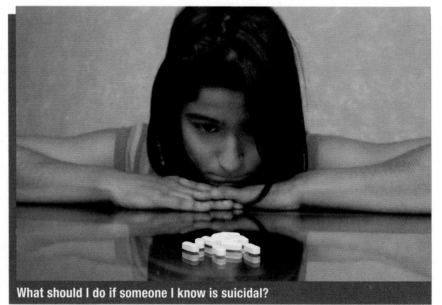

What should I do if someone I know is suicidal?

If you notice warning signs of suicide in someone you know, it is imperative that you take action. Suicidal people urgently need professional assistance; your willingness to talk to the person about depression and suicide in a nonjudgmental way can be the encouragement he or she needs to seek help. Remember: always take thoughts of or plans for suicide seriously; a life may depend on it.

- Recent loss and a seeming inability to let go of grief
- A history of depression
- Change in personality, such as sadness, withdrawal, irritability, anxiety, tiredness, indecisiveness, apathy
- Change in behavior, such as inability to concentrate, loss of interest in classes or work, unexplained demonstration of happiness following a period of depression
- Sexual dysfunction (such as impotence) or diminished sexual interest
- Expressions of self-hatred, excessive risk taking, or an "I don't care what happens to me" attitude
- Change in sleep patterns or eating habits

what do you think?

If your roommate showed warning signs of suicide, what action would you take? ● Whom would you contact first? ● Where on campus might your friend get help? ● What if someone in class whom you hardly know gave warning signs of suicide? What would you do then?

- A direct statement about committing suicide, such as, "I might as well end it all"
- An indirect statement, such as, "You won't have to worry about me anymore"
- Final preparations, such as writing a will, repairing poor relationships with family or friends, giving away prized possessions, or writing revealing letters
- A preoccupation with themes of death
- Marked changes in personal appearance

Preventing Suicide

Most people who attempt suicide really want to live but see suicide as the only way out of an intolerable situation. Crisis counselors and suicide hotlines may help temporarily, but the best way to prevent suicide is to get rid of conditions and substances that may precipitate attempts, including alcoholism, drugs, loneliness, isolation, and access to guns.

If someone you know threatens suicide or displays warning signs, get involved—ask questions and seek help. Specific actions you can take include the following:[58]

- **Monitor the warning signals.** Keep an eye on the person or see that there is someone around the person as much as possible. Don't leave him or her alone.
- **Take threats seriously.** Don't brush them off.
- **Let the person know how much you care about him or her.** State that you are there to help.
- **Listen.** Try not to discredit or be shocked by what the person says. Empathize, sympathize, and keep the person talking. Talk about stressors and listen to the responses.
- **Ask directly,** "Are you thinking of hurting or killing yourself?"
- **Do not belittle the person's feelings.** Don't say that he or she doesn't really mean it or couldn't succeed at suicide. To some people, these comments offer the challenge of proving you wrong.
- **Help the person think about alternatives to suicide.** Offer to go for help together. Call your local suicide hotline, and use

all available community and campus resources. Recommend a counselor or other person to talk to.
- **Tell your friend's spouse, partner, parents, siblings, or counselor.** Do not keep your suspicions to yourself. Don't let a suicidal friend talk you into keeping your discussions confidential. If your friend succeeds in a suicide attempt, you may find that others will question your decision, and you may blame yourself.

Seeking Professional Help for Psychosocial Problems

A physical ailment will readily send most of us to the nearest health professional, but many people view seeking professional help for psychosocial problems as an admission of personal failure. However, increasing numbers of Americans are turning to mental health professionals, and nearly one in five seeks such help. Researchers cite breakdown in support systems, high societal expectations of the individual, and dysfunctional families as three major reasons why more people are asking for assistance than ever before.

Consider seeking help if

- You feel like you need help.
- You experience wild mood swings or inappropriate emotional responses.
- Your fears or feelings of guilt frequently distract your attention.
- You begin to withdraw from others.
- You have hallucinations.
- You feel inadequate or worthless or feel that life is not worth living.
- Your daily life seems to be nothing but repeated crises.
- You are considering suicide.
- You turn to drugs or alcohol to escape from your problems.
- You feel out of control.

In addition to seeking professional help, there are other positive steps you can take now to help pull yourself out of negative thoughts and feelings (see the **Skills for Behavior Change** box on page 49).

Getting Evaluated for Treatment

If you are considering treatment for a psychosocial problem, schedule a complete evaluation first. Consult a credentialed health professional for a thorough examination, which should include three parts.

1. A physical checkup, which will rule out thyroid disorders, viral infections, and anemia—all of which can result in depressive-like symptoms—and a neurological check of coordination, reflexes, and balance to rule out brain disorders

2. **A psychiatric history,** which will attempt to trace the course of the apparent disorder, genetic or family factors, and any past treatments

3. **A mental status examination,** which will assess thoughts, speaking processes, and memory, and will include an in-depth interview with tests for other psychiatric symptoms.

Once physical factors have been ruled out, you may decide to consult a professional who specializes in psychosocial health.

Mental Health Professionals

Several types of mental health professionals are available to help you; Table 2.2 on page 50 compares several of the most common. When choosing a therapist to work with, the most important criterion is not how many degrees this person has, but whether you feel you can work together. A qualified mental health professional should be willing to answer all your questions during an initial consultation. Questions to ask the therapist and yourself include the following:

● **Can you interview the therapist before starting treatment?** An initial meeting will help you determine whether this person will be a good fit for you.

● **Do you like the therapist as a person?** Can you talk to him or her comfortably?

● **Is the therapist watching the clock or easily distracted?** You should be the main focus of the session.

● **Does the therapist demonstrate professionalism?** Be concerned if your therapist is frequently late or breaks appointments, suggests social interactions outside your therapy sessions, talks inappropriately about himself or herself, has questionable billing practices, or resists releasing you from therapy.

● **Will the therapist help you set your own goals?** A good professional should evaluate your general situation and help you set small goals to work on between sessions. The therapist should not tell you how to help yourself, but rather help you discover the steps.

Spending time in the fresh air with your best friend can boost your spirits and help you on the road to better psychosocial health.

Remember, in most states, the use of the titles *therapist* and *counselor* are unregulated. Make your choice carefully.

Dealing with and Defeating Depression

The first step in defeating depression is recognizing it. If you feel you have depression symptoms, setting up an appointment with a counselor is key. Depression is often a biological condition that you can't just get over on your own. Talk therapy, sometimes combined with antidepressant medication, may be necessary to help you reach a place where you are able to play a greater role in getting well. Once you've started along a path of therapy and healing, the following strategies may help you feel better faster.

✻ Set realistic goals in light of the depression and assume a reasonable amount of responsibility.

✻ Break large tasks into small ones, set some priorities, and do what you can as you can.

✻ Try to be with other people and to confide in someone; it is usually better than being alone and secretive.

✻ Participate in activities that may make you feel better.

✻ Mild exercise, going to a movie or a ballgame, or participating in religious or social activities may help.

✻ Take a course in meditation, yoga, tai chi, or some other mind–body practice. These disciplines can help you connect with your inner feelings, release tension, and empty your mind to make room for positive thoughts.

✻ Expect your mood to improve gradually, not immediately. Feeling better takes time.

✻ Consider postponing important decisions until the depression has lifted. Before deciding to make a significant transition, change jobs, or get married or divorced, discuss it with others who know you well and have a more objective view of your situation.

✻ Let your family and friends help you.

✻ Continue working with your counselor. If you find he or she isn't helpful, look for another one.

What to Expect in Therapy

Many different types of counseling exist, ranging from individual therapy, which involves one-on-one work between therapist and client, to group therapy, in which two or more clients meet with a therapist to discuss problems. The first trip to a therapist can be difficult. Most of us have misconceptions about what therapy is and what it can do. That first visit is a verbal and mental sizing up between you and the therapist. You may not accomplish much in that first hour. If you decide that this professional is not for you, you will at least have learned how to present your problem and what qualities you need in a therapist.

What are they called?	What kind of training do they have?	What kind of therapy do they do?	Professional association
Psychiatrist	Medical doctor (MD) degree, followed by 4 years of specialized mental health training	As a licensed MD, a psychiatrist can prescribe medications and may have admitting privileges at a local hospital. Some psychiatrists are affiliated with hospitals, while others are in private practice.	American Psychiatric Association www.psych.org
Psychologist	PhD degree in counseling or clinical psychology followed by several years of supervised practice to earn license	Psychologists are trained in various types of therapy, including behavior and insight therapy. Most can conduct both individual and group sessions. They may be trained in certain specialties, such as family counseling or sexual counseling.	American Psychological Association www.apa.org
Clinical/psychiatric social worker	Master's degree in social work (MSW) followed by 2 years of experience in a clinical setting to earn license	Social workers may be trained in certain specialties, such as substance abuse counseling or child counseling. Some social workers are employed in clinics, schools, or agencies; others have private practices.	National Association of Social Workers www.socialworkers.org
Counselor	Master's degree in counseling, psychology, educational psychology, or related human service. Generally must complete at least 2 years of supervised practice before obtaining a license	Many counselors are trained to do individual and group therapy. They often specialize in one type of counseling, such as family, marital, relationship, children, drug, divorce, behavioral, or personal counseling.	American Counseling Association www.counseling.org
Psychoanalyst	Postgraduate degree in psychology or psychiatry (PhD or MD), followed by 8 to 10 years of training in psychoanalysis, which includes undergoing analysis themselves	Psychoanalysis is a form of therapy based on the theories of Freud and his successors. It focuses on patterns of thinking and behavior and the recall of early traumas that have blocked personal growth. Treatment is intensive, lasting 5 to 10 years, with 3 or 4 sessions per week.	American Psychoanalytic Association www.apsa.org
Licensed marriage and family therapist (LMFT)	Master's or doctoral degree in psychology, social work, or counseling, specializing in family and interpersonal dynamics; generally must complete at least 2 years of supervised practice before obtaining a license	LMFTs treat individuals or families in the context of family relationships. Treatment is typically brief (20 sessions or less) and focused on finding solutions to specific relational problems. Some LMFTs work in clinics, schools, or agencies; others have private practices.	American Association for Marriage and Family Therapy www.aamft.org

Before meeting, briefly explain your needs. Ask what the fee is. Arrive on time, wear comfortable clothing, and expect to spend about an hour during your first visit. The therapist will want to take down your history and details about the problems that have brought you to therapy. Answer as honestly as possible. He or she may ask how you feel about aspects of your life. Do not be embarrassed to acknowledge your feelings. It is critical to the success of your treatment that you trust this person enough to be open and honest.

Do not expect the therapist to tell you what to do or how to behave. The responsibility for improved behavior lies with you. Ask if you can set your own therapeutic goals and timetables.

If after your first visit (or even after several visits) you feel you cannot work with this person, say so. You have the right to find a therapist with whom you feel comfortable.

What Is Your Psychosocial Health Status?

Being psychosocially healthy requires both introspection and the willingness to work on areas that need improvement. Begin by completing the following assessment scale. Use it to determine how much each statement describes you. When you're finished, ask someone who is very close to you to take the same test and respond with their perceptions of you. Carefully assess areas where your responses differ from those of your friend or family member. Which areas need some work? Which are in good shape?

	Never	Rarely	Fairly Frequently	Most of the Time	All of the Time
1. My actions and interactions indicate that I am confident in my abilities.	1	2	3	4	5
2. I am quick to blame others for things that go wrong in my life.	1	2	3	4	5
3. I am spontaneous and like to have fun with others.	1	2	3	4	5
4. I am able to give love and affection to others and show my feelings.	1	2	3	4	5
5. I am able to receive love and signs of affection from others without feeling uneasy.	1	2	3	4	5
6. I am generally positive and upbeat about things in my life.	1	2	3	4	5
7. I am cynical and tend to be critical of others.	1	2	3	4	5
8. I have a large group of people whom I consider to be good friends.	1	2	3	4	5
9. I make time for others in my life.	1	2	3	4	5
10. I take time each day for myself for quiet introspection, having fun, or just doing nothing.	1	2	3	4	5
11. I am compulsive and competitive in my actions.	1	2	3	4	5
12. I handle stress well and am seldom upset or stressed out by others.	1	2	3	4	5

	Never	Rarely	Fairly Frequently	Most of the Time	All of the Time
13. I try to look for the good in everyone and every situation before finding fault.	1	2	3	4	5
14. I am comfortable meeting new people and interact well in social settings.	1	2	3	4	5
15. I would rather stay in and watch TV or read than go out with friends or interact with others.	1	2	3	4	5
16. I am flexible and can adapt to most situations, even if I don't like them.	1	2	3	4	5
17. Nature, the environment, and other living things are important aspects of my life.	1	2	3	4	5
18. I think before responding to my emotions.	1	2	3	4	5
19. I am selfish and tend to think of my own needs before those of others.	1	2	3	4	5
20. I am consciously trying to be a "better person."	1	2	3	4	5
21. I like to plan ahead and set realistic goals for myself and others.	1	2	3	4	5
22. I accept others for who they are.	1	2	3	4	5
23. I value diversity and respect others' rights, regardless of culture, race, sexual orientation, religion, or other differences.	1	2	3	4	5

	Never	Rarely	Fairly Frequently	Most of the Time	All of the Time
24. I try to live each day as if it might be my last.	①	②	③	④	⑤
25. I have a great deal of energy and appreciate the little things in life.	①	②	③	④	⑤
26. I cope with stress in appropriate ways.	①	②	③	④	⑤
27. I get enough sleep each day and seldom feel tired.	①	②	③	④	⑤
28. I have healthy relationships with my family.	①	②	③	④	⑤

	Never	Rarely	Fairly Frequently	Most of the Time	All of the Time
29. I am confident that I can do most things if I put my mind to them.	①	②	③	④	⑤
30. I respect others' opinions and believe that others should be free to express their opinions, even when they differ from my own.	①	②	③	④	⑤

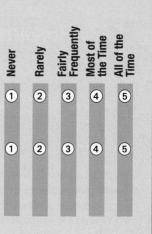

Interpreting Your Scores

Look at items 2, 7, 11, 15, and 19. Add up your score for these 5 items and divide by 5. Is your average for these items above or below 3? Did you score a 5 on any of these items? These may indicate areas where your attitudes and patterns of behavior and thought could use improvement. Now look at your scores for the remaining items (there should be 25 items). Total these scores and divide by 25. Is your average above or below 3? On which items did you score a 5? Obviously you're doing well in these areas. Now remove these items from this grouping of 25 (scores of 5), and add up your scores for the remaining items. Then divide your total by the number of items included. Now what is your average?

Do the same for the scores completed by your friend or family member. How do your scores compare? Which ones, if any, are different, and how do they differ? Which areas do you need to work on? What actions can you take now to improve your ratings in these areas?

YOUR PLAN FOR CHANGE

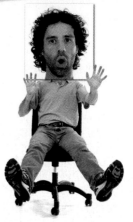

The **Assessyourself** activity gave you the chance to look at various aspects of your psychosocial health and compare your self-assessment with a friend's perceptions. Now that you have considered these results, you can take steps to change behaviors that may be detrimental to your psychosocial health.

Today, you can:

○ Develop a plan. Evaluate your behavior and identify patterns and specific things you are doing that negatively affect your psychosocial health. What can you change now? What can you change in the near future?

○ Start a journal in which you note changes in your mood. Look for trends and think about ways you can change your behavior to address them.

○ Make a list of the things that bring you joy—friends, family, activities, entertainment, nature. Commit yourself to making more room for these joy-givers in your life.

Within the next 2 weeks, you can:

○ Visit your campus health center and find out about the counseling services they offer. If you are feeling overwhelmed, depressed, or anxious, make an appointment with a counselor.

○ Pay attention to the negative thoughts that pop up throughout the day. Note times when you find yourself devaluing or undermining your abilities, and notice when you project negative attitudes on others. Bringing your awareness to these thoughts gives you an opportunity to stop and reevaluate them.

By the end of the semester, you can:

○ Make a commitment to an ongoing therapeutic practice aimed at improving your psychosocial health. Depending on your current situation, this could mean anything from seeing a counselor or joining a support group to practicing meditation or attending religious services.

○ Volunteer regularly with a local organization you care about. Focus your energy and gain satisfaction by helping to improve others' lives or the environment.

Summary

* Psychosocial health is a complex phenomenon involving mental, emotional, social, and spiritual health.
* Many factors influence psychosocial health, including life experiences, family, the environment, other people, self-esteem, self-efficacy, and personality. Some of these are modifiable; others are not.
* Developing self-esteem and self-efficacy, making healthy connections, having a positive outlook on life, enhancing your spiritual nature, and getting enough sleep are key to maintaining psychosocial health.
* Happiness is a key factor in determining overall reaction to life's challenges. The mind–body connection is an important link in overall health and well-being.
* Indicators of deteriorating psychosocial health include depression, difficulty sleeping, and emotional volatility. College life is a high-risk time for developing depression because of high stress and pressures for grades, financial problems, and other problems. Identifying symptoms of depression is the first step in treating this disorder.
* Other psychosocial problems are mood disorders, including major depressive disorder, dysthymic disorder, bipolar disorder, and seasonal affective disorder; anxiety disorders, including generalized anxiety disorder, panic attacks, social phobias, obsessive-compulsive disorder, and post-traumatic stress disorder; and personality disorders.
* Schizophrenia is a disorder once believed to be the result of environmental causes. Now brain function studies have shown that it is instead a biological disease of the brain.
* Suicide is a result of negative psychosocial reactions to life. People considering suicide often give warning signs of their intentions. Such people often can be helped.
* Mental health professionals include psychiatrists, psychologists, clinical/ psychiatric social workers, counselors, psychoanalysts, and licensed marriage and family therapists. Many therapy methods exist, including group and individual therapy. It is wise to interview a therapist carefully before beginning treatment.

Pop Quiz

1. A person with high self-esteem
   a. possesses feelings of self-respect and self-worth.
   b. believes he or she can successfully engage in a specific behavior.
   c. believes external influences shape one's psychosocial health.
   d. has a high altruistic capacity.

2. All of the following traits have been identified as characterizing psychosocially healthy people *except*
   a. conscientiousness.
   b. introversion.
   c. openness to experience.
   d. agreeableness.

3. Subjective well-being has all of the following components *except*
   a. psychological hardiness.
   b. satisfaction with present life.
   c. relative presence of positive emotions.
   d. relative absence of negative emotions.

4. People who have experienced repeated failures at the same task may eventually give up and quit trying altogether. This pattern of behavior is termed
   a. post-traumatic stress disorder.
   b. learned helplessness.
   c. self-efficacy.
   d. introversion.

5. The term that most accurately refers to the feelings or subjective side of psychosocial health is
   a. social health.
   b. mental health.
   c. emotional health.
   d. spiritual health.

6. Which statement below is false?
   a. One in four adults in the United States suffers from a diagnosable mental disorder in a given year.
   b. Mental disorders are the leading cause of disability in the United States.
   c. Dysthymia is an example of an anxiety disorder.
   d. Bipolar disorder can also be referred to as manic depression.

7. This disorder is characterized by a need to perform rituals over and over again; fear of dirt or contamination; or an unnatural concern with order, symmetry, and exactness.
   a. personality disorder
   b. obsessive-compulsive disorder
   c. phobic disorder
   d. post-traumatic stress disorder

8. What is the number-one mental health problem in the United States?
   a. depression
   b. anxiety disorders
   c. alcohol dependence
   d. schizophrenia

9. Every winter, Stan suffers from irritability, apathy, carbohydrate craving, weight gain, increased sleep time, and sadness. He most likely has
   a. panic disorder.
   b. generalized anxiety disorder.
   c. seasonal affective disorder.
   d. chronic mood disorder.

10. A person with a PhD in counseling psychology and training in various types of therapy is a
    a. psychiatrist.
    b. psychologist.
    c. social worker.
    d. psychoanalyst.

Answers to these questions can be found on page A-1.

Think about It!

1. What is psychosocial health? What indicates that you are or aren't psychosocially healthy? Why might the college environment provide a challenge to your psychosocial health?

2. Discuss the factors that influence your overall level of psychosocial health. Which factors can you change? Which ones may be more difficult to change?

3. What steps could you take today to improve your psychosocial health? Which steps require long-term effort?

4. Why is laughter therapeutic? How can humor help you better achieve wellness?

5. What factors appear to contribute to psychosocial difficulties and illnesses? Which of the common psychosocial illnesses is likely to affect people in your age group?

6. What are the warning signs of suicide? Of depression? Why is depression so pervasive among young Americans today? Why are some groups more vulnerable to suicide and depression than are others? What would you do if you heard a friend in the cafeteria say to no one in particular that he was going to "do the world a favor and end it all"?

7. Discuss the different types of health professionals and therapies. If you felt depressed about breaking off a long-term relationship, which professional therapy do you think would be most beneficial? Explain your answer. What services does your student health center provide? What fees are charged to students?

8. What psychosocial areas do you need to work on? Which are most important to you, and why? What actions can you take today?

Accessing Your Health on the Internet

The following websites explore further topics and issues related to personal health. For links to the websites below, visit the Companion Website for *Health: The Basics,* Green Edition at www.pearsonhighered.com/donatelle.

1. *American Foundation for Suicide Prevention.* Resources for suicide prevention and support for family and friends of those who have committed suicide. www.afsp.org

2. *American Psychological Association Help Center.* Includes information on psychology at work, the mind–body connection, psychological responses to war, and other topics. http://apahelpcenter.org

3. *Anxiety Disorders Association of America.* Offers links to treatment resources, self-help tools, information on clinical trials, and other information. www.adaa.org

4. *National Alliance on Mental Illness.* A support and advocacy organization of families and friends of people with severe mental illnesses. Over 1,200 state and local affiliates; local branches can often help with finding treatment. www.nami.org

5. *National Institute of Mental Health (NIMH).* Overview of mental health information and new research relating to mental health. www.nimh.nih.gov

6. *Mental Health America.* Works to promote mental health through advocacy, education, research, and services. www.nmha.org

7. *Helpguide.* Resources for improving mental and emotional health as well as specific information on topics such as self-injury, sleep, depressive disorders, and anxiety disorders. www.helpguide.org

References

1. H. Marano, "A Nation of Wimps," *Psychology Today* 37, no. 6 (2004): 58–68.

2. National Institute of Mental Health, National Survey of Counseling Center Directors, 2005.

3. A. H. Maslow, *Motivation and Personality.* 2nd ed. (New York: Harper and Row, 1970).

4. T. M. Chaplin, "Anger, Happiness, and Sadness: Association with Depressive Symptoms in Late Adolescence," *Journal of Youth and Adolescence* 35, no. 6 (2006): 977–86.

5. A. F. Jorm, "Social Networks and Health: It's Time for an Intervention Trial," *Journal of Epidemiology and Community Health* 59 (2005): 537–39; C. Huang, "Elderly Social Support System and Health Status in the Urban and Rural Areas," paper presented at the American Public Health Association Annual Meeting (New Orleans, 2005); C. Alarie, *Impact of Social Support on Women's Health: A Literature Review,* Women's Center of Excellence, www.pwhce.ca/limpactDuSupport.htm; A. Sherman, J. Lansford, and B. Volling, "Sibling Relationships and Best Friendships in Young Adulthood: Warmth, Conflict and Well-Being," *Personal Relationships* 13, no. 2 (2006): 151–65; N. Stevens, "Marriage, Social Integration, and Loneliness in the Second Half of Life," *Research on Aging* 28, no. 2 (2006): 713–29.

6. K. Karren et al., *Mind/Body Health.* 4th ed. (San Francisco: Benjamin Cummings, 2010).

7. NCCAM, "Prayer and Spirituality in Health: Ancient Practices, Modern Science," *CAM at the NIH: Focus on Complementary and Alternative Medicine* 12, no. 1 (2005), available at http://nccam.nih.gov/news/newsletter/pdf/2005winter.pdf. Updated October 2007.

8. M. Seligman and C. Peterson, "Learned Helplessness," in *International Encyclopedia for the Social and Behavioral Sciences,* vol. 13, ed. N. Smelser (New York: Elsevier, 2002), 8583–866.

9. M. Seligman, *Learned Optimism: How to Change Your Mind and Your Life* (New York: Free Press, 1998); J. H. Martin, "Motivation Processes and Performance: The Role of Global and Facet Personality," PhD dissertation, University of North Carolina at Chapel Hill, 2002.

10. M. Lemonick, "The Biology of Joy," *Time* (January 17, 2005): A12–A14; P. Herschberger, "Prescribing Happiness: Positive Psychology and Family Medicine," *Family Medicine* 37, no. 9 (2005): 630–34.

11. J. Kluger, "The Funny Thing about Laughter," *Time* (January 17, 2005): A25–A29.

12. Ibid.
13. R. Davidson et al., "The Privileged Status of Emotion in the Brain," *Proceedings of the National Academy of Sciences of the United States of America* 101, no. 33 (2004): 11915–16.
14. E. Diener and M. E. P. Seligman, "Beyond Money: Toward an Economy of Well-Being," *Psychological Science in the Public Interest* 5 (2004): 1–31; C. Peterson and M. Seligman, *Character Strengths and Virtues* (London: Oxford University Press, 2004).
15. D. Grady, "Think Right, Stay Well," *American Health* 11 (1992): 50–54.
16. Ibid.
17. D. Bazzini et al., "The Effect of Reminiscing about Laughter on Relationship Satisfaction," *Motivation and Emotion* 31, no. 1 (March 2007): 25–34; K. Taber et al., "Functional Anatomy of Humor: Positive Affect and Chronic Mental Illness," *Journal of Neuropsychiatry and Clinical Neuroscience* 19 (2007): 358–62.
18. B. Fredrickson, "Cultivating Positive Emotions to Optimize Health and Well-Being," *Prevention and Treatment* 3 (March 7, 2000), article 0001a.
19. N. Ross, "Health, Happiness, and Higher Levels of Social Organization," *Journal of Epidemiology and Community Health* 59 (2005): 614; A. J. Bishop, P. Martin, and L. Poon, "Happiness and Congruence in Older Adulthood: A Structural Model of Life Satisfaction," *Aging and Mental Health* 10, no. 5 (2006): 445–53.
20. E. Weiner, *The Geography of Bliss: One Grump's Search for the Happiest Places in the World* (New York: Hachette Book Group USA, 2008).
21. P. Herschberger, "Prescribing Happiness: Positive Psychology and Family Medicine," *Family Medicine* 37, no. 9 (2005): 630–34; M. E. Seligman et al., "Positive Psychology Progress: Empirical Validation of Interventions," *American Psychologist* 60, no. 5 (2005): 410–21.
22. M. Seligman, "Positive Interventions: More Evidence of Effectiveness," *Authentic Happiness Newsletter* (September 2004), www.authentichappiness.sas.upenn.edu/newsletter.aspx?id=45; S. I. Gable et al., "What Do You Do When Things Go Right? The Intrapersonal and Interpersonal Benefits of Sharing Positive Events," *Journal of Personal and Social Psychology* 87, no. 2 (2004): 228–45; B. Swartz, *The Paradox of Choice: Why More Is Less* (New York: HarperCollins, 2004); P. C. Seligman, *Character Strengths and Virtues: A Handbook and Classification* (New York: Oxford University Press, 2004).
23. MayoClinic.com, "Mental Health Definitions," 2008, www.mayoclinic.com.
24. National Institute of Mental Health, "The Numbers Count: Mental Disorders in America," www.nimh.nih.gov/health/publications/the-numbers-count-mental-disorders-in-america/index.shtml. Updated March 2008.
25. American College Health Association, *American College Health Association—National College Health Assessment (ACHA-NCHA): Reference Group Data Report Fall 2008* (Baltimore: American College Health Association, 2009).
26. National Institute of Mental Health, "The Numbers Count," 2008.
27. L. A. Lefton, *Psychology.* 8th ed. (Boston: Allyn & Bacon, 2002).
28. National Institute of Mental Health, "The Numbers Count," 2008.
29. R. C. Kessler et al., "Lifetime Prevalence and Age-of-Onset Distributions of *DSM-IV* Disorders in the National Comorbidity Survey Replication (NCS-R)," *Archives of General Psychiatry* 62, no. 6 (2005): 593–602.
30. National Institute of Mental Health, "Depression," www.nimh.nih.gov/publicat/depression.cfm, 2009.
31. National Institute of Mental Health, "The Numbers Count," 2008.
32. American Psychiatric Association, "Let's Talk about Seasonal Affective Disorder," www.healthyminds.org/Main-Topic/Seasonal-Affective-Disorder.aspx. Accessed October 2009.
33. American College Health Association, *ACHA-NCHA: Reference Group Data Report Fall 2008.*
34. National Institute of Mental Health, "Depression," 2009; N. Gavin et al., "Perinatal Depression: A Systematic Review of Prevalence and Incidence," *Obstetrics and Gynecology* 106 (2005): 1071–83.
35. National Sleep Foundation, "NSF's 2007 Sleep in America Poll: Stressed-Out American Women Have No Time for Sleep," March 6, 2007, www.sleepfoundation.org.
36. A. K. Ferketick et al., "Depression as an Antecedent to Heart Disease among Women and Men in the NHANES I Study," National Health and Nutrition Examination Survey," *Archives of Internal Medicine* 160, no. 9 (2002): 1261–68.
37. National Institute of Mental Health, "The Numbers Count," 2008.
38. A. K. Ferketick et al., "NHANES I Study," 2002.
39. National Institute of Mental Health, "Depression," 2009.
40. U.S. Food and Drug Administration (FDA), "Anti-depressant Drug Use in Pediatric Populations," September 23, 2004, www.fda.gov/NewsEvents/Testimony/ucm113265.htm; U.S. FDA, Center for Drug Evaluation and Research, "Antide-pressant Use in Children, Adolescents, and Adults," www.fda.gov/cder/drug/antidepressants/default.htm. Updated May 2007; National Institute of Mental Health, "The Numbers Count," 2008.
41. National Institute of Mental Health, "The Numbers Count," 2008.
42. National Institute of Mental Health, "Generalized Anxiety Disorder, GAD," www.nimh.nih.gov/health/publications/anxiety-disorders/generalized-anxiety-disorder-gad.shtml. Reviewed July 7, 2009.
43. MayoClinic.com, "Panic Attacks," www.mayoclinic.com/health/panic-attacks/DS00338. Updated July 1, 2008.
44. National Institute of Mental Health, "The Numbers Count," 2008.
45. C. W. Hoge, et al., "Combat Duty in Iraq and Afghanistan, Mental Health Problems, and Barriers to Care," *New England Journal of Medicine* 351 (2004): 13–22.
46. National Institute of Mental Health, "Generalized Anxiety Disorder, GAD," 2009.
47. W. T. O'Donohue, K. A. Fowler, and S. O. Lilienfeld, *Personality Disorders: Toward the DSM-V* (Thousand Oaks, CA: Sage, 2007).
48. National Institute of Mental Health, "National Survey Tracks Prevalence of Personality Disorders in U.S. Population" (October 18, 2007), www.nimh.nih.gov/science-news/2007/national-survey-tracks-prevalence-of-personality-disorders-in-us-population.shtml.
49. C. Wade and C. Tavries, *Invitation to Psychology.* 4th ed. (Upper Saddle River, NJ: Prentice Hall, 2008), 384–85.
50. Mayo Clinic Staff, "Borderline Personality Disorder" (May 14, 2008), www.mayoclinic.com/health/borderline-personality-disorder/DS00442.
51. J. Cole, "Facts," BPDWORLD (2009), www.bpdworld.org/demo-category/106-facts.
52. National Institute of Mental Health, "Schizophrenia," www.nimh.nih.gov/health/topics/schizophrenia/index.shtml. Updated March 2008.
53. Ibid.
54. National Institute of Mental Health, "Suicide in the U.S.: Statistics and Prevention," www.nimh.nih.gov/publicat/harmsway.cfm. Last reviewed May 18, 2009.
55. B. Hamilton et al., "Annual Summary of Vital Statistics: 2005," *Pediatrics* 119, no. 2 (2007): 336–37.
56. National Institute of Mental Health, "Suicide in the U.S.: Statistics and Prevention."
57. Ibid.
58. National Institute of Mental Health, "The Numbers Count," 2008.

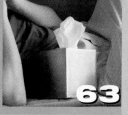
63
Why do I always get sick during finals week?

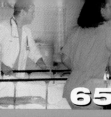
65
Who is most prone to stress?

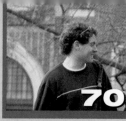
70
How can I cope with daily pressures and annoyances?

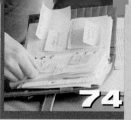
74
How can I manage my time more effectively?

3 Managing Your Stress

Objectives

✳ Define *stress*, and examine the potential impact of stress on health, relationships, and success in college.

✳ Explain the phases of the general adaptation syndrome and the physiological changes that occur.

✳ Examine the health risks that may occur with chronic stress.

✳ Discuss sources of stress, and examine the special stressors that affect college students.

✳ Explore techniques for coping with or reducing exposure to stress and using positive experiences and attitudes to enrich your life.

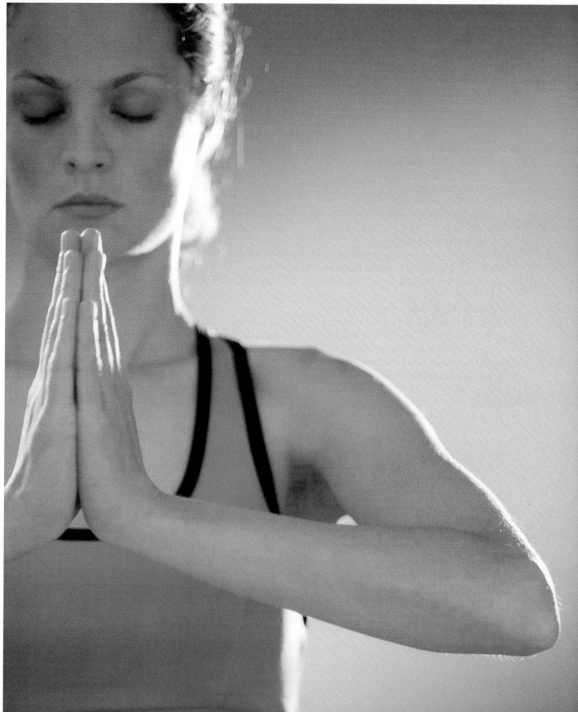

Rising tuition; roommates who bug you; social life drama; too much noise; no privacy; long lines at the bookstore; pressure to get good grades; never enough money; worries about the economy, terrorism, and natural disaster all add up to: STRESS! You can't run from it, you can't hide from it, and it can affect you in insidious ways that you aren't even aware of. When we try to sleep, it encroaches on our psyche through outside noise or internal worries over all the things that need to be done. While we work at the computer, stress may interfere in the form of noise from next door, strain on our eyes, and tension in our back. Even when we are out socializing with friends, we feel guilty, because there is just not enough time to do what needs to be accomplished. The precise toll that stress exacts from us over a lifetime is unknown, but increasingly, stress is recognized as a major threat to health. It can rob the body of needed nutrients; damage the cardiovascular system; raise blood pressure; increase risks for diabetes, cancer, and other chronic diseases; and dampen the immune system's defenses. In addition, it can drain emotional reserves; contribute to depression, anxiety, and irritability; and punctuate social interactions with hostility and anger. Although much has been written about stress, we are only now just beginning to understand the multifaceted nature of the stress response and its tremendous potential for harm or benefit.

The negative aspect of stress is a major concern in the United States, particularly among college students. Stress on America's college and university campuses appears to be a growing issue. Since students were first surveyed about their stress levels in the late 1970s and early 1980s, the stressors that students face have reached epidemic levels. According to a recent national survey of more than 1,900 colleges and universities, the *Annual Survey of Freshman 2008*, which gauges the academic climate, available resources, and health-related issues of more than 240,000 students, stress surfaces as the number one factor affecting student performance in college. In fact, more than 40 percent of first-year students indicated that they are "frequently overwhelmed" by all they have to do, up from a low of 16 percent when the question was first asked in 1985. Another 55 percent of first-year students reported that they are occasionally overwhelmed.[1] Consistent with those findings, students in a similar large-scale survey of college health conducted by the American College Health Association named stress as the most significant factor affecting their individual academic performance.[2] Regardless of geographical region, type of college or university, or rigor of programs, students are clearly stressed-out in record numbers!

stress The experience of a perceived threat (real or imagined) to one's well-being, resulting from a series of physiological responses and adaptations.

stressors A physical, social, or psychological event or condition that upsets homeostasis and produces a stress response.

strain The wear and tear sustained by the body and mind in adjusting to or resisting a stressor.

coping The act of managing events or conditions to lessen the physical or psychological effects of excess stress.

To deal more successfully with stress, there are things we can do, starting with learning to anticipate and recognize our personal stressors and developing skills to reduce or better manage those we cannot avoid or control. First, we must understand what stress is and what effects it has on the body.

What Is Stress?

Often we think of stress as an externally imposed factor. But for most of us, stress results from an internal state of emotional tension that occurs in response to the various demands of living. Most current definitions state that **stress** is the mental and physical response of our bodies to the changes and challenges in our lives. **Stressors** are demands made by the physical, social, or psychological environment that upset balance or homeostasis and cause our bodies to react or respond.[3] Several factors influence one's response to stressors, including characteristics of the stressor (Can you control it? Is it predictable? Does it occur often?), biological factors (such as your age or gender), and past experiences. Stressors may be tangible, such as an angry parent or a disgruntled roommate, or intangible, such as the mixed emotions associated with meeting your significant other's parents for the first time. **Strain** is the wear and tear the body and mind sustain during the stress process. **Coping** is the act of managing events or conditions to lessen the physical or psychological effects of excess stress.[4] Stress is in the eye of the beholder: Each person's unique combination of heredity, life experiences, personality, and ability to cope influences how the person perceives an event and what meaning he or she attaches to it.

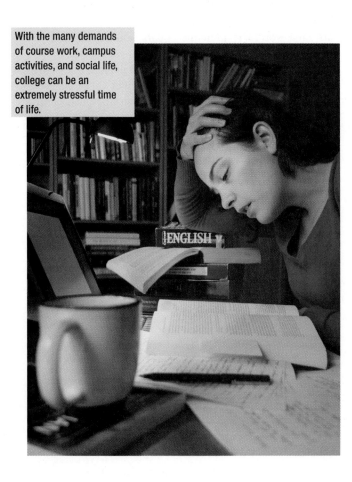

With the many demands of course work, campus activities, and social life, college can be an extremely stressful time of life.

Stress can be associated with most daily activities. Generally, positive stress—stress that presents the opportunity for personal growth and satisfaction—is termed **eustress.** Getting married, successfully kayaking Class II rapids, beginning a career, and developing new friends may all give rise to eustress. **Distress,** or negative stress, is caused by events that result in debilitative stress and strain, such as financial problems, the death of a loved one, academic difficulties, and the breakup of a relationship. Prolonged distress can have negative effects on health.

You cannot get rid of distress entirely: Like eustress, it is a part of life. However, you can train yourself to recognize the events that cause distress and to anticipate your reactions to them. You can learn coping skills and strategies that will help you manage stress more effectively.

The Body's Response to Stress

Being under stress is not just "all in your head." The body experiences very real physiological changes when it faces a situation that it perceives to be threatening. From the first days of human life on Earth, when our ancestors were faced with physical dangers, when these dangers were frequent, and when the need to respond quickly was a matter of life or death, the body's physiological responses were necessary. If you didn't respond by fighting or fleeing, you might have been eaten by a saber-toothed tiger or killed by a marauding enemy clan. Today, although we sometimes face real or perceived tigers in angry friends, vicious verbal attacks, or more insidious insults, these charged up physiological responses must be contained and/or repressed. Instead of lashing back or fighting physically, we are taught to resist fighting, to not show anger. We're all geared up for action, but our rational thoughts say, "STOP!" If these responses occur too frequently, they can harm your health over time.

eustress Stress that presents opportunities for personal growth; positive stress.

distress Stress that can have a detrimental effect on health; negative stress.

fight-or-flight response Physiological arousal response in which the body prepares to combat or escape a real or perceived threat.

homeostasis A balanced physical state in which all the body's systems function smoothly.

adaptive response Form of adjustment in which the body attempts to restore homeostasis.

general adaptation syndrome (GAS) The pattern followed in the physiological response to stress, consisting of the alarm, resistance, and exhaustion phases.

The Fight-or-Flight Response

Whenever we're confronted with a sudden stressor, such as someone swerving into our lane of traffic, our emotional reactions trigger the adrenal glands (two almond-sized glands sitting atop the kidneys) to secrete adrenaline and other hormones into the bloodstream. As a result, the heart speeds up, breathing rate increases, blood pressure elevates,

and blood flow to the muscles increases with a rapid release of blood sugars into the bloodstream. This sudden burst of energy and strength is believed to provide the extra edge that has helped generations of humans survive during adversity. Known as the **fight-or-flight response,** this physiological reaction is one of our most basic, innate survival instincts.[5] When activated, our bodies go on the alert either to fight danger or to escape from it.

The General Adaptation Syndrome

When a body is in **homeostasis,** the body's systems operate smoothly and maintain equilibrium. Stressors trigger a crisis-mode physiological response, after which the body attempts to return to homeostasis by means of an **adaptive response.** First characterized by Hans Selye in 1936, the internal fight to restore homeostasis in the face of a stressor is known as the **general adaptation syndrome (GAS)** (Figure 3.1). The GAS has three distinct phases: alarm, resistance, and exhaustion.[6]

Alarm Phase When the body is exposed to a real or perceived stressor, the fight-or-flight response kicks into gear. Stress hormones flow, and the body prepares to do battle. The subconscious perceptions and appraisal of the stressor stimulate the areas in the brain responsible for emotions. This emotional stimulation triggers the physical reactions we associate with stress (Figure 3.2). The entire process takes only a few seconds.

Suppose that you are walking to your residence hall after a night class on a dimly lit campus. As you pass a particularly dark area, you hear someone cough behind you, and you sense that this person is fairly close. You walk faster, only to hear the quickened footsteps of the other person. Your senses become increasingly alert, your breathing quickens, your heart races, and you begin to perspire. The stranger is getting

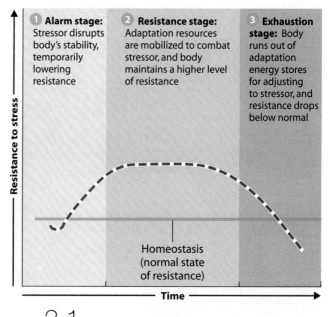

1. **Alarm stage:** Stressor disrupts body's stability, temporarily lowering resistance

2. **Resistance stage:** Adaptation resources are mobilized to combat stressor, and body maintains a higher level of resistance

3. **Exhaustion stage:** Body runs out of adaptation energy stores for adjusting to stressor, and resistance drops below normal

Resistance to stress

Homeostasis (normal state of resistance)

Time

FIGURE 3.1 **The General Adaptation Syndrome**

closer and closer. In desperation you stop, clutching your book bag in your hands, determined to use force if necessary to protect yourself. You turn around quickly and let out a blood-curdling yell. To your surprise, the only person you see is your classmate, who has been trying to stay close to you out of her own anxiety about walking alone in the dark. You look at her in startled embarrassment. You have just experienced the alarm phase of GAS.

When the mind perceives a real or imaginary stressor, the cerebral cortex, the region of the brain that interprets the nature of an event, triggers an **autonomic nervous system (ANS)** response that prepares the body for action. The ANS is the portion of the central nervous system regulating body functions that we do not normally consciously control, such as heart function, breathing, and glandular function.

The ANS has two branches: sympathetic and parasympathetic. The **sympathetic nervous system** energizes the body for fight or flight by signaling the release of several stress hormones that speed the heart rate, increase the breathing rate, and trigger many other stress responses. The **parasympathetic nervous system** functions to slow all the systems stimulated by the stress response—in effect, it counteracts the actions of the sympathetic branch. In a healthy person, these two branches work together in a balance that controls the negative effects of stress.

The responses of the sympathetic nervous system to stress involve a series of biochemical exchanges between different parts of the body. The **hypothalamus**, a structure in the brain, functions as the control center of the sympathetic nervous system and determines the overall reaction to stressors. When the hypothalamus perceives that extra energy is needed to fight a

autonomic nervous system (ANS) The portion of the central nervous system regulating body functions that a person does not normally consciously control.

sympathetic nervous system Branch of the autonomic nervous system responsible for stress arousal.

parasympathetic nervous system Branch of the autonomic nervous system responsible for slowing systems stimulated by the stress response.

hypothalamus A structure in the brain that controls the sympathetic nervous system and directs the stress response.

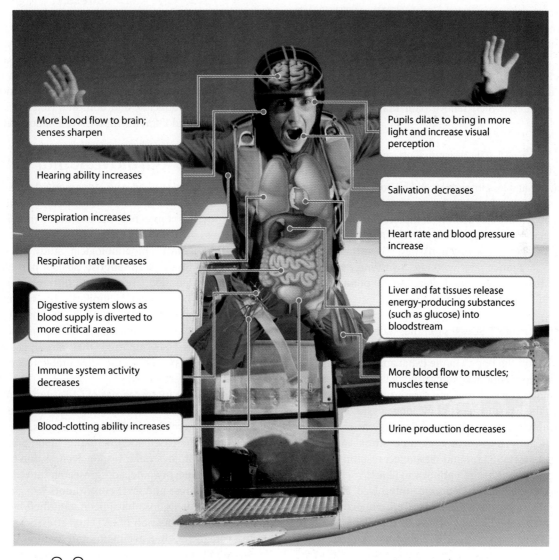

More blood flow to brain; senses sharpen

Hearing ability increases

Perspiration increases

Respiration rate increases

Digestive system slows as blood supply is diverted to more critical areas

Immune system activity decreases

Blood-clotting ability increases

Pupils dilate to bring in more light and increase visual perception

Salivation decreases

Heart rate and blood pressure increase

Liver and fat tissues release energy-producing substances (such as glucose) into bloodstream

More blood flow to muscles; muscles tense

Urine production decreases

FIGURE 3.2 **The Body's Acute Stress Response**

stressor, it stimulates the adrenal glands, located near the top of the kidneys, to release the hormone **epinephrine,** also called *adrenaline.* Epinephrine causes more blood to be pumped with each beat of the heart, dilates the airways in the lungs to increase oxygen intake, increases the breathing rate, stimulates the liver to release more glucose (which fuels muscular exertion), and dilates the pupils to improve visual sensitivity. The body is then poised to act immediately. As epinephrine secretion increases, blood is diverted away from the digestive system, possibly causing nausea and cramping if the distress occurs shortly after a meal and drying of nasal and salivary tissues, which produces dry mouth.

The alarm phase also provides for longer-term reaction to stress. The hypothalamus uses chemical messages to trigger the pituitary gland within the brain to release a powerful hormone, *adrenocorticotropic hormone (ACTH).* ACTH signals the adrenal glands to release **cortisol,** a hormone that makes stored nutrients more readily available to meet energy demands. (See the **Health Headlines** box on page 62 for more on how cortisol can affect the body.) Finally, other parts of the brain and body release endorphins, the body's naturally occurring opiates, which relieve pain that a stressor may cause.

Resistance Phase

The resistance phase of GAS is similar to the alarm phase in that the same organs and systems are mobilized, but at a less intense level. The body tries to return to homeostasis, but because some perceived stressor still exists, the body does not achieve complete rest. Instead, the body stays activated or aroused at a level that causes a higher metabolic rate in some organ tissues. These organs and systems of resistance are working "overtime" and after prolonged stress will become depleted to the point at which they cannot function effectively.

Exhaustion Phase

Stress promotes adaptation, but a prolonged response leads to **allostatic load,** or exhaustive wear and tear on the body.[7] In the exhaustion phase of GAS, the physical and emotional energy used to fight a stressor has been depleted. The toll that the stress takes on the body depends on the type of stress or how long it lasts. Short-term stress probably would not deplete all energy reserves in an otherwise healthy person, but chronic stress can create continuous states of alarm and resistance, resulting in total depletion of energy and susceptibility to illness.

As the body adjusts to chronic unresolved stress, the adrenal glands continue to release cortisol, which remains in the bloodstream for longer periods of time as a result of slower metabolic responsiveness. Over time, without relief, cortisol can reduce **immunocompetence,** or the ability of the immune system to respond to various assaults. Blood pressure can remain dangerously elevated, you may catch colds more easily, or your body's ability to control blood glucose levels can be affected.

Stress and Your Health

Although much has been written about the negative effects of stress, researchers have only recently begun to untangle the complex web of physical and emotional interactions that can break down the body over time. Stress is often described as a "disease of prolonged arousal" that leads to other negative health effects. Nearly all body systems become potential targets, and the long-term effects may be devastating. Look at the stress symptoms shown in **Figure 3.3.** Do you frequently experience any of these physical symptoms of stress?

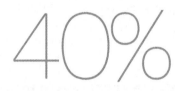

40% of deaths in the United States are related wholly or in part to stress.

Studies indicate that 40 percent of deaths and 70 percent of disease in the United States are related, in whole or in part, to stress.[8] The list of ailments related to chronic stress includes heart disease, diabetes, cancer, headaches, ulcers, low back pain, depression, and the common cold. Alarming increases in rates of suicide, homicide, and domestic violence across the United States are additional symptoms of a nation under stress.

Stress and Cardiovascular Disease

Perhaps the most studied and documented health consequence of unresolved stress is cardiovascular disease (CVD). Research on this topic has demonstrated the impact of chronic stress on heart rate, blood pressure, heart attack, and stroke.[9] The largest epidemiological study to date, the INTERHEART Study with almost 30,000 participants in 52 countries, identified stress as one of the key modifiable risk factors for heart attack.[10] Similarly, the National Health Interview Study, conducted annually by the Centers for Disease Control and Prevention (CDC) National Center for Health Statistics, has reported that stress accounts for approximately 30 percent of the attributable risk of myocardial infarction (heart attack).[11]

Historically, the increased risk of CVD from chronic stress has been linked to increased plaque buildup resulting from elevated cholesterol, hardening of the arteries, alterations in heart rhythm, increased and fluctuating blood pressure, and difficulties in cardiovascular responsiveness due to all of the above.[12] In the past two decades, research into the relationship between stress and CVD contributors has grown exponentially, and direct links have been identified between the incidence and progression of CVD and stressors such as job strain, caregiving, bereavement, and natural disasters.[13] Young people are not immune to these increased risks. (For more information about CVD, see Chapter 12.)

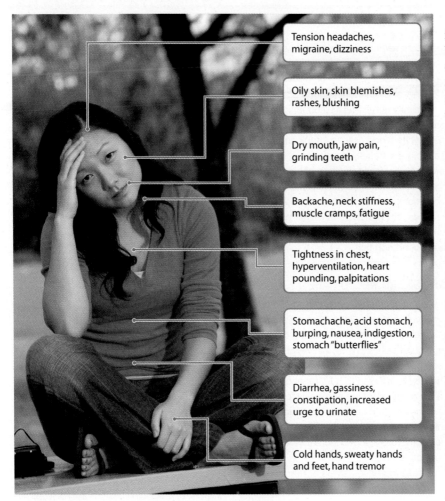

Tension headaches, migraine, dizziness

Oily skin, skin blemishes, rashes, blushing

Dry mouth, jaw pain, grinding teeth

Backache, neck stiffness, muscle cramps, fatigue

Tightness in chest, hyperventilation, heart pounding, palpitations

Stomachache, acid stomach, burping, nausea, indigestion, stomach "butterflies"

Diarrhea, gassiness, constipation, increased urge to urinate

Cold hands, sweaty hands and feet, hand tremor

FIGURE 3.3 **Common Physical Symptoms of Stress**

Stress and Impaired Immunity

As discussed in Chapter 2, a growing area of scientific investigation known as **psychoneuroimmunology (PNI)** analyzes the intricate relationship between the mind's response to stress and the immune system's ability to function effectively. A review of research linking stress to adverse health consequences suggests that too much stress over a long period can negatively regulate various aspects of the cellular immune response.[14] In particular, stress disrupts bidirectional communication networks between the nervous, endocrine, and immune systems. When these networks fail, messenger systems that regulate hormones, blood cell formation, and a host of other health-regulating systems begin to falter or send faulty information. Whereas the acute stress response is essentially protective and acute stress effects on health care controversial, *chronic stress* is a clear risk for a variety of health problems. Prolonged fight-or-flight response depresses the immune system, particularly through the actions of cortisol. During prolonged stress, elevated levels of adrenal hormones destroy or reduce the ability of certain white blood cells, known as *killer T cells*, to aid the immune response. When killer T cells are suppressed and other regulating systems aren't working correctly, illness may occur.

Loss of immune regulation can result in various disease states. The links between stress and physiological features of cancer, arthritis, HIV/AIDS, asthma, and many other ailments have been studied through PNI.[15] Although each of these diseases has distinct clinical consequences, the change in the immune system from balanced and flexible to unbalanced and inflexible suggests increased vulnerability to stress-related immune impairment. New research appears to support the theory that stress reduction, brought about through practicing mindfulness techniques (such as meditation, yoga, or tai chi), can reduce negative stress effects.[16]

How long do you have to be stressed to suffer from impaired immunity? A look at the research yields evidence of impaired immunity following acute stressors, such as arguments, public speaking, and academic examinations. More prolonged stressors, such as the loss of a spouse, exposure to natural disaster, caregiving, living with a handicap, and unemployment, also have been shown to impair the natural immune response among various populations.[17]

Other studies have linked stress with infectious diseases. More than 20 years of research have revealed that higher stress levels are associated with higher rates of viral infection and clinical cold symptoms.[18] Psychological stress and loneliness correlate to poorer immune responses following influenza vaccinations in college students.[19] Exposure to academic stressors and self-reported stress are associated with increased upper-respiratory-tract infection among students.[20]

Although strong indicators support the hypothesis of a relationship between high stress and increased risk for disease, we are only beginning to understand this link. Some research indicates that other factors, such as genetics and environmental stimuli, may be involved. Even so, studies supporting this relationship outnumber those that don't, and there is convincing evidence that susceptibility to disease is influenced by stress-induced alterations in immune functioning.[21]

psychoneuroimmunology (PNI) Science of the interaction between the mind and the immune system.

Stress and Digestive Problems

Although digestive disorders are physical conditions whose causes are often unknown, it is widely assumed that an underlying illness, pathogen, injury, or inflammation is already present and that stress can be a trigger that causes you to be nauseated, vomit, have stomach cramps and

Health
Headlines

THE LOOK OF STRESS

We've all seen that look: dark circles under the eyes, pained expression, furrowed brow, and deep lines along a downturned mouth. Usually these relate to too little sleep, too much worry, and a "too much to do and no end in sight" scenario. Although this situation can certainly make you look older, unhealthy, and wound up, prolonged stress poses very real threats to your appearance and health that can't simply be erased with a good night's sleep.

STRESS AND HAIR LOSS

Yes, it's true: Too much stress can lead to thinning, lackluster hair, exacerbate premature baldness in men, and encourage that all-too-common shiny scalp that glares through even the most attractive hairstyle for many women. The most common type of emotional or physical stress-induced hair loss is *telogen effluvium*. Often seen in individuals who have suffered a death in the family, had a difficult pregnancy, or experienced severe weight loss, this condition pushes colonies of hair to go on a long-term "vacation," or resting phase. Over time

(usually a few months), simply washing or combing your hair may cause clumps of hair to fall out, ending up on pillows, clothing, and other unintended places.

A similar stress-related condition known as *alopecia areata* occurs when stress triggers white blood cells to attack and destroy hair follicles, usually in patches. If stress is prolonged, varying degrees of baldness may occur. The good news is that for both conditions, you can reverse the hair loss process, not with expensive hair products, but rather with sleep, stress management, and sound nutrition.

STRESS AND WEIGHT GAIN

If a thinning crop of hair isn't bad enough, stress may pack an even bigger wallop to your appearance and your health by causing you to gain and maintain weight! In recent years, several studies have indicated that stress is linked to belly fat and that one of the most important strategies for weight loss may be to reduce stress. Exactly how this works is not clear; however, most theories point to prolonged increases in stress hormones.

Stress increases levels of hormones, such as *cortisol*, which help stimulate release of glucose into the bloodstream. When blood sugar levels rise, the body secretes insulin to help bring these levels down. However, when stress is chronic, insulin levels can remain high, causing fat cells to enlarge and fat to be more readily stored in the body. Prolonged rises in blood sugar and insulin increase risk for pre-diabetes and diabetes. There also is evidence that prolonged elevations of cortisol may slow your metabolism, thereby sabotaging efforts to lose weight.

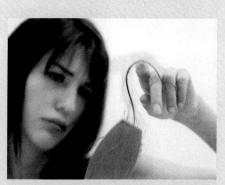

Losing hair? Maybe you need to de-stress!

As cortisol levels increase, you may find that you actually crave foods, particularly sweet foods made from refined carbohydrates. In addition, cortisol may cause you to feel hungry and eat more than you normally would. Rather than settling down and cooking a healthy meal, people who are frustrated, keyed up, angry, or depressed are more likely to eat fast foods, mindlessly munch entire bags of chips or candy, and nosh on junk food as they seek comfort in food. Ultimately, appearance is affected by out of control eating behaviors and your health also ends up suffering.

Sources: D. K. Hall-Flavin, "Stress and Hair Loss: Are They Related?" Mayo Clinic, October 4, 2008, www.mayoclinic.com/health/stress-and-hair-loss/AN01442; M. F. Dallman et al., "Minireview: Glucocorticoids, Food Intake, Abdominal Obesity and Wealthy Nations in 2004," *Endocrinology* 145, no. 6 (2004): 2633–38; T. Bray, "Diabetes," *LPI Research Newsletter*, Linus Pauling Institute, Oregon State University, May 2007; D. Eizirik, A. Cardozo, and M. Cnop, "The Role of Endoplasmic Reticular Stress in Diabetes Mellitus," *Endocrine Reviews* 29, no. 1 (2008): 42–61; R. Robertson, "Oxidative Stress and Impaired Insulin Resistance in Type 2 Diabetes," *Current Opinion in Pharmacology* 6, no. 6 (2007): 615–19.

related pain in the gut, or prompts you to make a mad dash for the bathroom. Although stress doesn't directly cause these symptoms, it is clearly related and, in fact, may actually make your risk of having symptoms even worse.[22] For example, people with depression or anxiety are more susceptible to irritable bowel syndrome (IBS), probably because stress stimulates colon spasms via the nervous system. If you are very nervous or upset, you might experience cramps, or you may just be more likely to be aware of problems with your stomach and gastrointestinal tract. Some relaxation techniques, such as progressive muscle relaxation, meditation, and guided imagery (discussed later in

this chapter), are particularly helpful in coping with stressors that make your digestive problems worse. These techniques promote relaxation by reducing the activity of the sympathetic nervous system, leading to decreases in heart rate, blood pressure, and other stress responses. They also appear to reduce gastrointestinal reactivity and decrease your risks of gastrointestinal tract flare-ups.[23]

Stress and the Mind

Stress may be one of the single greatest contributors to mental disability and emotional dysfunction in industrialized

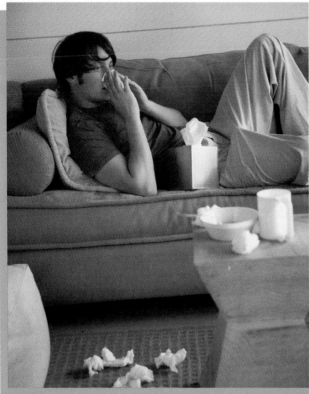

Why do I always get sick during finals week?

Prolonged stress can lower the functioning of your immune system, leaving you vulnerable to illness and infection. If you spend exam week in a state of high stress, sleeping too little, studying too hard, and worrying a lot, chances are you'll reduce your body's ability to fight off any cold or flu bugs you may encounter.

nations. Studies have shown that the rates of mental disorders, particularly depression and anxiety, are associated with various environmental stressors, including divorce, marital conflict, economic hardship, and stressful life events.[24] In particular, mental disorders are more prevalent among young people aged 15 to 24 than among other age groups. Based on this finding, researchers suggest that as individuals move from adolescence to adulthood, they face stressors of all kinds, from school to employment to relationships, that may challenge their mental health.[25]

Evidence suggests a strong relationship between stress and the potential for negative mental health reactions. Consider the following:[26]

- Stressful life events and inadequate sources of social support have been identified as predictors of psychiatric morbidity, including anxiety, insomnia, and depression.
- The high incidence of suicide among college students is assumed to indicate high personal and societal stress in the lives of young people.
- Eighty-five percent of college counseling centers report an increase in the number of students they see with severe psychological problems—problems largely related to stress and adjustment difficulties.

What Stresses You?

On any given day, we all experience eustress and distress, usually from a wide range of obvious and not-so-obvious sources. College students, in particular, face stressors that come from internal sources, as well as external pressures to succeed in a competitive environment that is often geographically far from the support of family and life-long friends. In a recent national survey of college students, more than two-thirds of the 81,000 students who responded said that they felt overwhelmed 1 to 10 times in the past year, with the remaining third indicating that they were overwhelmed 11 or more times. Not surprisingly, these same students indicated that they felt exhausted (not from physical activity) at approximately the same rates.[27] Ultimately, stressors can play a huge role in whether students stay in school, do well along their career path, or get involved in healthy or unhealthy behaviors. Awareness of the sources of stress can do much to help you develop a plan to avoid, prevent, and control the things that cause you stress.

Psychosocial Stressors

Psychosocial stressors refer to the factors in our daily macro- and social environment that cause us to experience stress. Interactions with others and the expectations we and others have of ourselves about our competence, our future careers, our personal characteristics and behaviors, and the social conditions we live in, force us to readjust continually. Key psychosocial stressors include adjustment to change, hassles, interpersonal relationships, academic and career pressures, frustrations and conflicts, overload, and stressful living environments.

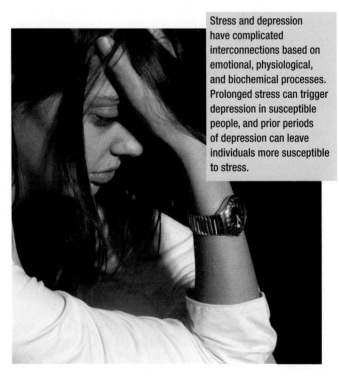

Stress and depression have complicated interconnections based on emotional, physiological, and biochemical processes. Prolonged stress can trigger depression in susceptible people, and prior periods of depression can leave individuals more susceptible to stress.

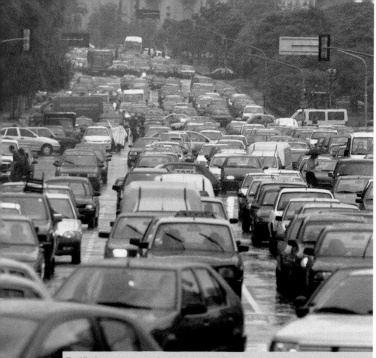
Traffic jams are a modern stressor and an example of one of the daily hassles that can add up and jeopardize our health.

Adjustment to Change

Anytime change occurs in your normal routine, whether good or bad, you will experience stress. The more changes you experience and the more adjustments you must make, the greater the chances that stress will take its toll on your health. Unfortunately, while your first days on campus can be exciting, they can also be among the most stressful you will face in your life. Moving away from home, trying to fit in on campus and make new friends from diverse backgrounds, adjusting to a new schedule, learning to live with strangers in housing that is often lacking in the comforts of home: all of these things can cause sleeplessness and anxiety and keep your body in a continual fight-or-flight mode. Four decades ago, Drs. Thomas Holmes and Richard Rahe developed the initial Social Readjustment Rating Scale (SRRS) to identify whether major life events preceded illness onset.[28] They determined that certain events (both positive and negative) were predictive of increased risk for illness. Since this time, the SRSS has served as the basis for similar scales used to study stressors among different populations. The **Assess Yourself** on page 79 includes a version of the SRSS that is specific to the unique stressors of college students. Although not perfect, this scale provides an indicator of the kinds of overall stressors that many students experience.

Hassles: The Little Things That Bug You

Although the SRSS provides an overview of major stressors, other psychologists have proposed that the little stressors, frustrations, and petty annoyances, known collectively as *hassles,* can be just as stressful.[29] In short, it isn't necessarily the big life changes that can do you in, but rather the daily barrage of little things that causes you to be continually uptight. Classmates who talk too much during lecture, not being able to get to class in time to score a good seat, waiting in long lines, enduring your neighbor's annoyingly loud music or TV while you are trying to study, encountering bad breath or body odor, and a host of other bothersome situations can push your buttons and result in frustration, anger, and fight-or-flight responses.[30] For many people, the fast pace of technology creates new hassles and adds to their stress; see the **Health Today** box on page 66 for more on "technostress."

The Toll of Relationships

Let's face it, relationships can trigger some of the biggest fight-or-flight reactions of all time. Remember that wild, exhilarating feeling of new love? You couldn't focus, you couldn't sleep, and you didn't get much work done while thinking about your *new* love interest. Likewise, remember when you ultimately broke up with someone you thought you were deeply in love with, or they broke up with you? You couldn't focus, you couldn't sleep, and you didn't get much done while thinking about your *former* love interest. Love relationships are the ones we often think of first; however, friends, family members, and coworkers can be the sources of overwhelming struggles, just as they can be sources of strength and support. Ironically, these relationships can make us strive to be the best that we can be and give us hope for the future, or they can diminish our self-esteem and leave us reeling from a destructive interaction.

Academic and Career Pressures

It isn't surprising that putting a group of top high school graduates into today's colleges and universities and telling them to compete for good grades, athletic positions, top jobs, and other future goals can cause mind-boggling amounts of pressure. Challenging classes can be tough enough, but many students also work at least part time to pay the bills, and juggle multiple responsibilities that parents may have taken care of in the past. Even in times of economic prosperity, students often have a tough time meeting all of their costs and obligations. Today's economic downturn can have major effects on college students and make distant dreams even harder to come true.

Frustrations and Conflicts

Whenever there is a disparity between our goals (what we hope to obtain in life) and our behaviors (actions that may or may not lead to these goals), frustration can occur. For example, you realize that you must get good grades in college to enter graduate school, which is your ultimate goal. If you know you should be getting good grades, but are having too much fun with friends when you should be studying, these inconsistencies between your goals and your behavior can cause significant stress. Determining whether behaviors are consistent with your goals is an important part of maintaining balance in your life.

Conflicts occur when we are forced to decide among competing motives, impulses, desires, and behaviors, or when we are forced to face pressures of demands that are incompatible with our own values and sense of importance. College students

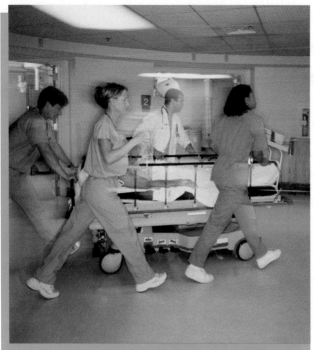

Who is most prone to stress?

Everyone experiences stress in his or her life, but some people have personalities and attitudes that leave them more susceptible, whereas others have careers or life circumstances that impose greater external pressures on them. Individuals such as doctors and nurses face long work hours and a high-stakes work environment, making them especially prone to stress, overload, and burnout.

who are away from their families for the first time may face a variety of conflicts among parental values, their own beliefs, and the beliefs of others who are very different from them. These situations can cause guilt and sleepless nights, and ultimately be very stressful.

Overload We've all experienced times in our lives when the demands of work, responsibilities, deadlines, and relationships all seem to be pulling us under water with a 200-pound weight tied to our feet. **Overload** occurs when, try as we might, there are not nearly enough hours in the day and our physical, mental, and emotional reserves are not sufficient to deal with all we have on our plate. Students suffering from overload may experience depression, sleeplessness, mood swings, frustration, anxiety, or a host of other symptoms. Taken together, these may make the likelihood of being productive even more remote. Binge drinking; high consumption of junk foods; and fighting with friends, family, and coworkers can all add fuel to the overload fire.[31] Unrelenting stress and overload can lead to a state of physical and mental exhaustion known as *burnout*.

9%
of college students report experiencing "tremendous stress" over the past 12 months.

Stressful Environments For many students, where they live and the environment around them can cause significant levels of stress. Many students cannot afford quality housing, and unscrupulous landlords have been known to exploit students by leasing them substandard, or even unhealthy, apartments. Fortunately, in more and more college and university communities, strictly enforced regulations governing student housing are being instituted. Increasing numbers of landlords are involved in these improvements, recognizing that in a competitive housing market, they must improve conditions to attract discriminating renters.

Although rare, natural disasters can wreak havoc on our lives, causing environmental distress. Flooding, earthquakes, hurricanes, blizzards, and tornadoes can all displace students from housing, and disrupt their ability to attend class and conduct their daily lives. Often as damaging as one-time disasters are **background distressors** in the environment, such as noise, air, and water pollution; allergy-aggravating pollen and dust; or environmental tobacco smoke. As with other challenges, our bodies respond to environmental distressors with GAS. People who cannot escape background distressors may exist in a constant resistance phase, which can contribute to stress-related disorders.

overload A condition in which a person feels overly pressured by demands.

background distressors Environmental stressors of which people are often unaware.

Stress and "-isms"

Today's racial and ethnic diversity of students, faculty members, and staff enriches everyone's educational experience yet also challenges everyone to deal with differences. Students come from vastly different contexts and life experiences. Imagine what it would be like to come to campus and find yourself isolated, lacking friends, and ridiculed on the basis of who you are or how you look. Often, those who act, speak, or dress differently face additional pressures that do not affect students considered more typical. Students perceived as different may become victims of subtle and not-so-subtle forms of bigotry, insensitivity, harassment, or hostility. Racism, ageism, sexism, or other "-*isms*"—different viewpoints and backgrounds—may hang like a dark cloud over these students.

Evidence of the health effects of excessive stress in minority groups abounds. For example, African Americans suffer higher rates of hypertension, CVD, and most cancers than do white people.[32] Although poverty and socioeconomic status have been blamed for much of the spike in hypertension rates for African Americans and other marginalized groups, chronic, physically debilitating stress may reflect real and perceived status in society more than it reflects actual poverty. Feeling that you occupy a position of low status because of your living conditions, financial security, or job status can be a source of stress. The problem is exacerbated for people who are socially disadvantaged early in life and grow up without a nurturing environment.[33]

TAMING TECHNOSTRESS

Are you "twittered out"? Is all that texting causing your thumbs to seize up in protest? If so, you're not alone. Like millions of others, you may find that all of the pressure for contact is more than enough stress for you! Known as *technostress*, this bombardment is defined as stress created by a dependence on technology and the constant state of being plugged in or wirelessly connected, which can include a perceived obligation to respond, chat, or tweet.

There is much good that comes from all that technological wizardry; however, for some, technomania can become obsessive—a situation in which people would rather hang out online, talking to strangers, than study, talk to friends, socialize in person, or generally connect in the real world. Although technology can allow us to multitask, work on the go, and communicate in new and different ways, there are some clear downsides to all of that "virtual" interaction.

✳ **Distracted driving.** Exact numbers are hard to come by, but some sources estimate that as much as 25 percent of distracted driving is the result of people either talking or texting on their cell phones or manipulating music devices. About 90 percent of the U.S. population, more than 270 million people, have cell phones and at any given moment, 11 percent of them are using those phones while driving. Because research indicates that doing so puts people at risk, more than 250 cities and several states have passed laws or are considering legislation that would either prohibit or restrict the use of cell phones by drivers.

✳ **Practice Safe Text!** This catchy website title emerged in 2008 and captured inter-

national attention. The truth behind the cleverness is a very real repetitive stress injury (RSI) known as *Blackberry thumb*. If you are one of a growing number of persons who have this malady, you already know that it refers to a problem experienced by too much thumb use on today's personal digital assistant (PDA) devices. It causes pain, swelling, or numbness of the thumb. There are exercises to strengthen thumb muscles and help stretch tight muscles and tendons, pain relievers, and more drastic treatments involving injections or surgery, but the best advice is to avoid the malady by stretching thumb muscles before texting and keeping messaging to a minimum.

✳ **Other repetitive stress injuries.** Sitting in front of a computer screen set at the wrong height, or working hunched over a laptop for hours can result in stressed muscles, ligaments, and tendons, often with painful consequences. Back pain, neck cramps, and carpal tunnel syndrome are all possible outcomes. Keeping sessions short, stretching muscles frequently, and getting an ergonomic check of your work station can all help prevent future problems.

✳ **Social distress.** Authors Michell Weil and Larry Rosen describe *technosis*, a very real syndrome in which people become so immersed in technology that they risk losing their own identity. Worrying about checking your voice mails, constantly switching to e-mail or Facebook to see who has left a message or is online, perpetually posting to Twitter, and so on can keep you distracted and take important minutes or hours from your day.

To avoid technosis and to prevent technostress, set time limits on your

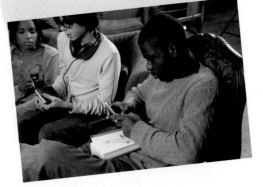

Technology may keep you in touch, but it can also add to your stress and take you away from real-world interactions.

technology usage, and make sure that you devote at least as much time to face-to-face interactions with people you care about as a means of cultivating and nurturing your relationships. Screen your contacts, especially when you are in public or engaged in face-to-face communication with someone. You don't always need to answer your phone or respond to a text or e-mail immediately.

Leave your devices at home or turn them off when you are out with others or on vacation. If you can't leave your PDA, laptop, or cell phone at home—or turned off—when you are out with others, or on vacation, then there is a problem. *Tune in* to your surroundings, your loved ones and friends, your job, and your classes by shutting off your devices.

Sources: AAA Foundation for Traffic Safety, "Safety Culture: Cell Phones and Driving: Research Update," 2008, www.aaafoundation.org/pdf/CellPhonesand DrivingFS.pdf; M. Weil and L. Rosen, "Technostress: Are You a Victim?" 2007, www.technostress.com.

Internal Stressors

Although stress can come from the environment and other external sources, it can also be a result of internal factors. Unsettling thoughts or feelings can be associated with internal stressors such as low self-esteem, low self-efficacy, and

negative appraisal.[34] It is important to address and manage these internal stressors.

Appraisal and Stress We encounter many different types of life demands and potential stressors—some biological, some psychological, and others sociological. In any case, it is

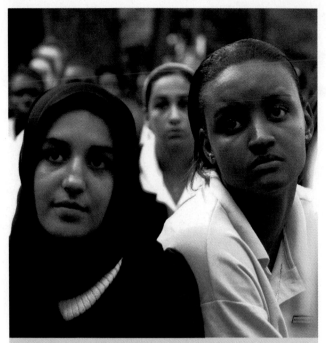

Language barriers, cultural conflicts, racial prejudices, and a reluctance to seek social support all contribute to a significantly higher rate of stress-related illnesses among international students studying in the United States.

our appraisal of these demands, not the demands themselves, that results in the experience of stress. **Appraisal** is defined as the interpretation and evaluation of information provided to the brain by the senses. Appraisal is not a conscious activity, but rather a natural process that the brain constantly performs. As new information becomes available, appraisal helps us recognize stressors, evaluate them on the basis of past experiences and emotions, and decide how to cope with them. When you perceive that your coping resources are sufficient to meet life's demands, you experience little or no stress. By contrast, when you perceive that life's demands exceed your coping resources, you are likely to feel strain and distress.

Self-Esteem and Self-Efficacy
As we learned in Chapter 2, *self-esteem* refers to a sense of positive self-regard, or how you feel about yourself. Self-esteem varies; it can and does continually change.[35] When you feel good about yourself, you are less likely to respond to or interpret an event as stressful. Conversely, if you place little or no value on yourself and believe you have inadequate coping skills, you become susceptible to stress and strain.[36]

Self-esteem is closely related to the emotions engendered by past experiences. Low self-esteem can lead to helpless anger. People suffering helpless anger usually have learned that they are wrong to feel anger, so instead of expressing it in healthy ways they turn it inward. They may swallow their rage in food, alcohol, or other drugs, or they may act in other self-destructive ways. Of particular concern, research with high school and college students has found that low self-esteem and stressful life events significantly predict **suicidal ideation,** a desire to die and thoughts about suicide. On a more positive note, research has also indicated that it is pos-

sible to increase an individual's ability to cope with stress by increasing self-esteem.[37] Chapter 2 discussed several ways to develop and maintain self-esteem.

Self-efficacy, also introduced in Chapter 2, is another important factor in the ability to cope with life's challenges. Self-efficacy refers to belief or confidence in personal skills and performance abilities.[38] Self-efficacy is considered one of the most important personality traits that influence psychological and physiological stress responses, and it has been found to predict a number of health behaviors in college students.[39]

Type A and Type B Personalities
It should come as no surprise to you that personality can have an impact on whether you are happy and socially well adjusted or sad and socially isolated. However, your personality may affect more than just your social interactions: It may be a critical factor in your stress level, as well as in your risk for CVD, cancer, and other chronic and infectious diseases.

Since 1974, when physicians Meyer Friedman and Ray Rosenman wrote a book indicating that Type A individuals had a greatly increased risk of heart disease, people have been labeling their friends and family members by their corresponding alphabet soup, heart disease characteristics.[40] *Type A* personalities are defined as hard-driving, competitive, time-driven perfectionists. In contrast, *Type B* personalities are described as being relaxed, noncompetitive, and more tolerant of others. Today, most researchers recognize that none of us will be wholly either a Type A or a Type B all of the time. We ebb and flow through these characteristics as we respond to the various challenges of our daily lives.

appraisal The interpretation and evaluation of information provided to the brain by the senses.
suicidal ideation A desire to die and thoughts about suicide.
hostility The cognitive, affective, and behavioral tendencies toward anger and cynicism.

In addition, recent research indicates that not all Type As experience negative health consequences; in fact, some hard-driving individuals seem to thrive on their supercharged lifestyles. Only those Type As who exhibit a "toxic core," or have disproportionate amounts of anger, are distrustful of others, and have a cynical, glass-half-empty approach to life—a set of characteristics referred to as **hostility**—are at increased risk for heart disease.[41] A hostile personality seems to make people more vulnerable to self-imposed stress, particularly if they also suffer from low self-esteem and lack social support. Hostility itself has three components: a cognitive component of negative beliefs about and attitudes toward others, including cynicism and mistrust, an affective component of anger that can range from irritation to rage; and a behavioral component of actions intended to harm others either verbally or physically, usually in an aggressive way. As such, hostility has been shown to increase risks for CVD in a variety of studies.[42]

Type C and Type D Personalities
In addition to CVD risks, personality types have been linked to increased risk for cancer. Psychologists have identified another personality type, *Type C* (cancer prone), as someone who may respond to stress with hopelessness and helplessness. Type C personalities tend

to be introverted, eager to please, and compliant. Those who are type C in nature may be less likely to respond with a "fighting spirit" after diagnosis of cancer and may more readily accept their fate.[43]

A more recently identified personality type is *Type D* (distressed), characterized by a tendency toward excessive negative worry, irritability, gloom, and social inhibition. Several recent studies have shown that type D people may be up to eight times more likely to die of a heart attack or sudden death.[44]

Psychological Hardiness According to psychologist Susanne Kobasa, **psychological hardiness** may negate self-imposed stress associated with Type A behavior. Psychologically hardy people are characterized by control, commitment, and an embrace of challenge.[45] People with a sense of control are able to accept responsibility for their behaviors and change those that they discover to be debilitating. People with a sense of commitment have good self-esteem and understand their purpose in life. People who embrace challenge see change as a stimulating opportunity for personal growth. The concept of hardiness has been studied extensively, and many researchers believe it is the foundation of an individual's ability to cope with stress and remain healthy.[46]

psychological hardiness A personality trait characterized by control, commitment, and the embrace of challenge.

psychological stress Stress caused by being in an environment perceived to be beyond one's resources and jeopardizing one's well-being.

Stress and the College Student

College students usually thrive under a certain amount of stress, but excessive stress can leave them overwhelmed and less than enthusiastic about their classes and social interactions. Students can experience numerous distressors, including changes related to being away from home, pressure to make friends, the feeling of anonymity imposed by large classes, and academic pressures and test-taking anxiety (for tips on how to overcome test-taking anxiety, see the **Skills for Behavior Change** box on the next page).[47] Some 32 percent of students surveyed for the National College Health Assessment reported that stress was the number one factor affecting their individual academic performance, followed closely by stress-related problems such as cold/flu/sore throat (26%) and sleep difficulties (23.9%).

The researchers at UCLA's Higher Education Research Institute define **psychological stress** as a relationship between a person and the environment that the person judges to be beyond his or her resources and jeopardizes his or her well-being. A 2005 study by the Higher Education Research

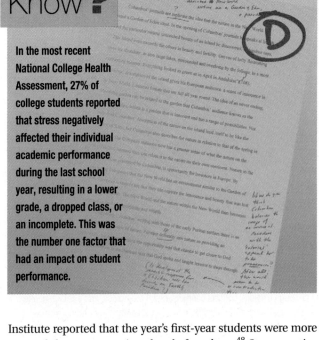

Institute reported that the year's first-year students were more stressed than any entering class before them.[48] Stress continues to be the number one factor affecting student performance.[49] First-year students seem to be the most vulnerable to the negative effects of psychological stress: Relationships, school events, safety, and feeling deviant from school norms have been noted as particularly distressful. In addition, first-year students have reported not only more problems with these issues, but also more emotional reactivity in the form of anger, hostility, frustration, and a greater sense of being out of control. Sophomores and juniors reported fewer problems with these issues, and seniors reported the fewest problems. The results may indicate students' progressive emotional growth through experience, maturity, increased awareness of support services, and more social connections.

Male and female students also report different stressors. Women indicate that among their most frequent stressors are being overweight, trying to diet, and managing an overload of schoolwork. Men, in contrast, tend to identify the following items as major stressors: being underweight, not having enough sex, being behind in schoolwork, and concerns about drug or alcohol use.

Differences in coping behaviors also have been identified. Women report greater use of time management techniques to deal with stress, whereas men tend to engage in more leisure activities to lessen academic stress. Students generally report using health-enhancing methods to combat stress, but research has found that students sometimes resort to health-compromising

reality of the situation may have absolutely nothing to do with your being liked or disliked. Perhaps party organizers didn't have your correct e-mail address, or the invitation was blocked by a spam filter, or they simply forgot or thought you wouldn't be in town.

In Chapter 1 we introduced the concept of self-talk. Stress management requires that you examine your self-talk and your emotional responses to interactions with others. With any emotional response to a stressor, you are responsible for the emotion and the resultant behaviors. Learning to tell the difference between normal emotions and those based on irrational beliefs or expressed and interpreted in an over-the-top manner can help you stop the emotion or express it in a healthy and appropriate way. The first reaction that comes to mind is not always the best. Stop before reacting so that you gain the time you need to find an appropriate response. Ask yourself, "What is to be gained from my response?"

Learn to Laugh, Be Joyful, and Cry If you've ever noticed that you feel better after a belly laugh or a good cry, you aren't alone. Old adages such as "laughter is the best medicine" and "smile and the world smiles with you" didn't just evolve out of the blue. Scientists have long recognized that smiling, laughing, singing, dancing, and other actions can elevate our moods, help us live longer, and help us improve our relationships. Crying can have similar positive physiological effects. Recent research has shown that laughter and joy can increase endorphin levels, increase oxygen levels in the blood, increase immune system functioning, decrease stress levels, relieve pain, enhance productivity, reduce risks of heart disease, and help fight cancer.[54] In a large study published recently, scientists indicated that happiness may be contagious and that happy people tend to spread their happiness to others.[55] For ideas on how to find more joy and laughter in your own life, see the **Health Today** box on page 72.

Fight the Anger Urge Anger usually results when we feel we have lost control of a situation or are frustrated by a situation that we can do little about. The five main sources of anger are related to threats to (1) safety and well-being, (2) power, (3) perfectionism and pride, (4) self-sufficiency and autonomy, and (5) self-esteem and status.[56]

Anger may vary in intensity from mild irritation to rage and may be acted out as cynicism, sarcasm, intimidation, frustration, impatience, quick flaring of temper, distrust, or anxiety. Not all anger is inherently bad. Sometimes, it can give us the energy we need to fight back if attacked or the resolve to work even harder to accomplish a goal. It is unresolved anger, the kind that festers and clouds our reasoning and our reactions, that we need to control.

Each of us has learned by this point in our lives that we have three main approaches to dealing with anger: expressing it, suppressing it, or calming it. You may be surprised to find out that *expressing* your anger is probably the healthiest thing to do in the long run, particularly if you express anger in an assertive rather than aggressive way. However, it's a

natural reaction to want to respond aggressively, and that is what we must learn to keep at bay. To accomplish this, there are several strategies you can use:[57]

- **Identify your anger style.** Do you express anger passively or actively? Do you hold anger in, or do you explode? Do you throw the phone, smash things, or scream at others?
- **Learn to recognize patterns in your anger responses and how to de-escalate them.** For 1 week, keep track of everything that angers you or keeps you "stewing." What thoughts or feelings lead up to your "boiling point"? Keep a journal and listen to your anger. Try to change your self-talk. Explore how you can interrupt patterns of anger, such as counting to 10, getting a drink of water, or taking some deep breaths.
- **Plan ahead.** Some situations (family get-togethers, long lines, traffic) can be foreseen as potentially provoking anger. Explore options to minimize your exposure to them.
- **Develop a support system.** Find a few close friends you can confide in or vent your frustration to. Don't force a person to agree with you, but allow him or her to listen and perhaps provide insight or another perspective that your anger has blinded you to. Don't wear down your supporter with continual rants.
- **Develop realistic expectations of yourself and others.** Anger is often the result of unmet expectations, frustrations, resentments, and impatience. Are your expectations of yourself and others realistic? Try talking with those involved about your feelings at a time when you are calm.
- **Turn complaints into requests.** When frustrated or angry with someone, try reworking the problem into a request. Instead of screaming and pounding on the floor because your downstairs neighbors' blaring music woke you up at 2:00 AM, have a conversation with them. Try to reach an agreement that works for everyone.
- **Leave past anger in the past.** Learn to resolve issues that have caused pain, frustration, or stress. If necessary, seek the counsel of a professional to make that happen.

Taking Physical Action

Physical activities can complement the emotional and mental strategies of stress management.

Exercise It is important to remember that the human stress response is intended to end in physical activity (fight or flight). The outpouring of sugar and fats into the blood is meant to nourish the muscles and brain. The heart and respiration rates speed up to meet the impending physical demands of the threat. If the threat persists, hormones are released into the bloodstream to maintain the response. Historically, most threats required physical responses. Today that is not true, yet our stress response has not changed to fit with the times. When we are stressed, this is not the time to sit and feel all those fight-or-flight sensations tearing away at our body's systems. This is the time to move and use up those products of the stress response. Exercise "burns off" existing

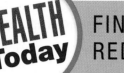
Don't we all just want to be happy? In the past few decades, a field of research—positive psychology, the study of positive emotions, positive individual traits, and positive institutions—has emerged to study the truth of that idea. Psychologists in this field believe that people *want* to lead meaningful and fulfilling lives, to cultivate what is best within themselves, and to enhance their life experiences in love, at work, and at play. In studying people's attitudes and choices, and evaluating the outcomes, some positive psychologists have found that people who are generally more optimistic or happier have fewer mental and physical health problems. If happiness and optimism are keys to health and stress reduction, how can you find the holy grail of all that is great and good? Experts have a range of opinions on how to achieve that glass-half-full attitude.

✳ **Set realistic goals.** In her best-selling book, *Be Happy without Being Perfect*, psychologist Alice Donner says that striving for a 100 percent dose of contentment and perfection is unrealistic. She suggests that managing your *expectations* is a key. Realize that both good and bad things in life will come to you. Expect them both and don't try to be that perfect friend, lover, partner, student, son or daughter, or career mogul. Decide what is realistic for you and work to get to a realistic place in your social structure, your classes, your relationships, and your career.

✳ **Remember that money doesn't buy happiness.** Although living in a posh neighborhood, driving a fancy car, and having all of the nicest "toys" might be important for some, these things do not ensure happiness. In fact, too much focus on the acquisition of things rather than a concentration on relationships and connections may be a major cause of discontent and result in loneliness and stress about paying for all of those possessions. Also, people who have all of those "toy" payments tend to work longer

hours, vacation less, and in general not take time for themselves.

✳ **Lose yourself in the moment.** According to Mihaly Csikszentmihalyi, a leading expert on positive psychology, finding your *flow,* a state of effortless concentration and enjoyment, should be a daily goal. What is it that energizes you, makes time fly by, and causes you to concentrate fully on the present? Find that and you'll be finding at least momentary happiness. Find it more often and you'll be closing in on a happier you.

✳ **Count your blessings.** Although we all can find time to be critical and complain, focusing on our many positive attributes and being thankful for all the good things in our lives should become a daily ritual. For some, this might include daily journaling, a time when they can contemplate all of the good things about their day, the things they've consciously tried to do to enrich the lives of others, and the good news they've heard on the Internet, on TV, or in newspaper. Telling your parents how much you appreciate them, telling your friends that they enrich your life, and bringing a smile to someone's face—even if you don't know them—are all important. Focusing more on the positives in our world and trying to add to the positives for others can help you find happiness and attract happier people to you.

✳ **Make changes and reinvigorate.** If you are finding that your life is pretty ho-hum, try to make changes. For example, try new recipes, find some new ways of exercising, plan at least one fun outing with someone you enjoy at least once a month, find a new place on campus to study, plan a trip somewhere different in the next 6 months, find a new place to walk, learn a new skill such as playing the guitar, learn a new meditation strategy, or help someone who needs it by volunteering your time.

✳ **Forgive and forget.** Rather than ruminating over some slight or indiscretion, try to think about what may have caused someone to act toward you in a hurtful manner.

Don't forget to make time for joy and beauty in your life.

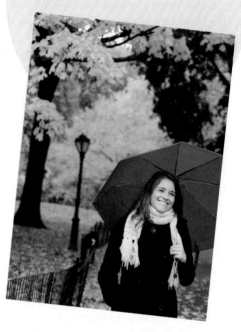

Is there something stressing that person? What may have motivated the person? Try to focus on the good things, rather than dwelling on the negative, and then move on. Forgive and get over it. Every moment you dwell on the negative is one less moment you are choosing to be happy.

✳ **Remember you are worth the time and energy.** Rather than letting yourself succumb to stress, force yourself to prioritize *you.* Your own happiness is as important as that of others in your life. Limit the time you spend with people who bring you down. Instead, find time for breaks, fun interludes, and alone time.

Sources: M. Csikszentmihalyi, *Flow: The Psychology of Optimal Experience* (New York: Harper & Row, 1990); The Positive Psychology Center at the University of Pennsylvania, "Frequently Asked Questions," 2007, www.ppc.sas.upenn.edu/faqs .htm; M. E. P. Seligman, *Authentic Happiness: Using the New Positive Psychology to Realize Your Potential for Lasting Fulfillment* (New York: Free Press/Simon & Schuster, 2002); A. Donner, *Be Happy without Being Perfect: How to Break Free from the Perfection Deception* (New York: Random House, 2008).

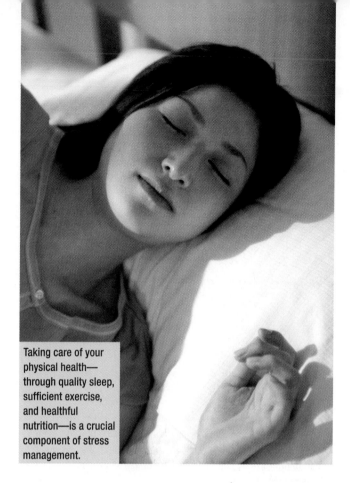

Taking care of your physical health—through quality sleep, sufficient exercise, and healthful nutrition—is a crucial component of stress management.

stress hormones by directing them toward their intended metabolic function.[58] In addition, exercise can help combat stress by raising levels of endorphins—mood-elevating, pain-killing hormones—in the bloodstream, increasing energy, reducing hostility, and improving mental alertness.

Most of us have relieved stress at some point by engaging in physical activity: talking a walk when we are feeling overwhelmed or even kicking a piece of furniture when we are angry. Although lashing out in anger is usually not a helpful response to stress, physical activity or exercise in general can reduce immediate stress symptoms. Even a quiet walk can refresh your mind, calm your stress response, and replenish your adaptation energy stores. However, a regular exercise program yields even more substantial benefits by conditioning the body to respond more efficiently. Plan walking breaks alone or with friends, or stretch after prolonged study periods at your desk. For more information on the beneficial effects of exercise, see Chapter 11.

Get Enough Sleep Increasingly, sleep is being recognized as one of the single greatest remedies for a host of potential threats to health. Adequate amounts of sleep allow you to refresh your vital energy, cope with multiple stressors more effectively, and be productive when you need to be. In fact, sleep is one of the biggest stress busters of them all. Perhaps even more important, sleep has been shown to increase the ability of the immune system to ward off infectious diseases, to help the body be more resilient and recover more readily from illness, and to prevent a wide range of chronic ailments,

ranging from CVD and hypertension to certain cancers and diabetes. These benefits are discussed in much more depth in **Focus On: Your Sleep** beginning on page 86.

Relax Like exercise, relaxation can help you cope with stressful feelings, preserve adaptation energy stores, and refocus your energies. The increasing numbers of spas popping up across the nation are testimony to Americans' growing need to relax and de-stress. But it isn't necessary to visit an expensive spa to experience the benefits of relaxation. A relaxation break could be as simple as taking a bath, listening to quiet music, practicing deep breathing, or spending 5 minutes stretching.

Once you have learned simple relaxation techniques, you can use them at any time—before or during a tough exam or when faced with a stressful confrontation or assignment, for example. As your body relaxes, your heart rate slows, your blood pressure and metabolic rate decrease, and many other body-calming effects occur, all of which allow you to channel energy appropriately. We discuss specific relaxation techniques later in the chapter.

Eat Right Is food really a de-stressor? Whether foods can calm us and nourish our psyches is a controversial question. High-potency supplements that are supposed to boost resistance against stress-related ailments are nothing more than gimmicks. However, it is clear that eating a balanced, healthful diet will help provide the stamina you need to get through problems and will stress-proof you in ways that are not fully understood. It also is known that undereating, overeating, and eating the wrong kinds of foods can create distress in the body. In particular, avoid **sympathomimetics**, food substances that produce (or mimic) stress-like responses. The most common sympathomimetic is caffeine, commonly found in sodas, coffee, tea, and chocolate. Sugar is often considered a sympathomimetic, but much of what has been published about hyperactivity and its relation to the consumption of sweets has been shown to be scientifically invalid. For more information about the benefits of sound nutrition, see Chapter 9.

Managing Your Time

Procrastination. If you're like 15 to 20 percent of all adults and up to 95 percent of all college students, you **procrastinate,** or voluntarily delay an intended course of action despite expecting to be worse off for the delay.[59] For college students, those voluntary delays—going to a party when exams loom or putting off writing a paper until the night before it is due—can result in academic difficulties, increased levels of stress, financial problems, relationship problems, and a multitude of stress-related ailments.[60] Procrastinators often put off seeing their doctors, avoid routine maintenance of their cars and bodies, and are perpetually late for appointments. For some, the reasons for

sympathomimetics Food substances that can produce stress-like physiological responses.

procrastinate To intentionally put off or avoid doing something that needs to be done.

procrastination may relate to a fear of failure and a wish to avoid being put on the spot. For others, distractions, such as a party down the street, can instantly send them off in pursuit of fun and excitement, rather than the steady course of studying. When the very real consequences of their dalliances loom, stress levels increase, and in a last-ditch attempt to finish projects that should have been started weeks ago, sleep goes by the wayside, coffee intake increases, and emotions flare.

How can you avoid the procrastination bug? According to psychologist Shane Owens and his colleagues at Hofstra University, setting clear "implementation intentions" specifying, for example, that you will do work on your paper from 6 PM to 7 PM each night for the next week, is one way of ensuring that you'll stay on task.[61] By making a clear plan of action with set deadlines and rewarding yourself for meeting these deadlines, you may be motivating yourself to follow steps along the path to project completion. Another strategy is to get started early and set a personal end date that is well ahead of the ultimate due date.

Learning to manage your time better overall is key to avoiding and overcoming procrastination. Keep a journal for 1 week to become aware of how you spend your time. Write down your activities every day—everything from going to class to doing your laundry to texting your friends—and the amount of time you spend doing each. Once you have kept track for several days, you can assess your activities. Are you completing the tasks you need to do on a daily basis? Are there any activities you can stop doing or that you would like to do more frequently? Use the following time-management tips in your stress management program:

- **Take on only one thing at a time.** Don't try to watch television, wash clothes, and write your term paper all at once. Stay focused.
- **Clean off your desk.** Go through the things on your desk, toss unnecessary papers, and put into folders the papers for tasks that you must do. Read your mail, recycle what you don't need, and file what you will need later.
- **Prioritize your tasks.** Make a daily "to do" list and try sticking to it. Categorize the things you must do today, the things that you must do but not immediately, and the things that it would be nice to do. Consider the "nice to do" items only if you finish the others or if they include something fun. Give yourself a reward as you finish each task.
- **Don't be afraid to say "no."** All too often we do things out of fear of what someone may think about us. Set your school and personal priorities and live according to your own agenda, values, and goals.
- **Find a clean, comfortable place to work, and avoid interruptions.** When you have a project that requires total concentration, schedule uninterrupted time. Don't answer the phone; close your door and post a "Do Not Disturb" sign; go to a quiet room in the library or student union where no one will find you.
- **Reward yourself for work completed.** Did you finish a task on your list? See a movie or go for a walk. Differentiate between rest breaks and work breaks. Work breaks simply

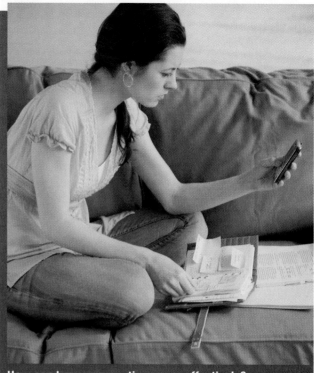

How can I manage my time more effectively?

Learning to manage your time involves recognizing that there are only 24 hours in a day and you can't do everything. Instead, you need to prioritize and set realistic time limits, while also identifying the things that cause you to "waste" time, and strategizing ways to deal with them. Establishing routines and using a calendar or other planning device to keep track of schedules and tasks can help you implement an effective time management plan.

mean switching tasks for a while. Rest breaks give you time to yourself to help you recharge and refresh your energy levels.
- **Use time to your advantage.** If you're a morning person, schedule activities to coincide with the time when you're at your best. Study and write papers in the morning, and take breaks when you start to slow down.
- **Break overwhelming tasks into small pieces, and allocate a certain amount of time to each.** If you are floundering in a task, move on and come back to it when you're refreshed.
- **Remember that time is precious.** Many people learn to value their time only when they face a terminal illness. Try to value each day. Time spent not enjoying life is a tremendous waste of potential.

Managing Your Money

Higher education can involve a huge financial burden on parents, students, and communities. In recent studies, nearly two-thirds of students have indicated that they have "some" or "major" concerns regarding their ability to finance the costs of their college education.[62] Some have already modified their list of possible college choices, believing that some of the more expensive or private schools may be out of their

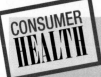

Lessen Your Financial Stress

Faced with the unusually high financial pressure of these tough economic times, students may find their performance in classes slipping and their health suffering. The following tips may help you better manage your money and reduce your finance-related stress.

✳ **Develop a realistic budget.** What are your monthly expenses? What types of "luxuries" do you regularly splurge on? Think about where you spend your money, what you really need, and what you could do without.

Remember that buying less also means generating less waste, both in the form of packaging and unwanted items that will ultimately need to be discarded.

✳ **Take care of bills immediately and consider electronic banking.** Late fees and other penalties are an unnecessary way of depleting your bank account and are easily avoided by paying bills as soon as you get them. Sign up for an online account to pay bills quickly and easily.

✳ **Educate yourself about how to manage your money.** Take advantage of campus workshops

on financial aid and money management. Take a course in personal financial planning.

✳ **Avoid those tempting credit card offers.** You need only one or two credit cards; more than that can be dangerous. If you get tons of offers in the mail, shred them and put them straight into the recycling bin.

✳ **Don't get into debt.** If you don't have the money for an item now, don't buy it on

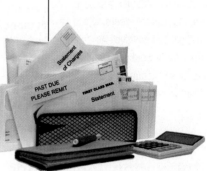

credit. If you want to buy a pricey item or pay for an expensive trip, put aside a certain amount toward that goal every month until you have enough to afford it.

---

reach. Regardless of where they go, one thing is certain: The recent economic downturn is likely to push already financially stressed students to the breaking point.

Several factors are converging to increase today's students' financial woes. First, a recession has caused many parents to lose their jobs. With parental job loss sometimes comes a loss of family health insurance, meaning that more and more students will either have to go without health insurance or find a low-cost plan through their respective schools. Faced with dwindling resources at home, many students are being forced to look for part-time or even full-time work. These students may encounter increasing competition for even the lowest paying jobs as displaced workers take these jobs to remain financially afloat. Already known to carry a disproportionate level of credit card debt, students are resorting to using plastic to pay for essentials, leading to more debt and higher stress. The **Consumer Health** box above offers tips on how to deal with financial woes in these tough times.

Consider Downshifting

Today's lifestyles are hectic and pressure packed, and stress often comes from trying to keep up. Many people are questioning whether "having it all" is worth it, and they are taking a step back and simplifying their lives. This trend has been labeled *downshifting,* or *voluntary simplicity.* Moving from a large urban area to a smaller town, leaving a high-paying, high-stress job for one that makes you happy, and a host of other changes in lifestyle typify downshifting.

35%

of college students report that their finances have been traumatic or very difficult to handle during the past 12 months.

Downshifting involves a fundamental alteration in values and honest introspection about what is important in life. When you contemplate any form of downshift or perhaps even start your career this way, it's important to move slowly and consider the following:

● **Determine your ultimate goal.** What is most important to you, and what will you need to reach that goal? What can you do without?

● **Make both short-term and long-term plans for simplifying your life.** Set up your plans in doable steps, and work slowly toward each step. Prioritize your time with others who are most important to you. Clear out clutter or material items you don't need or use.

● **Complete a financial inventory.** How much money will you need to do the things you want to do? Will you live alone or share costs with roommates? Do you need a car, or can you rely on public transportation? Pay off your debt, and get used to paying with cash. If you don't have the cash, don't buy.

● **Plan for health care costs.** Make sure that you budget for health insurance and basic preventive health services if you're not covered under your parents' plan. Understand your coverage. This should be a top priority.

- **Select the right career.** Look for work that you enjoy and that isn't necessarily driven by salary. Can you be happy taking a lower-paying job if it is less stressful?

What do you think?

Think about the changes you have made in the past few years. Which do you regard as positive? As negative? ● How did you initially react to these changes? ● Did your reactions change later?

- **Consider options for saving money.** Downshifting doesn't mean you renounce money; it means you choose not to let money dictate your life. Saving is still important. If you're just getting started, you need to prepare for emergencies and for future plans.

Relaxation Techniques for Stress Management

Relaxation techniques to reduce stress have been practiced for centuries, and there is a wide selection from which to choose. Some common stress management techniques include yoga, qigong, tai chi, deep breathing, meditation, visualization, progressive muscle relaxation, massage therapy, biofeedback, and hypnosis.

Yoga An estimated 20 million adults in America actively practice yoga, an ancient tradition that combines meditation, stretching, and breathing exercises designed to relax, refresh, and rejuvenate. Yoga began about 5,000 years ago in India and has been evolving ever since. There are many versions commonly practiced in the United States today.

Classical yoga is the ancestor of nearly all forms of yoga practiced today. Breathing, poses, and verbal mantras are often part of classical yoga. Of the many branches of classical yoga, *Hatha yoga* is the most well known because it is the most body focused. This style of yoga involves the practice of breath control and *asanas*—held postures and choreographed movements that enhance strength and flexibility.

Iyengar yoga is one of the most popular styles of Hatha yoga. Iyengar focuses on precise alignment in poses, breath control, meditation, and philosophy. *Kripalu yoga,* another modern style of Hatha yoga, is a gentle, introspective practice in which much emphasis is placed on breathing techniques, meditation, releasing emotional blockages, and practicing holistic health. Several other, more athletic, forms of yoga are discussed in Chapter 11.

Qigong *Qigong* (pronounced "chee-kong") is one of the fastest-growing and most widely accepted forms of mind–body health exercises. Even some of the country's largest health care organizations, such as Kaiser Permanente, have incorporated this relaxation technique into their system, particularly for people suffering from chronic pain or stress. Qigong is an ancient Chinese practice that involves becoming aware of and learning to control *qi* (or *chi,* pronounced "chee") or vital energy in your body. According to Chinese medicine, a complex system of internal pathways called *meridians* carry *qi* throughout your body. If your *qi* becomes stagnant or blocked, you'll feel sluggish or powerless. Thus, qigong incorporates a series of flowing movements, breath techniques, mental visualization exercises, and vocalizations of healing sounds designed to restore balance and integrate and refresh the mind and body.

Tai chi *Tai chi* (pronounced "ty-chee") is sometimes described as "mediation in motion." Originally developed in China as a form of self-defense, this graceful form of exercise has existed for about 2,000 years. Tai chi is noncompetitive and self-paced. To do tai chi, you perform a defined series of postures or movements in a slow, graceful manner. Each movement or posture flows into the next without pause. Tai chi has been widely practiced in China for centuries and is now becoming increasingly popular around the world, both as a basic exercise program and as a complement to other health care methods. Health benefits include stress reduction, greater balance, and increased flexibility.

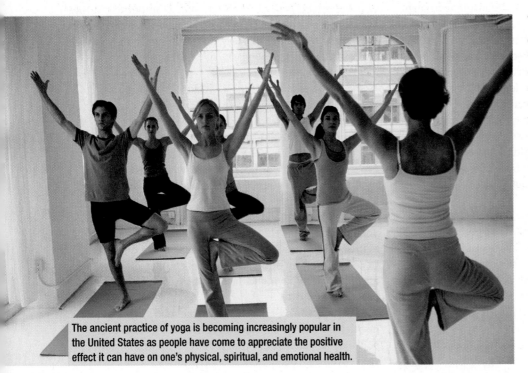

The ancient practice of yoga is becoming increasingly popular in the United States as people have come to appreciate the positive effect it can have on one's physical, spiritual, and emotional health.

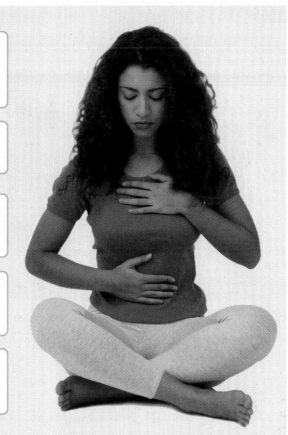

① Assume a natural, comfortable position either sitting up straight with your head, neck, and shoulders relaxed, or lying on your back with your knees bent and your head supported. Close your eyes and loosen binding clothes.

② In order to feel your abdomen moving as you breathe, place one hand on your upper chest and the other just below your rib cage.

③ Breathe in slowly and deeply through your nose. Feel your stomach expanding into your hand. The hand on your chest should move as little as possible.

④ Exhale slowly through your mouth. Feel the fall of your stomach away from your hand. Again, the hand on your chest should move as little as possible.

⑤ Concentrate on the act of breathing. Shut out external noise. Focus on inhaling and exhaling, the route the air is following, and the rise and fall of your stomach.

FIGURE 3.4 **Diaphragmatic Breathing**
This exercise will help you learn to breathe deeply as a way to relieve stress. Practice this for 5 to 10 minutes several times a day, and soon diaphragmatic breathing will become natural for you.

Diaphragmatic or Deep Breathing Typically, we breathe using only the upper chest and thoracic region rather than involving the abdominal region. Simply stated, diaphragmatic breathing is deep breathing that maximally fills the lungs by involving the movement of the diaphragm and lower abdomen. This technique is commonly used in yoga exercises and in other meditative practices. See Figure 3.4 for a description of a diaphragmatic breathing exercise you can try yourself.

Meditation and Mindfulness There are many different forms of **meditation.** Most involve sitting quietly for 15 to 20 minutes, focusing on a particular word or symbol, controlling breathing, and getting in touch with the inner

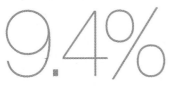 **9.4%** of American adults report having practiced some form of meditation in the past 12 months.

self. Practiced by Eastern religions for centuries, meditation is believed to be an important form of introspection and personal renewal. As a stress management tool, it can calm the body and quiet the mind, creating a sense of peace.

As a meditative technique, **mindfulness**—the ability to be fully present in the moment—can aid relaxation; reduce emotional and physical pain; and help us connect more effectively with ourselves, with others, and with nature.[63] Meditation, mindfulness, and other aspects of spiritual health are discussed in more detail in Focus On: Your Spiritual Health beginning on page 474.

Visualization Often it is our own thoughts and imagination that provoke distress by conjuring up worst-case scenarios and exaggerating the significance of situations. Our imagination, however, can also be an asset. **Visualization,** or the creation of mental scenes, works by engaging one's imagination of the physical senses of sight, sound, smell, taste, and touch to replace stressful stimuli with peaceful or pleasurable thoughts. The choice of mental images is unlimited, but natural settings such as ocean beaches and mountain lakes are often used, because they simulate vacation locations where people typically go to escape the stress of home, school, or work environments.

meditation A relaxation technique that involves deep breathing and concentration.
mindfulness The ability to be fully present in the moment.
visualization The creation of mental images to promote relaxation.

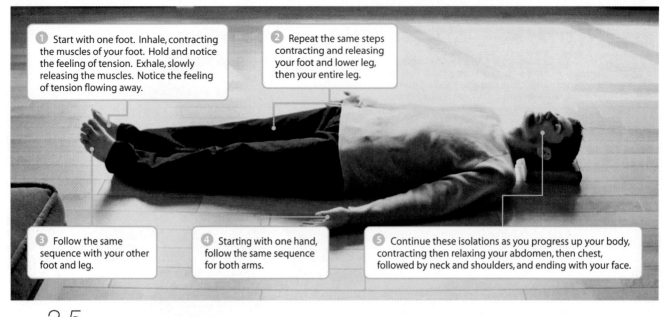

1. Start with one foot. Inhale, contracting the muscles of your foot. Hold and notice the feeling of tension. Exhale, slowly releasing the muscles. Notice the feeling of tension flowing away.

2. Repeat the same steps contracting and releasing your foot and lower leg, then your entire leg.

3. Follow the same sequence with your other foot and leg.

4. Starting with one hand, follow the same sequence for both arms.

5. Continue these isolations as you progress up your body, contracting then relaxing your abdomen, then chest, followed by neck and shoulders, and ending with your face.

FIGURE 3.5 **Progressive Muscle Relaxation**
Sit or lie down in a comfortable position and follow the steps described to increase your awareness of tension in your body.

Progressive Muscle Relaxation Progressive muscle relaxation involves systematically contracting and relaxing the different muscle groups in your body. The most standard pattern is to begin with the feet and work your way up your body, contracting and releasing as you go (see **Figure 3.5**). The process is designed to teach awareness of the different feelings of muscle tension and muscle release. With practice, you can quickly identify tension in your body when you are facing stressful situations and consciously release that tension to calm yourself.

Massage Therapy If you have ever had someone massage your stiff neck or aching feet, you know that massage is an excellent way to relax. Techniques vary from deep-tissue massage to vigorous Swedish massage to the gentler acupressure and Esalen massage. Chapter 17 provides more information about the benefits of massage as well as other body-based methods such as acupressure and shiatsu.

Biofeedback **Biofeedback** involves self-monitoring via machine of physical responses to stress and attempts to control these responses. The machine records perspiration, heart rate, respiration rate, blood pressure, surface body temperature, muscle tension, and other stress responses. Various relaxation techniques are employed while the person is hooked up to a biofeedback machine, and through trial and error and signals from the machine, the person learns to lower the stress response. Eventually, the person develops the ability to recognize and lower stress responses without using the machine.

biofeedback A technique using a machine to self-monitor physical responses to stress.
hypnosis A process that allows people to become unusually responsive to suggestion.

Hypnosis **Hypnosis** is a process that requires a person to focus on one thought, object, or voice, thereby freeing the right hemisphere of the brain to become more active. The person then becomes unusually responsive to suggestion. Whether self-induced or induced by someone else, hypnosis can reduce certain types of stress.

Assess yourself

What's Your Stress Level?

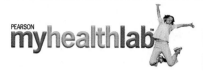

1 The Student Stress Scale

The Student Stress Scale represents an adaptation of Holmes and Rahe's Social Readjustment Rating Scale (SRRS). The SRRS has been modified for college-aged adults and provides a rough indication of stress levels and health consequences. In the scale, each event is given a score that represents the amount of readjustment a person must make as a result of the life change. To determine your stress score, check each event that you have experienced in the past 12 months, and then sum the number of points corresponding to each event.

1.	Death of a close family member	____	100
2.	Death of a close friend	____	73
3.	Divorce between parents	____	65
4.	Jail term	____	63
5.	Major personal injury or illness	____	63
6.	Marriage	____	58
7.	Firing from a job	____	50
8.	Failure of an important course	____	47
9.	Change in health of a family member	____	45
10.	Pregnancy	____	45
11.	Sex problems	____	44
12.	Serious argument with close friend	____	40
13.	Change in financial status	____	39
14.	Change of major	____	39
15.	Trouble with parents	____	39
16.	New girlfriend or boyfriend	____	37
17.	Increase in workload at school	____	37
18.	Outstanding personal achievement	____	36
19.	First quarter/semester in school	____	36
20.	Change in living conditions	____	31
21.	Serious argument with an instructor	____	30
22.	Lower grades than expected	____	29
23.	Change in sleeping habits	____	29
24.	Change in social activities	____	29
25.	Change in eating habits	____	28
26.	Chronic car trouble	____	26
27.	Change in number of family gatherings	____	26
28.	Too many missed classes	____	25
29.	Change of college	____	24
30.	Dropping of more than one class	____	23
31.	Minor traffic violations	____	20
	Total:	____	

Fill out this assessment online at www.pearsonhighered.com/myhealthlab or www.pearsonhighered.com/donatelle.

Scoring Part 1

If your score is 300 or higher, you may be at high risk for developing a stress-related illness. If your score is between 150 and 300, you have approximately a 50-50 chance of experiencing a serious health problem within the next 2 years. If your score is below 150, you have a 1 in 3 chance of experiencing a serious health change in the next few years.

Source: Adapted from T. Holmes and R. H. Rahe, "The Social Readjustment Rating Scale," *Journal of Psychosomatic Research* 11, no. 8 (1967): 213–18. Copyright © 1967 Elsevier, Inc. Used with permission.

2 What Is Stressing You Out?

Each of us reacts differently to life's little challenges. Faced with a long line at the bookstore, most of us will get anxious for a few seconds before we start grumbling or shrug and move on.

For others, a simple hassle such as getting stuck in a long line at the store can be part of a daily health assault. Completing the following assessment will help you evaluate how you respond to daily stressors. Although this survey is just an indicator of what your stressors might be and how stressful you find them, it will help you focus on the areas that you may need to work on to reduce stress.

For each statement, indicate how often the following stressful situations or feelings are a part of your daily life.

		Never	Rarely	Sometimes	Often	Always
1.	I find that there are not enough hours in the day to finish everything I have to do.	1	2	3	4	5
2.	I am anxious about how I am performing in my classes.	1	2	3	4	5
3.	People don't seem to notice whether or not I do a good job.	1	2	3	4	5
4.	I am tired and feel like I don't have the energy to do everything that I need to get done.	1	2	3	4	5

	Never	Rarely	Sometimes	Often	Always

5. I seem to be easily irritated by things that people do. 1 2 3 4 5

6. I worry about what is happening in my family (health of a loved one, financial problems, relationship problems, etc.). 1 2 3 4 5

7. I'm worried about my finances and having enough money to pay my bills. 1 2 3 4 5

8. I don't have enough time for fun. 1 2 3 4 5

9. I am unhappy with my body (weight, fitness level, etc.). 1 2 3 4 5

10. My family and friends count on me to help them with their problems. 1 2 3 4 5

11. I am concerned about my current relationship (or lack of a relationship). 1 2 3 4 5

12. I am impatient/intolerant of the weaknesses of others. 1 2 3 4 5

13. My house/apartment is a mess, and I'm embarrassed to have others see it. 1 2 3 4 5

14. I worry about whether I'll get a job and be able to support myself after graduation. 1 2 3 4 5

15. I worry that people don't like me. 1 2 3 4 5

Your Total Score: _____

Analyzing Part 2

Scores of 60–75:

Your stress level is probably quite high. Prioritize the areas where you scored 5s, and list two to three things for each area that you can do to reduce your stress level. Note any increase in headaches, backaches, or insomnia; your body is telling you to lighten your load. Plan at least one fun thing to do for yourself each day. Make yourself more of a daily priority.

Scores of 45–60:

Your stress level is moderate. Look at those areas that are 5s and list two to three things that you would like to change now to help yourself reduce stress. Practice at least one stress management technique each day. Make more time for yourself.

Scores of 30–45:

You seem to have a lower level of stress. This is good. However, there are still areas that you could work on. Think about what these are, and list things you could do now to reduce stress.

Scores below 30:

You seem to be doing a great job. Whatever your problems may be, stress isn't one of them. Even when stressful events do occur—and they will—your health probably won't suffer.

3 How Do You Respond to Stress?

Read the following scenarios and choose the most likely response you would have to these stressful events.

1. You've been waiting 20 minutes for a table in a crowded restaurant, and the hostess seats a group that arrived after you.
   a. You yell, "Hey! I was here first" in an irritated voice to the hostess.
   b. You say, "Excuse me" in a polite voice and inform the other group or the hostess that you were there first.
   c. You walk out of the restaurant in disgust. Obviously the hostess was willfully ignoring you.
2. You get to a movie theater early so that you and a friend can get great seats. You strategically pick a seat that will give you a good view. Although the theater is nearly empty, a tall man plops himself in the seat directly in front of you so that you cannot see the screen.
   a. You yell directly at the man, saying, "Can't you sit somewhere else? I can't see!"
   b. You calmly nudge your friend and suggest the two of you move over a few seats.
   c. You slump down in your seat and stew for the rest of the movie about how this always happens to you.
3. Your sister calls out of the blue and starts telling you how much you mean to her.
   a. Irritated for being put on the spot, you make fun of her for being sappy.
   b. You thank her and respond in kind.
   c. Uncomfortable, you dismiss her feelings for you as unfounded and change the subject.
4. You come home to find the kitchen looking like a disaster area and your spouse/roommate lounging in front of the TV.
   a. You pick a fight about how your spouse/roommate never does anything and always expects you to clean up after him or her.
   b. You sit down next to your spouse/roommate and ask if he or she would take a 5-minute break from the TV show to help you clean.
   c. You don't say anything but instead tense up and angrily start cleaning the kitchen, making as much noise as possible.
5. You have to present a paper in front of your class, and you are anxious about doing a good job.
   a. You get flustered during the presentation and snap at your fellow classmates when they ask questions about your topic.
   b. You ask a friend to help you practice the presentation ahead of time so you can feel confident going in to class.
   c. You lose sleep worrying about the presentation, and afterward you spend the rest of the day reliving all the mistakes you made.

6. Your partner is seen out with another person and appears to be acting more than just friendly to the person.
   a. You immediately assume your partner is cheating on you. Infuriated, you launch into him or her with accusations the next time you are together.
   b. The next time you see your partner, you calmly mention your concerns and describe your feelings, giving him or her a chance to explain the situation.
   c. You decide your partner no longer cares about you and spend the evening reproaching yourself for being so unlovable.
7. You aren't able to study as much as you'd like for an exam, and when you get it back, you find that you did horribly.
   a. You angrily bad-mouth your professor to your friends and anyone else who will listen.
   b. You make an appointment to talk with the professor and determine what you can do to improve on the next exam.
   c. You decide you're just crummy at the subject and don't even bother studying at all the next time.

Analyzing Part 3

Look carefully at each of these scenarios and your responses. Obviously, none of us is perfect, and we sometimes react in ways that we later regret. The key here is to assess how you react the majority of the time.

If you chose mostly "a" responses, you are probably a hot reactor who responds to mildly stressful situations with a fight-or-flight adrenaline rush that drives up blood pressure and can lead to heart rhythm disturbances, accelerated clotting, and damaged blood vessel linings. Before you honk or make obscene gestures at the guy who cuts you off in traffic, remember that getting angry can destroy thousands of heart muscle cells within minutes. Look at ways to change your perceptions and cope more effectively. Ponder the fact that the only thing you'll hasten by reacting is a decline in health.

If you chose mostly "b" responses, you are probably a cool reactor who tends to roll with the punches when a situation becomes stressful. This usually indicates a good level of coping; overall, you will suffer fewer health consequences when stressed. The key here is that you really are not stressed, and you really are calm and unworried about the situation—not just behaving as though you were.

If you chose mostly "c" responses, you have intense reactions to stress that you are prone to directing inward. This can negatively affect your health just as much as being explosive. Internalizing stressful situations can lead to headaches, stomachaches, and muscle tension. To change your approach to stress, work on ways of building your senses of self-efficacy and self-esteem. Changing the way you think about yourself and others can help you approach stress in a more balanced and productive way.

YOUR PLAN FOR CHANGE

The **Assessyourself** activity gave you the chance to look at your stress levels and identify particular situations in your life that cause stress. Now that you are aware of these patterns, you can change a behavior that leads to increased stress.

Today, you can:

◯ Practice one new stress management technique. For example, you could spend 10 minutes doing a deep-breathing exercise or find a good spot on campus to meditate.

◯ Purchase a journal and start writing down stressful events or symptoms of stress that you experience. Try to focus on intense emotional experiences and explore how they affect you.

Within the next 2 weeks, you can:

◯ Attend a class or workshop in yoga, tai chi, qigong, meditation, or some other stress-relieving activity. Look for beginner classes being offered both on campus and in the community.

◯ Make a list of the papers, projects, and tests that you have in store over the coming semester and create a schedule for them. Break projects and term papers into small, manageable tasks, and try to be realistic about how much time you'll need to get these tasks done.

◯ Keep track of the money you spend and where it goes. After 2 weeks, look over your records, and try to pinpoint places where you can economize.

By the end of the semester, you can:

◯ Establish a budget and follow it for at least 1 month.

◯ Commit to eating a healthy, balanced diet. See Chapter 9 for nutrition information.

◯ Find some form of exercise you can do regularly. You may consider joining a gym or just arranging regular "walk dates" or pickup basketball games with your friends. Try to exercise at least 30 minutes a day, every day. See Chapter 11 for more information about exercise and physical fitness.

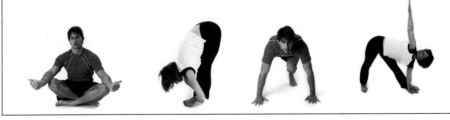

Summary

* Stress is an inevitable part of our lives. *Eustress* refers to stress associated with positive events, *distress* to negative events.

* The alarm, resistance, and exhaustion phases of the general adaptation syndrome involve physiological responses to both real and imagined stressors and cause a complex cascade of hormones to rush through the body. Prolonged arousal brought about by stress may be detrimental to health.

* Undue stress for extended periods of time can compromise the immune system and result in serious health consequences. Psychoneuroimmunology is the science that analyzes the relationship between the mind's reaction to stress and the function of the immune system. Stress has been linked to numerous health problems, including cardiovascular disease, diabetes, cancer, and increased susceptibility to infectious diseases.

* Multiple factors contribute to stress and the stress response. Psychosocial factors include change, hassles, relationships, pressure, conflict, overload, and burnout. Other factors are environmental stressors and self-imposed stress. Persons subjected to discrimination or bias due to "-isms" may face unusually high levels of stress.

* College can be especially stressful. Recognizing the signs of stress is the first step toward better health. Learning to reduce test anxiety and cope with multiple stressors is also important.

* Diet, adequate exercise, sleep, healthy relationships, social support, and stress-busting skills are all important factors in determining your stress level.

* Managing stress begins with learning simple coping mechanisms: assessing stressors, changing responses, and learning to cope.

Finding out what works best for you—probably some combination of managing emotional responses, taking mental or physical action, downshifting, learning time management, managing finances, or learning relaxation techniques—will help you better cope with stress in the long run.

Pop Quiz

1. Even though André experienced stress when he graduated from college and moved to a new city, he viewed these changes as an opportunity for growth. What is André's stress called?
   a. strain
   b. distress
   c. eustress
   d. adaptive response

2. The branch of the autonomic nervous system that is responsible for energizing the body for either fight or flight and for triggering many other stress responses is the
   a. central nervous system.
   b. parasympathetic nervous system.
   c. sympathetic nervous system.
   d. endocrine system.

3. During what phase of the general adaptation syndrome has the physical and psychological energy used to fight the stressors been depleted?
   a. alarm phase
   b. resistance phase
   c. endurance phase
   d. exhaustion phase

4. A state of physical and mental exhaustion caused by excessive stress is called
   a. conflict.
   b. overload.
   c. hassles.
   d. burnout.

5. Losing your keys is an example of what psychosocial source of stress?
   a. pressure
   b. inconsistent behaviors
   c. hassles
   d. conflict

6. After 5 years of 70-hour work weeks, Tom decided to leave his high-paying, high-stress law firm and lead a simpler lifestyle. What is this trend called?
   a. adaptation
   b. conflict resolution
   c. burnout reduction
   d. downshifting

7. Which of the following techniques is *not* recommended to reduce test-taking stress?
   a. Plan ahead and study over a period of time for the test.
   b. Take regular breaks to refresh the overstimulated brain.
   c. Do all of the studying the night before the exam so it is fresh in your mind.
   d. Practice by testing yourself with other classmates' sample test questions.

8. Which of the following is *not* an example of a time management technique?
   a. scheduling one's time with a calendar or day planner
   b. identifying time robbers
   c. practicing procrastination in completing homework assignments
   d. developing a game plan

9. Which of the following is an example of a chronic stressor?
   a. giving a talk in public
   b. meeting a deadline for a big project
   c. dealing with a permanent disability
   d. death of a family member or close friend

10. In which stage of the general adaptation syndrome does the fight-or-flight response occur?
   a. exhaustion stage
   b. alarm stage
   c. resistance stage
   d. response stage

Answers to these questions can be found on page A-1.

Think about It!

1. Describe the alarm, resistance, and exhaustion phases of the general adaptation syndrome and the body's physiological response to stress. Does stress lead to more irritability or emotionality, or does emotionality lead to stress? Provide examples.
2. What are some of the health risks that result from chronic stress? How does the study of psychoneuroimmunology link stress and illness?
3. Why are the college years often high-stress years for many? What factors increase stress risks?
4. Why are some students more vulnerable to stress than others? What services are available on your campus to help you deal with excessive stress?
5. What can college students do to inoculate themselves against negative stress effects? What actions can you take to manage your stressors? How can you help others manage their stressors more effectively?
6. How does anger affect the body? Discuss the steps you can take to manage your own anger and help your friends control theirs.
7. How much of a procrastinator are you? What can you do to reduce procrastination?

Accessing Your Health on the Internet

The following websites explore further topics and issues related to personal health. For links to the websites below, visit the Companion Website for *Health: The Basics,* Green Edition at www.pearsonhighered.com/donatelle.

1. *American College Counseling Association.* The website of the professional organization for college counselors; offers useful links and articles. www.collegecounseling.org
2. *American College Health Association.* Provides information and data from the National College Health Assessment survey. www.acha.org
3. *American Psychological Association, Topic: Stress.* Current information and research on stress and stress-related conditions. www.apa.org/topics/topicstress.html
4. *National Institute of Occupational Safety and Health, Stress at Work.* Excellent source for information and resources on workplace stress. www.cdc.gov/niosh/topics/stress
5. *National Institute of Mental Health.* A resource for information on all aspects of mental health, including the effects of stress. www.nimh.nih.gov

References

1. J. H. Pryor et al., *The American Freshman: National Norms for Fall 2008* (Los Angeles: Higher Education Research Institute, 2009).
2. American College Health Association, *American College Health Association—National College Health Assessment (ACHA-NCHA): Reference Group Data Report Fall 2008* (Baltimore: American College Health Association, 2009).
3. K. Glanz and M. Schwartz, "Stress, Coping and Health Behavior," in *Health Behavior and Health Education: Theory, Research and Practice,* 4th ed., eds. K. Glanz, B. Rimer, and K. Viswanath (San Francisco: Jossey Bass, 2002), 210–36.
4. Ibid.
5. W. B. Cannon, *The Wisdom of the Body* (New York: W. W. Norton, 1932).
6. H. Selye, *Stress without Distress* (New York: Lippincott, 1974), 28–29.
7. B. S. McEwen, "Mood Disorders and Allostatic Load," *Biological Psychiatry* 54 (2003): 200–207.
8. A. Mokdad et al., "Actual Causes of Death in the United States 2000," *Journal of the American Medical Association* 291 (2004): 1238–45.
9. S. Cohen, D. Janicki-Deverts, and G. Miller, "Psychological Stress and Cardiovascular Disease," *Journal of the American Medical Association* 298, no. 14 (2007): 1685–87; A. Väänänen et al., "Lack of Predictability at Work and Risk of Acute Myocardial Infarction: An 18-Year Prospective Study of Industrial Employees," *American Journal of Public Health* 98, no. 12 (2008): 2264–71; J. Bremner et al., *Stress and Health: Effects of a Cognitive Stress Challenge on Myocardial Perfusion and Plasma Cortisol in Coronary Heart Disease Patients with Depression* (San Francisco: John Wiley and Sons, 2009); A. Sgoifo, N. Montano, C. Shively, J. Thayer, and A. Stepto, "The Inevitable Link between Heart and Behavior: New Insights from Biomedical Research and Implications for Practice," *Neuroscience and Biobehavioral Reviews* 33, no. 2 (2008): 61–67; K. Monyeki and H. Kemper, "The Risk Factors for Elevated Blood Pressure and How to Address Cardiovascular Risk Factors: A Review in Pediatric Populations," *Journal of Human Hypertension* 22 (2008): 450–59; F. Sparrenberger et al., "Does Psychological Stress Cause Hypertension? A Systematic Review of Observational Studies," *Journal of Human Hypertension* 23 (2009): 12–19; M. Hamer, G. Molloy, and E. Stamatakis, "Psychological Distress as a Risk Factor for Cardiovascular Events," *Journal of the American College of Cardiology* 52 (2008): 2156–162.
10. S. Yusef et al., "Effect of Potentially Modifiable Risk Factors Associated with Myocardial Infarction in 52 Countries (the INTERHEART Study): Case-Control Study," *The Lancet* 364, no. 9438 (2004): 937–52.
11. J. Torpy, C. Lynm, and R. M. Glass, "Chronic Stress and the Heart," *Journal of the American Medical Association* 298, no. 14 (2007): 1722; Centers for Disease Control and Prevention, National Health Interview Survey (NHIS), www.cdc.gov/nchs/nhis.htm. Accessed April 2009.
12. J. Dimsdale, "Psychological Stress and Cardiovascular Disease," *Journal of the American College of Cardiology* 51 (2008): 1237–46.

13. B. Aggarwart, M. Liao, A. Christian, and L. Mosca, "Influence of Care-giving on Lifestyle and Psychosocial Risk Factors among Family Members of Patients Hospitalized with Cardiovascular Disease," *Journal of General Internal Medicine* 24, no. 1 (2009): 1497–1525; F. Sparrenberger et al., "Does Psychological Stress Cause Hypertension?" 2009; M. Kivimäki et al., "Socioeconomic Position, Psychosocial Work Environment, and Cerebrovascular Disease among Women: The Finnish Public Sector Study," *International Journal of Epidemiology* (January 20, 2009); A. Väänänen et al., "Lack of Predictability at Work and Risk of Acute Myocardial Infarction," 2008; A. Miller and B. Arquilla, "Chronic Disease and Natural Hazards: Impact of Disasters on Diabetes, Renal and Cardiac Patients," *Prehospital Disaster Medicine* 23, no. 2 (2008): 185–94; I. Weissbecker, S. Spehton, M. Martin, and D. Simpson, "Psychological and Physiological Correlates of Stress in Children Exposed to Disaster: Current Research and Recommendations for Intervention," *Children, Youth and Environments* 18, no. 1 (2008): 30–70.

14. S. Lightman, "Chronic Stress Can Significantly Damage Health," *Discover Health* (2008), http://health.discovery.com/centers/stress/interviews/liteman_int.html.

15. R. Ader, *Psychoneuroimmunology.* 4th ed. (Burlington, MA: Elsevier, 2007); E. Chen and G. Miller, "Stress and Inflammation in Exacerbations of Asthma," *Brain, Behavior, and Immunity* 21, no. 8 (2007): 993–99.

16. E. Pradham et al., "Effect of Mindfulness-Based Stress Reduction in Rheumatoid Arthritis Patients," *Arthritis and Rheumatism* 57, no. 7 (2007): 1116–18; L. Carlson, M. Speca, P. Faris, and K. Patel, "One Year Pre-Post Intervention Follow-Up of Psychological, Immune, Endocrine and Blood Pressure Outcomes of Mindfulness-Based Stress Reduction (MBSR) in Breast and Prostate Cancer Outpatients," *Brain, Behavior, and Immunity* 21, no. 8 (2007): 1038–49; J. Manikonda et al., "Contemplative Meditation Reduces Ambulatory Blood Pressure and Stress-Induced Hypertension: A Randomized Pilot Trial," *Journal of Human Hypertension* 22, no. 4 (2008): 139–40.

17. R. Ader, *Psychoneuroimmunology,* 2007.

18. S. Cohen, Keynote Presentation, Eighth International Congress of Behavioral Medicine: "The Pittsburgh Common Cold Studies: Psychosocial Predictors of Susceptibility to Respiratory Illness," *International Journal of Behavioral Medicine* 12, no. 3 (2005): 123–31; S. Cohen et al., "Reactivity and Vulnerability to Stress-Associated Risk for Upper Respiratory Illness," *Psychosomatic Medicine* 64 (2002): 302–10; B. Takkouche et al., "A Cohort Study of Stress and the Common Cold," *Epidemiology* 12, no. 3 (2001): 345–49.

19. S. D. Pressman et al., "Loneliness, Social Network Size, and Immune Responses to Influenza Vaccinations in College Freshmen," *Health Psychology* 24, no. 3 (2005): 297–306.

20. E. R. Volkman and N. Y. Weekes, "Basal SigA and Cortisol Levels Predict Stress-Related Health Outcomes," *Stress and Health* 22 (2006): 11–23.

21. R. Ader, *Psychoneuroimmunology,* 2007; E. V. Yang and R. Glaser, "Stress-Induced Immunomodulation and the Implications for Health," *International Immunopharmacology* 2 (2002): 15–24; R. Glaser, "Stress-Associated Immune Dysregulation and Its Importance for Human Health: A Personal History of Psychoneuroimmunology," *Brain, Behavior, and Immunity* 19 (2005): 3–11.

22. University of Maryland Medical Center, "Digestive Disorders: Irritable Bowel Syndrome," March 2009, www.umm.edu/digest/ibs.htm; National Digestive Diseases Information Clearinghouse (NDDIC), "Irritable Bowel Syndrome," NIH Publication No. 07-693, September 2007; Johns Hopkins Health Alerts, "Four Relaxation Techniques to Soothe Your Digestive Discomfort," 2008, www.johnshopkinshealthalerts.com/reports/digestive_health/2683-1.html?ty.

23. Johns Hopkins Health Alerts, "Four Relaxation Techniques to Soothe Your Digestive Discomfort," 2008.

24. D. A. Katerndahl and M. Parchman, "The Ability of the Stress Process Model to Explain Mental Health Outcomes," *Comprehensive Psychiatry* 43 (2002): 351–60; R. C. Kessler et al., "The Epidemiology of Major Depressive Disorder," *Journal of the American Medical Association* 289 (2003): 3095–105.

25. R. L. Turner and D. A. Lloyd, "Stress Burden and the Lifetime Incidence of Psychiatric Disorder in Young Adults: Racial and Ethnic Contrasts," *Archives of General Psychiatry* 61 (2004): 481–88.

26. V. R. Wilburn and D. E. Smith, "Stress, Self-Esteem, and Suicidal Ideation in Late Adolescence," *Adolescence* 40 (2005): 33–46; A. Väänänen et al., "Sources of Social Support as Determinants of Psychiatric Morbidity after Severe Life Events: Prospective Cohort Study of Female Employees," *Journal of Psychosomatic Research* 58 (2005): 459–67.

27. American College Health Association, *American College Health Association—National College Health Assessment,* 2009.

28. T. Holmes and R. Rahe, "The Social Readjustment Rating Scale," *Journal of Psychosocial Research* (1967): 213–17; B. P. Dohrenwend, "Inventorying Stressful Life Events as Risk Factors for Psychopathology: Toward Resolution of the Problem of Intracategory Variability," *Psychological Bulletin* 132, no. 3 (2006): 477–95.

29. R. Lazarus, "The Trivialization of Distress," in *Preventing Health Risk Behaviors and Promoting Coping with Illness,* ed. J. Rosen and L. Solomon (Hanover, NH: University Press of New England, 1985), 279–98.

30. D. J. Maybery and D. Graham, "Hassles and Uplifts: Including Interpersonal Events," *Stress and Health* 17 (2001): 91–104: R. Blonna, *Coping with Stress in a Changing World.* 4th ed. (New York: McGraw-Hill, 2006).

31. C. L. Park, S. Armeli, and H. Tennen, "The Daily Stress and Coping Process and Alcohol Use among College Students," *Journal of Studies on Alcohol* 65, no. 1 (2004): 126–30; B. E. Miller et al., "Alcohol Misuse among College Athletes: Self-Medication for Psychiatric Symptoms?" *Journal of Drug Education* 32 (2002): 41–52.

32. Z. Djuric et al., "Biomarkers of Psychological Stress in Health Disparities Research," *The Open Biomarkers Journal* 1 (2008): 7–19; J. Watson, H. Logan, and S. Tomar, "The Influence of Active Coping and Perceived Stress on Health Disparities in a Multi-Ethnic Low Income Sample," *BMC Public Health* 8 (2008): 41; C. M. Arthur, "A Little Bit of Rain Each Day: Psychological Stress and Health Disparities," *California Journal of Health Promotion* 5, Special Edition (2007): 58–67.

33. T. LaVeist, *Minority Populations and Health: An Introduction to Health Disparities* (San Francisco: Jossey-Bass, 2006); T. Lewis, "Discrimination, Black Americans, and Health: Results of the SWAN Study," paper presented at the annual meeting of the American Heart Association, Washington, D.C., 2005.

34. D. Stang, "Calming Down: An Introduction to Stress and Stress Solutions," *ScienceDaily,* 2006, http://sciencedaily.healthology.com/mental-health/article989.htm.

35. K. Karren et al., *Mind/Body Health: The Effects of Attitudes, Emotions, and Relationships.* 3d ed. (San Francisco: Benjamin Cummings, 2006).

36. K. Karren et al., *Mind/Body Health,* 2006; B. L. Seaward, *Managing Stress: Principles and Strategies for Health and Well-Being.* 5th ed. (Sudbury, MA: Jones and Bartlett, 2006); V. R. Wilburn and D. E. Smith, "Stress, Self-Esteem, and Suicidal Ideation in Late Adolescence," 2008.

37. V. R. Wilburn and D. E. Smith, "Stress, Self-Esteem, and Suicidal Ideation in Late Adolescence," 2005; D. Robotham and C. Julian, "Stress and the Higher Education Student: A Critical Review of the Literature," *Journal of Further and Higher Education* 30, no. 2 (2006): 107–17.

38. K. Glanz, B. Rimer, and F. Levis, eds., *Health Behavior and Health Education: Theory, Research, and Practice.* 3d ed. (San Francisco: Jossey-Bass, 2002).

39. A. D. Von et al., "Predictors of Health Behaviors in College Students," *Journal of Advanced Nursing* 48, no. 5 (2004): 463–74.

40. M. Friedman and R. H. Rosenman, *Type A Behavior and Your Heart* (New York: Knopf, 1974).

41. K. Karren et al., *Mind/Body Health,* 2006.

42. R. Niaura et al., "Hostility, Metabolic Syndrome, and Incident Coronary Heart Disease," *Health Psychology* 21, no. 6 (2002): 588–93.

43. Oral Cancer Foundation, "The Mind-Body Connection and Cancer," www.oralcancerfoundation.org/emotional/mind-body.htm. Accessed May 2008; St. Louis Psychologist and Counseling Referral Network, "Personality Types A, B and C and Disease," www.psychtreatment.com/personality_type_and_disease.htm. Revised March 19, 2006.

44. J. Denollet, "Prognostic Value of Type D Personality Compared with Depressive Symptoms," *Archives of Internal Medicine* 168, no. 4 (2008): 431–35; N. Kupper and J. Denollet, "Type D Personalities as a Prognostic Factor in Heart Disease: Assessment and Mediating Mechanisms," *Journal of Personality Assessment* 89, no. 3 (2007): 265–66; L. Williams et al., "Type D Personality Mechanisms of Effect: The Role of Health-related Behavior and Social Support," *Journal of Psychosomatic Research* 64, no. 1 (2008): 63–68.

45. S. Kobasa, "Stressful Life Events, Personality, and Health: An Inquiry into Hardiness," *Journal of Personality and Social Psychology* 37 (1979): 1–11.

46. B. J. Crowley, B. Hayslip, and J. Hobdy, "Psychological Hardiness and Adjustment to Life Events in Adulthood," *Journal of Adult Development* 10 (2003): 237–48; S. R. Maddi, "The Story of Hardiness: Twenty Years of Theorizing, Research, and Practice," *Consulting Psychology Journal: Practice and Research* 54 (2002): 173–86.

47. D. Robotham and C. Julian, "Stress and the Higher Education Student," 2006.

48. J. H. Pryor et al., *The American Freshman: National Norms for 2005* (Los Angeles: Higher Education Research Institute, 2006).

49. American College Health Association, *American College Health Association—National College Health Assessment,* 2009.

50. M. E. Pritchard and G. S. Wilson, "Do Coping Styles Change during the First Semester of College?" *Journal of Social Psychology* 146, no. 1 (2006): 125–27; C. L. Broman, "Stress, Race, and Substance Use in College," *College Student Journal* 39, no. 2 (2005): 340–52; D. Kariv, D. Heilman, and T. Heilman, "Task-Oriented versus Emotion-Oriented Coping Strategies: The Case of College Students," *College Student Journal* 39, no. 1 (2005): 72–84; K. M. Kieffer et al., "Test and Study Worry and Emotionality in the Prediction of College Students' Reasons for Drinking: An Exploratory Investigation," *Journal of Alcohol and Drug Education* 50, no. 1 (2006): 57–81.

51. P. A. Bovier, E. Chamot, and T. V. Perneger, "Perceived Stress, Internal Resources, and Social Support as Determinants of Mental Health among Young Adults," *Quality of Life Research* 13, no. 1 (2004): 161–70; E. Largo-Wright, P. M. Peterson, and W. W. Chen, "Perceived Problem Solving, Stress, and Health among College Students," *American Journal of Health Behavior* 29, no. 4 (2005): 360–70; C. L. Park, S. Armeli, and H. Tennen, "The Daily Stress and Coping Process and Alcohol Use among College Students," 2001.

52. B. L. Seaward, *Managing Stress,* 2006.

53. P. A. Bovier, E. Chamot, and T. V. Perneger, "Perceived Stress, Internal Resources, and Social Support as Determinants of Mental Health among Young Adults," 2004; E. Largo-Wright, P. M. Peterson, and W. W. Chen, "Perceived Problem Solving, Stress, and Health among College Students," 2005; C. L. Park., S. Armeli, and H. Tennen, "The Daily Stress and Coping Process and Alcohol Use among College Students," 2001; A. M. McLaughlin, L. Doane, A. Costiuc, and N. Feeny, *Determinants of Minority Mental Health and Wellness* (New York: Springer, 2009); L. Crockett et al., "Acculturative Stress, Social Support and Coping: Relations to Psychological Adjustment among Mexican American College Students," *Cultural Diversity and Ethnic*

Minority Psychology 13, no. 4 (2007): 347–55.

54. C. Hassed, "How Humor Keeps You Well," *Australian Family Physician* 30, no. 1 (2001): 25–28; A. Ong, C. Bergeman, T. Bisconti, and K. Wallace, "Psychological Resilience, Positive Emotions and Successful Adaptations to Stress in Later Life," *Journal of Personality and Social Psychology* 9, no. 14 (2006): 730–49; D. Lund, R. Utz, M. Caserta, and B. deVries, "Humor, Laughter and Happiness in the Daily Lives of Recently Bereaved Spouses," *OMEGA: Journal of Death and Dying* 58, no. 2 (2008–2009): 87–105; H. Bechman, N. Regier, and J. Young, "Effects of Workplace Laughter on Personal Efficacy Beliefs," *Journal of Primary Prevention* 28, no. 2 (2007): 1007–35; P. Devereux and K. Heffner, "Psychophysiological Approaches to the Study of Laughter," in *Oxford Handbook of Methods in Positive Psychology*, eds. A. Ong and M. Van Dulmen, (Oxford: Oxford University Press, 2007): 233–64.

55. J. Fowler and N. Christakis, "Dynamic Spread of Happiness in a Large Social Network: Longitudinal Analysis over 20 Years in the Framingham Heart Study," *BMJ* 337 (2008): a2338.

56. P. Holmes, "Managing Anger: Understanding the Dynamics of Violence, Abuse and Control," SIUC Mental Health, 2004, www.siu.edu.

57. P. Holmes, "Managing Anger," 2004; B. L. Seaward, *Managing Stress,* 2006.

58. D. A. Girdano, D. E. Dusek, and G. S. Everly, *Controlling Stress and Tension.* 8th ed. (San Francisco: Benjamin Cummings, 2009), 375.

59. P. Steel, "The Nature of Procrastination: A Meta-Analytic and Theoretical Review of Quintessential Self-Regulatory Failure," *Psychological Review* 133, no. 1 (2007): 65–94.

60. T. Gura, "Procrastinating Again? How to Kick the Habit," *Scientific American Mind*, December 2008, www.sciam.com/article.cfm?id=procrastinating-again.

61. Ibid.

62. H. Pryor et al., *The American Freshman: National Norms for Fall 2008*, 2009.

63. N. B. Allen, R. Chambers, and W. Knight, "Mindfulness-Based Psychotherapies: A Review of Conceptual Foundations, Empirical Evidence, and Practical Considerations," *Australian and New Zealand Journal of Psychiatry* 40 (2006): 285–94.

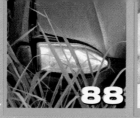

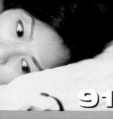

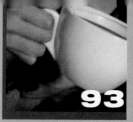

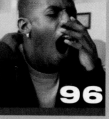

88 Is sleepiness dangerous?

91 What should I do if I can't fall asleep?

93 Why do caffeinated drinks keep me awake?

96 Are sleep disorders common?

FOCUS ON Your Sleep

Josh knew he wasn't ready for tomorrow's physics exam, but he went to his roommate's basketball game anyway. By the time it was over and he hit the books, it was past 11:00 PM. The exam would cover four chapters, and he hadn't even read the last two. To keep himself awake, he drank a can of Mountain Dew, an energy drink, and finally a cup of instant coffee as he plowed through the text, his notes, the online study guide, . . . Just before 4:00 AM, he fell into bed exhausted. But instead of drifting into sleep, his mind kept racing. Dynamics, inertia, action and reaction tumbled around with disjointed memories of all the stressful situations he'd been through in the past few days . . . losing his cell phone, his girlfriend dumping him, the argument he'd had with his dad. . . . He glanced at the clock: It was 5:30 AM. The exam was in 3 hours.

If you've ever tackled an exam on way too little sleep, you can probably predict what happened to Josh: He flunked.

In a recent survey from the American College Health Association (ACHA), 10 percent of students reported that in the past week they did not get enough sleep to feel rested on even a single day. And nearly 42 percent of students reported that, in the past week, they felt rested on fewer than

3 days.[1] It's widely acknowledged that college students are among the most sleep-deprived age group in the United States.[2] Today's students are going to bed an average of 1 to 2 hours later and sleeping 1 to 1.6 fewer hours than students of their parents' generation did.[3]

One factor commonly implicated in reduced sleep time among college students is the Internet and the 24-hour access to online games, videos, news, and virtual friendships it provides. Other things keeping students awake include academic pressures, an underlying sleep disorder, chronic pain and other disease symptoms, anxiety or depression, the use of drugs (including alcohol), and stress from a variety of sources, including the stress of juggling classes and

What with papers and exams, classes and caffeine, extracurricular events and social lives, today's college students are largely a sleep-deprived bunch—and their health may be in jeopardy as a result.

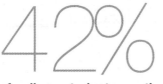

42%
of college students say they don't feel rested most days of the week.

homework with a job or responsibilities at home. When there just aren't enough hours in the day, what typically gets shortchanged is sleep.

Unfortunately, the statistics don't improve much for adults out in the workforce. The most recent *Sleep in America* poll from the National Sleep Foundation (NSF) found that nearly a third (32%) of Americans get a good night's sleep on only a few nights per month.[4] Reasons for less sleep among working adults include working longer hours at the job, taking work home, and having greater access to work and work colleagues at home via the Internet and other technologies.

Since Americans are managing to function on campus and on the job with less sleep, you might conclude that sleep is somewhat dispensable. In fact, sleep deprivation is a real problem. Let's look at the benefits of sleep, and find out what happens when you don't get enough.

Why Do You Need to Sleep?

Sleep serves at least two biological purposes: (1) It conserves body energy. When you sleep, your core body temperature and the rate at which you burn calories drop. This leaves you with more energy to perform activities throughout your waking hours. (2) It restores you both physically and mentally. For example, certain reparative chemicals are released while you sleep. And there is some evidence, discussed shortly, that during sleep the brain is cleared of daily minutiae, learning is synthesized, and memories are consolidated, allowing you to prepare for morning

"with a clean slate." In short, getting enough sleep to feel ready to meet daily challenges is essential.

Sleep Maintains Your Physical Health

Sleep has beneficial effects on most body systems. That's why, when you consistently don't get a good night's rest, your body doesn't function as well, and you become more vulnerable to a wide variety of health problems.[5] Researchers are only just beginning to explore the physical benefits of sleep. The following is a brief summary of what we've learned so far.

● **Sleep helps maintain your immune system.** The common cold, strep throat, the flu, mononucleosis, cold sores, and a variety of other ailments are more common when your immune system is depressed. And that's more likely to happen if you're not getting enough sleep. For instance, one recent study found that poor sleep quality and shorter sleep duration increased susceptibility to the common cold.[6]

● **Sleep helps reduce your risk for high blood pressure and cardiovascular disease.** A study of more than 5,000 adults suggested that high blood pressure is more common in people who get fewer than 7 hours of sleep a night.[7] The association was particularly strong in people getting fewer than 6 hours of sleep per night. In addition, two separate studies found that poor sleep quality or reduced sleep time increased the prevalence of high levels in the blood of a substance called C-reactive protein (CRP), which is a risk factor for heart disease.[8] Sleep also seems to influence the risk of stroke (a blockage affecting a blood vessel in the brain): A study of more than 93,000 women suggested that sleep duration of 6 or fewer hours a night increases the risk of stroke.[9]

● **Sleep contributes to a healthy metabolism and body weight.** Every moment of your life your body's cells are participating in chemical reactions, many of which involve the breakdown of food and the synthesis of new compounds that the body needs. The sum of all these reactions is called *metabolism*.

People who routinely sleep fewer than 7 hours a night are at increased risk for obesity.

Several recent studies suggest that sleep contributes to healthy metabolism and thus helps you maintain a healthy body weight. In contrast, inadequate sleep may play a role in our population's increased prevalence of *type 2 diabetes*, a disorder of glucose metabolism, as well as obesity.[10]

The relationship between sleep and obesity might be due, in part, to disturbances in **hormones,** chemicals that help regulate body functions: One study found that participants who habitually slept only 5 hours a night had higher blood levels of a hormone that increases appetite and lower levels of a hormone that suppresses appetite than did participants who got 8 hours of sleep. Not surprisingly, the so-called "short sleepers" also weighed significantly more than the people who got adequate sleep.[11] And in still another study, short sleepers were shown to be at higher risk for *metabolic syndrome*, a cluster of risk factors including obesity, poor glucose metabolism, high blood pressure, and unhealthful levels of certain types of cholesterol in the blood.[12]

hormone A "chemical messenger" that is released from one of the many endocrine glands of the body and travels in the bloodstream to a distant site where it helps to regulate body functions.

Sleep Affects Your Ability to Function

If you routinely shortchange yourself on sleep, you could be sabotaging your grades and, if you drive while drowsy, endangering your life. Let's look at what the research reveals about how sleep helps you to function.

● **Sleep contributes to neurological functioning.** Restricting sleep below what your body needs can cause a wide range of neurological problems, including lapses of attention, slowed or poor memory, reduced cognitive ability, and a tendency for your thinking to get "stuck in a rut."[13] Your ability not only to remember facts but also to integrate those facts, make meaningful generalizations about them, and consolidate what you've learned into lasting memories requires adequate sleep time.[14] So when you don't get enough sleep, your academic performance deteriorates: Studies have shown that college students who pull all-nighters, as well as students who are short sleepers, have significantly lower overall grade-point averages compared with classmates who get adequate sleep.[15]

● **Sleep improves motor tasks.** Sleep also has a restorative effect on motor function, that is, the ability to perform tasks such as shooting a basket, playing a musical instrument, or driving a car.[16] It's one thing to mess up on a Schubert sonata, but the consequences get a lot more serious when sleep deprivation makes you mess up behind the wheel. Some sleep researchers contend that a night without sleep impairs your motor skills and reaction time as much as if you were driving drunk.[17] As Americans have become more and more sleep-deprived, the incidence of drowsy driving and so-called "fall-asleep crashes" has become a national concern. The NSF reports that 37 percent of Americans admit to having fallen asleep at the wheel in the past year, and more than 1,500 Americans die in fatigue-related crashes annually.[18]

Sleep Promotes Your Psychosocial Health

Research suggests that certain brain regions, including the cerebral cortex (your "master mind"), can achieve some form of essential rest only during sleep.[19] So if your roommate says you're acting like a jerk after you've gone for a few nights without enough sleep, don't take it too personally: Your irritability is actually just a sign of brain fatigue.

In addition, you're more likely to feel stressed-out, worried, or sad when you're sleep-deprived. The relationship between sleep and stress is highly complex: Stress can cause or contribute to sleep problems, and sleep problems can cause or increase your level of stress! The same is true of clinical psychiatric conditions such as depression and anxiety disorders: Reduced or poor quality sleep can trigger these disorders, but it's also a common symptom resulting from them.[20] Still, if you've been burning the midnight oil lately and you find yourself feeling unusually anxious or down,

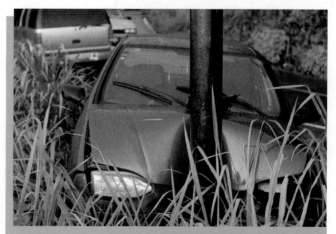

Is sleepiness dangerous?

Lack of sleep impairs your reflexes, cognitive functioning, and motor skills, all of which you need to safely ride a bike or operate a car. The National Sleep Foundation estimates that 100,000 sleep-related auto accidents, resulting in 1,500 deaths, occur in the United States every year.

getting to bed earlier each night is a smart strategy.

What Goes on When You Sleep?

If you've ever taken a flight that crossed two or more time zones, you've probably experienced *jet lag*, a feeling that your body's "internal clock" is out of sync with the hours of daylight and darkness at your destination. Jet lag happens because the new day/night pattern disrupts your **circadian rhythm,** the 24-hour cycle by which you are accustomed to going to sleep, waking up, and performing habitual behaviors throughout your day. Your circadian rhythm is regulated in part by a tiny gland in your brain called the *pineal body*: It releases a hormone called *melatonin* that induces drowsiness.

You can fight the effects of melatonin for hours—even days!—especially if, like Josh in our opening story, you load up on caffeine. But like all human beings, and in fact all mammals, you will eventually succumb to **sleep,** which is clinically defined as a readily reversible state of reduced responsiveness to, and interaction with, the environment.[21] Sleep researchers generally distinguish between two primary sleep states: A state that is not characterized by rapid eye movement, called **non-REM (NREM) sleep,** and a state in which rapid eye movement does occur, called **REM sleep.** During the night, you slide through the stages of NREM sleep, then into REM, then back through NREM again, repeating one full cycle about once every 90 minutes.[22] Overall, you spend about 75 percent of each night in NREM sleep, and 25 percent in REM (Figure 1).

Non-REM Sleep Is Restorative

During non-REM sleep the body rests. Movement can occur, for instance, to shift your position in bed, but muscle tension is reduced. Both your body temperature and your energy use drop, sensation is dulled, and your brain waves, heart rate, and breathing slow. In contrast, digestive processes speed up, and your body stores nutrients. During NREM sleep, you do not typically dream. Four distinct stages of NREM sleep have been distinguished by their characteristic brain-wave patterns.

Stage 1. You're out of it. Your eyes may be open or closed, but essentially, you're drifting off. Stage 1 lasts only a few minutes, and is the lightest stage of sleep from which you are most easily awakened. For instance, if you've nodded off during class, but the instructor says, "This will be on the test," you might suddenly wake up!

Stage 2. This stage is slightly deeper and lasts from 5 to 15 minutes. Your eyes are closed, eye and body movements gradually cease, and you disengage from your environment.

circadian rhythm The 24-hour cycle by which you are accustomed to going to sleep, waking up, and performing habitual behaviors.
sleep A readily reversible state of reduced responsiveness to, and interaction with, the environment.
non-REM (NREM) sleep A period of restful sleep dominated by slow brain waves; during non-REM sleep, rapid eye movement is rare.
REM sleep A period of sleep characterized by brain-wave activity similar to that seen in wakefulness; rapid eye movement and dreaming occur during REM sleep.

Stage 3. NREM sleep is also called *slow-wave sleep*, because during stages 3 and 4, a sleeper's brain generates slow, large-amplitude delta waves on an electroencephalogram (EEG). Your blood pressure drops, your heart rate and respiration slow considerably, and you enter deep sleep.

Stage 4. This is the deepest stage of sleep. Human growth hormone is released and signals your body to repair worn tissues. Speech and movement are rare during this stage, but can and do sometimes occur. For example, sleepwalking typically occurs during the first stage 4 period of the night. You've probably heard that it's difficult to awaken a sleepwalker, and that's true of anyone in stage 4 sleep.

REM Sleep Is Energizing

Dreaming takes place primarily during REM sleep. On an EEG, a REM sleeper's brain-wave activity is almost undistinguishable from that of someone who is

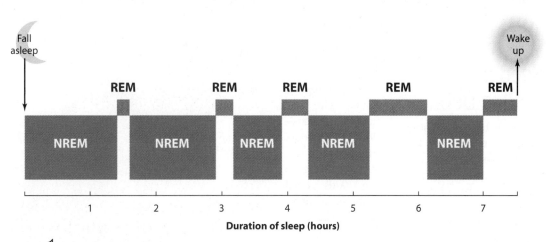

FIGURE 1 **The Nightly Sleep Cycle**
As the number of hours you sleep increases, your brain spends more and more time in REM sleep.
Thus, sleeping for too few hours could mean you're depriving yourself primarily of needed REM sleep.

wide awake, and the brain's energy use is higher than that of a person performing a difficult math problem![23] Your muscles are paralyzed during REM sleep: You may dream that you're rock climbing, but your body is incapable of movement. Almost the only exceptions are your respiratory muscles, which allow you to breathe, and the tiny muscles of your eyes, which move your eyes rapidly as if you were following the scenario of your dream. This rapid eye movement gives REM sleep its name.

During REM sleep, your brain processes the experiences you've had and consolidates the information you've learned during the day. Some researchers theorize that, if you are deprived of REM sleep, you may lose information or skills learned in the previous 24 to 48 hours. Other scientists believe that REM sleep has little effect on memory.[24] As the night progresses, the duration of NREM sleep declines and you spend more and more time in REM. That's why a full night's sleep is important for getting as much REM sleep as you need.

How Much Sleep Do You Really Need?

Given the importance of adequate sleep, especially REM sleep, you're probably asking yourself how much you really need. Unfortunately, there's no magic number. Let's find out why.

Sleep Need Includes Baseline Plus Debt

The short answer to how much sleep you need is about 7 to 8 hours. This recommendation is used by researchers as the standard for "average" sleep time, and is supported by a variety of studies over many years.[25] For instance, one classic study showed that men and

sleep debt The difference between the number of hours of sleep an individual needed in a given time period and the number of hours he or she actually slept.

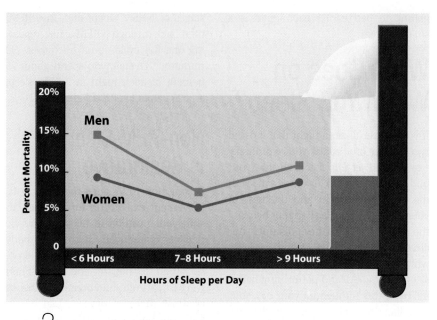

FIGURE 2 **Death Rate Linked to Sleep Duration**
In one classic study that is still supported by recent research, risk of death during the 9-year follow-up period was highest in people who got fewer than 6 hours of sleep a night and lowest in people who got 7 to 8 hours.

Source: Adapted from D. L. Wingard and L. F. Berkman, "Mortality Risk Associated with Sleeping Patterns among Adults," *Sleep* 6, no. 2 (1983): 102–07. © 1983 American Academy of Sleep Medicine.

women who slept 7 to 8 hours a night had a lower risk of death during the follow-up period than men and women who got fewer than 7 or more than 8 hours of sleep (Figure 2).[26]

But what if you're absolutely certain that you get by just fine on 5 or 6 hours a night? Then you might be interested in the results of another study in which young people who claimed they needed less sleep were found to need the average 7 to 8 hours when monitored in a sleep lab![27]

Still, sleep is not a "one size fits all" proposition. Individual variations do occur according to age (kids need more sleep), gender (women need more sleep), and many other factors. In addition, when trying to

figure out your sleep needs, you have to consider two aspects: your body's physiological need plus your current **sleep debt.** That's the total number of hours of missed sleep you're carrying around with you, either because you got up before your body was fully rested, or because your sleep was inter-

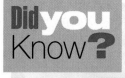

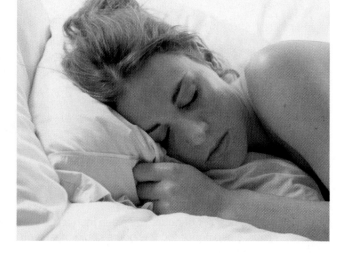

Every night you don't get 8 hours of sleep creates a "sleep debt." The average college student gets 5 hours of sleep a night. In just one semester, that's a sleep debt of 336 hours, or 14 days!

rupted. Let's say that last week you managed just 5 hours of sleep a night Monday through Thursday. Even if you get 7 to 8 hours a night Friday through Sunday, that unresolved sleep debt of 8 to 12 hours will still leave you feeling tired and groggy when you start the week again. So that means you need *more than* 8 hours a night for the next several nights to "catch up."

Still, the good news is that you *can* catch up if you go about it sensibly. Getting 5 hours of sleep a night all semester long, then sleeping 48 hours the first weekend you're home on break won't restore your functioning, and it's likely to disrupt your circadian rhythm. Instead, whittle away at that sleep debt by sleeping 9 hours a night throughout your break—then start the new term resolved to sleep 7 to 8 hours a night.

Do Naps Count?

Speaking of catching up, do naps count? While naps can't entirely cancel out a significant sleep debt, they can help to improve your mood, alertness, and performance.[28] It's best to nap in the early to mid-afternoon, when the pineal body in your brain releases a small amount of melatonin and your body experiences a natural dip in its circadian rhythm. Never nap in the late afternoon, as it could interfere with your ability to fall asleep that night. Keep your naps short, because a nap of more than 30 minutes can leave you in a state of **sleep inertia,** which is characterized by cognitive impairment, grogginess, and a disoriented feeling. In short, getting adequate sleep each night is the best way to feel alert and energized throughout the day, but a quick nap can help you recharge.

How Can You Get a Good Night's Sleep?

Do you need a jolt of caffeine to get you jump-started in the morning? Do you find it hard to stay awake in class? Have you ever nodded off behind the wheel? These are all signs of inade-

7 to 8

hours is the sleep duration associated with optimal health and functioning.

quate or poor quality sleep. To find out whether or not you're sleep-deprived, take the **Assess Yourself** questionnaire on page 97.

To Promote Restful Sleep, Try These Tips

The following tips can help you get a longer and more restful night's sleep.

● **Let there be light.** Throughout the day, stay in sync with your circadian rhythm by spending time in the sunlight. If you live in an area where the sun seldom shines for weeks at a time, invest in special LED lighting designed to mimic the sun's rays. Exposure to natural light outdoors is most beneficial, but opening the

shades indoors and, on overcast days, turning on room lights can also help keep you alert.
● **Stay active.** It's hard to feel sleepy if you've been sedentary all day, so make sure you get plenty of physical activity during the day. Resist the temptation to postpone exercise until you're sleeping better. Start gently, but start now, because regular exercise may help you maintain regular sleep habits.
● **Create a sleep "cave."** Take a lesson from bats, bears, and burrowing animals! As bedtime approaches, keep your bedroom quiet, cool, and dark. Start by turning off your computer and cell phone. If you live in an apartment or dorm where there's noise outside or in the halls, wear ear plugs or get an electronic device that produces "white noise" such as the sound of gentle rain. Turn down the thermostat or, on hot nights, run a quiet electric fan. Install room-darkening shades or curtains if necessary to block out any light from the street.

sleep inertia A state characterized by cognitive impairment, grogginess, and disorientation that is experienced upon rising from short sleep or an overly long nap.

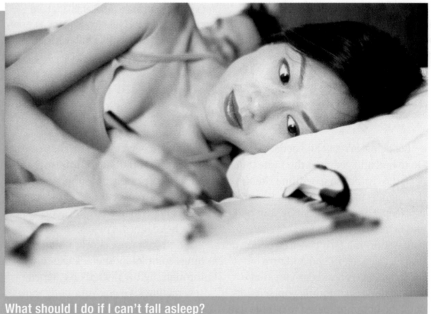

What should I do if I can't fall asleep?

If you have difficulty falling asleep, it may be that noises, lights, interruptions, or persistent worries are keeping you awake. Use ear plugs or a white noise machine to block out noise, wear an eye shade to block out light, and turn off your phone and computer to prevent interruptions. If a worry keeps you awake, jot it down in a journal. You'll be better prepared to handle it in the morning after you've had a good night's sleep.

GREEN GUIDE

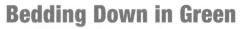

Bedding Down in Green

We may not lie awake thinking about our bed's impact on the environment, but we can still make healthier and environmentally sound choices through the bedding products we buy. To begin with, ecofriendly choices for most textile products—including sheets and blankets—have become widely available. Organic cotton and bamboo are both gaining popularity, and they offer comfortable advantages.

During the production of conventional cotton, or nonorganic cotton, synthetic pesticides and other environmentally harmful chemicals are used. Conversely, organic cotton reduces global pesticide use and is grown using organic farming techniques, such as crop rotation and biological pest control. These techniques are aimed at producing crops without exhausting the soil or polluting the environment.

After harvest, there are other aspects of nonorganic cotton production that can be environmentally harmful. The conventional cotton industry uses a large number of chemicals, including bleach and petroleum-based dyes. In contrast, organic cotton products are typically processed without bleach and use natural dyes.

Bamboo is another useful fiber that has environmental benefits. The use of bamboo fiber in textiles offers a soft fabric from a rapidly renewable resource. Bamboo is actually a type of grass that can grow extremely fast, up to several feet per day! Further, bamboo does not require replanting and helps offset greenhouse gases by absorbing CO_2 from the atmosphere. This plant is naturally resistant to pests and infection, so no pesticides are used in its cultivation, and its natural antibacterial and antifungal properties are an added bonus of using bamboo bedding.

For most people, a mattress is an extremely important purchase: The bed you choose can affect the quality of your rest and can impact your overall health for years. Your choice of mattress can impact the planet's health, too. Synthetic materials used in conventional mattresses, such as polyurethane foam, can emit volatile organic compounds that have been associated with poor respiratory function. Moreover, conventional mattresses are often treated with synthetic chemicals (e.g., formaldehyde, fire retardants, and stain repellants) that are known to "off-gas," affecting indoor air quality and potentially causing future negative health consequences.

More healthful and environmentally responsible mattress materials include organic cotton, wool, and natural latex. Some ecofriendly mattresses combine organic cotton with wool, a natural fire retardant. Wool is also nonabsorbent and, consequently, is less hospitable to microorganisms than more absorbent materials, meaning no antimicrobial chemicals are necessary on wool products.

Similarly, natural latex mattresses and pillows can offer a comfortable night's sleep without the company of mold or bacteria. Natural latex products, derived from the resin of the rubber tree, are hypoallergenic, mold and mildew resistant, and breathable. They are also biodegradable and are produced from a renewable resource—rubber trees are not killed or damaged by the process of tapping them for their resin, so they can continue producing resin and contributing to counterbalancing greenhouse gases for years.

With ecofriendly beds and bedding, you can sleep easily knowing that your choices are healthier for you and for the environment, both inside and outside your home.

● **Condition yourself into better sleep.** Go to bed and get up at the same time each day. Establish a bedtime ritual that signals to your body that it's time for sleep. For instance, sit by your bed and listen to a quiet song; meditate; or read a short magazine article, poem, or prayer. Then get in bed and turn out the light. If a worry keeps you awake, write it down, reminding yourself that you'll be better prepared to handle it in the morning after a good night's sleep.
● **Sleep tight.** Don't let a pancake pillow, pilled sheets, or a threadbare blanket keep you from sleeping soundly. If your mattress is uncomfortable and you can't replace it, try

putting an egg crate foam mattress overlay on top of it. For information about ecofriendly bedding, see the **Green Guide** above.
● **Breathe.** Do it deeply, as soon as your head hits the pillow. Inhale through your nose slowly, filling your lungs completely, then exhale slowly through slightly pursed lips. Repeat several times. Giving your body the oxygen it needs, deep breathing can also decrease anxiety and tension that sometimes make it difficult to fall asleep.
● **Don't toss and turn.** If you're not asleep after 20 minutes, get up. Turn on a low light, and read something

relaxing, not stimulating, or listen to some gentle music. Once you feel sleepy, go back to bed.

To Prevent Sleep Problems, Avoid These Behaviors

Maybe you're already doing most of the actions suggested above, and you still can't sleep. If so, perhaps it's time to learn what *not* to do:

● Don't nap in the late afternoon or evening, and don't nap for longer than 30 minutes.

- Don't engage in strenuous exercise within 6 hours of bedtime. Activity speeds up your metabolism and makes it harder to fall asleep.
- Don't read, study, watch TV, use your laptop, talk on the phone, eat, or smoke in bed. In fact, don't smoke at all: Besides promoting cancer and heart disease, smoking is known to disturb your sleep.
- Don't try to sleep if you're starving or stuffed. Allow at least 3 hours between your evening meal and bedtime and, as already noted, if you feel hungry before bed, have a light snack.
- Don't drink coffee, energy drinks, or anything else that contains caffeine within several hours of bedtime. Once you consume caffeine, which is a

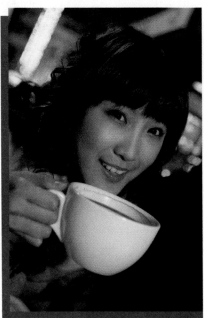

Why do caffeinated drinks keep me awake?

After-dinner coffee? Not unless it's decaf. Caffeine promotes alertness by blocking the neurotransmitter adenosine in your brain—a useful thing when you are studying, but a potential problem when you are trying to sleep. The stimulant effects of caffeine can be felt quickly, but they also last a long time: Your body needs 6 hours to process half of the caffeine you drink (and another 6 to process half of what remains, and so on). So coffee at 8 PM means you won't be sleeping soundly until well after midnight.

powerful stimulant, it takes your body about 6 hours to clear just *half* of it from your system.[29]
- Don't drink alcohol within several hours of bedtime. Although initially it can make you drowsy, it interferes with your natural sleep stages and can cause you to awaken in the middle of the night, unable to get back to sleep.
- Don't drink large amounts of any liquid before bed, to prevent having to get up in the night to use the bathroom.
- Don't take sleeping pills or night-time pain medications unless they have been prescribed by your health care provider. Casual use of over-the-counter sleeping aids can interfere with your brain's natural progression through the healthy stages of sleep. You may also experience "payback" later when you try to stop using the drug and your sleep challenges return, worse than they were before you started using the medication.
- Don't get triggered. Remember the earlier advice about turning off your cell phone as you begin to prepare for bed? One reason is to avoid those late-night phone calls that can end up in arguments, disappointments, and other emotional stressors. If something—or someone—does trigger you shortly before bed, journal about it briefly, then promise yourself that you'll make time the next day to explore your feelings more deeply.

Beat Jet Lag

Insomnia, fatigue, stomachache, or headache: These are symptoms of jet lag and not a great way to spend a spring break vacation. In general, the more time zones you cross, the worse the jet lag will be. There are ways to avoid or reduce jet lag. Here's how:

* Begin the trip rested (preexisting sleep deprivation intensifies jet lag).
* Plan a daytime flight.
* Reset your watch as soon as you depart.
* Avoid alcohol, caffeine, and nicotine.
* Eat small meals at the appropriate mealtime for your destination.
* Several days before going west, go to bed and wake up 1 hour later each day.
* Once in the west, seek morning light and avoid afternoon light.
* Several days before going east, go to bed and wake up 1 hour earlier each day.
* Once in the east, seek evening light and avoid morning light.
* If you take an overnight flight, avoid sleeping too much on the day of your arrival. You'll find it hard to fight the fatigue, but sleeping during the day will make it harder for you to adjust to your new time zone's schedule.

What special steps should you take to prevent sleep problems when you travel? The **Skills for Behavior Change** box above identifies some important things you can do to beat jet lag.

What If You're Still Not Sleeping Well?

If you're following the advice in this chapter and you still aren't sleeping well, then it's time to see your health care provider, as you may be one of the estimated 50 to 70 million Americans who have a clinical sleep disorder.[30] To aid in diagnosis, you will probably be asked to keep a sleep diary like the one in **Figure 3**, and you may be referred to a sleep disorders center for an overnight stay. This type of evaluation is known

	Day 1	Day 2	Day 3	Day 4	Day 5	Day 6	Day 7
Complete in morning							
Bedtime	11 pm	11:30 pm					
Wake time	7:30 am	8:30 am					
Time to fall asleep	45 min	30 min					
Awakenings (how many and how long?)	2 times 1 hour	1 time 45 min					
Total sleep time	6.75 hrs	7.75 hrs					
Feeling at waking (refreshed, groggy, etc.)	Still tired	Energized					
Complete at bedtime							
Exercise (what, when, how long?)	Jog at 2 pm 30 min	Soccer practice at 4 pm; 2 hrs					
Naps (when, where, how long?)	4 pm, my bed 30 min	2 pm, library 1 hour					
Caffeine (what, when, how much?)	2 cups coffee at 8 am	1 latte at 10 am; 1 soda at 9 pm					
Alcohol (what, when, how much?)	1 beer at 8 pm	None					
Evening snacks (what, when, how much?)	Bag of popcorn at 10 pm	Chips and soda at 9 pm					
Medications (what, when, how much?)	None	None					
Feelings (happiness, anxiety, major cause, etc.)	Stressed about paper	Worried about sister					
Activities 1 hour before bed (what and how long?)	Wrote paper	Watched TV					

FIGURE 3 **Sample Sleep Diary**
Using a sleep diary such as this one can help you and your health care provider discover any behavioral factors that might be contributing to your sleep problem.

as a clinical **sleep study.** While you are asleep in the sleep center, sensors and electrodes record data that will be reviewed by a sleep specialist who will help your primary health care provider determine the precise nature of your sleep problem.

The American Academy of Sleep Medicine identifies more than 80 specific sleep disorders. The following are a few of the most common. Did you know that the reasons for sleep disorders differ somewhat in men and women? Check out the **Gender & Health** box on page 95.

sleep study A clinical assessment of sleep in which the patient is monitored while spending the night in a sleep disorders center.
insomnia A disorder characterized by difficulty in falling asleep quickly, frequent arousals during sleep, or early morning awakening.
sleep apnea A disorder in which breathing is briefly and repeatedly interrupted during sleep.

Insomnia

Insomnia—difficulty in falling asleep quickly, frequent arousals during sleep, or early morning awakening—is the most common sleep complaint. Annual *Sleep in America* polls dating back at least 10 years reveal that more than 50 percent of Americans experience insomnia at least a few nights a week. About 10 to 15 percent of Americans report that they have chronic insomnia, that is, insomnia that persists longer than a month. Insomnia is more common among women than men, and its prevalence increases with age.[31]

Sleep Apnea

Sleep apnea is a disorder in which breathing is briefly and repeatedly interrupted during sleep.[32] *Apnea* refers to a breathing pause that lasts at least 10 seconds. During that time, the chest may rise and fall, but little or no air may be exchanged, or the person may actually not breathe until the brain triggers a gasping inhalation. Sleep apnea affects more than 18 million Americans, or 1 in every 15 people.[33]

There are two major types of sleep apnea: central and obstructive. *Central sleep apnea* occurs when the brain fails to tell the respiratory muscles to initiate breathing. Consumption of alcohol, certain illegal drugs, and certain medications can contribute to this condition. *Obstructive sleep apnea (OSA),* which is the more common form, occurs when air cannot move in and out of a person's nose or mouth, even though the body tries to breathe.

Typically, OSA occurs when a person's throat muscles and tongue relax

Gender Differences in Sleep Disorders

Women and men each face a unique set of issues that can affect sleep. In recent years, researchers have started recognizing that women are much more likely than men to suffer from sleep disorders. In a major study conducted by the National Sleep Foundation, 70 percent of menstruating women of all age groups reported sleep disruptions during their period, and women were also more likely than men to suffer from insomnia in general. The table explores the most common sources of sleep problems for women and men, and what can be done to treat them.

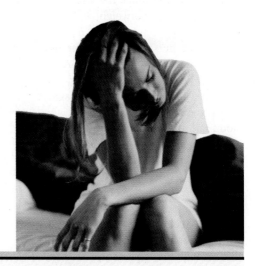

Biological Reasons for Sleep Disorders

Women

	Symptoms	Causes	Remedies
Menstruation	Bloating, soreness, cramps, and headaches disturb 2 or 3 nights of sleep per month.	Hormonal fluctuation that affects the body and nervous system can disrupt normal sleep patterns.	Most symptoms improve with time. Otherwise, try over-the-counter painkillers and reduce caffeine intake.
Pregnancy	At first, frequent bathroom trips and daytime sleepiness may occur. Later, restlessness, heartburn, and back pain often appear.	Rising progesterone levels cause sleepiness. Other symptoms are caused by pressure placed on the internal organs by the baby.	Short naps in the early afternoon, supportive pillows, and lying on the side to sleep all help. Avoid spicy foods to prevent heartburn.
Menopause	Hot flashes, insomnia, and sleep apnea, in which the airway is briefly but repeatedly blocked during sleep, may occur.	There may be drops in progesterone and estrogen levels (the exact cause of hot flashes is still unclear) and weight gain.	Hormone therapy works for some but may increase the risk of blood clots or aggravate certain types of cancer.

Men

	Symptoms	Causes	Remedies
Sleep apnea	May experience daytime exhaustion, snoring, and gasping sounds.	Overweight, fat around the neck, and abnormal facial structure are all potential factors.	Continuous positive airway pressure (CPAP), weight loss, and sleeping on one's side can all provide relief.
Prostatism	Frequent bathroom trips through the night are an indication of presence of condition.	Enlarged prostate is the cause.	Surgery to remove obstructing prostate tissue and medication provide relief.

Mental and Physical Reasons for Sleep Disorders

Both Genders

	Symptoms	Causes	Remedies
Stress	Insomnia, a "racing" mind, restlessness, headaches, and nightmares are all indicators.	Tension brought on by stressful situations, such as marital troubles or financial problems, can trigger insomnia.	Learn relaxation techniques and exercise early in the day; hypnotics are a short-term option.
Depression	Early-morning waking, fatigue, and excessive sleepiness during the day and insomnia at night are all indicators associated with depression.	Depression can change brain chemical levels and disrupt sleep.	Antidepressants (consult a doctor) and psychotherapy can help.
Anxiety	Nighttime panic attacks can wake the sleeper; insomnia from chronic fear and worrying can also cause sleep deprivation.	Anxiety triggers the release of chemicals that speed up breathing and heart rate; caffeine may also contribute.	Exercise regularly and avoid caffeine. If that isn't enough, antianxiety drugs may help.

Sources: M. Kryger, *A Woman's Guide to Sleep Disorders* (Boston: McGraw-Hill, 2004); National Sleep Foundation, "Sleep in America," 2009, www.sleepfoundation.org; L. R. McKnight-Eily et al., "Perceived Insufficient Rest or Sleep-Four States, 2006," *Morbidity and Mortality Weekly Report* 57, no. 8 (2008): 200–03.

during sleep and block the airways.[34] People who are overweight or obese often have more tissue that flaps or sags, which puts them at higher risk for sleep apnea. People with OSA are prone to heavy snoring, snorting, and gasping. These sounds occur because, as oxygen saturation levels in the blood fall, the body's autonomic nervous system is stimulated to trigger inhalation, often via a sudden gasp of breath. This response may wake the person, preventing deep sleep and causing the person to wake up in the morning feeling tired and unwell. More serious risks of OSA include chronic high blood pressure, irregular heartbeats, heart attack, and stroke. Apnea-associated sleeplessness may be a factor in an increased risk of type 2 diabetes, immune system deficiencies, and a host of other problems.

Parasomnias

A **parasomnia** is a disorder in which undesired events occur while sleeping. Two common parasomnias are REM sleep behavior disorder and sleepwalking.

REM sleep behavior disorder (RBD) occurs when a person acts out vivid dreams during REM sleep. The activity involved may be mild, such as moving the hands, or violent, such as tackling an imaginary attacker. People with RBD do not have their eyes open and rarely get up and walk. The episodes may begin in the first cycle of REM sleep and continue to occur during subsequent REM stages until the sleeper awakes in the morning. RBD occurs most commonly in adult men, often after age 50.[35]

Sleepwalking is a parasomnia in which a sleeper gets up and walks around, typically with eyes open, all the while entirely asleep. Unlike RBD, it typically occurs in stage 3 or 4 of NREM sleep. The sleepwalker may eat, perform a chore, urinate, or even get in a car and drive. Sleepwalking is more common in children, but up to 4 percent of adults sleepwalk.[36]

parasomnia A disorder characterized by the occurrence of undesirable events while sleeping.
narcolepsy Excessive, intrusive sleepiness.

Narcolepsy

Narcolepsy is excessive, intrusive sleepiness. The person affected can fall asleep quite suddenly—in class, at work, driving, or in any other situation. Narcolepsy occurs in about 1 of every 2,000 people, and affects men and women equally. The condition is apparently due to a dramatic reduction in the number of nerve cells containing a substance called hypocretin in the brains of narcoleptics. Hypocretin plays a role in sleep regulation. There appears to be a genetic basis for the disorder.[37]

Clinical Treatments Are Available

If you are diagnosed with a sleep disorder, the good news is that help is available, and new therapies are being developed all the time. Primary sleep therapies include the following:

● **Medications.** If you suffer from insomnia, you may be prescribed a type of drug called a *hypnotic* (or *sedative*). These drugs induce sleep, and some may help relieve anxiety. However, some have undesirable side effects ranging from daytime sleepiness and hallucinations to sleepwalking and other strange nighttime behaviors. Some can actually promote anxiety and/or depression. Antidepressants are also commonly prescribed for insomnia.

● **Melatonin.** The hormone melatonin is sometimes prescribed as a nutritional supplement to treat certain sleep disorders involving disruption in circadian rhythm. Some people take melatonin-based sleep aids to prevent jet lag.

● **Continuous positive airway pressure (CPAP).** The most commonly prescribed therapy for obstructive sleep apnea is use of a continuous positive airway pressure (CPAP) device, which consists of an airflow device, long tube, and mask. People with sleep apnea wear this mask during sleep, and air is forced into the nose to keep the airway open. Snoring and sleep disturbances generally stop with the use of this machine.

● **Cognitive behavioral therapy.** In cognitive behavioral therapy, a therapist assists a patient in identifying thought and behavioral patterns that contribute to a problem such as inability to fall asleep. Once these patterns are recognized, the patient practices new habits that produce positive change.

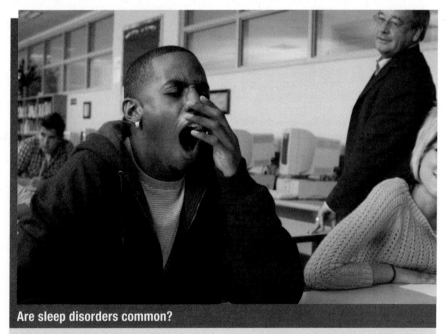

Are sleep disorders common?

From insomnia to sleepwalking to narcolepsy, sleep disorders are more common than you might think. There are more than 80 different clinical sleep disorders, and it is estimated that between 50 and 70 million Americans—children and adults—suffer from one. Many aren't even aware of their disorder, and many others never seek treatment.

Assess yourself

Are You Sleeping Well?

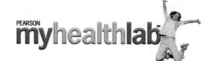

Read each statement below, then circle True of False according to whether or not it applies to you in the current school term.

Fill out this assessment online at www.pearsonhighered.com/myhealthlab or www.pearsonhighered.com/donatelle.

1. I sometimes doze off in my morning classes.   True   False

2. I sometimes doze off in my last class of the day.   True   False

3. I go through most of the day feeling tired.   True   False

4. I feel drowsy when I'm a passenger in a bus or car.   True   False

5. I often fall asleep while reading or studying.   True   False

6. I often fall asleep at the computer or watching TV.   True   False

7. It usually takes me a long time to fall asleep.   True   False

8. My roommate tells me I snore.   True   False

9. I wake up frequently throughout the night.   True   False

10. I have fallen asleep while driving.   True   False

If you answer true more than once, you may be sleep-deprived. Try the strategies in this chapter for getting more or better quality sleep, but if you still experience sleepiness, see your health care provider.

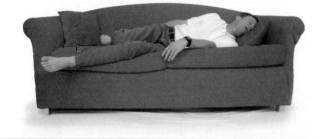

YOUR PLAN FOR CHANGE

The **Assess yourself** activity gave you the chance to determine whether you are sleep-deprived. Now that you have considered your answers, you can take steps to improve your sleep, starting tonight.

Today, you can:

◯ Evaluate your behaviors and identify things you're doing that get in the way of a good night's sleep. Develop a plan. What can you do differently starting today?

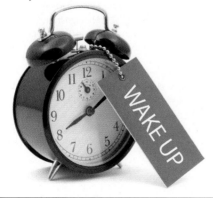

◯ Write a list of personal Dos and Don'ts. For instance: *Do* turn off your cell phone after 11:00 PM. *Don't* drink anything with caffeine after 3:00 PM.

Within the next 2 weeks, you can:

◯ Keep a sleep diary, noting not only how many hours of sleep you get each night, but also how you feel and how you function the next day.

◯ Arrange your room to promote restful sleep. Remember the "cave": Keep it quiet, cool, and dark, and replace any uncomfortable bedding.

◯ Visit your campus health center and ask for more information about getting a good night's sleep.

By the end of the semester, you can:

◯ Establish a regular sleep schedule. Get in the habit of going to bed and waking up at the same time, even on weekends.

◯ Create a ritual, such as stretching, meditation, light reading, or listening to music, that you follow each night to help your body ease from the activity of the day into restful sleep.

◯ If you are still having difficulty sleeping and feel you may have a sleep disorder or an underlying health problem disrupting your sleep, contact your health care provider.

References

1. *American College Health Association—National College Health Assessment (ACHA-NCHA): Reference Group Executive Summary Fall 2008* (Baltimore: American College Health Association, 2009).

2. Central Michigan University, "College Student Sleep Patterns Could Be Detrimental," *ScienceDaily* (May 13, 2008). www.sciencedaily.com/releases/2008/05/080512145824.htm. Accessed March 18, 2009.

3. D. Law, "Exhaustion in University Students and the Effect of Coursework Involvement," *Journal of American College Health* 55, no. 4 (2007): 239–45.

4. National Sleep Foundation, *Longer Work Days Leave Americans Nodding Off on the Job,* Press Release (March 3, 2008), www.sleepfoundation.org.

5. S. Banks and D. F. Dinges, "Behavioral and Physiological Consequences of Sleep Restriction," *Journal of Clinical Sleep Medicine* 3, no. 5 (2007): 519–28.

6. S. Cohen et al., "Sleep Habits and Susceptibility to the Common Cold," *Archives of Internal Medicine* 169, no. 1 (2009): 62–67.

7. D. J. Gottlieb et al., "Association of Usual Sleep Duration with Hypertension: The Sleep Heart Health Study," *Sleep* 29, no. 8 (2006): 1009–14.

8. S. R. Patel et al., "Sleep Duration and Biomarkers of Inflammation," *Sleep* 32, no. 2 (2009): 200–04; M. L. Okun, M. Coussons-Read, and M. Hall, "Disturbed Sleep Is Associated with Increased C-Reactive Protein in Young Women," *Brain, Behavior, and Immunity* 23, no. 3 (2009): 351–54.

9. J-C. Chen et al., "Sleep Duration and Risk of Ischemic Stroke in Postmenopausal Women," *Stroke* 30, no. 12 (2008): 3185–92.

10. K. L. Knutson, K. Spiegel, P. Penev, and E. Van Cauter, "The Metabolic Consequences of Sleep Deprivation," *Sleep Medicine Reviews* 11, no. 3 (2007): 163–78; National Sleep Foundation, *Obesity and Sleep,* 2009, www.sleepfoundation.org.

11. S. Taheri et al., "Short Sleep Duration Is Associated with Reduced Leptin, Elevated Ghrelin, and Increased Body Mass Index," *PLoS Medicine* 1, no. 3 (2004): 362.

12. M. H. Hall et al., "Self-Reported Sleep Duration Is Associated with the Metabolic Syndrome in Midlife Adults," *Sleep* 31, no. 5 (2008): 635–43.

13. S. Banks and D. F. Dinges, "Behavioral and Physiological Consequences of Sleep Restriction," *Journal of Clinical Sleep Medicine* 3, no. 5 (2007): 519–28.

14. H. Eichenbaum, "To Sleep, Perchance to Integrate," *Proceedings of the National Academy of Sciences of the United States of America* 104, no. 18 (2007): 7317–18; J. M. Ellenbogen, P. T. Hu, D. Titone, and M. P. Walker, "Human Relational Memory Requires Time and Sleep," *Proceedings of the National Academy of Sciences of the United States of America* 104, no. 18 (2007): 7723–28; J. M. Ellenbogen, J. C. Hulbert, Y. Jiang, and R. Stickgold, "The Sleeping Brain's Influence on Verbal Memory: Boosting Resistance to Interference," *PLoS ONE* 4, no. 1 (2009): e4117.

15. P. V. Thacher, "University Students and the 'All-Nighter': Correlates and Patterns of Students' Engagement in a Single Night of Total Sleep Deprivation," *Behavioral Sleep Medicine* 6, no. 1 (2008): 16–31; W. E. Kelly, K. E. Kelly, and R. C. Clanton, "The Relationship between Sleep Length and Grade-Point Average among College Students—Statistical Data Included," *College Student Journal* (March 2001): 84–87.

16. B. R. Sheth, D. Janvelyan, and M. Khan, "Practice Makes Imperfect: Restorative Effects of Sleep on Motor Learning," *PLoS ONE* 3, no. 9 (2008): e3190.

17. T. Jan, "Colleges Calling Sleep a Success Prerequisite," *Boston Globe* (September 30, 2008), www.boston.com/news/education/higher/articles/2008/09/30/colleges_calling_sleep_a_success_prerequisite. Accessed March 2009.

18. National Sleep Foundation, *State of the States Report on Drowsy Driving: Summary of Findings,* (Washington, DC: National Sleep Foundation, 2008) Executive Summary, p. 2, www.sleepfoundation.org.

19. M. F. Bear, B.W. Connors, and M. A. Paradiso, *Neuroscience: Exploring the Brain.* 3d ed. (Baltimore: Lippincott Williams & Wilkins, 2007), 600.

20. National Sleep Foundation, "Depression and Sleep," www.sleepfoundation.org/article/sleep-topics/depression-and-sleep, Accessed March 2009; T. Roth, "Expert Column-Stress, Anxiety, and Insomnia: What Every PCP Should Know," *Current Perspectives in Insomnia* 4 (2004) http://cme.medscape.com/viewarticle/495354; A. Gregory, F. V. Rijsdijk, J. Y. F. Lau, R. E. Dahl, and T. C. Eley, "The Direction of Longitudinal Associations between Sleep Problems and Depression Symptoms: A Study of Twins Aged 8 and 10 Years," *Sleep* 32, no. 2 (2009): 189–99.

21. M. F. Bear, B.W. Connors, and M. A. Paradiso, *Neuroscience,* 594.

22. Ibid., 596.

23. Ibid., 596.

24. L. Genzel et al., "Slow Wave Sleep and REM Sleep Awakenings Do Not Affect Sleep Dependent Memory Consolidation," *Sleep* 32, no 3. (2009): 302–10.

25. J. Ferrie et al., "A Prospective Study of Change in Sleep Duration: Associations with Mortality in the Whitehall II Cohort," *Sleep* 30, no. 12 (2007): 1659–66; C. Hublin et al., "Sleep and Mortality: A Population-Based 22-Year Follow-Up Study," *Sleep* 30, no. 12 (2007): 1614–15.

26. D. L. Wingard and L. F. Berkman, "Mortality Risk Associated with Sleeping Patterns among Adults," *Sleep* 6, no. 2 (1983): 102–07.

27. E. B. Klerman and D. Dijk, "Interindividual Variation in Sleep Duration and Its Association with Sleep Debt in Young Adults," *Sleep* 28, no. 10 (2005): 1253–59.

28. National Sleep Foundation, "Napping," 2009, www.sleepfoundation.org/article/sleep-topics/napping.

29. National Sleep Foundation, "Caffeine and Sleep," 2009, www.sleepfoundation.org/article/sleep-topics/caffeine-and-sleep.

30. American Academy of Sleep Medicine, "A Sleep Study May Be Your Best Investment for Long-Term Health," *AASM* (2008), www.sleepeducation.com/Article.aspx?id=1083.

31. National Sleep Foundation, "Can't Sleep? What to Know about Insomnia," 2009, www.sleepfoundation.org/article/sleep-related-problems/insomnia-and-sleep.

32. National Sleep Foundation, "Obstructive Sleep Apnea and Sleep," 2009, www.sleepfoundation.org/article/sleep-related-problems/obstructive-sleep-apnea-and-sleep.

33. Sleep Disorders Guide, "Sleep Apnea Statistics," 2009, www.sleepdisordersguide.com/sleepapnea/sleep-apnea-statistics.html.

34. National Sleep Foundation, "Obstructive Sleep Apnea and Sleep," 2009; American Sleep Apnea Association, "Sleep Apnea Information," 2008, www.sleepapnea.org/info/index.html.

35. American Academy of Sleep Medicine, "REM Sleep Behavior Disorder," AASM. October 21, 2005, www.sleepeducation.com/Disorder.aspx?id=29.

36. American Academy of Sleep Medicine, "Sleepwalking," *AASM.* August 31, 2007, www.sleepeducation.com/Disorder.aspx?id=14. Accessed March 2009.

37. American Academy of Sleep Medicine, "Narcolepsy," *AASM.* May 16, 2006, www.sleepeducation.com/Disorder.aspx?id=5. Accessed March 2009.

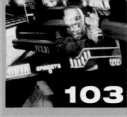
103 Does violence in the media cause violence in real life?

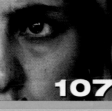
107 Why do people stay in abusive relationships?

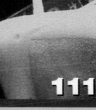
111 What is meant by *date rape*?

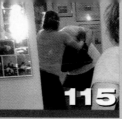
115 How can I protect myself from becoming a victim of violence?

Preventing Violence and Injury

4

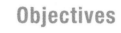

Objectives

✴ Differentiate between intentional and unintentional injuries, and discuss societal and personal factors that contribute to violence in American society.

✴ Discuss factors that contribute to homicide, domestic violence, sexual victimization, and other intentional acts of violence.

✴ Describe strategies to prevent intentional injuries and reduce their risk of occurrence.

✴ Explain potential risks to students on campus and potential strategies that campus leaders, law enforcement officials, and individuals can develop to prevent students from becoming victims.

Crime is increasing. Confidence in rigid and speedy justice is decreasing.[1]

Innocent and unoffending persons are shot, stabbed and otherwise shamefully maltreated, and not infrequently the offender is not even arrested.[2]

To millions of Americans few things are more pervasive, more frightening, more real today than violent crime. . . . The fear of being victimized by criminal attack has touched us all in some way.[3]

Although these quotes may seem as though they were spoken by today's news makers, you may be surprised to learn that they describe the violence that was part of everyday life for many of your ancestors. The first quotation comes from President Herbert Hoover's 1929 inauguration speech; the second comes from an 1860 Senate report on crime in Washington, D.C., and the third comes from a 1968 staff report to the National Commission on the Causes and Prevention of Violence. Life may have been less technologically advanced in the late 1800s and early 1900s in the United States; however, it was far from easy and even further from the safe haven that many idealize. Today, we seem fascinated by a steady stream of blood and gore on prime-time television, by murder mysteries that depict heinous crimes, by our worry over terrorist threats, and by our fears about identity thefts and crimes against our property. However, violence has been a part of American culture since our earliest beginnings.

Before we can discuss the nature and extent of violence in the United States or in the global population today, it's important that we have an understanding of what the word *violence* really means. Any definition of **violence** implicitly includes the use of force, regardless of the intent, but some forms of violence are extremely subtle. Typically, the word refers to a set of behaviors that produces injuries, such as those inflicted by gunshot wounds, physical force, projectile forces, or other assaults against the body. However, most experts today realize that emotional and psychological forms of violence can be as devastating as physical blows to the body. The U.S. Public Health Service has categorized violence resulting in injuries into either intentional injuries or unintentional injuries. **Intentional injuries**—those committed with intent to harm—typically include assaults, homicides, self-inflected injuries, and suicides. **Unintentional injuries**—those committed without intent to harm, often accidentally—typically include motor vehicle crashes, fires, and drownings.[4]

You may wonder why we would devote an entire chapter to violence in an introductory health text for college and university students. The answer is simple: Unintentional injuries, particularly those including drug- and alcohol-related vehicle crashes, are the number one cause of death among 15- to 24-year-olds in the United States today, whereas two forms of intentional injuries, homicide and suicide, are the second and third leading causes of death in young adults.[5]

violence A set of behaviors that produces injuries, as well as the outcomes of these behaviors (the injuries themselves).
intentional injuries Injury, death, psychological harm, maldevelopment, or deprivation that involves the intentional use of physical force or power, threatened or actual, against oneself, another person, or against a group or community.
unintentional injuries Injury, death, or harm that involves accidents committed without intent to harm, often as a result of circumstances, or without premeditation.

Violence in the United States

If you think that violence is a new phenomenon in the United States, think again. In fact, think back to our earliest days of colonization, when wife beatings, witch hunts, decimations of Native American tribes, brutal attacks against immigrants, rapes, and other violent acts were commonplace. Ironically, it wasn't until the 1980s that the U.S. Public Health Service identified violence as a leading cause of death and disability and gave it chronic disease status, indicating that it was a pervasive threat to society.[6] People from around the world often indicate that they fear travel to the United States because of their perception of gun-toting murderers on our streets, but, while violence is indeed pervasive in our country, the statistics don't support the blood-soaked images portrayed again and again in the media.

In fact, statistics from the Federal Bureau of Investigation (FBI) have shown that, after steadily increasing from 1973 to 2006, the rates of overall crime and certain types of violent crime have begun showing yearly decreases. Beginning in 2007, violent crimes and property crimes have decreased in many regions of the country.[7] Nationwide, violent crime rates fell 3.5 percent and property crime rates 2.5 percent during the first 6 months of 2008 (see **Figure 4.1** for percent change and **Figure 4.2** for the frequency of different types of crimes).[8] So why should we be concerned about violence, if government statistics seem to indicate a downward trend in some of the most lethal forms? The answer is that none of us is immune to the potentially devastating effects of violence. Whereas direct victims may suffer physical signs, others suffer from the climate of fear that violence generates. Even if we have never been victimized personally, we all are victimized by violent acts that cause us to be fearful, impinge on our liberty, and damage our nation's reputation in the international community.

Violence on U.S. Campuses

On April 16, 2007, Americans were horrified by news of the most deadly mass shooting in U.S. history at Virginia Tech University. Later, many would comment on the seemingly obvious shooter profile—a loner student who had enough trouble in classes that he was sent to counseling, who had interactions with law enforcement for his behavior, and who displayed an abnormal amount of anger in his written work and interactions with others. Why did faculty and student concerns about this student go largely unnoticed?

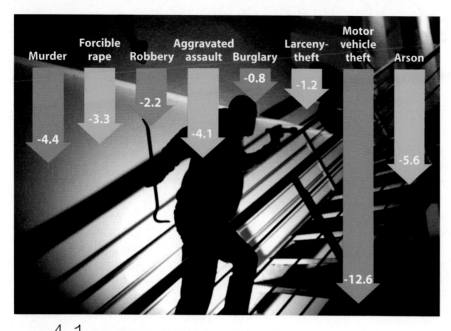

FIGURE 4.1 **Declining Crime Rates**
According to the FBI's Preliminary Semiannual Uniform Crime Report, violent crime in the nation dropped 3.5 percent and property crime declined 2.5 percent during the first 6 months of 2008, compared to the same period in 2007.

Source: Adapted from Federal Bureau of Investigation, *Crime in the United States, Preliminary Semiannual Uniform Crime Report 2008,* 2009, www.fbi.gov/ucr/2008prelim.

Why didn't administrators and members of the law enforcement community act more quickly to prevent large numbers of fatalities? The tragedy shocked the nation and left an indelible mark on our collective thoughts, but it also sparked dialogue and action on campuses across the nation and throughout the world. A year later, when the February 14, 2008, shootings at Northern Illinois University sent another shock wave through college campuses, increased priorities were put on campus security and student and faculty safety.

Campuses may be relatively safe, but they are by no means immune from acts of violence. Relationship violence is an especially prevalent problem on college campuses. In the most recent American College Health Association's survey, 12 percent of women and 7 percent of men reported being emotionally abused in the past 12 months by a significant other. Two percent of men and 2 percent of women reported being involved in a physically abusive relationship. Another 1 percent of men and 2 percent of women reported being in a sexually abusive relationship.[9]

Consider the following facts about campus violence:[10]

- Simple assault (attack without a weapon resulting either in no injury or in minor injuries) accounts for 63 percent of college student violent crimes, while rape or sexual assault accounts for 6 percent.
- Only about 5 percent of completed and attempted rapes committed against students are ever reported to the police.
- Nearly 80 percent of all rapes on campus are committed by persons the victim knows.
- Alcohol and other drugs are implicated in 55 to 74 percent of sexual assaults on campus.
- More than 36 percent of lesbian, gay, bisexual, and transgender (LGBT) students have experienced harassment within the past year.
- White college students experience higher rates of violent victimization than students of other races.

These statistics represent only a glimpse of the big picture. The sad fact is that fewer than 25 percent of campus crimes are reported to *any* authority.[11] Why would students fail to report such crimes? Typical reasons include concerns over privacy, embarrassment or shame, lack of support, perception that the crime was too minor, or uncertainty that it was a crime.

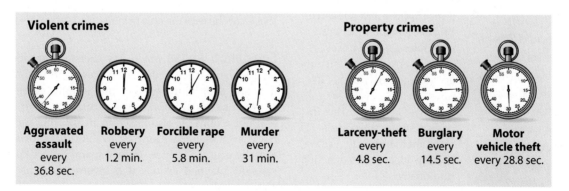

FIGURE 4.2 **Crime Clock**
The Crime Clock represents the annual ratio of crime to fixed time intervals. The Crime Clock should not be taken to imply a regularity in the commission of crime.

Source: Adapted from Federal Bureau of Investigation, "Crime in the United States, 2007," 2008, www.fbi.gov/ucr/cius2007/about/crime_clock.html.

Factors Contributing to Violence

Several social, cultural, environmental, and individual factors increase the likelihood of violent acts:

- **Poverty.** Low socioeconomic status and poor living conditions can create an environment of hopelessness in which people view violence as the only way to obtain what they want.
- **Unemployment.** It is a well-documented fact that when the economy goes sour, violent and nonviolent crimes increase.
- **Parental influence.** Children raised in environments in which shouting, hitting, and other forms of violence are commonplace are more apt to act out these behaviors as adults. Recent research has substantiated this cycle of violence.[12]

primary aggression Goal-directed, hostile self-assertion that is destructive in character.

reactive aggression Hostile emotional reaction brought about by frustrating life experiences.

- **Cultural beliefs.** Cultures that objectify women and empower men to be tough and aggressive show higher rates of violence in the home.
- **Discrimination or oppression.** Whenever one group is oppressed or perceives that its members are oppressed by those of another group, seeds of discontent are sown, and violence against others is more likely.
- **Religious beliefs and differences.** Religious persecution has been a part of the human experience since earliest times. Strong beliefs can lead people to think violence against others is justified by religious doctrine. Such beliefs also foster martyrdom, often expressed in such actions as suicide bombings.
- **Political differences.** Civil unrest and differences in political party affiliations and beliefs have historically been triggers for violent acts.

what do you think?

Why do you think rates of violence in the United States are so much higher than those of other nations, such as Great Britain and Japan? ● Which of the factors listed here do you think is the single greatest cause of violence, and why? ● What could be done to reduce risk from this factor?

- **Breakdowns in the criminal justice system.** Overcrowded prisons, lenient sentences, early releases from prison, and trial errors subtly encourage violence in a number of ways.
- **Stress.** People who are in crisis or under stress are more apt to be highly reactive, striking out at others or acting irrationally.
- **Heavy use of alcohol and other substances.** Alcohol and drug abuse are often catalysts for violence and other crimes.

In addition to these broad, societally based factors, many personal factors also can increase risks for violence.

93%

of crimes against college students occur at off-campus locations.

Personal Precipitators of Violence

If you are like most people, you probably acted out your anger more readily as a child than you do today. With increasing maturity, most people learn to control outbursts of anger in a socially acceptable and rational manner. However, some people go through life acting out their aggressive tendencies in much the same ways they did as children or as their families did. There are several predictors of future aggressive behavior.[13]

Anger *Anger* is a spontaneous, usually temporary, biological feeling or emotional state of displeasure that occurs most frequently during times of personal frustration. Because life is stressful, anger becomes a part of daily experience. Anger can range from slight irritation to *rage*, a violent and extreme form of anger. When a person acts out on his or her rage at home or in public, the consequences can be deadly.

What makes some people flare up at the slightest provocation? Often, people who are quick to anger have a low tolerance for frustration, believing that they should not have to put up with inconvenience or petty annoyances. They feel entitled and seek instant gratification. The cause may be genetic or physiological; there is evidence that some people are born unstable, touchy, or easily angered. Another cause of anger is sociocultural. People who are taught not to express anger in public do not know how to handle it when it reaches a level where they can no longer hide it. Family background may be the most important factor. Typically, anger-prone people come from families that are disruptive, chaotic, and unskilled in emotional expression.[14]

Aggressive behavior is often a key aspect of violent interactions. **Primary aggression** is goal-directed, hostile self-assertion that is destructive in nature. **Reactive aggression** is more often part of an emotional reaction brought about by frustrating life experiences. Whether aggression is reactive or primary, it is most likely to flare up in times of acute stress, during relationship difficulties or loss, or when a person is so frustrated that he or she feels the only recourse is to strike out at others.

Substance Abuse Much has been written about a link between substance abuse and violence. In fact, drinking is a major contributor to the fifth leading cause of death in America today: accidents—particularly auto accidents. Substance abuse is also linked to many other forms of violence, even though we have yet to show that substance abuse actually causes violence. In fact, many violent episodes are carefully planned actions that involve no alcohol or drug abuse. In some situations, however, psychoactive substances appear to be a form of ignition for violence:[15]

- Consumption of alcohol—by perpetrators of the crime, the victim, or both—immediately precedes more than half of all violent crimes, including murder.

- Chronic drinkers are more likely than others to have histories of violent behavior.
- Criminals using illegal drugs commit robberies and assaults more frequently than nonusing criminals and do so especially during periods of heavy drug use.
- In domestic assault cases, more than 86 percent of the assailants and 42 percent of victims report using alcohol at the time of the attack. Nearly 15 percent of victims and assailants report using cocaine at the time of the attack.
- Substance abuse markedly increases the risk of both homicide and suicide. The combination of depression and alcohol or other drugs increases homicide and suicide rates threefold.

The Impact of the Media

Although the media are often cited as contributing to the epidemic of violence in the world today, this association is not as clear as you might suspect. Does the teenager who plays the most gory video games run an increased risk of shooting his classmates and teachers compared to the game player who prefers less violent games? Do violent movies trigger violence and mayhem in the streets? Do sexually explicit videos and Internet sites promote rape on campus?

Over the past decade, there have been countless calls for limitations in what we view on television, what we see online, and what video games we play. The profile of the rapist, the school shooter, the domestic abuser, the gang member, and others has seemed to be inextricably linked to a history of excessive exposure to violent media. Several early studies in which people were surveyed about self-reported media use and involvement in various forms of violence seemed to support this link, and a recent study of the self-reported perceived behavior of nearly 1,600 youth, aged 10 to 15, indicated that there was a perception of significantly higher levels of shootings, stabbings, assault, robbery, and sexual assault among students who had watched higher amounts of violence in the media.[16]

Not so fast, say critics of such studies. Arguing that perceptions and reality are not the same when it comes to violence, and that the media itself can distort perceptions of what is really happening, they point out that today's youth are being exposed to more media violence than any previous generation without any measurable negative impact on crime rates. Fifteen years ago the Internet was in its infancy; now it is omnipresent and offers access to an ever-increasing number of violent and sexually explicit sites. At the same time cable and satellite TV hookups have been bringing a much wider range of violence into homes, making violent programs standard fare. Yet, over the same time period, just as media violence seems to

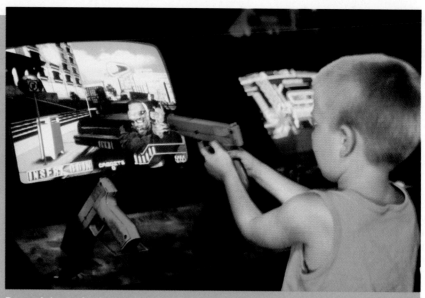

Does violence in the media cause violence in real life?

Evidence of the real-world effects of violence in the media is inconclusive. Arguably, Americans today—especially children—are exposed to more depictions of violence in the news, movies, music, and games than ever before, but research has not shown a clear link between a person's exposure to violent media and his or her propensity to engage in violent acts. Regardless, many people are concerned that children today are being exposed to more violence than they have the emotional or cognitive maturity to handle.

have exploded into our homes and lives, rates of violent crime and victimization among teens aged 10 to 17 have plummeted to the lowest rates ever recorded:[17]

- According to the National Crime Victimization Survey, which looks at offenses committed that did not lead to actual arrest, a 58 percent decline in violence has been noted overall, with teen violence down at greater levels than in any other population.
- A meta-analysis of 26 studies examining the relationship between exposure to media violence and violent aggression did not support the idea that media violence and criminal aggression are positively associated.

Overall, there is increasing evidence that media violence is not the main culprit in societal violence; in fact, many experts believe that its influence has been overstated through time. However, debate continues over whether a person who sees so much violence enacted in the media becomes *desensitized* to violence. Most experts believe that there are many more factors involved in whether a person becomes violent than just viewing too much violence in various media.

what do you think?

Do you think the media influence your behavior? In what ways?
- Do you believe that watching violent TV shows, playing violent video games, or viewing violent websites will make someone more likely to perform violent acts?
- Are there instances where curtailing violent viewing or restricting the nature and extent of violence and sex in the media is warranted? If so, under what circumstances?

Intentional Injuries

Any time someone sets out to harm other people or their property, the incident may be referred to as *intentional* violence. Although nonviolent crime is more common, violent crime occurs all too often. The resulting intentional injuries cause pain and suffering at the very least, and death and disability at the worst.

Homicide

Homicide, defined as murder or non-negligent manslaughter, is the 15th leading cause of death in the United States, but the second leading cause of death for persons aged 15 to 24. It accounts for more than 18,000 premature deaths in the United States annually.[18] Homicide rates reveal particularly clear disparities among races. For an American, the average lifetime probability of being murdered is 1 in 153—but this average masks large differences for specific segments of the population. Asian/Pacific Islanders, Hispanic or Latino, and African American groups all list homicide among the top ten causes of death, but homicide is not among the top ten killers of white Americans. Homicide rates for African American men are higher than those for any other group. For African American men of any age, the risk of murder is 1 in 28; for a black man aged 20 to 22 years the risk is 1 in 3. See the **Health Headlines** box at right for a discussion of the role guns play in the high rates of homicide in the United States.

Most homicides are not random acts of violence. Over half of all homicides occur among people who know one another. In two-thirds of these cases, the perpetrator and the victim are friends or acquaintances; in one-third, they belong to the same family.[19]

Hate and Bias-Motivated Crimes

A **hate crime** is a crime committed against a person, property, or group of people that is motivated by the offender's bias against a race, religion, disability, sexual orientation, or ethnicity. In spite of national efforts to promote understanding and appreciation of diversity in workplaces, schools, and communities, intolerance of differences continues to smolder in many parts of U.S. society. According to the FBI's most recent Hate Crime Statistics Report, there were 9,006 reported victims of hate crimes in 2007 (Figure 4.3).[20]

Since the 2001 terrorist attacks in the United States and the conflicts in Iraq and Afghanistan, reports of hate-related incidents, beatings, and other physical and verbal assaults have

homicide Death that results from intent to injure or kill.
hate crime A crime targeted against a particular societal group and motivated by bias against that group.
ethnoviolence Violence directed randomly at persons affiliated with a particular, usually ethnic, group.
prejudice A negative evaluation of an entire group of people that is typically based on unfavorable and often wrong ideas about the group.
discrimination Actions that deny equal treatment or opportunities to a group, often based on prejudice.

70%

of all hate crimes are committed against a person or persons; the rest are crimes against property.

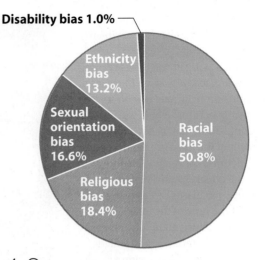

FIGURE 4.3 **Bias-Motivated Crimes, 2007**
Source: Federal Bureau of Investigation, "Hate Crime Statistics, 2007," www.fbi.gov/ucr/hc2007, 2008.

escalated. In particular, persons of Muslim or Middle Eastern descent have reported civil rights violations at work, in mass transit, and in communities throughout the United States.

Bias-related crime, both on campus and in the community, is sometimes referred to as **ethnoviolence,** a term that describes violence among groups in the larger society that is based on prejudice and discrimination. Although ethnoviolence often is directed randomly at persons affiliated with a particular group, the group itself is specifically targeted apart from other people, and that differentiation is usually ethnic in nature.

Prejudice and discrimination are always at the base of hate crimes and ethnoviolence. **Prejudice** is a set of negative attitudes toward a group of people; a person who is prejudiced against some group holds a set of beliefs about the group, has an emotional reaction to the group, and is motivated to behave in a certain way toward the group. **Discrimination** constitutes actions that deny equal treatment or opportunities to a group of people, often based on prejudice. Often prejudice and discrimination stem from a fear of change and a desire to blame others when forces such as the economy and crime seem to be out of control.

Hate crimes and ethnoviolence vary along two dimensions: (1) the way they are carried out and (2) their effects on victims. Recent studies have identified three additional characteristics of hate crimes: They are excessively brutal, perpetrated at random on total strangers, and perpetrated by multiple offenders.[21]

Academic settings are not immune to hatred and bias. In fact, with nearly 13 percent of all bias-related and hate crimes occurring on campuses, schools and colleges have the fastest-growing risks for such crimes. Campuses have responded to reports of hate crimes by offering courses that emphasize diversity, training faculty appropriately, and developing policies that strictly enforce punishment for hate crimes.[22] Sadly, many

Health Headlines

THE GUN DEBATE

According to the most recent statistics, more than 100,000 people in the United States were shot in murders, assaults, suicides, accidents, or by police intervention in 2007. Nearly 31,000 died from gun violence, whereas many who survived experienced significant physical and emotional repercussions.

✻ In 2007, firearm homicide was the second leading cause of injury death for men and women aged 10 to 24, second only to motor vehicle crashes.
✻ Handguns are consistently responsible for more murders than any other single type of weapon (see figure below).
✻ Today, 35 percent of American homes have a gun on the premises, with more than 283 million privately owned guns registered—40 percent of which are handguns.
✻ The presence of a gun in the home triples the risk of a homicide there. The presence of a gun in the home increases suicide risk by more than five times.

What factors contribute to excessive gun deaths in the United States? Of course, by sheer numbers, if you have more guns, the likelihood of people using them in inappropriate ways increases. However, the number of guns available doesn't tell the entire story. Countries such as Canada with similar household possessions of guns have much different gun-related crime rates than does the United States: In 2004, there were 11,344 murders by firearms in the United States, compared to only 184 in Canada. Critics of gun control argue that guns don't murder people; it's the person pulling the trigger on the gun who is ultimately the problem. In addition, the argument about the "right to bear arms" as a constitutional right is a difficult area of debate.

Shootings at Columbine and Springfield high schools, and high-profile shootings of faculty and students at the University of Iowa, Virginia Tech, and other campuses have moved school administrators to take action to protect students. Nationwide, 24 states have passed laws prohibiting or restricting guns on college campuses. States frequently have had legislation proposed that would allow students with permits to carry weapons to "protect" themselves and others—there were at least 14 such bills in 2009. As of this writing, only one state—Utah—prohibits colleges from setting their own rules regarding guns on campus, thus effectively allowing them. Although guns on campus are just a microcosm of larger society, concern over bans, restriction of gun ownership, and movements to allow guns on campus have raised tensions to a new high.

Sources: J. Fox and M. Zawitz, *Homicide Trends in the United States*, U.S. Department of Justice, Office of Justice Programs, Bureau of Justice Statistics, www.ojp.usdoj.gov/bjs/homicide/homtrnd.htm. Revised 2007; Brady Campaign to Prevent Gun Violence, "Facts: Gun Violence," www .bradycampaign.org/facts/gunviolence. Revised 2009; Brady Campaign to Prevent Gun Violence, "Guns in Colleges and Schools," www .bradycampaign.org/stateleg/publicplaces/ gunsoncampus. Revised 2009; National Center for Injury Prevention and Control, "WISQARS Injury Mortality Reports," http://webapp.cdc.gov/sasweb/ ncipc/mortrate.html. Updated 2007; L. Hepburn, M. Miller, and D. Hemenway, "The U.S. Gun Stock: Results from the 2004 National Firearms Survey," *Injury Prevention* 13 (2007): 15–19; T. Smith, *Public Attitudes towards the Regulation of Firearms* (Chicago: National Opinion Research Center, 2007); M. Miller and D. Hemenway, "Guns and Suicide in the United States," *New England Journal of Medicine* 359 (2008): 989–91.

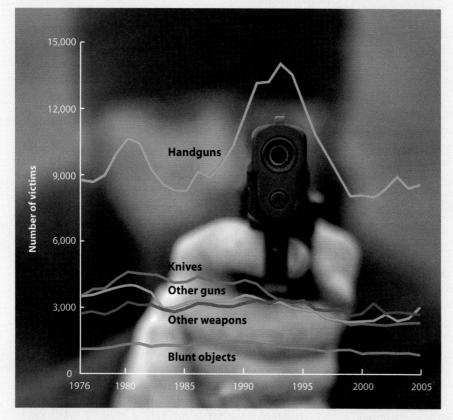

Homicide in the United States by Weapon Type, 1976–2005
Like the homicide rate generally, gun-involved incidents increased sharply in the late 1980s and early 1990s before falling to a low in 1999. The number of gun-involved homicides increased thereafter to levels experienced in the mid-1980s. During this same time period, homicides involving weapons other than firearms have declined slightly.

Source: Adapted from J. Fox and M. Zawitz, *Homicide Trends in the United States,* U.S. Department of Justice, Office of Justice Programs, Bureau of Justice Statistics, www.ojp.usdoj.gov/bjs/homicide/homtrnd.htm. Revised 2007.

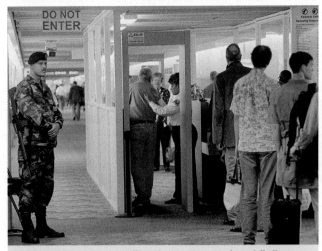

The threat of terrorism has affected many aspects of our daily lives.

minor assaults do go unreported, because the victims fear retaliation or continued stigmatization; underreporting is a major impediment to reducing the rate of hate crimes on campus.

Gang Violence

The growing influence of street gangs has had a harmful impact on our country, even though the media do not highlight gang violence as often today as they did some years ago. Drug abuse, gang shootings, beatings, thefts, carjackings, and the possibility of being caught in the crossfire have caused entire neighborhoods to live in fear. Once thought to occur only in urban areas, gang violence now also appears in rural and suburban communities, particularly in southeastern, southwestern, and western states.

terrorism The unlawful use of force or violence against persons or property to intimidate or coerce a government, the civilian population, or any segment thereof, in furtherance of political or social objectives.
domestic violence The use of force to control and maintain power over another person in the home environment, including both actual harm and the threat of harm.

Why do young people join gangs? Although the reasons are complex, gangs seem to meet many of their needs. Gangs provide a sense of belonging to a family that gives them self-worth, companionship, security, and excitement. In other cases, gangs provide economic security through criminal activity, drug sales, or prostitution. Once young people become involved in the gang subculture, it is difficult for them to leave. Threats of violence or fear of not making it on their own dissuade even those who are most seriously trying to get out.

Who is at risk for gang membership? The age range of gang members is typically 12 to 22 years. Risk factors include low self-esteem, academic problems, low socioeconomic status, alienation from family and society, a history of family violence, and living in gang-controlled neighborhoods.[23]

Terrorism

Not so long ago, Americans thought terrorism occurred only in distant cities, seldom amounting to more than a blip on the evening news. Since September 11, 2001, times have changed dramatically. Terrorist attacks on the World Trade Center and Pentagon revealed our nation's vulnerability to domestic and international threats. Today, the specter of a terrorist attack looms ever present.

According to the Code of Federal Regulations, **terrorism** is "the unlawful use of force or violence against persons or property to intimidate or coerce a government, the civilian population, or any segment thereof, in furtherance of political or social objectives."[24] Typically, terrorism is of two major types:

1. Domestic terrorism, which involves groups or individuals whose terrorist activities are directed at elements of our government or population without foreign direction

2. International terrorism, which involves groups or individuals whose terrorist activities are foreign based, transcend national boundaries, and are directed by countries or groups outside the United States

Clearly, terrorist activities may have immediate impact in loss of lives and resources. However, the 2001 attacks also had far-reaching effects on the U.S. economy, airlines, and transportation systems. Perhaps most damaging in the aftermath of the attacks was the fear, anxiety, and altered behavior of countless Americans.

The Centers for Disease Control and Prevention (CDC) has a wide range of ongoing programs and services to help Americans respond to terrorist threats and prepare for possible attacks. The Department of Homeland Security has been established to prevent future attacks, and the FBI and other government agencies have also prepared a sweeping set of procedures and guidelines for ensuring citizen safety.

Domestic Violence

Domestic violence refers to the use of force to control and maintain power over another person in the home environment. It can occur between parent and child, between spouses or intimate partners, or between siblings or other family members and may involve emotional abuse, verbal abuse, threats of physical harm, and actual physical violence ranging from slapping and shoving to beatings, rape, and homicide.

Today, domestic violence is at epidemic levels in America. The National Crime Victimization Survey found that in 2005, 14 percent of U.S. households experienced one or more violent or property victimizations.[25] Fewer than one-half of these crimes are reported to law enforcement. Nearly 5.2 million intimate partner victimizations occur each year among U.S. women aged 18 and older, resulting in more than 2 million injuries and nearly 1,300 deaths.[26] Homicide by a current or former intimate partner is the leading cause of injury death among pregnant women in the United States.[27] In addition, 74 percent of all murder-suicides in the United States involve an intimate partner. Of these, 96 percent involve women killed by their intimate partners and 75 percent of those incidents occur in the home.[28] And women are not the only victims of intimate partner violence; the Gender & Health box on page 108 explores some of the issues surrounding male victimization.

Although the ultimate result of domestic violence assaults can be murder, there are other devastating effects as well.

Depression, panic attacks, eating disorders, chronic neck or back pain, migraine and other headaches, sexually transmitted infections, ulcers, and social isolation can all result from domestic violence.

Intimate Partner Violence and Women

Although young men are more apt to become victims of violence from strangers, women are much more likely to become victims of intimate partner violence, violent acts perpetrated by spouses, lovers, ex-spouses, and ex-lovers. This aggression often includes pushing, slapping, and shoving, but it can take more severe forms. In reported assaults, only 31 percent of the men who attack women are "strangers." In fact, six of every ten women in the United States will be assaulted at some time in their lives by someone they know.[29] Worldwide, one out of every three women will be abused during her lifetime. In some countries, rates of abused women reach 70 percent.

How many times have you heard of a woman who is repeatedly beaten by her partner and wondered, "Why doesn't she just leave him?" There are many reasons why some women find it difficult to break their ties with their abusers. Many women, particularly those with small children, are financially dependent on their partners. Others fear retaliation against themselves or their children. Some hope the situation will change with time (it rarely does), and others stay because cultural or religious beliefs forbid divorce. Finally, some women still love the abusive partner and are concerned about what will happen to him if they leave.

Psychologist Lenore Walker developed a theory known as the *cycle of violence* to explain how women can get caught in a downward spiral without realizing it.[30] The cycle has three phases:

1. **Tension building.** In this phase, minor battering occurs. To forestall further violence, the woman may become more nurturing, more pleasing, and more intent on anticipating the abuser's needs. She assumes guilt for doing something to provoke him and tries hard to avoid doing it again.

2. **Acute battering.** At this stage, pleasing her man doesn't help, and she can no longer control or predict the abuse. Usually, the spouse is trying to "teach her a lesson," and when he feels he has inflicted enough pain, he'll stop. When the acute attack is over, he may respond with shock and denial about his own behavior. Both batterer and victim may soft-pedal the seriousness of the attacks.

3. **Remorse/reconciliation.** During this "honeymoon" period, the batterer may be kind, loving, and apologetic, swearing

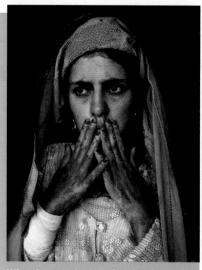

Why do people stay in abusive relationships?

People who stay with their abusers may do so because they are dependent on the abuser, because they fear the abuser, or even because they love the abuser. In some cultures, women may not be free to leave an abusive relationship because of restrictive laws, religious beliefs, or social mores. Such women sometimes turn to drastic measures in order to escape; this young Afghani woman bears burn scars from when she set herself on fire in an attempt to end her life with an abusive husband.

he will never act violently again. He may "behave" for several weeks or months, and the woman may come to question whether she overreacted. However, when the tension that precipitated past abuse resurfaces, the man beats her again.

Unless some form of intervention breaks this downward cycle of abuse—contrition, further abuse, denial, and contrition—it will repeat itself again and again, perhaps ending only in the woman's (or, rarely, the man's) death. For most women who get caught in this cycle (which may include forced sexual relations and psychological and economic abuse as well as beatings), it is very hard to summon the resolution to extricate themselves. Most need effective outside intervention.

Causes of Domestic Violence

There is no single explanation for why people tend to be abusive in relationships. Although alcohol abuse is often associated with such violence, marital dissatisfaction is also a predictor. Numerous studies also point to differences in the communication patterns between abusive and nonabusive relationships. Although some researchers argue that the hormone testosterone causes male aggression, studies have failed to show a strong association between physical abuse in relationships and this hormone. Many experts believe that men who engage in severe violence are more likely than other men to suffer from personality disorders.[31]

Regardless of the cause, it is the dynamics that both people bring to a relationship that result in violence and allow it to continue. Community support and counseling services can help determine underlying problems and allow the victim and batterer to break the cycle. The **Assess Yourself** box on page 120 may help you determine whether you are involved in an abusive relationship. The **Green Guide** on page 109 provides information on one type of domestic violence program that also has positive environmental impact.

child abuse The systematic harming of a child by a caregiver, typically a parent.

neglect Failure to provide for a child's basic needs such as food, shelter, medical care, and clothing.

Child Abuse and Neglect

Children raised in families in which domestic violence and/or sexual abuse occur are at great risk for damage to personal health and well-being. The effects of such violent acts are powerful and long lasting. **Child abuse** refers to the systematic harm of a child by a caregiver, generally a parent. The abuse may be sexual, psychological, physical, or any combination of these. **Neglect** includes failure to provide for a child's basic needs for food, shelter, clothing, medical care, education, or proper supervision.

Intimate Partner Violence against Men

Although we tend to think of intimate partner violence as something that happens only to women, every year in the United States about 3.2 million men are victims of an assault by an intimate partner. While women's assaults on men are usually not as life threatening as the assaults that stronger men perpetrate against women, they can be physically and psychologically damaging, result in destruction of property, exact an emotional toll that affects health, and, in rare instances, lead to life-threatening injuries. Intimate partner violence within gay relationships is a recognized health problem and gay men appear to be just as susceptible to male-perpetrated violence as women in heterosexual populations. Unfortunately, we may never really know the exact nature and extent of man-against-man intimate partner violence or woman-against-man intimate partner violence because of the stigma associated with a man reporting that he has been brutalized—either by a male partner or by a woman. However, several studies have indicated that between 20 and 24 percent of men have experienced physical, sexual, or psychological intimate partner violence

during their lifetime. Why don't men report? Probably the biggest reason is that when women assault men, the injuries are usually emotional or psychological in nature and hard to identify. Injuries tend to be minor in nature and consist of scratches, bruises, or property damage. Other possible reasons include the following:

* Fear that no one will believe them
* Societal judgment about what it means if a woman hits a man
* Belief that "taking it" and never hitting back is a badge of honor, strength, and masculinity
* Humiliation and fear of being found out, machismo attitude
* Belief that they deserve bad treatment because they are so emotionally abused
* Lack of awareness and support services for men in abusive relationships.

Recognizing that a real problem exists, communities across the nation are responding with education and awareness about various forms of violence, support groups, resources, and options potential victims can take to protect themselves.

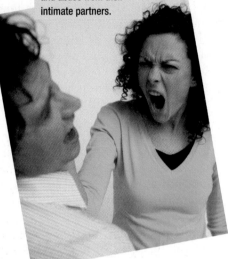

Both men and women are subject to violence and abuse from their intimate partners.

Sources: National Domestic Violence Hotline, "Abuse In America," www.ndvh.org/get-educated/abuse-in-america. Accessed June 2009; Medical Review Board, "Men as Victims of Abusive Relationships," http://menshealth.about.com/od/relationships/a/Battered_Men.htm. Updated January 2007; Oregon Counseling Center, "About Domestic Violence against Men," www.oregoncounseling.org/Handouts/DomesticViolenceMen.htm. Revised May 2007.

How serious are the problems of child abuse and neglect? Although exact figures are lacking, many experts believe that nearly a million cases of child abuse and neglect occur every year in the United States, involving severe injury, permanent disability, or death (see **Figure 4.4**).[32] In 2007, 3.2 million allegations of child abuse and neglect concerning the welfare of approximately 5.8 million children were made to child protective service agencies in the United States. In about 62 percent of these cases, sufficient abuse was detected to prompt investigation, resulting in an estimated 905,000 cases, or 2,479 cases per day![33]

There is no single profile of a perpetrator of child abuse. Frequently, the perpetrator is a young adult in his or her mid-twenties without a high school diploma, living at or below the poverty level, depressed, socially isolated, with a poor self-image, and with difficulty coping with stressful situations. In many instances, the perpetrator has experienced violence and is frustrated by life. Although it is difficult to measure long-term consequences of abuse, an average of nearly five children die every day as a result of abuse or

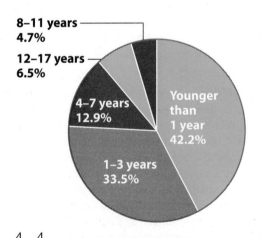

8–11 years 4.7%
12–17 years 6.5%
4–7 years 12.9%
Younger than 1 year 42.2%
1–3 years 33.5%

FIGURE 4.4 **Child Abuse and Neglect Fatalities, by Age, 2007**

Source: U.S. Department of Health and Human Services, Administration on Children, Youth and Families, *Child Maltreatment 2007* (Washington, DC: U.S. Government Printing Office, 2009). www.acf.hhs.gov/programs/cb/pubs/cm07/index.htm.

GREEN GUIDE

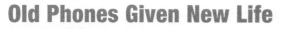

Old Phones Given New Life

In today's technocentric world, cell phones, BlackBerries, computers, and other electronic goods quickly become outdated. However, while a cell phone might be outdated for you, it could be a lifeline for a family in need of protective services or an emergency 911 call. Before you donate your e-goods for general e-recycling, consider donating them to a violence prevention agency—it's an ecofriendly way to contribute to the safety of your community. Cell phones are particularly needed for domestic violence shelters and family violence prevention shelters around the nation. Check your regional and local violence prevention agencies to determine if and when they accept recycled cell phones.

This idea is catching on with larger corporations as well. Some companies are collecting recycled cell phones to deliver to domestic and family violence shelters. In addition to accepting cell phones, many agencies also accept cell phone chargers, batteries, and other accessories to maximize the use of the phones provided.

The National Coalition against Domestic Violence has partnered with The Wireless Foundation to create their "Call to Protect" program (www.wirelessfoundation.org/CallToProtect). Check out this and other websites to donate your used phone to help prevent domestic violence:

* www.recellular.com/recycling
* www.collectivegood.com
* http://aboutus.vzw.com/communityservice/hopeLine.html

SAFETY REMINDER: Before donating or recycling your cell phone, erase all data and remove the SIM card and identifying information. Download free instructions for erasing this information specific to your phone's manufacturer and model at www.recellular.com/recycling/data_eraser.

---

neglect.[34] Most fatalities from *physical abuse* are caused by fathers and other male caretakers. Mothers are most often held responsible for deaths resulting from *neglect*. However, in some cases the reason may be that it is women who spend the most time with the children and whom society deems responsible for their care.

Not all violence against children is physical. Health can be severely affected by psychological violence—assaults on personality, character, competence, independence, or general dignity as a human being. The negative consequences of this kind of victimization can be harder to discern and therefore harder to combat. They include depression, low self-esteem, and a pervasive fear of offending the abuser.

Elder Abuse With the aging of the baby-boomer generation comes a population of people over the age of 65 that will exceed 71 million by 2030—nearly double the number of that in 2000. By all estimates, these elderly will need increasing levels of care in the coming decades, and there will be fewer and fewer people who are willing and able to provide it. That means that your parents and grandparents may be increasingly likely to become victims—of domestic violence; of caregiver abuse in assisted living and long-term care facilities; of financial scams and business scams; and of sexual, physical, and emotional abuse, neglect, abandonment, and exploitation at all levels of society.

Between 2000 and 2006, elder abuse statistics rose nearly 18 percent.[35] However, it is difficult to determine the full extent of elder abuse. It is estimated that, of the millions of elder abuse crimes that occur in our society, as few as 1 in 14 are ever reported. These vulnerable individuals don't report incidents because they fear retaliation, abandonment by family members, and worsening conditions as a result of registering complaints.[36] Today, a variety of social service and public health groups are exploring options for protecting our elderly citizens in much the same way as we protect children in our society. Policies, programs, and education are among their priorities, as is respite care for caregivers who often face difficult challenges in caring for their disabled family members.

Sexual Victimization

The term *sexual victimization* refers to any situation in which an individual is coerced or forced to comply with or endure another's sexual acts or overtures. It can run the gamut from harassment to stalking to assault and rape. As with all forms of violence, both men and women are susceptible to sexual victimization. Young people are especially vulnerable: 60.4 percent of female victims of sexual violence and 69.2 percent of male victims were first raped before the age of 18.[37] In some cases, people who are victimized at a young age later become perpetrators themselves.[38] Sexual victimization and violence can have devastating and far-reaching effects on people of any age. Depression, suicide risks, drug and alcohol abuse, traumatic stress disorders, self-harm, and a host of interpersonal problems often increase among women and men who have been victimized sexually.[39]

Sexual Assault and Rape

Sexual assault is any act in which one person is sexually intimate with another person without that person's consent. This act may range from simple touching to forceful penetration and may include, for example, ignoring indications that intimacy is not wanted, threatening force or other negative consequences, and actually using force.

Rape Considered to be the most extreme form of sexual assault, **rape** is defined as "penetration without the victim's consent."[40] Incidents of rape generally fall into one of two types—aggravated or simple. An **aggravated rape** is any rape involving one or multiple attackers, strangers, weapons, or physical beatings. A **simple rape** is a rape perpetrated by one person, whom the victim knows, and does not involve a physical beating or use of a weapon. Most rapes are classified as simple rape, but that terminology should not be taken to mean a "simple" rape is any less violent or criminal. The FBI ranks rape as the second most violent crime, trailing only murder.[41]

> **sexual assault** Any act in which one person is sexually intimate with another person without that person's consent.
> **rape** Sexual penetration without the victim's consent.
> **aggravated rape** Rape that involves one or multiple attackers, strangers, weapons, or physical beating.
> **simple rape** Rape by one person, usually known to the victim, that does not involve a physical beating or use of a weapon.

How serious a problem is sexual assault and rape in the United States? According to the latest National Crime Victimization Survey, there were an estimated 248,300 sexual assaults in 2007 against victims aged 12 and older. Every 2 minutes, another American is sexually assaulted, and one in six American women is sexually assaulted at some point in her lifetime. An estimated 63 percent of all sexual assaults reported in 2007 were committed by someone the victim knew: 38 percent of perpetrators were the victim's friend or acquaintance; 22 percent were an intimate; and 3 percent were relatives.[42]

Men are also victims of rape and sexual assault, and a growing number have come forward to report their abusers. Recent surveys indicate that between 2 to 3 percent, or 1 out of every 33 men, have experienced forced sex or been sexually assaulted at some time in their lives, usually by acquaintances (32.3%), family members (17.7%), friends (17.6%), and intimate partners (15.9%). Over 41 percent of male victims were first raped before the age of 12, and 27.9 percent were first raped between the ages of 12 and 17.[43]

By most indicators, reported cases of rape appear to have declined in the United States since the early 1990s, even as reports of other forms of sexual assault have increased. This decline is thought to be due to shifts in public awareness and attitudes about rape, combined with tougher crime policies, major educational campaigns, and media attention. These changes enforce the idea that rape is a violent crime and should be treated as such.

While these declines in reported cases may seem encouraging, studies show that only 16 percent of all rapes are actually reported to law enforcement![44] Why do so many victims never report their crimes? Reasons vary, but typically major barriers include not wanting others to know about the rape, fear of retaliation, perception of insufficient evidence, uncertainty about how to report, and uncertainty whether a crime was committed or whether harm was intended.

Acquaintance or Date Rape Whether perpetrated by a stranger, acquaintance, relative, friend, or intimate partner, any rape is harmful to the victim. Although the terms *date rape* and *acquaintance rape* have become standard terminology, they are often misunderstood. Not all "date rapes" occur on dates, and sometimes the word *acquaintance* is used all too loosely. Many acquaintance rapes occur as the result of incidental contact at a party or when groups of people congregate at one person's house. These are crimes of opportunity, not necessarily a prearranged date. Although most date or acquaintance rapes happen to women aged 15 to 24 years, the 18-year-old new college student is the most likely victim.[45]

Date rape is not simply miscommunication; it is an act of violence. Well-known expert on interpersonal relationships Susan Jacoby puts it this way:

> Some women (especially the young) initially resist sex not out of real conviction, but as part of the elaborate persuasion and seduction rituals accompanying what was once called courtship. And it is true that many men (again, especially the young) take pride in their ability to coax a woman further than she intended to go. But these mating rituals do not justify or even explain date rape. Even the most callow youth is capable of understanding the difference between resistance and genuine fear; between a halfhearted "no, we shouldn't" and tears or screams.[46]

Rape on U.S. Campuses An estimated 673,000 of the nearly 6 million women (about 12%) currently attending college in the United States have been raped. During the past year alone, over 300,000 college women were raped, nearly two-thirds of them by forcible means that resulted in injury.[47] By some estimates these rates may be as high as 25 percent of college women who have reported an attempted or completed rape in college.[48] Over 80 percent of these rapes were committed by persons the victim knew, most occurred on campus, and alcohol was commonly involved, as were the two most commonly used rape-facilitating drugs, Rohypnol and GHB.[49]

Usually, alcohol serves as a catalyst for aggressive behavior in perpetrators and lowers normal resistance behaviors in victims. Sometimes specific drugs are used to immobilize victims and make them unable to defend themselves. These drugs are typically slipped into the drinks of unsuspecting people, who wake up later and can remember few details of the assault. See the

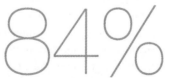

84%

of sexual assaults that occur on college campuses are acquaintance rapes.

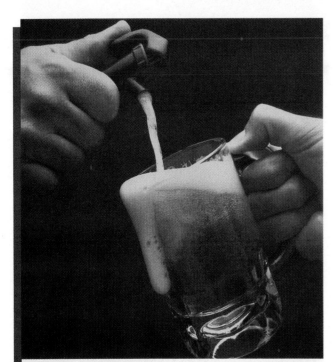

A lot of campus rapes start here.

Whenever there's drinking or drugs, things can get out of hand. So it's no surprise that many campus rapes involve alcohol.

But you should know that under any circumstances, sex without the other person's consent is considered rape. A felony, punishable by prison. And drinking is no excuse.

That's why, when you party, it's good to know what your limits are. You see, a little sobering thought now can save you from a big problem later.

What is meant by *date rape*?

The term *date rape* used to be applied to sexual assault (coercive, nonconsensual sexual activity) occurring in the context of a "dating" relationship. However, the term has fallen out of favor because the word *date* implies something reciprocal or arranged, thus minimizing the crime. The term *acquaintance rape* is now more commonly used, referring to any rape in which the rapist is known to the victim, even if only minimally. Acquaintance rape is particularly common on college campuses, where alcohol and drug use can impair young people's judgment and self-control.

Avoiding Drug-Facilitated Crimes

✳ Do not accept beverages or open-container drinks from anyone you do not know well and trust. At a bar or a club, accept drinks only from the bartender or wait staff.

✳ Never leave a drink or food unattended. If you get up to dance, have someone you trust watch your drink or take it with you.

✳ Go with friends and leave with friends. Never leave a bar or a party with someone you don't know well.

✳ If you think someone slipped something into your drink, tell a friend and have him or her get you to an emergency room.

✳ If a friend seems disproportionately intoxicated in relation to what he or she has had to drink, stay with your friend and watch him or her carefully. Call 911 if anyone experiences seizures, vomits, passes out, has difficulty breathing, or experiences other complications.

---

spouses obtained by force, by threat of force, or when the wife is unable to consent. Some researchers estimate that marital rape may account for 25 percent of all rapes.

Although this problem has undoubtedly existed since the origin of marriage as a social institution, it is noteworthy that marital rape did not become a crime in all 50 states until 1993. Even more noteworthy is the fact that 30 states still allow exemptions from rape prosecution, meaning that the judicial system may treat it as a lesser crime.

Who is most vulnerable to marital rape? In general, women under the age of 25 and those from lower socioeconomic groups are at highest risk. Women from homes where other forms of domestic violence are common and where alcoholism and/or substance abuse are prevalent also tend to be victimized at greater rates. Women who are subjected to marital rape often report multiple offenses over a period of time; these events are likely to be forced anal and oral experiences.[50]

Child Sexual Abuse

Sexual abuse of children by adults or older children includes sexually suggestive conversations; inappropriate kissing; touching; petting; oral, anal, or vaginal intercourse; and other kinds of sexual interaction. Girls are more commonly abused than boys, although young boys are also frequent victims, usually of male family members. Between 20 and 30 percent of all adult women report having had an unwanted childhood sexual encounter with an adult male, usually a father, uncle, brother, or grandfather.[51]

sexual abuse of children Sexual interaction between a child and an adult or older child.

The most frequent abusers are a child's parent or a parent's companion or spouse. The next most frequent abusers are grandfathers and siblings. Unfortunately, the "stranger

Skills for Behavior Change box at right for tips on reducing your risk of becoming a victim of a drug-facilitated crime.

In 1992, Congress passed the Campus Sexual Assault Victim's Bill of Rights, known as the *Ramstad Act*. The act gives victims the right to call in off-campus authorities to investigate serious campus crimes. In addition, it requires universities to set up educational programs and to notify students of available counseling. More recent provisions of the act specify received notification procedures and options for victims, rights of victims and the accused perpetrators, and consequences if schools do not comply. It also requires the Department of Education to publish campus crime statistics annually.

Marital Rape Although the legal definition varies within the United States, *marital rape* can be defined as any unwanted intercourse or penetration (vaginal, anal, or oral) between

danger" programs taught in some schools may give children the false impression that they are more likely to be assaulted by some seedy-looking character lurking in the bushes. They may not recognize that they are being victimized by the very people whom they trust and love.

Most sexual abuse occurs in the child's home. The following situations raise the risk:[52]

- The child lives without one of his or her biological parents.
- The mother is unavailable because she is disabled, ill, or working outside the home.
- The parents' marriage is unhappy.
- The child has a poor relationship with his or her parents or is subjected to extremely punitive discipline.
- The child lives with a stepfather.

People who were abused as children often bear spiritual, psychological, and physical scars. To appreciate the impact of child abuse on later life, studies have shown that children who experience maltreatment and abuse are at increased risk later in life for smoking, alcoholism, drug abuse, eating disorders, mental health problems, and suicide.[53]

Parents and caretakers of children should be aware of the following behavioral changes that may signal sexual abuse:

- Noticeable fear of a certain person or place
- Unusual or unexpected response when the child is asked whether he or she has been touched by someone
- Unreasonable fear of a physical exam
- Drawings that show sexual acts
- Abrupt changes in behavior, such as bed-wetting
- Sudden or unusual awareness of genitals or sexual acts
- Attempts to get other children to perform sexual acts

Other Forms of Sexual Victimization

Not all sexual victimization is as overtly violent as rape or child sexual abuse. There are other more subtle acts of sexual aggression that are still harmful and illegal. College students in particular can be subject to victimization in the form of harassment, stalking, or emotionally abusive relationships.

sexual harassment Any form of unwanted sexual attention related to any condition of employment or performance evaluation.

Sexual Harassment **Sexual harassment** is
defined as unwelcome sexual conduct that is related to any condition of employment or evaluation of student performance. Typically, it has one or more of the following components: (1) submission to such conduct is a condition of employment, academic progress, or participation in a university program; (2) submission to or rejection of such conduct influences employment, academic or university program decisions, or

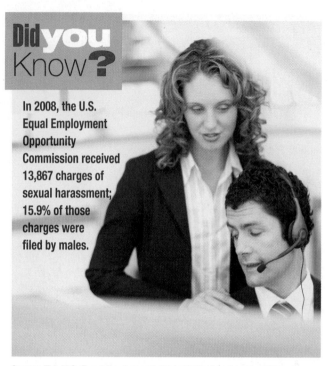

grades; and (3) the conduct interferes with an employee's work or a student's academic career, or creates an intimidating, hostile, or offensive work, learning, or program environment.[54]

Commonly, people think of harassment as involving only faculty members or persons in power, where sex is used to exhibit control of a situation. However, peers can harass one another too. Although definitions vary, for actions to be labeled as "sexual harassment" in this context, they would typically have one or more of the following characteristics:

1. The behavior is unwelcome and unwanted. It does not stop when challenged and often occurs when others aren't around to witness it.
2. The behavior is sexual in nature or is gender directed.
3. The behavior interferes with the ability of someone to pursue an education; perform professional duties; or feel safe or comfortable at his or her school, work, or living environment.

Harassment can occur at many levels and can lead the victim to experience shame, fear, self-doubt, embarrassment, guilt, anger, powerlessness, stress, isolation, reduced productivity, academic difficulties, and suicide. Sexual harassment may include unwanted touching; unwarranted sex-related comments or subtle pressure for sexual favors; deliberate or repeated humiliation or intimidation based on sex; and gratuitous comments, jokes, questions, or remarks about clothing or bodies, sexuality or past sexual relationships. Making derogatory jokes based on sex or appearance, speaking in crude or offensive language, spreading

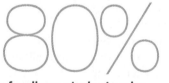

80%

of college students who have experienced sexual harassment report being harassed by another student or former student.

rumors about a person's sexuality, placing compromising photos on the Web, or ogling are all forms of sexual harassment as well.

It's always important to watch what you say and how you say it. Learning now what constitutes sexual harassment may save you embarrassment or worse in the future. A simple compliment on someone's appearance can be offensive if stated without sensitivity, regardless of the intent. Also, the context in which such comments are made can make a huge difference in interpretation.

Most schools and companies have sexual harassment policies in place, as well as procedures for dealing with harassment problems. If you feel you are being harassed, the most important thing you can do is be assertive:

● Tell the harasser to stop. Be clear and direct about what is bothering you and why you are upset. Tell the person if it continues that you will report it to the proper legal authorities. If harassing is via phone or Internet, block the person from your listings.
● Document the harassment. Make a record of the incident. If the harassment becomes intolerable, a record of exactly what occurred (and when and where) will help make your case. Save copies of all communication that the harasser sends you.
● Try to make sure you aren't alone in the harasser's presence. Witnesses to harassment can ensure appropriate validation of the event.

what do you think?

What policies does your school have regarding consensual relationships between faculty members and students? ● Should consenting adults have the right to become intimate or interact socially, regardless of their positions within a school or workplace? ● What are the potential dangers of such interactions? ● Are there ever situations when such interactions are okay?

● Complain to a higher authority. Talk to your instructor, adviser, or counseling center about what happened. If they don't take you seriously, investigate your school's internal grievance procedures.
● Remember that you have not done anything wrong. You will likely feel awful after being harassed (especially if you have to complain to superiors). However, feel proud that you are not keeping silent.

Stalking The crime of **stalking** can be defined as a course of conduct directed at a specific person that would cause a reasonable person to feel fear. This may include repeated visual or physical proximity, nonconsensual written or verbal communication, and implied or explicit threats. Stalking can even occur online (see the **Health Today** box on page 114 about the risks of social networking sites). Although tremendous underreporting is the norm, millions of women and men are stalked annually in the United States, and the vast majority of stalkers are persons involved in relationship breakups or other dating acquaintances. Stalking is particularly prevalent on college campuses; in fact, between 25 and 30 percent of college women and between 11 and 17 percent of college men have been stalked.[55] Researchers suggest several reasons for stalking: (1) Stalkers may have deficits in social skills; (2) they are young and have not yet learned how to deal with complex social relationships and situations; (3) they may not realize their behavior is stalking; (4) they have a flexible schedule and free time; and (5) they are not accountable to authority figures for their daily activities.[56]

Often, students do not report a stalking incident because they do not think it is serious enough or they worry that the police will not take it seriously. But this crime should be taken more seriously, and the best way for that to happen is by educating students about the subtle forms that stalking may take, whether calling a person constantly to monitor their actions, following them to bars or parties to see whom they are with, or going on "stealth" drive-bys to see what a former intimate is doing. Student stalkers may not view such behaviors as criminal in nature, or they may be surprised to find out that their showing "interest and persistence" is causing the other party to be anxious and fearful. Any time that happens, stalking charges are possible. Knowing what is appropriate behavior, being able to tell people when they are making you uncomfortable, and knowing what options are available for involving authorities are key ways of reducing risks.

Emotional and Psychological Abuse A common and insidious form of violence between intimate partners is emotional or psychological abuse. Emotional abuse can occur in any intimate relationship but is particularly prevalent in romantic and sexual relationships, between both same-sex and opposite-sex partners. This abuse can take the form of constant criticisms, personal verbal attacks, displays of explosive anger meant to intimidate, and controlling behavior. Psychological abusers seek to intimidate, denigrate, and debase their partners, thereby gaining control over the partner and the relationship. Often this form of abuse can lead to or accompany physical abuse and sexual coercion. If you note that your friend's or a family member's intimate partner is verbally or emotionally abusive or controlling, encourage them to seek counseling before the situation escalates further.

stalking The willful, repeated, and malicious following, harassing, or threatening of another person.

Social Contributors to Sexual Violence

Sexual violence and intimate partner violence share common factors that increase the likelihood of their occurrence as well as their continued acceptance in modern society. Even as we do our best to demonstrate more progressive thinking and actions, certain assumptions and traditions in our society continue to be present, including the following:[57]

● **Minimization.** Although one out of every six women in the United States has been a victim of a sexual assault, the

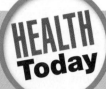
Social Networking Safety

Social networking sites such as Facebook, MySpace, Bebo, Xanga, and Twitter; dating services; personal blogs; and other such virtual arenas have come of age in recent years. At any given time, millions of people are chatting away with friends, family, and strangers, and posting photos and personal information that may be available to people they barely know, sometimes placing them at considerable risk. These sites raise some concerns about potential risks—from stalking and identity theft to gossip and slander to embarrassment and defamation. For example:

✳ A first-year student at Virginia Commonwealth University was murdered by someone she met on MySpace.
✳ A student at the University of Kansas learned the consequences of revealing too much information on Facebook when she was stalked by a man who encountered her class schedule online.
✳ In Britain, 4.5 million Web users between ages 14 and 21 were vulnerable to identity fraud because of information provided on their social networking sites when security measures were hacked.
✳ Hiring and firing decisions have been influenced by information employees and job applicants made publicly available on Facebook and Twitter.
✳ Underage users may pose as adults, leading to claims of inappropriate sexual contact with minors and other criminal

To stay safe online, think before you tweet.

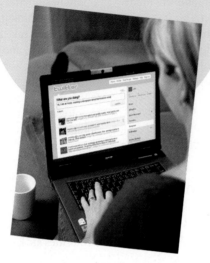

offenses on the part of people interacting with them online.

Although very real threats to health, reputation, financial security, and future employment lie in wait for those who post indiscriminately and unwisely to the Web, social networking sites are far from wholly dangerous. Social networking forums also have many benefits, particularly for college students. Social networking sites provide a quick and easy way to meet new people, to engage in interesting conversations, and to stay connected with friends and relatives who are far away. It's often easy to make friends and communicate at a deeper level online than one might be

able to do in a loud party environment or on a large, impersonal campus.

To safely enjoy the benefits and to avoid the risks of social networking sites, you'll need to practice a little caution and use some common sense. The following tips will help you to remain safe, protect your identity, and feel free to express yourself without fear of repercussions:

✳ Don't post anything on the Web that you wouldn't want someone to pick out of your trashcan and read. Your address, phone numbers, banking information, calendar, family secrets, and other information should be kept off the sites. Assume that out of all the people who view your information, there will be at least one unscrupulous person who poses a potential threat.
✳ Don't post compromising pictures, videos, or other things that you wouldn't want your mother or coworkers to see. Would potential employers or older family members think your photos were cute? Or would they wonder about your judgment, values, and trustworthiness?
✳ Never meet a stranger in person whom you've met only online without bringing a trusted friend along, or at the very least, notifying a close friend of where you will be and when you will return. Arrange a ride home with a friend in advance and choose a well-established, public place to meet during daylight hours. Don't give your address or traceable phone numbers to the person you are meeting.

Uniform Crime Reports of the FBI show rape crimes as a rate per thousand. Many do not understand what these numbers mean.

● **Trivialization.** Since rape is underreported, many are not aware that they know rape victims and may consider rape by a husband or intimate partner not to count or not to be serious. Often rape and sexual assault are the subjects of jokes and ridicule.

● **Blaming the victim.** In spite of massive efforts to combat this type of thinking, there is still a subtle suggestion that a scantily clad woman "asks" for sexual advances.

● **Gender roles.** Males are taught from a young age that "big boys don't cry"; that showing emotions is a sign of weakness; and that they must put on a macho persona to the outside

world. This portrayal often depicts men as aggressive and predatory and females as passive targets.

● **Male socialization.** Many still believe that "sowing wild oats" and "boys will be boys" are merely normal parts of development to adulthood in males. Women are often *objectified,* or treated like sexual objects, in the media, which contributes to the idea that it's only natural for men to be predatory.

● **Male misperceptions.** With media implying that sex is the focus of life, it's not surprising that some men believe that when a woman says no, she is really asking to be seduced. Later, these same men may be surprised when the woman says she was raped.

● **Situational factors.** Several factors increase the likelihood of sexual assaults. Dates in which the male makes all the decisions, pays for everything, and generally controls the entire situation are more likely to end in an aggressive sexual scenario. Alcohol and other drugs increase the risk and severity of assaults. If two people have been seeing each other for a long time, the chances of aggression escalate, particularly if there has already been a sexual incident that didn't turn out as the male expected.

Strategies for Preventing Intentional Injuries

After a violent act is committed against someone we know, we acknowledge the horror of the event, express sympathy, and go on with our lives—but the person who has been brutalized may take months or years to recover. It is far better to prevent a violent act than to recover from it. Both individuals and communities can play important roles in the prevention of violence and intentional injuries.

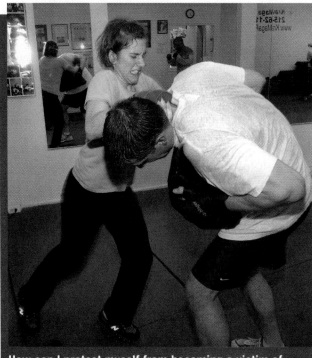

How can I protect myself from becoming a victim of violence?

One of the best ways to protect yourself from violence is to avoid situations or circumstances that could lead to it: keep to lighted paths instead of dark alleys, pay attention to your surroundings, don't let strangers into your home, don't become intoxicated when at parties or social events, and arrange rides home beforehand with trusted friends who will remain sober. Another way to protect yourself is to learn self-defense techniques. College campuses often offer safety workshops and self-defense classes to arm students with physical and mental skills that may help them repel or deter an assailant.

Self-Defense against Personal Assault and Rape

Assault can occur no matter what preventive actions you take, but commonsense self-defense tactics can lower the risk. Self-defense is a process that includes increasing your awareness, developing self-defense skills, taking reasonable precautions, and having the judgment necessary to respond to different situations. Because rape and assault on campus often occur in social or dating settings, it is important to know ways to avoid and extract yourself from potentially dangerous situations. The **Skills for Behavior Change** box below identifies practical tips for preventing dating violence.

Most attacks by unknown assailants are planned in advance. Many rapists use certain ploys to initiate their attacks. Examples include asking for help, offering help, staging a deliberate "accident" such as bumping into you, or posing as a police officer or other authority figure. Sexual assault frequently begins with a casual, friendly conversation.

Reducing Your Risk of Dating Violence

Remember that if a potential romantic partner truly cares for you and respects you, that person will respect your wishes and feelings. Here are some tips for dealing with sexual pressure or unwanted advances when dating and socializing:

✳ Prior to your date, think about your values, and set personal boundaries before you walk out the door.
✳ Set limits. If the situation feels like it is getting out of control, stop and talk, say no directly, and don't be coy or worry about hurting feelings. Be firm.
✳ Watch your alcohol consumption. Drinking might get you into situations you'd otherwise avoid.
✳ Pay attention to your date's actions. If there is too much teasing and all the decisions are made for you, it may mean trouble. Trust your intuition.
✳ Go out in couples or groups when dating someone new.
✳ Stick with your friends. Agree to keep an eye out for one another at parties, and have a plan for leaving together and checking in with each other. Never leave a bar or party alone with a stranger.
✳ Practice what you will say to your date if things go in an uncomfortable direction. You have the right to express your feelings, and it is okay to be assertive. Do not be swayed by arguments such as, "What about my feelings?" "You were leading me on," and "If you really cared about me, you would."

Skills for Behavior Change

Listen to your feelings, and trust your intuition. Be assertive and direct to someone who is getting out of line or threatening—this may convince the would-be rapist or attacker to back off. Stifle your tendency to be nice, and don't fear making a scene. Use the following tips to let a potential assailant know that you mean what you say and are prepared to defend yourself:

- **Speak in a strong voice.** Use statements such as, "Leave me alone" rather than questions such as, "Will you please leave me alone?" Avoid apologies and excuses. Sound like you mean it.
- **Maintain eye contact with the would-be attacker.** This keeps you aware of the person's movements and conveys an aura of strength and confidence.
- **Stand up straight, act confident, and remain alert.** Walk as though you owned the sidewalk.

If you are attacked, act immediately. Draw attention to yourself and your assailant. Scream, "Fire!" loudly. Research has shown that passersby are much more likely to help if they hear the word *fire* rather than just a scream.

What to Do If Rape Occurs

If you are a rape victim, report the attack. This gives you a sense of control. Follow these steps:

- Call 911 (if a phone is available).
- Do not bathe, shower, douche, clean up, or touch anything the attacker may have touched.
- Save the clothes you were wearing, and do not launder them. They will be needed as evidence. Bring a clean change of clothes to the clinic or hospital.
- Contact the rape assistance hotline in your area, and ask for advice on therapists or counseling if you need additional help.

If a friend is raped, here's how you can help:

- Believe her, and don't ask questions that may appear to implicate her in the assault.
- Recognize that rape is a violent act and that the victim was not looking for this to happen.
- Encourage your friend to see a doctor immediately because she may have medical needs but feel too embarrassed to seek help on her own. Offer to go with her.
- Encourage her to report the crime.
- Be understanding, and let her know you will be there for her.
- Recognize that this is an emotional recovery, and it may take 6 months to a year for her to bounce back.
- Encourage your friend to seek counseling.

Campuswide Responses to Violence

Increasingly, campuses have become microcosms of the greater society, complete with the risks, hazards, and dangers people face in the world. Many college administrators have

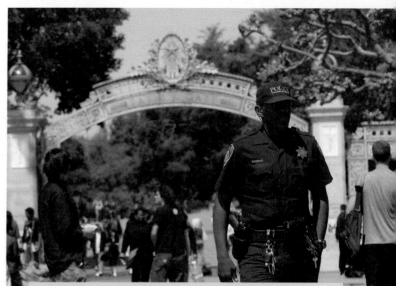
The presence and visibility of campus law enforcement have increased in recent years.

been proactive in establishing violence prevention policies, programs, and services. They have also begun to examine the culture that promotes violent acts and tolerance for them.[58]

Campus Law Enforcement Campus law enforcement has changed over the years in both numbers and authority to prosecute student offenders. Campus police are responsible for emergency responses to situations that threaten safety, human resources, the general campus environment, traffic and bicycle safety, and other dangers. They have the power to enforce laws with students in the same way they are handled in the general community. In fact, many campuses now hire state troopers or local law enforcement officers to deal with campus issues rather than maintain a separate police staff.

Many of these law enforcement groups follow a community policing model in which officers have specific responsibilities for certain areas of campus, departments, or events. By narrowing the scope of each officer's territory, officers get to know people in the area and are better able to anticipate and prevent risks. In the wake of major campus tragedies in the past few years, schools around the country are also enhancing the ability of campus law enforcement to respond in case of an emergency. Many officers are receiving special training in handling crisis and hostage situations, as well as being issued stun guns and other equipment meant to disable potential offenders.

Prevention and Early Response Efforts The Virginia Tech and Northern Illinois tragedies of 2007 and 2008 prompted vast restructuring of existing policies and strategies for prevention, as well as implementation of methods for notifying students and faculty of immediate risk. Historically, prevention efforts have focused on rape-awareness programs; safety workshops; antitheft programs; and grounds safety measures such as good lighting, escort services, and emergency call boxes. Newer programs being developed include emergency response drills that enable campus police, campus administration, members of community law enforcement, and emergency medical teams to practice how they would respond in the event of a major threat, such as a shooter on campus.

Campuses are reviewing the effectiveness of campus e-mail for emergency messaging. E-mail alerts can only reach campus community members who are either at their computers or who receive e-mail updates on their cell phones or PDAs, so campuses are also working to implement cell phone alert systems. The REVERSE 911 system uses database and geographic information system (GIS) mapping technologies to notify campus police and community members in the event of problems, whereas systems developed by companies such as Rave Wireless allow campus administrators to send out alerts in text, voice, e-mail, or instant message formats. Some campuses are programming the phone numbers, photographs, and basic student information for all incoming first-year students into a university security system, so that, in the event of a threat, students need only hit a button on their phones, whereupon campus police will be notified and tracking devices will pinpoint their location.

what do you think?

What types of safety and violence response resources are available to you on your campus? ● Does your school have a system for sending campus alerts to all students? ● Does it have an emergency plan in the event of a biological or physical threat to students?

Community Strategies for Preventing Violence

There are many steps you can take to ensure your own personal safety (see the **Skills for Behavior Change** box at right); however, it is also necessary to address the issues of violence and safety on a community level. Because the factors that contribute to violence are complex and interrelated, community strategies for prevention must also be multidimensional, focusing on individuals, schools, families, communities, policies, programs, and services designed to reduce risk. As part of the CDC's Injury Response initiatives, recommended strategies include a variety of interventions designed to prevent violence before it begins:

● Inoculate children against violence in the home. Youth exposed to physical and emotional abuse in their families are much more likely to victimize others. Teaching youth principles of respect and responsibility, and ensuring that their basic needs for safety, love, and security are met are fundamental to the health and well-being of future generations.

● Develop policies, intervention programs, and laws that prevent violence, such as counseling services, education programs focused on parenting skills or dating behavior, and assistance in giving individuals the confidence to protect themselves against physical and emotional assaults.

Stay Safe on All Fronts

There are many steps you can take to protect yourself from assault. Follow these tips to increase your awareness and reduce your risk of a violent attack.

OUTSIDE ALONE:

✳ Carry a cell phone, but stay off it. Be aware of what is happening around you.
✳ If you are being followed, don't go home. Head for a location where there are other people. If you decide to run, run fast and scream loudly to attract attention.
✳ Vary your routes; walk or jog with others at a steady pace. Stay close to others.
✳ Park near lights; avoid dark areas where people could hide.
✳ Carry pepper spray or other deterrents. Consider using your campus escort service.
✳ Tell others where you are going and when you expect to be back.

IN YOUR CAR:

✳ Lock your doors. Do not open your doors or windows to strangers.
✳ If someone hits you while you are driving, drive to the nearest gas station or other public place. Call the police or road service for help, and stay in your car until help comes.
✳ If a car appears to be following you, do not drive home. Drive to the nearest police station.

IN YOUR HOME:

✳ Install dead bolts on all doors and locks on all windows. Make sure the locks work, and don't leave a spare key outside. Consider installing a home alarm system.
✳ Lock doors when at home, even during the day. Close blinds and drapes whenever you are away and in the evening when you are home.
✳ Rent apartments that require a security code or clearance to gain entry, and avoid easily accessible apartments, such as first-floor units. When you move into a new residence, pay a locksmith to change the keys and locks.
✳ Don't let repair people in without asking for their identification, and have someone else with you when repairs are being made in your home or apartment.
✳ Keep a cell phone near your bed and program it to dial 911.
✳ If you return home to find your residence has been broken into, don't enter. Call the police. If you encounter an intruder, it is better to give up your money than to fight.

- Work with individuals and develop skills-based educational programs teaching basics of interpersonal communication and symptoms of healthy relationships, anger management, conflict resolution, peaceful negotiation, appropriate assertiveness, healthy coping, stress management, and other health-based behaviors.
- Begin early and through families, schools, community programs, athletics, music, faith-based groups, or wherever feasible, provide experiences that help youth develop self-esteem and confidence (self-efficacy).
- Promote tolerance and acceptance, and establish and enforce policies that forbid discrimination on the basis of religion, gender, race, sexual orientation, age, marital status, income, or other differences.
- Improve community services focused on family planning, mental health services, day care and respite care, alcohol, and substance abuse prevention.
- Improve community-based support and treatment for victims. Ensure that support services are available and that individuals have choices available when trying to stop the violence in their lives.

Unintentional Injuries

As stated at the beginning of the chapter, unintentional injuries occur without planning or intention to harm. Examples include car accidents, falls, boating accidents, accidental gunshots, recreational accidents, and workplace accidents. None of these injuries happen on purpose, yet they may result in pain, suffering, and possibly even death. Most efforts to prevent unintentional injuries focus on changing something about the person, the environment, or the circumstances (policies, procedures) that put people in harm's way. The **Health Today** box at right discusses the danger of unintentional hearing loss through noise exposure.

Two types of unintentional injuries that cause numerous deaths and injuries among young adults every year are motor vehicle crashes and cycling incidents. Motor vehicle accidents account for the most unintentional injury deaths, and bicycle injuries account for more than 500,000 emergency room visits every year. If you drive a car or ride a bicycle, you must be aware of what generally causes accidents and the steps you can take to help ensure your safety.

Vehicle Safety

Each year, about 40,000 Americans die in automobile crashes and another 1.9 million are disabled, 140,000 permanently. The risk of dying in an automobile crash is related to age. Young drivers (aged 16 to 24) have the highest death rate, owing to their inexperience and immaturity. However, driving drunk is the single greatest risk for drivers of all ages. Most car crashes are avoidable. The best way to prevent crashes is to avoid distracted or impaired driving, practice risk-management driving, and learn accident-avoidance techniques.

Risk-Management Driving Risk-management driving techniques, which help reduce the chances of being involved in a collision, include the following:

- Don't drink and drive
- Don't drive when tired or when in a highly emotional or stressed state
- Avoid distractions while driving, such as eating, using cell phones, or fiddling with stereo equipment.
- Surround your car with a safety "bubble." The rear bumper of the car ahead of you should be at least 3 seconds away.
- Scan the road ahead of you and to both sides.
- Drive with your low-beam headlights on, *day and night*, to make your car more visible to other drivers.
- Anticipate the actions of other drivers as much as you can, and be on the alert for unsignaled lane changes, sudden braking, or other unexpected manuevers.
- Obey all traffic laws.
- Whether you are the driver or a passenger, always wear a seat belt.

Accident-Avoidance Techniques To avoid a serious accident, you may need to steer into another, less severe collision. Here are the Automobile Association of America's (AAA) rules for accident avoidance:

- Generally, veer to the right.
- Steer, don't skid, off the road to avoid rolling your vehicle.
- If you have to hit a vehicle, hit one moving in the same direction as your own.
- If you have to hit a stationary object, try to hit a soft one (bushes, small trees) rather than a hard one (boulders, brick walls, giant trees).
- If you have to hit a hard object, hit it with a glancing blow.
- Avoid hitting pedestrians, motorcyclists, and bicyclists at all costs.

Wearing a helmet while biking can reduce the risk of head injury by 85%.

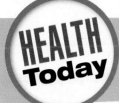

YOUNG BODIES, OLD EARS

It probably shouldn't surprise you that in a world where excess noise is a part of our daily existence, hearing loss is becoming increasingly common. In fact, more than 29 million U.S. adults have hearing loss. Noise-induced hearing loss results from high-decibel (dB) noise exposure, usually over extended periods of time, that damages sensory receptors in the cochlea, or inner ear. Common levels of noise for various exposures include normal conversation (60 dB); lawnmower (90 db); rock concert (115–150 dB+); bar/nightclub (110 dB); sporting event (110–140 dB); and portable listening devices such as MP3 players (90–120 dB). In general, noise levels above 85 dB increase risks for hearing loss. Hearing loss can be temporary or permanent, and in general worsens with age.

One of the highest rates of noise-induced hearing loss is among young adults aged 20 to 29. Hearing loss may be caused by one evening in front of huge speakers at a rock concert, or it may be the result of prolonged lower-level exposure from an iPod. Increasingly, teens and young adults are exposing themselves to dangerous noise levels through frequent use of earphones to listen to MP3 players and talk on cell phones. In-ear products such as earbuds and phone headsets are notably worse for long-term exposure than are over-ear headphones.

Ironically, although in a recent study many students (more than 75%) reported being aware that there is a danger of permanent hearing loss from exposure to hazardous noise, more than 50 percent continued to expose themselves. More than 66 percent of these students reported having experienced tinnitus (ringing in the ears), but most said they weren't worried about it. However, tinnitus can be a precursor to hearing loss, and students who experience it or find themselves frequently in noisy settings should take steps to avoid prolonged exposure. Most rock musicians use earplugs when performing or rehearsing, and their audiences would be wise to do the same. In addition, young adults should turn down the volumes on their stereos and MP3 players, and rest their ears in between nights out partying, or attending concerts

Earplugs let you enjoy the concert without risking permanent hearing loss.

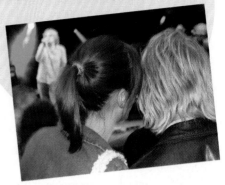

or sporting events. If other people can hear the music through your headset, it is too loud, and if you can't hear the person standing next to you at the concert, then you should put in earplugs or look for a quieter spot.

Sources: Y. Agrawal, E. Plaz, and J. Naparko, "Prevalence of Hearing Loss and Differences by Demographic Characteristics among U.S. Adults," *Archives of Internal Medicine* 168, no. 14 (2008): 1522–30; V. Rawool and L. Colligon-Wayne, "Auditory Lifestyles and Beliefs Related to Hearing Loss among College Students in the USA," *Noise and Health* 10, no. 38 (2008): 1–10.

Cycling Safety

Currently, more than 63 million Americans of all ages ride bicycles for transportation, recreation, and fitness. The Consumer Product Safety Commission reports about 800 deaths per year from cycling accidents. Approximately 87 percent of fatal collisions were due to cyclists' errors, usually failure to yield at intersections. Alcohol also plays a significant role in bicycle deaths and injuries. Cyclists should consider the following suggestions:

- Wear a helmet. It should be approved by American National Standards Institute (ANSI) or Snell.
- Don't drink and ride.
- Follow traffic laws and ride with the flow of traffic.
- Wear light reflective clothing that is easily seen at night and during the day.
- Avoid riding after dark.
- Know and use proper hand signals.
- Keep your bicycle in good working condition.
- Use bike paths whenever possible.
- Stop at stop signs and traffic lights.

Assess yourself

Are You at Risk for Violence?

How often are you at risk for sustaining an intentional or unintentional injury? Answer the questions below to find out.

PEARSON **myhealthlab**

Fill out this assessment online at www.pearsonhighered.com/myhealthlab or www.pearsonhighered.com/donatelle.

1 Relationship Risk

How often does your partner:

	Never	Sometimes	Often
1. Criticize you for your appearance (weight, dress, hair, etc.)?	○	○	○
2. Embarrass you in front of others by putting you down?	○	○	○
3. Blame you or others for his or her mistakes?	○	○	○
4. Curse at you, shout at you, say mean things, insult, or mock you?	○	○	○
5. Demonstrate uncontrollable anger?	○	○	○
6. Criticize your friends, family, or others who are close to you?	○	○	○
7. Threaten to leave you if you don't behave in a certain way?	○	○	○
8. Manipulate you to prevent you from spending time with friends or family?	○	○	○
9. Express jealousy, distrust, and anger when you spend time with other people?	○	○	○
10. Make all the significant decisions in your relationship?	○	○	○
11. Intimidate or threaten you, making you fearful or anxious?	○	○	○
12. Make threats to harm others you care about?	○	○	○
13. Control your telephone calls, listen in on your messages, or read your e-mail?	○	○	○
14. Punch, hit, slap, or kick you?	○	○	○
15. Gossip about you to turn others against you or make them think bad things about you?	○	○	○
16. Make you feel guilty about something?	○	○	○
17. Use money or possessions to control you?	○	○	○
18. Force you to have sex or perform sexual acts that make you uncomfortable?	○	○	○
19. Threaten to kill himself or herself if you leave?	○	○	○
20. Follow you, call to check on you, or demonstrate a constant obsession with what you are doing?	○	○	○

2 Risk for Assault or Rape

How often do you:

	Never	Sometimes	Often
1. Drink more than 1 or 2 drinks while out with friends or at a party?	○	○	○
2. Leave your drinks unattended while you get up to dance or go to the bathroom?	○	○	○
3. Accept drinks from strangers while out at a bar or party?	○	○	○
4. Leave parties with people you barely know or just met?	○	○	○
5. Walk alone in poorly lit or unfamiliar places?	○	○	○
6. Open the door to strangers?	○	○	○
7. Leave your car or home door unlocked?	○	○	○

3 Risk for Vehicular Injuries

How often do you:

	Never	Sometimes	Often
1. Drive after you have had one or two drinks?	○	○	○
2. Drive after you have had three or more drinks?	○	○	○
3. Drive when you are tired?	○	○	○
4. Drive while you are extremely upset?	○	○	○
5. Drive while talking on your cell phone?	○	○	○
6. Drive or ride in a car while not wearing a seat belt?	○	○	○
7. Drive faster than the speed limit?	○	○	○
8. Accept rides from friends who have been drinking?	○	○	○

120 | PART ONE | FINDING THE RIGHT BALANCE

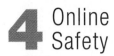

4 Online Safety

How often do you:

	Never	Sometimes	Often
1. Give out your name/address on the Internet?	○	○	○
2. Put personal identifying information on your blog, Web page, or networking sites?	○	○	○
3. Post personal pictures and other private material on networking sites like Facebook or MySpace?	○	○	○
4. Date people you meet online?	○	○	○
5. Use a shared or public computer to check e-mail without clearing the browser cache?	○	○	○
6. Make financial transactions online without confirming security measures?	○	○	○

Analyzing Your Responses

Now look at your responses to the list of questions in each of these sections. Part 1 focused on relationships—if you answered "sometimes" to one or more of these questions, you may be at risk for emotional or physical abuse. Typically, such potentially abusive patterns only get worse over time as a person gains control and power in a relationship. If you are anxious about talking to your partner, seek counseling through your campus counseling center, student health center, or community services. If you don't know where to go, ask your professor for possible options. In each of the other sections, if you answered "often" to any question, you may need to adjust your behavior and educate yourself about steps you can take to remain safe.

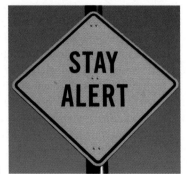

YOUR PLAN FOR CHANGE

The **Assess yourself** activity gave you a chance to consider symptoms of abuse in your relationships and signs of unsafe behavior in other realms of your life. Now that you are aware of these signs and symptoms, you can work on changing behaviors to reduce your risk.

Today, you can:

○ Pay attention as you walk your normal route around campus, and think about whether you are taking the safest route. Is it well lit? Do you walk in areas that receive little foot traffic? Are there any emergency phone boxes along your route? Does campus security patrol the area? If part of your route seems unsafe, look around for alternate routes.

○ Look at your residence's safety features. Is there a secure lock, dead bolt, or keycard entry system on all outer doors? Can windows be shut and locked? Is there a working smoke alarm in every room and hallway? Are the outside areas well lit? If you live in a dorm or apartment building, is there a security guard at the main entrance? If you notice any potential safety hazards, report them to your landlord or campus residential life administrator right away.

Within the next 2 weeks, you can:

○ If you are worried about potentially abusive behavior in a partner or in a friend's partner, visit the campus counseling center and ask about resources on campus or in your community to help you deal with potential relationship abuse. Consider talking to a counselor about your concerns or sitting in on a support group.

○ Next time you attend a party, set limits for yourself in order to remain in control of your behavior and to avoid putting yourself in a dangerous or compromising position. Decide ahead of time on the number of drinks you will have, arrange with a friend to monitor each other's behavior during the party, and be sure you have a reliable, safe way of getting home.

○ Purchase a hands-free device for your cell phone. Talking on a cell phone while driving is unsafe (and illegal in some states), but if you must make and answer calls while driving, a hands-free device will enable you to keep your hands on the wheel and your eyes on the road.

By the end of the semester, you can:

○ Learn ways to protect yourself by signing up for a self-defense workshop on campus or in the community.

○ Get involved in an on-campus or community group dedicated to promoting safety. You might want to attend a meeting of an antiviolence group, join in a Take Back the Night rally, or volunteer at a local rape crisis center or battered women's shelter.

Summary

✳ Violence in the form of intentional and unintentional injuries continues to be a major problem in the United States today, even though rates of homicide and other violent crimes seem to be on the decrease. Intentional injuries result from actions committed with the intent to do harm.

✳ Violence affects everyone in society—from the direct victims, to children and families who witness it, and those who modify their behaviors because they are fearful. Shootings and extreme acts of violence on campuses have resulted in a groundswell of activities that are designed to protect students and ensure their safety.

✳ Factors that lead people to be violent include anger, alcohol and substance abuse, discrimination, mental health problems, stress, poor coping skills, economic difficulties, fear/anxiety/insecurity at home, and a history of violence.

✳ Potential terrorist threats continue to result in fear, anxiety, and issues with discrimination enacted against people we regard as different. Bias-related and hate crimes divide people, but teaching tolerance can reduce risks. Gang violence continues to grow but can be combated by programs that reduce the problems that lead to gang membership.

✳ Sexual assault occurs in many forms; each form, including unwanted touching, stalking, harassment, and rape, can result in severe physical and emotional trauma or death. Recognizing how to protect yourself and your friends; knowing where to turn for help; and having honest, straightforward dialogue about sexual matters in dating situations are sound strategies to reduce risk. Alcohol moderation is another key factor in reducing your risks.

✳ Preventing violence is a public health priority. It means community activism; prioritizing mental and emotional health; and providing skills training in anger management, coping, parenting, and other key areas.

Pop Quiz

1. For an African American man aged 20 to 22 years, the probability of being murdered is
   a. 1 in 3.
   b. 1 in 28.
   c. 1 in 153.
   d. 1 in 450.

2. Emotional reaction brought about by frustrating life experiences is called
   a. reactive aggression.
   b. primary aggression.
   c. secondary aggression.
   d. tertiary aggression.

3. When Jane began her new job with all male coworkers, her supervisor told her that he enjoyed having an attractive woman in the workplace, and he winked at her. His comment constitutes
   a. acquaintance rape.
   b. sexual assault.
   c. sexual harassment.
   d. sexual battering.

4. Psychologist Lenore Walker developed a theory known as the
   a. aggression cycle.
   b. sexual harassment cycle.
   c. cycle of child abuse.
   d. cycle of violence.

5. What is the single greatest cause of injury to women?
   a. rape
   b. mugging
   c. auto accidents
   d. domestic violence

6. In a sociology class, a group of students was discussing sexual assault. One student commented that some women dress too provocatively. The social assumption this student made is
   a. minimization.
   b. trivialization.
   c. blaming the victim.
   d. "boys will be boys."

7. Rape by a person known to the victim and that does not involve a physical beating or use of a weapon is called
   a. simple rape.
   b. sexual assault.
   c. simple assault.
   d. aggravated rape.

8. Which of the following is not a cause of violence?
   a. cultural beliefs
   b. poverty
   c. lack of education
   d. unemployment

9. Which of the following is an example of stalking?
   a. making intimate and personal sexually charged comments to another person
   b. repeated visual or physical seeking out of another person
   c. an unwelcome sexual conduct by the perpetrator
   d. sexual abuse upon a child

10. Jack beats his wife Melissa "to teach her a lesson." Afterward, he denies attacking her. The phase of the cycle of violence that this illustrates is
    a. acute battering.
    b. chronic battering.
    c. remorse/reconciliation.
    d. tension building.

Answers to these questions can be found on page A-1.

Think about It!

1. What forms of violence do you think are most significant or prevalent in the United States today? Why? Are there some populations that are more susceptible than others to these forms of violence?

2. How do you think campus violence affects students at your school? Are there differences in how men and women respond to news that there has been a rape or violent assault on campus? If so, why?

3. Have you known anyone personally who has been sexually assaulted on campus? What actions were taken to help them cope with their assault? What campus services, if any, were utilized?

4. How worried are you that you will become a victim of a violent attack? Be accused of perpetrating a violent attack? What things are you worried about and why?

5. Should students be able to obtain licenses to carry concealed weapons on your campus? Why or why not? How would you feel if you were sitting next to someone with a handgun in his or her belt? How do you think your instructors would feel about having gun-toting students in their classes?

6. Why do some people develop into violent or abusive adults and others become pacifists or peaceful adults? What key factors influence violent offenders to be violent?

7. What actions need to be taken to stem the tide of violence in America? At the individual level? At the community level? In schools? On college campuses? Nationally?

Accessing Your Health on the Internet

The following websites explore further topics and issues related to personal health. For links to the websites below, visit the Companion Website for *Health: The Basics*, Green Edition at www.pearsonhighered.com/donatelle.

1. *Communities against Violence Network.* An extensive, searchable database for information about violence against women, with articles, legal information, and statistics. www.cavnet2.org

2. *Higher Education Center for Alcohol and Other Drug Abuse and Violence Prevention.* This division of the U.S. Department of Education helps college and community leaders create and implement programs and policies to address problems of violence and substance abuse on campuses. www.higheredcenter.org

3. *Men Can Stop Rape.* Practical suggestions for men interested in helping to protect women from sexual predators and assault. www.mencanstoprape.org

4. *National Center for Injury Prevention and Control.* The WISQARS database of this CDC section provides statistics and information on fatal and nonfatal injuries, both intentional and unintentional. www.cdc.gov/injury

5. *National Center for Victims of Crime.* Provides information and resources for victims of crimes ranging from hate crimes to sexual assault. www.ncvc.org

6. *National Sexual Violence Resource Center.* An excellent resource for victims of sexual violence. www.nsvrc.org

References

1. Herbert Hoover, Inaugural Address, March 4, 1929.
2. C. Silberman, *Criminal Violence, Criminal Justice* (New York, 1978), 22. The quotation is taken from a report by a U.S. Senate committee investigating crime in the city.
3. D. Mulvihillft, M. Tummin, and L. Curtis, *Crimes of Violence: A Staff Report to the National Commission on the Causes and Prevention of Violence*, U.S. Government Printing Office: 1 970 O 399-809, June 10, 1968.
4. World Health Organization, "World Report on Violence and Health," www.who.int/violence_injury_prevention/violence/world_report/en, 2009.
5. Society of Public Health Educators (SOPHE) Unintentional Injury and Violence Prevention, "Injury 101: Violence/Intentional Injury," www.sophe.org/ui/injury-violence.shtml, 2009.
6. Centers for Disease Control and Prevention (CDC), National Center for Health Statistics, *Health, United States, 2008, with Special Feature on the Health of Young Adults* (Hyattsville, MD: National Center for Health Statistics, 2009), figure 37.
7. Federal Bureau of Investigation, *Crime in the United States, Preliminary Semiannual Uniform Crime Report, 2008*, www.fbi.gov/ucr/2008prelim, 2009.
8. Ibid.
9. American College Health Association, *American College Health Association—National College Health Assessment II: Reference Group Data Report Fall 2008* (Baltimore: American College Health Association, 2009).
10. J. Carr, *American College Health Association Campus Violence White Paper* (Baltimore: American College Health Association, 2005).
11. A. Hoffman et al., eds., *Violence on Campus: Defining the Problems, Strategies for Action* (Gaithersburg, MD: Aspen, 1998), 1–40.
12. A. Gover, C. Kaukinen, and K. Fox, "The Relationship between Violence in the Family of Origin and Dating Violence among College Students," *Journal of Interpersonal Violence* 23, no. 12 (2008): 1667–1693.
13. Ibid.
14. Ibid.
15. M. Randolph, H. Torres, C. Gore-Felton, B. Lloyd, and E. McGarvey, "Alcohol Use and Sexual Risk Behavior among College Students: Understanding Gender and Ethnic Differences," *American Journal of Drug & Alcohol Abuse* 35, no. 2 (2009): 80–84; E. Reed, H. Amaro, A. Matsumoto, and D. Kaysen, "The Relation between Interpersonal Violence and Substance Use among a Sample of University Students: Examination of the Role of Victim and Perpetrator Substance Use," *Addictive Behaviors* 34, no. 3 (2009): 316–318; T. Messman-Moore, R. Ward, and A. Brown, "Substance Use and PTSD Symptoms Impact the Likelihood of Rape and Revictimization in College Women," *Journal of Interpersonal Violence* 24, no. 3 (2009): 499–521; H. Foley et al., "Adolescent Sexual Victimization, Use of Alcohol and Other Substances, and Other Health Risk Behaviors," *Journal of Adolescent Health* 4 (2004): 321–28.
16. M. Ybares, M. Diner-West, D. Markow, and P. Leaf, "Linkages between Internet and Other Media Violence with Serious Violent Behavior by Youth," *Pediatrics* 122, no. 5 (2008): 929–937; C. Anderson, A. Sakamoto, D. Gentile, N. Ihori, A. Shibuya, S. Yukawa, M. Naito, and K. Kobayashi, "Longitudinal Effects of Violent Video Games on Aggression in Japan and the United States," *Pediatrics* 122 (2008): e1067–e1072; J. Savage, "The Effects of Media Violence Exposure on Criminal Aggression," *Criminal Justice and Behavior* 35, no. 6 (2008): 772–791.
17. M. Ferguson, "Weak Results: Misleading Conclusions—Response to Anderson Article," *Pediatrics*, "eLetters," http://pediatrics.aappublications.org/cgi/eletters/122/5/e1067, 2008; C. Ferguson et al., "Personality, Parental and Media Influences on

Aggressive Personality and Violent Crime in Youth," *Journal of Aggression, Maltreatment and Trauma* 17, no. 4 (2008): 395–414; B. Wilson, "Media and Children's Aggression, Fear, and Altruism," *The Future of Children* 18, no. 1 (2008): 1550–54.

18. CDC, National Center for Health Statistics, *Health, United States, 2008*, 2009; National Center for Health Statistics, "Deaths: Final Data for 2006," *National Vital Statistics Report* 57, no. 14 (2009): table 10.

19. U.S. Department of Justice, Federal Bureau of Investigation (FBI), *Crime in the United States, Preliminary Semiannual Uniform Crime Report, 2008*, www.fbi.gov/ucr/2008prelim, 2009.

20. Federal Bureau of Investigation, "Hate Crime Statistics, 2007," www.fbi.gov/ucr/hc2007/index.html, November 2008.

21. C. Berlet, "Hate, Repression and the Apocalyptic Style: Facing Complex Questions and Challenges," *Journal of Hate Studies* 3 (2004): 145–58.

22. J. Carr, *American College Health Association Campus Violence White Paper*, 2005; U.S. Department of Justice, FBI, "Hate Crime Statistics, 2007," November 2008.

23. National Youth Violence Prevention Resource Center, "Youth Gangs and Violence," www.safeyouth.org/scripts/faq/youthgang.asp. Updated January 4, 2008.

24. U.S. Code of Federal Regulations, Title 28CFRO.85.

25. P. Klaus, *National Crime Victimization Survey: Crime and the Nation's Households, 2005* (Washington DC: Bureau of Justice Statistics, 2007), DOJ (US) NCJ217198.

26. M. Rand and S. Catalano, *National Crime Victimization Survey: Criminal Victimization, 2007* (Washington DC: Bureau of Justice Statistics, 2008), DOJ (US) NCJ224390.

27. J. Chang, C. Berg, L. Saltzman, and J. Herndon, "Homicide: A Leading Cause of Injury Deaths among Pregnant and Postpartum Women in the United States, 1991–1999," *American Journal of Public Health* 96, no. 3 (2005): 471–77.

28. Violence Policy Center, *American Roulette: Murder-Suicide in the United States*. 3d ed. (Washington, DC: Violence Policy Center, 2008).

29. L. Rosen and J. Fontaine, *Compendium of Research on Violence Against Women, 1993–2008* (Washington, DC: National Institute of Justice, 2008).

30. N. West, "Crimes against Women," *Community Safety Quarterly* 5 (1992): 3.

31. L. Rosen and J. Fontaine, *Compendium of Research on Violence against Women* 2008.

32. National Center for Injury Prevention and Control, "Child Maltreatment: Facts at a Glance," www.cdc.gov/ViolencePrevention/pdf/CM_Data_Sheet-Spring09-a.pdf, 2009.

33. U.S. Department of Health and Human Services, Administration on Children, Youth and Families, *Child Maltreatment 2007* (Washington, DC: U.S. Government Printing Office, 2009).

34. Ibid.

35. E. F. Wood, "The Availability and Utility of Interdisciplinary Data on Elder Abuse: A White Paper for the National Center on Elder Abuse," National Center on Elder Abuse and American Bar Association Commission on Law and Aging, www.ncea.aoa.gov/NCEAroot/Main_Site/pdf/publication/WhitePaper060404.pdf, May 2006.

36. D. Dancy and B. Uekert, "The Aging of America, the Rise of Elder Abuse and Its Impact on Judicial Education," *NASJENewsQuarterly*, http://nasje.org/news/newsletter0703/resources02.htm, July 2007.

37. CDC, National Center for Injury Prevention and Control, "Sexual Violence: Facts at a Glance," www.cdc.gov/ncipc/dvp/SV/SVDataSheet.pdf, Spring 2008.

38. Ibid.

39. D. Kilpatrick et al., "Drug-Facilitated, Incapacitated, and Forcible Rape: A National Study," National Crime Victims Research and Treatment Center, www.ncjrs.gov/pdffiles1/nij/grants/219181.pdf, February 1, 2007.

40. CDC, National Center for Injury Prevention and Control, "Sexual Violence," 2008.

41. M. Rand and S. Catalano, *National Crime Victimization Survey: Criminal Victimization, 2007*, 2008.

42. Ibid.

43. CDC, National Center for Injury Prevention and Control, "Sexual Violence," 2008; L. Schneider, L. Mori, P. Lambert, and A. Wong, "The Role of Gender and Ethnicity in Perceptions of Rape and Its Aftereffects," *Sex Roles*, 60, no. 5/6 (2009): 410–21.

44. Ibid.

45. J. Carr, *American College Health Association Campus Violence White Paper*, 2005.

46. J. Butcher, S. Mineka, and J. Hooley, *Abnormal Psychology*. 13th ed. (Boston: Allyn & Bacon, 2007).

47. D. Kilpatrick et al., "Drug-Facilitated, Incapacitated, and Forcible Rape," 2007.

48. CDC, National Center for Injury Prevention and Control, "Sexual Violence," 2008.

49. University of Illinois at Chicago, "Most Sexual Assaults Drug Facilitated, Study Claims," *ScienceDaily*, www.sciencedaily.com/releases/2006/05/060513122928.htm, May 13, 2006. Retrieved May 18, 2008.

50. R. Bergen and E. Barnhill, "Marital Rape," 2006.

51. World Health Organization, "Prevention of Child Maltreatment," www.who.int/violence_injury_prevention/violence/neglect/en, 2006.

52. CDC, National Center for Injury Prevention and Control, "Sexual Violence," 2009.

53. A. Gover, C. Kaukinen, and K. Fox, "The Relationship between Violence in the Family of Origin and Dating Violence among College Students," *Journal of Interpersonal Violence* 23, no. 12 (2008): 1667–93.

54. University of Wisconsin-Madison, "Sexual Harassment Information and Resources," www.oed.wisc.edu/sexualharassment/what.html, Updated February 2, 2007.

55. K. Baum, S. Catalano, M. Rand, and K. Rose. *National Crime Victimization Survey: Stalking Victimization in the United States* (Washington DC: Bureau of Justice Statistics, 2008), DOJ (US) NCJ224527.

56. Ibid.

57. CDC Injury Center, "Preventing Intimate Partner Violence, Sexual Violence and Child Maltreatment," www.cdc.gov/ncipc/pub-res/research_agenda/07_violence.htm, 2006; P. Benson et al., "Acquaintance Rape on Campus," *Journal of American College Health* 40 (1992): 157–65; M. M. York, "Traditional Gender Role Attitudes and Violence against Women: A Test of Feminist Theory," Paper presented at the annual meeting of the American Society of Criminology, www.allacademic.com/meta/p200649_index.html, November 13, 2007. Accessed June 2008.

58. J. Carr, *American College Health Association Campus Violence White Paper*, 2005.

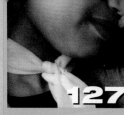
127

Does an intimate relationship have to be sexual?

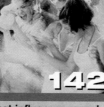
132

To what extent do people communicate without words?

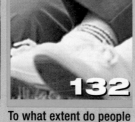
142

What influences sexual identity besides biology?

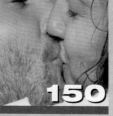
150

What is "normal" sexual behavior?

Healthy Relationships and Sexuality

5

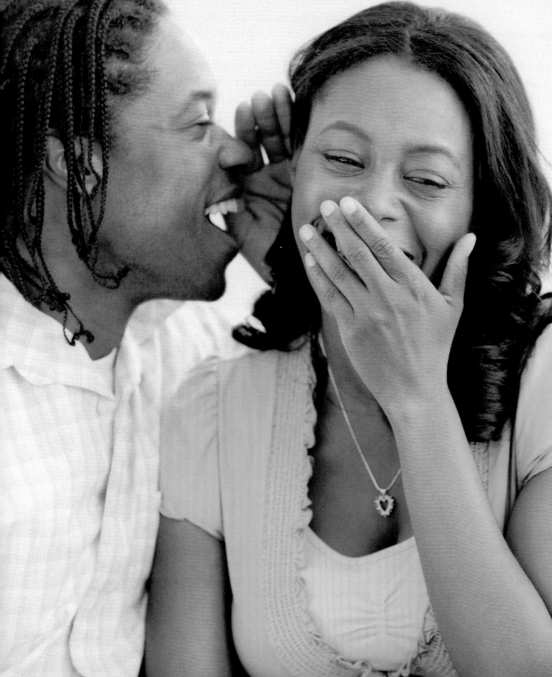

Objectives

✳ Discuss ways to improve communication skills and interpersonal interactions.

✳ Identify the characteristics of successful relationships, including how to maintain them and overcome common barriers.

✳ Examine factors that affect life decisions, such as whether to have children.

✳ Define *sexual identity,* and discuss its major components, including biology, gender identity, gender roles, and sexual orientation.

✳ Identify major features and functions of sexual anatomy and physiology.

✳ Classify sexual dysfunctions, and describe major disorders.

✳ Explain the nature of human sexual response and the variety of sexual expression.

Humans are social beings—we have a basic need to belong and to feel loved, appreciated, and wanted. We can't live without relating to and interacting with others in some way. In fact, some research suggests that the ability to relate well with people, as well as give and receive love and support throughout your life, can have almost as much impact on your health as exercise and good nutrition.[1]

All relationships involve a degree of risk. However, only by taking these risks can we grow and truly experience all that life has to offer. By looking at our intimate and nonintimate relationships, components of sexual identity, gender roles, and sexual orientation, we will come to better understand who we are.

Characterizing and Forming Intimate Relationships

We can define **intimate relationships** in terms of four characteristics: behavioral interdependence, need fulfillment, emotional attachment, and emotional availability. Each of these characteristics may be related to interactions with family, close friends, and romantic partners.

Behavioral interdependence refers to the mutual impact that people have on each other as their lives and daily activities intertwine. What one person does influences what the other person wants to do and can do. Behavioral interdependence may become stronger over time to the point that each person would feel a great void if the other were gone.

intimate relationships
Relationships with family members, friends, and romantic partners, characterized by behavioral interdependence, need fulfillment, emotional attachment, and emotional availability.

Intimate relationships also fulfill psychological needs and so are a means of *need fulfillment*. Through relationships with others, we fulfill our needs for

- **Intimacy**—someone with whom we can share our feelings freely

- **Social integration**—someone with whom we can share worries and concerns
- **Nurturance**—someone whom we can take care of and who will take care of us
- **Assistance**—someone to help us in times of need
- **Affirmation**—someone who will reassure us of our own worth and tell us that we matter

In intimate relationships that are mutually rewarding, partners and friends meet each other's needs. They disclose feelings, share confidences, and provide support and reassurance. Each person comes away from interactions feeling better for the experience and validated by the other person.

In addition to behavioral interdependence and need fulfillment, intimate relationships involve strong bonds of *emotional attachment,* or feelings of love. When we hear the word *intimacy,* we often think of a sexual relationship. Although sex can play an important role in emotional attachment, a relationship can be very intimate and yet not sexual. Two people can be emotionally intimate (share feelings) or spiritually intimate (share spiritual beliefs and meanings), or they can be intimate friends. With such a range of possibilities, the intimacy level that two people experience cannot be judged easily by those outside the relationship (Figure 5.1).

Emotional availability, the ability to give to and receive from others emotionally without fear of being hurt or rejected, is the fourth characteristic of intimate relationships. At times, all of us may limit our emotional availability. For example, after a painful breakup we may decide not to jump into another relationship immediately, or we may decide not to talk about it with every friend. Holding back can offer time for introspection and healing, as well as for considering the lessons learned. However, some people who have experienced intense trauma find it difficult ever to be fully available emotionally. This limits their ability to experience intimate relationships.

In the early years of life, families provide the most significant relationships. Gradually, the circle widens to include friends, coworkers, and acquaintances. Ultimately, most of us develop romantic or sexual relationships with significant others. Each of these relationships plays a significant role in psychological, social, spiritual, and physical health.

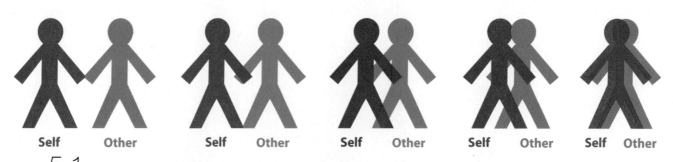

Self **Other**   **Self** **Other**   **Self** **Other**   **Self** **Other**   **Self** **Other**

FIGURE 5.1 **How Intimate Is a Relationship?**
Relationships can exist on a continuum of closeness and inclusion. Asking people to choose the diagram that best portrays a particular relationship of theirs does a remarkably good job of assessing the closeness they feel.
Source: Adapted from A. Aron, D. J. Mashek, and E. N. Aron, "Closeness as Including the Other in the Self," in *Handbook of Closeness and Intimacy,* eds. D. J. Mashek and A. Aron (Mahwah, NJ: Erlbaum, 2004), 27–41. Copyright © Taylor & Francis. Used with permission.

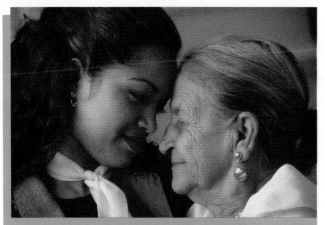

Does an intimate relationship have to be sexual?

We may be accustomed to hearing "intimacy" used to describe romantic or sexual relationships, but intimate relationships can take many forms. The emotional bonds that characterize intimate relationships often span the generations and help individuals gain insight and understanding into each other's worlds.

Being Self-Nurturant

You have probably heard the notion that you must love yourself before you can love someone else. What does this mean? Learning how you function emotionally and how to nurture yourself through all life's situations is a lifelong task. You should certainly not postpone intimate connections with others until you achieve this state. However, a certain level of individual maturity helps in maintaining a committed relationship.

Two concepts that are especially important to any good relationship are *accountability* and *self-nurturance*. **Accountability** means that both partners see themselves as responsible for their own decisions, choices, and actions. They don't hold the other person responsible for positive or negative experiences. **Self-nurturance,** which goes hand in hand with accountability, means developing individual potential through a balanced and realistic appreciation of self-worth and ability. To make good choices in life, a person must balance many physical and emotional needs, including sleeping, eating, exercising, working, relaxing, and socializing. When the balance is disrupted, as inevitably it will be at times, self-nurturing people are patient with themselves and try to put things back on course. It is a lifelong process to learn to live in a balanced and healthy way. Partners who are both on a path of accountability and self-nurturance have a much better chance of maintaining a satisfying relationship with each other.

Families: The Ties That Bind

A family is a recognizable group of people with roles, tasks, boundaries, and personalities whose central focus is to protect, care for, love, and socialize one another (Figure 5.2). Because the family is a dynamic institution that changes as society changes, the definition of *family*, and those individuals believed to constitute family membership, changes over time as well. Who are members of today's families? Historically, most families have been made up of people related by blood, marriage or long-term committed relationships, or adoption.[2] Yet today, many other groups of people are being recognized and are functioning as family units. Although there is no "best" family type, we do know that a healthy family's key roles and tasks are to nurture and support.

Healthy families foster a sense of security and feelings of belonging that are central to growth and development. It is from our **family of origin,** the people present in our household during our first years of life, that we initially learn about feelings, problem solving, love, intimacy, and gender roles. We learn to negotiate relationships and have opportunities to communicate effectively; develop attitudes and values; and explore spiritual belief systems. It is not uncommon when we establish relationships outside the family to rely on these initial experiences and on skills modeled by our family of origin.

accountability Accepting responsibility for personal decisions, choices, and actions.

self-nurturance Developing individual potential through a balanced and realistic appreciation of self-worth and ability.

family of origin People present in the household during a child's first years of life—usually parents and siblings.

Establishing Friendships

Good friends—they can make a boring day fun, a cold day warm, or a gut-wrenching worry disappear. They can make us feel that we matter and that we have the strength to get through just about anything. They can also make us angry,

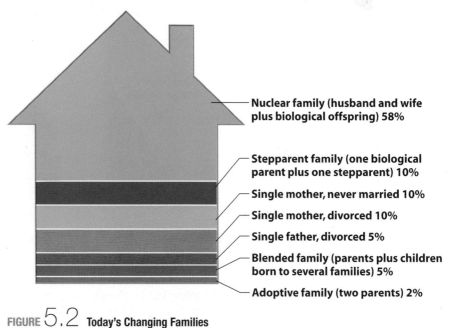

- Nuclear family (husband and wife plus biological offspring) 58%
- Stepparent family (one biological parent plus one stepparent) 10%
- Single mother, never married 10%
- Single mother, divorced 10%
- Single father, divorced 5%
- Blended family (parents plus children born to several families) 5%
- Adoptive family (two parents) 2%

FIGURE 5.2 **Today's Changing Families**

Source: Based on data from the U.S. Census Bureau, 2000.

disappoint us, or seriously jolt our comfortable ideas about right and wrong.

Friendships are relationships between two or more people that involve mutual respect, trust, support, and intimacy that may or may not include sexual intimacy. Like our family relationships, our friendships should have identified roles and boundaries. Persons in friendships should communicate their understandings, needs, expectations, limitations, and affections.[3]

Psychologists believe that people are attracted to and form relationships with people who give them positive reinforcement and that they dislike those who punish or overcriticize them. The basic idea is simple: You like people who like you. Another factor that affects the development of a friendship is a real or perceived similarity in attitudes, opinions, and background.[4] In addition, true friends have a sense of equity in which they share confidences, contribute fairly and equally to maintaining the friendship, and consistently try to give as much as they get back from the interactions.[5]

Take a few minutes to examine one of your current friendships. What characteristics can you identify in that relationship that keep your friendship intact?

Significant Others, Partners, and Couples

Most people choose at some point to enter into an intimate sexual relationship with another person. Most committed partners fit into one of four categories: married heterosexual couples, cohabitating heterosexual couples, lesbian couples, and gay male couples. These groups are discussed in greater detail later in this chapter.

Love relationships in each of these four groups typically include all the characteristics of friendship as well as the following characteristics related to passion and caring:[6]

● **Fascination.** Lovers tend to pay attention to the other person even when they should be involved in other activities. They are preoccupied with the other and want to think about, talk to, or be with the other.

● **Exclusiveness.** Lovers have a special relationship that usually precludes having the same relationship with a third party. The love relationship often takes priority over all others.

● **Sexual desire.** Lovers desire physical intimacy and want to touch, hold, and engage in sexual activities with the other.

● **Giving the utmost.** Lovers care enough to give the utmost when the other is in need, sometimes to the point of extreme sacrifice.

● **Being a champion or advocate.** Lovers actively champion each other's interests and attempt to ensure that the other succeeds.

This Thing Called Love

What is love? This four-letter word has been written about and sung about; it has been the theme of countless novels, movies, and plays. There is no single definition of *love*, and the word may mean different things to people, depending on cultural values, age, gender, and situation. Yet, we all know what it is when it strikes.

Many social scientists maintain that love may be of two kinds: companionate and passionate. Companionate love is a secure, trusting attachment, similar to what we may feel for family members or close friends. In companionate love, two people are attracted, have much in common, care about each other's well-being, and express reciprocal liking and respect. Passionate love, in contrast, is a state of high arousal filled with the ecstasy of being loved and the potential agony of being rejected.[7]

Theories of Love

How and why love develops are not easy questions to answer. Several theories have been proposed to help provide insight into the process. Sternberg's classic Triangular Theory of Love (Figure 5.3) suggests that there are three key components to loving relationships:[8]

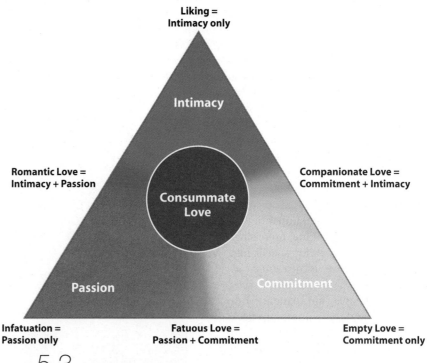

FIGURE 5.3 **Sternberg's Triangular Theory of Love**
According to Sternberg's model, three elements—intimacy, passion, and commitment—existing alone or in combination form different types of love. The most complete, ideal type of love in the model is consummate love, which combines balanced amounts of all three elements.

1. **Intimacy**—the emotional component, which involves closeness, sharing, and mutual support
2. **Passion**—the motivational component, which includes lust, attraction, and sexual arousal
3. **Commitment**—the cognitive component, which includes the decision to be open to love in the short term and the commitment to the relationship in the long term

The quality of love relationships is reflected by the level of intimacy, passion, and commitment each person brings to the relationship over time.

A second theory of love and attraction, based on brain circuitry and chemistry, is quite different from that of Sternberg. Anthropologist Helen Fisher, among others, hypothesizes that attraction and falling in love follow a fairly predictable pattern based on (1) *imprinting,* in which our evolutionary patterns, genetic predispositions, and past experiences trigger a romantic reaction; (2) *attraction,* in which neurochemicals produce feelings of euphoria and elation; (3) *attachment,* in which endorphins—natural opiates—cause lovers to feel peaceful, secure, and calm; and (4) *production of a cuddle chemical,* in which the brain secretes the hormone *oxytocin,* thereby stimulating sensations during lovemaking and eliciting feelings of satisfaction and attachment.[9]

Lovers who claim that they are swept away by passion may not be far from the truth. Why? Because the love-smitten person's endocrine system secretes chemical substances such as dopamine, norepinephrine, and phenylethylamine (PEA), which are chemical cousins to amphetamines.[10] Although attraction may in fact be a "natural high," this hit of passion loses effectiveness over time as the body builds up tolerance. Many people may become attraction junkies, seeking the intoxication of love much as the drug user seeks a chemical high. Fisher speculates that PEA levels drop significantly over a 3- to 4-year period, leading to the "4-year itch" that shows up in the peaking fourth-year divorce rates present in over 60 cultures. Romances that last beyond the 4-year mark are influenced by another set of chemicals, known as endorphins, soothing substances that give lovers a sense of security, peace, and calm.[11]

Picking Partners

For both men and women, choosing a relationship partner is influenced by more than just chemical and psychological processes. One important factor is *proximity,* or being in the same place at the same time. The more often that you see a person in your hometown, at social gatherings, or at work, the more likely that interaction will occur. Thus, if you live in New York, you'll probably end up with another New Yorker. With the advent of the Internet, however, geographic proximity has become less important.

You also choose a partner based on *similarities* (in attitudes, values, intellect, interests, education, and socioeconomic status); the old adage that "opposites attract" usually isn't true. If your potential partner expresses interest or liking, you may react with mutual regard known as *reciprocity.* The more you express interest, the safer it is for someone else to return the regard, and the cycle spirals onward.

A final factor that plays a significant role in selecting a partner is *physical attraction.* Whether such attraction is caused by a chemical reaction or a socially learned behavior, men and women appear to have different attraction criteria. When selecting mates, men tend to be attracted primarily to youth and beauty, while women tend to be attracted to older mates and to place higher emphasis on partners who have good financial prospects and who appear to be dependable and industrious.[12]

what do you think?

What factors do you consider most important in a potential partner? ● Which are absolute musts? ● Are there any differences between what you believe to be important in a relationship and the things your parents feel are important?

Communicating: A Key to Good Relationships

From the moment of birth, we struggle to be understood. We flail our arms, cry, scream, smile, frown, and make sounds and gestures to attract attention, get a reaction from someone we care about, or have someone understand what we want or need from him or her. By the time we enter adulthood, each of us has developed a unique way of communicating to others with gestures, words, expressions, and body positions. No two of us communicate in the exact same way or have the same need for connecting with others. Some of us are outgoing and quick to express our emotions and thoughts. Others are quiet, are reluctant to talk about feelings, and may prefer to spend time alone rather than with others.

Different cultures have unique languages and dialects, as well as different ways of expressing feelings and using body language. Some cultures gesture wildly; others maintain a closed and rigid means of speaking. Some are offended by direct eye contact; others welcome a steady look in the eyes. Men and women also tend to have different styles of communication, which are often largely dictated by culture and socialization (see the **Gender & Health** box on page 130).

There's more to good communication than just the ability to gab.

He Says/She Says

Women

FACIAL EXPRESSIONS
Smile and nod more often
Maintain better eye contact

SPEECH PATTERNS
Higher pitched, softer voices
Use approximately 5 speech tones
May sound more emotional
Make more tentative statements
Interrupt less often

BODY LANGUAGE
Take up less space
Gesture toward the body
Lean forward when listening
More gentle when touching others
More feedback via body language

BEHAVIORAL DIFFERENCES
More emotional approach
Express intimate feelings more readily
Tendency to hold grudges
Give more compliments
Gossip more
More likely to ask for help
Tend to take rejection more personally
Apologize more frequently
Talk is primarily a means of rapport, establishing connections, and negotiating relationships

Men

FACIAL EXPRESSIONS
Frown more often
Often avoid eye contact

SPEECH PATTERNS
Lower pitched, louder voices
Use approximately 3 speech tones
May sound more abrupt
Make more direct statements
More likely to interrupt

BODY LANGUAGE
Occupy more space
Gesture away from the body
Lean back when listening
More forceful gestures
Less feedback via body language

BEHAVIORAL DIFFERENCES
More inclined to be analytical
Have more difficulty in expressing intimate feelings
Hold fewer grudges
Give fewer compliments
Gossip less
Less likely to ask for help
Tend to take rejection less personally
Apologize less often
Talk is primarily a means of preserving independence and negotiating and maintaining status

Although men and women may make decisions differently, act differently in terms of their sexual and partnering behaviors, and act in ways that are somewhat distinctive to their genders, these lines have begun to blur over time. Books such as *Men Are from Mars, Women Are from Venus* that focus on these differences capture media attention, but they also have their critics.

According to Dr. Cynthia Burggraf Torppa at Ohio State University, differences in communication between men and women are really quite minor. What is most important, she says, is the way in which men and women interpret or process the same message. She indicates that studies support the idea that women, to a greater extent than men, are sensitive to the interpersonal meanings that lie between the lines in the messages they exchange with their mates. This is because societal expectations often make women responsible for regulating intimacy. Men, on the other hand, are more sensitive than women to subtle messages about status. For them, societal expectations dictate that they negotiate hierarchy, or who's the captain and who's the crew.

Within our society and in light of these general trends, there are some gender-specific communication patterns and behaviors that are obvious to the casual observer (see the figure). Recognizing these differences and how they make us unique is a good first step in avoiding unnecessary frustrations and irritations.

Sources: C. Burggraf Torppa, "Gender Issues: Communication Differences in Interpersonal Relationships," Family Life Packet, 2002, http://ohioline.osu.edu/flm02/FS04.html; J. Wood, *Gendered Lives: Communication, Gender, and Culture.* 8th ed. (Belmont, CA: Wadsworth, 2008); M. L. Knapp and A. L. Vangelisti, *Interpersonal Communication and Human Relationships.* 5th ed. (Boston: Allyn & Bacon, 2004).

Although people differ in the way they communicate, this doesn't mean that one sex, culture, or group is better at it than another. We have to be willing to accept differences and work to keep communication lines open and fluid. Remaining interested, actively engaged in the interaction, and open and willing to exchange ideas and thoughts is something that we typically learn with practice and hard work.

Self-Esteem and Self-Acceptance

Important factors that affect your communication effectiveness include the way you define yourself (*self-concept*) and the way you evaluate yourself (*self-esteem*). Your self-concept is like a mental mirror that reflects how you view your physical features, emotional states, talents, likes and dislikes, values, and roles.[13] Are you an athlete, a mother, an honor student, an activist, a pianist? How you define yourself is your self-concept. How you feel about yourself or evaluate yourself constitutes your self-esteem. You might consider yourself an excellent student, a horrible singer, a great lover, or a "10" in terms of appearance—such judgments indicate your level of self-esteem or self-evaluation.

When two people begin a relationship, they bring their past communication styles with them. How often have you heard someone say, "We just can't communicate" or "You're sending me mixed messages"? These exchanges occur regularly as people start relationships or work through ongoing communication problems in an existing relationship. Because communication is a process, our every action, word, facial expression, gesture, or body posture becomes part of our shared experience and part of the evolving impression we make on others. If we are angry in our responses, others will be reluctant to interact with us. If we bring "baggage" from past bad interactions to new relationships, we may be cynical, distrustful, and guarded in our exchanges with others. If we are positive, happy, and share openly with others, they will be more likely to communicate openly with us. This ability to communicate assertively is an important skill in relationships. Assertive communicators are in touch with their feelings and values and can communicate their needs directly and honestly to defend choices in a positive manner.

Self-perceptions influence communication choices. If you feel unattractive, uncomfortable, or inferior to others, you may choose not to interact with them or to avoid social events. If you are self-conscious and ill at ease around people who seem different, you might avoid or be suspicious of them. Conversely, if you are secure about your unique characteristics and talents, that positive self-concept will make it easier to interact with a variety of people in a healthy, balanced way.

Learning Appropriate Self-Disclosure

Sharing personal information with others is called **self-disclosure.** If you are willing to share personal information with others, they will likely share personal information with you. In other words, if you want to learn more about someone, you have to be willing to share parts of your personal self with that person. Self-disclosure is not storytelling or sharing secrets; rather, it is revealing how you are reacting to the present situation and giving any information about the past that is relevant to the other person's understanding of your current reactions.

Self-disclosure can be a double-edged sword, for there is risk in divulging personal insights and feelings. If you sense that sharing feelings and personal thoughts will result in a closer relationship, you will likely take

self-disclosure Sharing personal feelings or information with others.

such a risk. But if you believe that the disclosure may result in rejection or alienation, you may not open up so easily. If the confidentiality of previously shared information has been violated, you may hesitate to disclose yourself in the future.

However, the risk in not disclosing yourself to others is that you will lack intimacy in relationships. Psychologist Carl Rogers stressed the importance of understanding yourself and others through self-disclosure. Rogers believed that weak relationships were characterized by inhibited self-disclosure.[14]

If self-disclosure is a key element in creating healthy communication, but fear is a barrier to that process, what can we do? The following suggestions can help:

- **Get to know yourself.** Remember that your self includes your feelings, beliefs, thoughts, and concerns. The more you know about yourself, the more likely you will be able to communicate with others about yourself.
- **Become more accepting of yourself.** No one is perfect or has to be.
- **Be willing to discuss your sexual history.** In a culture that puts many taboos on discussions of sex in everyday conversation, it's no wonder we find it hard to disclose our sexual feelings to those with whom we are intimate. However, with the soaring rate of sexually transmitted infections and the ever-looming threat of AIDS, there has never been a more important time to disclose sexual feelings and history. The life-altering effects of an unwanted pregnancy or contracting HIV underscore the need to communicate about sex before you become intimate.
- **Choose a safe context for self-disclosure.** When and where you make such disclosures and to whom may greatly influence the response. Choose a setting in which you feel safe to let yourself be known.

Are You Really Listening?

Most of us have lamented the fact that someone "never listens" and seems to monopolize the entire conversation. Although we are quick to recognize such flaws in others, we are often less likely to spot listening problems of our own. What does it take to be an excellent listener? Try practicing the following skills and consciously using them on a daily basis:

✽ Be present in the moment. Good listeners participate and acknowledge what the other person is saying. Nodding, smiling, saying "yes" or "uh-huh," and asking questions at appropriate times all convey that you are attentive. Use positive body language and voice tone.

✽ Show empathy and sympathy. Watch for verbal and nonverbal clues to the other person's feelings and try to relate.

✽ Ask for clarification. If you aren't sure what the speaker means, indicate that you're not sure you understand, or paraphrase what you think you heard.

✽ Control that deadly desire to interrupt. Try taking a deep breath for 2 seconds, then hold your breath for another second and really listen to what is being said as you slowly exhale.

✽ Avoid snap judgments based on what other people look like or are saying.

✽ Resist the temptation to "set the other person straight."

✽ Try to focus on the speaker. Hold back the temptation to launch into your own rendition of a similar situation.

✽ Be tenacious. Stick with the speaker and try to stay on topic. If the person seems to wander, gently bring the topic back by saying, "You were just saying . . . ".

✽ Offer your thoughts and suggestions, but remember that you should advise only up to a certain point. Clarify statements with "This is my opinion" as a reminder that it is only a viewpoint rather than a fact.

we are in the mood to listen (free of distractions and worries). When we really listen effectively, we try to understand what people are thinking and feeling from their perspective. We not only hear the words, but also try to understand what is really being said. How many times have you been caught pretending to listen when you were not? After several moments of nodding and saying, "Uh-huh," your friend finally asks you a question, and you haven't a clue what she has been saying. Sometimes this tuned-out behavior is due to lack of sleep, stress overload, being preoccupied, having had too much to drink, or being under the influence of drugs. Other times the reason is that the speaker is a motormouth who talks for the sake of talking, or that you find the speaker or topic of conversation boring. Some of the most common listening difficulties are things that we can work to improve. See the **Skills for Behavior Change** box at left for suggestions to improve your listening.

Using Nonverbal Communication

Understanding what someone is saying often involves much more than listening and speaking. Often, what is not actually said may speak louder than any words. Rolling the eyes, looking at the floor or ceiling rather than maintaining eye contact, making body movements and hand gestures—all these nonverbal clues influence the way we interpret messages. **Nonverbal communication** includes all unwritten and unspoken messages, both intentional and unintentional. Ideally, our nonverbal communication matches and

Becoming a Better Listener

Listening is a vital part of interpersonal communication; it allows us to share feelings, express concerns, communicate wants and needs, and let our thoughts and opinions be known. We must do the necessary work to improve both our speaking and listening skills, which will enhance our relationships, improve our grasp of information, and allow us to interpret more effectively what others say. We listen best when (1) we believe that the message is somehow important and relevant to us; (2) the speaker holds our attention through humor, dramatic effect, use of media, or other techniques; and (3)

nonverbal communication All unwritten and unspoken messages, both intentional and unintentional.

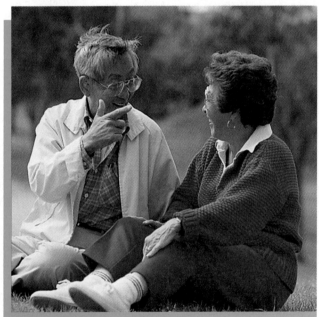

To what extent do people communicate without words?

Researchers have found that 93% of communication effectiveness is determined by nonverbal cues. Positive communication means using positive body language. Laughing, smiling, and gesturing all help convey meaning and assure your partner you are engaged.

supports our verbal communication. This is not always the case. Research shows that when verbal and nonverbal communications don't match, we are more likely to believe the nonverbal cues.[15] This is one reason why it is important to be aware of all the nonverbal cues we use regularly and to understand how others might interpret them.

Nonverbal communication can include the following:[16]

- **Touch.** This can be a handshake, a warm hug, a hand on the shoulder, or a kiss on the cheek.
- **Gestures.** These can include physical mannerisms that replace words, such as a thumbs-up or a wave hello or good-bye, or movements that augment verbal communication, such as fanning your face when you are hot or indicating with your hands the size of the fish that got away. Gestures can also be rude, such as glancing at one's watch, shifting weight from foot to foot, and evasive eye movements.
- **Interpersonal space.** This is the amount of physical space that separates two people.
- **Facial expressions.** These can signal moods and emotions and often have universal meaning.
- **Body language.** This includes things like folding your arms across your chest, crossing your legs, or leaning forward in your chair.
- **Tone of voice.** This refers not to what you say, but how you say it—the elements of speaking that color the use of words, such as pitch, volume, and speed.

To communicate as effectively as possible, it is important to recognize and use nonverbal cues that support and help clarify your verbal messages. Awareness and practice of your verbal and nonverbal communication will also enhance your skills in interpreting others' messages.

Committed Relationships

Commitment in a relationship means that one intends to act over time in a way that perpetuates the well-being of the other person, oneself, and the relationship. Polls show that the majority of Americans—as many as 96 percent—strive to develop a committed relationship, even though many have difficulty maintaining them. These relationships can take several forms, including marriage, cohabitation, and gay and lesbian partnerships.

Marriage

In many societies around the world, traditional committed relationships take the form of marriage. In the United States, marriage means entering into a legal agreement that includes shared financial plans, property, and responsibility for raising children. Many Americans also view marriage as a religious sacrament that emphasizes certain rights and obligations for each spouse.

Historically, close to 90 percent of Americans marry at least once during their lifetime, although in recent years Americans have become less likely to marry. From 1960 to 2005, annual

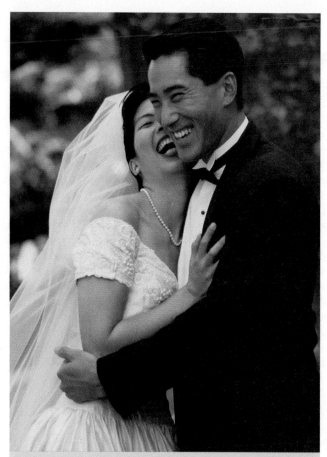

For many people, weddings or commitment ceremonies serve as the ultimate symbol of commitment between two people and validate their love for each other.

marriages of adult women declined by 45 percent.[17] This decrease may be due to several factors, including delay of first marriages, increase in cohabitation, and a small decrease in the number of divorced persons who remarry. In 1960, the median age for first marriage was 23 years for men and 20 years for women; by 2005, the median age of first marriage had risen to 27 years for men and 26 years for women.[18]

Many Americans believe that marriage involves **monogamy,** or exclusive sexual involvement with one partner. In fact, the lifetime pattern for many Americans appears to be **serial monogamy,** which means that a person has a monogamous sexual relationship with one partner before moving on to another monogamous relationship. However, some people prefer to have an **open relationship,** or open marriage, in which the partners agree that there may be sexual involvement for each person outside their relationship.

Marriage is socially sanctioned and highly celebrated in our culture, so there are numerous incentives for couples to formalize their relationship with a wedding ceremony. (See the **Green Guide** on page 134 for ideas on how to make such a celebration greener.) A healthy marriage provides emotional support by combining the benefits of friendship

monogamy Exclusive sexual involvement with one partner.
serial monogamy A series of monogamous sexual relationships.
open relationship A relationship in which partners agree that sexual involvement can occur outside the relationship.

GREEN GUIDE

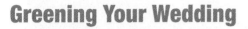

Greening Your Wedding

According to recent Census calculations, more than 2 million couples get married in the United States every year. That is a lot of invitations, photographs, bouquets, dresses, flowers, and rice!

Just as the wedding industry is booming, so is the movement toward green weddings. Many wedding service suppliers are providing green services, products, and options for an ecofriendly event. Entire organizations are devoted to promoting an ecofriendly approach to the "biggest day of your life," and numerous websites support and advocate green weddings; two of our favorites are www.greatgreenwedding.com and www.thegreenbrideguide.com.

With only a little additional planning, research, and thoughtful consideration, your big event can have great personal significance while leaving hardly a trace on the environment. Here are just a few ideas:

✳ Invitations, save-the-date cards, wedding programs, and RSVP cards mailed to your friends and loved ones can add up to a lot of paper consumption. To make these more environmentally friendly, have them printed on recycled paper, using soy inks and making sure that the printed goods can be recycled after the event. Take this a step further and consider using electronic RSVPs and save-the-date services or other electronic options to minimize the use of paper goods.

✳ When selecting wedding and engagement rings, do a little research and be well informed before you buy. Several environmentally responsible jewelry designers are using ecofriendly techniques in the design of wedding and engagement rings, including using recycled metals and stones, as well as avoiding diamonds and other gems that have been cultivated under socially and environmentally irresponsible conditions. Also consider purchasing and resizing vintage or antique rings. These ideas can lead to unique and personal wedding jewelry that reflects your commitment to environmental responsibility and to each other.

✳ What about the gowns and the tuxedos? Look for designs that are crafted with organic fabrics and textiles. If organic wedding couture is not for you, consider purchasing preworn, classic, recycled vintage wedding attire for bride, groom, and attendants. Don't like vintage? Work with a seamstress and use materials from another wedding dress for your own. Some brides use dresses handed down through families or use previously worn dresses to redesign their own look without using entirely new materials.

✳ Most couples want to preserve memories of their special day with photographs and videography. Interview photographers and videographers to find agents who provide environmentally responsible services. Ask about paperless imagery, 100 percent electronic image exchange, and environmentally responsible techniques such as digital approaches that avoid the toxic chemicals used in creating negatives. Also, consider printing or having printed *only* the images that are particularly important, and save the others on a computer or other electronic source—just don't forget to back up your files!

✳ Flowers are a big part of many wedding ceremonies. When selecting floral arrangements, find a retailer that provides flowers grown and harvested organically in pesticide-free soil. Also consider using live plants and arrangements instead of flowers harvested for the event. These living floral arrangements can be wedding favors for your guests and serve as a metaphor for the future growth of the celebrated relationship. Finally, when selecting a florist, opt for those that provide arrangements and services using environmentally responsible products such as petroleum-free containers and floral foams. Ask florists whether they recycle, compost, and reuse materials. With a little extra research, every dollar you spend on your wedding can support your commitment to environmental responsibility while also creating a day you will remember forever.

---

and a loving committed relationship. A happy marriage also provides stability for both the couple and for those involved in the couple's life. Considerable research indicates that married people live longer, feel happier, remain mentally alert longer, and suffer fewer physical and mental health problems.[19] Couples in healthy marriages have less stress, which in turn contributes to better overall health. Healthy marriage contributes to lower levels of stress in three important ways: financial stability, expanded support networks, and improved personal behaviors. Married adults are about half as likely to be smokers as are single, divorced, or separated adults. They are also less likely to be heavy drinkers or to engage in risky sexual behavior. The one negative health indicator for married people is body weight. Married adults, particularly men, weigh more than do single adults.[20]

However, traditional marriage does not work for everyone, and it is not the only path to a happy and successful committed relationship. See the **Health Headlines** box at right for some common misperceptions about marriage.

Cohabitation

Cohabitation is defined as a relationship in which two unmarried people with an intimate connection live together in the same household. For a variety of reasons, increasing numbers

cohabitation Living together without being married.

Health Headlines

MARRIAGE DEMYSTIFIED

What does marriage mean to you? It is the great unknown for many young people, and you may wonder when Mr. or Ms. Right will come along, where you'll find your lifetime partner, or if there is such a thing as the "perfect" marriage. The National Marriage Project studies the state of marriage in the United States and world-wide and educates the public on marital status and child well-being. The following facts and myths are from the National Marriage Project's research findings:

FACT—*The most likely way to find a future marriage partner is through an introduction by family, friends, or acquaintances.* Despite the romantic notion that people meet and fall in love through chance or fate, the evidence suggests that social networks are important in bringing together individuals of similar interests and backgrounds, especially when it comes to selecting a marriage partner.

FACT—*The more similar people are in their values, backgrounds, and life goals, the more likely they are to have a successful marriage.* Opposites may attract but they may not live together harmoniously as married couples. People who share common backgrounds and similar social networks are better suited as marriage partners than people who are very different in their backgrounds and networks.

MYTH—*Couples who live together before marriage, and are thus able to test how well suited they are for each other, have more satisfying and longer-lasting marriages than couples who do not.*
FACT—*Many studies have found that those who live together before marriage* have less satisfying marriages and a considerably higher chance of eventually breaking up. One reason is that people who cohabit may be more skittish of commitment and more likely to call it quits when problems arise. But in addition, the very act of living together may lead to attitudes that make happy marriages more difficult. The findings of one recent study, for example, suggest "there may be less motivation for cohabiting partners to develop their conflict resolution and support skills." (One important exception: cohabiting couples who are already planning to marry each other in the near future have just as good a chance of staying together as couples who don't live together before marriage.)

FACT—*For large segments of the population, the risk of divorce is far below 50 percent.* Although the overall divorce rate in America remains close to 50 percent of all marriages, it has been dropping gradually over the past two decades. Also, the risk of divorce is far below 50 percent for educated people marrying for the first time, and lower still for people who wait to marry until at least their mid-twenties, who haven't lived with many different partners prior to marriage, or who are strongly religious and marry someone of the same faith.

MYTH—*Having a child together will help a couple improve their marital satisfaction and prevent a divorce.*
FACT—*Many studies have shown that the most stressful time in a marriage is after the first child is born.* Couples who have children together have a slightly decreased risk of divorce compared to couples without children, but the decreased risk is far less than it used to be when parents with marital problems were more likely to stay together "for the sake of the children."

MYTH—*Married people have less satisfying sex lives, and less sex, than single people.*
FACT—*Contrary to the popular belief that married sex is boring and infrequent, married people report higher levels of sexual satisfaction than both sexually active singles and cohabiting couples.* The

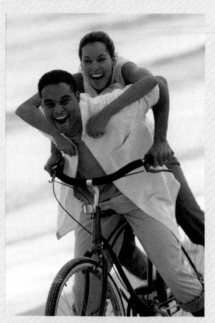

Sharing common interests and taking pleasure in each other's company are two keys to marital success.

higher level of commitment in marriage is probably the reason for the high level of reported sexual satisfaction; marital commitment contributes to a greater sense of trust and security, less drug- and alcohol-infused sex, and more mutual communication.

MYTH—*The keys to long-term marital success are good luck and romantic love.*
FACT—*Rather than luck and love, the most common reasons that couples give for their long-term marital success are commitment and companionship.* They define their marriage as a creation that has taken hard work, dedication, and commitment (to each other and to the institution of marriage). The happiest couples are friends who share lives and have compatible interests and values.

Sources: D. Popenoe, "Top Ten Myths of Marriage," 2002, Copyright © 2002 by the National Marriage Project at Rutgers University; D. Popenoe, "Top Ten Myths of Divorce," 2001, Copyright © 2001 by the National Marriage Project at Rutgers University; and D. Popenoe and B. D. Whitehead, "Ten Important Research Findings on Marriage and Choosing a Marriage Partner," 2004, Copyright © 2004 by the National Marriage Project at Rutgers University. Reprinted by permission of the National Marriage Project.

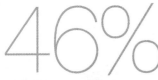

46% of couples living together in a given year are doing so as a precursor to marriage, according to one study. Within 5 to 7 years, 52% of those couples will have actually married and 31% will have split up.

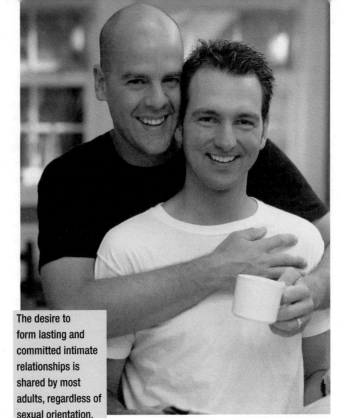

The desire to form lasting and committed intimate relationships is shared by most adults, regardless of sexual orientation.

of Americans are choosing cohabitation. In some states, cohabitation that lasts a designated number of years (usually 7) legally constitutes a **common-law marriage** for purposes of purchasing real estate and sharing other financial obligations.

Between 1960 and 2004, the number of cohabiting adults in America increased by over 1,000 percent. In fact, today over half of all first marriages are preceded by cohabitation.[21] Cohabitation can serve as a prelude to marriage, but for some people it is an alternative to marriage. Cohabitation is more common among people of lower socioeconomic status, people who are less religious, people who have been divorced, and people who have experienced parental divorce or high levels of parental conflict during childhood. Many people believe that living together before marriage is a good way to find out how compatible you are with your partner and possibly avoid a bad marriage; however, current data do not support this belief.[22] The long-term outcomes or implications of living together may be related more to who chooses to cohabit rather than the experience of cohabiting itself.

Although cohabitation has its advantages, it also has some drawbacks. Perhaps the greatest disadvantage is the lack of societal validation for the relationship, especially if the couple then has children. Many cohabitors must deal with pressures from parents and friends, difficulties in obtaining insurance and tax benefits, and legal issues over property. In 1996, the U.S. Congress reaffirmed tax advantages for married couples and effectively blocked cohabiting heterosexual and homosexual couples from these benefits through the Defense of Marriage Act (DOMA). The purpose of DOMA was to normalize heterosexual marriage on a federal level and permit each state to decide for itself whether to recognize same-sex unions or not.

common-law marriage Cohabitation lasting a designated period of time (usually 7 years) that is considered legally binding in some states.

Gay and Lesbian Partnerships

Most adults want intimate, committed relationships, whether they are gay or straight, men or women. Lesbians and gay men seek the same things in primary relationships that heterosexual partners do: friendship, communication, validation, companionship, and a sense of stability.

The 2000 U.S. Census revealed a significant increase in the number of same-sex partner households across the country—more than three times the total reported in the 1990 Census. The states with the most reported same-sex households are California, New York, Florida, Illinois, and Georgia. According to Lee Badgett, research director of the Institute for Gay and Lesbian Strategic Studies, the actual number of households is probably much higher. Many gay and lesbian partners hesitate to report their relationship because of concerns about discrimination.[23]

Challenges to successful lesbian and gay relationships often stem from discrimination and difficulties dealing with social, legal, and religious doctrines. For lesbian and gay couples, obtaining the same level of "marriage benefits," such as tax deductions, power-of-attorney rights, child custody rights, and other rights, continues to be a challenge. At the time of this writing in late 2009, Massachusetts, Connecticut, Iowa, New Hampshire, and Vermont are the only states to grant same-sex couples marriage equality, while New York and the District of Columbia recognize same-sex marriages performed in other states. Five other states currently have broad family-recognition laws that extend to same-sex couples all, or nearly all, the state rights and responsibilities of married heterosexual couples. More limited rights and protections for same-sex couples are legislated in five additional states.[24] Worldwide, same-sex marriages are legal in the Netherlands, Belgium, Spain, South Africa, Canada, Norway, and Sweden. Seventeen additional countries around the world approve civil unions or registered domestic partnerships for same-sex couples.

Staying Single

Increasing numbers of adults of all ages are electing to marry later or to remain single altogether. Data from 2007 indicate that 76.4 percent of women aged 20 to 24 have never been

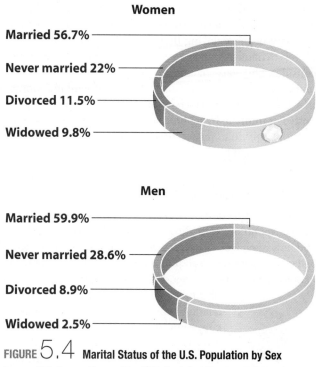

Women

Married 56.7%

Never married 22%

Divorced 11.5%

Widowed 9.8%

Men

Married 59.9%

Never married 28.6%

Divorced 8.9%

Widowed 2.5%

FIGURE 5.4 **Marital Status of the U.S. Population by Sex**

Source: U.S. Census Bureau, *The 2009 Statistical Abstract,* Table 56, "Marital Status of the Population by Sex and Age: 2007," 2008.

married. Likewise, men in this age group postponed marriage in increasing numbers, with 86.9 percent remaining unmarried in 2007.[25] According to the most recent figures from the Census Bureau and the National Center for Health Statistics, the number of unmarried women aged 15 and older may soon surpass the number of married women.[26] The number of unmarried men is also increasing (Figure 5.4).

Today, large numbers of people prefer to remain single or to delay marriage. Singles clubs, social outings arranged by communities and religious groups, extended family environments, and many social services support the single lifestyle.

what do you think?
What are the advantages to remaining single? ● What are the potential disadvantages? ● What societal or organizational supports are available for the single lifestyle?

Many singles live rich, rewarding lives and maintain a large network of close friends and family. Although sexual intimacy may or may not be present, the intimacy achieved through other interactions with loved ones is a key aspect of the single lifestyle.

Confronting Couples Issues

Our definition of success in a relationship tends to be based on whether a couple stays together over the years. Couples seeking a long-term relationship have to confront a number of issues that can enhance or ruin their chances of success. Learning to communicate, respecting each other, and sharing a genuine fondness are crucial to relationship success. Many social scientists agree that the happiest committed relationships are flexible enough to allow the partners to grow throughout their lives.

Jealousy in Relationships

"Jealousy is like a San Andreas fault running beneath the surface of an intimate relationship. Most of the time, its eruptive potential lies hidden. But when it begins to rumble, the destruction can be enormous."[27] **Jealousy** has been described as an aversive reaction evoked by a real or imagined relationship involving one's partner and a third person.

Contrary to what many of us believe, jealousy is not a sign of intense devotion. Instead, jealousy often indicates underlying problems, such as insecurity or possessiveness, that may prove to be a significant barrier to a healthy intimate relationship. Often, jealousy is rooted in a past relationship in which an individual experienced deception and loss. Other causes of jealousy typically include the following:

jealousy An aversive reaction evoked by a real or imagined relationship involving a person's partner and a third person.

- **Overdependence on the relationship.** People who have few social ties and who rely exclusively on their significant other tend to be fearful of losing them.
- **Severity of the threat.** People may feel uneasy if someone with stunning good looks and a great personality appears interested in their partner.
- **High value on sexual exclusivity.** People who believe that sexual exclusivity is a crucial indicator of love are more likely to become jealous.
- **Low self-esteem.** People who feel good about themselves are less likely to feel unworthy or fear that someone is going to snatch their partner away.
- **Fear of losing control.** Some people need to feel in control of every situation. Feeling that they may be losing the attachment of or control over a partner can cause jealousy.

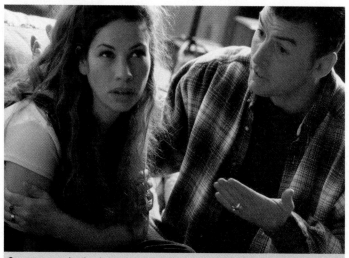

Open communication is key in addressing relationship problems. When one person shuts down, the argument can spin out of control.

In both sexes, jealousy is related to believing it would be difficult to find another relationship if the current one ends. For men, jealousy is positively correlated with the degree to which the man's self-esteem is affected by his partner's judgments. Though a certain amount of jealousy can be expected in any loving relationship, it doesn't have to threaten a relationship as long as partners communicate openly about it.[28]

what do you think?

Have you ever experienced jealousy in a relationship? ● Can you identify what actions or events caused you to feel this way? ● Did you have actual facts to support your feelings, or was your response based on suspicions?

Changing Gender Roles

Throughout history, women and men have taken on various roles in their relationships. In agricultural America, gender roles were determined by tradition, and each task within a family unit held equal importance. Our modern society has very few gender-specific roles. Women and men alike drive cars, care for children, operate computers, manage finances, and perform equally well in the tasks of daily living. Rather than taking on traditional female and male roles, many couples find it makes more sense to divide tasks on the basis of schedule, convenience, and preference. However, it rarely works out that the division is equal. Today's working woman, living in a dual-career family and coping with the responsibilities of being a partner, a mother, and a professional, is often stressed and frustrated. Even when women work full time, they tend to bear heavy family and household responsibilities. Men, who may have expected a more traditional role for their partners, may experience difficulties. Over time, if couples are unable to communicate how they feel about performing certain tasks, the relationship may suffer.

All couples have conflicts. Learning to handle them maturely is vital to relationship success.

Sharing Power

Power can be defined as the ability to make and implement decisions. There are many ways to exercise power, but powerful people are those who know what they want and have the ability to attain it. In traditional relationships, men were the wage earners and consequently had decision-making power. Women exerted much influence,

power The ability to make and implement decisions.

but in the final analysis they needed a man's income for survival. As women became wage earners in increasing numbers and began enjoying their own financial resources, the power dynamics between women and men have shifted considerably. Part of the increase in the divorce rate undoubtedly reflects the recognition by working women that they can leave bad relationships in which they previously felt trapped. In general, successful couples have power relationships that reflect their unique needs rather than popular stereotypes.

Unmet Expectations

We all have expectations of ourselves and our partners—how we will spend our time, how we will spend our money, how and how often we will express love and intimacy, and how we will grow together as a couple. Expectations are an extension of our values, beliefs, hopes, and dreams for the future. When communicated and agreed upon, these help relationships thrive. If we are unable to communicate our expectations, we set ourselves up for disappointment and hurt. Partners in healthy relationships can communicate wants and needs and have honest discussions when things aren't going as expected or as planned.

Having Children . . . Or Not?

When a couple decides to raise children, their relationship changes. Resources of time, energy, and money are split many ways, and the partners no longer have each other's undivided attention. Babies and young children do not time their requests for food, sleep, and care to the convenience of adults. Therefore, individuals or couples whose own basic needs for security, love, and purpose are already met make better parents. Any stresses existing in a relationship will be further accentuated when parenting is added to the responsibilities. Having a child does not save a bad relationship—in fact, it seems only to compound the problems that already exist. A child cannot and should not be expected to provide the parents with self-esteem and security.

Changing patterns in family life affect the way children are raised. In modern society, it is not always clear which partner will adjust his or her work schedule to provide the primary care of children. Nearly half a million children each year become part of a blended family when their parents remarry; remarriage creates a new family of stepparents and stepsiblings. In addition, increasing numbers of individuals are choosing to have children in a family structure other than a heterosexual marriage. Single women or lesbian couples can choose adoption or alternative insemination as a way to create a family. Single men or gay couples can choose to adopt or obtain the services of a surrogate mother. According to the 2000 Census, over 25 percent of all school-aged children were living in families headed by a man or woman raising a child alone, reflecting a growing trend in America and in the international community.[29] Regardless of the structure of the family, certain factors remain important to the well-being of the unit: consistency, communication, affection, and mutual respect. Good parenting does not necessarily come naturally. Many people parent as they were parented (see Table 5.1). This strategy may or may not follow sound child-rearing principles. Establishing a positive, respectful parenting style sets the stage for healthy family growth and development.

Finally, potential parents must consider the financial implications of deciding to have a child. It is estimated that a family that had a child in 2005 will spend close to $250,000 to raise the child over the following 17 years, and this does not take into account the costs of college.[30] Today, many families find that two incomes are needed just to make ends meet. Indeed, more than 80 percent of all mothers with children under the age of 5 work outside the home. Day care workers, family members, friends, grandparents, neighbors, and nannies "mind the kids." Some employers offer family leave arrangements that allow parents more latitude in taking time away from work.

Some people become parents without a lot of forethought. Some children are born into a relationship that was supposed to last and didn't. This does not mean it is too late to do a good job of parenting. Children are amazingly resilient and forgiving if parents show respect and communicate about household activities that affect their lives. Even children who grew up in a household of conflict can feel loved and respected if the parents treat them fairly. This means that parents must take responsibility for their own emotions and make it clear to children that they are not the reason for the conflict.

When Relationships Falter

Breakdowns in relationships usually begin with a change in communication, however subtle. Either partner may stop listening and cease to be emotionally present for the other. In turn, the other feels ignored, unappreciated, or unwanted. Unresolved conflicts increase, and unresolved anger can cause problems in sexual relations.

When a couple who previously enjoyed spending time together find themselves continually in the company of others, spending time apart, or preferring to stay home alone, it may

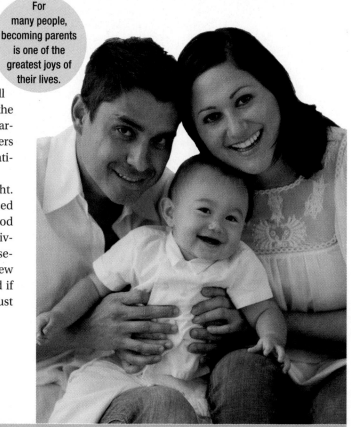

For many people, becoming parents is one of the greatest joys of their lives.

TABLE 5.1 | **Common Parenting Styles**

Authoritarian "giving orders"	Parents use a set of rules that are clear and unbending. Obedience is highly valued and rewarded. Misbehavior is punished. Children may behave for a reward or out of fear of punishment. Children are not encouraged to think for themselves or to question those in authority.
Permissive "giving in"	Parents take a hands-off approach. Children are allowed great freedom with few boundaries, minimal guidance, and little discipline. Without limits and expectations, children often struggle with impulse control, poor choices, and insecurity, and have trouble taking responsibility for their actions.
Assertive–Democratic "giving choices"	Parents have clear expectations for children, clarify issues, and give reasons for limits. Children are given lots of practice in making choices and are guided to see the consequences of their decisions. Encouragement and acknowledgment of good behavior form the focal point of this style. Misbehavior is handled with an appropriate consequence or by problem solving with the child.

Source: S. Dinwiddie, *Effective Parenting Styles: Why Yesterday's Models Won't Work Today.* Retrieved January 12, 2009, from www.kidsource.com/better.world .press/parenting.html. Copyright © Sue Dinwiddie. Used with permission.

In an unhealthy relationship...	In a healthy relationship...
You care for and focus on another person only and neglect yourself or you focus only on yourself and neglect the other person.	Partners love and take care of themselves before and while in a relationship.
One of you feels pressure to change to meet the other person's standards and is afraid to disagree or voice ideas.	Partners respect individuality, embrace differences, and allow each person to "be themselves."
One of you has to justify what you do, where you go, and whom you see.	Partners do things with friends and family and have activities independent of each other.
One of you makes all the decisions and controls everything without listening to the other's input.	Partners discuss things, allow for differences of opinion, and compromise equally.
One of you feels unheard and is unable to communicate what you want.	Partners express and listen to each other's feelings, needs, and desires.
You lie to each other and find yourself making excuses for the other person.	Partners trust and are honest with themselves and each other.
You don't have any personal space and have to share everything with the other person.	Partners respect each other's need for privacy.
Your partner keeps his or her sexual history a secret or hides a sexually transmitted infection from you, or you do not disclose your history to your partner.	Partners share sexual histories and sexual health with each other.
One of you is scared of asking the other to use protection or has refused the other's requests for safer sex.	Partners practice safer sex methods.
One of you has forced or coerced the other to have sex.	Partners respect sexual boundaries and are able to say no to sex.
One of you yells and hits, shoves, or throws things at the other in an argument.	Partners resolve conflicts in a rational, peaceful, and mutually agreed upon way.
You feel stifled, trapped, and stagnant. You are unable to escape the pressures of the relationship.	Partners have room for positive growth and learn more about each other as they develop and mature.

FIGURE 5.5 **Healthy versus Unhealthy Relationships**

Source: Reprinted with permission from Advocates for Youth, www.advocatesforyouth.org. Copyright © 2000, Washington, D.C. 20036.

be a sign that the relationship is in trouble. Of course, the need for individual privacy is not a cause for worry—it's essential to health. If, however, a partner decides to change the amount and quality of time spent together without the input or understanding of the other, it may be a sign of hidden problems. Figure 5.5 illustrates some of the factors that signal a healthy or unhealthy relationship.

College students, particularly those who are socially isolated and far from family and hometown friends, may be particularly vulnerable to staying in unhealthy relationships. They may become emotionally dependent on a partner for everything from eating meals to spending recreational and study time. Mutual obligations, such as shared rental arrangements, transportation, and child care, can make it tough to leave. It's also easy to mistake sexual advances for physical attraction or love. Without a network of friends and supporters to talk with, to

obtain validation for feelings, or to share concerns, a student may feel stuck in a relationship that is headed nowhere.

Honesty and verbal affection are usually positive aspects of a relationship. In a troubled relationship, however, they can be used to cover up irresponsible or hurtful behavior. "At least I was honest" is not an acceptable substitute for acting in a trustworthy way. "But I really do love you" is not a license for being inconsiderate or rude.

When and Why Relationships End

Often we hear in the news that 50 percent of American marriages end in divorce. This number is based on the annual marriage rate compared with the annual divorce rate. This is misleading because in any given year, the people who are divorcing are mostly not the same as those who are marrying. The preferred method to determine the divorce rate is to calculate how many people who have ever married subsequently divorce. Using this calculation, the divorce rate in the United States has never exceeded 41 percent.[31] Although this number is still high, the divorce rate in this country has declined slightly from previous decades. This decrease may be related to an increase in the age at which persons first marry and also a higher level of education among those who are marrying—both contribute to marital stability.[32]

The divorce rate represents only a portion of the actual number of failed relationships. Many people never go through a legal divorce process so are not counted in these statistics. Cohabitors and unmarried partners who raise children, own homes together, and exhibit all the outward appearances of marriage without the license are also not included.

Why do relationships end? There are many reasons, including illness, financial concerns, and career problems. Other breakups arise from unmet expectations. Many people enter a relationship with certain expectations about how they and their partner will behave. Failure to communicate these beliefs can lead to resentment and disappointment. Differences in sexual needs may also contribute to the demise of a relationship. Under stress, communication and cooperation between partners can break down. Conflict, negative interactions, and a general lack of respect between partners can erode even the most loving relationship.

Coping with Failed Relationships

No relationship comes with a guarantee, no matter how many promises partners make to be together forever. Losing a love is as much a part of life as falling in love. That being said, the uncoupling process can be very painful (see the **Skills for Behavior Change** box at right for advice on approaching this difficult process). Whenever we risk getting close to another, we also risk being hurt if things don't work out. Remember that knowing, understanding, and feeling good about oneself before entering the relationship is very important. Consider these tips for coping with a failed relationship.[33]

- **Recognize and acknowledge your feelings.** These may include grief, loneliness, rejection, anger, guilt, relief, or sadness. Seek professional help and support as needed.
- **Find healthful ways to express your emotions, rather than turning them inward.** Go for a walk, talk to friends, listen to music, work out at the gym, volunteer with a community organization, or write in a journal.
- **Spend time with current friends, or reconnect with old friends.** Get reacquainted with yourself, what you enjoy doing, and the people whose company you enjoy.
- **Don't rush into a "rebound" relationship.** You need time to resolve your past experience rather than escape from it. You can't be trusting and intimate in a new relationship if you are still working on getting over a past relationship.

Skills for Behavior Change

How Do You End It?

Relationship endings are just as important as their beginnings. Healthy closure affords both parties the opportunity to move on without wondering or worrying about what went wrong and whose fault it was. If you need to end a relationship, do so in a manner that preserves and respects the dignity of both partners. If you are the person "breaking up," you probably have had time to think about the process and may be at a different stage than your partner.

Here are some tips for ending a relationship in a respectful and caring way:

✳ Arrange a time and quiet place where you can talk without interruption.
✳ Say in advance that there is something important you want to discuss.
✳ Accept that your partner may express strong feelings and be prepared to listen quietly.
✳ Consider in advance if you might also become upset and what support you might need.
✳ Communicate honestly using "I" messages and without personal attacks. Explain your reasons as much as you can without being cruel or insensitive.
✳ Don't let things escalate into a fight, even if you have very strong feelings.
✳ Provide another opportunity to talk about the end of the relationship when you both have had time to reflect.

Your Sexual Identity: More Than Biology

Sexual identity, the recognition and acknowledgment of oneself as a sexual being, is determined by a complex interaction of genetic, physiological, environmental, and social factors. The beginning of sexual identity occurs at conception with the combining of chromosomes that determine sex. All eggs carry an X sex chromosome; sperm may carry either an X or a Y chromosome. If a sperm carrying an X chromosome fertilizes an egg, the resulting combination of sex chromosomes (XX) provides the blueprint to produce a female. If a sperm carrying a Y chromosome fertilizes an egg, the XY combination produces a male.

Not all people, however, have XX or XY chromosomes, nor do they all necessarily exhibit exclusively female or male sexual anatomy. **Intersexuality** may occur as often as 1 in 100 live births. Intersexuality

sexual identity Recognition of oneself as a sexual being; a composite of biological sex characteristics, gender identity, gender roles, and sexual orientation.

intersexuality Not exhibiting exclusively male or female primary and secondary sex characteristics.

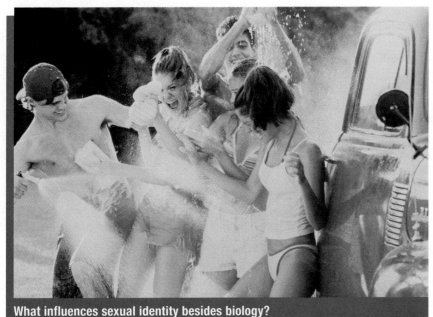

What influences sexual identity besides biology?

How you perceive yourself as a sexual being is influenced by socialization and personal experience. Your understanding of gender roles, your contact with people of various gender identities or sexual orientations, and your own degree of emotional maturity can all affect your sense of sexual identity.

gonads The reproductive organs that produce germ cells and sex hormones in a man (testes) or woman (ovaries).

puberty The period of sexual maturation.

pituitary gland The endocrine gland controlling the release of hormones from the gonads.

secondary sex characteristics Characteristics associated with sex but not directly related to reproduction, such as vocal pitch, degree of body hair, and location of fat deposits.

gender The psychological condition of being feminine or masculine as defined by the society in which one lives.

socialization Process by which a society communicates behavioral expectations to its individual members.

gender roles Expression of maleness or femaleness in everyday life.

gender identity Personal sense or awareness of being masculine or feminine, a male or a female.

transgendered When one's gender identity does not match one's biological sex.

transsexual A person who is psychologically of one sex but physically of the other.

gender-role stereotypes Generalizations concerning how men and women should express themselves and the characteristics each possesses.

is a biological condition in which a person is born with sex chromosomes, external genitalia, and/or an internal reproductive system that have both male and female components.

The genetic instructions included in the sex chromosomes lead to the differential development of male and female **gonads** (reproductive organs) at about the eighth week of fetal life. Once the male gonads (testes) and the female gonads (ovaries) develop, they play a key role in all future sexual development because the gonads are responsible for the production of sex hormones. The primary female sex hormones are estrogen and progesterone. The primary male sex hormone is testosterone. The release of testosterone in a maturing fetus signals the development of a penis and other male genitals. If no testosterone is produced, female genitals form.

At the time of **puberty,** sex hormones again play major roles in development. Hormones released by the **pituitary gland,** called *gonadotropins*, stimulate the testes

and ovaries to make appropriate sex hormones. The increase of estrogen production in females and testosterone production in males leads to the development of **secondary sex characteristics.** Male secondary sex characteristics include deepening of the voice, development of facial and body hair, and growth of the skeleton and musculature. Female secondary sex characteristics include growth of the breasts, widening of the hips, and the development of pubic and underarm hair.

Thus far, we have described sexual identity only in terms of a person's biology. Although biology is an important facet of sexual identity, the relationship between biology and culture is much more complicated than the popular notion that *sex* refers to biology and *gender* to social issues. Biological factors are themselves always understood and interpreted within the cultural framework that gives meaning to those facts.

Gender is the practice of behaving in masculine or feminine ways as defined by the society in which one lives and as a component of one's identity. Sex, in contrast, is more related to physical form and function. In this sense, gender is a performance, something we do rather than something we have, and we learn gender through the process of **socialization.** Through interactions with family, peers, teachers, media, and other social organizations, we learn to act in ways that society deems appropriate.

Each of us expresses our maleness or femaleness on a daily basis by the **gender roles** we play. **Gender identity** refers to the personal sense or awareness of being masculine or feminine, a male or a female. A person's gender identity does not always match his or her biological sex—this is called being **transgendered.** There is a broad spectrum of expression among transgendered persons that reflects the degree of dissatisfaction or disassociation they have with their sexual anatomy. Some transgendered persons are very comfortable with their bodies and are content simply to dress and live as the other gender. At the other end of the spectrum are **transsexuals,** who feel extremely trapped in their bodies and may opt for therapeutic interventions, such as sex reassignment surgery. Being transgendered or transsexual is not related to sexual orientation, nor should it be confused with transvestism, or cross-dressing.

It may sometimes be difficult to express one's true sexual identity because of the bounds established by **gender-role stereotypes,** or generalizations about how men and women should express themselves and the characteristics each possesses. Our traditional sex roles are an example of gender-role stereotyping. Men, on the one hand, are traditionally expected to be independent, aggressive, logical, and always in control of their emotions. Women, on the other hand, are

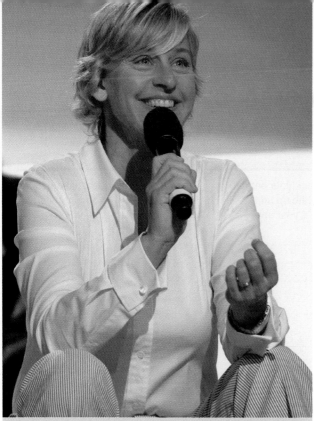

The presence of gay and lesbian celebrities in the media contributes to the increasing acceptance of gay relationships in everyday life. Talk show host Ellen DeGeneres is an openly gay comedian whose character in the 1990s sitcom *Ellen* famously came out as a lesbian on network television.

traditionally expected to be passive, nurturing, intuitive, sensitive, and emotional. **Androgyny** refers to the combination of traditional masculine and feminine traits in a single person. Androgynous people do not always follow traditional sex roles but instead choose behaviors based on a given situation.

By now you can see that defining sexual identity is not a simple matter. It is a lifelong process of growing and learning. Your sexual identity is made up of the unique combination of your biology, gender identity, chosen gender roles, sexual orientation, and personal experiences. It is up to you to take every opportunity to get to know and like yourself so that you may enjoy your life to the fullest.

Sexual Orientation

Sexual orientation refers to a person's enduring emotional, romantic, sexual, or affectionate attraction to others. You may be primarily attracted to members of the other sex **(heterosexual)**, your same sex **(homosexual)**, or both sexes **(bisexual).**

Many homosexuals prefer the terms **gay** and **lesbian** to describe their sexual orientations, because these terms go beyond the exclusively sexual connotation of the term *homosexual*. *Gay* can apply to both men and women, but *lesbian* refers specifically to women.

Gay, lesbian, and bisexual persons are repeatedly the targets of **sexual prejudice.** Sexual prejudice refers to negative attitudes and hostile actions directed at a social group and its members.[34] Hate crimes, discrimination, and hostility target-

ing sexual minorities are evidence of ongoing sexual prejudice. Recent data from the Federal Bureau of Investigation indicated that bias regarding sexual orientation was the motivation for over 16 percent of all hate crimes reported.[35]

Most researchers today agree that sexual orientation is best understood using a multifactorial model, which incorporates biological, psychological, and socioenvironmental factors. Biological explanations focus on research into genetics, hormones, and differences in brain anatomy, whereas psychological and socioenvironmental explanations examine parent–child interactions, sex roles, and early sexual and interpersonal interactions. Collectively, this growing body of research suggests that the origins of homosexuality, like heterosexuality, are complex. To diminish the complexity of sexual orientation to "a choice" is a clear misrepresentation of current research. Homosexuals do not "choose" their sexual orientation any more than heterosexuals do.

Sexual orientation is often viewed as a concept based entirely on whom one has sex with, but this is an inaccurate and overly simplistic idea. Researcher F. Klein developed a questionnaire that not only looks at who you are sexually attracted to, fantasize about, and actually have sex with, but also considers factors such as who you feel close to emotionally and in which "community" you feel most comfortable. You can find this questionnaire in the **Gender & Health** box on page 144. After completing it, you may realize that there are not just two or three orientations, but a whole range of complex, interacting, and fluid factors influencing your sexuality over time.

androgyny Combination of traditional masculine and feminine traits in a single person.
sexual orientation A person's enduring emotional, romantic, sexual, or affectionate attraction to other persons.
heterosexual Experiencing primary attraction to and preference for sexual activity with people of the other sex.
homosexual Experiencing primary attraction to and preference for sexual activity with people of the same sex.
bisexual Experiencing attraction to and preference for sexual activity with people of both sexes.
gay Sexual orientation involving primary attraction to people of the same sex; usually but not always applies to men attracted to men.
lesbian Sexual orientation involving attraction of women to other women.
sexual prejudice Negative attitudes and hostile actions directed at social groups.

Sexual Anatomy and Physiology

An understanding of the functions of the male and female reproductive systems will help you derive pleasure and satisfaction from your sexual relationships, be sensitive to your partner's wants and needs, and make responsible choices regarding your own sexual health.

Female Sexual Anatomy and Physiology

The female reproductive system includes two major groups of structures, the external genitals and the internal organs (Figure 5.6). The external female genitals are collectively

Gender&Health

Analyzing Your Sexual Preferences

To complete this worksheet, use the scales provided below and choose a number for each of the three aspects of your life: your past, your present, and your ideal. Remember that there are no right or wrong answers.

Variable	Past (your entire life up until 1 year ago)	Present (the past 12 months)	Ideal (if you could order your life any way you wanted)
A. SEXUAL ATTRACTION: To whom are you sexually attracted?	_____	_____	_____
B. SEXUAL BEHAVIOR: With whom do you have sex?	_____	_____	_____
C. SEXUAL FANTASIES: Whom do you fantasize about?	_____	_____	_____
D. EMOTIONAL PREFERENCE: Whom do you feel more drawn to or close to emotionally?	_____	_____	_____
E. SOCIAL PREFERENCE: With whom do you spend most of your social life?	_____	_____	_____
F. LIFESTYLE PREFERENCE: In which community (gay, straight, mixed) do you prefer to spend your time or feel most comfortable?	_____	_____	_____
G. SELF-IDENTIFICATION: How do you label or identify yourself?	_____	_____	_____

SCALE FOR A–E	SCALE FOR F AND G
0 = other sex only	0 = heterosexual only
1 = other sex mostly	1 = heterosexual mostly
2 = other sex somewhat more	2 = heterosexual somewhat more
3 = both sexes equally	3 = equally heterosexual and homosexual
4 = same sex somewhat more	4 = homosexual somewhat more
5 = same sex mostly	5 = homosexual mostly
6 = same sex only	6 = homosexual only

Source: From F. Klein, *The Bisexual Option.* Copyright © 1978 The Haworth Press, Inc. Used with permission.

---

vulva Region that encloses the female's external genitalia.

mons pubis Fatty tissue covering the pubic bone in females; in physically mature women, the mons is covered with coarse hair.

labia majora "Outer lips," or folds of tissue covering the female sexual organs.

labia minora "Inner lips," or folds of tissue just inside the labia majora.

clitoris A pea-sized nodule of tissue located at the top of the labia minora; central to sexual arousal in women.

urethral opening The opening through which urine is expelled.

hymen Thin tissue covering the vaginal opening in some women.

perineum Tissue that forms the "floor" of the pelvic region.

known as the **vulva** and include all structures that are outwardly visible, specifically, the mons pubis, the labia minora and majora, the clitoris, the urethral and vaginal openings, and the vestibule of the vagina and its glands. The **mons pubis** is a pad of fatty tissue covering and protecting the pubic bone; after the onset of puberty, it becomes covered with coarse hair. The **labia majora** are folds of skin and erectile tissue that enclose the urethral and vaginal openings; the **labia minora,** or inner lips, are folds of mucous membrane found just inside the labia majora.

The **clitoris** is located at the upper end of the labia minora and beneath the mons pubis, and its only known function is to provide sexual pleasure. Directly below the clitoris is the **urethral opening** through which urine is expelled from the body. Below the urethral opening is the vaginal opening. In some women, the vaginal opening is covered by a thin membrane called the **hymen.** It is a myth that an intact hymen is proof of virginity, as the hymen can be stretched or torn by physical activity, and is not present in all women to begin with.

The **perineum** is the area of smooth tissue found between the vulva and the anus. Although not technically part of the external genitalia, the tissue in this area has many nerve endings and is sensitive to touch; it can play a part in sexual excitement.

The internal female genitals include the vagina, uterus, fallopian tubes, and ovaries. The **vagina** is a tubular organ

External Anatomy

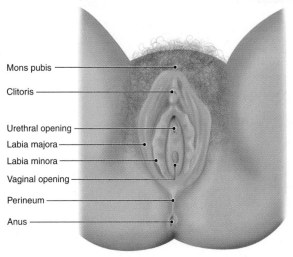

Mons pubis
Clitoris
Urethral opening
Labia majora
Labia minora
Vaginal opening
Perineum
Anus

Internal Organs

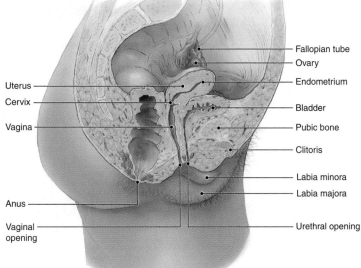

Uterus
Cervix
Vagina
Anus
Vaginal opening

Fallopian tube
Ovary
Endometrium
Bladder
Pubic bone
Clitoris
Labia minora
Labia majora
Urethral opening

FIGURE 5.6 **Female Reproductive System**

that serves as a passageway from the uterus to the outside of the body. This passage allows menstrual flow to exit from the uterus during a woman's monthly cycle, receives the penis during intercourse, and serves as the birth canal during childbirth. The **uterus (womb)** is a hollow, muscular, pear-shaped organ. Hormones acting on the inner lining of the uterus (the **endometrium**), either prepare the uterus for implantation and development of a fertilized egg or signal that no fertilization has taken place, in which case the endometrium deteriorates and becomes menstrual flow.

The lower end of the uterus, the **cervix,** extends down into the vagina. The **ovaries,** almond-sized organs suspended on either side of the uterus, produce the hormones estrogen and progesterone and are also the reservoir for immature eggs. All the eggs a woman will ever have are present in her ovaries at birth. Eggs mature and are released from the ovaries in response to hormone levels. Extending from the upper end of the uterus are two thin, flexible tubes called the **fallopian tubes.** The fallopian tubes, which do not actually touch the ovaries, capture eggs as they are released from the ovaries during ovulation, and they are the site where sperm and egg meet and fertilization takes place. The fallopian tubes then serve as the passageway to the uterus, where the fertilized egg becomes implanted and development continues.

The Onset of Puberty and the Menstrual Cycle With the onset of puberty, the female reproductive system matures, and the development of secondary sex characteristics transforms young girls into young women. The first sign of puberty is the beginning of breast development, which generally occurs around age 11. The pituitary gland, the **hypothalamus,** and the ovaries all secrete hormones that act

as chemical messengers among them. Working in a feedback system, hormonal levels in the bloodstream act as the trigger mechanism for release of more or different hormones.

Around age $9\frac{1}{2}$ to $11\frac{1}{2}$, the hypothalamus receives the message to begin secreting *gonadotropin-releasing hormone (GnRH)*. The release of GnRH in turn signals the pituitary gland to release hormones called *gonadotropins.* Two gonadotropins, *follicle-stimulating hormone (FSH)* and *luteinizing hormone (LH),* signal the ovaries to start producing **estrogens** and **progesterone.** Estrogens regulate the menstrual cycle, and increased estrogen levels assist in the development of female secondary sex characteristics. Progesterone helps the endometrium to develop in preparation to nourish a fertilized egg and helps maintain pregnancy.

The normal age range for the onset of the first menstrual period, termed **menarche,** is 9 to 17 years, with the average age being $11\frac{1}{2}$ to $13\frac{1}{2}$ years. Body fat heavily influences the onset of puberty, and increasing rates of obesity in children may account for the fact that girls here and in other countries seem to be reaching puberty much earlier than they used to.[36] Very thin girls, such as young athletes, tend to start menstruating later.

vagina The passage in females leading from the vulva into the uterus.
uterus (womb) Hollow, muscular, pear-shaped organ whose function is to contain the developing fetus.
endometrium Soft, spongy matter that makes up the uterine lining.
cervix Lower end of the uterus that opens into the vagina.
ovaries Almond-size organs that house developing eggs and produce hormones.
fallopian tubes Tubes that extend from near the ovaries to the uterus; site of fertilization and passageway for fertilized eggs.
hypothalamus An area of the brain located near the pituitary gland; works in conjunction with the pituitary gland to control reproductive functions.
estrogens Hormones secreted by the ovaries, which control the menstrual cycle.
progesterone Hormone secreted by the ovaries; helps the endometrium develop and helps maintain pregnancy.
menarche The first menstrual period.

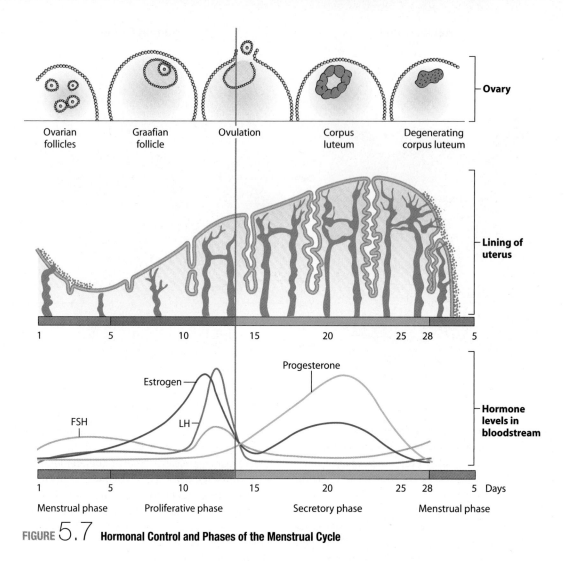

Ovary

Ovarian follicles   Graafian follicle   Ovulation   Corpus luteum   Degenerating corpus luteum

Lining of uterus

1 5 10 15 20 25 28 5

Progesterone

Estrogen

FSH

LH

Hormone levels in bloodstream

1 5 10 15 20 25 28 5 Days

Menstrual phase   Proliferative phase   Secretory phase   Menstrual phase

FIGURE 5.7 **Hormonal Control and Phases of the Menstrual Cycle**

The average menstrual cycle lasts 28 days and consists of three phases: the proliferative phase, the secretory phase, and the menstrual phase. The *proliferative phase* begins with the end of menstruation. During this time, the endometrium develops, or "proliferates." How does this process work? By the end of menstruation, the hypothalamus senses very low levels of estrogen and progesterone in the blood. In response, it increases its secretions of GnRH, which in turn triggers the pituitary gland to release FSH. When FSH reaches the ovaries, it signals several **ovarian follicles** to begin maturing (Figure 5.7). Normally, only one of the follicles, the **graafian follicle,** reaches full maturity in the days preceding ovulation. While the follicles mature, they begin producing estrogen, which in turn signals the endometrium to proliferate. If fertilization occurs, the endometrium will become a nesting place for the developing embryo. High estrogen levels signal the pituitary to slow down FSH production and in-

crease release of LH. Under the influence of LH, the ovarian follicle ruptures and releases a mature **ovum** (plural: *ova*), a single mature egg cell, near a fallopian tube (around day 14). This is the process of **ovulation.** The other ripening follicles degenerate and are reabsorbed by the body. Occasionally, two ova mature and are released during ovulation. If both are fertilized, fraternal (nonidentical) twins develop. Identical twins develop when one fertilized ovum (called a *zygote*) divides into two separate zygotes.

The phase following ovulation is called the *secretory phase.* The ruptured graafian follicle, which has remained in the ovary, is transformed into the **corpus luteum** and begins secreting large amounts of estrogen and progesterone. These hormone secretions peak around the twentieth or twenty-first days of the average cycle and cause the endometrium to thicken and continue preparing for a potential fertilized ovum. If fertilization and implantation take place, cells surrounding the developing embryo release a hormone called *human chorionic gonadotropin (HCG),* increasing estrogen and progesterone secretions that maintain the endometrium and signal the pituitary not to start a new menstrual cycle. If no implantation occurs, the hypothalamus responds by signaling the pituitary to stop producing FSH and LH, thus

ovarian follicles Areas within the ovary in which individual eggs develop.
graafian follicle Mature ovarian follicle that contains a fully developed ovum, or egg.
ovum A single mature egg cell.
ovulation The point of the menstrual cycle at which a mature egg ruptures through the ovarian wall.
corpus luteum A body of cells that forms from the remains of the graafian follicle following ovulation; it secretes estrogen and progesterone during the second half of the menstrual cycle.

peaking the levels of progesterone in the blood. The corpus luteum begins to decompose, leading to rapid declines in estrogen and progesterone levels. These hormones are needed to sustain the lining of the uterus. Without them, the endometrium is sloughed off in the menstrual flow, and this begins the *menstrual phase*. The low estrogen levels of the menstrual phase signal the hypothalamus to release GnRH, which acts on the pituitary to secrete FSH, and the cycle begins again.

Menstrual Problems **Premenstrual syndrome (PMS)** is a term used for a collection of physical, emotional, and behavioral symptoms that many women experience 7 to 14 days prior to their menstrual period. The most common symptoms are tender breasts, food cravings, fatigue, irritability, and depression. It is estimated that 75 percent of menstruating women experience some signs and symptoms of PMS each month. For the majority of women, these disappear as their period begins, but for a small subset of women (3 to 5 percent), their symptoms are severe enough to affect their daily routines and activities to the point of being disabling. This severe form of PMS has its own psychiatric designation, **premenstrual dysphoric disorder (PMDD),** with symptoms that include severe depression, hopelessness, anger, anxiety, low self-esteem, difficulty concentrating, irritability, and tension.

There are several natural approaches to managing PMS that can also help PMDD. These strategies include eating more carbohydrates (grains, fruits, and vegetables), reducing caffeine and salt intake, exercising regularly, and taking measures to reduce stress. Recent investigation into methods of controlling the severe emotional swings has led to the use of antidepressants for treating PMDD, primarily selective serotonin reuptake inhibitors (SSRIs; e.g., Prozac, Paxil, and Zoloft).

Dysmenorrhea is a medical term for menstrual cramps, the pain or discomfort in the lower abdomen that many women experience just before or after menstruation. Along with cramps, some women can experience nausea and vomiting, loose stools, sweating, and dizziness. Menstrual cramps can be classified as primary or secondary dysmenorrhea. Primary dysmenorrhea doesn't involve any physical abnormality and usually begins 6 months to a year after a woman's first period, while secondary dysmenorrhea has an underlying physical cause such as endometriosis or uterine fibroids.[37] If you experience primary dysmenorrhea, you can reduce your discomfort by using over-the-counter nonsteroidal anti-inflammatory drugs (NSAIDS) such as aspirin, ibuprofen (Advil or Motrin), and naproxen (Aleve). Other self-care strategies such as soaking in a hot bath or using a heating pad on your abdomen may also ease your cramps. For severe cramping, your health care provider may recommend a low-dose oral contraceptive to prevent ovulation, which in turn may reduce the production of prostaglandins and therefore the severity of your cramps. Managing secondary dysmenorrhea involves treating the underlying cause.

Toxic shock syndrome (TSS), although rare today, is still something women should be aware of. It is caused by a bacterial infection facilitated by tampon or diaphragm use (see Chapter 6). Symptoms are sometimes hard to recognize because they mimic the flu and include sudden high fever, vomiting, diarrhea, dizziness, fainting, or a rash that looks like sunburn during one's period or a few days after. Proper treatment usually assures recovery in 2 to 3 weeks.

Menopause Just as menarche signals the beginning of a woman's reproductive years, **menopause**—the permanent cessation of menstruation—signals the end. Generally occurring between the ages of 40 and 60, and at age 51 on average in the United States, menopause results in decreased estrogen levels, which may produce troublesome symptoms in some women. Decreased vaginal lubrication, hot flashes, headaches, dizziness, and joint pain all have been associated with the onset of menopause.

Hormones, such as estrogen and progesterone, have long been prescribed as **hormone replacement therapy** to relieve menopausal symptoms and reduce the risk of heart disease and osteoporosis. (The National Institutes of Health prefers the term **menopausal hormone therapy,** because this hormone treatment is not a replacement and does not restore the physiology of youth.) However, recent studies, including results from the Women's Health Initiative (WHI), suggest that hormone therapy may actually do more harm than good. In fact, the WHI terminated this research ahead of schedule because of concerns about participants' increased risk of breast cancer, heart attack, stroke, blood clots, and other health problems.[38] All women need to discuss the risks and benefits of menopausal hormone therapy with their health care provider and come to an informed decision. It is crucial to find a doctor who specializes in women's health and keeps up to date with the latest research findings. Certainly a healthy lifestyle, such as regular exercise, a balanced diet, and adequate calcium intake, can also help protect postmenopausal women from heart disease and osteoporosis.

premenstrual syndrome (PMS) Comprises the mood changes and physical symptoms that occur in some women during the 1 or 2 weeks prior to menstruation.

premenstrual dysphoric disorder (PMDD) Collective name for a group of negative symptoms similar to but more severe than PMS, including severe mood disturbances.

dysmenorrhea Condition of pain or discomfort in the lower abdomen just before or after menstruation.

menopause The permanent cessation of menstruation, generally occurring between the ages of 40 and 60.

hormone replacement therapy, menopausal hormone therapy Use of synthetic or animal estrogens and progesterone to compensate for decreases in estrogens in a woman's body during menopause.

Male Sexual Anatomy and Physiology

The structures of the male reproductive system are divided into external and internal genitals (Figure 5.8). The external genitals are the penis and the scrotum. The internal male genitals include the testes, epididymides, vasa deferentia, ejaculatory ducts, urethra, and three other structures—the seminal vesicles, the prostate gland, and the Cowper's glands—that secrete components that, with sperm, make up semen. These three structures are sometimes referred to as the *accessory glands*.

External Anatomy

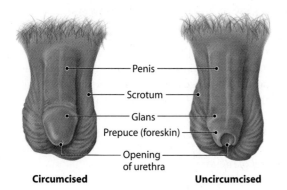

Penis
Scrotum
Glans
Prepuce (foreskin)
Opening of urethra

Circumcised   **Uncircumcised**

Internal Organs

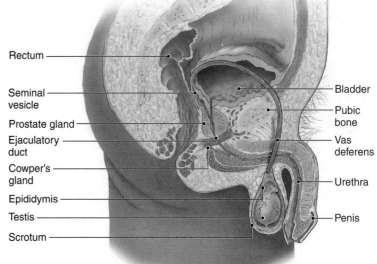

Rectum
Seminal vesicle
Prostate gland
Ejaculatory duct
Cowper's gland
Epididymis
Testis
Scrotum

Bladder
Pubic bone
Vas deferens
Urethra
Penis

FIGURE 5.8 **Male Reproductive System**

penis Male sexual organ that releases sperm into the vagina.

ejaculation The propulsion of semen from the penis.

scrotum Sac of tissue that encloses the testes.

testes Two organs, located in the scrotum, that manufacture sperm and produce hormones.

testosterone The male sex hormone manufactured in the testes.

spermatogenesis The development of sperm.

epididymis A comma-shaped structure atop the testis, where sperm mature.

vas deferens A tube that stores and transports sperm toward the penis.

seminal vesicles Storage areas for sperm where nutrient fluids are added to them.

semen Fluid containing sperm and nutrient fluids that increase sperm viability and neutralize vaginal acid.

prostate gland Gland that secretes nutrients and neutralizing fluids into the semen.

Cowper's glands Glands that secrete a fluid that lubricates the urethra and neutralizes any acid remaining in the urethra after urination.

vasocongestion The engorgement of the genital organs with blood.

The **penis** is the organ that deposits sperm in the vagina during intercourse. The urethra, which passes through the center of the penis, acts as the passageway for both semen and urine to exit the body. During sexual arousal, the spongy tissue in the penis becomes filled with blood, making the organ stiff (erect). Further sexual excitement leads to **ejaculation,** a series of rapid, spasmodic contractions that propel semen out of the penis.

Debate continues over the practice of *circumcision,* the surgical removal of a fold of skin covering the end of the penis known as the *foreskin.* Most circumcisions are performed for religious or cultural reasons or because of hygiene concerns. However, recent research supports the claim that circumcision yields medical benefits, including decreased risk of urinary tract infections in the first year, decreased risk of penile cancer (although cancer of the penis is very rare to begin with), and decreased risk of sexual transmission of human papillomavirus (HPV) and human immunodeficiency virus (HIV).[39]

Situated behind the penis and also outside the body is a sac called the **scrotum.** The scrotum protects the testes and also helps control the temperature within the testes, which is vital to proper sperm production. The **testes** (singular: *testis*) manufacture sperm and **testosterone,** the hormone responsible for the development of male secondary sex characteristics.

The development of sperm is referred to as **spermatogenesis.** Like the maturation of eggs in the female, this process is governed by the pituitary gland. Follicle-stimulating hormone (FSH) is secreted into the bloodstream to stimulate the testes to manufacture sperm. Immature sperm are released into a comma-shaped structure on the back of each testis called the **epididymis** (plural: *epididymides*), where they ripen and reach full maturity.

Each epididymis contains coiled tubules that gradually "unwind" and straighten out to become the **vas deferens.** The two vasa deferentia, as they are called in the plural, make up the tubular transportation system whose sole function is to store and move sperm. Along the way, the **seminal vesicles** provide sperm with nutrients and other fluids that compose **semen.**

The vasa deferentia eventually connect each epididymis to the ejaculatory ducts, which pass through the prostate gland and empty into the urethra. The **prostate gland** contributes more fluids to the semen, including chemicals that help the sperm fertilize an ovum and neutralize the acidic environment of the vagina to make it more conducive to sperm motility (ability to move) and potency (potential for fertilizing an ovum).

Just below the prostate gland are two pea-shaped nodules called the **Cowper's glands.** The Cowper's glands secrete a fluid that lubricates the urethra and neutralizes any acid that may remain in the urethra after urination. Urine and semen do not come into contact with each other. During ejaculation of semen, a small valve closes off the tube to the urinary bladder.

Human Sexual Response

Psychological traits greatly influence sexual response and sexual desire. Thus, you may find a relationship with one partner vastly different from experiences with other partners.

Sexual response is a physiological process that generally follows a pattern. Sexual responses in both men and women are somewhat arbitrarily divided into four stages: excitement/arousal, plateau, orgasm, and resolution. Researchers agree that each individual has a personal response pattern that may or may not conform to these phases. Regardless of the type of sexual activity (stimulation by a partner or self-stimulation), the response stages for an individual are the same.

During the first stage, *excitement/arousal*, **vasocongestion** (increased blood flow that causes swelling in the genitals) stimulates male and female genital responses. The vagina begins to lubricate in preparation for penile penetration, and the penis becomes partially erect. Both sexes may exhibit a "sex flush," or light blush all over their bodies. Excitement/arousal can be generated through fantasy or by touching parts of the body, kissing, viewing films or videos, or reading erotic literature.

During the *plateau phase,* the initial responses intensify. Voluntary and involuntary muscle tensions increase. The woman's nipples and the man's penis become erect. The penis secretes a few drops of preejaculatory fluid, which may contain sperm.

During the *orgasmic phase,* vasocongestion and muscle tensions reach their peak, and rhythmic contractions occur through the genital regions. In women, these contractions are centered in the uterus, outer vagina, and anal sphincter.

In men, the contractions occur in two stages. First, contractions within the prostate gland begin propelling semen through the urethra. In the second stage, the muscles of the pelvic floor, urethra, and anal sphincter contract. Semen usually, but not always, is ejaculated from the penis. In both sexes, spasms in other major muscle groups also occur, particularly in the buttocks and abdomen. In both men and women, feet and hands may also contract, and facial features often contort.

Muscle tension and congested blood subside in the *resolution phase,* as the genital organs return to their pre-arousal states. Both sexes usually experience deep feelings of well-being and profound relaxation. Following orgasm and resolution, many women can become aroused again and experience additional orgasms. However, some men experience a refractory period, during which their systems are incapable of subsequent arousal. This refractory period may last from a few minutes to several hours and tends to lengthen with age.

Men and women experience the same stages in the sexual response cycle; however, the length of time spent in any one stage varies. Thus, one partner may be in the plateau phase while the other is in the excitement or orgasmic phase. Such variations in response rates are entirely normal. Some couples believe that simultaneous orgasm is desirable for sexual satisfaction. Although simultaneous orgasm is pleasant, so are orgasms achieved at different times.

Sexual pleasure and satisfaction are also possible without orgasm or even intercourse. Expressing sexual feelings for another person involves many pleasurable activities, of which intercourse and orgasm may be only a part.

what do you think?

Why do we place so much importance on orgasm? ● Can sexual pleasure and satisfaction be achieved without orgasm? ● What is the role of desire in sexual response?

Expressing Your Sexuality

Finding healthy ways to express your sexuality is an important part of developing sexual maturity. Many avenues of sexual expression are available.

Sexual Behavior: What Is "Normal"?

Most of us want to fit in and be identified as normal, but how do we know which sexual behaviors are considered normal? What or whose criteria should we use? These are not easy questions.

Every society sets standards and attempts to regulate sexual behavior. Boundaries arise that distinguish good from bad, acceptable from unacceptable, and they result in criteria used to establish what is viewed as normal or abnormal. Some of the common sociocultural standards for sexual behavior commonly held in Western culture today include the following:[40]

- **The coital standard.** Penile-vaginal intercourse (coitus) is viewed as the ultimate sex act.
- **The orgasmic standard.** Sexual interaction should lead to orgasm.
- **The two-person standard.** Sex is an activity to be experienced by two.
- **The romantic standard.** Sex should be related to love.
- **The safer sex standard.** If we choose to be sexually active, we should act to prevent unintended pregnancy or disease transmission.

These are not laws or rules, but rather social scripts that have been adopted over time. Sexual standards often shift through the years, and many people choose not to follow them. We are a pluralistic nation, and that pluralism extends to our sexual practices. Rather than making blanket judgments about normal versus abnormal, we might ask the following questions:[41]

- Is a sexual behavior healthy and fulfilling for a particular person?
- Is it safe?
- Does it lead to the exploitation of others?
- Does it take place between responsible, consenting adults?

23.3% of college students report having had more than one sex partner in the past 12 months.

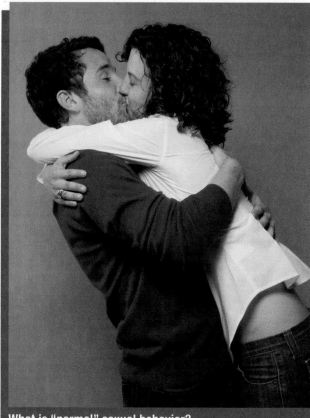

What is "normal" sexual behavior?

As with any other human behavior, the idea of "normal" sexual behavior varies from person to person and from society to society, usually along a spectrum of perceived acceptability or appropriateness. For example, in most modern cultures kissing is a common way to express affection; however, societies have different standards—and individuals have different comfort levels—for the circumstances in which a full-on smack is considered appropriate.

In this way, we can view behavior along a continuum that takes into account many individual factors. As you read about the options for sexual expression in the pages ahead, use these questions to explore your feelings about what is normal for you.

Options for Sexual Expression

celibacy State of not being involved in a sexual relationship.
autoerotic behaviors Sexual self-stimulation.
sexual fantasies Sexually arousing thoughts and dreams.
masturbation Self-stimulation of genitals.
erogenous zones Areas of the body of both men and women that, when touched, lead to sexual arousal.
cunnilingus Oral stimulation of a woman's genitals.
fellatio Oral stimulation of a man's genitals.

The range of human sexual expression is virtually infinite. What you find enjoyable may not be an option for someone else. The ways you choose to meet your sexual needs today may be very different from what they were two weeks ago, or will be two years from now. Accepting yourself as a sexual person with individual desires and preferences is the first step in achieving sexual satisfaction. Curious about your college peers' sexual behavior? See the

Health Today box on the next page—you may be surprised by what it says!

Celibacy Celibacy is avoidance of or abstention from sexual activities with others. Some individuals choose celibacy for religious or moral reasons. Others may be celibate for a period of time because of illness, the breakup of a long-term relationship, or lack of an acceptable partner. For some, celibacy is a lonely, agonizing state, but others find it an opportunity for introspection, values assessment, and personal growth.

Autoerotic Behaviors Autoerotic behaviors involve sexual self-stimulation. The two most common are sexual fantasy and masturbation.

Sexual fantasies are sexually arousing thoughts and dreams. Fantasies may reflect real-life experiences, forbidden desires, or the opportunity to practice new or anticipated sexual experiences. The fact that you may fantasize about a particular sexual experience does not mean that you want to, or have to, act that experience out. Sexual fantasies are just that—fantasy.

Masturbation is self-stimulation of the genitals. Although many people feel uncomfortable discussing masturbation, it is a common sexual practice across the life span. Masturbation is a natural pleasure-seeking behavior in infants and children. It is a valuable and important means for adolescents, as well as adults, to explore sexual feelings and responsiveness. In a recent survey of college students, 64 percent of women and 98 percent of men reported that they had ever masturbated.[42]

Kissing and Erotic Touching Kissing and erotic touching are two very common forms of nonverbal sexual communication. Both men and women have **erogenous zones,** areas of the body that when touched lead to sexual arousal. Erogenous zones may include genital as well as nongenital areas, such as the earlobes, mouth, breasts, and inner thighs. Almost any area of the body can be conditioned to respond erotically to touch. Spending time with your partner to explore and learn about his or her erogenous areas is another pleasurable, safe, and satisfying means of sexual expression.

Manual Stimulation Both men and women can be sexually aroused and achieve orgasm through manual stimulation of the genitals by a partner. For many women, orgasm is more likely to be achieved through manual stimulation than through intercourse. *Sex toys* include a wide variety of objects that can be used for sexual stimulation alone or with a partner. Vibrators and dildos are two common types of toys and can be found in a variety of shapes, styles, and sizes. Sex toys can add zest to sexual experiences and, for women who may not reach orgasm by intercourse, may provide another option for satisfaction. Toys must be cleaned after each use.

Oral–Genital Stimulation Cunnilingus refers to oral stimulation of a woman's genitals, and **fellatio** to oral stimulation of a man's genitals. Many partners find oral–genital stimulation intensely pleasurable. In one study, 43 percent of college

College students often think everyone is having more sex than they are and with numerous partners. These perceptions may cause them to feel self-conscious about their own lack of sexual activity or encourage increased promiscuity in order to "measure up." In reality, college students' opinions about sex, relationships, contraception, and attitudes toward sexual activity vary greatly. Results from a survey answered by college students nationwide might help you sort through some of these misperceptions:

✳ Approximately 77 percent of college students reported having had no or one

sexual (oral, anal, or vaginal) partners within the past school year. However, 83 percent thought the typical student at their school had more than one sexual partner in the past school year.

✳ 43 percent of students reported having had oral sex one or more times in the past 30 days, but 93 percent thought the typical student had oral sex at least once during that time.

✳ 49.5 percent of students reported having had vaginal intercourse one or more times in the past 30 days, yet 94.5 percent thought the typical student had vaginal intercourse at least once during that time.

✳ 5 percent of students reported having anal intercourse one or more times in the past 30 days, whereas 63.5 percent

thought the typical student had anal sex at least once during that time.

✳ 2.6 percent of college students who had vaginal intercourse within the past school year reported experiencing an unintentional pregnancy during that time.

✳ Approximately 28 percent of students reported ever being tested for HIV.

✳ The most common methods of birth control used by sexually active students or their partners the last time they had vaginal intercourse were: birth control pill, 34 percent, and condoms, 36 percent.

Source: American College Health Association, *American College Health Association—National College Health Assessment: Reference Group Data Report Fall 2007* (Baltimore: American College Health Association, 2008).

---

students reported having oral sex in the past month.[43] For some people, oral sex is not an option because of moral or religious beliefs. Remember, HIV (human immunodeficiency virus) and other sexually transmitted infections (STIs) can be transmitted via unprotected oral–genital sex, just as they can through intercourse. Use of an appropriate barrier device is strongly recommended if either partner's health status is in question.

Vaginal Intercourse The term *intercourse* generally refers to **vaginal intercourse** (*coitus,* or insertion of the penis into the vagina), which is the most often practiced form of sexual expression. Coitus can involve a variety of positions, including the missionary position (man on top facing the woman), woman on top, side by side, or man behind (rear entry). Many partners enjoy experimenting with different positions. Knowledge of yourself and your body, along with your ability to communicate effectively, will play a large part in determining the enjoyment or meaning of intercourse for you and your partner. Whatever your circumstance, you should practice safer sex to avoid disease and unwanted pregnancy.

Anal Intercourse The anal area is highly sensitive to touch, and some couples find pleasure in the stimulation of this area. **Anal intercourse** is insertion of the penis into the anus. Research indicates that over 26 percent of college-aged men and women

have had anal sex.[44] Stimulation of the anus by mouth or with the fingers also is practiced. As with all forms of sexual expression, anal stimulation or intercourse is not for everyone. If you do enjoy this form of sexual expression, remember to use condoms to avoid transmitting disease. Also, anything inserted into the anus should not be then directly inserted into the vagina, because bacteria commonly found in the anus can cause vaginal infections.

Variant Sexual Behavior

Although attitudes toward sexuality have changed radically since the Victorian era, some people still believe that any sexual behavior other than heterosexual intercourse is abnormal or perverted. People who study sexuality prefer the neutral term **variant sexual behavior** to describe sexual activities that most people do not engage in, for example:

When used properly, latex condoms can play a significant role in preventing STI transmission.

● **Group sex**—sexual activity involving more than two people. Participants in group sex run a higher risk of exposure to HIV and other STIs.

● **Transvestism**—wearing the clothing of the opposite sex. Most transvestites are male, heterosexual, and married.

vaginal intercourse The insertion of the penis into the vagina.
anal intercourse The insertion of the penis into the anus.
variant sexual behavior A sexual behavior that most people do not engage in.

TABLE
5.2 Types of Sexual Dysfunction

	Basic Description	Examples
Desire Disorders	When you are not interested in sexual activity When you have phobias (fears) or anxiety about sexual contact	Inhibited sexual desire Sexual aversion disorder
Arousal Disorders	When you don't feel a sexual response in your body When you cannot stay sexually aroused	Erectile dysfunction Female sexual arousal disorder
Orgasmic Disorders	When you reach orgasm rapidly or prematurely When you can't have an orgasm or have difficulty or delay in reaching orgasm	Premature ejaculation Female orgasmic disorder
Pain Disorders	When you have pain during or after sex	Dyspareunia Vaginismus

● **Fetishism**—sexual arousal achieved by looking at or touching inanimate objects, such as underclothing or shoes.

Some variant sexual behaviors can be harmful to the individual, to others, or to both. Many of the following activities are illegal in at least some states:

● **Exhibitionism**—exposing one's genitals to strangers in public places. Most exhibitionists are seeking a reaction of shock or fear from their victims. Exhibitionism is a minor felony in most states.
● **Voyeurism**—observing other people for sexual gratification. Most voyeurs are men who attempt to watch women undressing or bathing. Voyeurism is an invasion of privacy and is illegal in most states.
● **Sadomasochism**—sexual activities in which gratification is received by inflicting pain (verbal or physical abuse) on a partner or by being the object of such infliction. A sadist is a person who enjoys inflicting pain, and a masochist is a person who enjoys experiencing it.
● **Pedophilia**—sexual activity or attraction between an adult and a child. Any sexual activity involving a minor, including possession of child pornography, is illegal.
● **Autoerotic asphyxiation**—practice of reducing or eliminating oxygen to the brain, usually by tying a cord around one's neck, while masturbating to orgasm. Tragically, some individuals accidentally strangle themselves.

Sexual Dysfunction

Research indicates that *sexual dysfunction,* the term used to describe problems that can hinder sexual functioning, is quite common. Sexual dysfunction can be divided into four major categories: desire disorders, arousal disorders, orgasmic disorders, and pain disorders (see Table 5.2). All of them can be treated successfully.

Don't feel embarrassed if you experience sexual dysfunction at some point in your life. The sexual part of you does not come with a lifetime guarantee. You can have breakdowns involving your sexual functioning just as in any other body system. If you experience a problem with your sexual function, an important first step is to seek out a qualified health care provider to investigate the possible causes. The causes of a person's sexual problem can be varied and overlapping. Common causes include biological/medical factors, substance-induced factors (recreational, over-the-counter, or prescription drug use), psychological factors (stress, performance pressure), and factors related to social context (relationship tensions, poor communication).[45]

what do you think?

Why do we find it so difficult to discuss sexual dysfunction?
● Do you think it is more difficult for men than for women to talk about dysfunction? Or vice versa?
● Have you ever used alcohol or some other drug to enhance your sexual performance?

Responsible and Satisfying Sexual Behavior

Our sexuality is a fascinating, complex, contradictory, and sometimes frustrating aspect of our lives. Healthy sexuality doesn't happen by chance. It is a product of assimilating information and skills, of exploring values and beliefs, and of making responsible and informed choices. Healthy and responsible sexuality includes the following:

● **Good communication as the foundation.** Open and honest communication with your partner is the basis for establishing respect, trust, and intimacy. Do you communicate with your partner in caring and respectful ways? Can you share your thoughts and emotions freely with your partner? Do you talk about being sexually active and what that means? Can you share your sexual history with your partner? Do you discuss contraception and disease prevention? Are you able to communicate what you like and don't like? All of these are components of open communication that accompany healthy responsible sexuality.

● **Acknowledging that you are a sexual person.** People who can see and accept themselves as sexual beings are more likely to make informed decisions and take responsible actions. If you see yourself as a potentially sexual person, you will plan ahead for contraception and disease prevention. If you are comfortable being a sexually active person, you will not need or want your sexual experiences clouded by alcohol or other drug use. If you choose not to be sexually active, you do so consciously, as a personal decision based on your convictions. Even if you are not sexually active, it is important to acknowledge that sex is a natural aspect of everyone's life and to recognize that you are in charge of your own decisions about your sexuality.

● **Understanding sexual structures and their functions.** If you understand how your body works, sexual pleasure and response will not be mysterious events. You will be able to pleasure yourself as well as communicate to your partner how best to pleasure you. You will understand how pregnancy and sexually transmitted infections can be prevented. You will be able to recognize sexual dysfunction and take responsible actions to address the problem.

● **Accepting and embracing your gender identity and your sexual orientation.** "Being comfortable in your own skin" is an old saying that is particularly relevant when it comes to sexuality. It is difficult to feel sexually satisfied if you are conflicted about your gender identity or sexual orientation. You should explore and address questions and feelings you may have about either your gender identity or your sexual orientation. Good communication skills, acknowledging that you are a sexual person, and understanding your sexual structures and their functions will allow you to complete this task.

Drugs and Sex

Because psychoactive drugs affect the body's entire physiological functioning, it is only logical that they affect sexual behavior. Promises of increased pleasure make drugs very tempting to people seeking greater sexual satisfaction. Too often, however, drugs become central to sexual activities and damage the relationship. Drug use can also lead to undesired sexual activity.

Alcohol is notorious for reducing inhibitions and promoting feelings of well-being and desirability. At the same time, alcohol inhibits sexual response; thus, the mind may be willing, but not the body. An increasing number of young men have begun experimenting with the recreational use of drugs intended to treat erectile dysfunction, including Viagra, Cialis, and Levitra. These drugs work by relaxing the smooth muscle cells in the penis, allowing for increased blood flow to the erectile tissues. Young men who take this type of medication are hoping to increase their sexual stamina, or counteract sexual performance anxiety or the effects of alcohol or other drugs. However, these drugs probably have only a placebo effect in men with normal erections, and combining them with other drugs, such as ketamine, amyl nitrate, and methamphetamine, can lead to potentially fatal drug interactions. In particular, when combined with amyl nitrate these drugs can lead to a sudden drop in blood pressure, and possible cardiac arrest.[46]

"Date rape" drugs have been a growing concern in recent decades. They have become prevalent on college campuses, where they are often used in combination with alcohol. Rohypnol ("roofies," "rope," "forget pill"), GHB (gamma-hydroxybutyrate, or "liquid X," "Grievous Bodily Harm," "easy lay," "Mickey Finn"), and ketamine ("K," "Special K," "cat valium") have been used to facilitate rape. GHB and Rohypnol are difficult-to-detect drugs that depress the central nervous system. Ketamine can cause dreamlike states, hallucinations, delirium, amnesia, and impaired motor function. These drugs are often introduced to unsuspecting women through alcoholic drinks to render them unconscious and vulnerable to rape. This problem is so serious that the U.S. Congress passed the Drug-Induced Rape Prevention and Punishment Act of 1996 to increase federal penalties for using drugs to facilitate sexual assault. The dangers of these drugs are discussed in more detail in Chapter 7.

Perhaps the most common danger associated with use of drugs during sex is the tendency to blame the drug for negative behavior or unsafe sexual activities. "I can't help what I did last night because I was drunk" is a statement that demonstrates sexual immaturity. A sexually mature person carefully examines risks and benefits and makes decisions accordingly. If drugs are necessary to increase erotic feelings, it is likely that the partners are being dishonest about their feelings for each other. Good sex should not depend on chemical substances.

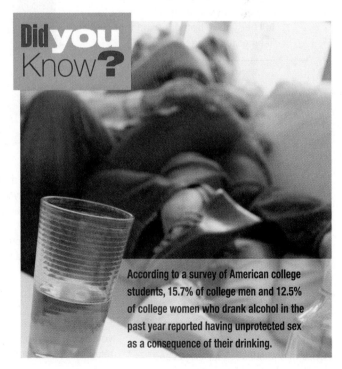

Did you Know?

According to a survey of American college students, 15.7% of college men and 12.5% of college women who drank alcohol in the past year reported having unprotected sex as a consequence of their drinking.

Assess yourself

How Well Do You Communicate?

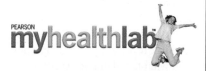

Fill out this assessment online at
www.pearsonhighered.com/myhealthlab or
www.pearsonhighered.com/donatelle.

Imagine that you are in each of the situations below, and indicate how confident and satisfied you are that you could communicate competently using the following scale.

1. Very dissatisfied with my ability to communicate
2. Somewhat dissatisfied with my ability to communicate
3. Not sure how effectively I could communicate
4. Somewhat satisfied that I could communicate competently
5. Very satisfied that I could communicate competently

____ 1. Someone asks you personal questions that you feel uncomfortable answering. You'd like to tell the person that you don't want to answer.

____ 2. You think a friend is drinking more alcohol than is healthy, and you want to bring it up with her.

____ 3. Your colleague asks you to write him a letter of recommendation. You don't think he is well suited for the position to which he's applying.

____ 4. During a heated discussion about social issues, the person with whom you are talking says, "You're not listening to anything I'm saying!"

____ 5. A friend shares his creative writing with you. You don't think the writing is very good, but you need to respond to his request for an opinion.

____ 6. Your roommate's habits are really getting on your nerves. You want to tell her you're bothered and that you'd like her to change the habit.

____ 7. You arrive at a party and discover that you don't know anyone there.

____ 8. A classmate asks you for notes for the classes he missed, but you realize he has missed half the classes and expects you to bail him out.

____ 9. The person you have been dating declares, "I love you." You care about her, but you don't love her, at least not yet.

____ 10. A friend comes to you with his problems, and you give him attention and advice. However, when you want to discuss your problems, he doesn't seem to have the time. You value the friendship, but you don't like feeling it's one-way.

____ TOTAL

Interpreting Your Score

If your score indicates that you are moderately satisfied (25–39) or dissatisfied (10–24) with your communication skills, notice whether your answers are extremes (1s and 5s). Focus on improving your skills in the situations that make you uneasy.

Source: Based on Julia Wood and Stephanie Coopman's Instructor's Resource Manual for Wood's text, *Interpersonal Communication: Everyday Encounters,* 5th ed. Copyright © 2006, Cengage Learning.

YOUR PLAN FOR CHANGE

The **Assess yourself** activity gave you the chance to look at how you communicate. Now that you have considered your responses, you can take steps toward becoming a better communicator and improving your relationships.

Today, you can:

◯ Call a friend you haven't talked to in a while or arrange a coffee date with a new acquaintance you'd like to get to know better.

◯ Start a journal in which you keep track of communication and relationship issues that arise. Look for trends and think about ways you can change your behavior to address them.

Within the next 2 weeks, you can:

◯ Spend some time letting the people you care about know how important their relationship is to you.

◯ If there is someone with whom you have a conflict, arrange a time to sit down with that person in a neutral setting away from distractions to talk about the issues.

By the end of the semester, you can:

◯ Practice being an active listener and notice when your mind wanders while you are listening to someone.

◯ Take note of your nonverbal messages. Work on maintaining good eye contact and using open body language and inviting facial expressions.

Summary

* Characteristics of intimate relationships include behavioral interdependence, need fulfillment, emotional attachment, and emotional availability. These characteristics influence how we interact with others and the types of intimate relationships we form. Family, friends, and partners or lovers provide the most common opportunities for intimacy. Each relationship may include healthy and unhealthy characteristics that affect daily functioning.

* To improve our ability to communicate with others, we need to address several factors, including learning how to use self-disclosure, listening effectively, conveying and interpreting nonverbal communication, establishing a proper climate for communicating, and managing and resolving conflicts.

* For most people, commitment is an important ingredient in successful relationships. The major types of committed relationships include marriage, cohabitation, and gay and lesbian partnerships.

* Success in committed relationships requires understanding the elements of a good relationship, including open communication and mutual respect, and coping with conflicts such as jealousy, gender roles, power sharing, and unmet expectations.

* Life decisions such as whether to marry or whether to have children require serious consideration. Remaining single is more common than ever. Most single people lead healthy, happy, and well-adjusted lives. Those who decide to have or not to have children also can lead rewarding, productive lives as long as they have given this decision the utmost thought and weighed the pros and cons of each alternative in the context of their lifestyle.

* Before relationships fail, often many warning signs appear. By recognizing these signs and taking action to change behaviors, partners may save and enhance their relationships.

* Sexual identity is determined by a complex interaction of genetic, physiological, and environmental factors. Biological sex, gender identity, gender roles, and sexual orientation all are blended into our sexual identity.

* Sexual orientation refers to a person's enduring emotional, romantic, sexual, or affectionate attraction to other persons. Gay, lesbian, and bisexual persons are repeatedly the targets of sexual prejudice. Sexual prejudice refers to negative attitudes and hostile actions directed at a social group and its members.

* The major components of the female sexual anatomy include the mons pubis, labia minora and majora, clitoris, urethral and vaginal openings, vagina, cervix, fallopian tubes, and ovaries. The major components of the male sexual anatomy are the penis, scrotum, testes, epididymides, vasa deferentia, ejaculatory ducts, and urethra.

* Physiologically, men and women experience the same four phases of sexual response: excitement/arousal, plateau, orgasm, and resolution.

* People can express their sexual selves in a variety of ways, including celibacy, autoerotic behaviors, kissing and erotic touch, manual stimulation, oral–genital stimulation, vaginal intercourse, and anal intercourse.

* Sexual dysfunctions can be classified into disorders of sexual desire, sexual arousal, orgasm, and sexual pain, and can be caused by biological factors, substance use, psychological factors, or social factors. All are treatable.

* Responsible and satisfying sexuality involves good communication, recognition of yourself as a sexual being, understanding sexual structures and functions, and acceptance of your gender identity and sexual orientation.

* Alcohol and other psychoactive drugs can affect sexual behavior. Drug use can decrease inhibitions and lead people to engage in unsafe or undesired sexual activity. "Date rape" drugs are illicit substances used to incapacitate a person in order to facilitate rape.

Pop Quiz

1. Intimate relationships fulfill our psychological need for someone to listen to our worries and concerns. This is known as our need for
   a. dependence.
   b. social integration.
   c. enjoyment.
   d. spontaneity.

2. Lovers tend to pay attention to the other person even when they should be involved in other activities. This is called
   a. inclusion.
   b. exclusivity.
   c. fascination.
   d. authentic intimacy.

3. Intense feelings of elation, sexual desire, and ecstasy in being with a partner are characteristic of
   a. companionate love.
   b. mature love.
   c. passionate love.
   d. intimacy.

4. According to anthropologist Helen Fisher, attraction and falling in love follow a pattern based on
   a. lust, attraction, and attachment.
   b. intimacy, passion, and commitment.
   c. imprinting, attraction, attachment, and the production of a cuddle chemical.
   d. fascination, exclusiveness, sexual desire, giving the utmost, and being a champion.

5. One of the most important ways to express difficult feelings with another person is to
   a. be specific rather than general about how you feel.
   b. express anger and resentment so the other person feels your heartache.

c. point your finger at the other person.

d. blame the other person for the difficulty you are experiencing.

6. Terms such as *behavioral interdependence, need fulfillment,* and *emotional availability* describe which type of relationship?
   a. dysfunctional relationship
   b. sexual relationship
   c. intimate relationship
   d. behavioral relationship

7. One factor in choosing a partner is *proximity,* which refers to
   a. mutual regard.
   b. attitudes and values.
   c. physical attraction.
   d. being in the same place at the same time.

8. Your personal inner sense of maleness or femaleness is known as your
   a. sexual identity.
   b. sexual orientation.
   c. gender identity.
   d. gender.

9. Individuals who are sexually attracted to both sexes are identified as
   a. heterosexual.
   b. bisexual.
   c. homosexual.
   d. intersexual.

10. The most sensitive or erotic spot in the female genital region is the
    a. mons pubis.
    b. vagina.
    c. clitoris.
    d. labia.

Answers to these questions can be found on page A-1.

Think about It!

1. What are the characteristics of intimate relationships? What are behavioral interdependence, need fulfillment, emotional attachment, and emotional availability, and why is each important in relationship development?

2. Why are relationships with family important? Explain how your family unit was similar to or different from the traditional family unit in early America. Who made up your family of origin?

3. What problems can form barriers to intimacy? What actions can you take to reduce or remove these barriers?

4. What are the common elements of good relationships? What are some common warning signs of trouble? What actions can you take to improve your own interpersonal relationships?

5. How have gender roles changed over your lifetime? Do you view the changes as positive for both men and women?

6. What is "normal" sexual behavior? What criteria should we use to determine healthy sexual practices?

7. If scientists ever establish the combination of factors that interact to produce homosexual, heterosexual, or bisexual orientation, will that put an end to antigay prejudice? Why or why not?

Accessing Your Health on the Internet

The following websites explore further topics and issues related to personal health. For links to the websites below, visit the Companion Website for *Health: The Basics,* Green Edition at www.pearsonhighered.com/donatelle.

1. *American Association of Sexuality Educators, Counselors, and Therapists (AASECT).* Professional organization providing standards of practice for treating sexual issues and disorders. www.aasect.org

2. *The BACCHUS Network.* Student-friendly source of information about sexual and other health issues.
   www.bacchusgamma.org

3. *Go Ask Alice!.* An interactive question-and-answer resource from the Columbia University Health Services. "Alice" is available to answer questions about any health-related issues, including relationships, nutrition and diet, exercise, drugs, sex, alcohol, and stress. www.goaskalice.columbia.edu

4. *Sexuality Information and Education Council of the United States (SIECUS).* Information, guidelines, and materials for advancement of healthy and proper sex education.
   www.siecus.org

5. *Advocates for Youth.* Current news, policy updates, research, and other resources about the sexual health of and choices particular to high-school and college-aged students.
   www.advocatesforyouth.org

References

1. MayoClinic.com, "Nurture Relationships: A Healthy Habit for Healthy Aging," 2003, Mayo Foundation for Medical Education and Research (MFMER), www.mayohealth.org; K. Uberg et al., "Supportive Relationships as a Moderator of the Effects of Peer Drinking on Adolescents," *Journal of Research on Adolescents* 15, no. 1 (2005): 1–20.
2. E. Weinstein and E. Rosen, *Teaching about Human Sexuality and Family: A Skills-Based Approach* (Belmont, CA: Thomson Higher Education, 2006).
3. Ibid.
4. L. Lefton and L. Brannon, *Psychology,* 9th ed. (Boston: Allyn & Bacon, 2005), 474.
5. Ibid.
6. H. Fisher, *Why We Love: The Nature and Chemistry of Romantic Love* (New York: Henry Holt, 2004).
7. E. Hatfield and R. L. Rapson, *Love, Sex, and Intimacy: Their Psychology, Biology, and History* (New York: Harper Collins, 1993).
8. R. Sternberg, "Construct Validation of a Triangular Love Scale," *European Journal of Social Psychology* 27 (1997): 313–35.
9. H. Fisher, *Why We Love;* H. Fisher, A. Aron, D. Mashek, H. Li, and L. L. Brown, "Defining the Brain System of Lust, Romantic Attraction, and Attachment," *Archives of Sexual Behavior* 31, no. 5 (2002): 413–19.
10. A. Toufexis and P. Gray, "What Is Love? The Right Chemistry," *Time,* February 15, 1993, 47–52.

11. H. Fisher et al., "Defining the Brain System," 413–19.
12. S. A. Rathus, J. Nevid, and L. Fichner-Rathus, *Human Sexuality in a World of Diversity.* 6th ed. (Boston: Allyn & Bacon, 2005).
13. R. Adler and G. Rodman, "Perceiving the Self," in *Making Connections*, eds. K. Galvin and P. Cooper (Los Angeles: Roxbury Press, 2000), 23.
14. B. L. Seaward, *Managing Stress: Principles and Practices for Health and Well-Being.* 4th ed. (Boston: Jones & Bartlett, 2004), 100.
15. J. K. Burgoon, C. Segrin, and N. E. Dunbar, "Nonverbal Communication and Social Influence," in *Persuasion: Developments in Theory and Practice*, eds. J. P. Dillard and M. Pfau (Thousand Oaks, CA: Sage, 2002), 445–76.
16. R. S. Miller, D. Perlman, and S. S. Brehm, *Intimate Relationships.* 4th ed. (New York: McGraw-Hill, 2007), 150–56.
17. The National Marriage Project, Rutgers, the State University of New Jersey, "The State of Our Unions," 2007, http://marriage.rutgers.edu/Publications/SOOU/TEXTSOOU2007.htm.
18. Ibid.
19. Mayo Clinic Staff, "Healthy Marriage: Why Love Is Good for You," Mayo Foundation for Medical Education and Research (MFMER), February 6, 2006, www.mayoclinic.com.
20. C. A. Schoenborn, "Marital Status and Health: United States, 1999–2002," December 15, 2004, Advance Data from Vital and Health Statistics, Centers for Disease Control and Prevention.
21. Ibid.
22. J. Teachman, "Premarital Sex, Premarital Cohabitation, and the Risk of Subsequent Marital Dissolution among Women," *Journal of Marriage and Family* 65, no. 2 (2002): 444–55; C. L. Cohan and S. Kleinbaum, "Toward a Greater Understanding of the Cohabitation Effect: Premarital Cohabitation and Marital Communication," *Journal of Marriage and Family* 64, no. 1 (2002): 180–92.
23. C. A. Schoenborn, "Marital Status and Health," 2004.
24. National Gay and Lesbian Task Force, "Relationship Recognition Map for Same-Sex Couples in the U.S.," November 2009, www.thetaskforce.org/reports_and_research/relationship_recognition.
25. U.S. Census Bureau, Housing and Household Economic Statistics Division, Fertility & Family Statistics Branch, "America's Families and Living Arrangements: 2007," 2008, www.census.gov/population/www/socdemo/hh-fam/cps2007.html.
26. U.S. Census Bureau; Centers for Disease Control and Prevention, "National Survey of Family Growth," Updated June 2009, www.cdc.gov/nchs/nsfg.htm.
27. S. Brehm et al., *Intimate Relationships.* 3d ed. (New York: McGraw-Hill, 2002), 263.
28. G. F. Kelly, *Sexuality Today: The Human Perspective.* 8th ed. (Boston: McGraw-Hill, 2006), 270; B. Strong et al., *Human Sexuality: Diversity in Contemporary America.* 5th ed. (New York: McGraw-Hill, 2005).
29. National Center for Health Statistics, *National Vital Statistics Report* 49, no. 6 (August 2001).
30. U.S. Department of Labor Statistics, "Consumer Expenditure Survey Anthology, 2005," May 6, 2005, www.bls.gov/cex/csxanthol05.htm.
31. D. Hurley, "Divorce Rate: It's Not as High as You Think," *New York Times*, April 19, 2005.
32. The National Marriage Project, Rutgers, "The State of Our Unions," 2007.
33. G. F. Kelly, *Sexuality Today*, 2006.
34. G. M. Herek, "The Psychology of Sexual Prejudice," *Current Directions in Psychological Science* 9 (2000): 12–22.
35. Federal Bureau of Investigation, "Hate Crime Statistics, 2007," November 2008, www.fbi.gov/ucr/hc2007/index.html.
36. S. E. Anderson, G. E. Dallal, and A. Must, "Relative Weight and Race Influence Average Age at Menarche: Results from Two Nationally Representative Surveys of U.S. Girls Studied 25 Years Apart," *Pediatrics* 111, no. 4 (2003): 844–50.
37. Mayo Clinic Staff, "Menstrual Cramps," 2007, www.mayoclinic.com/Health/Menstrual-Cramps/Ds00506/Dsection=1.
38. Writing Group for the Women's Health Initiative Investigators, "Risk and Benefits of Estrogen Plus Progestin in Healthy Postmenopausal Women: Principal Results from the Women's Health Initiative Randomized Controlled Trial," *Journal of the American Medical Association* 288, no. 3 (2002): 321–33.
39. N. Siegfried et al., "HIV and Male Circumcision—A Systematic Review with the Assessment of Quality of Studies," *The Lancet—Infectious Diseases* 5, no. 3 (2005): 165–73; A. Bertran et al., "Randomized, Controlled Intervention Trial of Male Circumcision for Reduction of HIV Transmission Risk: The ANRS 1265 Trial," *PLoS Medicine* 2, no. 11 (2005): 1112–22; B. G. Williams et al., "The Potential Impact of Male Circumcision on HIV in Sub-Saharan Africa," *PLoS Medicine* 3, no. 7 (2006): e262; B. P. Homeier, "Circumcision," Paper presented at KidsHealth for Parents, Nemours Foundation, January 2005, http://kidshealth.org/parent/system/surgical/circumcision.html; Mayo Clinic Staff, "Circumcision for Baby Boys: Weighing the Pros and Cons," MayoClinic.com, March 2006, www.mayoclinic.com/health/circumcision/PR00040.
40. G. F. Kelly, "Sexual Individuality and Sexual Values," in *Sexuality Today.* 2006.
41. Ibid.
42. S. D. Pinkerton et al., "Factors Associated with Masturbation in a Collegiate Sample," *Journal of Psychology and Human Sexuality* 14, no. 2 (2002): 103–21.
43. American College Health Association, *American College Health Association—National College Health Assessment (ACHA-NCHA) Reference Group Data Report Fall 2007* (Baltimore: American College Health Association, 2008).
44. Ibid.
45. G. F. Kelly, "Sexual Dysfunctions and Their Treatment," in *Sexuality Today.* 9th ed. (New York: McGraw-Hill, 2008), 528.
46. K. M. Smith and F. Romanelli, "Recreational Use and Misuse of Phosphodiesterase 5 Inhibitors," *Journal of the American Pharmacists Association* 45, no. 1 (2005): 63–75; R. Kloner, "Erectile Dysfunction and Hypertension," *International Journal of Impotence Research* 19, no. 3 (2007): 296–302.

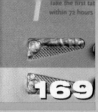
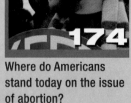

166
Does the birth control pill cause any side effects?

169
What is emergency contraception?

174
Where do Americans stand today on the issue of abortion?

178
How can I prepare to be a parent?

6 Your Reproductive Choices

Objectives

* Compare the different types of contraceptive methods and their effectiveness in preventing pregnancy and sexually transmitted infections.

* Summarize the legal decisions surrounding abortion and the various types of abortion procedures.

* Discuss key issues to consider when planning a pregnancy.

* Explain the importance of prenatal care and the physical and emotional aspects of pregnancy.

* Describe the basic stages of childbirth and complications that can arise during labor and delivery.

* Explain primary causes of and possible solutions to infertility.

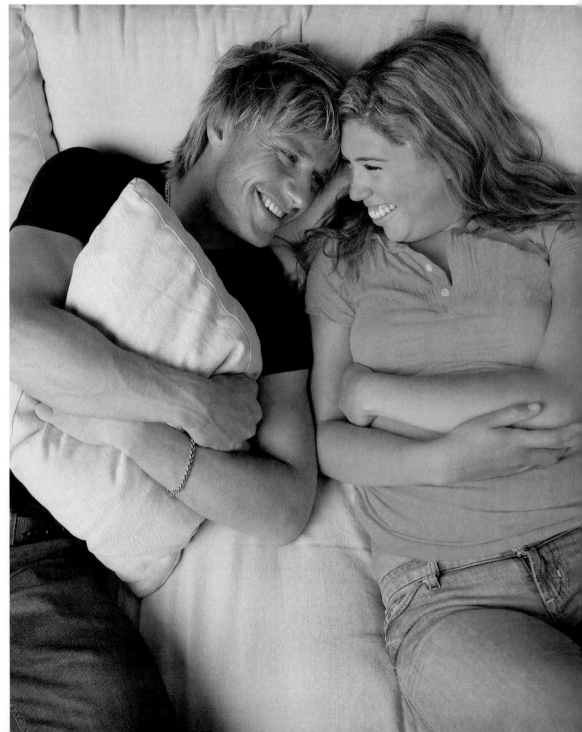

Today we not only understand the intimate details of reproduction, but also possess technologies that control or enhance our **fertility,** our ability to reproduce. Along with information and technological advances comes choice, and choice goes hand in hand with responsibility. Choosing whether and when to have children is one of our greatest responsibilities. A woman and her partner have much to consider before planning or risking a pregnancy. Children transform people's lives. They require a lifelong personal commitment of love and nurturing. Are you physically, emotionally, and financially prepared to care for another human being?

One measure of maturity is the ability to discuss reproduction and birth control with one's sexual partner before engaging in sexual activity. Men often assume that their partners are taking care of birth control. Women often feel that bringing up the subject implies they are promiscuous. Both may feel that this discussion interferes with romance and spontaneity. You will find discussion easier and less embarrassing if you understand human reproduction and contraception and honestly consider your attitudes toward these matters.

Methods of Fertility Management

Conception refers to the fertilization of an ovum by a sperm. The following conditions are necessary for conception:

1. A viable egg (ovum)
2. A viable sperm
3. Access to the egg by the sperm

The term **contraception** (sometimes called **birth control**) refers to methods of preventing conception. These methods offer varying degrees of control over when and whether pregnancies occur. Society has searched for a simple, infallible, and risk-free way to prevent pregnancy since people first associated sexual activity with pregnancy. We have not yet found one.

To evaluate the effectiveness of a particular contraceptive method, you must be familiar with two concepts: perfect failure rate and typical use failure rate. *Perfect failure rate* refers to the number of pregnancies that are likely to occur in the first year of use (per 100 users of the method) if the method is used absolutely perfectly, that is, without any error. The *typical use failure rate* refers to the number of pregnancies that are likely to occur during the first year of use with typical use—that is, with the normal number of errors, memory lapses, and incorrect or incomplete use. The typical use information is much more practical in helping people make informed decisions about contraceptive methods.

Present methods of contraception fall into several categories. **Barrier methods** block the egg and sperm from joining. **Hormonal methods** introduce synthetic hormones into the woman's system that prevent ovulation, thicken cervical mucus, or prevent a fertilized egg from implanting. Surgical methods can prevent pregnancy permanently. Other methods may involve temporary or permanent abstinence or planning intercourse in accordance with fertility patterns. Some contraceptive methods can also protect, to some degree, against **sexually transmitted infections (STIs),** which you'll learn more about in Chapter 13. This is an important factor to consider in choosing a contraceptive. Table 6.1 on page 160 summarizes the effectiveness, STI protection, frequency of use, and costs of various methods.

Barrier Methods

Barrier methods work on the simple principle of preventing sperm from ever reaching the egg by use of a physical or chemical barrier during intercourse. Some barrier methods prevent semen from having any contact with the woman's body, and others prevent sperm from going past the cervix. In addition, many barrier methods contain or are used in combination with a substance that kills sperm.

The Male Condom

The **male condom** is a thin sheath designed to cover the erect penis and catch semen before it enters the vagina. The majority of male condoms are made of latex, although condoms made of polyurethane or lambskin are also available. Condoms come in a wide variety of styles. All may be purchased in pharmacies, supermarkets, public bathrooms, and many health clinics. A new condom must be used for each act of vaginal, oral, or anal intercourse.

A condom must be rolled onto the penis before the penis touches the vagina and held in place when removing the penis from the vagina after ejaculation (see Figure 6.1 on page 161). Condoms come with or without spermicide and with or without lubrication. Spermicides can cause irritation for some users, and there is no evidence that using a spermicide with condoms reduces the risk of pregnancy. If desired, users can lubricate their own condoms with contraceptive foams, creams, and jellies or other water-based lubricants. Never use products such as baby oil, cold cream, petroleum jelly, vaginal yeast infection medications, or hand or body lotion with a condom. These products contain mineral oil and will cause the latex to disintegrate.

Condoms are less effective and more likely to break during intercourse if they are old or poorly stored. To maintain effectiveness, store them in a cool place (not in a

fertility A person's ability to reproduce.
conception The fertilization of an ovum by a sperm.
contraception (birth control) Methods of preventing conception.
barrier methods Contraceptive methods that block the meeting of egg and sperm by means of a physical barrier (such as condom, diaphragm, or cervical cap), a chemical barrier (such as spermicide), or both.
hormonal methods Contraceptive methods that introduce synthetic hormones into the woman's system to prevent ovulation, thicken cervical mucus, or prevent a fertilized egg from implanting.
sexually transmitted infections (STIs) A variety of infections that can be acquired through sexual contact.
male condom A single-use sheath of thin latex or other material designed to fit over an erect penis and to catch semen on ejaculation.

Contraceptive Effectiveness, STI Protection, Frequency of Use, and Costs

Method	Failure Rate Typical Use	Failure Rate Perfect Use	STI Protection	Frequency of Use	Cost
Continuous abstinence	0	0	Yes	N/A	None
Female sterilization	0.5	0.5	No	Done once	$1,500–$6,000/interview, counseling, examination, operation, and follow-up
Male sterilization	0.15	0.1	No	Done once	$350–$1,000/interview, counseling, examination, operation, and follow-up sperm count
Implanon	0.05	0.05	No	Inserted every 3 years	$400–$600/exam, device, and insertion; $75–$250 for removal
IUD (intrauterine device)					
ParaGard (copper T)	0.8	0.6	No	Inserted every 10 years	$175–$500/exam, insertion, and follow-up visit
Mirena (LNG-IUS)	0.2	0.2	No	Inserted every 5 years	$175–$500/exam, insertion, and follow-up visit
Depo-Provera	3	0.3	No	Injected every 12 weeks	$30–$75/3-month injection; $35–$175 for initial exam; $20–$40 for further visits to clinician for shots
Oral contraceptives (combined pill and progestin-only pill)	8	0.3	No	Taken daily	$15–$35 for monthly pill pack at drugstores, often less at clinics; $35–$175 for initial exam
Ortho Evra patch	8	0.3	No	Applied weekly	$30–$40/month at drugstores; often less at clinics, $35–$175 for initial exam
NuvaRing	8	0.3	No	Inserted every 4 weeks	$30–$35/month at drugstores, often less at clinics; $35–$175 for initial exam
Male condom (without spermicides)	15	2	Some	Used every time	$0.50 and up/condom—some family planning centers give them away or charge very little; available in drugstores, family planning clinics, some supermarkets, and from vending machines
Diaphragm (with spermicidal cream or jelly)	16	6	Some	Used every time	$15–$75 for diaphragms, caps, and shields; $50–$200 for initial exam; $8–$17/supplies of spermicide jelly or cream
Today sponge					
Women who have never given birth	16	9	No	Used every time	$7.50–$9/package of three sponges; available at family planning centers, drugstores, online, and in some supermarkets
Women who have given birth	32	20	No	Used every time	
Female condom (without spermicides)	21	5	Some	Used every time	$2.50/condom; available at family planning centers, drugstores, and in some supermarkets
Fertility awareness–based methods	25	12	No	Followed every month	$10–$12 for temperature kits; charts and classes often free in health centers and churches
Withdrawal	27	4	No	Used every time	None
Spermicides (foams, creams, gels, vaginal suppositories, and vaginal film)	29	18	No	Used every time	$8–$17/applicator kits of foam and gel ($4–$8 refills); film and suppositories are priced similarly; available at family planning clinics, drugstores, and some supermarkets
No method	85	85	No	N/A	None
Emergency contraceptive pill	Treatment initiated within 72 hours after unprotected intercourse reduces the risk of pregnancy by 75%–89% (with no protection against STIs). Costs depend on what services are needed: $10–$45/Plan B, available OTC to women 18 and older; $20–$50/one pack of combination pills; $50–$70/two packs of progestin-only pills; $35–$150/visit with health care provider; $10–$20/pregnancy test				

Note: "Failure Rate" refers to the number of unintended pregnancies per 100 women during the first year of use. "Typical Use" refers to failure rates for men and women whose use is not consistent or always correct. "Perfect Use" refers to failure rates for those whose use is consistent and always correct.

Some family planning clinics charge for services and supplies on a sliding scale according to income.

Source: Adapted from R. Hatcher et al., *Contraceptive Technology*. 19th rev. ed. Copyright © 2007 Contraceptive Technology Communications, Inc. Used with permission.

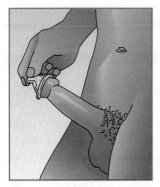

1 Pinch the air out of the top half-inch of the condom to allow room for semen.

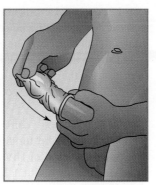

2 Holding the tip of the condom with one hand, use the other hand to unroll it onto the penis.

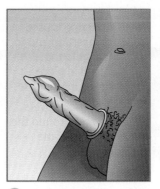

3 Unroll the condom all the way to the base of the penis, smoothing out any air bubbles.

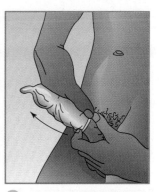

4 After ejaculation, hold the condom around the base until the penis is totally withdrawn to avoid spilling any semen.

FIGURE 6.1　**How to Use a Male Condom**

wallet or hip pocket), and inspect them for small tears before use. Discard all condoms that have passed their expiration date.

Advantages When used consistently and correctly, condoms can be up to 98 percent effective. The condom is the only temporary means of birth control available for men, and latex and polyurethane condoms are the only barriers that effectively prevent the spread of some STIs and HIV. ("Skin" condoms, made from lamb intestines, are not effective against STIs.) Many people choose condoms as their form of birth control because they are inexpensive, readily available without a prescription, and their use is limited to times of sexual activity, with no negative health effects. Some

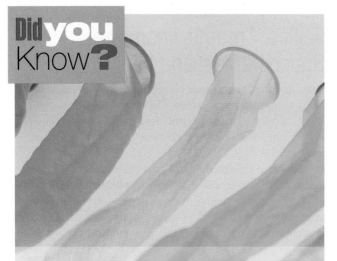

Did you Know?

Condoms have been protecting people for millennia. The ancient Egyptians used linen sheaths and animal intestines as condoms back in 1220 BC. The oldest evidence of condom use in Europe is said to come from cave paintings at the Grotte des Combarelles in France, dating from AD 100–200!

80–90%

That's the reduction in risk of STI transmission provided by latex condoms, according to several research studies.

men find that condoms help them stay erect longer or help prevent premature ejaculation.

Disadvantages The easy availability of condoms is accompanied by considerable potential for user error; as a result, the typical use effectiveness of condoms in preventing pregnancy is around 85 percent. Improper use of a condom can lead to breakage, leakage, or slipping, potentially exposing the users to STI transmission or an unintended pregnancy. Even when used perfectly, a condom doesn't protect against transmission of STIs that may have external areas of infection (e.g., herpes).

For some people, a condom ruins the spontaneity of sex because stopping to put it on may break the mood. Others report that the condom decreases sensation. These inconveniences and perceptions contribute to improper use or avoidance of condoms altogether. Partners who apply a condom as part of foreplay are generally more successful with this form of birth control. As a new condom is required for each act of intercourse, some users find it difficult to be sure to have a condom available when needed.

The Female Condom

The **female condom** (brand name, Reality Condom) is a single-use, soft, loose-fitting polyurethane sheath meant for internal vaginal

female condom A single-use polyurethane sheath for internal use during vaginal or anal intercourse to catch semen on ejaculation.

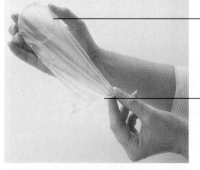

Inner ring is used for insertion and to help hold the sheath in place during intercourse

Outer ring covers the area around the opening of the vagina

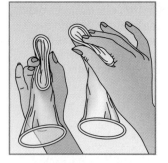

1 Grasp the flexible inner ring at the closed end of the condom, and squeeze it between your thumb and second or middle finger so it becomes long and narrow.

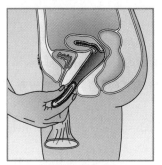

2 Choose a comfortable position for insertion: squatting, with one leg raised, or sitting or lying down. While squeezing the ring, insert the closed end of the condom into your vagina.

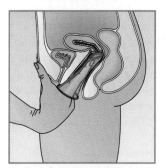

3 Placing your index finger inside of the condom, gently push the inner ring up as far as it will go. Be sure the sheath is not twisted. The outer ring should remain outside of the vagina.

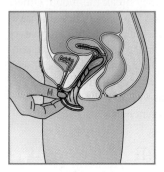

4 During intercourse, be sure that the penis is not entering on the side, between the sheath and the vaginal wall. When removing the condom, twist the outer ring so that no semen leaks out.

FIGURE 6.2 **How to Use a Female Condom**

use. It is designed as one unit with two flexible rings. One ring lies inside the sheath and serves as an insertion mechanism and internal anchor. The other ring remains outside the vagina once the device is inserted and protects the labia and the base of the penis from infection. Figure 6.2 shows the proper use of the female condom.

Advantages Used consistently and correctly, female condoms can be up to 95 percent effective. They also can prevent the spread of HIV and other STIs, including those that can be transmitted by external genital contact. The female condom can be inserted up to 8 hours in advance, so its use doesn't have to interrupt lovemaking. Some women choose to use the female condom because it gives them more personal control over pregnancy prevention and STI protection, or because they cannot rely on their partner to use a male condom. Because the polyurethane is thin and pliable, there is less loss of sensation with the female condom than there is with the latex male condom. The female condom is relatively inexpensive, readily available without a prescription, and causes no negative health effects. It can also be used by either gender for anal intercourse.

Disadvantages As with the male condom, there is potential for user error with the female condom, including possible breaking, slipping, or leaking, all of which could lead to STI transmission or an unintended pregnancy. Because of the potential problems, the typical use effectiveness of the female condom is 79 percent. Some people dislike using the female condom because they feel it is disruptive, noisy, odd looking, or difficult to use. Some women have reported external or vaginal irritation from using the female condom. A new condom is required for each act of intercourse, so users may not always have one available when needed.

Jellies, Creams, Foams, Suppositories, and Film

Like condoms, some other barrier methods—jellies, creams, foam, suppositories, and film—do not require a prescription. They are referred to as **spermicides**—substances designed to kill sperm. The active ingredient in most of them is nonoxynol-9 (N-9).

Jellies and creams are packaged in tubes, and foams are available in aerosol cans. All have applicators designed for insertion into the vagina. They must be inserted far enough to cover the cervix, thus providing both a chemical barrier that kills sperm and a physical barrier that stops sperm from continuing toward an egg.

Suppositories are waxy capsules that are inserted deep in the vagina, where they melt. They must be inserted 10 to 20 minutes before intercourse to have time to melt, but no longer than 1 hour prior to intercourse, or they lose their effectiveness. Additional contraceptive chemicals must be applied for each subsequent act of intercourse.

Vaginal contraceptive film is another method of spermicide delivery. A thin film infused with spermicidal gel is inserted into the vagina, so that it covers the cervix. The film dissolves into a spermicidal gel that is effective for up to 3 hours. As with other spermicides, a new film must be inserted for each act of intercourse.

Advantages Spermicides are most effective when used in conjunction with another barrier method (condom, diaphragm, etc.); used alone they offer only 71 percent (typical use) to 82 percent (perfect use) effectiveness at preventing pregnancy. Like condoms, spermicides are inexpensive and readily available, and their use is limited to the time of sexual activity.

Disadvantages Spermicides can be messy and must be reapplied for each act of intercourse. Some people experience irritation or allergic reactions to spermicides, and recent studies indicate that spermicides containing N-9 are not effective in preventing transmission of STIs such as gonorrhea, chlamydia, and HIV. In fact, frequent use of N-9 spermicides has been shown to cause irritation and breaks in the mucous layer or skin of the genital tract, creating a point of entry for viruses and bacteria that cause disease.[1] Spermicides containing N-9 have also been associated with increased risk of urinary tract infection.

The Diaphragm with Spermicidal Jelly or Cream

Invented in the mid-nineteenth century, the **diaphragm** was the first widely used birth control method for women. This device is a soft, shallow cup made of thin latex rubber. Its flexible, rubber-coated ring is designed to fit snugly behind the pubic bone in front of the cervix and over the back of the cervix on the other side so it blocks access to the uterus. Diaphragms must be used with spermicidal cream or jelly, which is applied to the inside of the diaphragm before it is inserted, up to 6 hours before intercourse. The diaphragm holds the spermicide in place, creating a physical and chemical barrier against sperm (Figure 6.3). Diaphragms are manufactured in different sizes and must be fitted to the woman by a trained practitioner, who should make sure the user knows how to insert her diaphragm correctly before leaving the practitioner's office.

Advantages If used consistently and correctly, diaphragms can be 94 percent effective in preventing pregnancy. When used with spermicidal jelly or cream, the diaphragm also offers significant protection against gonorrhea and possibly chlamydia and human papillomavirus (HPV). After the initial prescription and fitting, the only ongoing expense involved with diaphragm use is spermicide. Because the diaphragm can be inserted up to 6 hours in advance and used for multiple acts of intercourse, some users may find it less disruptive than other barrier methods.

Disadvantages Although the diaphragm can be left in place for multiple acts of intercourse, additional spermicide must be applied before each time, and the diaphragm must then stay in place for 6 to 8 hours after intercourse to allow the chemical to kill any sperm remaining in the vagina. Some women find inserting the device can be awkward, especially if the woman is rushed. When inserted incorrectly, diaphragms are much less effective. It is also possible for a diaphragm to slip out of place, be difficult to remove, or require refitting by a physician (e.g., following a pregnancy or a significant weight gain or loss).

> **spermicides** Substances designed to kill sperm.
> **diaphragm** A latex, cup-shaped device designed to cover the cervix and block access to the uterus; should always be used with spermicide.

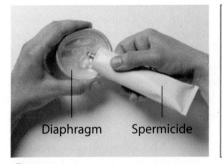

① Place spermicidal jelly or cream inside the diaphragm and all around the rim.

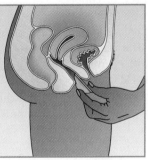

② Fold the diaphragm in half and insert dome-side down (spermicide-side up) into the vagina, pushing it along the back wall as far as it will go.

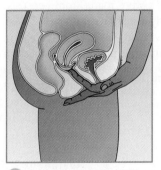

③ Position the diaphragm with the cervix completely covered and the front rim tucked up against your pubic bone; you should be able to feel your cervix through the rubber dome.

FIGURE 6.3 **The Proper Use and Placement of a Diaphragm**

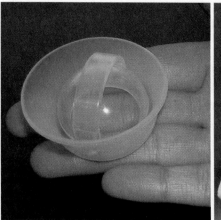

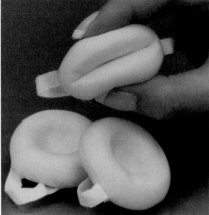

a FemCap is used in conjunction with spermicide and is positioned to cover the cervix. It is shaped like a sailor's cap and has a loop for easier removal.

b The Today sponge is a combination barrier method and spermicide that is most effective when used in conjunction with male condoms.

FIGURE 6.4 **Two Types of Barrier Contraceptive Methods**

Using the diaphragm during the menstrual period or leaving it in place longer than 24 hours slightly increases the user's risk of **toxic shock syndrome (TSS).** To reduce the risk of TSS, women should wash their hands carefully with soap and water before inserting or removing a diaphragm. Another potential health problem with the diaphragm is that it can put undue pressure on the urethra, blocking urinary flow and predisposing the user to bladder infections.

The Cervical Cap with Spermicidal Jelly or Cream

One of the oldest methods used to prevent pregnancy, early **cervical caps** were made from beeswax, silver, or copper. The currently available FemCap **(Figure 6.4a)** is a clear silicone cup that fits snugly over the entire cervix. It comes in three sizes and must be fitted by a practitioner. The FemCap is designed for use with spermicidal jelly or cream. It is held in place by suction created during application and works by blocking sperm from the uterus.

Advantages Cervical caps can be reasonably effective if used consistently and correctly (23 percent failure rate). They also may offer some protection against transmission of gonorrhea, HPV, and possibly chlamydia. They are relatively inexpensive, as the only ongoing cost is for the spermicide.

toxic shock syndrome (TSS) A potentially life-threatening disease that occurs when specific bacterial toxins multiply and spread to the bloodstream, most commonly through improper use of tampons or diaphragms.
cervical cap A small cup made of latex that is designed to fit snugly over the entire cervix.
Today sponge A contraceptive device, made of polyurethane foam and containing nonoxynol-9, that fits over the cervix to create a barrier against sperm.

The FemCap can be inserted up to 6 hours prior to intercourse, making it potentially less disruptive than other barrier methods. The device must be left in place for 6 to 8 hours afterward, but after that time period, if removed and cleaned, it can be reinserted immediately. Because the FemCap is made of silicon rubber, not latex, it is a suitable alternative for people who are allergic to latex.

Disadvantages The FemCap is somewhat more difficult to insert than a diaphragm because of its smaller size. Like a diaphragm, it requires an initial fitting and may require subsequent refitting if a woman's cervix size changes, as after giving birth. Because the FemCap can become dislodged during intercourse, placement must be checked frequently. The device cannot be used during the menstrual period or for longer than 48 hours because of the risk of TSS. Some women report unpleasant vaginal odors after use.

The Sponge

The **Today sponge** is made of polyurethane foam and contains N-9 **(Figure 6.4b)**. Prior to insertion, the sponge must be moistened with water to activate the spermicide. It is then folded and inserted deep into the vagina, where it fits over the cervix and creates a barrier against sperm.

Advantages The sponge is fairly effective (91 percent perfect use; 84 percent typical use) when used consistently and correctly. A main advantage of the sponge is convenience, because it does not require a trip to the doctor for fitting. Protection begins immediately on insertion and lasts for up to 24 hours. There is no need to reapply spermicide or insert a new sponge for any subsequent acts of intercourse within the same 24-hour period; it must be left in place for at least 6 hours after the last intercourse. Like the diaphragm and cervical cap, the sponge offers limited protection from some STIs.

Disadvantages The sponge is less effective for women who have previously given birth (80 percent perfect use; 68 percent typical use). Allergic reactions, such as irritations of the vagina, are more common with the sponge than with other barrier methods. Should the vaginal lining become irritated, the risk of yeast infections and other STIs may increase. Some cases of TSS have been reported in women using the sponge; the same precautions should be taken as with the diaphragm and cervical cap. In addition, some women find the sponge difficult or messy to remove.

Hormonal Methods

The term *hormonal contraception* refers to birth control that contains synthetic estrogen and/or progestin. These ingredients are similar to the hormones estrogen and progesterone, which a woman's ovaries produce naturally for the process of ovulation and the menstrual cycle. In recent years, hormonal contraception has become available in a variety of forms (transdermal, injection, and oral). All forms require a prescription from a health care provider.

Hormonal contraception alters a woman's biochemistry, preventing ovulation (release of the egg) from taking place and producing changes that make it more difficult for the sperm to reach the egg if ovulation does occur. Some hormonal contraceptives contain both estrogen and progestin (synthetic progesterone), and several methods contain just progestin. Synthetic estrogen works to prevent the ovaries from releasing an egg. If no egg is released, there is nothing to be fertilized by sperm and pregnancy cannot occur. Synthetic progesterone works to thicken the cervical mucus, which hinders the movement of the sperm, inhibits the egg's ability to travel through the fallopian tubes, and suppresses the sperm's ability to unite with the egg. Progestin also alters the uterine lining, which renders the egg unlikely to implant in the uterine wall.

Oral Contraceptives

Oral contraceptive pills were first marketed in the United States in 1960. Their convenience quickly made them the most widely used reversible method of fertility control. Most modern pills are up to 99 percent effective at preventing pregnancy with perfect use. Today, oral contraceptives are the most commonly used contraceptive among college-aged women (Figure 6.5).

Most oral contraceptives work through the combined effects of synthetic estrogen and progesterone (*combination pills*). Combination pills are taken in a cycle. At the end of each 3-week cycle, the user discontinues the drug or takes placebo pills for 1 week. The resultant drop in hormones causes the uterine lining to disintegrate, and the user will have a menstrual period, usually within 1 to 3 days. Menstrual flow is generally lighter than it is for women who don't use the pill because the hormones in the pill prevent thick endometrial buildup.

Several new types of pills have extended cycles, such as the 91-day

Seasonale. A woman using this type of regimen takes active pills for 12 weeks, followed by 1 week of placebos. Under this cycle, women can expect to have a menstrual period every 3 months. Data indicate that women do have an increased occurrence of spotting or bleeding in the first few cycles.[2] Lybrel, another extended-cycle pill, is taken continuously for 365 days a year with no placebo pills, thus eliminating menstruation completely.

Advantages Combination pills are highly effective at preventing pregnancy: 99.7 percent with perfect use and 92 percent with typical use. It is easier to achieve perfect use with pills than with barrier contraceptives, as there is less room for user error. Aside from its effectiveness, much of the pill's popularity is due to its convenience and discreetness. Users like that it does not interrupt or interfere with lovemaking, which can lead to enhanced sexual enjoyment.

oral contraceptives Pills containing synthetic hormones that prevent ovulation by regulating hormones.

In addition to preventing pregnancy, the pill may lessen menstrual difficulties, such as cramps and premenstrual syndrome (PMS). Oral contraceptives also lower the risk of several health conditions, including endometrial and ovarian cancers, noncancerous breast disease, osteoporosis, ovarian cysts, pelvic inflammatory disease (PID), and iron-deficiency

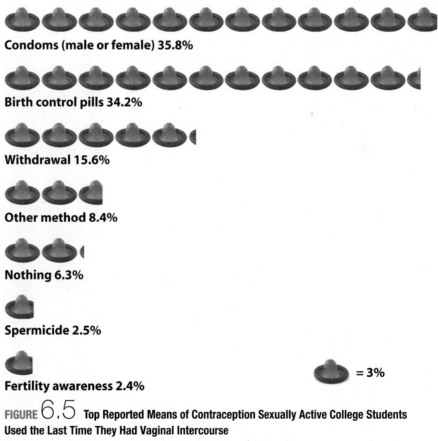

Condoms (male or female) 35.8%

Birth control pills 34.2%

Withdrawal 15.6%

Other method 8.4%

Nothing 6.3%

Spermicide 2.5%

Fertility awareness 2.4%

= 3%

FIGURE 6.5 **Top Reported Means of Contraception Sexually Active College Students Used the Last Time They Had Vaginal Intercourse**

Source: Data are from American College Health Association (ACHA), "ACHA-National College Health Assessment, Reference Group Data Report, Spring 2007," *Journal of American College Health* 56, no. 5 (2008).

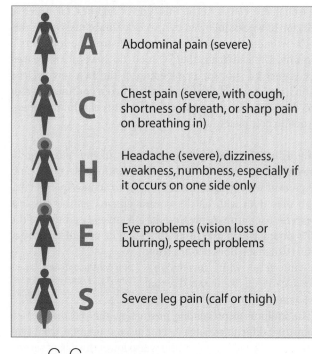

	A	Abdominal pain (severe)
	C	Chest pain (severe, with cough, shortness of breath, or sharp pain on breathing in)
	H	Headache (severe), dizziness, weakness, numbness, especially if it occurs on one side only
	E	Eye problems (vision loss or blurring), speech problems
	S	Severe leg pain (calf or thigh)

FIGURE 6.6 **Early Warning Signs of Medical Complications for Users of the Birth Control Pill**

Source: Adapted from R. A. Hatcher et al., *Contraceptive Technology*, 19th rev. ed. Copyright © 2007 Contraceptive Technology Communications, Inc. Used with permission.

anemia.[3] There are many different brands of combination pills on the market, some of which contain progestins that offer additional benefits, such as reducing acne or minimizing fluid retention. Less-expensive generic versions are also available for many brands. With the extended-cycle pills, the major additional benefit is the reduction in or absence of menstruation and any cramps or PMS symptoms associated with it. Users of these pills also like that they don't need to remember when to stop or start a cycle of pills, or when to use placebos.

Disadvantages The estrogen in combination pills is associated with the risk of several serious health problems, including blood clots (which can lead to strokes or heart attacks) and an increased risk of high blood pressure. The risk is low for most healthy women under the age of 35 who do not smoke; it increases with age and especially with cigarette smoking. See Figure 6.6 for early warning signs of complications associated with oral contraceptives.

Different brands of pills can cause varying minor side effects. Some of the most common are spotting between periods (particularly with extended cycle regimens), breast tenderness, and nausea and vomiting. With most pills, these side effects clear up within a few months. Other, less common potential side effects include a change in sexual desire, acne, weight gain, and hair loss or growth. Because there are so many brands available, most women who wish to use the pill are able to find one that works for them without causing unpleasant side effects.

Apart from the risk factors and potential side effects associated with the pill, its greatest disadvantage is that it must be taken every day. If a woman misses one pill, she should use an alternative form of contraception for the remainder of that cycle. A backup method of birth control is also necessary during the first week of use. After a woman discontinues the pill, return of fertility may be delayed, but the pill is not known to cause infertility. Another drawback is that the pill does not protect against STIs. Cost may also be a problem for some women, whereas some teenagers report that the requirement to have a complete gynecological examination in order to get a prescription for the pill is a huge obstacle.

Progestin-Only Pills

Progestin-only pills (or minipills) contain small doses of synthetic progesterone and no estrogen. These pills are taken continuously (there are no placebo pills included in each pack). Because these pills do not contain estrogen, women taking them may ovulate, but the progestin prevents pregnancy by thickening cervical mucus and by interfering with implantation.

Advantages Progestin-only pills are a good choice for women who are at high risk for estrogen-related side effects or who cannot take estrogen-containing pills because of diabetes, high blood pressure, or other cardiovascular conditions. They also can be used safely by women who are older than age 35 and by women who are currently breastfeeding. The effectiveness rate of these pills is 96 percent with perfect use, which is slightly lower than that of estrogen-

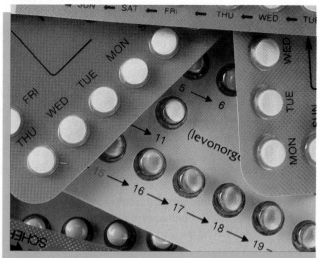

Does the birth control pill cause any side effects?

There are many different brands and regimens of oral contraceptives available to women today, some of which are associated with various health benefits such as acne reduction or lessening of PMS symptoms. Some women experience minor side effects from pill use—the most common being headaches, breast tenderness, nausea, and breakthrough bleeding—but these usually clear up within 2 to 3 months. If you experience any side effects from pill use, talk to your health care provider about them, as she may be able to recommend another brand of pill or method of birth control that will work better for you.

containing pills. Progestin-only pills share some of the health benefits associated with combination pills, and they carry no estrogen-related cardiovascular risks. Also, some of the typical side effects of combination pills, including nausea and breast tenderness, usually do not occur with progestin-only pills. With progestin-only pills, women's menstrual periods generally become lighter or stop altogether.

Disadvantages Because of the lower dose of hormones in progestin-only pills, it is especially important that they be taken at the same time each day. If a woman takes a pill three or more hours later than usual, she will need to use a backup method of contraception for the next 48 hours. The most common side effect of progestin-only pills is irregular menstrual bleeding or spotting. Less common side effects include mood changes, changes in sex drive, and headaches. As with all oral contraceptives, progestin-only pills do not protect against STI transmission.

Ortho Evra (the Patch)

Ortho Evra is a square, transdermal adhesive patch. It is as thin as a plastic strip bandage, is worn for 1 week, and is replaced on the same day of the week for 3 consecutive weeks; the fourth week is patch-free. Ortho Evra works by delivering continuous levels of estrogen and progestin through the skin and into the bloodstream. The patch can be worn on one of four areas of the body: buttocks, abdomen, upper torso (front and back, excluding the breasts), or upper outer arm.

Advantages Ortho Evra is 99.7 percent effective with perfect use. As with other hormonal methods, there is less room for user error than there is with barrier methods. Women who choose to use the patch often do so because they find it easier to remember than taking a daily pill, and they like that they need to change the patch only once a week. Ortho Evra probably offers similar potential health benefits as combination pills (reduction in risk of certain cancers and diseases, lessening of PMS symptoms, etc.). Like other hormonal methods, the patch regulates a woman's menstrual cycle.

Disadvantages Using the patch requires an initial exam and prescription, weekly patch changes, and the ongoing monthly expense of patch purchase. There is currently no generic version. A backup method is required during the first week of use. Similar to other hormonal methods of birth control, the patch offers no protection against HIV or other STIs. Some women experience minor side effects like those associated with combination pills. The estrogen in the patch is associated with cardiovascular risks, particularly in women who smoke and women who are over the age of 35. In 2005, amidst evidence that the patch may increase a woman's risk for life-threatening blood clots, the FDA mandated an additional warning label explaining that patch use exposes women to about 60 percent more total

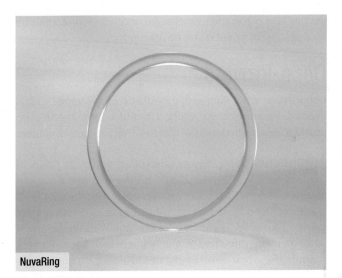

NuvaRing

estrogen than if they were taking a typical combination pill. While studies on this health concern continue, the FDA will monitor the safety of Ortho Evra.[4]

NuvaRing

NuvaRing is a soft, flexible plastic hormonal contraceptive ring about 2 inches in diameter. The user inserts the ring into her vagina, leaves it in place for 3 weeks, and removes it for 1 week for her menstrual period. Once the ring is inserted, it releases a steady flow of estrogen and progestin.

Advantages When used properly, the ring is 99.7 percent effective. Advantages of NuvaRing include less likelihood of user error, protection against pregnancy for 1 month, no pill to take daily or patch to change weekly, no need to be fitted by a clinician, no requirement to use spermicide, and rapid return of fertility when use is stopped. It also exposes the user to a lower dosage of estrogen than do the patch and some combination pills, so it may have fewer estrogen-related side effects. It probably offers some of the same potential health benefits as combination pills, and, like other hormonal contraceptives, it regulates a woman's menstrual cycle.

Ortho Evra A patch that releases hormones similar to those in oral contraceptives; each patch is worn for 1 week.
NuvaRing A soft, flexible ring inserted into the vagina that releases hormones, preventing pregnancy.

Disadvantages NuvaRing requires an initial exam and prescription, monthly ring changes, and the ongoing monthly expense of purchasing the ring (there is currently no generic version). A backup method must be used during the first week, and the ring provides no protection against STI transmission. Like combination pills, the ring poses possible minor side effects, and potentially more serious health risks for some women. Possible side effects unique to the ring include increased vaginal discharge and vaginal irritation or infection. Oil-based vaginal medicines to treat yeast infections cannot be used when

Ortho Evra, the contraceptive patch

the ring is in place; and a diaphragm or cervical cap cannot be used as a backup method for contraception.

Depo-Provera

Depo-Provera is a long-acting synthetic progesterone that is injected intramuscularly every 3 months by a health care provider. Researchers believe that the drug prevents ovulation.

Advantages Depo-Provera takes effect within 24 hours of the first shot so there is usually no need to use a backup method. There is little room for user error with the shot (as it is administered by a clinician every 3 months): with perfect use the shot is 99.7 percent effective, and with typical use it is 97 percent effective. Some women feel Depo-Provera encourages sexual spontaneity, because they do not have to remember to take a pill or insert a device. With continued use of this method, a woman's menstrual periods become lighter and may eventually stop altogether. There are no estrogen-related health risks associated with Depo-Provera, and it offers the same potential health benefits as progestin-only pills. Unlike estrogen-containing hormonal methods, Depo-Provera can be used by women who are breast-feeding.

Disadvantages Using Depo-Provera requires an initial exam and prescription, as well as follow-up visits every 3 months to have the shot administered. It offers no protection against transmission of STIs. The main disadvantage of Depo-Provera use is irregular bleeding, which can be troublesome at first, but within a year, most women are amenorrheic (have no menstrual periods). Weight gain (an average of 5 pounds in the first year) is common. Depo-Provera comes with a warning that prolonged use is linked with loss of bone density. Other possible side effects include dizziness, nervousness, and head-ache. Unlike other methods of contraception, this method cannot be stopped immediately if problems arise, and the drug and its side effects may linger for up to 6 months after the last shot. Also, after the final injection, it may take women who wish to get pregnant up to a year to conceive.

Depo-Provera An injectable method of birth control that lasts for 3 months.

intrauterine device (IUD) A device, often T-shaped, that is implanted in the uterus to prevent pregnancy.

Implanon and Other Implants

A new single-rod implantable contraceptive, Implanon, is a small (about the size of a matchstick), soft plastic capsule that is inserted just beneath the skin on the inner side of a woman's upper underarm by a health care provider. Implanon continually releases a low, steady dose of progestin for up to 3 years, suppressing ovulation during that time. Jadelle, a two-rod implant, is currently waiting approval by the FDA to enter the market in the United States.

Advantages After insertion, Implanon is generally not visible, making it a discreet method of birth control. The main advantages of Implanon are that it is highly effective (99.95 percent), it is not subject to user error, and it needs to be replaced only every 3 years. It has similar benefits as other progestin-only forms of contraception, including the lightening or cessation of menstrual periods, the lack of estrogen-related side effects, and safety for use by breast-feeding women. Fertility usually returns quickly after removal of the implant.

Disadvantages Insertion and removal of Implanon must be performed by a clinician. There is a higher initial cost for this method, and it may not be covered by all health plans. Potential minor side effects include irritation, swelling, or scarring around the area of insertion, and there is also a possibility of difficulty or complications with removal. As with other progestin-only contraceptives, users can experience irregular bleeding. Implanon offers no protection against transmission of STIs, and it may require a backup method during the first week of use.

Intrauterine Contraceptives

Women have been using **intrauterine devices (IUDs)** since 1909, and they are currently the most popular form of reversible contraception throughout the world. However, in the United States, the number of IUD users is relatively small. The IUD is a small plastic, flexible device that is placed in the uterus and left there for up to 10 years at a time. The exact mechanism by which it works is not clearly understood, but researchers believe IUDs affect the way sperm and egg move, thereby preventing fertilization and/or affecting the lining of the uterus to prevent a fertilized ovum from implanting.

ParaGard and Mirena IUDs

Two IUDs are currently available in the United States. *ParaGard* is a T-shaped plastic device with copper wrapped around the shaft. It does not contain any hormones and can be left in place for 10 years before replacement. A newer IUD, *Mirena,* is effective for 5 years and releases small amounts of progestin. A physician must fit and insert an IUD. One or two strings extend from the IUD into the vagina so the user can check to make sure that her IUD is in place. The device is removed by a practitioner when desired.

ParaGard IUD

Advantages The IUD is a safe, discreet, and highly effective method of birth control (99.4%). It is effective immediately and needs to be replaced only every 10 years (ParaGard) or every 5 years

(Mirena). ParaGard has the benefit of containing no hormones at all, whereas Mirena probably offers some of the same potential health benefits as other progestin-only methods. Both IUDs can be used by breast-feeding women. With Mirena, periods become lighter or stop altogether. IUDs are fully reversible; after removal, there is usually no delay in return of fertility.

Disadvantages Disadvantages of IUDs include possible discomfort, cost of insertion, and potential complications. Also, the IUD does not protect against STIs. In some women, the device can cause heavy menstrual flow and severe cramps for the first few months. Women using IUDs have a higher risk of uterine perforation, ectopic pregnancy, pelvic inflammatory disease, infertility, and tubal infections. If a pregnancy occurs while the IUD is in place, the device should be removed as soon as possible, because the chance of miscarriage is 25 to 50 percent. Doctors often offer therapeutic abortion to women who become pregnant while using an IUD because of the serious risks (including premature delivery, infection, and congenital abnormalities) associated with continuing the pregnancy. IUDs are usually not recommended for use by women who have never had children because of an increased incidence of side effects and risk of infection with possible resultant infertility.

Emergency Contraception

Emergency contraception is the use of a contraceptive to prevent pregnancy after unprotected intercourse, a sexual assault, or the failure of another birth control method. Combination estrogen–progestin pills and progestin-only pills are two common types of **emergency contraceptive pills (ECPs).** The copper-bearing IUD has also been used as emergency contraception for years.

Pills used for emergency contraception are sometimes referred to as "morning-after pills." They are not the same as the "abortion pill," although the two are often confused. Emergency contraception is used after unprotected intercourse but before a woman misses her period. A woman taking ECPs does so to prevent pregnancy; the method will not work if she is already pregnant. In contrast, Mifeprex or mifepristone (formerly known as RU-486), the early abortion pill, is taken after a woman is sure she is pregnant, having already taken a pregnancy test with a positive result. It and other methods of abortion are discussed in more detail later in the chapter.

ECPs prevent pregnancy the same way as other hormonal contraceptives: They delay or inhibit ovulation, inhibit fertilization, or block implantation of a fertilized egg, depending on the phase of the woman's menstrual cycle. Although ECPs use the same hormones as birth control pills, not all brands of birth control pills can be used for emergency contraception. When taken within 24 hours, ECPs are up to 95 percent effective; when taken 2 to 5 days later, ECPs are 75 to 89 percent effective.

In August 2006, the FDA approved the over-the-counter sale of Plan B, one brand of emergency contraceptive pills, in the United States to women aged 18 and older. For women under 18, a prescription is still required. Nine states have enacted laws that permit a pharmacist to provide emergency contraception to customers under 18, if they are working in collaboration with a physician under state-approved protocols.[5]

emergency contraceptive pills (ECPs) Drugs taken within 3 days after unprotected intercourse to prevent fertilization or implantation.

Plan B is a progestin-only pill whose first dose should be taken as soon as possible (but not later than 120 hours, or 5 days) after unprotected intercourse. A second pill follows 12 hours after the first pill. Overall, Plan B reduces pregnancy risk by about as much as other ECPs that require a prescription.

There are 6.4 million pregnancies every year in the United States. Half of these are unintended, and ECPs have the potential to reduce this number by at least half. Researchers estimate that widespread availability of ECPs could prevent 1.7 million unintended pregnancies and 800,000 abortions each year in the United States.[6] Although ECPs are no substitute for taking proper precautions before having sex (such as using latex condoms with a spermicide), their potential for reducing the rate of unintended pregnancy and ultimately abortion is very strong. According to the American College

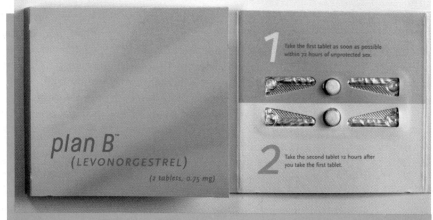

What is emergency contraception?

Emergency contraception is the use of a contraceptive—either hormone-containing pills or an IUD—after an act of unprotected intercourse. Plan B is the only brand of emergency contraceptive currently available to American consumers 18 or older without a prescription. When taken within 72 hours of unprotected intercourse, Plan B reduces the risk of pregnancy by 89%. It carries less risk of nausea and vomiting than most combination pills prescribed by a physician for the purpose of emergency contraception.

Health Association's National College Health Assessment (ACHA-NCHA), 67 percent of all college health centers provide emergency contraception and approximately 14 percent of sexually active college students reported using (or reported their partner had used) it within the past school year.[7]

Behavioral Methods

Some methods of contraception rely on one or both partners altering their sexual behavior. In general, these methods require more self-control, diligence, and commitment, making them more prone to user error than hormonal and barrier methods.

Withdrawal

Withdrawal, also called *coitus interruptus*, involves removing the penis from the vagina just prior to ejaculation. In the 2008 ACHA-NCHA, approximately 27 percent of respondents reported that withdrawal was their method of birth control the last time they had sexual intercourse.[8] This statistic is startlingly high, considering the very high risk of pregnancy or contracting an STI associated with this method of birth control.

Advantages and Disadvantages While withdrawal can be practiced when there is absolutely no other contraceptive available, it is highly unreliable, even with "perfect" use, because there can be up to half a million sperm in the drop of fluid at the tip of the penis *before* ejaculation. Timing withdrawal is also difficult, and males concentrating on accurate timing may not be able to relax and enjoy intercourse. Withdrawal offers no protection against the transmission of STIs and requires a high degree of self-control, experience, and trust.

Abstinence and "Outercourse"

Strictly defined, *abstinence* means deliberately avoiding intercourse. This strict definition would allow one to engage in such forms of sexual intimacy as massage, kissing, and solitary masturbation. But many people today have broadened the definition of abstinence to include all forms of sexual contact, even those that do not culminate in sexual intercourse. Couples who go a step further than massage and kissing and engage in activities such as oral–genital sex and mutual masturbation are sometimes said to be engaging in "outercourse."

withdrawal A method of contraception that involves withdrawing the penis from the vagina before ejaculation; also called *coitus interruptus*.

fertility awareness methods (FAMs) Several types of birth control that require alteration of sexual behavior rather than chemical or physical intervention in the reproductive process.

Advantages and Disadvantages Abstinence is the only method of avoiding pregnancy that is 100 percent effective. It is also the only method that is 100 percent effective against transmitting disease. Like abstinence, outercourse can be

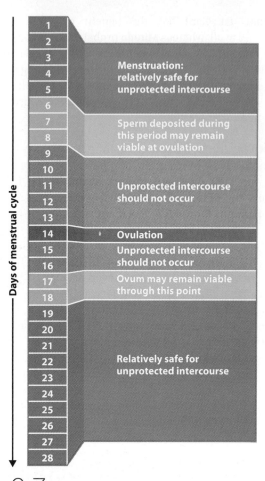

FIGURE 6.7 **The Fertility Cycle**
Fertility awareness methods, or FAMs, can combine the use of a calendar, the cervical mucus method, and body temperature measurements to identify the fertile period. It is important to remember that most women do not have a consistent 28-day cycle.

100 percent effective for birth control as long as the male does not ejaculate near the vaginal opening. Unlike abstinence, however, outercourse is not 100 percent effective against STIs. Oral–genital contact can transmit disease, although the practice can be made safer by using a condom on the penis or a latex barrier, such as a dental dam, on the vaginal opening. Both abstinence and outercourse may be difficult for couples to sustain over long periods of time.

Fertility Awareness Methods

Fertility awareness methods (FAMs) of birth control rely on altering sexual behavior during certain times of the month (Figure 6.7). These techniques require observing female fertile periods and abstaining from sexual intercourse (or any penis–vagina contact) during these times.

Fertility awareness methods rely on a knowledge of basic physiology. A released ovum can survive for up to 48 hours after ovulation. Sperm can live for as long as 5 days in the vagina. Natural methods of birth control teach women to recognize their fertile times.

- **Cervical mucus method.** The cervical mucus method requires women to examine the consistency and color of their normal vaginal secretions. Prior to ovulation, vaginal mucus becomes gelatinous and stretchy, and normal vaginal secretions may increase. To prevent pregnancy, partners must avoid sexual activity involving penis–vagina contact while this mucus is present and for several days afterward.
- **Body temperature method.** The body temperature method relies on the fact that the woman's basal body temperature rises between 0.4 and 0.8 degrees after ovulation has occurred. For this method to be effective, the woman must chart her temperature for several months to learn to recognize her body's temperature fluctuations. To prevent pregnancy, partners must abstain from penis–vagina contact before the temperature rise until several days after the temperature rise is observed.
- **Calendar method.** The calendar method requires the woman to record the exact number of days in her menstrual cycle. Because few women menstruate with complete regularity, this method involves keeping a record of the menstrual cycle for 12 months, during which time some other method of birth control must be used. This method assumes that ovulation occurs during the midpoint of the cycle. To prevent pregnancy, the couple must abstain from penis–vagina contact during the fertile time.

Advantages and Disadvantages Fertility awareness methods are the only forms of birth control that comply with certain religious teachings, including those of the Roman Catholic Church. They don't require a medical visit or prescription, and there are no negative health effects. Women who are untrained in these techniques run a high risk of unintended pregnancy; anyone interested in using them is advised to take a class. Classes are often offered for free by health centers and churches, and there is only minimal expense for supplies. The effectiveness of fertility awareness methods depends on diligence, commitment, and self-discipline; they are not very effective with typical use (25 percent failure rate). These methods offer no STI protection, and they may not work for women with irregular menstrual cycles.

Surgical Methods

In the United States, **sterilization** has become the second leading method of contraception for women of all ages and the leading method of contraception among married women.[9] Because sterilization is permanent, anyone considering it should think through possibilities such as divorce and remarriage or a future improvement in financial status that might make a pregnancy realistic or desirable.

Female Sterilization

One method of sterilization for women is **tubal ligation,** a surgical procedure in which the fallopian tubes are sealed shut to block sperm's access to released eggs (see **Figure 6.8a**

on page 172). The operation is usually done laparoscopically in a hospital on an outpatient basis. The procedure usually takes less than an hour, and the patient is generally allowed to return home within a short time.

A tubal ligation does not affect ovarian and uterine function. The woman's menstrual cycle continues, and released eggs simply disintegrate and are absorbed by the lymphatic system. As soon as her incision heals, the woman may resume sexual intercourse with no fear of pregnancy.

A new sterilization procedure, Essure, involves the placement of small microcoils into the fallopian tubes via the vagina. Once in place, the microcoils expand to the shape of the fallopian tubes. The coils promote the growth of scar tissue around the device and lead to the fallopian tubes becoming blocked. Like traditional forms of tubal ligation, Essure is permanent.

A **hysterectomy,** or removal of the uterus, is a method of sterilization requiring major surgery. It is usually done only when the patient's uterus is diseased or damaged.

Advantages The main advantage to female sterilization is that it is highly effective and permanent. After the one-time expense and operation, there is no other cost or ongoing action required. Sterilization has no negative effect on a woman's sex drive. A potential advantage of the Essure method is that it does not require an incision. The entire procedure takes only 35 minutes and can be performed in a physician's office. It is recommended for women who cannot have a tubal ligation because of chronic health conditions such as obesity or heart disease.

Disadvantages As with any surgery, there are risks involved with a tubal ligation. Although rare, possible complications include infection, pulmonary embolism, hemorrhage, anesthesia complications, and ectopic pregnancy. Essure does not require an incision, so the immediate risks are lower; however, because Essure is a relatively new technique, the long-term risks are unknown. Sterilization offers no protection against STI transmission, and is initially expensive. The procedure is permanent and should be used only if both partners are certain they do not want more children.

> **sterilization** Permanent fertility control achieved through surgical procedures.
> **tubal ligation** Sterilization of the woman that involves the cutting and tying off or cauterizing of the fallopian tubes.
> **hysterectomy** Surgical removal of the uterus.
> **vasectomy** Sterilization of the man that involves the cutting and tying off of both vasa deferentia.

Male Sterilization

Sterilization in men is less complicated than it is in women. A **vasectomy** is frequently done on an outpatient basis, using a local anesthetic (see **Figure 6.8b**). This procedure involves making a small incision in the side of the scrotum to expose a vas deferens, cutting the vas deferens and either tying off or cauterizing the ends, then repeating this on the other side.

Many men are reluctant to consider sterilization because they fear the operation will affect their sexual performance.

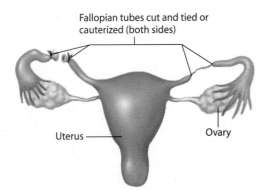

Fallopian tubes cut and tied or cauterized (both sides)

Uterus

Ovary

a In a tubal ligation, both fallopian tubes are cut and tied or sealed shut. This surgery is usually performed laparoscopically.

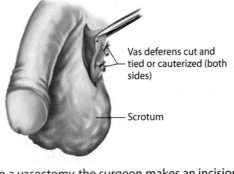

Vas deferens cut and tied or cauterized (both sides)

Scrotum

b In a vasectomy, the surgeon makes an incision in the scrotum, then locates and cuts the vasa deferentia, either sealing or tying both sides shut.

FIGURE 6.8 **Female and Male Sterilization**

However, a vasectomy in no way affects sexual response. Because sperm constitute only a small percentage of the semen, the amount of ejaculate is not changed significantly. The testes continue to produce sperm, but the sperm can no longer enter the ejaculatory duct. Any sperm that are manufactured disintegrate and are absorbed into the lymphatic system.

Advantages A vasectomy is a highly effective and permanent means of preventing pregnancy: The pregnancy rate in women whose partners have had vasectomies after 1 year is 0.15 percent.[10] A vasectomy is a fairly simple outpatient procedure requiring minimal recovery time, and after the one-time expense and operation, there is no other cost or ongoing action required. A vasectomy has no negative effect on a man's sex drive or sexual performance.

Disadvantages In addition to its initial expense, male sterilization offers no protection against STI transmission. Also, a vasectomy is not immediately effective in preventing pregnancy. Because sperm are stored in other areas of the reproductive system beside the vasa deferentia, couples must use alternative methods of birth control for at least 1 month after the vasectomy. The man must check with his physician (who will do a semen analysis) to determine when unprotected intercourse can take place. As with any surgery, there are some

risks involved with a vasectomy. In a small percentage of cases, serious complications occur, such as formation of a blood clot in the scrotum, infection, or inflammatory reactions. Very infrequently the vas deferens may create a new path, negating the procedure.

Choosing a Method of Contraception

With all the options available, how does a person or a couple decide what method of contraception is best? Take some time to research the various methods, ask questions of your health care provider, and be honest with yourself about your own preferences. Some questions to ask yourself include:

● **How comfortable would I be using a particular method?** If you aren't at ease with a method, you may not use it consistently, and it probably will not be a reliable choice for you. Think about whether the method may cause discomfort for you or your partner, and consider your own comfort level with touching your body. For women, some methods, such as the diaphragm, sponge, or NuvaRing, require inserting an apparatus into the vagina and taking it out. For men, using a condom requires rolling it onto the penis.

● **Will this method be convenient for me and my partner?** Some methods require more effort than others. Be honest with yourself about how likely you are to use the method consistently. Are you willing to interrupt lovemaking, to abstain from sex during certain times of the month, or to take a pill every day? You may feel condoms are easy and convenient to use, or you may prefer something that requires little ongoing thought, such as Depo-Provera or an IUD.

● **Am I at risk for the transmission of sexually transmitted infections?** If you have multiple sex partners or are uncertain about the sexual history or disease status of your current sex partner, then you are at risk for transmission of sexually transmitted infections and HIV (the virus that causes AIDS). Condoms (both male and female) are the *only* birth control method that protects against STIs and HIV (although some other barrier methods offer limited protection). They reduce your risk of STIs as well as HIV. Condoms alone are not a highly effective birth control method; to avoid both STI infection and pregnancy, combine a condom with a more effective birth control method.

● **Do I want to have a biological child in the future?** If you are unsure about your plans for future childbearing, you should use a temporary birth control method, rather than a permanent one such as sterilization. Keep in mind that you may regret choosing a permanent method if you are young, if you have few or no children, if you are choosing this method because your partner wants you to, or if you believe this option will fix relationship problems. If you know you want to have children in the future, consider how soon that will be, as some methods, such as Depo-Provera, will cause a delay in return to fertility.

- **How would an unplanned pregnancy affect my life?** If an unplanned pregnancy would be a potentially devastating event for you, or would have a serious impact on your plans for the future, then you should choose a highly effective birth control method, for example, the pill, patch, ring, implant, or IUD. If, however, you are in a stable relationship, have a reliable source of income, are planning to have children in the future, and would embrace a pregnancy should it occur now, then you may be comfortable with a less reliable method such as the diaphragm, cervical cap, or spermicides.
- **What are my religious and moral values?** Fertility awareness methods are a good option if you are morally or spiritually opposed to using certain other birth control methods. When both partners are motivated to use these methods, they can be successful at preventing unintended pregnancy. If you are considering this option, sign up for a class to get specific training using the method effectively.
- **How much will the birth control method cost?** Some contraceptive methods involve an initial outlay of money and few continuing costs (e.g., sterilization, IUD), whereas others are fairly inexpensive but must be purchased repeatedly (e.g., condoms, spermicides, monthly pill prescriptions). You should consider whether a method will be cost effective for you in the long run. Remember that any prescription methods require routine checkups, which may involve some cost to you.
- **Do I have any health factors that could limit my choice?** Hormonal birth control methods can pose potential health risks to women with certain preexisting conditions, such as high blood pressure, a history of stroke or blood clots, liver disease, migraines, or diabetes. You should discuss this issue with your health care provider when considering birth control methods. In addition, women who smoke or are over the age of 35 are at risk from complications of combination hormonal contraceptives. Breast-feeding women can use progestin-only methods, but should avoid methods containing estrogen. Men and women with latex allergies may need to use polyurethane or plastic barrier methods.
- **Are there any additional benefits I'd like to get from my contraceptive?** Hormonal birth control methods can have desirable secondary effects, such as the reduction of acne and the lessening of premenstrual symptoms. Certain pills are marketed as having specific effects, so it is possible to choose one that is known to clear skin or reduce mood changes caused by menstruation. Hormonal birth control methods are also associated with reduced risks of certain cancers. Extended-cycle pills and some progestin-only methods cause menstrual periods to be less frequent or to stop altogether, which

some women find desirable. Condoms carry the added health benefit of protecting against STIs.

Abortion

Unintended pregnancies can occur despite every possible precaution. Even the best birth control methods can fail. Women may be raped. When an unintended pregnancy does occur, a woman must decide whether to terminate it, carry it to term and keep the baby, or carry it to term and give the baby up for adoption. This is a personal decision that each woman must make, based on her personal beliefs, values, and resources, and after carefully considering all alternatives.

In 1973, the landmark U.S. Supreme Court decision in *Roe v. Wade* stated that the "right to privacy . . . founded on the Fourteenth Amendment's concept of personal liberty . . . is broad

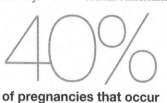

40%
of pregnancies that occur each year are unintended.

enough to encompass a woman's decision whether or not to terminate her pregnancy."[11] The decision maintained that during the first trimester of pregnancy, a woman and her practitioner have the right to terminate the pregnancy through **abortion** without legal restrictions. It allowed individual states to set conditions for second-trimester abortions. Third-trimester abortions were ruled illegal unless the mother's life or health was in danger. Prior to the legalization of first- and second-trimester abortions, women wishing to terminate a pregnancy had to travel to a country where the procedure was legal, consult an illegal abortionist, or perform their own abortions. These procedures sometimes led to death from hemorrhage or infection or to infertility from internal scarring.

abortion The expulsion or removal of an embryo or fetus from the uterus.

The Debate over Abortion

Abortion is a highly charged and politically thorny issue in American society. Pro-choice individuals feel that it is a woman's right to make decisions about her own body and health, including the decision to continue or terminate a pregnancy. On the other side of the issue, pro-life individuals believe that the embryo or fetus is a human being with rights that must be protected. The political debate continues as pro-life groups lobby for laws prohibiting the use of public funds for abortion and abortion counseling at the same time that pro-choice groups lobby for laws that make abortions more widely available. At times, violence has arisen as a result of this controversy, in the form of attacks on clinics or on individual physicians who perform abortions.

In recent years, new legislation has given states the right to impose certain restrictions on abortions. The procedure cannot be performed in publicly funded clinics in some states, and other states have laws requiring parental notification before a teenager can obtain an abortion. In 2008 alone, 20 states enacted 33 new sexual and reproductive health laws, half of which were related to abortion access. However,

what do you think?

Who do you think is responsible for deciding which method of contraception should be used in a sexual relationship? ● What are some examples of good opportunities for you and your partner to discuss contraceptives? ● What do you think are the biggest barriers in our society to the use of condoms?

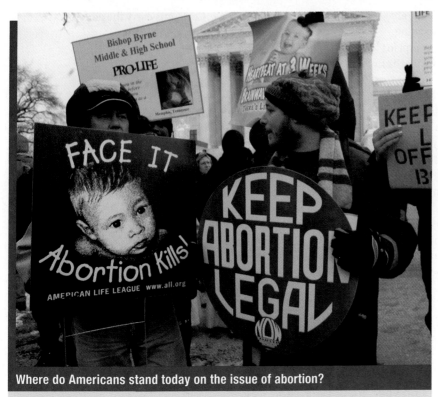

Where do Americans stand today on the issue of abortion?

Abortion continues to be a controversial and emotional issue in the United States. In recent polls, roughly 20% of the population have favored unrestricted access, 20% have favored a complete ban, and 60% have fallen somewhere between these two extremes.

an abortion causes long-term psychological trauma. In a longitudinal study of more than 5,000 women who had had abortions, researchers found that the best predictor of a woman's emotional well-being following an abortion was her emotional well-being prior to the procedure. Even factors such as marital status or affiliation with a religion that strongly opposes abortion were found to have no effect on a woman's later sense of self-esteem and well-being.[15]

Methods of Abortion

The choice of abortion procedure is determined by how many weeks the woman has been pregnant. Length of pregnancy is calculated from the first day of her last menstrual period.

Surgical Abortions If performed during the first trimester of pregnancy, abortion presents a relatively low risk to the woman. About 89 percent of abortions are performed during the first 12 weeks of pregnancy (see **Figure 6.9**).[16] The most commonly used method of first-trimester abortion is **suction curettage (Figure 6.10)**. Approximately 90 percent of abortions in the United States are done with this procedure, which is usually performed under a local anesthetic. The cervix is dilated with instruments or by placing laminaria, a sterile seaweed product, in the cervical canal. The laminaria is left in place for a few hours or overnight and slowly dilates the cervix. After it is removed, a long tube is inserted into the uterus through the cervix, and gentle suction removes fetal tissue from the uterine walls.

17 states currently do appropriate public funds for women in poverty who seek an abortion.[12]

On the federal level, the U.S. Congress has banned access to abortion for virtually all women who receive health care through the federal government. Since the Federal Abortion Ban was signed in 2003, it has been challenged by the American Civil Liberties Union (ACLU), the National Abortion Federation, Planned Parenthood, and the Center for Reproductive Rights in federal courts across the country on the grounds that it is unconstitutional. The two main reasons for these claims are that the broad language could ban abortion as early as the twelfth week in pregnancy and that it does not include exceptions to protect women's health.[13] The U.S. Supreme Court struck down an identical law as unconstitutional in 2000, and the 2003 law has been declared unconstitutional by all the federal courts of appeals that have heard challenges to it. However, in April of 2007, the U.S. Supreme Court handed down a decision to uphold the Federal Abortion Ban.[14] For a discussion on how contraception and abortion are perceived in different countries, see the **Health in a Diverse World** box on page 176.

suction curettage The use of gentle suction to remove fetal tissue from the uterus.
dilation and evacuation (D&E) An abortion technique that uses a combination of instruments and vacuum aspiration; fetal tissue is both sucked and scraped out of the uterus.

Emotional Aspects of Abortion

Although a variety of feelings such as regret, guilt, sadness, relief, and happiness are normal, no evidence has shown that

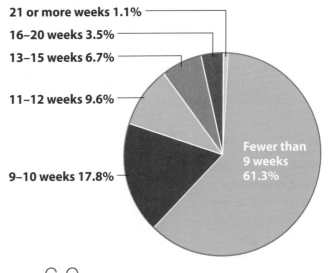

21 or more weeks 1.1%
16–20 weeks 3.5%
13–15 weeks 6.7%
11–12 weeks 9.6%
9–10 weeks 17.8%

Fewer than 9 weeks 61.3%

FIGURE 6.9 **When Women Have Abortions (in weeks from the last menstrual period)**

Source: Data are from *Facts on Induced Abortions in the United States*. Guttmacher Institute, 2008. Accessed October 5, 2009, www.guttmacher.org/pubs/fb_induced_abortion.html.

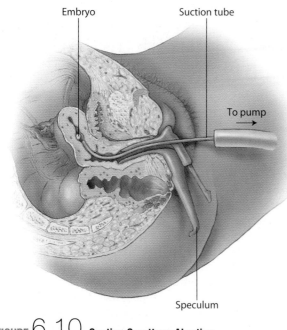

Embryo   Suction tube

To pump →

Speculum

FIGURE 6.10 **Suction Curettage Abortion**

Pregnancies that progress into the second trimester can be terminated through **dilation and evacuation (D&E).** For this procedure, the cervix is dilated for 1 to 2 days, and a combination of instruments and suction curetage is used to empty the uterus. Second-trimester abortions may be done under general anesthetic. The D&E can be performed on an outpatient basis (usually in the physician's office), with or without pain medication. Generally, however, the woman is given a mild tranquilizer to help her relax. This procedure may cause moderate to severe uterine cramping and blood loss. After a D&E, a return visit to the clinician is an important follow-up procedure.

Two other methods used in second-trimester abortions, though less common than the D&E, are prostaglandin or saline **induction abortions.** Prostaglandin hormones or saline solution is injected into the uterus, which kills the fetus and initiates labor contractions. After 24 to 48 hours, the fetus and placenta are expelled from the uterus. The **hysterotomy,** or surgical removal of the fetus from the uterus, may be used during emergencies, when the mother's life is in danger, or when other types of abortions are deemed too dangerous.

One surgical method of performing abortion that has been the target of abortion opponents is **intact dilation and extraction (D&X),** sometimes referred to by the nonmedical term *partial-birth abortion.* This procedure is rarely performed, but it is considered when other abortion methods could injure the mother and when there are severe fetal abnormalities. The dilation and extraction procedure is used after 21 weeks' gestation. Two days before the procedure, laminaria is inserted vaginally to dilate the cervix. The water should break on the third day, at which time the woman should return to the clinic. The fetus is rotated to a breech (feet first) position, and forceps are used to pull the legs, shoulders, and arms through the birth canal. The head is

collapsed to allow it to pass through the cervix. Then the fetus is completely removed.

The risks associated with surgical abortion include infection, incomplete abortion (when parts of the placenta remain in the uterus), excessive bleeding, and cervical and uterine trauma. Follow-up and attention to danger signs decrease the chances of long-term problems.

The mortality rate for women undergoing first-trimester abortions in the United States averages 1 death per every 1,000,000 procedures at 8 or fewer weeks. The risk of death increases with the length of pregnancy. At 16 to 20 weeks, the mortality rate is 1 per 29,000; at 21 weeks or more, it increases to 1 per 11,000.[17] This higher rate later in the pregnancy is due to the increased risk of uterine perforation, bleeding, infection, and incomplete abortion; these things can happen because the uterine wall becomes thinner as the pregnancy progresses.

Medical Abortions Unlike surgical abortions, **medical abortions** are performed without entering the uterus. Mifepristone, formerly known as RU-486 and currently sold in the United States under the brand name Mifeprex, is a steroid hormone that induces abortion by blocking the action of progesterone, a hormone produced by the ovaries and placenta that maintains the lining of the uterus. As a result, the uterine lining and the embryo are expelled from the uterus, terminating the pregnancy.

Mifepristone's nickname, the "abortion pill," may imply an easy process. However, this treatment actually involves more steps than a surgical abortion, which takes approximately 15 minutes followed by a physical recovery of about 1 day. With mifepristone, a first visit to the clinic involves a physical exam and a dose of three tablets, which may cause minor side effects such as nausea, headaches, weakness, and fatigue. The patient returns 2 days later for a dose of prostaglandins (misoprostol; brand name: Cytotec), which cause uterine contractions that expel the fertilized egg. The patient is required to stay under observation at the clinic for 4 hours and to make a follow-up visit 12 days later.[18]

Ninety-six percent of women who take mifepristone and prostaglandins during the first 9 weeks of pregnancy will experience a complete abortion. The side effects of this treatment are similar to those reported during heavy menstruation and include cramping, minor pain, and nausea. Approximately 1 in 1,000 women requires a blood transfusion because of severe bleeding. The procedure does not require hospitalization; women may be treated on an outpatient basis.

induction abortion Abortion technique in which chemicals are injected into the uterus through the uterine wall; labor begins, and the woman delivers a dead fetus.

hysterotomy The surgical removal of the fetus from the uterus.

intact dilation and extraction (D&X) A late-term abortion procedure in which the body of the fetus is extracted up to the head and then the contents of the cranium are aspirated.

medical abortion The termination of a pregnancy during its first 9 weeks using hormonal medications that cause the embryo to be expelled from the uterus.

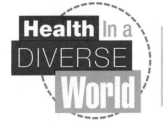

CONTRACEPTIVE USE AND THE INCIDENCE OF ABORTION WORLDWIDE

Approximately 208 million pregnancies occur throughout the world every year, more than a third of which are unintended. Worldwide, about one-fifth of all pregnancies end in induced abortion, although reports have indicated a decline in the overall number of abortions in recent decades. This decline has been greater in developed nations than in developing ones. In developed nations, where almost all abortions are safe and legal, the incidence of the procedure dropped from 39 per 1,000 women aged 15 to 44 in 1995 to 26 per 1,000 women aged 15 to 44 in 2003. In developing nations, the rate declined from 34 to 29 in the same period of time. The world's population is largely concentrated in developing nations, and consequently most abortions occur in those countries—36 million annually—often in places where abortion is illegal and access to contraception is limited.

The primary cause of abortion is unplanned pregnancy. Whether abortion is legal or not has little to do with its overall incidence. The abortion rate in Africa, where abortion is illegal in most countries, is the same as the rate in Europe, where abortion is generally legal. Abortions performed illegally are usually unsafe; 67,000 women die of complications from unsafe abortions each year, nearly all in developing nations where abortion is illegal. Worldwide, 48 percent of all abortions are unsafe; however, only 8 percent of abortions in developed nations are unsafe, compared to 55 percent in developing nations.

When abortion is legalized in a country, it also becomes safer. For example, after expanding the legalization of abortion in 1996, South Africa experienced a 52 percent reduction in the incidence of infection resulting from abortion. The general global trend is to remove legal restrictions on abortion: Since 1995, 17 countries have liberalized their abortion laws, compared to only 3 countries that have tightened them.

Access to voluntary family planning services, including contraception, is essential in helping to reduce the number of unintended pregnancies and, consequently, the incidence of abortion. When modern contraceptives are unavailable, women often turn to abortion to end unwanted pregnancy. Countries where contraceptive use is most prevalent usually have lower abortion rates.

The lowest abortion rates are in western Europe, where abortion is legal and contraceptives are widely accepted and available at low cost. In eastern Europe and the former Soviet Union, abortion rates were high throughout the cold war, when it was free and was the only reliable method of fertility control available to most women. Modern contraceptives manufactured in the West were not available to these women until the fall of the Soviet Union. Since that time, contraceptives have become prevalent in eastern Europe and the former Soviet bloc countries, such that the abortion rate dropped 50 percent between 1995 and 2003. However, because of economic pressure to keep families small, the ratio of abortions to live births in eastern Europe is still the highest in the world: 105 abortions for every 100 live births.

Sources: S. Cohen, "New Data on Abortion Incidence, Safety Illuminate Key Aspects of Worldwide Abortion Rate," *Guttmacher Policy Review* 10, no. 4 (2007); Alan Guttmacher Institute and WHO, "Issues in Brief: Facts on Induced Abortion Worldwide," 2009, www.guttmacher.org/pubs/fb_IAW.pdf; G. Sedgh et al., "Legal Abortions Worldwide: Incidence and Recent Trends," *International Family Planning Perspectives* 33, no. 3 (2007).

Planning a Pregnancy

The many methods available to control fertility give you choices that did not exist when your parents—and even you—were born. If you are in the process of deciding whether to have children, take the time to evaluate your emotions, finances, and physical health.

Emotional Health

preconception care Medical care received prior to becoming pregnant that helps a woman assess and address potential maternal health issues.

First and foremost, consider why you want to have a child: To fulfill an inner need to carry on the family? To escape loneliness? Other reasons? Are you ready to make all the sacrifices necessary to bear and raise a child? Can you care for this new human being in a loving and nurturing manner?

If you feel that you are ready to be a parent, the next step is preparation. You can prepare for this change in your life in several ways: read about parenthood, take classes, talk to parents of children of all ages, and join a support group. If you choose to adopt, you will find many support groups available as well.

Maternal Health

Before becoming pregnant, a woman should have a thorough medical examination. **Preconception care** should include assessment of potential complications that could occur during pregnancy. Medical problems such as diabetes and high blood

Preparing for Pregnancy

Before becoming pregnant, parents-to-be should take stock of, and possibly improve, their own health to help ensure the health of their child. Among the most important factors to consider are the following:

FOR WOMEN:

* If you smoke, drink alcohol, or use drugs, stop.
* Reduce or eliminate your caffeine intake.
* Maintain a healthy weight; lose or gain weight if necessary.
* Avoid X rays and environmental chemicals, such as lawn and garden chemicals.
* Take prenatal vitamins, which are especially important in providing adequate folic acid.

FOR MEN:

* If you smoke, quit.
* Drink alcohol only in moderation, and avoid drug use.
* Get checked for STIs and seek treatment if you have one.
* Avoid exposure to toxic chemicals in your work or home environment.
* Maintain a healthy weight; lose or gain weight if necessary.

pressure should be discussed, as well as any genetic disorders that run in the family. Additional suggestions for preparing for a healthy pregnancy can be found in the **Skills for Behavior Change** box above.

Paternal Health

It is common wisdom that mothers-to-be should steer clear of toxic chemicals that can cause birth defects, should eat a healthy diet, and should stop smoking and drinking alcohol. Now, similar precautions are recommended for fathers-to-be. New research suggests that a man's exposure to chemicals influences not only his ability to father a child, but also the future health of his child.

Fathers-to-be have been overlooked in past preconception and prenatal studies for several reasons. Researchers assumed that the genetic damage leading to birth defects and other health problems occurred while a child was in the mother's womb or were caused by random errors of nature. However, it now appears that some disorders can be traced to sperm damaged by chemicals. Sperm are naturally vulnerable to toxic assault and genetic damage. Many drugs and ingested chemicals can readily invade the testes from the bloodstream; others ambush sperm after they leave the testes and pass through the epididymides, where they mature and are stored. By one route or another, half of 100 chemicals studied so far (including by-products of cigarette smoke) apparently harm sperm.

Financial Evaluation

Finances are another important consideration. Are you prepared to go out to dinner less often, forgo a new pair of shoes, or drive an older car? These are important questions to ask yourself when considering the financial aspects of being a parent. Can you afford to give your child the life you would like him or her to enjoy?

First, check your medical insurance: Does it provide pregnancy benefits? If not, you can expect to pay, on average, $7,000 for a normal delivery and up to $11,500 for a cesarean section. These costs don't include prenatal medical care, and complications can also increase the cost substantially. Both partners should investigate their employers' policies concerning parental leave, including length of leave available and conditions for returning to work.

The U.S. Department of Agriculture estimates that it can cost as much as $250,000 for a middle-class married couple to raise a child to the age of 17 (housing costs and food are the two largest expenditures).[19] That figure does not include college, which can now run over $40,000 per year at a private institution, with room and board. Also consider the cost and availability of quality child care. How much does full-time child care cost? Prices vary by region and type of care. According to statistics gathered in the last U.S. Census, families with young children spent 10 percent of their total income on child care in 2002.[20]

what do you think?

Have you thought about whether and when to have children? ● Is there a certain age at which you feel you will be ready to be a parent? ● What goals do you hope to achieve before undertaking parenthood? ● What are your biggest concerns about parenthood?

Pregnancy

Pregnancy is an important event in a woman's life. The actions taken before a pregnancy begins, as well as behaviors during pregnancy, can have a significant effect on the health of both infant and mother.

Prenatal Care

A successful pregnancy depends on a mother who takes good care of herself and the fetus. Good nutrition; exercise; avoiding drugs, alcohol, and other harmful substances; and regular medical checkups beginning early in the pregnancy are essential. Early detection of fetal abnormalities, identification of high-risk mothers and infants, and a complication-free pregnancy are the major purposes of prenatal care.

Several different types of practitioners are qualified to care for a woman through pregnancy, birth, and the postpartum period, including obstetrician-gynecologists, family practioners, and midwives. A woman should carefully choose a practitioner to oversee her pregnancy and delivery. If possible, she should make this choice before she becomes pregnant. Recommendations from friends and from one's family physician are a good starting point. Also consider a practitioner's philosophy about pain management during labor, experience handling complications, and willingness to accommodate your personal beliefs on these issues.

On the first visit, the practitioner should obtain a complete medical history of the mother and her family and note any hereditary conditions that could put a woman or her fetus at risk. Additional concerns include the mother's physical condition, her level of nutrition, her confidence in her ability to give birth, her use of drugs and medications, and the availability of a skilled practitioner who can oversee the pregnancy and delivery. A woman planning a pregnancy also needs a support system (spouse or partner, family, friends, community groups) that is available to provide love and emotional assistance during and after her pregnancy.

Nutrition and Exercise Pregnant women need additional protein, calories, vitamins, and minerals, so their diets should be carefully monitored by a qualified practitioner. Special attention should be paid to getting enough folic acid (found in dark, leafy greens), iron (found in dried fruits, meats, legumes, liver, and egg yolks), calcium (found in nonfat or low-fat dairy products and some canned fish), and fluids.

Vitamin supplements can correct some deficiencies, but there is no substitute for a well-balanced diet. Babies born to poorly nourished mothers run high risks of substandard mental and physical development. Folic acid, when consumed before and during early pregnancy, reduces the risk of spina bifida, a disabling birth condition that results from failure of the spinal column to close. Manufacturers of breads, pastas, rice, and other grain products now are required to add folic acid to their products to reduce neural tube defects in newborns.

Weight gain during pregnancy helps nourish a growing baby. For a woman of normal weight before pregnancy, the recommended weight gain during pregnancy is 25 to 35 pounds. For obese or overweight women, weight gain of 15 to 25 pounds is recommended. Underweight women can gain 28 to 40 pounds, and women carrying twins should gain about 35 to 45 pounds. Gaining too much or too little weight can lead to complications. With higher weight gains, women may develop gestational diabetes, hypertension, or increased risk for delivery complications. Gaining too little weight increases the chance of a low-birth-weight baby.

Of the total number of pounds gained during pregnancy, about 6 to 8 are the baby. The baby's birth weight is important because low weight can mean health problems during labor and the baby's first few months. Pregnancy is not the time for a woman to think about losing weight—doing so may endanger the fetus.

As in all other stages of life, exercise is an important factor in weight control during pregnancy and in overall maternal

teratogenic Causing birth defects; may refer to drugs, environmental chemicals, X rays, or diseases.

fetal alcohol syndrome (FAS) A collection of symptoms, including mental retardation, that can appear in infants of women who drink alcohol during pregnancy.

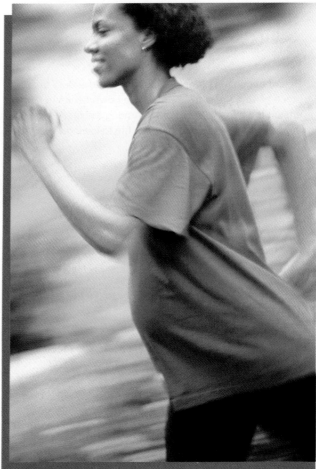

How can I prepare to be a parent?

Following a doctor-approved exercise program during pregnancy is just one aspect of healthy preparation for parenthood. Even before they conceive, prospective mothers and fathers should evaluate their emotional, physical, social, and financial well-being, and implement healthy change where needed to better ready themselves for bringing a child into the world.

health. Pregnant women should consult their physicians before starting any exercise program.

Drugs and Alcohol A woman should avoid all types of drugs during pregnancy. Even common over-the-counter medications, such as aspirin, and some beverages, such as coffee and tea, can damage a developing fetus.

During the first 3 months of pregnancy, the fetus is especially subject to the **teratogenic** (birth defect–causing) effects of drugs, environmental chemicals, X rays, or diseases. The fetus also can develop an addiction to or tolerance for drugs that the mother is using. Of particular concern to medical professionals is the use of tobacco and alcohol during pregnancy.

Consumption of alcohol is detrimental to a growing fetus. Symptoms of **fetal alcohol syndrome (FAS)** include mental retardation, slowed nerve reflexes, and small head size. The exact amount of alcohol necessary to cause FAS is not known, but researchers doubt that it is safe to consume any alcohol. Therefore, they recommend total abstinence from alcohol during pregnancy.

Smoking Tobacco use, in particular smoking, harms every phase of reproduction. Women who smoke have more difficulty becoming pregnant and a higher risk of being infertile. Women who smoke during pregnancy have a greater chance of complications, premature births, low-birth-weight infants, stillbirth, and infant mortality.[21] Tobacco use by the mother appears to be a significant factor in the development of cleft lip and palate in fetuses. Studies are now revealing that secondhand smoke is also detrimental. The exposed fetus is likely to experience low birth weight, increased susceptibility to childhood diseases, and sudden infant death syndrome.[22]

Other Teratogens A pregnant woman should avoid exposure to X rays, toxic chemicals, heavy metals, pesticides, gases, and other hazardous compounds. She should not clean cat-litter boxes because cat feces can contain organisms that cause a disease called **toxoplasmosis.**

If a pregnant woman has never had rubella (German measles), she should be immunized for it prior to becoming pregnant. A rubella infection can kill the fetus or cause blindness or hearing disorders in the infant. Sexually transmitted infections such as genital herpes or HIV are also risk factors. A woman should inform her physician of any infectious condition so that proper precautions and treatment options can be taken. The physician may want to deliver the baby by cesarean section, especially if a woman has active lesions. Contact with an active herpes infection during birth can be fatal to the baby.

According to new research, caffeine can significantly increase the risk of miscarriage.[23] Women in this study who consumed 200 milligrams of caffeine or more a day were about twice as likely to miscarry. That's about the amount of caffeine in two 5-ounce cups of coffee, five 12-ounce cans of soda, or six 5-ounce cups of tea.

Maternal Age The average age at which a woman has her first child has been creeping up, and today, a woman who becomes pregnant after age 35 has plenty of company. Although births to women in their twenties are declining, the rate of first births to women between the ages of 30 and 39 has doubled in the past decade, and births to women over 39 have increased by more than 50 percent. Many doctors note that older mothers tend to be more conscientious about following medical advice during pregnancy and are more psychologically mature and ready to include an infant in their family than are some younger women.

Statistically, the chances of having a baby with birth defects do rise after the age of 35. Researchers believe that there is a decline in both the quality and viability of eggs after this age. The incidence of **Down syndrome** increases with the mother's age.[24] An-

other concern is that a woman's fertility begins to decline as she ages. Fewer than 10 percent of women in their early twenties have issues with infertility, compared to nearly 30 percent in their early forties.

Prenatal Testing and Screening Modern technology enables medical practitioners to detect health defects in a fetus as early as the fourteenth to eighteenth weeks of pregnancy. One common test is **ultrasonography** or **ultrasound,** which uses high-frequency sound waves to create a *sonogram,* or visual image, of the fetus in the uterus. The sonogram is used to determine the fetus's size and position. Knowing the baby's position helps health care providers perform other tests and deliver the infant. Sonograms can also detect birth defects in the central nervous and digestive systems.

The **triple marker screen (TMS)** is a maternal blood test that is optimally conducted between the sixteenth and eighteenth weeks of pregnancy. TMS is a screening test, not a diagnostic tool; it can detect susceptibility for a birth defect or genetic abnormality but is not meant to confirm a diagnosis of any condition.

Amniocentesis is a common testing procedure that is strongly recommended for women over age 35. This test involves inserting a long needle through the mother's abdominal and uterine walls into the **amniotic sac,** the protective pouch surrounding the fetus. The needle draws out 3 to 4 teaspoons of fluid, which is analyzed for genetic information about the baby. Although widely used, amniocentesis is not without risk. The chance of miscarriage as a result of testing is 1 in 200, or less.

Another procedure, **chorionic villus sampling (CVS),** involves snipping tissue from the developing fetal sac. CVS can be used at 10 to 12 weeks of pregnancy. CVS is an attractive option for couples who are at high risk for having a baby with Down syndrome or a debilitating hereditary disease.

If any of these tests reveals a serious birth defect, parents

toxoplasmosis A disease caused by an organism found in cat feces that, when contracted by a pregnant woman, may result in stillbirth or an infant with mental retardation or birth defects.

Down syndrome A genetic disorder characterized by mental retardation and a variety of physical abnormalities.

ultrasonography (ultrasound) A common prenatal test that uses high-frequency sound waves to create a visual image of the fetus.

triple marker screen (TMS) A maternal blood test that can be used to help identify fetuses with certain birth defects and genetic abnormalities.

amniocentesis A medical test in which a small amount of fluid is drawn from the amniotic sac to test for Down syndrome and other genetic diseases.

amniotic sac The protective pouch surrounding the fetus.

chorionic villus sampling (CVS) A prenatal test that involves snipping tissue from the fetal sac to be analyzed for genetic defects.

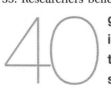

40 genetic abnormalities can be identified through amniocentesis, the most common being Down syndrome.

what do you think?
Would you want to know if you or your partner were carrying a child with a genetic birth defect or other abnormality? ● Would you consider having your own genes tested before starting a family? ● What would you do if both you and your partner were carriers of a genetic disorder that could be passed to your children?

are advised to undergo genetic counseling. In the case of a chromosomal abnormality such as Down syndrome, the parents are usually offered the option of a therapeutic abortion. Some parents choose this option; others research the disability and decide to go ahead with the pregnancy.

Pregnancy Testing

A woman may suspect she is pregnant before she takes any pregnancy tests. A pregnancy test scheduled in a medical office or birth control clinic will confirm the pregnancy. Women who wish to know immediately can purchase home pregnancy test kits sold over the counter in drugstores. A positive test is based on the secretion of human chorionic gonadotropin (HCG), which is found in the woman's urine (HCG is also detectable in blood).

human chorionic gonadotropin (HCG) Hormone detectable in blood or urine samples of a mother within the first few weeks of pregnancy.

Home pregnancy test kits are about 85 to 95 percent reliable. Instructions must be followed carefully. If the test is done too early in the pregnancy, it may show a false negative. Other causes of false negatives are unclean test tubes, ingestion of certain drugs, and vaginal or urinary tract infections. Accuracy also depends on the quality of the test itself and the user's ability to perform it and interpret the results. Blood tests administered and analyzed by a medical laboratory are more accurate.

The Process of Pregnancy

The process of pregnancy begins the moment a sperm fertilizes an ovum in the fallopian tubes (Figure 6.11). From there, the single fertilized cell, now called a *zygote*, multiplies and becomes a sphere-shaped cluster of cells called a *blastocyst*, as it travels toward the uterus, a journey that may take 3 to 4 days. On arrival, the embryo burrows into the thick, spongy endometrium (implantation) and is nourished from this carefully prepared lining.

Early Signs of Pregnancy A woman's body undergoes substantial changes during the course of a pregnancy (Figure 6.12). The first sign of pregnancy is usually a missed menstrual period (although some women "spot" in early pregnancy, which may be mistaken for a period). Other signs include breast tenderness, emotional upset, extreme fatigue, nausea, sleeplessness, and vomiting (especially in the morning).

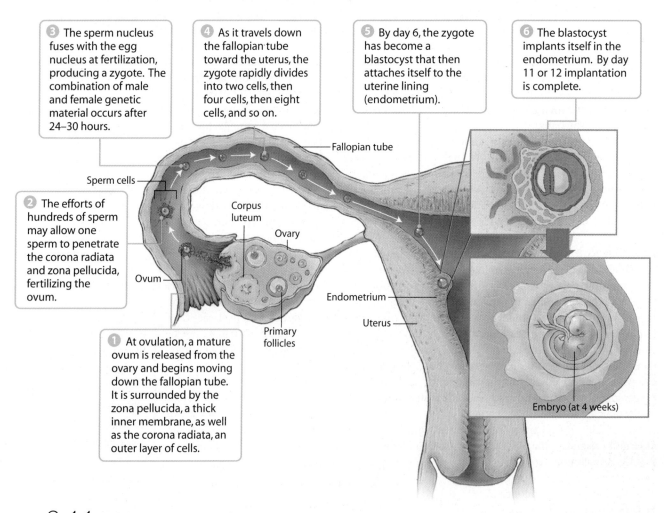

❸ The sperm nucleus fuses with the egg nucleus at fertilization, producing a zygote. The combination of male and female genetic material occurs after 24–30 hours.

❹ As it travels down the fallopian tube toward the uterus, the zygote rapidly divides into two cells, then four cells, then eight cells, and so on.

❺ By day 6, the zygote has become a blastocyst that then attaches itself to the uterine lining (endometrium).

❻ The blastocyst implants itself in the endometrium. By day 11 or 12 implantation is complete.

❷ The efforts of hundreds of sperm may allow one sperm to penetrate the corona radiata and zona pellucida, fertilizing the ovum.

❶ At ovulation, a mature ovum is released from the ovary and begins moving down the fallopian tube. It is surrounded by the zona pellucida, a thick inner membrane, as well as the corona radiata, an outer layer of cells.

Fallopian tube

Sperm cells

Corpus luteum

Ovary

Ovum

Primary follicles

Endometrium

Uterus

Embryo (at 4 weeks)

FIGURE 6.11 **Fertilization**

Pregnancy typically lasts 40 weeks. The due date is calculated from the expectant mother's last menstrual period. Pregnancy is typically divided into three phases, or **trimesters,** of approximately 3 months each.

The First Trimester

During the first trimester, few noticeable changes occur in the mother's body. She may urinate more frequently and experience morning sickness, swollen breasts, or undue fatigue. These symptoms may not be frequent or severe, so she may not even realize she is pregnant unless she has a pregnancy test.

During the first 2 months after conception, the **embryo** differentiates and develops its various organ systems, beginning with the nervous and circulatory systems. At the start of the third month, the embryo is called a **fetus,** which indicates that all organ systems are in place. For the rest of the pregnancy, growth and refinement occur in each major body system so that they can function independently, yet in coordination, at birth. The photos in **Figure 6.13** on the next page illustrate physical changes during fetal development.

The Second Trimester At the beginning of the second trimester, physical changes in the mother become more visible. During this time, the fetus makes greater demands on the mother's body. In particular, the **placenta,** the network of blood vessels connected to the umbilical cord that carry nutrients and oxygen to the fetus and fetal waste products to the mother, becomes well established.

The Third Trimester From the end of the sixth month through the ninth is considered the third trimester. This is the period of greatest fetal growth, when the fetus gains most of its weight. During the third trimester, the fetus must get large amounts of calcium, iron, and nitrogen from the food the mother eats.

Although the fetus may live if it is born during the seventh month, it needs the layer of fat it acquires during the eighth

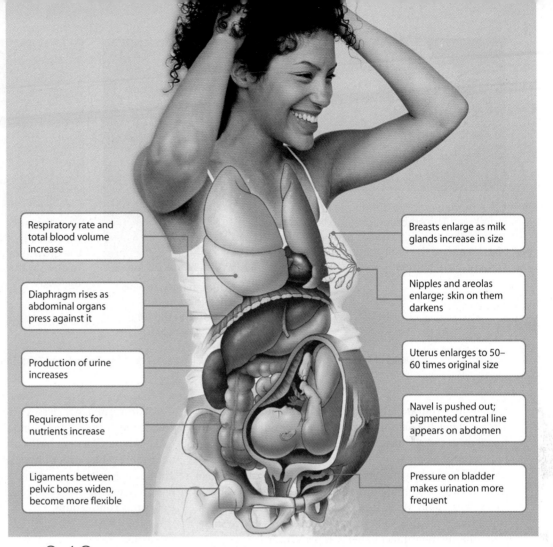

Respiratory rate and total blood volume increase

Diaphragm rises as abdominal organs press against it

Production of urine increases

Requirements for nutrients increase

Ligaments between pelvic bones widen, become more flexible

Breasts enlarge as milk glands increase in size

Nipples and areolas enlarge; skin on them darkens

Uterus enlarges to 50–60 times original size

Navel is pushed out; pigmented central line appears on abdomen

Pressure on bladder makes urination more frequent

FIGURE 6.12 **Changes in a Woman's Body during Pregnancy**

month and time for the organs (especially the respiratory and digestive organs) to develop to their full potential. Babies born prematurely usually require intensive medical care.

Childbirth

Prospective parents need to make a number of key decisions long before the baby is born. These include where to have the baby, whether to use drugs during labor and delivery, which childbirth method to choose, and whether to breast-feed or bottle-feed. Answering these questions will ensure a smoother passage into parenthood.

Labor and Delivery

During the few weeks preceding delivery, the baby normally shifts to a head-down position, and the cervix begins to dilate (widen). The junction of the pubic bones

trimester A 3-month segment of pregnancy; used to describe specific developmental changes that occur in the embryo or fetus.

embryo The fertilized egg from conception until the end of 2 months' development.

fetus The term for a developing baby from the third month of pregnancy until birth.

placenta The network of blood vessels connected to the umbilical cord that carries nutrients, oxygen, and wastes between the developing infant and the mother.

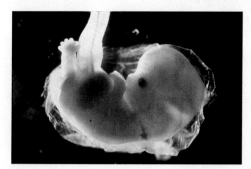

a A human embryo during the first trimester. The embryonic period lasts from the third to the eighth week of development. By the end of the embryonic period, all organs have formed.

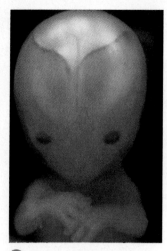

b A human fetus during the second trimester. Growth during the fetal period is very rapid.

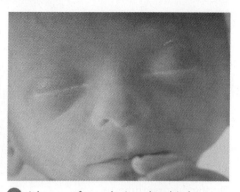

c A human fetus during the third trimester. By the end of the fetal period, the growth rate of the head has slowed relative to the growth rate of the rest of the body.

FIGURE 6.13 **Series of Fetoscopic Photographs Showing Development in the First, Second, and Third Trimesters of Pregnancy**

loosens to permit expansion of the pelvic girdle during birth. The exact mechanisms that initiate labor are unknown. Contractions in the abdomen and lower back usually signal the beginning of labor. Another common early signal of labor is the breaking of the amniotic sac, which causes a rush of fluid from the vagina (commonly referred to as "water breaking").

The birth process has three stages, described in **Figure 6.14**, which can last from several hours to more than a day. In some cases, the attending practitioner may perform an *episiotomy*, a straight incision in the mother's perineum (the area between the vulva and the anus), toward the end of the second stage to prevent the baby's head from tearing vaginal tissues and to speed the baby's exit from the vagina. Upon exit, the baby takes its first breath, which is generally accompanied by a loud wail. After delivery, the attending practitioner assesses the baby's overall condition, cleans the baby's mucus-filled breathing passages, and ties and severs the umbilical cord.

Managing Labor Painkilling drugs given to the mother during labor can cause sluggish responses in the newborn and other complications. For this reason, many women choose drug-free labor and delivery—but it is important to keep a flexible attitude about pain relief, because each labor is different. Use of painkilling medication during a delivery is not a sign of weakness. One person is not a "success" for delivering without medication and another a "failure" for using medical measures. Remember, pain is to be expected. In fact, many experts say that the pain of labor is the most difficult in the human experience. There is no one right answer for managing that pain.

The Lamaze method is the most popular technique of childbirth preparation in the United States. It discourages the use of drugs; prelabor classes teach the mother to control her pain through special breathing patterns, focusing exercises, and relaxation. Lamaze births usually take place in a hospital or birthing center with a physician or midwife in attendance. The partner (or labor coach) assists by giving emotional support, physical comfort, and coaching for proper breath control during contractions.

Cesarean Section (C-section) If labor lasts too long or if a baby is in physiological distress or is about to exit the uterus any way but headfirst, a **cesarean section (C-section)** may be necessary. This surgical procedure involves making an incision across the mother's abdomen and through the uterus to remove the baby. A C-section may also be performed if labor is extremely difficult, maternal blood pressure falls rapidly, the placenta separates from the uterus too soon, the mother has diabetes, or other problems occur. A C-section can be traumatic for the mother if she is not prepared for it. Risks are the same as for any major abdominal surgery, and recovery from birth takes considerably longer after a C-section.

The rate of delivery by C-section in the United States has increased from 5 percent in the mid-1960s to 31.1 percent in 2006.[25] Although this procedure is necessary in certain cases, some physicians and critics, including the Centers for Disease Control and Prevention (CDC), feel that C-sections are performed too frequently in this country. Natural birth advocates suggest that hospitals driven by profits and worried about malpractice are too quick to intervene in the birth process. Some doctors say that the increase is due to maternal demand: busy mothers who want to schedule their deliveries. It has also been reported that late preterm delivery (34 to 36 weeks) increased from 7.3 to 8.9 percent between 1990 and 2004 in the United States.[26] It is not clear how much of that is because of maternal choice.

cesarean section (C-section) A surgical birthing procedure in which a baby is removed through an incision made in the mother's abdominal and uterine walls.

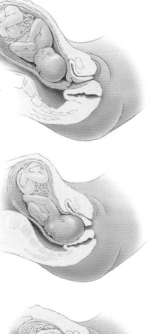

1 Stage I: Dilation of the cervix Contractions in the abdomen and lower back push the baby downward, putting pressure on the cervix and dilating it. The first stage of labor may last from a couple of hours to more than a day for a first birth, but it is usually much shorter during subsequent births.

2 End of Stage I: Transition The cervix becomes fully dilated, and the baby's head begins to move into the vagina (birth canal). Contractions usually come quickly during transition, which generally lasts 30 minutes or less.

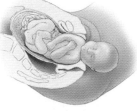

3 Stage II: Expulsion Once the cervix has become fully dilated, contractions become rhythmic, strong, and more intense as the uterus pushes the baby headfirst through the birth canal. The expulsion stage lasts 1 to 4 hours and concludes when the infant is finally pushed out of the mother's body.

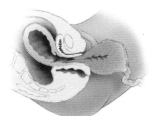

4 Stage III: Delivery of the placenta In the third stage, the placenta detaches from the uterus and is expelled through the birth canal. This stage is usually completed within 30 minutes after delivery.

FIGURE 6.14 **The Birth Process**

The Postpartum Period

The postpartum period typically lasts 4 to 6 weeks after delivery. During this period, many women experience fluctuating emotions. For many new mothers, the physical stress of labor, dehydration and blood loss, and other stresses challenge their stamina. About 50 to 80 percent of new mothers experience what is called the "baby blues," characterized by periods of sadness, anxiety, headache, sleep disturbances, and irritability. For most women, these symptoms disappear after a short while. About 10 percent of new mothers experience **postpartum depression,** a more disabling syndrome characterized by mood swings, lack of energy, crying, guilt, and depression. It can happen anytime within the first year after childbirth. Mothers experiencing postpartum depression should be encouraged to seek professional treatment.

Counseling and in some cases medication are two of the most common types of treatment.[27]

Breast-Feeding

Although the new mother's milk will not begin to flow for 2 or more days, her breasts secrete a thick yellow substance called *colostrum.* Because this fluid contains vital antibodies to help fight infection, the newborn baby should be allowed to suckle.

The American Academy of Pediatrics strongly recommends that infants be breast-fed for at least 6 months and ideally for 12 months. Scientific findings indicate there are many advantages to breast-feeding. Breast-fed babies have fewer illnesses and a much lower hospitalization rate, because breast milk contains maternal antibodies and immunological cells that stimulate the infant's immune system. When breast-fed babies do get sick, they recover more quickly. They are also less likely to be obese than babies fed on formulas, and they have fewer allergies. They may even be more intelligent: a recent study found that the longer a baby was breast-fed, the higher the IQ in adulthood. Researchers theorize that breast milk contains substances that enhance brain development.[28] There is also a potential environmental advantage to breast-feeding. Compounds found in baby bottles, including bisphenol-A, are under intense scrutiny following research suggesting they can lead to health problems. (See the **Green Guide** on page 184 for more environmental parenting concerns.)

This does not mean that breast milk is the only way to nourish a baby. Some women are unable or unwilling to breast-feed; women with certain medical conditions or who are receiving certain medications are advised not to breast-feed. Prepared formulas can provide nourishment that allows a baby to grow and thrive. When deciding whether to breast- or bottle-feed, mothers must consider their own desires and preferences, too. Both feeding methods can supply the physical and emotional closeness so essential to the parent–child relationship.

Complications of Pregnancy and Childbirth

Pregnancy carries the risk for potential complications and problems that can interfere with the proper development of the fetus or threaten the health of the mother and child. Some complications may result from a preexisting health condition of the mother, such as diabetes or an STI, whereas others can develop during pregnancy and may result from physiological problems, genetic abnormalities, or exposure to teratogens.

postpartum depression Energy depletion, anxiety, mood swings, and depression that women may feel during the postpartum period.
preeclampsia A complication in pregnancy characterized by high blood pressure, protein in the urine, and edema.

Preeclampsia and Eclampsia **Preeclampsia** is a condition that is characterized by high blood pressure, protein in the urine, and edema (fluid retention), which usually causes swelling of the hands and face. This condition complicates

GREEN GUIDE

Diaper Dilemma: Cloth or Disposable?

There are a million things you can do to be "green" when raising a baby. You can choose furniture and toys made out of ecofriendly materials, look for organic baby foods, and dress your child in hand-me-downs, just to name a few. However, one of the most environmentally significant decisions you'll make is whether to use disposable or cloth diapers. A baby will spend around 25,000 hours in a diaper and need about 6,000 diaper changes in its first few years of life. The decision to use disposable or cloth diapers will not only greatly impact your baby's comfort and health, but it can also impact the environment and your finances. Of course, there are pros and cons for each type of diaper.

One of the main benefits to disposable diapers is ease of use. These are the easy choice to use when traveling, largely because they are considered to be more absorbent and leak-proof. Also, because they are not washed and reused, disposable diapers use about 29 percent less energy than home-laundered or commercially washed diapers. However, the environmental impact is significant. An estimated 5 million tons of untreated human waste is deposited into landfills via disposable diapers every year. Disposable diapers can also expose a baby's skin to harsh chemicals that may be used on the diaper material. One chemical of concern is sodium polyacrylate, which has been linked to toxic shock syndrome (TSS) and can cause allergic reactions.

Cloth diapers require the ongoing energy use of commercial laundering or home laundering. Depending on how the diapers are washed (temperature of water, method of drying, and so forth), this energy expenditure may actually involve more depletion of fossil fuels and a greater output of carbon dioxide than does the creation and use of disposable diapers. Because they are cleaned and reused, cloth diapers do not end up in landfills in the same numbers as disposable diapers. Cloth diapers can also be gentler on your baby's skin: Diaper rash is much less common with cloth diapers, due to the natural cotton fibers breathing more easily. In spite of these benefits, some people may find cloth diapers difficult or inconvenient to use, and they are generally less absorbent and messier than disposables.

---

approximately 10 percent of pregnancies and is responsible for 18 percent of U.S. maternal deaths each year. Symptoms may include sudden weight gain, headache, nausea or vomiting, changes in vision, racing pulse, mental confusion, and stomach or right shoulder pain. If preeclampsia is not treated, it can cause strokes and seizures, a condition called eclampsia. Potential problems can include liver and kidney damage, internal bleeding, stroke, poor fetal growth, and fetal and maternal death.

This condition tends to occur in the late second or third trimester. The cause is not known; however, the incidence of preeclampsia is higher in first-time mothers; women over 40 or under 18 years of age; women carrying multiple fetuses; and women with a history of chronic hypertension, diabetes, kidney disorder, or previous history of preeclampsia. Family history of preeclampsia is also a risk factor, whether the history is on the man's or woman's side. Treatment for preeclampsia ranges from bed rest and monitoring for women with mild cases, to hospitalization and close monitoring for more severe cases, which have the potential to be life threatening for the woman and her fetus.

miscarriage Loss of the fetus before it is viable; also called *spontaneous abortion*.

ectopic pregnancy Implantation of a fertilized egg outside the uterus, usually in a fallopian tube; a medical emergency that can end in death from hemorrhage or peritonitis.

stillbirth The birth of a dead baby.

Miscarriage
One in ten pregnancies does not end in delivery. Loss of the fetus before it is viable is called a **miscarriage** (also referred to as *spontaneous abortion*). An estimated 70 to 90 percent of women who miscarry eventually become pregnant again.

Reasons for miscarriage vary. In some cases, the fertilized egg has failed to divide correctly. In others, genetic abnormalities, maternal illness, or infections are responsible. Maternal hormonal imbalance also may cause a miscarriage, as may a weak cervix, toxic chemicals in the environment, or physical trauma to the mother. In most cases, the cause is not known.

Ectopic Pregnancy
The implantation of a fertilized egg outside the uterus, usually in the fallopian tube or occasionally in the pelvic cavity, is called an **ectopic pregnancy.** Because these structures are not capable of expanding and nourishing a developing fetus, the pregnancy must be terminated surgically, or a miscarriage will occur. If an ectopic pregnancy goes undiagnosed and untreated, the fallopian tube will rupture, putting the woman at great risk of hemorrhage, peritonitis (infection in the abdomen), and even death.

Infant Mortality
One of the most traumatic events a couple can face is a **stillbirth.** Stillbirth is death of a fetus *after* the *twentieth* week of pregnancy, but before delivery. A stillborn baby is born dead, often for no apparent reason. Each year in the United States, about 25,000 babies, or 68 babies every day, are stillborn. Birth defects, placental problems, poor fetal growth, infections, and umbilical cord accidents are all factors that may contribute to the baby's death.

After birth, infant death can be caused by birth defects, low birth weight, injuries, or unknown causes. The infant mortality rate in the United States is currently the lowest it has been since 2000; however, it is far higher than that of most of the developed world. In the United States, the unexpected death of a child under 1 year old for no apparent reason is called **sudden infant death syndrome (SIDS).** SIDS is the leading cause of death for children age 1 month to 1 year and affects about 1 in 1,000 infants each year. It is not a specific disease; rather, it is ruled a cause of death after all other possibilities are ruled out. A SIDS death is sudden and silent; death occurs quickly, often during sleep, with no signs of suffering.

Doctors do not know what causes SIDS. However, research done in countries such as England, New Zealand, Australia, and Norway has shown that placing children on their backs or sides to sleep cuts the rate of SIDS by as much as half. The American Academy of Pediatrics advises parents to lay infants on their backs and is a sponsor of the Back to Sleep educational campaign urging parents to do so. The use of a pacifier is also recommended and should be offered to an infant up to 1 year old during daytime naps and at night. Research has shown that this practice reduces the risk of SIDS.[29]

Infertility

For the couple desperately wishing to conceive, the road to parenthood may be frustrating. An estimated one in six American couples experiences **infertility,** usually defined as the inability to conceive after trying for a year or more. In the United States, it affects about 10 to 20 percent of the reproductive-age population. Although the focus is often on women, 30 to 40 percent of the factors contributing to infertility are associated with men, and in 10 to 30 percent of infertile couples, both partners have problems. Because of the likelihood of this, it is important for both partners to be evaluated.

Reasons for the high level of infertility in the United States today include the trend toward delaying childbirth (as a woman gets older, she is less likely to conceive), endometriosis, the rising incidence of pelvic inflammatory disease, and low sperm count. Environmental contaminants known as *endocrine disrupters,* such as some pesticides and emissions from burning plastics, appear to affect fertility in both men and women. Stress and anxiety, both in general and about fertility, can also interfere with getting pregnant. The linked diseases of obesity and diabetes also have reproductive implications.

Causes in Women

Endometriosis is the leading cause of infertility in women in the United States. With this very painful disorder, parts of the endometrial lining of the uterus implant themselves outside the uterus and block the fallopian tubes. The disorder can be treated surgically or with hormonal therapy.

Another cause of infertility is **pelvic inflammatory disease (PID),** a serious infection that scars the fallopian tubes and blocks sperm migration. PID often results from

chlamydia or gonorrheal infections that spread to the fallopian tubes or ovaries. (See Chapter 13 for more on PID.) The past 30 years have brought a tremendous increase in the annual number of PID cases, from 17,800 to about 1 million per year. One episode of PID causes sterility in 10 to 15 percent of women, and 50 to 75 percent become sterile after three or four infections.[30]

Causes in Men

Among men, the single largest fertility problem is **low sperm count**. Although only one viable sperm is needed for fertilization, research has shown that all the other sperm in the ejaculate aid in the fertilization process. There are normally 60 to 80 million sperm per milliliter of semen. When the count drops below 20 million, fertility declines.

Low sperm count may be attributable to environmental factors (such as exposure of the scrotum to intense heat or cold, radiation, or altitude) or even to wearing excessively tight underwear or outerwear. However, other factors, such as the mumps virus, can damage the cells that make sperm.

sudden infant death syndrome (SIDS) The sudden death of an infant under 1 year of age for no apparent reason.

infertility Difficulties in conceiving.

endometriosis A disorder in which uterine lining tissue establishes itself outside the uterus; the leading cause of infertility in women in the United States.

pelvic inflammatory disease (PID) An infection that scars the fallopian tubes and consequently blocks sperm migration, causing infertility.

low sperm count A sperm count below 20 million sperm per milliliter of semen; the leading cause of infertility in men.

10% of infertility cases have no known cause. About 35% of infertility cases arise from problems with the man's system, whereas another 35% arise from problems with the woman's system. In 20% of cases both the man and woman have fertility problems.

Infertility Treatments

Medical treatment can identify the cause of infertility in about 90 percent of cases. The chances of becoming pregnant range from 30 to 70 percent, depending on the reason for infertility. The countless tests and the invasion of privacy that characterize some couples' efforts to conceive can put stress on an otherwise strong, healthy relationship. A good physician or fertility team will take the time to ascertain the couple's level of motivation.

Workups to determine the cause of infertility can be expensive, and the costs are not usually covered by insurance companies. Fertility workups for men include a sperm count, a test for sperm motility, and analysis of any disease processes present. Women are thoroughly examined by an obstetrician-gynecologist for the composition of cervical mucus and evidence of problems such as tubal scarring or endometriosis.

Fertility Drugs Fertility drugs stimulate ovulation in women who are not ovulating. Ninety percent of women who use these drugs will begin to ovulate, and half will conceive. Fertility drugs can have many side effects, including headaches, irritability, restlessness, depression, fatigue, edema (fluid retention), abnormal uterine bleeding, breast tenderness, vasomotor flushes (hot flashes), and visual difficulties. Women using fertility drugs are also at increased risk of developing multiple ovarian cysts (fluid-filled growths) and liver damage. The drugs sometimes trigger the release of more than one egg—a woman treated with one of these drugs has a one in ten chance of having multiple births. Most such births are twins, but triplets and even quadruplets are not uncommon.

Alternative Insemination Another treatment option is **alternative insemination** of a woman with her partner's sperm. The couple may also choose insemination by an anonymous donor through a sperm bank. The sperm are medically screened, classified according to the physical characteristics of the donor (for example, blond hair, blue eyes), and then frozen for future use.

Assisted Reproductive Technology (ART) Assisted reproductive technology (ART) describes several different medical procedures that help a woman become pregnant. The most common type of ART is **in vitro fertilization (IVF);** during IVF, eggs and sperm are mixed in a laboratory dish to fertilize, and some of the fertilized eggs (zygotes) are then transferred to the woman's uterus.

Other types of assisted reproductive technologies include:

alternative insemination
Fertilization accomplished by depositing a partner's or a donor's semen into a woman's vagina via a thin tube; almost always done in a doctor's office.
in vitro fertilization (IVF)
Fertilization of an egg in a nutrient medium and subsequent transfer back to the mother's body.

- Intracytoplasmic sperm injection (ICSI), which involves the injection of a single sperm into an egg. The fertilized egg is then placed in the woman's uterus or fallopian tube. Used with IVF, ICSI is often a successful treatment for men with impaired sperm.
- Gamete intrafallopian transfer (GIFT), which involves collecting eggs from the ovaries, then placing them into a thin flexible tube with the sperm. This is then injected into the woman's fallopian tubes, where fertilization takes place.
- Zygote intrafallopian transfer (ZIFT), which combines IVF and GIFT. Eggs and sperm are mixed outside of the body. The fertilized eggs (zygotes) are then returned to the fallopian tubes, through which they travel to the uterus.

Nonsurgical Embryo Transfer and Other Techniques

In nonsurgical embryo transfer, a donor egg is fertilized by the man's sperm and implanted in the woman's uterus. In embryo transfer, an ovum from a donor is artificially inseminated by the man's sperm, allowed to stay in the donor's body for a time, and then transplanted into the woman's body. Infertile couples have another alternative— embryo adoption programs. Fertility treatments such as IVF often produce excess fertilized eggs that a couple may choose to donate for other infertile couples to adopt.

The ethical and moral questions surrounding experimental infertility treatments are staggering. Before moving forward with any of these treatments, individuals need to ask themselves a few important questions. Has infertility been absolutely confirmed? Are reputable infertility counseling services accessible? Have they explored all possible alternatives and considered potential risks? Have all parties examined their attitudes, values, and beliefs about conceiving a child in this manner? Finally, they need to consider what and how they will tell the child about their method of conception.

Surrogate Motherhood

Sixty to 70 percent of infertile couples are able to conceive after treatment. The rest decide to live without children, to adopt, or to attempt surrogate motherhood. In this option, the couple hires a woman to be alternatively inseminated by the male partner. The surrogate then carries the baby to term and surrenders it to the couple at birth. Surrogate mothers are reportedly paid about $10,000 for their services and are reimbursed for medical expenses. Legal and medical expenses can run as high as $30,000 for the infertile couple.

Couples considering surrogate motherhood are advised to consult a lawyer regarding contracts. Most of these legal documents stipulate that the surrogate mother undergo amniocentesis and that if the fetus is defective, she must consent to an abortion. In that case, or if the surrogate miscarries, she is reimbursed for her time and expenses. The prospective parents must also agree to take the baby if it is carried to term, even if it is unhealthy or has physical abnormalities.

Adoption

For couples who have decided that biological childbirth is not an option, adoption provides an alternative. About 50,000 children are available for adoption in the United States every year. This is far fewer than the number of couples seeking adoptions. By some estimates, only 1 in 30 couples receives the child they want. On average, couples spend 2 years and $100,000 on the adoption process.

Increasingly, couples are choosing to adopt children from other countries. In 2008, U.S. families adopted over 17,400 foreign-born children.[31] The cost of intercountry adoption varies from approximately $10,000 to more than $30,000, including agency fees, dossier and immigration processing fees, and court costs. However, it may be a good alternative for many couples, especially those who want to adopt an infant rather than an older child.

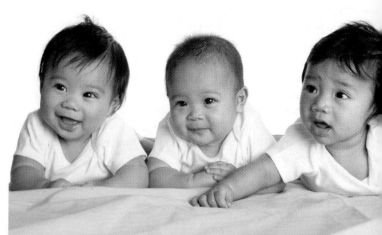

Are You Comfortable with Your Contraception?

PEARSON
myhealthlab™

Fill out this assessment online at www.pearsonhighered.com/myhealthlab or www.pearsonhighered.com/donatelle.

These questions will help you assess whether your current method of contraception or one you may consider using in the future will be effective for you. Answering yes to any of these questions predicts potential problems. If you have more than a few yes responses, consider talking to a health care provider, counselor, partner, or friend to decide whether to use this method or how to use it so that it will really be effective.

Method of contraception you use now or are considering:

_____

1. Have I or my partner ever become pregnant while using this method? Ⓨ Ⓝ

2. Am I afraid of using this method? Ⓨ Ⓝ

3. Would I really rather not use this method? Ⓨ Ⓝ

4. Will I have trouble remembering to use this method? Ⓨ Ⓝ

5. Will I have trouble using this method correctly? Ⓨ Ⓝ

6. Does this method make menstrual periods longer or more painful for me or my partner? Ⓨ Ⓝ

7. Does this method cost more than I can afford? Ⓨ Ⓝ

8. Could this method cause serious complications? Ⓨ Ⓝ

9. Am I, or is my partner, opposed to this method because of any religious or moral beliefs? Ⓨ Ⓝ

10. Will using this method embarrass me or my partner? Ⓨ Ⓝ

11. Will I enjoy intercourse less because of this method? Ⓨ Ⓝ

12. Am I at risk of being exposed to HIV or other sexually transmitted infections if I use this method? Ⓨ Ⓝ

Total number of yes answers: _____

Source: Adapted from R. A. Hatcher et al., *Contraceptive Technology.* 19th ed. Copyright © 2007 Contraceptive Technology Communications, Inc. Used with permission.

YOUR PLAN FOR CHANGE

The **Assess yourself** activity gave you the chance to assess your comfort and confidence with a contraceptive method you are using now or may use in the future. Depending on the results, you may consider changing your birth control method.

Today, you can:

◯ Visit your local drugstore and study the forms of contraception that are available without a prescription. Think about which of them you would consider using and why.

◯ If you are not currently using any contraception or are not in a sexual relationship but might become sexually active, purchase a package of condoms (or pick up a few free samples from your campus health center) to keep on hand just in case.

Within the next 2 weeks, you can:

◯ Make an appointment for a checkup with your health care provider. Be sure to ask him or her any questions you have about contraception.

◯ Sit down with your partner and discuss contraception. Decide who will be responsible and which form will work best for you.

By the end of the semester, you can:

◯ Periodically reevaluate whether your new or continued contraception is still effective for you. Review your experiences, and take note of any consistent problems you may have encountered.

◯ Always keep a backup form of contraception on hand. Check this supply periodically and throw out and replace any supplies that have expired.

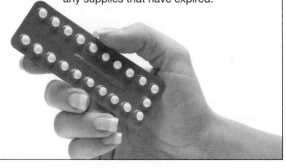

Summary

* Latex male condoms and the female condom, when used correctly for oral sex or intercourse, provide the most effective protection in preventing sexually transmitted infections (STIs). Other contraceptive methods include abstinence, outercourse, oral contraceptives, spermicides, the diaphragm, the cervical cap, the Today sponge, Ortho Evra, NuvaRing, intrauterine devices, Depo-Provera, and withdrawal. Emergency contraception may be used within 72 hours of unprotected intercourse or the failure of another contraceptive method. Fertility awareness methods rely on altering sexual practices to avoid pregnancy. Whereas all these methods of contraception are reversible, sterilization is permanent.

* Abortion is legal in the United States through the second trimester. Abortion methods include suction curretage, dilation and evacuation (D&E), intact dilation and extraction (D&X), hysterectomy, induction abortion, and medical abortions.

* Parenting is a demanding job that requires careful planning. Prospective parents need to take into account emotional health, maternal and paternal health, and financial plans.

* Prenatal care includes a complete physical exam within the first trimester and avoidance of all substances that could have teratogenic effects on the fetus, such as alcohol and drugs, smoking, X rays, and harmful chemicals. Full-term pregnancy covers three trimesters.

* Childbirth occurs in three stages. Partners should jointly choose a labor method early in the pregnancy to be better prepared for labor when it occurs. Possible complications of pregnancy and childbirth include preeclampsia and eclampsia, miscarriage, ectopic pregnancy, stillbirth, and the need for a C-section.

* Infertility in women may be caused by pelvic inflammatory disease (PID) or endometriosis. In men, it may be caused by low sperm count. Treatments may include alternative insemination, in vitro fertilization (IVF), assisted reproductive technology (ART), embryo transfer, and embryo adoption programs. Surrogate motherhood and adoption are also options.

Pop Quiz

1. What type of contraceptive method involves long-acting synthetic progesterone injected intramuscularly every 3 months?
   a. Seasonale
   b. Ortho Evra
   c. Depo-Provera
   d. Lea's Shield

2. Which of the following is *not* a barrier contraceptive?
   a. cervical cap
   b. condom
   c. diaphragm
   d. contraceptive patch

3. What is the most commonly used method of first-trimester abortion?
   a. suction curretage
   b. dilation and evacuation (D&E)
   c. medical abortion
   d. induction abortions

4. What is meant by the *failure rate* of contraceptive use?
   a. the number of times a woman fails to get pregnant when she wanted to
   b. the number of times a woman gets pregnant when she did not want to
   c. the number of pregnancies that occur for women using a particular method of birth control
   d. the reliability of alternative methods of birth control that do not use condoms

5. Toxic chemicals, pesticides, X rays, and other hazardous compounds that cause birth defects are known as
   a. carcinogens.
   b. teratogens.
   c. mutants.
   d. environmental assaults.

6. In an ectopic pregnancy, the fertilized egg usually implants in the woman's
   a. fallopian tube.
   b. uterus.
   c. vagina.
   d. ovaries.

7. What is the recommended pregnancy weight gain for a woman who is at a healthy weight before pregnancy?
   a. 15 to 20 pounds
   b. 20 to 30 pounds
   c. 25 to 35 pounds
   d. 30 to 45 pounds

8. What prenatal test involves snipping tissue from the developing fetal sac?
   a. fetoscopy
   b. ultrasound
   c. amniocentesis
   d. chorionic villus sampling

9. Why is it recommended not to use condoms made of lambskin?
   a. They are less elastic than latex condoms.
   b. They cannot be stored for as long as latex condoms.
   c. They do not protect against the transmission of STIs.
   d. They are likely to cause allergic reactions.

10. The number of American couples who experience infertility is
    a. 1 in 6.
    b. 1 in 24.
    c. 1 in 60.
    d. 1 in 100.

Answers to these questions can be found on page A-1.

1. List the most effective contraceptive methods. What are their drawbacks? What medical conditions would keep a person from using each one? What are the characteristics of the methods that you think would be most effective for you? Why do you consider them most effective for you personally?

2. What are the various methods of abortion? What are the two opposing viewpoints concerning abortion? What is *Roe v. Wade,* and what impact did it have on the abortion debate?

3. What are the most important considerations in deciding whether the time is right to become a parent? If you choose to have children, what factors will you consider regarding the number of children to have?

4. Discuss the growth of the fetus through the three trimesters. What medical checkups or tests should be done during each trimester?

5. Discuss the emotional aspects of pregnancy. What types of emotional reactions are common in each trimester and the postpartum period (the "fourth trimester")?

6. If you and your partner are unable to have children, what alternative methods of conception would you consider? Is adoption an option you would consider?

Accessing Your Health on the Internet

The following websites explore further topics and issues related to personal health. For links to the websites below, visit the Companion Website for *Health: The Basics,* Green Edition at www.pearsonhighered.com/donatelle.

1. *Guttmacher Institute.* This is a non-profit organization focused on sexual and reproductive health research, policy analysis, and public education. www.guttmacher.org

2. *Association of Reproductive Health Professionals.* This organization was originally founded by Alan Guttmacher as the educational arm of Planned Parenthood. Now an independent organization, it provides education for health care professionals and the general public. The Patient Resources portion of the website includes information on various methods of birth control and an interactive tool to help you choose a method that will work for you. www.arhp.org

3. *The American Pregnancy Association.* A national organization offering a wealth of resources to promote reproductive and pregnancy wellness. The website includes educational materials and information on the latest in research. www.americanpregnancy.org

4. *Choosing Wisely birth control selection tool.* This interactive tool provided by the Society of Obstetricians and Gynaecologists of Canada helps you evaluate what type of birth control would best suit your needs. The questionnaire is quick and easy to use, and provides thorough information about the available contraceptive methods. www.sexualityandu.ca/trialdp/index.aspx

5. *Planned Parenthood.* This site offers a range of up-to-date information on sexual health issues, such as birth control, deciding when and whether to have a child, sexually transmitted infections, and safer sex. www.plannedparenthood.org

6. *Sexuality Information and Education Council of the United States.* Information, guidelines, and materials for the advancement of sexuality education. The site advocates the right of individuals to make responsible sexual choices. www.siecus.org

References

1. World Health Organization, "Nonoxynol-9 Ineffective in Preventing HIV Infection," June 28, 2002, www.who.int/mediacentre/news/releases/who55/en.

2. U.S. Department of Health and Human Services, "FDA Approves Seasonale Oral Contraceptive," FDA Talk Paper TO3–65, September 5, 2003, www.fda.gov.

3. R. A. Hatcher et al., *Contraceptive Technology.* 19th rev ed. (New York: Ardent Media, 2007); R. Burkman et al., "Safety Concerns and Health Benefits Associated with Oral Contraception," *American Journal of Obstetrics and Gynecology* 190 (4 Suppl S; 2004): S5–S22.

4. Food and Drug Administration, "FDA Approves Update to Label on Birth Control Patch," FDA News, January 18, 2008, www.fda.gov/NewsEvents/Newsroom/PressAnnouncements/2008/ucm116842.htm.

5. National Conference of State Legislatures, "50 State Summary of Emergency Contraception Laws," www.ncsl.org/programs/health/ecleg.htm. Updated September 2009.

6. S. J. Ventura, J. C. Abma, W. D. Mosher, and S. Henshaw, "Estimated Pregnancy Rates for the United States, 1990–2000: An Update," *National Vital Statistic Reports* 52 (2004): 1–2; H. Boonstra, "Emergency Contraception: The Need to Increase Public Awareness," *Guttmacher Rep Public Policy* 5 (2002): 3–6; Planned Parenthood Federation of America, "Emergency Contraception (Morning After Pill)," www.plannedparenthood.org/health-topics/emergency-contraception-morning-after-pill-4363.htm. Accessed November 2009.

7. American College Health Association—National College Health Assessment (ACHA-NCHA), "Spring 2007 Reference Group Data Report," *Journal of American College Health* 56, no. 5 (2008).

8. American College Health Association, *American College Health Association—National College Health Assessment II: Reference Group Data Report Fall 2008* (Baltimore: American College Health Association, 2009).

9. D. Bensyl et al., "Contraceptive Use—United States and Territories, Behavioral Risk Factor Surveillance System, 2002," *Morbidity and Mortality Weekly Report* 54 (SS6; November 18, 2005): 1–72.

10. K. N. Anderson, L. E. Anderson, and W. D. Glanze, eds., *Mosby's Medical, Nursing and Allied Health Dictionary* (Philadelphia: W. B. Saunders, 2002); R. A. Hatcher et al., *Contraceptive Technology,* 2007.

11. Boston Women's Health Collective, *Our Bodies, Ourselves: A New Edition for a New Era* (New York: Simon & Schuster, 2005).

12. The Alan Guttmacher Institute, "State Policies in Brief: State Funding of Abortion under Medicaid," October 1, 2009, www.guttmacher.org/statecenter/spibs/spib_SFAM.pdf; The Alan Guttmacher Institute, "Sexual and Reproductive Health Issues in the States: Major Trends in 2005," www.guttmacher.org.

13. NARAL, Pro Choice America, "The Bush Administration's Federal Abortion Ban," December 1, 2007, www.prochoiceamerica.org/assets/files/Abortion-Abortion-Bans-Federal-Abortion-Ban.pdf.

14. Ibid.

15. N. F. Russo and A. J. Dabul, "The Relationship of Abortion to Well-Being: Do Race and Religion Make a Difference?" *Professional Psychology: Research and Practice* 28, no. 1 (2000): 23–31.

16. *Facts on Induced Abortions in the United States.* Allan Guttmacher Institute, July 2008, Accessed October 5, 2009. www.guttmacher.org/pubs/fb_induced_abortion.html.

17. Ibid.

18. Planned Parenthood, "The Difference between Emergency Contraception Pills and Medication Abortion," December 13, 2006, www.plannedparenthoodaction.org/files/ecmedab1206.pdf.

19. Center for Policy and Promotion, "Expenditures on Children by Families, 2006," April 2007, www.cnpp.usda.gov/Publications/CRC/crc2006.pdf.

20. J. Overturf-Johnson, "Who's Minding the Kids? Child Care Arrangements: Winter 2002," *Current Population Reports,* Publication no. 70–101 (Washington, DC: U.S. Census Bureau, 2005).

21. National Center for Chronic Disease Prevention and Health Promotion, "Tobacco Use and Pregnancy," www.cdc.gov/reproductivehealth/TobaccoUsePregnancy/index.htm. Updated October 2, 2007.

22. M. Kharrazi et al., "Environmental Tobacco Smoke and Pregnancy Outcome," *Epidemiology* 15, no. 6 (November 2006): 660–70.

23. X. Weng et al., "Maternal Caffeine Consumption during Pregnancy and the Risk of Miscarriage: A Prospect Cohort Study," *American Journal of Obstetrics and Gynecology* 198, no. 3 (2008): e1–e8.

24. National Institute of Child Health and Human Development, "Down Syndrome," www.nichd.nih.gov/health/topics/down_syndrome.cfm. Updated February 16, 2007.

25. J. Yabroff, "Birth the American Way," *Newsweek* 151, no. 4 (2008): 46.

26. Ibid.

27. National Women's Health Information Center, "Frequently Asked Questions: Depression during and after Pregnancy," Updated March 2009, www.4woman.gov/faq/postpartum.pdf.

28. E. de Lisser, "Breast Feeding Boosts Adult I.Q., Research Suggests," *Wall Street Journal*, May 2, 2002, D2; American Pregnancy Association, "What's in Breast Milk?" www.americanpregnancy.org/firstyearoflife/whatsinbreastmilk.html. Updated August 2006.

29. F. R. Hawk et al., "Do Pacifiers Reduce the Risk of Sudden Infant Death Syndrome? A Meta-Analysis," *Pediatrics* 116, no. 5 (2005): e716–e723.

30. Centers for Disease Control and Prevention, "Pelvic Inflammatory Disease—Fact Sheet," www.cdc.gov/std/PID/STDFact-PID.htm. Updated April 7, 2008.

31. Bureau of Consular Affairs, "Total Adoptions to the United States," 2009, http://adoption.state.gov/news/total_chart.html.

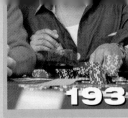

193

What makes an addiction different from a habit?

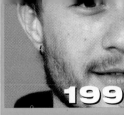

199

Why is prescription drug abuse on the rise?

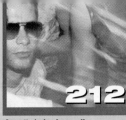

212

Are "club drugs" dangerous?

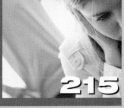

215

How can I help someone who I think has a problem with addiction?

7

Addiction and Drug Abuse

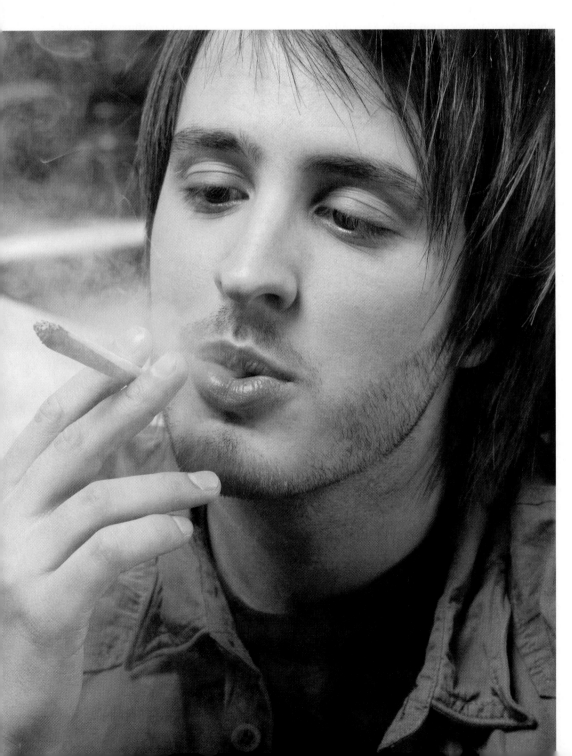

Objectives

✴ Identify the signs of addiction and discuss types of addictions, including compulsive behaviors such as gambling and shopping.

✴ Identify the six categories of drugs and distinguish between drug misuse and drug abuse.

✴ Discuss the issues of over-the-counter and prescription drug misuse and abuse, including their impact on college campuses.

✴ Profile illicit drug use in the United States, including who uses illicit drugs, financial impact, and prevalence on college campuses.

✴ Discuss the use and abuse of controlled substances, including cocaine, amphetamines, marijuana, opioids, hallucinogens, inhalants, and steroids.

✴ Discuss treatment and recovery options for addicts, and discuss public health approaches to preventing drug abuse and reducing the impact of addiction on our society.

It isn't difficult these days to find high-profile cases of compulsive and destructive behavior. Stories of celebrities and politicians struggling with addictions to alcohol, drugs, and sex are splashed in the headlines and profiled on television news programs. But millions of "everyday" people throughout the world are staging their own battles with addiction as well. Addictions can be perplexing, because many potentially addictive activities may actually enhance the lives of those who engage in them moderately. In addition to alcohol and drugs, commonly recognized objects of addiction include gambling, shopping, Internet use, technology, and exercise.

Defining Addiction

Addiction is defined as continued involvement with a substance or activity despite its ongoing negative consequences. It is classified by the American Psychiatric Association (APA) as a mental disorder. Addictive behaviors initially provide a sense of pleasure or stability that is beyond an individual's power to achieve in other ways. Eventually, the individual needs to consume the addictive substance or enact the behavior to feel normal.

To be addictive, a substance or behavior must have the potential to produce positive mood changes, such as euphoria or anxiety or pain reduction. The danger comes when people become dependent on these substances or behaviors to feel normal or to function on a daily basis. Signs of addiction become apparent when people continue to use the substance despite knowing the harm that it causes to themselves and others, such as deterioration in work or school performance or impaired relationships and social interactions. People with **physiological dependence** to a substance, such as an addictive drug, experience **tolerance** when increased amounts of the drug are required to achieve the desired effect. They also experience **withdrawal,** a series of temporary physical and psychological symptoms that occurs when substance use stops. Tolerance and withdrawal are important criteria for determining whether or not someone is addicted.

Psychological dependence can also play an important role in addiction, which explains why behaviors not related to the use of chemicals, such as gambling, can lead to dependence and addiction. Some researchers believe that compulsive behaviors, such as overeating, overexercising, and gambling, may produce the same feelings of euphoria as an addictive drug, along with a strong desire to repeat the behavior and a craving for the behavior when it stops.

Signs of Addiction

Studies show that all animals share the same basic pleasure and reward circuits in the brain that turn on when they engage in something pleasurable. We all engage in potentially addictive behaviors to some extent because some are essential to our survival and are highly reinforcing, such as eating, drinking, and sex. At some point along the continuum, however, some individuals are not able to engage in these behaviors moderately, and they become addicted.

Addictions are characterized by four common symptoms: (1) **compulsion,** which is characterized by **obsession,** or excessive preoccupation, with the behavior and an overwhelming need to perform it; (2) **loss of control,** or the inability to predict reliably whether any isolated occurrence of the behavior will be healthy or damaging; (3) **negative consequences,** such as physical damage, legal trouble, finan-

addiction Continued involvement with a substance or activity despite ongoing negative consequences.

physiological dependence The adaptive state of brain and body processes that occurs with regular addictive behavior and results in withdrawal if the addictive behavior stops.

tolerance Phenomenon in which progressively larger doses of a drug or more intense involvement in a behavior are needed to produce the desired effects.

withdrawal A series of temporary physical and psychological symptoms that occur when an addict abruptly abstains from an addictive chemical or behavior.

psychological dependence Dependency of the mind on a substance or behavior, which can lead to psychological withdrawal symptoms, such as anxiety, irritability, or cravings.

compulsion Preoccupation with a behavior and an overwhelming need to perform it.

obsession Excessive preoccupation with an addictive object or behavior.

loss of control Inability to predict reliably whether a particular instance of involvement with an addictive substance or behavior will be healthy or damaging.

negative consequences Physical damage, legal trouble, financial ruin, academic failure, family dissolution, and other severe problems associated with addiction.

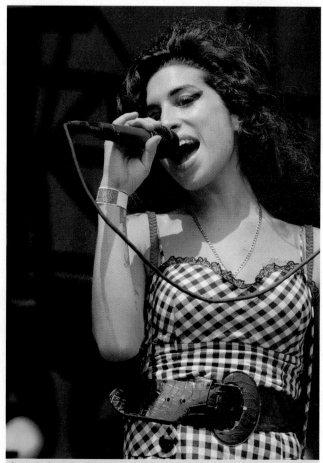

Grammy Award–winning singer Amy Winehouse is well known for her struggles with substance abuse.

cial problems, academic failure, or family dissolution, which do not occur with healthy involvement in any behavior; and (4) **denial,** the inability to perceive that the behavior is self-destructive. These four components are present in all addictions, whether chemical or behavioral.

Addictive Behaviors

Clearly, tobacco, alcohol, and other drugs are addictive, and addictions to them create multiple problems for addicted individuals, their families, and society. We have examined the fundamental concepts and process of addiction and its associated problems; later in this chapter we will discuss specific drugs that are addictive or commonly abused. Alcohol and tobacco use and addiction are discussed in detail in Chapter 8. Here we will look at what are commonly called **process addictions**—behaviors known to be addictive because they are mood altering. Traditionally, the word *addiction* has been confined to use mainly with alcohol and other psychoactive substances. However, this is changing. New knowledge about the brain's reward system suggests that, as far as the brain is concerned, a reward is a reward, whether it is brought on by a chemical or a behavior. When there is a reward, there is a risk that a vulnerable brain might get trapped in a compulsion. Examples of process addictions include pathological gambling, compulsive spending, compulsive exercise, and compulsive Internet or technology use.

Compulsive or Pathological Gambling

Gambling is a form of recreation and entertainment for millions of Americans. Most people who gamble do so casually and moderately to experience the excitement of anticipating a win. However, more than 2 million Americans are **compulsive,** or **pathological, gamblers,** and 6 million more are considered to be at risk for developing a gambling addiction.[1] The APA recognizes pathological gambling as a mental disorder and lists ten characteristic behaviors, including preoccupation with gambling, unsuccessful efforts to cut back or quit, using gambling to escape problems, and lying to family members to conceal the extent of involvement with gambling.

Gamblers and drug addicts describe many similar cravings and highs. A recent study supports what many experts believe to be true: that compulsive gambling is like drug addiction. Compulsive gamblers in this study were found to have decreased blood flow to a key section of the brain's reward system. Much as with people who abuse drugs, it is thought that compulsive gamblers compensate for this deficiency in their brain's reward system by overdoing it and getting hooked.[2] Most compulsive gamblers state that they seek excitement even more than money. They place increasingly larger bets to obtain the desired level of excitement. Like drug addicts, compulsive gamblers live from fix to fix. Their subjective cravings can be as intense as those of drug abusers; they show tolerance

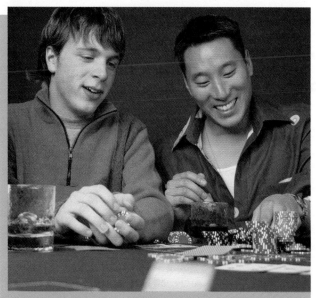

What makes an addiction different from a habit?

Once a person recognizes a habit and decides to change it, the habit can usually be broken. With an addiction, however, there is a sense of compulsion so strong that the addict is no longer in control of his or her behavior. For example, you may be in the habit of playing a few hands of video poker every night before you study, or getting together for a weekly game with your buddies, but your gambling isn't considered an addiction unless you have lost control over where and when you gamble—and how much—and you are experiencing negative impacts on the rest of your life as a result.

in their need to increase the amount of their bets; and they experience highs rivaling that of a drug high. Up to half of pathological gamblers show withdrawal symptoms similar to a mild form of drug withdrawal, including sleep disturbance, sweating, irritability, and craving.

Who is at risk for getting hooked on the rush of gambling? Men are more likely to have gambling problems than women are. Gambling prevalence is also higher among lower-income individuals, those who are divorced, African Americans, older adults, and individuals residing within 50 miles of a casino. Residents in southern states, where opportunities to gamble have increased significantly over the past 20 years, also have higher gambling rates.[3]

Gambling among college students appears to be on the rise across the nation. In a 2005 telephone poll conducted by University of Pennsylvania's Annenburg Public Policy Center, 15.5 percent of college students reported gambling once a week, up from 8.3 percent in 2002, an 87 percent increase.[4] What accounts for this trend? College students have easier access to gambling opportunities than ever before with the advent of online gambling, and a growing number of casinos, scratch tickets, lotteries, and sports betting networks. In particular, the largest boost has

denial Inability to perceive or accurately interpret the self-destructive effects of an addictive behavior.

process addiction A condition in which a person is dependent on (addicted to) some mood-altering behavior or process, such as gambling, eating, or exercise.

compulsive (pathological) gambler A person addicted to gambling.

come from the increasing popularity of poker. Access to poker on the Internet and televised poker tournaments have revived the game, causing many young people to spend an unhealthy amount of time and money playing it. Some characteristics associated with gambling among college students include spending more time watching TV; using computers for nonacademic purposes; spending less time studying; earning lower grades; participating in intercollegiate athletics; and engaging in heavy, episodic drinking and using illicit drugs.[5]

Whereas casual gamblers can stop anytime they wish and are capable of seeing the necessity to do so, compulsive gamblers are unable to control the urge to gamble even in the face of devastating consequences: high debt; legal problems; and the loss of everything meaningful, including homes, families, jobs, health, and even their lives. Gambling can also have a detrimental effect on health: Cardiovascular problems affect 38 percent of compulsive gamblers, and their suicide rate is 20 times higher than that of the general population.

Compulsive Spending

People who "shop till they drop" and run their credit cards to the limit often have a shopping addiction. Since the credit card's introduction, millions of Americans have found themselves mired in consumer debt. There are 400 million Master-Cards and Visas out there, and on average, **compulsive spenders** are $23,000 in debt, usually in the form of credit card debt or mortgages against their homes.[6] College students may be particularly vulnerable to spending problems because advertisers and credit card companies aggressively target them.

In our society, people often use shopping as a way to make themselves feel better. However, for compulsive shoppers, it does not make them feel any better but actually worse. Compulsive spending has many of the same characteristics as alcoholism, gambling, and other addictions. Symptoms that a spender has crossed the line into addiction include buying more than one of the same item, keeping items in the closet with the tags still attached, repeatedly buying much more than they need or can afford, hiding purchases from relatives and loved ones, and experiencing feelings of euphoria and excitement when shopping.[7]

Compulsive gambling and spending can frequently lead to compulsive borrowing to help support the addiction. Irresponsible investments and purchases lead to debts that the addict tries to repay by borrowing more. Compulsive spenders often borrow money repeatedly from family, friends, or institutions in spite of the problems this causes.

compulsive spenders People who shop on impulse as a way of coping and find it difficult to control their spending behaviors.
addictive exercisers People who exercise compulsively to try to meet needs of nurturance, intimacy, self-esteem, and self-competency.
Internet addiction Compulsive use of the computer, PDA, cell phone, or other form of technology to access the Internet for activities such as e-mail, games, shopping, and blogging.
codependence A self-defeating relationship pattern in which a person is "addicted to the addict."
enablers People who knowingly or unknowingly protect addicts from the consequences of their behavior.

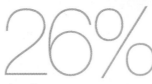

26% of college men report gambling at least once a week, compared to 5.5% of college women.

Exercise Addiction

It may seem odd that a personal health text that advocates exercise would also identify it as a potential addiction. Yet, as a powerful mood enhancer, exercise can be addictive. Firm statistics on the incidence of this addiction are not available, but one indication of its prevalence is that a large portion of America's 2 million people with the eating disorders anorexia nervosa and bulimia nervosa use exercise to purge instead of, or in addition to, self-induced vomiting. **Addictive exercisers** use exercise compulsively to try to meet needs—for nurturance, intimacy, self-esteem, and self-competency—that an object or activity cannot truly meet. Consequently, addictive exercise results in negative consequences similar to those found in other addictions: alienation of family and friends, injuries from overdoing it, and a craving for more.

Traditionally, women have been perceived as being more at risk for exercise addiction. However, evidence is growing that more men are developing unhealthy exercise patterns. Media images promoting six-pack abs and lean, muscular bodies have influenced society's view of the masculine ideal. Meanwhile, more men are abusing steroids and overexercising to attain an ideal frame. *Muscle dysmorphia*, sometimes referred to as *bigarexia*, is a pathological preoccupation with being larger and more muscular.[8] Sufferers view themselves as small and weak even though they may be quite the opposite.[9] Consequences of muscle dysmorphia include excessive weight lifting and exercising as well as steroid or supplement abuse. See Focus On: Your Body Image begining on page 314 for further discussion of these disorders and the body image issues associated with them.

Technology Addictions

As technology becomes an ever larger part of our daily lives, the risk of overexposure grows for people of all ages. Some people, in fact, become addicted to new technologies, such as cell phones, video games, PDAs, networking sites, and the Internet in general. Have you ever opened your Web browser to quickly check something, and an hour later found yourself still blogging or checking your Facebook page?

For compulsive spenders, shopping is an exhilarating experience.

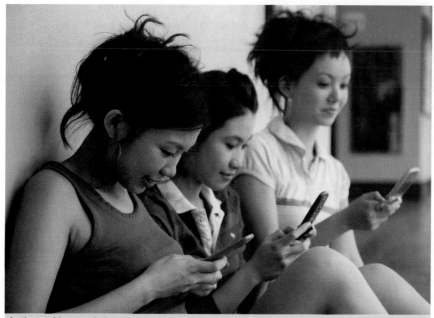
As the world goes wireless, many of us are becoming increasingly dependent on—and compulsive about—our technology.

Do you have friends who seem more concerned with texting or surfing the Internet than with eating, going out, studying, or watching TV? These attitudes and behaviors are not unusual; many experts suggest that technology addiction is real and can present serious problems for those addicted. An estimated 5 to 10 percent of Internet users will likely experience **Internet addiction.**[10] Approximately 11 percent of college students report that Internet use and computer games have interfered with their academic performance.[11]

What is normal Internet use? Because the Internet has been around a relatively short time, it is difficult to say. Studies suggest that some college students average 8 hours or so per week, and Web surfers can average 20 hours online without having major problems. What you do online may be as important as how long you spend there. Some online activities, such as gaming and cybersex, seem to be more compelling and potentially addictive than others.

Internet addicts have multiple signs and symptoms, including general disregard for one's health, sleep deprivation, neglecting family and friends, lack of physical activity, euphoria when online, lower grades in school, and poor job performance. Internet addicts may feel moody or uncomfortable when they are not online. These addicts may be using their behavior to compensate for feelings of loneliness, marital or work problems, a poor social life, or financial problems.

Addiction Affects Family and Friends

The family and friends of an addicted person also suffer many negative consequences. Often they struggle with **codependence,** a self-defeating relationship pattern in which a person is "addicted to the addict." It is the primary outcome of dysfunctional relationships or families.

Codependence is defined by a pattern of behavior. Codependents find it hard to set healthy boundaries and often live in the chaotic, crisis-oriented mode that naturally occurs around addicts. They assume responsibility for meeting others' needs to the point that they subordinate or even cease being aware of their own needs. They may be unable to perceive their needs because they have repeatedly been taught that their needs are inappropriate or less important than someone else's. Although the word *codependent* is used less frequently today, treatment professionals still recognize the importance of helping addicts see how their behavior affects those around them and of working with family and friends to establish healthier relationships and boundaries.

Family and friends can play an important role in getting an addict to seek treatment. They are most helpful when they refuse to be enablers. **Enablers** are people who knowingly or unknowingly protect addicts from the natural consequences of their behavior. If they don't have to deal with the consequences, addicts cannot see the self-destructive nature of their behavior and will therefore continue it. Codependents are the primary enablers of their addicted loved ones, although anyone who has contact with an addict can be an enabler and thus contribute (perhaps powerfully) to continuation of the addictive behavior. Enablers are generally unaware that their behavior has this effect. In fact, enabling is rarely conscious and certainly not intentional.

what do you think?

Why do we tend to protect others from the natural consequences of their destructive behaviors? ● Have you ever confronted someone you were concerned about? If so, was the confrontation successful? ● What tips would you give someone who wants to confront a loved one about an addiction?

Drug Dynamics

Although drug abuse is usually referred to in connection with illicit psychoactive drugs, many people also abuse and misuse prescription, over-the-counter (OTC) medications, and recreational drugs. **Drug misuse** involves using a drug for a purpose for which it was not intended. For example, taking a friend's high-powered prescription painkiller for your headache is a misuse of that drug. This is not too far removed from **drug abuse,**

drug misuse Use of a drug for a purpose for which it was not intended.
drug abuse Excessive use of a drug.

or the excessive use of any drug, and may cause serious harm.

Drug misuse and abuse are problems of staggering proportions in our society. Each year, drug and alcohol abuse contributes to the destruction of families and jobs and to the deaths of more than 120,000 Americans. Drug abuse costs taxpayers more than $294 billion annually in preventable health care costs, extra law enforcement, vehicle crashes, crime, and lost productivity.[12] It's impossible to put a dollar amount on the pain, suffering, and dysfunction that drugs cause in our everyday lives.

Although overall use of drugs in the United States has fallen by 50 percent in the past 20 years, the past 10 years have shown an increase in the use of certain drugs by adolescents.[13] It is important to understand how drugs work and why people use them. Humans appear to have a need to alter their consciousness, or mental state. We like to feel good or escape the normal. Consciousness can be altered in many ways: Children spinning until they become dizzy and adults enjoying the rush of thrilling extreme sports are examples. To change our awareness, many of us listen to music, skydive, ski, read, daydream, meditate, pray, or have sexual relations. Others turn to drugs to alter consciousness.

Drugs work because they physically resemble the chemicals produced naturally within the body. Most bodily processes result from chemical reactions or from changes in electrical charge. Because drugs possess an electrical charge and chemical structure similar to those of chemicals that occur naturally in the body, they can affect physical functions in many different ways.

How Drugs Affect the Brain

Pleasure, which scientists call *reward*, is a very powerful biological force for survival. If you do something experienced as pleasurable, the brain is wired in such a way that you tend to do it again. Life-sustaining activities, such as eating, activate a circuit of specialized nerve cells devoted to producing and regulating pleasure. One important set of these nerve cells, which uses a chemical **neurotransmitter** called *dopamine*, sits at the very top of the brainstem in the *ventral tegmental area (VTA)*. These dopamine-containing neurons relay messages about pleasure through their nerve fibers to nerve cells in the limbic system, structures in the brain regulating emotions. Still other fibers connect to a related part of the frontal region of the cerebral cortex, the area of the brain that plays a key role in memory, perception, thought, and consciousness. So, this "pleasure circuit," known as the *mesolimbic dopamine* system, spans the survival-oriented brainstem, the emotional limbic system, and the thinking frontal cerebral cortex.

All drugs that are addicting can activate the brain's pleasure circuit. Drug addiction is a biological, pathological process that alters the way in which the pleasure center, as well as other parts of

neurotransmitter A chemical that relays messages between nerve cells or from nerve cells to other body cells.

psychoactive drugs Drugs that affect brain chemistry and have the potential to alter mood or behavior.

the brain, functions. Almost all **psychoactive drugs** (those that change the way the brain works) do so by affecting chemical neurotransmission, either enhancing it, suppressing it, or interfering with it. Some drugs, such as heroin and LSD, mimic the effects of a natural neurotransmitter. Others, such as PCP, block receptors and thereby prevent neuronal messages from getting through. Still others, such as cocaine, block the *reuptake* of neurotransmitters by neurons, thus producing an increased concentration of the neurotransmitters in the synaptic gap, the space between individual neurons (Figure 7.1). Finally, some drugs, such as methamphetamine, act by causing neurotransmitters to be released in greater amounts than is normal.

Types of Drugs

Scientists divide drugs into 6 categories: prescription, over-the-counter (OTC), recreational, herbal, illicit, and commercial drugs. These classifications are based primarily on drug action, although some are based on the source of the chemical in question. Each category includes some drugs that stimulate the body, some that depress body functions, and others that produce hallucinations (images, auditory or visual, that are perceived but are not real). Each category also includes psychoactive drugs.

- **Prescription drugs.** These can be obtained only with a prescription from a licensed physician. More than 10,000 types of prescription drugs are sold in the United States.
- **OTC drugs.** These can be purchased without a prescription. More than 300,000 OTC products are available, and an estimated three out of four people routinely self-medicate with them.[14] (See Chapter 16 for a discussion of the OTC label and common types of OTC drugs.)
- **Recreational drugs.** These belong to a somewhat vague category whose boundaries depend upon how the term *recreation* is defined. Generally, recreational drugs contain chemicals used to help people relax or socialize. Most of them are legal even though they are psychoactive. Alcohol, tobacco, and caffeine products are included in this category.
- **Herbal preparations.** These encompass approximately 750 substances, including herbal teas and other products of botanical (plant) origin that are believed to have medicinal properties. (See Chapter 17 for more on herbal preparations.)
- **Illicit (illegal) drugs.** These are the most notorious type of drug. Although laws governing their use, possession, cultivation, manufacture, and sale differ from state to state, illicit drugs are generally recognized as harmful. All of them are psychoactive.
- **Commercial preparations.** These are the most universally used yet least commonly recognized chemical substances. More than 1,000 of them exist, including seemingly benign items such as perfumes, cosmetics, household cleansers, paints, glues, inks, dyes, and pesticides.

Routes of Drug Administration

Route of administration refers to the way in which a given drug is taken into the body. The most common method is by

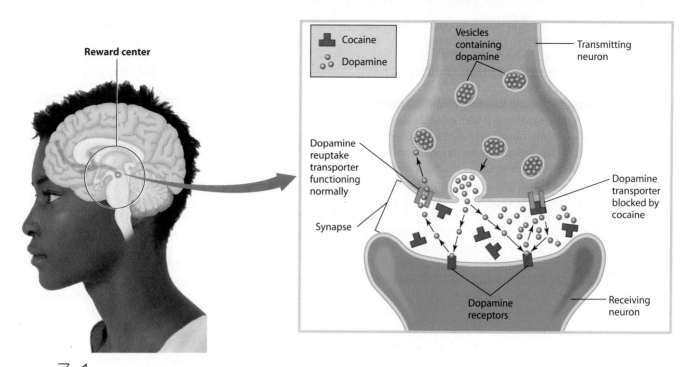

FIGURE 7.1 **The Action of Cocaine at Dopamine Receptors in the Brain, an Example of Psychoactive Drug Action**

In normal neural communication, dopamine is released into the synapse between neurons. It binds temporarily to dopamine receptors on the receiving neuron, and then is recycled back into the transmitting neuron by a transporter. When cocaine molecules are present, they attach to the dopamine transporter and block the recycling process. Too much dopamine remains active in the synaptic gaps between neurons, creating feelings of excitement and euphoria.

Source: Adapted from NIDA Research Report—Cocaine Abuse and Addiction (NIH Publication no. 99-4342, printed May 1999, revised November 2004).

swallowing a tablet, capsule, or liquid (**oral ingestion**). Drugs taken in this manner don't reach the bloodstream as quickly as drugs introduced to the body by other means. A drug taken orally may not reach the bloodstream for as long as 30 minutes.

Drugs can also enter the body through the respiratory tract via sniffing, snorting, smoking, or inhaling (**inhalation).** Inhaling cigarettes, marijuana, gases, and aerosol sprays are a few examples of ways drugs reach the brain very quickly. Drugs that are inhaled and absorbed by the lungs travel the most rapidly of all the routes of drug administration.

Another rapid form of drug administration is by **injection** into the muscles, bloodstream, or just under the skin. Intravenous injection, which involves inserting a hypodermic needle directly into a vein, is the most common method of injection for drug users, owing to the rapid speed (within seconds in most cases) in which a drug's effect is felt. It is also the most dangerous method of administration because of the risk of damaging blood vessels and contracting HIV (human immunodeficiency virus) and hepatitis B.

Drugs can also be absorbed through the skin or tissue linings (**inunction**)—the nicotine patch is a common example of a drug that is administered in this manner—or through the vagina or anus in the form of **suppositories.** Suppositories are typically mixed with a waxy medium that

melts at body temperature so the drug can be released into the bloodstream. However the drug enters the system, most drugs remain active in the body for several hours.

Drug Interactions

Polydrug use, taking several medications, vitamins, recreational drugs, or illegal drugs simultaneously, can lead to dangerous health problems. Alcohol in particular frequently has dangerous interactions with other drugs. The most hazardous interactions are synergism, antagonism, inhibition, intolerance, and cross-tolerance.

Synergism, also called *potentiation*, is an interaction of two or more drugs in which the effects of the individual drugs are multiplied beyond what would normally be expected if they were taken alone. You might think of synergism as 2 + 2 = 10.

A synergistic reaction can be very dangerous and even deadly. Prescription and OTC medications carry labels that

oral ingestion Intake of drugs through the mouth.
inhalation The introduction of drugs through the respiratory tract.
injection The introduction of drugs into the body via a hypodermic needle.
inunction The introduction of drugs through the skin.
suppositories Mixtures of drugs and a waxy medium designed to melt at body temperature that are inserted into the anus or vagina.
polydrug use Use of multiple medications, vitamins, or illicit drugs simultaneously.
synergism Interaction of two or more drugs that produces more profound effects than would be expected if the drugs were taken separately; also called *potentiation*.

warn the user not to combine the drug with certain other drugs or with alcohol. You should always verify any possible drug interactions before using a prescribed or OTC drug. Pharmacists, physicians, drug information centers, or community drug education centers can answer your questions. Even if one of the drugs in question is illegal, you should attempt to determine the dangers involved in combining it with other drugs. Health care professionals are legally bound to maintain confidentiality even when they know that a client is using illegal substances.

Antagonism, although usually less serious than synergism, can also produce unwanted and unpleasant effects. In an antagonistic reaction, drugs work at the same receptor site so that one drug blocks the action of the other. The blocking drug occupies the receptor site and prevents the other drug from attaching, thus altering its absorption and action.

antagonism A type of interaction in which two or more drugs work at the same receptor site so that one blocks the action of the other.

inhibition A type of drug interaction in which the effects of one drug are eliminated or reduced by the presence of another drug at the receptor site.

intolerance A type of interaction in which two or more drugs produce extremely uncomfortable symptoms.

cross-tolerance Development of a tolerance to one drug that reduces the effects of another, similar drug.

With **inhibition,** the effects of one drug are eliminated or reduced by the presence of another drug at the receptor site. One common inhibitory reaction occurs between antacid tablets and aspirin. The antacid inhibits the absorption of aspirin and makes it less effective as a pain reliever.

Intolerance occurs when drugs combine in the body to produce extremely uncomfortable reactions. The drug Antabuse, used to help alcoholics give up alcohol, works by producing this type of interaction. It binds liver enzymes (the chemicals the liver produces to break down alcohol), making it impossible for the body to metabolize alcohol. As a result, an Antabuse user who drinks alcohol experiences nausea, vomiting, and, occasionally, fever.

Cross-tolerance occurs when a person develops a physiological tolerance to one drug and shows a similar tolerance to selected other drugs as a result. Taking one drug may actually increase the body's tolerance to another substance. For example, cross-tolerance can develop between alcohol and barbiturates, two depressant drugs.

Abuse of Over-the-Counter (OTC) Drugs

OTC medications are drugs that do not require a prescription and can simply be bought in drug stores, supermarkets, and the like. They come in many different forms, including pills, liquids, nasal sprays, and topical creams. Although many people assume that no harm can come from drugs that are not illegal and for which a prescription is not needed, OTC medications can be abused, with resultant health complications and potential addiction. Depending on the medication, when high doses of OTC drugs are taken, hallucinations, bizarre sleep patterns, and mood changes can occur. In extreme cases, abuse of OTC drugs can lead to death. People who appear to be most vulnerable to abusing OTC drugs are teenagers and young adults and people over the age of 65.

OTC drugs are abused when the drug is taken in more than the recommended dosage or over a longer period of time than is recommended. Abuse of and addiction to OTC drugs can be accidental. A person may develop tolerance from continued use, creating an unintended dependence. Teenagers and young adults sometimes intentionally abuse OTC medications in search of a cheap high, by drinking large amounts of cough medicine, for instance. The following are a few types of OTC drugs that are subject to misuse and abuse:

● **Sleep aids.** These drugs may be harmful in excess as they can cause problems with the sleep cycle, weaken areas of the body, or induce narcolepsy (a condition of excessive, intrusive sleepiness). Continued use of these products can lead to tolerance and dependence.

● **Cold medicines (cough syrups and tablets).** There are many different ingredients in cough and cold medicines, but one of particular concern is dextromethorphan (DXM), which is present in about 125 different types of OTC medications. As many as 6 percent of high school seniors report taking drugs containing DXM in order to get high.[15] Large doses of products containing DXM can cause hallucinations, loss of motor control, and "out-of-body" (disassociative) sensations. Other possible side effects of DXM abuse include confusion, impaired judgment, blurred vision, dizziness, paranoia, excessive sweating, slurred speech, nausea, vomiting, abdominal pain, irregular heartbeat, high blood pressure, headache, lethargy, numbness of fingers and toes, facial redness, and dry and itchy skin. In extreme cases, abuse of DXM can lead to loss of consciousness, seizures, brain damage, and even death. Some states have passed laws limiting the amount of products containing DXM a person can purchase, or prohibiting sale to individuals under age 18.[16]

Pseudoephedrine is another cold and allergy medication ingredient that is frequently abused, most commonly by being used to illegally manufacture methamphetamine. U.S. law limits the amount of products containing this drug that an individual may purchase in a month, and requires that it be sold "behind the counter" (i.e., without a prescription, but only through a pharmacist), and that photo identification be presented and recorded. Pharmacists are required to keep a record of purchasers for at least 2 years.[17]

Over-the-counter cough syrup is frequently abused by young people seeking a high from the ingredient DXM.

- **Diet pills.** Some teens use diet pills as a way of getting high, whereas other people use these drugs in an attempt to lose weight. Diet pills often contain a stimulant such as caffeine (discussed later in this chapter) or an herbal ingredient claimed to promote weight loss, such as *Hoodia gordonii.* Many diet pills are marketed as "dietary supplements" and so are regulated by the Food and Drug Administration (FDA) as "food," not as "drugs." This means their manufacturers may make unsubstantiated claims of effectiveness or use untested and unsafe ingredients. One such ingredient, ephedra, was banned by the FDA in 2004 after a major study reported more than 16,000 adverse side effects, including heart palpitations, tremors, and insomnia.[18]

A number of people who use diet pills have some form of an eating disorder. In these cases, both treatment at a drug rehab facility and an eating disorder treatment center may be necessary for full recovery. See Chapter 10 for information on specific diet aids and Focus On: Your Body Image beginning on page 314 for further discussion of eating disorders.

Prescription Drug Abuse

In the United States today, the abuse of prescription medications is at an all-time high. Only marijuana is more widely abused.[19] The prescription drugs that are commonly abused in the United States fall under several broad categories (described in detail later): opioids/narcotics, depressants, and stimulants. Individuals abuse these drugs because they are an easily accessible and inexpensive means of altering a user's mental and physical state; the effects vary depending on the drugs.

The latest data available indicate that 15.2 million people over the age of 12 (6.2%) report abusing controlled prescription drugs in the past year. Prescription drug abuse is particularly common among teenagers. In 2007, more than 2.1 million teenagers 12 to 17 reported abusing prescription drugs.[20]

The risks associated with prescription drug abuse vary depending on the drugs that are abused. Abuse of opioids, narcotics, and pain relievers can result in life-threatening respiratory depression (reduced breathing). Individuals who abuse depressants place themselves at risk of seizures, respiratory depression, and decreased heart rate. Stimulant abuse can cause elevated body temperature, irregular heart rate, cardiovascular system failure, and fatal seizures. It can also result in hostility or feelings of paranoia. Individuals who abuse prescription drugs by injecting them expose themselves to additional risks, including contracting HIV, hepatitis B and C, and other bloodborne viruses.

Unfortunately, prescription drugs are often easier to obtain than illegal ones. In some cases, unscrupulous pharmacists or other medical professionals either steal the drugs or sell fraudulent pre-

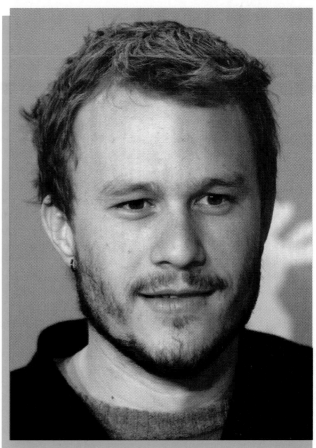

Why is prescription drug abuse on the rise?

Because there are legitimate, legal applications of prescription drugs, they are more readily available and easier to obtain than illicit drugs. As more and more people—especially students—turn to these medications to help them study or to get high, the more socially acceptable their usage becomes and the rate of use continues to rise. In addition, the fact that prescription drugs are regulated and approved by the FDA leads to the impression that they are safer than illicit drugs. This is a fallacy, as was tragically demonstrated by the 2008 death of actor Heath Ledger from an accidental overdose of prescription painkillers, sleeping pills, and antianxiety medication.

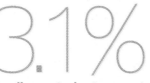

3.1% of college students report having abused prescription painkillers such as Percocet, Vicodin, and OxyContin in the past month.

scriptions. In a process called *doctor shopping,* abusers visit several doctors to obtain multiple prescriptions. Some may fake or exaggerate symptoms in order to persuade physicians to write prescriptions. Individuals may also call pharmacies with fraudulent prescriptions. Young people typically obtain prescription drugs from peers, friends, or family members. Some teenagers and college students who have legitimate prescriptions sell or give away their medications to other students, or trade them for others. Others order from suspicious Internet pharmacies where prescriptions are not always required. (See the Consumer Health box on the next page for tips on safe online drug shopping.)

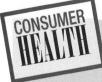

CONSUMER HEALTH

MEDICATIONS ONLINE: BUYER BEWARE

The Food and Drug Administration (FDA) cannot warn people enough about the possible dangers of buying medications online. Buying prescription and over-the-counter drugs online from a company you don't recognize means you may not know exactly what you're getting.

While many websites are operating legally and offering convenience, privacy, and the safeguards of traditional procedures for dispensing drugs, consumers must be wary of "rogue websites" that often sell unapproved drugs, or sidestep required practices meant to protect consumers.

Some websites sell counterfeit drugs. Counterfeit drugs are of unknown quality and safety and may be contaminated, contain the wrong active ingredient, or be made with the wrong amounts of ingredients. Sometimes they contain no active ingredients at all or contain too much of an active ingredient. As a result of these inconsistencies, they may not help the condition or disease that the medicine is intended to treat, and may even cause dangerous side effects.

The National Association of Boards of Pharmacy's (NABP) Verified Internet Pharmacy Practice Sites seal, also known as the VIPPS seal, is given to Internet pharmacy sites that apply and meet state licensure requirements and other VIPPS criteria.

Follow these tips to protect yourself from fraudulent sites:

✱ Buy only from state-licensed pharmacy sites based in the United States (preferably from VIPPS-certified sites, when possible).

✱ Don't buy from sites that sell prescription drugs without a prescription or that offer to prescribe a medication for the first time without a physical exam by your doctor.

✱ Check with your state board of pharmacy or the NABP to see if an online pharmacy has a valid pharmacy license and meets state quality standards.

✱ Use legitimate websites that have a licensed pharmacist to answer your questions.

✱ Look for privacy and security policies that are easy to find and easy to understand.

✱ Don't provide any personal information, such as a Social Security number, credit card information, or medical or health history, unless you are sure the website will keep your information safe and private.

Source: U.S. Food and Drug Administration, "The Possible Dangers of Buying Medicine over the Internet," 2009, www.fda.gov/ForConsumers/ConsumerUpdates/ucm048396.htm.

College Students and Prescription Drug Abuse

Similar to the rest of the U.S. population, college student prescription drug abuse has increased dramatically over the past decade. Because they are prescribed by doctors and approved by the FDA, many college students seem to perceive prescription drugs as safer than illicit drugs. However, nothing could be further from the truth when these drugs are misused. Many students also perceive the misuse of prescription drugs to be more socially acceptable than other forms of drug use. Some students who abuse prescription drugs believe that such use will enhance their well-being or performance. The major reasons students report abusing prescription stimulants such as Adderal and Ritalin are to help them concentrate, study, and to increase alertness. Students who abuse prescription painkillers such as Vicodin, OxyContin, or Percocet, say they do so to relax or get high.[21]

From 1993 to 2005, the rate of student abuse of prescription painkillers rose 343 percent; this equals approximately 240,000 full-time students. Over the same period, abuse of prescription stimulants rose 93 percent; abuse of prescription tranquilizers rose 450 percent and there was a 225 percent increase in abuse of sedatives.[22] Undergraduates who use or abuse prescription medications are much more likely to report heavy drinking and use of illicit drugs. This poses another set of problems, as combining any of these medications with alcohol can make a dangerous cocktail.

Illicit Drugs

The problem of illicit (illegal) drug use touches us all. We may use illicit substances ourselves, watch someone we love struggle with drug abuse, or become the victim of a drug-related crime. At the very least, we are forced to pay increasing taxes for law enforcement and drug rehabilitation. When our coworkers use drugs, the effectiveness of our own work is diminished. If the car we drive was assembled by drug-using workers at the plant, we are in danger. A drug-using bus driver, train engineer, or pilot jeopardizes our safety.

Many of us have stereotyped notions of illicit drug users but it is difficult to generalize. Illicit drug users span all

Women and Drug Abuse

According to the 2007 National Survey on Drug Use and Health, approximately 50 million women report having used an illicit drug at some point in their lives, representing 41.8 percent of all females (compared to 50.6% for men) aged 12 and older. Approximately 11.6 percent of females aged 12 and older reported past-year use of an illicit drug versus 17.4 percent for men; 5.8 percent of women reported past-month use of an illicit drug versus 10.4 percent of men.

Data have revealed that women are at particular risk for prescription drug abuse, with higher rates of abuse among teen girls. More emergency room visits related to drug use occur for women than men: 55 percent versus 45 percent. Currently, 56 percent of those being treated for dependence on sedatives and 53 percent of those being treated for dependence on tranquilizers are women. This is a disturbing new trend that runs counter to traditional drug use patterns, where males typically exceed females.

While men often abuse drugs to cope with pressures, women may turn to drug misuse and abuse to "escape" an abusive home life or because they see a parent or other loved one abusing drugs or alcohol. Studies show that at least 70 percent of female drug users were sexually abused by the age of 16. Most of them had at least one parent who abused alcohol or drugs. Furthermore, they often have little self-esteem or self-confidence. They frequently feel lonely, powerless, and isolated from support networks.

Unfortunately, many female drug users are unable to seek help. Some may be unable to find or afford child care during treatment, while others worry that the courts will take away their children once the drug problem is known. Others may fear violence from their husbands, boyfriends, or partners.

Research has shown that female drug abusers have a better chance of recovery when treatment takes care of their basic needs, such as food, shelter, and clothing. Others also need transportation, child care, and training in parenting. The most successful treatments also teach reading, basic education, and vocational skills. As a woman's self-esteem increases, so do her chances of remaining drug free.

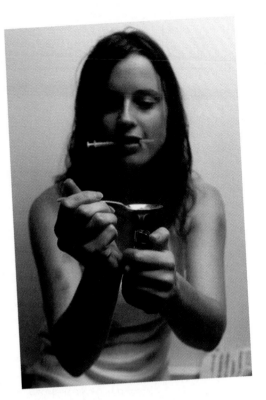

Sources: Office of National Drug Control Policy, *Drug Facts: Women and Drugs,* 2008, www .whitehousedrugpolicy.gov/drugfact/women/index .html; Office of National Drug Control Policy, "Women and Prescription Drugs," April 2007; Substance Abuse and Mental Health Services Administration, *Results from the 2007 National Survey on Drug Use and Health: National Findings* (Office of Applied Studies, NSDUH Series H-34, DHHS Publication no. SMA 08-4343, Rockville, MD, 2008).

age groups, genders, ethnicities, occupations, and socioeconomic groups (see the **Gender & Health** box above). No matter the group, illicit drug use has a devastating effect on users and their families in the United States and in many other countries.

The good news is that the use of illicit drugs has leveled off and is not increasing for most groups of people. Use of most drugs increased from the early 1970s to the late 1970s, peaked between 1979 and 1986, and declined until 1992, from which point it has not changed. In 2004, an estimated 20.4 million Americans were illicit drug users, about three-quarters the 1979 peak level of 25 million users. Among youth, however, illicit drug use, notably of marijuana, has been rising in recent years.[23]

Drug Use on Campus

In 2006, the number of college students nationwide who had tried any drug stood at almost 51 percent; a third had smoked marijuana in the past year, and 20 percent had done so in the past month (see Table 7.1 on page 202). Daily use of marijuana is at its highest point since 1989.[24] Cocaine use is down sharply, but LSD use has more than doubled. These figures vary from school to school.

For many students, their college environment coupled with our culture's societal mores regarding substance use on college campuses may make substance use and abuse seem like the norm. Drugs are present on most campuses, though perhaps not to the degree that students perceive. College administrators, staff, and faculty are aware of substance abuse on their campuses and of the link between substance abuse and poor academic performance, depression, anxiety, suicide, property damage, vandalism, fights, serious medical problems, and death.[25]

Why Do Some College Students Use Drugs? There are many factors that influence a college student's decision to use drugs. Research has identified the following factors in a student's life that increase the risk of substance abuse; the more factors, the greater the risk:

TABLE

7.1

Annual Drug Use Prevalence, Full-Time College Students vs. Respondents 1–4 Years beyond High School

	Full-Time College (%)	Others (%)		Full-Time College (%)	Others (%)
Any illicit drug	35.0	35.4	Amphetamines, adjusted	6.9	7.5
Any illicit drug other than marijuana	17.3	21.1	Ritalin	3.7	2.3
Marijuana	31.8	31.8	Methamphetamine	0.4	1.9
Inhalants	1.5	1.2	Crystal methamphetamine	0.7	1.1
Hallucinogens	4.9	5.5	Sedatives (barbiturates)	3.6	5.3
LSD	1.3	1.5	Tranquilizers	5.5	8.4
Hallucinogens other than LCD	4.7	5.3	Rohypnol	0.1	1.2
Ecstasy (MDMA)	2.2	3.8	GHB	0.1	0.9
Cocaine	5.4	8.3	Ketamine	0.2	0.9
Crack	0.6	1.2	Alcohol	80.9	79.3
Other cocaine	5.3	7.8	Been drunk	64.8	60.9
Heroin	0.2	0.8	Flavored alcoholic beverage	62.6	63.5
With a needle	*	0.4	Cigarettes	30.7	44.1
Without a needle	0.2	0.7	Steroids	0.6	1.2
Narcotics other than heroin	7.7	10.5	*Approximate*		
OxyContin	2.8	4.5	*weighted N =*	*1,250*	*730*
Vicodin	6.7	10.6			

Source: L. D. Johnson et al., *Monitoring the Future National Survey Results on Drug Use, 1975–2007: Volume II, College Students and Adults* (Bethesda, MD: National Institute on Drug Abuse, 2008).

- **Genetics and family history.** Genetics and family history play a significant role in the risk for developing an addiction.
- **Substance use in high school.** Two-thirds of college students who use illicit drugs began doing so in high school.
- **Positive expectations.** The most common reason students give to explain why they drink, smoke, or use drugs is to relax, reduce stress, or forget about problems (Figure 7.2). Students also report using drugs such as Adderall and Ritalin as study aids, because they believe the drugs will allow them to concentrate better and make them more alert.
- **Mental health problems.** Students who report being diagnosed with depression are more likely to have abused prescription drugs, to have used marijuana or other illicit drugs, and to be current or frequent smokers.
- **Sorority and fraternity membership.** Being a member of a sorority or fraternity increases the likelihood of using alcohol, marijuana, or cocaine and makes one twice as likely to abuse prescription drugs.

Why Do Some College Students *Not* Use Drugs?

There can be many factors influencing a student to avoid

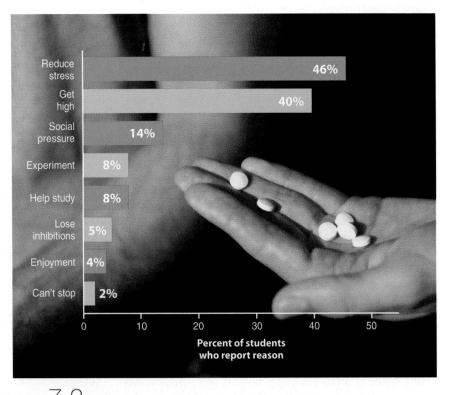

FIGURE 7.2 **Reasons Why College Students Use Illicit Drugs or Controlled Prescription Drugs**

Source: Adapted from *Wasting the Best and the Brightest: Substance Abuse at America's Colleges and Universities.* New York: National Center on Addiction and Substance Abuse at Columbia University, March 2007, page 47. Copyright © 2007. Used with permission.

drugs; some of the most commonly reported include the following:[26]

- **Parental attitudes and behavior.** Those students who say they are more influenced by their parents' concerns or expectations drink, use marijuana, and smoke significantly less than those students less influenced by parents.
- **Religion and spirituality.** The greater the student's level of religiosity (hours in prayer, attendance at services), the less likely they are to drink, smoke, or use other drugs.
- **Student engagement.** The more a student is involved in the learning process and other extracurricular activities, the less likely he or she is to binge drink, use marijuana, or abuse prescription drugs.
- **College athletics.** College athletes drink at higher rates than nonathletes but are less likely to use illicit drugs.

what do you think?

What is the attitude toward drug use on your campus? ● Are some substances considered more acceptable than others? ● Is drug use considered more acceptable at certain times or occasions?

Common Drugs of Abuse

Hundreds of drugs are subject to abuse—some are legal, such as recreational drugs and prescription medications, while many others are illegal and classified as "controlled substances." For general purposes, drugs can be divided into the following categories: *stimulants, marijuana and other cannabis products, opioids, depressants, hallucinogens, inhalants,* and *steroids.* These categories are discussed in subsequent sections; Table 7.2 on pages 204–205 summarizes the categorization, uses, and effects of various drugs of abuse, both licit (prescription) and illicit.

Stimulants

A **stimulant** is a drug that increases activity of the central nervous system. Its effects, therefore, usually involve increased activity, anxiety, and agitation; users often seem jittery or nervous while high. Commonly used stimulants include cocaine, amphetamines, methamphetamine, and caffeine. See Chapter 8 for a discussion of nicotine, the addictive substance in tobacco products, which is another common stimulant.

Cocaine A white crystalline powder derived from the leaves of the south American coca shrub (not related to cocoa plants), *cocaine* ("coke") has been described as one of the most powerful naturally occurring stimulants.

Methods of Use and Physical Effects Cocaine can be taken in several ways, including snorting, smoking, and injecting. The powdered form is snorted through the nose, which can damage mucous membranes and cause sinusitis. It can destroy the user's sense of smell, and occasionally it even

eats a hole through the septum. The effects of cocaine are felt rapidly. When snorted, the drug enters the bloodstream through the lungs in less than 1 minute and reaches the brain in less than 3 minutes. Cocaine binds at receptor sites in the central nervous system, producing intense pleasure. The euphoria quickly abates, however, and the desire to regain the pleasurable feelings makes the user want more cocaine.

Cocaine alkaloid, or *freebase,* is obtained from removing the hydrochloride salt from cocaine powder. In this base form, the cocaine is much more suitable for smoking. Smoked freebase cocaine reaches the brain within seconds and produces an intense high that disappears quickly, leaving a powerful craving for more. *Crack* is identical pharmacologically to freebase, but the hydrochloride salt is still present and is processed with baking soda and water. It is a cheap, widely available drug that is smokable and very potent. Because crack is such a pure drug, it takes little time to achieve the desired high, and a crack user can become addicted quickly.

Many cocaine users occasionally inject the drug intravenously, which introduces large amounts into the body rapidly, creating a brief, intense high, and a subsequent crash. Injecting users place themselves at risk not only for contracting HIV and hepatitis (a severe liver disease) through shared needles, but also for skin infections, vein damage, inflamed arteries, and infection of the heart lining.

Cocaine is both an anesthetic and a central nervous system stimulant. In tiny doses, it can slow the heart rate. In larger doses, the physical effects are dramatic: increased heart rate and blood pressure, loss of appetite that can lead to dramatic weight loss, convulsions, muscle twitching, irregular heartbeat, and even death resulting from an overdose. Other effects of cocaine include temporary relief of depression, decreased fatigue, talkativeness, increased alertness, and heightened self-confidence. However, as the dose increases, users become irritable and apprehensive, and their behavior may turn paranoid or violent.

stimulants Drugs that increase activity of the central nervous system.
amphetamines A large and varied group of synthetic agents that stimulate the central nervous system.

Treatment for Cocaine Addiction Treatment for cocaine addiction involves mainly psychiatric counseling and 12-step programs. Currently, a promising new cocaine vaccine is in development. The vaccine does not eliminate the desire for cocaine; instead, it keeps the user from getting high by stimulating the immune system to attack the drug when it's taken. Clinical human trials are expected to begin soon, and vaccines against nicotine, heroin, and methamphetamine are also in development.

Amphetamines The **amphetamines** include a large and varied group of synthetic agents that stimulate the central nervous system. Small doses of amphetamines improve

7%

of college students reported smoking crack at least once in 2006.

TABLE

7.2   **Drugs of Abuse: Uses and Effects**

Category	Drugs	Trade or Street Names	Dependence	Usual Method	Possible Effects	Effects of Overdose	Withdrawal Syndrome
Stimulants	Cocaine	Coke, Flake, Snow, Crack, Coca, Blanca, *Perico*	*Physical:* Possible *Psychological:* High *Tolerance:* Yes	Snorted, smoked, injected	Increased alertness, excitation, euphoria, increased pulse rate and blood pressure, insomnia, loss of appetite	Agitation, increased body temperature, hallucinations, convulsions, possible death	Apathy, long periods of sleep, irritability, depression, disorientation
	Amphetamine, Methamphetamine	Crank, Ice, Cristal, Krystal Meth, Speed, Adderall, Dexedrine	*Physical:* Possible *Psychological:* High *Tolerance:* Yes	Oral, injected, smoked			
	Methylphenidate	Ritalin (Illy's), Concerta, Focalin, Metadate	*Physical:* Possible *Psychological:* High *Tolerance:* Yes	Oral, injected, snorted, smoked			
Cannabis	Marijuana	Pot, Grass, Sinsemilla, Blunts, *Mota, Yerba, Grifa*	*Physical:* Possible *Psychological:* High *Tolerance:* Yes	Oral, injected, smoked	Euphoria, relaxed inhibitions, increased appetite, disorientation	Fatigue, paranoia, possible psychosis	Occasional reports of insomnia, hyperactivity, decreased appetite
	Hashish, Hashish Oil	Hash, Hash oil	*Physical:* Unknown *Psychological:* Moderate *Tolerance:* Yes	Smoked, oral			
Narcotics	Heroin	Diamorphine, Horse, Smack, Black tar, *Chiva*	*Physical:* High *Psychological:* High *Tolerance:* Yes	Injected, snorted, smoked	Euphoria, drowsiness, respiratory depression, constricted pupils, nausea	Slow and shallow breathing, clammy skin, convulsions, coma, possible death	Watery eyes, runny nose, yawning, loss of appetite, irritability, tremors, panic, cramps, nausea, chills and sweating
	Morphine	MS-Contin, Roxanol	*Physical:* High *Psychological:* High *Tolerance:* Yes	Oral, injected			
	Hydrocodone, Oxycodone	Vicodin, OxyContin, Percocet, Percodan	*Physical:* High *Psychological:* High *Tolerance:* Yes	Oral			
	Codeine	Acetaminophen w/ Codeine, Tylenol w/ Codeine	*Physical:* Moderate *Psychological:* Moderate *Tolerance:* Yes	Oral, injected			
Depressants	Gamma-hydroxybutrate	GHB, Liquid Ecstasy, Liquid X	*Physical:* Moderate *Psychological:* Moderate *Tolerance:* Yes	Oral	Slurred speech, disorientation, drunken behavior without odor of alcohol, impaired memory of events, interacts with alcohol	Shallow respiration, clammy skin, dilated pupils, weak and rapid pulse, coma, possible death	Anxiety, insomnia, tremors, delirium, convulsions, possible death
	Benzodiazepines	Valium, Xanax, Halcion, Ativan, Rohypnol (Roofies, R-2), Klonopin	*Physical:* Moderate *Psychological:* Moderate *Tolerance:* Yes	Oral, injected			
	Other Depressants	Ambien, Sonata, Barbiturates, Methaqualone (Quaalude)	*Physical:* Moderate *Psychological:* Moderate *Tolerance:* Yes	Oral			
Hallucinogens	MDMA, Analogs	Ecstasy, XTC, Adam, MDA (Love Drug), MDEA (Eve)	*Physical:* None *Psychological:* Moderate *Tolerance:* Yes	Oral, snorted, smoked	Heightened senses, teeth grinding, dehydration	Increased body temperature, electrolyte imbalance, cardiac arrest	Muscle aches, drowsiness, depression, acne
	LSD	Acid, Microdot, Sunshine, Boomers	*Physical:* None *Psychological:* Unknown *Tolerance:* Yes	Oral	Illusions and hallucinations, altered perception of time and distance	Longer, more intense "trips"	None
	Phencyclidine, Analogs	PCP, Angel Dust, Hog, Ketamine (Special K)	*Physical:* Possible *Psychological:* High *Tolerance:* Yes	Smoked, oral, injected, snorted		Unable to direct movement, feel pain, or remember	Drug-seeking behavior
	Other Hallucinogens	Psilocybe mushrooms, Mescaline, Peyote, Dextromethorphan	*Physical:* None *Psychological:* None *Tolerance:* Possible	Oral			

Continued on next page

TABLE
7.2 | (continued)

Category	Drugs	Trade or Street Names	Dependence	Usual Method	Possible Effects	Effects of Overdose	Withdrawal Syndrome
Inhalants	Amyl and Butyl Nitrite	Pearls, Poppers, Rush, Locker Room	*Physical:* Unknown *Psychological:* Unknown *Tolerance:* No	Inhaled	Flushing, hypotension, headache	Methemoglobinemia	Agitation
	Nitrous Oxide	Laughing gas, balloons, Whippets	*Physical:* Unknown *Psychological:* Low *Tolerance:* No	Inhaled	Impaired memory, slurred speech, drunken behavior, slow-onset vitamin deficiency, organ damage	Vomiting, respiratory depression, loss of consciousness, possible death	Trembling, anxiety, insomnia, vitamin deficiency, confusion, hallucinations, convulsions
	Other Inhalants	Adhesives, spray paint, hairspray, lighter fluid	*Physical:* Unknown *Psychological:* High *Tolerance:* No	Inhaled			
Anabolic Steroids	Testosterone	Depo Testosterone, Sustanon, Sten, Cypt	*Physical:* Unknown *Psychological:* Unknown *Tolerance:* Unknown	Injected	Virilization, edema, testicular atrophy, gynecomastia, acne, aggressive behavior	Unknown	Possible depression
	Other Anabolic Steroids	Parabolan, Winstrol, Equipose, Anadrol, Dianabol	*Physical:* Unknown *Psychological:* Yes *Tolerance:* Unknown	Oral, injected			

Source: U.S. Department of Justice Drug Enforcement Administration, www.usdoj.gov/dea/pubs/abuse/chart.htm.

alertness, lessen fatigue, and generally elevate mood. With repeated use, however, physical and psychological dependence develops. Sleep patterns are affected (insomnia); heart rate, breathing rate, and blood pressure increase; and restlessness, anxiety, appetite suppression, and vision problems are common. High doses over long time periods can produce hallucinations, delusions, and disorganized behavior.

Certain types of amphetamines or amphetamine-like drugs are used for medicinal purposes. Drugs such as Adder-

all and Ritalin are used to treat children with attention deficit/hyperactivity disorder (ADHD). However, in recent years, these drugs have become popular on college campuses. In fact, Ritalin is on the Drug Enforcement Administration's top-ten list of most often stolen prescription drugs. The drugs are generally sold or given by other students—some of them prescription holders, others not.

Students primarily report using ADHD drugs for academic gains (Figure 7.3). A recent study on two university campuses

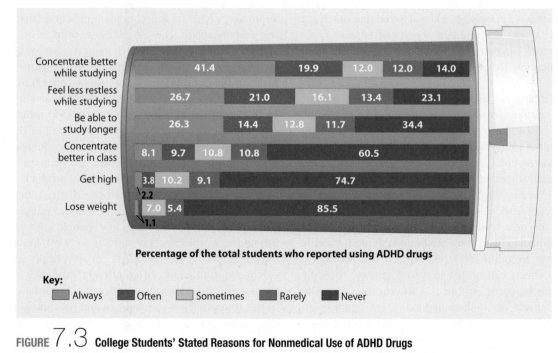

Percentage of the total students who reported using ADHD drugs

Key:
☐ Always ■ Often ☐ Sometimes ■ Rarely ■ Never

FIGURE 7.3 **College Students' Stated Reasons for Nonmedical Use of ADHD Drugs**
While a small percentage of students in this study used ADHD drugs to get high or to lose weight, the majority of students reported using the drugs to enhance their academic performance.
Source: Data are from D. L. Rabiner et al, "Motives and Perceived Consequences of Nonmedical ADHD Medication Use by College Students: Are Students Treating Themselves for Attention Problems?" *Journal of Attention Disorders*, 13, no. 3 (2009); 259–70.

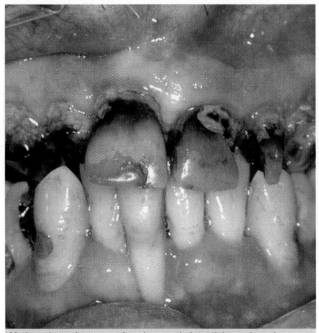
Methamphetamine users often damage their teeth beyond repair because of the toxic chemicals in the substance. This condition is commonly referred to as "meth mouth."

revealed that 9 percent of students had used ADHD drugs without a prescription at some point in their college careers, while 5.4 percent had done so in the past 6 months.[27] ADHD drug use was found to be more common among white students and members of fraternities or sororities. ADHD drug users in the study also tended to have lower grade point averages than nonusers and to engage in illegal substance use or other risky behaviors. Users generally believed that the drugs were beneficial, despite frequent reports of adverse reactions. The most commonly reported adverse effects were sleeping difficulties, irritability, and reduced appetite.

Methamphetamine An increasingly common form of amphetamine, *methamphetamine* (commonly called simply "meth") is a potent, long-acting, addictive drug that strongly activates the brain's reward center by producing a sense of euphoria. Methamphetamine can be snorted, smoked, injected, or orally ingested. Small doses of methamphetamine produce increased physical activity, alertness, and a decreased appetite; however, the drug's effects quickly wear off, leaving the user seeking more. Users often experience tolerance immediately, making methamphetamine a highly addictive drug from the very first time it is used. When snorted, the effects can be felt in 3 to 5 minutes; if orally ingested, effects occur within 15 to 20 minutes. The pleasurable effects of methamphetamine are typically an intense rush lasting only a few minutes when snorted; in contrast, smoking the drug can produce a high lasting more than 8 hours. Large doses can lead to convulsions, irregular heartbeat, hallucinations, and even death, while long-term use can cause dependence, psychosis, paranoia, aggression, weight loss, and stroke. Abusers often do not sleep or eat for

days. A high state of irritability and agitation has been associated with violent behavior among some users.

Like other amphetamines, the downside of this drug is devastating. Prolonged use can cause fatal lung and kidney damage as well as long-lasting psychological damage. In some instances, major psychological dysfunction can persist as long as 2.5 years after last use. Methamphetamine can cause psychosis, increased risk for heart attack and stroke, and brain damage that results in impaired motor skills and cognitive functions.

Methamphetamine abuse is an increasingly serious problem, especially in rural areas of the United States, in Hawaii, and on the West Coast. In 2005, 4.5 percent of high school seniors reported using methamphetamine in their lifetime. Rates among adults are difficult to determine, but it is believed that more than 12 million Americans have tried methamphetamine.[28] A possible contributing factor to the increasing rate of methamphetamine use is that it is relatively easy to make. It is produced by "cookers" using recipes that often include common OTC ingredients such as ephedrine and pseudoephedrine, found in cold and allergy medications.

Caffeine What is the most popular and widely consumed drug in the United States? Caffeine. Almost half of all Americans drink coffee every day, and many others consume caffeine in some other form, mainly for its well-known "wake-up" effect. Drinking coffee, tea, soft drinks, and other caffeine-containing products is legal, even socially encouraged. Caffeine may seem harmless, but excessive consumption is associated with addiction and certain health problems.

Caffeine is derived from the chemical family called *xanthines,* which are found in plant products such as coffee, tea, and chocolate. The xanthines are mild, central nervous system stimulants that enhance mental alertness and reduce feelings of fatigue. Other stimulant effects include increased heart muscle contractions, oxygen consumption, metabolism, and urinary output. A person feels these effects within 15 to 45 minutes of ingesting a caffeinated product. It takes 4 to 6 hours for the body to metabolize half of the caffeine ingested, so, depending on the amount of caffeine taken in, it may continue to exert effects for a day or longer. Figure 7.4 compares the caffeine content of various products.

Side effects of the xanthines include wakefulness, insomnia, irregular heartbeat, dizziness, nausea, indigestion, and sometimes mild delirium. Some people also experience heartburn. As the effects of caffeine wear off, frequent users may feel let down—mentally or physically depressed, exhausted, and weak. To counteract this, they commonly choose to drink another cup of coffee. Habitually engaging in this practice leads to tolerance and psychological dependence. Symptoms of excessive caffeine consumption include chronic insomnia, jitters, irritability, nervousness, anxiety, and involuntary muscle twitches. Withdrawing from caffeine may compound the effects and produce severe headaches, fatigue, and nausea. Because caffeine meets the requirements for addiction—tolerance, psychological

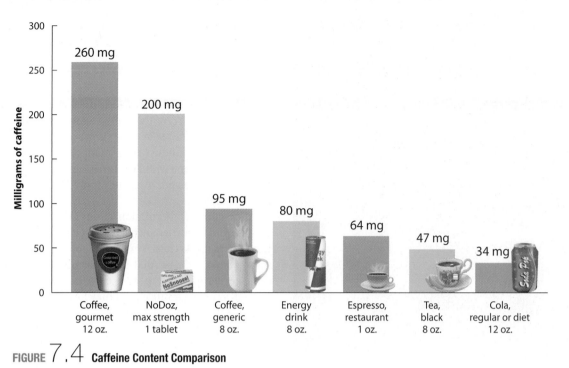

FIGURE 7.4 **Caffeine Content Comparison**

Source: Data are from USDA National Nutrient Database for Standard Reference, Release 20 (2007).

dependence, and withdrawal symptoms—it can be classified as addictive.

Long-term caffeine use has been suspected of being linked to several serious health problems. However, no strong evidence exists to suggest that moderate caffeine use (less than 300 mg daily, approximately 3 cups of regular coffee) produces harmful effects in healthy, nonpregnant people. Caffeine does not appear to cause long-term high blood pressure. It has not been linked to strokes, nor is there any evidence of a relationship between caffeine and heart disease.[29] However, people who suffer from irregular heartbeat are cautioned against using caffeine, because the resultant increase in heart rate might be life threatening.

what do you think?

How much caffeine do you consume regularly, and why? ● What is your pattern of caffeine consumption for the day? ● Have you ever experienced any ill effects after going without caffeine for a period of time?

Marijuana and Other Cannabinoids

Although archaeological evidence documents the use of *marijuana* ("grass," "weed," "pot") as far back as 6,000 years, the drug did not become popular in the United States until the 1960s. Today marijuana is the most commonly used illicit drug in the United States. Nearly one of every three Americans over the age of 12 has tried marijuana at least once. Some 12 million Americans have used it; more than 1 million cannot control their use of it.

Methods of Use and Physical Effects Marijuana is derived from either the *Cannabis sativa* or *Cannabis indica* (hemp) plant. Most of the time, marijuana is smoked, although it can also be ingested, as in brownies baked with marijuana in them. When marijuana is smoked, it is usually rolled into cigarettes (joints) or placed in a pipe or water pipe (bong). Current American-grown marijuana is a turbocharged version of that grown in the late 1960s. **Tetrahydrocannabinol (THC)** is the psychoactive substance in marijuana and the key to determining how powerful a high it will produce. More potent forms of the drug can contain up to 27 percent THC, but most average 12 percent.[30] *Hashish*, a potent cannabis preparation derived mainly from the plant's thick, sticky resin, contains high THC concentrations. Hash oil, a substance produced by percolating a solvent such as ether through dried marijuana to extract the THC, is a tarlike liquid that may contain up to 300 mg of THC in a dose.

tetrahydrocannabinol (THC) The chemical name for the active ingredient in marijuana.

One common way of smoking marijuana is to use a pipe.

The effects of smoking marijuana are generally felt within 10 to 30 minutes and usually wear off within 3 hours. The most noticeable effect of THC is the dilation of the eyes' blood vessels, which produces the smoker's characteristic bloodshot eyes. Marijuana smokers also exhibit coughing; dry mouth and throat ("cotton mouth"); increased thirst and appetite; lowered blood pressure; and mild muscular weakness,

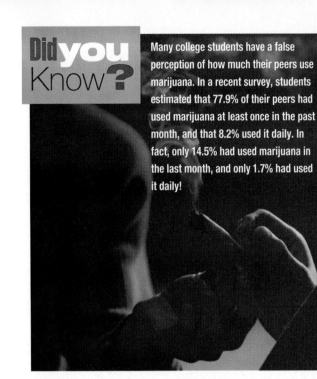
primarily exhibited in drooping eyelids. Users can also experience severe anxiety, panic, paranoia, and psychosis, and may have intensified reactions to various stimuli—colors, sounds, and the speed at which things move may seem altered. High doses of hashish may produce vivid visual hallucinations.

Marijuana use presents clear hazards for drivers of motor vehicles and others on the road with them. The drug substantially reduces a driver's ability to react and make quick decisions. In a study by the National Highway Traffic Safety Administration, a moderate dose of marijuana alone was shown to impair driving performance; however, the effects of even a low dose of marijuana combined with alcohol were markedly greater than for either drug alone. Studies show that approximately 6 to 11 percent of fatally injured drivers in motor vehicle accidents test positive for THC.[31] In many of these cases, alcohol is detected as well. Perceptual and other performance deficits resulting from marijuana use may persist for some time after the high subsides. Users who attempt to drive, fly, or operate heavy machinery often fail to recognize their impairment.

Marijuana and Medicine Although recognized as a dangerous drug by the U.S. government, marijuana has several medical purposes. It helps control such side effects as the severe nausea and vomiting produced by chemotherapy, the chemical treatment for cancer. It improves appetite and forestalls the loss of lean muscle mass associated with AIDS-wasting syndrome. Marijuana reduces the muscle pain and spasticity caused by diseases such as multiple sclerosis. It

also temporarily relieves the eye pressure of glaucoma, although it is unclear whether it is more effective than legal glaucoma drugs.[32] Marijuana's legal status for medicinal purposes continues to be hotly debated.

Effects of Chronic Marijuana Use Because marijuana is illegal in most parts of the United States and has been widely used only since the 1960s, long-term studies of its effects have been difficult to conduct. Also, studies conducted in the 1960s involved marijuana with THC levels only a fraction of those of today, so their results may not apply to the stronger forms now available.

Most current information about chronic marijuana use comes from countries such as Jamaica and Costa Rica, where the drug is legal. These studies of long-term users (for 10 or more years) indicate that smoking marijuana causes lung damage comparable to that caused by smoking tobacco. Indeed, smoking a single joint may be as bad for the lungs as smoking three tobacco cigarettes.

Inhaling marijuana smoke introduces carbon monoxide into the bloodstream. Because the blood has a greater affinity for carbon monoxide than it does for oxygen, its oxygen-carrying capacity is diminished, and the heart must work harder to pump oxygen to oxygen-starved tissues. Furthermore, the tar from cannabis contains higher levels of carcinogens than does tobacco smoke. Smoking marijuana results in three times more tar inhalation and retention in the respiratory tract than smoking tobacco.

Recent research has found that frequent and/or long-term marijuana use may significantly increase a man's risk of developing testicular cancer. The researchers found that being a marijuana smoker at the time of diagnosis was associated with a 70 percent increased risk of testicular cancer. The risk was particularly elevated (about twice that of those who never smoked marijuana) for those who used marijuana at least weekly or who had long-term exposure to the substance beginning in adolescence. The results also suggested that the association with marijuana use might be limited to *nonseminoma*, an aggressive, fast-growing testicular malignancy that tends to strike early, between ages 20 and 35, and accounts for about 40 percent of all testicular cancer cases.[33]

According to the National Survey on Drug Use and Health, teens and young adults who use marijuana are more likely to develop serious mental health problems. A number of studies have shown an association between marijuana use and increased rates of anxiety, depression, suicidal ideation, and schizophrenia. Some of these studies have shown age at first use as an indicator of vulnerability to later problems. Among individuals 18 and older, those who used marijuana before the age of 12 were twice as likely to have a serious mental illness as those who first used marijuana at age 18 or older.[34]

Other risks associated with marijuana use include suppression of the immune system, blood pressure changes, and impaired memory function. Recent studies suggest that pregnant women who smoke marijuana are at a higher risk for

what do you think?

Why do you think that marijuana is the most popular illicit drug on college campuses? ● How widespread is marijuana use at your school?

stillbirth or miscarriage and for delivering low-birth-weight babies and babies with abnormalities of the nervous system.[35] Babies born to marijuana smokers are five times more likely to exhibit features similar to those of children with fetal alcohol syndrome.

Depressants

Whereas central nervous system stimulants increase muscular and nervous system activity, **depressants** have the opposite effect. These drugs slow down neuromuscular activity and cause sleepiness or calmness. If the dose is high enough, brain function can be slowed to the point of causing death. Alcohol is the most widely used central nervous system depressant (see Chapter 8), but other forms include opioids, benzodiazepines, and barbiturates.

Opioids

Opioids cause drowsiness, relieve pain, and induce euphoria. Also called *narcotics,* opioids are derived from the parent drug *opium,* a dark, resinous substance made from the milky juice of the opium poppy seed pod.

The word *narcotic* comes from the Greek word for "stupor" and generally is used to describe sleep-inducing substances. Until the early twentieth century, many patent medicines contained opioids and were advertised as cures for everything from menstrual cramps to teething pains. More powerful than opium, *morphine* (named after Morpheus, the Greek god of sleep) was widely used as a painkiller during the Civil War. *Codeine,* a less powerful analgesic (pain reliever) derived from morphine, also became popular.

As opioids became more common, physicians noted that patients tended to become dependent on them. Growing concern about addiction led to government controls of narcotic use. The Harrison Act of 1914 prohibited the production, dispensation, and sale of opioid products unless prescribed by a physician. Subsequent legislation required physicians prescribing opioids to keep careful records. Today, physicians remain subject to audits of their prescriptions.

Some opioids are still used for medical purposes. Morphine is sometimes prescribed for severe pain, and codeine is found in prescription cough syrups and other painkillers. Several prescription drugs, including Vicodin, Percodan, Oxycontin, Demerol, and Dilaudid, contain synthetic opioids.

Opioids are powerful depressants of the central nervous system. In addition to relieving pain, these

Opium is extracted from opium poppy seed pods like this one.

drugs lower heart rate, respiration, and blood pressure. Side effects include weakness, dizziness, nausea, vomiting, euphoria, decreased sex drive, visual disturbances, and lack of coordination. Of all the opioids, heroin has the greatest notoriety as an addictive drug. The following section discusses the progression of heroin addiction; addiction to any opioid follows a similar path.

Heroin Addiction *Heroin* is a white powder derived from morphine. *Black tar heroin* is a sticky, dark brown, foul-smelling form of heroin that is relatively pure and inexpensive. Once considered a cure for morphine dependence, heroin was later discovered to be even more addictive and potent than morphine. Today, heroin has no medical use.

Heroin is a depressant that produces drowsiness and a dreamy, mentally slow feeling. It can cause drastic mood swings, with euphoric highs followed by depressive lows. Heroin slows respiration and urinary output and constricts the pupils of the eyes. Symptoms of tolerance and withdrawal can appear within 3 weeks of first use.

An estimated 3.7 million people have used heroin at one time in their lives. The highest number of users are adults aged 26 or older.[36] While heroin is usually injected, the contemporary version of heroin is so potent that users can get high by snorting or smoking the drug. This has attracted a more affluent group of users who may not want to inject, for reasons such as the increased risk of contracting diseases such as HIV.

The most common route of administration for heroin addicts is "mainlining"—intravenous injection of powdered heroin mixed in a solution. Many users describe the "rush" they feel when injecting themselves as intensely pleasurable, whereas others report unpredictable and unpleasant side effects. The temporary nature of the rush contributes to the drug's high potential for addiction—many addicts shoot up four or five times a day. Mainlining can cause veins to scar and eventually collapse. Once a vein has collapsed, it can no longer be used to introduce heroin into the bloodstream. Addicts become expert at locating new veins to use: in the feet, the legs, the temples, under the tongue, or in the groin.

The human body's physiology could be said to encourage opioid addiction. Opioid-like substances called **endorphins** are manufactured in the body and have multiple receptor sites, particularly in the central nervous system. When endorphins attach themselves at these points, they create feelings of painless well-being; medical researchers refer to them as "the body's own opioids." When endorphin levels are high, people feel euphoric. The same euphoria occurs when opioids or related chemicals are active at the endorphin receptor sites.

Treatment for Heroin Addiction Programs to help people addicted to heroin and other opioids have not been very successful. Some addicts resume drug use even after years of

depressants Drugs that slow down the activity of the central nervous system.

opioids Drugs that induce sleep and relieve pain; includes derivatives of opium and synthetics with similar chemical properties; also called *narcotics.*

endorphins Opioid-like hormones that are manufactured in the human body and contribute to natural feelings of well-being.

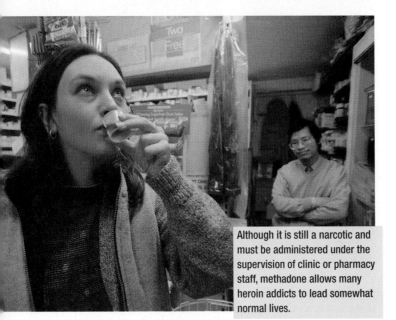

Although it is still a narcotic and must be administered under the supervision of clinic or pharmacy staff, methadone allows many heroin addicts to lead somewhat normal lives.

addicts do not have the compulsion to use heroin, and if they do use it, they don't get high, so there is no point in using the drug. More recently, researchers have reported promising results with Temgesic (buprenorphine), a mild, nonaddicting synthetic opioid that, like heroin and methadone, bonds to certain receptors in the brain, blocks pain messages, and persuades the brain that its cravings for heroin have been satisfied.

Benzodiazepines and Barbiturates A sedative drug promotes mental calmness and reduces anxiety, whereas a hypnotic drug promotes sleep or drowsiness. The most common sedative-hypnotic drugs are **benzodiazepines,** more commonly known as *tranquilizers.* These include prescription drugs such as Valium, Ativan, and Xanax. Benzodiazepines are most commonly prescribed for tension, muscular strain, sleep problems, anxiety, panic attacks, and alcohol withdrawal. **Barbiturates** are sedative-hypnotic drugs that include Amytal and Seconal. Because they are less safe than benzodiazepines, barbiturates are not typically prescribed for medical conditions that call for sedative-hypnotic drug therapy. Today, benzodiazepines have largely replaced barbiturates, which were used medically in the past for relieving tension and inducing relaxation and sleep.

One benzodiazepine of concern is Rohypnol, a potent tranquilizer similar in nature to Valium but many times stronger. The drug produces a sedative effect, amnesia, muscle relaxation, and slowed psychomotor responses. The most publicized "date rape" drug, Rohypnol has gained notoriety as a growing problem on college campuses. The drug has been added to punch and other drinks at parties, where it is reportedly given to women in hopes of lowering their inhibitions and facilitating potential sexual conquests. The manufacturer changed the formula to give the drug a bright blue color that would make it easy to detect in most drinks, so would-be perpetrators are now using blue tropical drinks and punches to disguise the drug. See Chapter 4 for more information about drug-facilitated rape.

Sedative-hypnotics have a synergistic effect when combined with alcohol, another central nervous system depressant. Taken together, these drugs can lead to respiratory failure and death. All sedative or hypnotic drugs can produce physical and psychological dependence in several weeks. A complication specific to sedatives is cross-tolerance, which occurs when users develop tolerance for one sedative or become dependent on it and develop tolerance for others as well. Withdrawal from sedative or hypnotic drugs may range from mild discomfort to severe symptoms, depending on the degree of dependence.

GHB *Gamma-hydroxybutyrate (GHB)* is a central nervous system depressant known to have euphoric, sedative, and anabolic (bodybuilding) effects. It was originally sold over the counter to bodybuilders to help reduce body fat and build muscle. Concerns about GHB led the FDA to ban OTC sales in 1992, and GHB is now a Schedule I controlled substance.[37] GHB is an odorless, tasteless fluid that can be made easily at home or in a chemistry lab. Like Rohypnol, GHB has been

drug-free living because the craving for the injection rush is very strong. It takes a great deal of discipline to seek alternative, nondrug highs.

Heroin addicts experience a distinct pattern of withdrawal. Symptoms of withdrawal include intense desire for the drug, sleep disturbance, dilated pupils, loss of appetite, irritability, goose bumps, and muscle tremors. The most difficult time in the withdrawal process occurs 24 to 72 hours following last use. All of the preceding symptoms continue, along with nausea, abdominal cramps, restlessness, insomnia, vomiting, diarrhea, extreme anxiety, hot and cold flashes, elevated blood pressure, and rapid heartbeat and respiration. Once the peak of withdrawal has passed, all these symptoms begin to subside. Still, the recovering addict has many hurdles to jump.

Methadone maintenance is one treatment available for people addicted to heroin or other opioids. This synthetic narcotic blocks the effects of opioid withdrawal. It is chemically similar enough to opioids to control the tremors, chills, vomiting, diarrhea, and severe abdominal pains of withdrawal. Methadone dosage is decreased over a period of time until the addict is weaned off it.

Methadone maintenance is controversial because of the drug's own potential for addiction. Critics contend that the program merely substitutes one addiction for another. Proponents argue that people on methadone maintenance are less likely to engage in criminal activities to support their habits than heroin addicts are. For this reason, many methadone maintenance programs are financed by state or federal government and are available free of charge or at reduced cost.

A number of new drug therapies for opioid dependence are emerging. Naltrexone (Trexan), an opioid antagonist, has been approved as a treatment. While on naltrexone, recovering

benzodiazepines A class of central nervous system depressant drugs with sedative, hypnotic, and muscle relaxant effects; also called *tranquilizers.*
barbiturates Drugs that depress the central nervous system and have sedative and hypnotic effects.

slipped into drinks without being detected, resulting in loss of memory, unconsciousness, amnesia, and even death. Other dangerous side effects include nausea, vomiting, seizures, hallucinations, coma, and respiratory distress.

Hallucinogens

Hallucinogens, or *psychedelics,* are substances that are capable of creating auditory or visual hallucinations and unusual changes in mood, thoughts, and feelings. The major receptor sites for most of these drugs are in the reticular formation (located in the brain stem at the upper end of the spinal cord), which is responsible for interpreting outside stimuli before allowing these signals to travel to other parts of the brain. When a hallucinogen is present at a reticular formation site, messages become scrambled, and the user may see wavy walls instead of straight ones or may "smell" colors and "hear" tastes. This mixing of sensory messages is known as **synesthesia.** Users may also become less inhibited or recall events long buried in the subconscious mind.

The most widely recognized hallucinogens are LSD, Ecstasy, PCP, mescaline, psilocybin, and ketamine. All are illegal and carry severe penalties for manufacture, possession, transportation, or sale.

LSD Of all the psychedelics, *lysergic acid diethylamide (LSD)* is the most notorious. First synthesized in the late 1930s, LSD resulted from experiments to derive medically useful drugs from the ergot fungus found on rye and other cereal grains. Because LSD seemed capable of unlocking the secrets of the mind, psychiatrists initially felt it could be beneficial to patients unable to remember suppressed traumas. From 1950 through 1968, the drug was used for such purposes.

Media attention focused on LSD in the 1960s. Young people used the drug to "turn on" and "tune out." In 1970, federal authorities placed LSD on the list of controlled substances. LSD's popularity peaked in 1972 then tapered off, primarily because of users' inability to control dosages accurately.

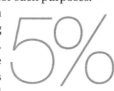

Because of recent waves of nostalgia for the 1960s, this dangerous psychedelic drug, known on the street as "acid," has been making a comeback. More than 11 million Americans, most of them under age 35, have tried LSD at least once. LSD especially attracts younger users. A national survey of college students showed that 1.3 percent had used the drug in the past year.[38]

The most common and most popular form of LSD is blotter acid—small squares of blotterlike paper that have been impregnated with a liquid LSD mixture. The blotter is swallowed or chewed briefly. LSD also comes in tiny thin squares of gelatin called *windowpane* and in tablets called *microdots,* which are less than an eighth of an inch across (it would take 10 or more to add up to the size of an aspirin tablet). As with any illegal drug, purchasers run the risk of buying an impure product.

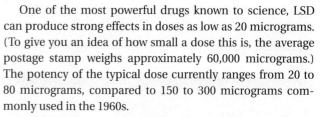

One of the most powerful drugs known to science, LSD can produce strong effects in doses as low as 20 micrograms. (To give you an idea of how small a dose this is, the average postage stamp weighs approximately 60,000 micrograms.) The potency of the typical dose currently ranges from 20 to 80 micrograms, compared to 150 to 300 micrograms commonly used in the 1960s.

In addition to its psychedelic effects, LSD produces several physical effects, including increased heart rate, elevated blood pressure and temperature, gooseflesh (roughened skin), increased reflex speeds, muscle tremors and twitches, perspiration, increased salivation, chills, headaches, and mild nausea. The drug also stimulates uterine muscle contractions, so it can lead to premature labor and miscarriage in pregnant women. Research into long-term effects has been inconclusive.

> **hallucinogens** Substances capable of creating auditory or visual distortions and heightened states.
> **synesthesia** A drug-created effect in which sensory messages are incorrectly assigned—for example, the user "hears" a taste or "smells" a sound.

The psychological effects of LSD vary. Euphoria is the common psychological state produced by the drug, but *dysphoria* (a sense of evil and foreboding) may also be experienced. The drug also shortens attention span, causing the mind to wander. Thoughts may be interposed and juxtaposed, so the user experiences several different thoughts simultaneously. Users become introspective, and suppressed memories may surface, often taking on bizarre symbolism. Many more effects are possible, including decreased aggressiveness and enhanced sensory experiences.

LSD causes distortions of ordinary perceptions, such as the movement of stationary objects. "Bad trips," the most publicized risk of LSD, are commonly related to the user's mood. The person, for example, may interpret increased heart rate as a heart attack (a "bad body trip").

Although there is no evidence that LSD creates physical dependence, it may well create psychological dependence. Many LSD users become depressed for 1 or 2 days following a trip and turn to the drug to relieve this depression. The result is a cycle of LSD use to relieve post-LSD depression, which often leads to psychological addiction.

Ecstasy *Ecstasy* is the most common street name for the drug *methylene-dioxymethamphetamine (MDMA),* a synthetic compound with both stimulant and mildly hallucinogenic effects. It is one of the most well-known "club drugs" or "designer drugs," a term applied to synthetic analogs of existing illicit drugs that tend to be popular among teens and young adults at nightclubs, bars, raves, and other all-night parties. Ecstasy creates feelings of extreme euphoria, openness and warmth, an increased willingness to communicate, feelings of love and empathy, increased awareness, and heightened appreciation for music. Young people may use Ecstasy initially to improve their mood or get energized. Like other hallucinogenic drugs Ecstasy can

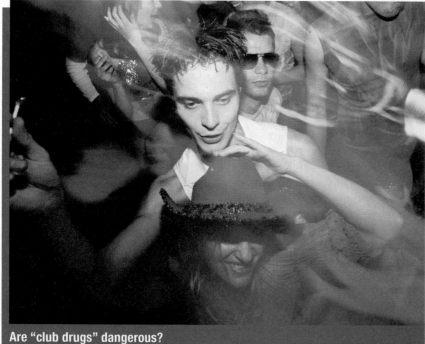

Are "club drugs" dangerous?

So-called club drugs are a varied group of synthetic drugs including Ecstasy, GHB, ketamine, Rohypnol, and meth that are often abused by teens and young adults at nightclubs, bars, or all-night dances. The sources and chemicals used to make these drugs vary, so dosages are unpredictable and drugs may not be "pure." Although users may think them relatively harmless, research has shown that club drugs can produce hallucinations, paranoia, amnesia, dangerous increases in heart rate and blood pressure, coma, and, in some cases, death. Some club drugs work on the same brain mechanisms as alcohol and can be particularly dangerous when used in combination with alcohol. In addition, some club drugs can be easily slipped into unsuspecting partygoers' drinks, thus facilitating sexual assault and other crimes.

emotion, memory, sleep, and pain. Combined with alcohol, Ecstasy can be extremely dangerous and sometimes fatal. Some studies indicate that the drug may cause long-lasting neurotoxic effects by damaging brain cells that produce serotonin.[39]

PCP *Phencyclidine,* or *PCP,* is a synthetic substance that became a black-market drug in the early 1970s. PCP was originally developed as a dissociative anesthetic, which means that patients receiving this drug could keep their eyes open and apparently remain conscious but feel no pain during a medical procedure. Afterward, patients would experience amnesia for the time the drug was in their system. Such a drug had obvious advantages as an anesthetic, but its unpredictability and drastic effects (postoperative delirium, confusion, and agitation) made doctors abandon it, and it was withdrawn from the legal market.

On the illegal market, PCP is a white, crystalline powder that users often sprinkle onto marijuana cigarettes. It is dangerous and unpredictable regardless of the method of administration. Common street names for PCP are "angel dust" for the crystalline powdered form and "peace pill" and "horse tranquilizer" for the tablet form.

enhance the sensory experience and distort perceptions, but it does not create visual hallucinations. Effects begin within 20 to 90 minutes and can last for 3 to 5 hours.

Some of the risks associated with Ecstasy use are similar to those of other stimulants. Because of the nature of the drug, Ecstasy users are at greater risk of inappropriate and/or unintended emotional bonding and have a tendency to say things they might feel uncomfortable about later. More physical consequences of Ecstasy use may include such things as mild to extreme jaw clenching, tongue and cheek chewing; short-term memory loss or confusion; increased body temperature as a result of dehydration and heat stroke; and increased heart rate and blood pressure. Individuals with high blood pressure, heart disease, or liver trouble are at greatest danger when using this drug. As the effects of Ecstasy begin to wear off the user can experience mild depression, fatigue, and a hangover that can last from days to weeks. Chronic use appears to damage the brain's ability to think and to regulate

The effects of PCP depend on the dose. A dose as small as 5 mg will produce effects similar to those of strong central nervous system depressants—slurred speech, impaired coordination, reduced sensitivity to pain, and reduced heart and respiratory rate. Doses between 5 and 10 mg cause fever, salivation, nausea, vomiting, and total loss of sensitivity to pain. Doses greater than 10 mg result in a drastic drop in blood pressure, coma, muscular rigidity, violent outbursts, and possible convulsions and death.

Psychologically, PCP may produce either euphoria or dysphoria. It also is known to produce hallucinations as well as delusions and overall delirium. Some users experience a prolonged state of "nothingness." The long-term effects of PCP use are unknown.

Mescaline *Mescaline* is one of hundreds of chemicals derived from the peyote cactus, a small, buttonlike plant that grows in the southwestern United States and in Latin America. Natives of these regions have long used the dried peyote "buttons" for religious purposes.

Mescaline comes from "buttons" of the peyote cactus, like this one.

Users typically swallow 10 to 12 buttons. They taste bitter and generally induce immediate nausea or vomiting. Long-time users claim that the nausea becomes less noticeable with frequent use. Those who are able to keep the drug down begin to feel the effects within 30 to 90 minutes, when mescaline reaches maximum concentration in the brain. (It may persist for up to 9 or 10 hours.) Mescaline is both a powerful hallucinogen and a central nervous system stimulant.

Psilocybe mushrooms produce hallucinogenic effects when ingested.

Products sold on the street as mescaline are likely to be synthetic chemical relatives of the true drug. Street names of these products include DOM, STP, TMA, and MMDA. Any of these can be toxic in small quantities.

Psilocybin *Psilocybin* and *psilocin* are the active chemicals in a group of mushrooms sometimes called "magic mushrooms." Psilocybe mushrooms, which grow throughout the world, can be cultivated from spores or harvested wild. When consumed, these mushrooms can cause hallucinations. Because many mushrooms resemble the psilocybe variety, people who harvest wild mushrooms for any purpose should be certain of what they are doing. Mushroom varieties can be easily misidentified, and mistakes can be fatal. Psilocybin is similar to LSD in its physical effects, which generally wear off in 4 to 6 hours.

Ketamine The liquid form of *ketamine,* or Special K, as it is commonly called, is used as an anesthetic in some hospital and veterinary clinics. After stealing it from hospitals or medical suppliers, dealers typically dry the liquid (usually by cooking it) and grind the residue into powder. Special K causes hallucinations, as it inhibits the relay of sensory input; the brain fills the resulting void with visions, dreams, memories, and sensory distortions. The aftereffects of Special K are less severe than those of Ecstasy, so it has grown in popularity as a club drug among people who must go to work or school after a night of partying.

Inhalants

Inhalants are chemicals that produce vapors that, when inhaled, can cause hallucinations and create intoxicating and euphoric effects. Not commonly recognized as drugs, inhalants are legal to purchase and universally available but dangerous when used incorrectly. They generally appeal to young people who can't afford or obtain illicit substances. Some products often misused as inhalants include rubber cement, model glue, paint thinner, lighter fluid, varnish, wax, spot removers, and gasoline. Most of these substances are sniffed or "huffed" by users in search of a quick, cheap high.

Amyl nitrite and nitrous oxide ("laughing gas") are also sometimes abused.

Because they are inhaled, the volatile chemicals in these products reach the bloodstream within seconds. An inhaled substance is not diluted or buffered by stomach acids or other body fluids and thus is more potent than it would be if swallowed. This characteristic, along with the fact that dosages are extremely difficult to control because everyone has unique lung and breathing capacities, makes inhalants particularly dangerous.

The effects of inhalants usually last fewer than 15 minutes and resemble those of central nervous system depressants. Combining inhalants with alcohol produces a synergistic effect and can cause severe liver damage that can be fatal. Users may experience dizziness, disorientation, impaired coordination, reduced judgment, and slowed reaction times.

An overdose of fumes from inhalants can cause unconsciousness. If the user's oxygen intake is reduced during the inhaling process, death can result within 5 minutes. Whether a user is a first-time or chronic user, sudden sniffing death (SSD) syndrome can be a fatal consequence. This syndrome can occur if a user inhales deeply and then participates in physical activity or is startled.

Anabolic Steroids

Anabolic steroids are artificial forms of the male hormone testosterone that promote muscle growth and strength. These **ergogenic drugs** are used primarily by people who believe the drugs will increase their strength, power, bulk (weight), speed, and athletic performance.

Most steroids are obtained through the black market. It was once estimated that approximately 17 to 20 percent of college athletes used them. Now that stricter drug-testing policies have been instituted by the National Collegiate Athletic Association (NCAA), reported use of anabolic steroids among intercollegiate athletes has dropped to 1.1 percent. However, a recent survey among high school students found a significant increase in the use of anabolic steroids since 1991.[40] Few data exist on the extent of steroid abuse by adults. It has been estimated that hundreds of thousands of people aged 18 and older abuse anabolic steroids at least once a year. Among both adolescents and adults, steroid abuse is higher among men than women. However, steroid abuse is growing most rapidly among young women.[41] Some young women report using steroids to improve their looks, while others are looking to gain an extra edge in athletics. Other steroid users—both women and men—may suffer from body image problems, including muscle dysmorphia (a distorted

inhalants Products that are sniffed or inhaled to produce highs.
anabolic steroids Artificial forms of the hormone testosterone that promote muscle growth and strength.
ergogenic drugs Substances believed to enhance athletic performance.

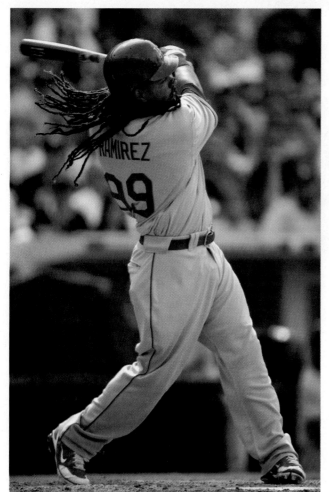

In May 2009, L.A. Dodgers slugger Manny Ramirez became the first major star suspended by the Major League Baseball Player Association (MLBPA) under its stricter drug-testing policy implemented in 2003.

hair, and male-pattern baldness; they may also result in an enlarged clitoris, smaller breasts, and changes in or absence of menstruation. When taken by healthy men, anabolic steroids shut down the body's production of testosterone, causing men's breasts to grow and testicles to atrophy.

Steroid Use and Society To combat the growing problem of steroid use, Congress passed the Anabolic Steroids Control Act (ASCA) of 1990. This law makes it a crime to possess, prescribe, or distribute anabolic steroids for any use other than the treatment of specific diseases. Penalties for their illegal use include up to 5 years' imprisonment and a $250,000 fine for the first offense and up to 10 years' imprisonment and a $500,000 fine for subsequent offenses.

The use of steroids and related substances among professional athletes periodically makes the news. In recent years, high-profile athletes in sports such as cycling, track and field, swimming, and baseball have all garnered media attention for suspected use of steroids or other banned performance-enhancing drugs. The Mitchell Report released in December 2007 was an investigation into the history of steroid and human growth hormone use by Major League Baseball players, 89 of whom are alleged by the report to have used steroids or other ergogenic drugs.

Among the most talked about ergogenic drugs are supplements containing androstenedione (andro), an adrenal hormone that is produced naturally in both men and women. Andro raises levels of the male hormone testosterone, which helps build lean muscle mass and promotes quicker recovery after injury. This supplement was available for purchase over the counter throughout the 1990s but was reclassified as a controlled substance by the Anabolic Steroid Control Act of 2004.

Other drugs are also sometimes used to achieve the effects of steroids. The two most common steroid alternatives are GHB and clenbuterol. GHB, discussed earlier, is a primary ingredient in many "performance-enhancing" formulas. In ergogenic preparations, GHB does not produce a high. It does, however, cause headaches, nausea, vomiting, diarrhea, seizures, and other central nervous system disorders, and possibly death. Clenbuterol is used in some countries for veterinary treatments but is not approved for any use—in animals or humans—in the United States.

perception of lack of muscle size; see **Focus On: Your Body Image** beginning on page 314).

Physical Effects of Steroids Steroids are available in two forms: injectable solutions and pills. Although their primary effects are not psychotropic, anabolic steroids can produce a state of euphoria, and diminished fatigue, in addition to increased bulk and power in both sexes. These qualities give steroids an addictive quality. When users stop, they can experience psychological withdrawal and sometimes severe depression, in some cases leading to suicide attempts. If untreated, depression associated with steroid withdrawal has been known to last for a year or more after steroid use stops.

Men and women who use steroids experience a variety of adverse effects. These drugs cause mood swings (aggression and violence), sometimes known as "'roid rage"; acne; liver tumors; elevated cholesterol levels; hypertension; kidney disease; and immune system disturbances. There is also a danger of transmitting AIDS and hepatitis (a serious liver disease) through shared needles. In women, large doses of anabolic steroids may trigger the development of masculine attributes such as lowered voice, increased facial and body

what do you think?

Do you believe an athlete's admission of steroid use invalidates his or her athletic achievements? ● How do you think professional athletes who have used steroids or other performance enhancers should be disciplined? ● If you are an athlete, have you ever considered using some type of ergogenic aid to improve your performance?

Treatment and Recovery

An estimated 23.6 million Americans aged 12 or older needed treatment for an illicit drug or alcohol use problem in 2007. Of these, only 2.5 million—approximately

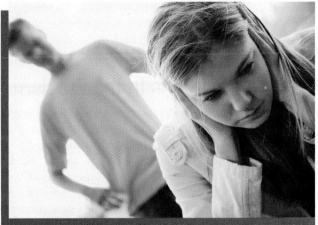

How can I help someone who I think has a problem with addiction?

The process of acknowledging and overcoming an addiction is a long and difficult journey for everyone involved. One way of beginning the recovery process is to stage an intervention, a planned process of confrontation by people who are important to the addict, with a goal of breaking down the addict's denial compassionately and getting him or her to see the addiction's destructive nature. Intervention is a serious step that should be well planned and rehearsed. Most addiction treatment centers have specialists who can help plan an intervention.

10 percent—received treatment. The most difficult step in the recovery process is for the substance abuser to admit that he or she is an addict. This can be difficult because of the power of *denial*—the inability to see the truth. Denial is the hallmark of addiction. It can be so powerful that a planned intervention is sometimes necessary to break down the addict's defenses against recognizing the problem.

Recovery from drug addiction is a long-term process and frequently requires multiple episodes of treatment. The first step generally begins with abstinence—refraining from the behavior. Whereas complete abstinence is possible for people addicted to chemicals, it is obviously not feasible for people addicted to behaviors such as work, exercise, or sex. For those addicts, abstinence means restoring balance to their lives through noncompulsive engagement in behaviors and avoiding certain addiction-triggering activities.

Detoxification refers to an early abstinence period during which an addict adjusts physically and cognitively to being free from the addiction's influence. It occurs in virtually every recovering addict, and, whereas it is uncomfortable for most addicts, it can be dangerous for some. This is primarily true for those addicted to chemicals, especially alcohol and heroin, and painkillers such as OxyContin. For these people, early abstinence may involve profound withdrawals that require medical supervision. Because of this, most inpatient treatment programs provide a pretreatment component of supervised detoxification to achieve abstinence safely before treatment begins.

Treatment Approaches

Outpatient behavioral treatment encompasses a wide variety of programs for addicts who visit a clinic at regular intervals. Most of the programs involve individual or group drug counseling. Some programs also offer other forms of behavioral treatment, such as the following:

- Cognitive behavioral therapy, which seeks to help patients recognize, avoid, and cope with the situations in which they are most likely to abuse drugs
- Multidimensional family therapy, which addresses a range of influences on the drug abuse patterns of adolescents and is designed for them and their families
- Motivational interviewing, which is a client-centered, direct method for enhancing intrinsic motivation to change by exploring and resolving ambivalence
- Motivational incentives (contingency management), which uses positive reinforcement to encourage abstinence from drugs

Residential treatment programs can also be very effective, especially for those with more severe problems. For example, therapeutic communities (TCs) are highly structured programs in which addicts remain at a residence, typically for 6 to 12 months. The focus of the TC is on the resocialization of the addict to a drug-free lifestyle.

12-Step Programs The first 12-step program was Alcoholics Anonymous (AA), begun in 1935 in Akron, Ohio. The 12-step program has since become the most widely used approach to dealing with not only alcoholism, but also drug abuse and various other addictive or dysfunctional behaviors. There are more than 200 different recovery programs based on the program, including Narcotics Anonymous, Cocaine Anonymous, Crystal Meth Anonymous, Gamblers Anonymous, and Pills Anonymous.

The 12-step program is nonjudgmental and based on the idea that a program's only purpose is to work on personal recovery. Working the 12 steps involves admitting to having a serious problem, recognizing there is an outside power that could help, consciously relying on that power, admitting and listing character defects, seeking deliverance from defects, apologizing to those individuals one has harmed in the past, and helping others with the same problem. The 12-step meetings are held at a variety of times and locations

21.1 million people who needed treatment for an illicit drug or alcohol use problem in 2007 did not receive that treatment.

detoxification The process of freeing a drug user from an intoxicating or addictive substance in the body or from dependence on such a substance.

in almost every city. There is no membership cost and the meetings are open to anyone who wishes to attend.

College Students' Treatment and Recovery

For college students who have developed substance or behavioral addictions, early intervention increases the likelihood of successful treatment, successful sobriety, and completion of a college education. Depending on the severity of the abuse or dependence, college students undergoing drug treatment may be required to spend time away from school in a residential drug rehabilitation inpatient facility. The needs of college students seeking drug treatment in rehab do not differ greatly from other adult recovering addicts, but for best results, the community of addicts should include others of a similar age and educational background. Private therapy, group therapy, cognitive training, nutrition counseling, and health therapies can all be used to help with recovery.

A growing number of colleges and universities offer special services to students who are recovering from alcohol and other drug addiction and want to stay in school without being exposed to excessive drinking or drug use. For example, the University of Texas at Austin opened its Center for Students in Recovery, which provides students with a support system and a for-credit academic course called "Complete Recovery 101." Another campus, Texas Tech University, recently received a $250,000 federal grant to create a national model of its students-in-recovery program. The program offers scholarships to students in recovery, as well as on-campus 12-step meetings and academic support.

Addressing Drug Misuse and Abuse in the United States

Stories of people who have tried illegal drugs, enjoyed them, and suffered no consequences may tempt you to try them yourself. You may convince yourself that one-time use is harmless. Given the dangers surrounding these substances, however, you should think twice. The risks associated with drug use extend beyond the personal. The decision to try any illicit substance encourages illicit drug manufacture and transport, thus contributing to the national drug problem.

The financial burden of illegal drug use on the U.S. economy is staggering, with an estimated cost of around $180.9 billion per year.[42] This estimate includes costs associated with substance abuse treatment and prevention, health care, reduced job productivity and lost earnings, and social consequences such as crime and social welfare. In addition, roughly half of all expenditures to combat crime are related to illegal drugs. The burden of these costs is absorbed primarily by the government (46%), followed by people who abuse drugs and members of their households (44%).

Possible Solutions to the Problem

Americans are alarmed by the increasing use of illegal drugs. Respondents in public opinion polls feel that the most important strategy for fighting drug abuse is educating young people. They also endorse strategies such as stricter border surveillance to reduce drug trafficking; longer prison sentences for drug dealers; increased government spending on prevention; antidrug law enforcment; and greater cooperation among government agencies, private groups, and individuals providing treatment assistance. All of these approaches will probably help up to a point, but they do not offer a total solution to the problem. Drug abuse has been a part of human behavior for thousands of years, and it is not likely to disappear in the near future. For this reason, it is necessary to educate ourselves and to develop the self-discipline necessary to avoid dangerous drug dependence.

For many years, the most popular antidrug strategies were total prohibition and "scare tactics." Both approaches proved ineffective. Prohibition of alcohol during the 1920s created more problems than it solved, as did prohibition of opioids in 1914. A more recent prohibition campaign is commonly referred to as the "War on Drugs," undertaken by the U.S. government with the assistance of participating countries. This campaign includes laws and policies that are intended to reduce the illegal drug trade and to diminish and discourage the production, distribution, and consumption of illicit substances.

In general, researchers in the field of drug education agree that a multimodal approach is best. Young people should be taught the difference between drug use, misuse, and abuse. Factual information that is free of scare tactics must be presented; lecturing and moralizing have proven not to work.

Harm Reduction Strategies Harm reduction is a set of practical approaches to reducing negative consequences of drug use, incorporating a spectrum of strategies from safer use to managed use to abstinence. Harm reduction approaches have been widely used in needle exchange programs, where injection drug users receive clean needles and syringes, and bleach for cleaning needles; these efforts help reduce the number of HIV and hepatitis B cases. Harm reduction may involve changing the legal sanctions associated with drug use, increasing the availability of treatment services to drug abusers, and/or attempting to change drug users' behavior through education. Harm reduction strategies meet drug users "where they're at," addressing conditions of use along with the use itself. This strategy recognizes that people always have and always will use drugs and, therefore, attempts to minimize the potential hazards associated with drug use rather than the use itself.

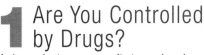

Do You Have a Problem with Drugs?

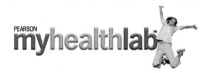

Fill out this assessment online at www.pearsonhighered.com/myhealthlab or www.pearsonhighered.com/donatelle.

1 Are You Controlled by Drugs?

A dependent person can't stop using drugs. This abuse hurts the user and everyone around him or her. The more "yes" checks you make below, the more likely it is that you have a problem.

	Yes	No
1. Do you use drugs to handle stress or escape from life's problems?	○	○
2. Have you unsuccessfully tried to cut down on or quit using your drug?	○	○
3. Have you ever been in trouble with the law or been arrested because of your drug use?	○	○
4. Do you think a party or social gathering isn't fun unless drugs are available?	○	○
5. Do you avoid people or places that do not support your usage?	○	○
6. Do you neglect your responsibilities because you'd rather use your drug?	○	○
7. Have your friends, family, or employer expressed concern about your drug use?	○	○
8. Do you do things under the influence of drugs that you would not normally do?	○	○
9. Have you seriously thought that you might have a chemical dependency problem?	○	○

Source: Reprinted by permission of Krames Communications, 1100 Grundy Lane, San Bruno, CA 94066-3030, www.krames.com.

2 Are You Controlled by a Drug User?

Your love and care may actually be enabling another person to continue chemical abuse, hurting you and others. The more "yes" checks you make below, the more likely there's a problem.

	Yes	No
1. Do you often have to lie or cover up for the chemical abuser?	○	○
2. Do you spend time counseling the person about the problem?	○	○
3. Have you taken on additional financial or family responsibilities?	○	○
4. Do you feel that you have to control the chemical abuser's behavior?	○	○
5. At the office, have you done work or attended meetings for the abuser?	○	○
6. Do you often put your own needs and desires after the user's?	○	○
7. Do you spend time each day worrying about your situation?	○	○
8. Do you analyze your behavior to find clues to how it might affect the chemical abuser?	○	○
9. Do you feel powerless and at your wit's end about the abuser's problem?	○	○

YOUR PLAN FOR CHANGE

The **Assess Yourself** activity describes signs of being controlled by drugs or by a drug user. Depending on your results, you may need to change certain behaviors that may be detrimental to your health.

Today, you can:

○ Imagine a situation in which someone offers you a drug and think of several different ways of refusing. Rehearse these scenarios in your head.

○ Stop by your campus health center to find out about any drug treatment programs or support groups they may have.

Within the next 2 weeks, you can:

○ Think about the drug use patterns among your social group. Are you ever uncomfortable with these people because of their drug use? Is it difficult to avoid using drugs when you are with them? If the answers are yes, begin exploring ways to expand your social circle.

○ If you are concerned about your own drug use or the drug use of a close friend, make an appointment with a counselor to talk about the issue.

By the end of the semester, you can:

○ Participate in clubs, activities, and social groups that do not rely on substance abuse for their amusement.

○ If you have a drug problem, make a commitment to enter a treatment program. Acknowledge that you have a problem and that you need the assistance of others to help you overcome it.

Summary

* Addiction is the continued involvement with a substance or activity despite ongoing negative consequences of that involvement. Habits are repeated behaviors, whereas addiction is behavior resulting from compulsion; without the behavior, the addict experiences withdrawal. All addictions share four common symptoms: compulsion, loss of control, negative consequences, and denial.
* Addictive behaviors include compulsive gambling, compulsive spending, exercise addiction, and Internet and technology addiction. Codependents are typically friends or family members who are "addicted to the addict." Enablers are people who knowingly or unknowingly protect addicts from the consequences of their behavior.
* Mood-altering substances and experiences produce biochemical reactions that make the body feel good; when absent, the person feels the effects of withdrawal.
* The six categories of drugs are prescription drugs, over-the-counter (OTC) drugs, recreational drugs, herbal preparations, illicit (illegal) drugs, and commercial preparations. Routes of administration include oral ingestion, inhalation, injection (intravenous, intramuscular, and subcutaneous), inunction, and suppositories.
* OTC medications are drugs that do not require a prescription. Some OTC medications, including sleep aids, cold medicines, and diet pills, can be addictive.
* Prescription drug abuse is at an all-time high, particularly among college students. Only marijuana is more commonly abused. The most commonly abused prescription drugs fall into the following classifications: opioids/narcotics, depressants, and stimulants.
* People from all walks of life use illicit drugs, although college students report higher usage rates than do the general population. Drug use declined from the mid-1980s to the early 1990s but has remained steady since then. However, among young people, use of drugs has been rising in recent years.
* Controlled substances include cocaine and its derivatives, amphetamines, methamphetamine, marijuana, opioids, depressants, hallucinogens/psychedelics, inhalants, and steroids. Each has its own set of risks and effects.
* Treatment begins with abstinence from the drug or addictive behavior, usually instituted through intervention by close family, friends, or other loved ones. Treatment programs may include individual, group, or family therapy, as well as 12-step programs.
* The drug problem reaches everyone through crime and elevated health care costs. Public health and governmental approaches to the problem involve regulation, enforcement, education, and harm reduction.

Pop Quiz

1. Which of the following is not a characteristic of addiction?
   a. denial
   b. tolerance
   c. loss of control
   d. habit

2. An individual who knowingly tries to protect an addict from natural consequences of his or her destructive behaviors is
   a. enabling.
   b. coddling.
   c. practicing intervention.
   d. controlling.

3. Chemical dependence *relapse* refers to
   a. a person who is experiencing a blackout memory loss.
   b. a gap in one's drinking or drugging patterns.
   c. a full return to addictive behavior.
   d. the failure to change one's behavior.

4. Taking excessive drugs on a continual basis, even when it is not necessary to, describes
   a. drug misuse.
   b. drug addiction.
   c. drug tolerance.
   d. drug abuse.

5. Cross-tolerance occurs when
   a. drugs work at the same receptor site so that one blocks the action of the other.
   b. the effects of one drug are eliminated or reduced by the presence of another drug at the receptor site.
   c. a person develops a physiological tolerance to one drug and shows a similar tolerance to selected other drugs as a result.
   d. two or more drugs interact and the effects of the individual drugs are multiplied beyond what normally would be expected if they were taken alone.

6. Rebecca takes a number of medications for various conditions, including Prinivil (an antihypertensive drug), insulin (a diabetic medication), and Claritin (an antihistamine). This is an example of
   a. synergism.
   b. illegal drug use.
   c. polydrug use.
   d. antagonism.

7. Which of the following is not an example of drug misuse?
   a. excessive use of and dependency on a drug
   b. taking a friend's prescription medicine
   c. taking medicine more often than is recommended
   d. not following the instructions when taking a medicine

8. Which of the following is classified as a stimulant drug?
   a. methamphetamine
   b. alcohol
   c. marijuana
   d. LSD

9. Freebasing is
   a. mixing cocaine with heroin.
   b. inhaling heroin fumes.
   c. injecting a drug into the veins.
   d. smoking the fumes of cocaine.

10. The psychoactive drug mescaline is found in what plant?
    a. mushrooms
    b. peyote cactus
    c. marijuana
    d. belladonna

Answers to these questions can be found on page A-1.

Think about It!

1. What is the current theory that explains how drugs work in the body?
2. Explain the terms *synergism, antagonism,* and *inhibition.*
3. Why do you think many people today feel that marijuana use is not dangerous? What are the arguments in favor of legalizing marijuana? What are the arguments against legalization?
4. What could you do to help a friend who is fighting a substance abuse problem? What resources on your campus could help you?
5. What types of programs do you think would be effective in preventing drug abuse among high school and college students? How would programs for high school students differ from those for college students?
6. Discuss how addiction affects family and friends. What role do family and friends play in helping the addict get help and maintain recovery?

Accessing Your Health on the Internet

The following websites explore further topics and issues related to personal health. For links to the websites below, visit the Companion Website for *Health: The Basics,* Green Edition at www.pearsonhighered.com/donatelle.

1. *Join Together.* An excellent site for the most current information related to substance abuse. Also includes information on alcohol and drug policy and provides advice on organizing and taking political action. www.jointogether.org
2. *National Institute on Drug Abuse (NIDA).* The home page of this U.S. government agency has information on the latest statistics and findings in drug research. www.nida.nih.gov
3. *Substance Abuse and Mental Health Services Administration (SAMHSA).* Outstanding resource for information about national surveys, ongoing research, and national drug interventions. www.samhsa.gov
4. *National Council on Problem Gambling.* Provides information and help for people with gambling problems and their families, including a searchable directory for counselors. www.ncpgambling.org

References

1. National Council on Problem Gambling, "FAQs—Problem Gamblers," www.ncpgambling.org/i4a/pages/index.cfm?pageid=3390. Accessed June 2009.
2. C. Holden, "Gambling as Addiction," *Science* 307, no. 5708 (2005): 349, www.sciencemag.org.
3. J. W. Welte et al., "Gambling Participation and Pathology in the United States," *Addictive Behaviors* 29, no. 5 (2004): 983–89.
4. The Annenburg Public Policy Center, "Card-Playing Trend in Young People Continues," Press Release, September 28, 2005, www.annenbergpublicpolicycenter.org.
5. W. DeJong et al., "Gambling: The New Addiction Crisis in Higher Education," *Prevention Profile* (March 2006): 11–13.
6. S. Durling, "Conquer the Compulsive Shopping Blues," *Women's Wall Street* (June 19, 2004).
7. R. Engs, "How Can I Manage Compulsive Shopping and Spending Addiction?" www.indiana.edu/~engs/hints/shop.html. Updated December 2007.
8. J. Leone et al., "Recognition and Treatment of Muscle Dysmorphia and Related Body Image Disorders," *Journal of Athletic Training* 40, no. 4 (2005): 352–59.
9. M. Maine, *Body Wars: Making Peace with Women's Bodies* (Carlsbad, CA: Gurze, 2000), 282.
10. D. M. Wieland, "Computer Addiction: Implications for Nursing Psychotherapy Practice," *Perspectives in Psychiatric Care* 41, no. 4 (2005): 153–61.
11. American College Health Association, *American College Health Association—National College Health Assessment: Reference Group Data Report Fall 2008* (Baltimore: American College Health Association, 2009).
12. U.S. Department of Health and Human Services, "Substance Abuse—A National Challenge: Prevention, Treatment, and Research at HHS," January 13, 2006, www.hhs.gov/news/factsheet/subabuse.html.
13. Ibid.
14. P. Kittenger and D. Herron, "Patient Power: Over-the-Counter Drugs—Brief Analysis," National Center for Policy Analysis, 2005, www.ncpa.org/pub/ba/ba524.
15. L. D. Johnston et al., *Monitoring the Future National Survey Results on Drug Use, 1975–2007: Volume I, Secondary School Students* (NIH Publication No. 08-6418A, Bethesda, MD: National Institute on Drug Abuse, 2008).
16. The U.S. Department of Justice's National Drug Intelligence Center, *Intelligence Bulletin: DXM (Dextromethorphan)* (DOJ Publication no. 2004-L0424-029, Johnstown, PA: National Drug Intelligence Center, 2004).
17. U.S. Food and Drug Administration, "Legal Requirements for the Sale and Purchase of Drug Products Containing Pseudoephedrine, Ephedrine, and Phenylpropanolamine," www.fda.gov/Drugs/DrugSafety/InformationbyDrugClass/ucm072423.htm. Updated May 2006.
18. U.S. Food and Drug Administration, "Press Release: FDA Announces Rule Prohibiting Sale of Dietary Supplements Containing Ephedrine Alkaloids Effective April 12," April 2004, www.fda.gov/NewsEvents/Newsroom/PressAnnouncements/2004/ucm108281.htm.

19. National Youth Anti-Drug Media Campaign, "Prescription Drug Abuse," 2009, www.theantidrug.com/drug_info/prescription_drugs.asp.

20. Substance Abuse and Mental Health Services Administration, *Results from the 2007 National Survey on Drug Use and Health: National Findings* (Office of Applied Studies, NSDUH Series H-32, DHHS Publication no. SMA 07-4293, Rockville, MD, 2008).

21. National Center on Addiction and Substance Abuse at Columbia University, *Wasting the Best and the Brightest: Substance Abuse at America's Colleges and Universities* (New York: National Center on Addiction and Substance Abuse at Columbia University, 2007).

22. Ibid.

23. Substance Abuse and Mental Health Services Administration, *Results from the 2007 National Survey on Drug Use and Health,* 2008.

24. L. D. Johnston et al., *Monitoring the Future National Survey Results on Drug Use, 1975–2007: Volume II, College Students and Adults* (NIH Publication no. 08-6418B, Bethesda, MD: National Institute on Drug Abuse, 2008).

25. National Center on Addiction and Substance Abuse at Columbia University, *Wasting the Best and the Brightest,* 2007.

26. Ibid.

27. D. L. Rabiner et al., "Motives and Perceived Consequences of Nonmedical ADHD Medication Use by College Students: Are Students Treating Themselves for Attention Problems?" *Journal of Attention Disorders,* 13, no. 3 (2009): 259–70.

28. L. D. Johnston et al., *Monitoring the Future National Survey Results on Drug Use, 1975–2007: Volume II,* 2008.

29. D. Schardt, "Caffeine: The Good, the Bad, and the Maybe," *Nutrition Action Healthletter,* (March 2008): 6.

30. U.S. Department of Health and Human Services, *Marijuana: Facts for Teens* (NIH Publication no. 04–4037, 2004).

31. U.S. Department of Health and Human Services, National Institute on Drug Abuse Research Report Series, *Marijuana Abuse* (NIH Publication no. 05-3859, 2005).

32. EyeCare America, The Foundation of the American Academy of Ophthalmology, "The Use of Marijuana in the Treatment of Glaucoma," 2003, www.aao.org/eyecare/treatment/alternative-therapies/marijuana-glaucoma.cfm.

33. J. Daling et al., "Association of Marijuana Use and the Incidence of Testicular Germ Cell Tumors," *Cancer* 115, no. 6 (2009): 1215–23.

34. Substance Abuse and Mental Health Services Administration, *Results from the 2007 National Survey on Drug Use and Health,* 2008.

35. U.S. Department of Health and Human Services, *Marijuana: Facts Parents Need to Know* (NIH Publication no. 07-4036, 2007).

36. U.S. Department of Health and Human Services, National Institute on Drug Abuse Research Report Series, *Heroin: Abuse and Addiction* (Publication no. 05-4165), 2005.

37. National Institute on Drug Abuse, "NIDA InfoFacts: Drugs (GHB, Ketamine, and Rohypnol)." Revised August 2008, www.drugabuse.gov/infofacts/clubdrugs.html.

38. L. D. Johnston et al., *Monitoring the Future National Survey Results on Drug Use, 1975–2007: Volume II,* 2008.

39. National Institute on Drug Abuse, "NIDA InfoFacts: Club Drugs," 2006.

40. L. D. Johnston et al., *Monitoring the Future National Survey Results on Drug Use, 1975–2007: Volume I,* 2008.

41. National Institute on Drug Abuse, "Anabolic Steroids," *NIDA for Teens,* 2005, http://teens.drugabuse.gov/drnida/drnida_ster1.asp.

42. National Drug Intelligence Center, "National Drug Threat Assessment, 2006: The Impact of Drugs on Society," 2006, www.justice.gov/ndic/pubs11/18862/impact.htm.

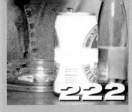
222
Are the majority of college students heavy drinkers?

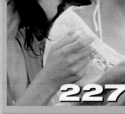
227
Why do some people feel the effects of alcohol more quickly than others?

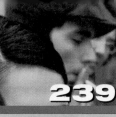
239
Is social smoking really that bad for me?

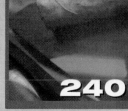
240
Are cigars as harmful as cigarettes?

Alcohol and Tobacco

8

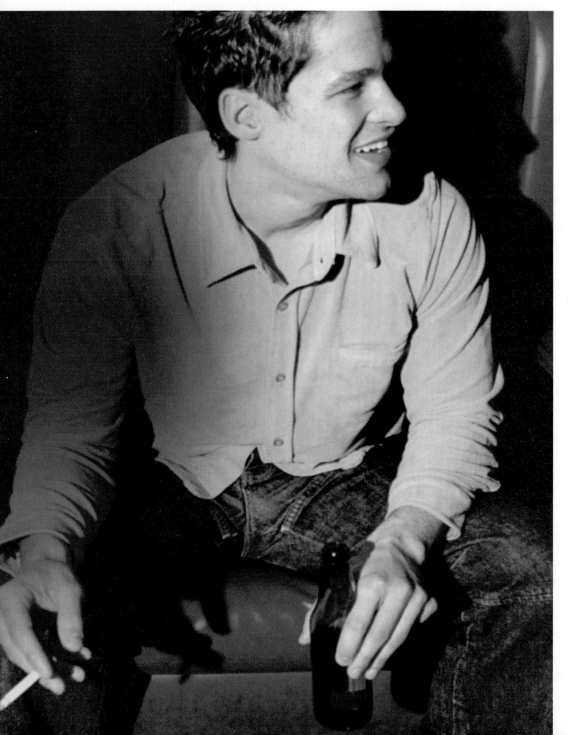

Objectives

✱ Discuss the alcohol use patterns of college students and overall trends in consumption.

✱ Explain the physiological and behavioral effects of alcohol, including blood alcohol concentration, absorption, metabolism, and immediate and long-term effects of alcohol consumption.

✱ Explain the symptoms and causes of alcoholism, its cost to society, effects on the family, and treatment options.

✱ Discuss the social and political issues involved in tobacco use.

✱ Discuss the health risks of smoking, smokeless tobacco, and environmental tobacco smoke, and describe how the chemicals in tobacco products affect the body.

Usually the word *drug* conjures up images of people abusing illegal substances. We use the term to describe dangerous chemicals such as heroin or cocaine, without recognizing that socially accepted substances can be drugs, too—for example, alcohol and tobacco.

Alcohol: An Overview

People all over the world and throughout history have used alcohol for everything from social gatherings to religious ceremonies. The consumption of alcoholic beverages is interwoven with many traditions, and moderate use of alcohol can enhance celebrations or special times. Research even shows that very low levels of alcohol consumption may actually lower some health risks. However, while alcohol can sometimes play a positive role in some people's lives, we need to remember that it is first and foremost a chemical substance that affects your physical and mental behavior. The fact is, alcohol is a drug, and if it is not used responsibly, it can become dangerous.

An estimated 61 percent of Americans consume alcoholic beverages regularly, while about 25 percent abstain from drinking alcohol altogether.[1] Among those who drink, consumption patterns vary. Ten percent are heavy drinkers, and they account for half of all the alcohol consumed.

heavy episodic (binge) drinking
A "binge" is a pattern of drinking alcohol that brings blood alcohol concentration (BAC) to 0.08 grampercent or above; for a typical adult, this pattern corresponds to consuming five or more drinks (male), or four or more drinks (female), in about 2 hours.

Alcohol and College Students

Alcohol is the most widely used and abused recreational drug in our society. It is also the most popular drug on college campuses, where approximately 63 percent of students report having consumed alcoholic beverages in the past 30 days.[2] In a new trend on college campuses, women's consumption of alcohol has come close to equaling men's. Almost half of all college students engage in **heavy episodic (binge) drinking.** Over the years, there has been a lack of uniformity in defining this term; recognizing this, in 2007, the National Advisory Council of the National Institute on Alcohol Abuse and Alcoholism (NIAAA) approved a new definition: "A binge is pattern of drinking alcohol that brings blood alcohol concentration (BAC) to 0.08 gram-percent or

90%

of the drinking population are infrequent, light, or moderate drinkers.

above. For a typical adult, this pattern corresponds to consuming 5 or more drinks (male), or 4 or more drinks (female), in about 2 hours."[3] Therefore, students who might go out and drink only once a week are considered heavy episodic drinkers (binge drinkers) if they consume 5 or more drinks (for men) or 4 or more drinks (for women) within 2 hours. (See the **Health Today** box on the next page for more on alcohol and college students.)

College is a critical time to become aware of and responsible for drinking. There is little doubt that drinking is a part of campus culture and tradition. Many students are away from home, often for the first time, and are excited by their newfound independence. For some students, this independence and the rite of passage into the college culture are symbolized alcohol use. It provides the answer to one of the most commonly heard statements on any college campus: "There is nothing to do." Additionally, many students say they drink to have fun. "Having fun," which often means drinking simply to get drunk, may really be a way of coping with stress, boredom, anxiety, or pressures created by academic and social demands.

A significant number of students experience negative consequences as a result of their alcohol consumption. In the American College Health Association's National College Health Assessment, 34 percent of students reported doing something they regretted after drinking; 29 percent forgot where they were or what they did; 15 percent

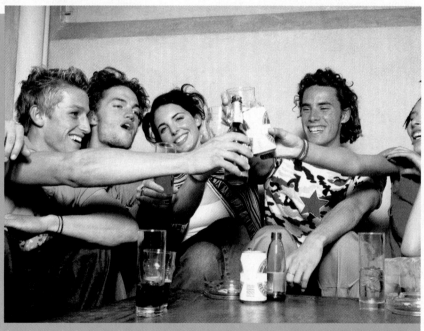

Are the majority of college students heavy drinkers?

It may sometimes seem like your campus is crowded with heavy drinkers, but, in fact, most college students—about 63%—drink only occasionally, and 23% don't drink at all. However, college students have high rates of "binge" drinking; when they do drink, they tend to drink a lot. Irresponsible consumption of alcohol can easily result in disaster, so it is important for you to take control of when you drink, and how much.

Alcohol in Academia

There is no doubt that many students on America's college and university campuses drink alcohol. But how much and with what consequences do they do so? Some of the following facts about students and alcohol consumption may surprise you:

* Alcohol kills more people under age 21 than cocaine, marijuana, and heroin combined.

* Each year, half a million students between ages 15 and 24 are unintentionally injured while intoxicated.

* Of today's first-year college students, 159,000 will drop out of school next year for alcohol- or other drug-related reasons.

* About 5 percent of four-year-college students are involved with the police or campus security as a result of their drinking, and an estimated 110,000 students are arrested for an alcohol-related violation such as public drunkenness or driving under the influence.

* Areas of a college campus offering cheap beer prices have more crime, including trouble between students and police or other campus authorities, arguments, physical fighting, property damage, false fire alarms, and sexual misconduct.

* Male students at a beach destination on spring break average 18 drinks a day; females, 10.

* It is estimated that 300,000 of today's college students will eventually die of alcohol-related causes such as drunk-driving accidents, cirrhosis of the liver, various cancers, and heart disease.

* Approximately 71 percent of drinkers have reported *pregaming*, meaning heavy alcohol consumption prior to attending a party, sporting event, or school-sponsored activity, and report drinking 4.9 drinks per session.

* Alcohol is involved in more than two-thirds of suicides among college students, 90 percent of campus rapes and sexual assaults, and 95 percent of violent crimes on campus.

* Each year, more than 100,000 students between the ages of 18 and 24 report having been too intoxicated to know if they consented to having sex.

* College students under the age of 21 are more prone to binge drinking and pay less for their alcohol than do their older classmates. Though underage students drink less often, they consume more per occasion than students age 21 and older who are allowed to drink legally.

* Nearly half of first-year college students who drink alcohol spend more time drinking each week than they do studying. Students who said they had at least one drink in the past 14 days spent an average 10.2 hours a week drinking and averaged about 8.4 hours a week studying.

* Among college students, non-Latino whites and Latinos report the highest rates of alcohol use in the past 30 days (75%), compared to 73 percent of Native Americans, 59 percent of Asian Americans and Pacific Islanders, and 52 percent of African Americans. Reported rates of heavy episodic drinking follow a similar breakdown.

Sources: Data were compiled from the numerous studies cited throughout this chapter and from

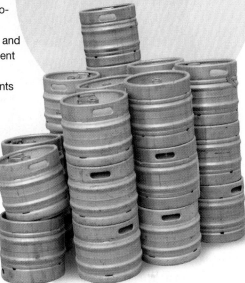

From keggers to tailgate parties, alcohol is a frequent part of college life.

M. Mohler-Kuo et al., "College Rapes Linked to Binge-Drinking Rates," *Journal of Studies on Alcohol* 65, no. 1 (2004); Facts on Tap, "The College Experience: Alcohol and Student Life," 2009, www.factsontap.org/factsontap/alcohol_and_student_life/index.htm; B. DeRicco et al., "Pregaming: A New Challenge for Campus Alcohol Efforts," *Student Health Spectrum* (2007). P. Greenbaum et al., "Variation in the Drinking Trajectories of Freshmen College Students," *Journal of Counseling and Clinical Psychology* 73, no. 2 (2005): 229–38; M. B. Marklein, "College Freshmen Study Booze More Than Books," *USA Today*, March 11, 2009, www.usatoday.com/news/education/2009-03-11-college-drinking_N.htm; The U.S. Department of Education's Higher Education Center for Alcohol and Other Drug Abuse and Violence Prevention, "Prevalence and Problems among Different Populations," *Catalyst* 8, no. 3 (2007): 2.

physically injured themselves; and 15 percent had unprotected sex. Women were more likely to have someone use force or use the threat of force to have sex with them after they had been drinking.[4]

In the same survey, many college students reported always or usually practicing protective behaviors when consuming alcohol to reduce the risk of negative consequences as a result of their alcohol use. Seventy-seven percent of students reported eating before or during drinking, 85 percent

reported using a designated driver, 67 percent kept track of how many drinks they consumed, and 40 percent determined in advance a set number of drinks they would not exceed.[5] It is important for students to recognize that if they consume alcohol, choices such as these can help reduce the risk of experiencing a negative consequence as a result of their drinking.

What are colleges currently doing to address the problem of drinking on campus? The NIAAA has studied interventions

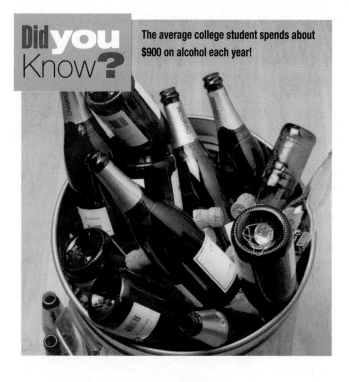
that effectively deal with the problem. Programs that have proven particularly effective use cognitive-behavioral skills training with *motivational interviewing.*[6] This is a nonjudgmental approach to working with students to change behavior. Brief interventions with health educators, counselors, or health care providers trained in motivational interviewing help build students' belief in their ability to change their drinking behavior.

Other effective programs use data to counter student misperceptions about peer drinking patterns and to increase students' motivation to change their drinking habits. Many colleges and universities are trying this *social norms* approach to reduce alcohol consumption. There is growing research that college students' drinking behavior is strongly influenced by the incorrect perception that their peers drink more than they actually do. This misperception includes inaccurately estimating the frequency and amount that students drink, and the actual consequences students experience as a result of their drinking.

Today, many campuses are working to change misperceptions of normal drinking behavior. As a result, heavy episodic alcohol consumption—"binge drinking"—has declined at campuses across the country. For example, Michigan State University, Florida State University, and the University of Arizona all reported 20 to 30 percent reductions in heavy episodic alcohol consumption within 3 years of implementing social norms campaigns, while Hobart and William Smith Colleges saw a 40 percent reduction in 5 years and Northern Illinois University saw a 44 percent reduction in 10 years.[7]

High-Risk Drinking and College Students

There are, however, some students who indulge in binge drinking. The stakes of binge drinking are high because it poses high risk for alcohol-related injuries and death. According to a recent study, 1,700 college students die each year because of alcohol-related unintentional injuries, including car accidents. Binge drinking is the number one cause of preventable death among undergraduate college students in the United States today.[8]

A study by the Harvard School of Public Health found that 44.4 percent of students were binge drinkers, and, of those, 22.8 percent were frequent bingers (people who binge drink three times or more in a 2-week period; Figure 8.1).[9] Compared with nonbinge drinkers, frequent binge drinkers are 16 times more likely to miss class, 8 times more likely to get behind in their school work, and more apt to get into trouble with campus or local police.[10] Figure 8.2 shows other negative consequences that frequent binge drinkers are more likely experience.

Although everyone is at some risk for alcohol-related problems, college students seem to be particularly vulnerable for the following reasons:

- Alcohol exacerbates their already high risk for suicide, automobile crashes, and falls.
- Many college and university students' customs (e.g., greek rush or initiations), norms (e.g., reputation as party schools, tailgating), and traditional celebrations (e.g., St. Patrick's Day, 21st birthday, Mardi Gras) encourage certain dangerous practices and patterns of alcohol use.

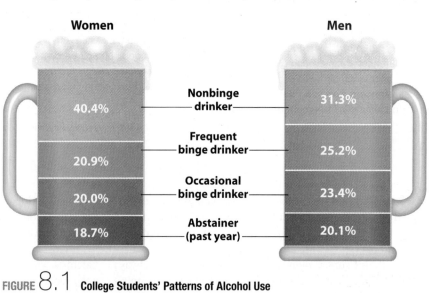

Women		Men
40.4%	Nonbinge drinker	31.3%
20.9%	Frequent binge drinker	25.2%
20.0%	Occasional binge drinker	23.4%
18.7%	Abstainer (past year)	20.1%

FIGURE 8.1 **College Students' Patterns of Alcohol Use**

Source: Data are from H. Wechsler et al., "Trends in College Binge Drinking During a Period of Increased Prevention Efforts: Findings from Four Harvard School of Public Health College Study Surveys: 1993–2001," *Journal of American College Health* 50, no. 5 (2002): 203–17.

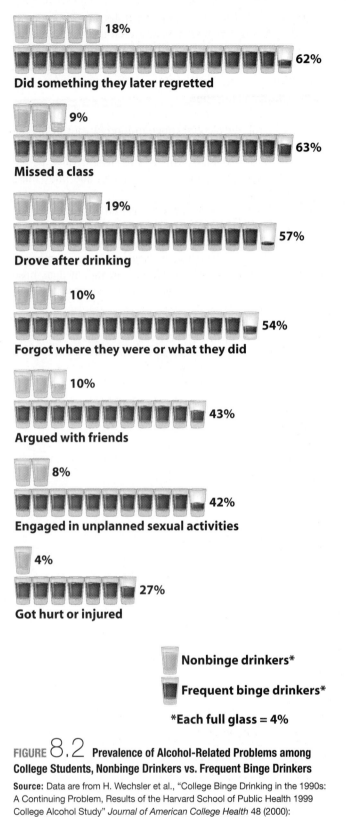

Did something they later regretted — Nonbinge: 18%, Frequent binge: 62%

Missed a class — Nonbinge: 9%, Frequent binge: 63%

Drove after drinking — Nonbinge: 19%, Frequent binge: 57%

Forgot where they were or what they did — Nonbinge: 10%, Frequent binge: 54%

Argued with friends — Nonbinge: 10%, Frequent binge: 43%

Engaged in unplanned sexual activities — Nonbinge: 8%, Frequent binge: 42%

Got hurt or injured — Nonbinge: 4%, Frequent binge: 27%

Nonbinge drinkers*

Frequent binge drinkers*

*Each full glass = 4%

FIGURE 8.2 Prevalence of Alcohol-Related Problems among College Students, Nonbinge Drinkers vs. Frequent Binge Drinkers

Source: Data are from H. Wechsler et al., "College Binge Drinking in the 1990s: A Continuing Problem, Results of the Harvard School of Public Health 1999 College Alcohol Study" *Journal of American College Health* 48 (2000): 199–210.

- Advertising and promotions from the alcoholic beverage industry heavily target university campuses.
- College students are more likely than their noncollegiate peers to drink recklessly and to engage in drinking games and other dangerous drinking practices.

- College students are particularly vulnerable to peer influence and have a strong need to be accepted by their peers.
- College administrators often deny that alcohol problems exist on their campuses.

Binge drinking is especially dangerous because it often involves drinking a lot of alcohol in a very short period of time. This type of consumption can quickly lead to extreme intoxication, involving unconsciousness, alcohol poisoning, and even death. Often, drinking competitions or games and hazing rituals encourage this type of drinking. To see whether your alcohol consumption is a problem, complete the quiz in the **Assess Yourself** box on page 250.

Unfortunately, recent studies confirm what students have been experiencing for a long time—binge drinkers cause problems not only for themselves, but also for those around them. One study indicated that more than 696,000 students between the ages of 18 and 24 were assaulted by another student who had been drinking.[11] Other students report sleep and study disruptions, vandalism of personal property, and sexual abuse and other unwanted sexual advances. There is significant evidence that campus rape is linked to binge drinking. Women from colleges with medium to high binge-drinking rates are 1.5 times more at risk of being raped than those from schools with low binge-drinking rates. Seventy-two percent of campus rapes occur when the victim is so intoxicated that she is unable to either consent or refuse.[12] The laws regarding sexual consent are clear: A person who is drunk or passed out cannot consent to sex. If you have sex with someone who is drunk or unconscious (passed out), you are committing rape. Claiming you were also drunk when you had sex with someone who is intoxicated or unconscious will not absolve you of your legal and moral responsibility for this crime. For more on rape, see Chapter 4.

what do you think?

Why do some college students drink excessive amounts of alcohol? ● Are there particular traditions or norms related to when and why students drink on your campus? ● Have you ever had your sleep or studies interrupted, or have you had to babysit a friend because he or she had been drinking?

Trends in Consumption

In general, alcohol consumption levels among Americans have declined steadily since the late 1970s. In 2007, the estimated per capita consumption was the equivalent of 2.31 gallons of pure alcohol per person.[13] This represents a substantial decline from 2.64 gallons reported for 1977. (This measure is the amount of alcohol that a person would obtain by drinking approximately 50 gallons of beer, 20 gallons of wine, or more than 4 gallons of distilled spirits.)

This downward trend has been tied to a growing attention to weight, personal health, and physical activity. The alcohol industry has responded by introducing beer and wines with fewer calories and carbohydrates and with reduced alcohol content.

Alcohol in the Body

Learning about the amount of alcohol found in different beverages and how alcohol is metabolized and absorbed in the body can help you understand how it affects each person differently. It is also key in understanding how it is possible to drink safely and how to avoid life-threatening circumstances such as alcohol poisoning. This information can be critical for your safety and that of your friends.

The Chemistry and Potency of Alcohol

The intoxicating substance found in beer, wine, liquor, and liqueurs is **ethyl alcohol,** or **ethanol.** It is produced during a process called **fermentation,** in which yeast organisms break down plant sugars, yielding ethanol and carbon dioxide. Manufacturers then add other ingredients that dilute the alcohol content of the beverage. Hard liquor is produced through further processing called **distillation,** during which alcohol vapors are condensed and mixed with water to make the final product.

The **proof** of an alcoholic drink is a measure of the percentage of alcohol in the beverage and therefore the strength of the drink. Alcohol percentage is half of the given proof. For example, 80 proof whiskey or scotch is 40 percent alcohol by volume, and 100 proof vodka is 50 percent alcohol by volume. Lower-proof drinks will produce fewer alcohol effects than the same amount of higher-proof drinks. Most wines are between 12 and 15 percent alcohol, and most beers are between 2 and 8 percent, depending on state laws and type of beer.

When discussing alcohol consumption, researchers usually talk in terms of "standard drinks." As defined by the NIAAA, a **standard drink** is any drink that contains about 14 grams of pure alcohol (about 0.6 fluid ounce or 1.2 tablespoons; see **Figure 8.3**). The actual size of a standard drink depends on the proof: a 12-oz can of beer and a 1.5-oz shot of vodka are both considered one standard drink because they contain the same amount of alcohol—about 0.6 fluid ounce. If you are estimating your blood alcohol concentration using standard drinks as a measure (see the following sections), you need to keep in mind the size of your drinks as well as their proof. For example, you may have bought only one beer while you were at the ballpark last weekend, but if that beer came in a 22-oz glass, then you actually consumed two standard drinks.

ethyl alcohol (ethanol) An addictive drug produced by fermentation and found in many beverages.
fermentation The process whereby yeast organisms break down plant sugars to yield ethanol.
distillation The process whereby mash is subjected to high temperatures to release alcohol vapors, which are then condensed and mixed with water to make the final product.
proof A measure of the percentage of alcohol in a beverage.
standard drink The amount of any beverage that contains about 14 grams of pure alcohol (about 0.6 fluid ounce or 1.2 tablespoons).

Absorption and Metabolism

Unlike the molecules found in most foods and drugs, alcohol molecules are sufficiently small and fat soluble to be absorbed throughout the entire gastrointestinal system. A negligible amount of alcohol is absorbed through the lining of the mouth. Approximately 20 percent of ingested alcohol diffuses through the stomach lining into the bloodstream, and nearly 80 percent passes through the lining of the upper third of the small intestine.

Several factors influence how quickly your body will absorb alcohol: the alcohol concentration in your drink, the amount of alcohol you consume, the amount of food in your stomach, pylorospasm (spasm of the pyloric valve in the digestive system), your metabolism, weight and body mass index, and your mood.

The higher the concentration of alcohol in your drink, the more rapidly it will be absorbed in your digestive tract. As a rule, wine and beer are absorbed more slowly than distilled beverages. "Fizzy" alcoholic beverages—such as champagne and carbonated wines—are absorbed more rapidly than those containing no sparkling additives. Carbonated beverages and

Standard drink equivalent (and % alcohol)		Approximate number of standard drinks in:
	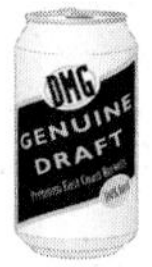 Beer = 12 oz (~5% alcohol)	12 oz = 1 16 oz = 1.3 22 oz = 2 40 oz = 3.3
	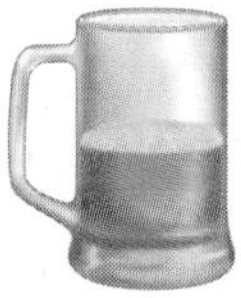 Malt liquor = 8.5 oz (~7% alcohol)	12 oz = 1.5 16 oz = 2 22 oz = 2.5 40 oz = 4.5
	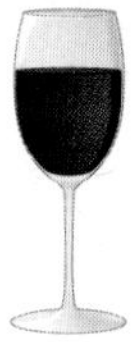 Table wine = 5 oz (~12% alcohol)	750-mL (25-oz) bottle = 5
	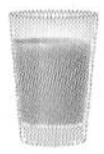 80 proof spirits (gin, vodka, etc.) = 1.5 oz (~40% alcohol)	mixed drink = 1 or more* pint (16 oz) = 11 fifth (25 oz) = 17 1.75 L (59 oz) = 39

FIGURE 8.3 What Is a Standard Drink?
*Note: It can be difficult to estimate the number of standard drinks in a single mixed drink made with hard liquor. Depending on factors such as the type of spirits and the recipe, a mixed drink can contain from one to three or more standard drinks.
Source: Adapted from National Institute on Alcohol Abuse and Alcoholism, *Tips for Cutting Down on Drinking* NIH Publication no. 07–3769, (Bethesda, MD: National Institute of Health, 2007) http://pubs.niaaa.nih.gov/publications/Tips/tips.htm.

drinks served with mixers cause the pyloric valve—the opening from the stomach into the small intestine—to relax, thereby emptying the contents of the stomach more rapidly into the small intestine. Because the small intestine is the site of the greatest absorption of alcohol, carbonated beverages increase the rate of absorption.

The more alcohol you consume, the longer absorption takes. Alcohol can irritate the digestive system, which causes pylorospasm. When the pyloric valve is closed, nothing can move from the stomach to the upper third of the small intestine, which slows absorption. If the irritation continues, it can cause vomiting. Alcohol also takes longer to absorb if there is food in your stomach, because the surface area exposed to alcohol is smaller, and because a full stomach retards the emptying of alcoholic beverages into the small intestine.

Mood is another factor, because emotions affect how long it takes for the contents of the stomach to empty into the intestine. Powerful moods, such as stress and tension, are likely to cause the stomach to dump its contents into the small intestine. That is why alcohol is absorbed much more rapidly when people are tense than when they are relaxed.

Alcohol is metabolized in the liver, where it is converted to *acetaldehyde* by the enzyme *alcohol dehydrogenase.* It is then rapidly oxidized to *acetate,* converted to carbon dioxide and water, and eventually excreted from the body. Acetaldehyde is a toxic chemical that can cause immediate symptoms, such as nausea and vomiting, as well as long-term effects, such as liver damage. A very small portion of alcohol is excreted unchanged by the kidneys, lungs, and skin.

Alcohol contains 7 calories (kcal) per gram (you will learn more about calories in Chapter 9). This means that the average regular beer contains about 150 calories. Mixed drinks may contain more if they are combined with sugary soda or fruit juice. The body uses the calories in alcohol in the same manner it uses those found in carbohydrates: for immediate energy or for storage as fat if not immediately needed.

The breakdown of alcohol occurs at a fairly constant rate of 0.5 ounce per hour (approximately equivalent to one standard drink). This amount of alcohol is equivalent to 12 ounces of 5 percent beer, 5 ounces of 12 percent wine, or 1.5 ounces of 40 percent (80 proof) liquor. Unmetabolized alcohol circulates in the bloodstream until enough time passes for the body to break it down.

Blood Alcohol Concentration

Blood alcohol concentration (BAC) is the ratio of alcohol to total blood volume. It is the factor used to measure the

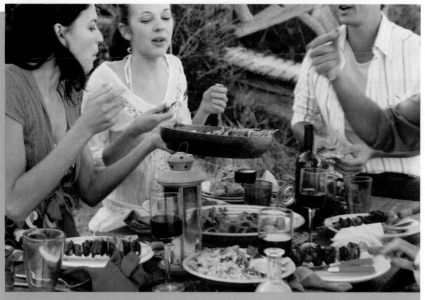

Why do some people feel the effects of alcohol more quickly than others?

Many factors influence how rapidly a person's body absorbs alcohol, and thus how quickly that person feels the effects of the alcohol. For example, eating while drinking slows down the absorption of alcohol into your bloodstream. Other relevant factors include gender, body weight, body composition, and mood.

physiological and behavioral effects of alcohol. Despite individual differences, alcohol produces some general behavioral effects, depending on BAC (see **Figure 8.4** on the next page). At a BAC of 0.02 percent, a person feels slightly relaxed and in a good mood. At 0.05, relaxation increases, there is some motor impairment, and a willingness to talk becomes apparent. At 0.08, the person feels euphoric, and there is further motor impairment. The legal limit for BAC is 0.08 percent in all states and the District of Columbia. At 0.10, the depressant effects of alcohol become apparent, drowsiness sets in, and motor skills are further impaired, followed by a loss of judgment. Thus, a driver may not be able to estimate distance or speed, and some drinkers may do things they would not do when sober. As BAC increases, the drinker suffers increased physiological and psychological effects. All these changes are negative. Alcohol ingestion does not enhance any physical skills or mental functions.

A drinker's BAC depends on weight and body fat, the water content in body tissues, the concentration of alcohol in the beverage consumed, the rate of consumption, and the volume of alcohol consumed. Heavier people have larger body surfaces through which to diffuse alcohol; therefore, they have lower concentrations of alcohol in their blood than do thin people after drinking the same amount. Because alcohol does not diffuse as rapidly into body fat as into water, alcohol concentration is higher in a person with more body fat. Because a woman is likely to have proportionately more body fat and less water in her body tissues than a man of the same weight, she will be more intoxicated than a man after drinking the

blood alcohol concentration (BAC) The ratio of alcohol to total blood volume; the factor used to measure the physiological and behavioral effects of alcohol.

Blood Alcohol Concentration (BAC)	Psychological and Physical Effects
Not Impaired	
<0.01%	Negligible
Sometimes Impaired	
0.01–0.04%	Slight muscle relaxation, mild euphoria, slight body warmth, increased sociability and talkativeness
Usually Impaired	
0.05–0.07%	Lowered alertness, impaired judgment, lowered inhibitions, exaggerated behavior, loss of small muscle control
Always Impaired	
0.08–0.14%	Slowed reaction time, poor muscle coordination, short-term memory loss, judgment impaired, inability to focus
0.15–0.24%	Blurred vision, lack of motor skills, sedation, slowed reactions, difficulty standing and walking, passing out
0.25–0.34%	Impaired consciousness, disorientation, loss of motor function, severely impaired or no reflexes, impaired circulation and respiration, uncontrolled urination, slurred speech, possible death
0.35% and up	Unconsciousness, coma, extremely slow heartbeat and respiration, non-responsiveness, probable death

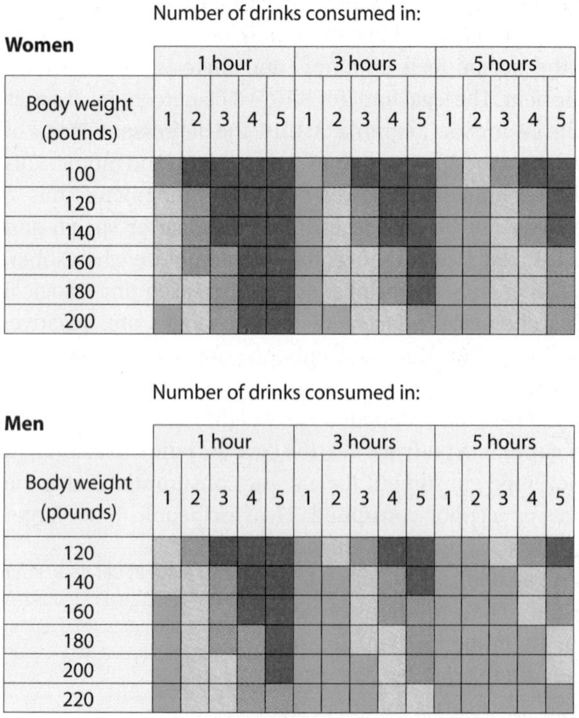

Number of drinks consumed in:

Women

Body weight (pounds)	1 hour					3 hours					5 hours				
	1	2	3	4	5	1	2	3	4	5	1	2	3	4	5
100															
120															
140															
160															
180															
200															

Number of drinks consumed in:

Men

Body weight (pounds)	1 hour					3 hours					5 hours				
	1	2	3	4	5	1	2	3	4	5	1	2	3	4	5
120															
140															
160															
180															
200															
220															

FIGURE 8.4 **Approximate Blood Alcohol Concentration (BAC) and the Physiological and Behavioral Effects**
Remember that there are many variables that can affect BAC, so this is only an estimate of what your BAC would be.

same amount of alcohol See the **Gender & Health** box on page 230 for more on the differences in alcohol's effects on women and men.

Both breath analysis (Breathalyzer tests) and urinalysis are used to determine whether an individual is legally intoxicated, but blood tests are more accurate measures of BAC. An increasing number of states are requiring blood tests for people suspected of driving under the influence of alcohol. In some states, refusal to take the breath or urine test results in immediate revocation of the person's driver's license.

People can acquire physical and psychological tolerance to the effects of alcohol through regular use. The nervous system adapts over time, so greater amounts of alcohol are required to produce the same physiological and psychological effects. Though BAC may be quite high, the individual has learned to modify his behavior to appear sober. This ability is called **learned behavioral tolerance.**

Alcohol and Your Health

The immediate and long-term effects of alcohol consumption can vary greatly (see **Figure 8.5**). Whether or not you experience any immediate or long-term consequences as a result of your alcohol use depends on you as an individual, the amount of alcohol you consume, and your circumstances.

Immediate and Short-Term Effects of Alcohol

The most dramatic effects produced by ethanol occur within the central nervous system (CNS). Alcohol depresses CNS functions, which decreases respiratory rate, pulse rate, and blood pressure. As CNS depression deepens, vital functions become noticeably affected. In extreme cases, coma and death can result.

Alcohol is a diuretic that causes increased urinary output. Although this effect might be expected to lead to automatic **dehydration** (loss of water), the body actually retains water, most of it in the muscles or in the cerebral tissues. The reason is that water is usually pulled out of the *cerebrospinal fluid* (fluid within the brain and spinal cord). This results in symptoms that include the "morning-after" headaches some drinkers suffer.

Alcohol irritates the gastrointestinal system and may cause indigestion and heartburn if taken on an empty stomach. In addition, people who engage in brief drinking sprees during which they consume unusually high amounts of alcohol put themselves at risk for irregular heartbeat or even total loss of heart rhythm, which can disrupt blood flow and damage the heart muscle.

Hangover A **hangover** is often experienced the morning after a drinking spree. The symptoms of a hangover are familiar to most people who drink: headache, muscle aches, upset stomach, anxiety, depression, diarrhea, and thirst. **Congeners,** forms of alcohol that are metabolized more

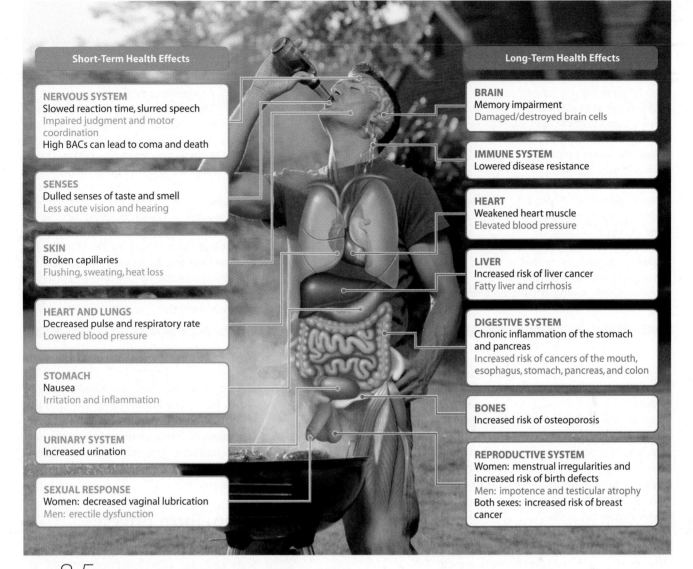

Short-Term Health Effects	Long-Term Health Effects

NERVOUS SYSTEM
Slowed reaction time, slurred speech
Impaired judgment and motor coordination
High BACs can lead to coma and death

SENSES
Dulled senses of taste and smell
Less acute vision and hearing

SKIN
Broken capillaries
Flushing, sweating, heat loss

HEART AND LUNGS
Decreased pulse and respiratory rate
Lowered blood pressure

STOMACH
Nausea
Irritation and inflammation

URINARY SYSTEM
Increased urination

SEXUAL RESPONSE
Women: decreased vaginal lubrication
Men: erectile dysfunction

BRAIN
Memory impairment
Damaged/destroyed brain cells

IMMUNE SYSTEM
Lowered disease resistance

HEART
Weakened heart muscle
Elevated blood pressure

LIVER
Increased risk of liver cancer
Fatty liver and cirrhosis

DIGESTIVE SYSTEM
Chronic inflammation of the stomach and pancreas
Increased risk of cancers of the mouth, esophagus, stomach, pancreas, and colon

BONES
Increased risk of osteoporosis

REPRODUCTIVE SYSTEM
Women: menstrual irregularities and increased risk of birth defects
Men: impotence and testicular atrophy
Both sexes: increased risk of breast cancer

FIGURE 8.5 **Effects of Alcohol on the Body and Health**

slowly than ethanol and are more toxic, are thought to play a role in the development of a hangover. The body metabolizes the congeners after the ethanol is gone from the system, and their toxic by-products may contribute to the hangover. Alcohol also upsets the water balance in the body, which results in excess urination, dehydration, and thirst the next day. Increased production of hydrochloric acid can irritate the stomach lining and cause nausea. It usually takes 12 hours to recover from a hangover. Bed rest, solid food, and aspirin may help relieve a hangover's discomforts, but the only sure way to avoid one is to abstain from excessive alcohol use in the first place. Drinking less and drinking slowly, and consuming water or other nonalcoholic beverages between drinks, will also help in avoiding a hangover.

Alcohol and Injuries Alcohol use plays a significant role in the types of injuries people experience. Thirteen percent of emergency room visits by undergraduates are related to alcohol; of this total, 34 percent are the result of acute intoxication. A recent study found that injured patients with a BAC over 0.08 percent who were treated in emergency rooms were 3.2 times more likely to have a violent intentional injury than an unintentional injury.[14] Most people admitted to emergency rooms are men 21 years or older, mostly as the result of accidents or fights where alcohol was involved.[15]

Alcohol and Sexual Decision Making Alcohol has a clear influence on one's ability to make good decisions about sex, because it lowers inhibitions, and you may do things you

learned behavioral tolerance The ability of heavy drinkers to modify behavior so that they appear to be sober even when they have high BAC levels.

dehydration Loss of fluids from body tissues.

hangover The physiological reaction to excessive drinking, including symptoms such as headache, upset stomach, anxiety, depression, diarrhea, and thirst.

congeners Forms of alcohol that are metabolized more slowly than ethanol and produce toxic by-products.

Women and Alcohol

Body fat is not the only contributor to the differences in alcohol's effects on men and women. Compared with men, women have half as much *alcohol dehydro-genase,* the enzyme that breaks down alcohol in the stomach before it reaches the blood-stream and the brain. Therefore, if a man and a woman drink the same amount of alcohol, the woman's BAC will be approximately 30 percent higher than the man's, leaving her more vulnerable to slurred speech, careless driving, and other drinking-related impairments.

Cosmopolitans and other drinks popular among women may be sweet and fruity, but the alcohol in them still packs a punch.

Hormonal differences can also affect a woman's BAC. Certain times in the menstrual cycle and the use of oral contraceptives are likely to contribute to longer periods of intoxication. This prolonged peak appears to be related to estrogen levels.

Women who consume alcohol need to pay close atten-tion to how much they drink. A woman matching her male friend drink for drink could become twice as intoxicated. For example, if a 180-pound college-aged man and a 120-pound college-aged woman each have three drinks within 1 hour, the BAC for the male would be 0.06 percent and for the female 0.11 percent, almost double that of her male friend.

---

might not do when sober. Students who are intoxicated are less likely to use safer sex practices and are more likely to engage in high-risk sexual activity. The chance of acquiring a sexually transmitted infection or experiencing an unplanned pregnancy also increases among students who drink more heavily, compared with those who drink moderately or not at all.

Alcohol Poisoning Alcohol poisoning oc-curs much more frequently than people realize, and all too often it can be fatal. Drinking large amounts of alcohol in a short period of time can cause the blood alcohol level to quickly reach the lethal range. Alcohol, used either alone or in combination with other drugs, is responsible for more toxic overdose deaths than any other substance.

The amount of alcohol that causes a person to lose con-sciousness is dangerously close to the lethal dose. Death from alcohol poisoning can be caused by either CNS and respiratory depression or by the inhalation of vomit or fluid into the lungs. Alcohol depresses the nerves that control involuntary actions such as breathing and the gag reflex (which prevents choking). As BAC levels reach higher concentrations, eventually these functions can be completely suppressed. If a drinker becomes unconscious and vomits, there is a danger of asphyxiation, through choking to death on one's own vomit. It is important to realize that blood alcohol concentration can continue rising even after a drinker becomes unconscious, because alcohol in the stomach and intestine continues to empty into the blood-stream. Signs of alcohol poisoning include inability to be roused; a weak, rapid pulse; an unusual or irregular breathing

70%
of college students admit to having engaged in sexual activity primarily as a result of being under the influence of alcohol.

pattern; and cool (possibly damp), pale, or bluish skin. If you are with someone who has been drinking heavily and who exhibits these symptoms, or if you are unsure about the per-son's condition, call your local emergency number (911 in most areas) for immediate assistance.

Long-Term Effects

Alcohol is distributed throughout most of the body and may affect many organs and tis-sues. Problems associated with long-term, habitual use of alcohol include diseases of the nervous system, cardiovascu-lar system, and liver, as well as some cancers.

Effects on the Nervous System The nervous system is especially sensitive to alcohol. Even people who drink moderately experience shrinkage in brain size and weight and a loss of some degree of intellectual ability.

Research suggests that developing brains in adolescents are much more prone to brain damage than was previously thought. Alcohol appears to damage the frontal areas of the adolescent brain, which are crucial for controlling impulses and thinking through consequences of intended actions.[16] In addition, researchers suggest that people who begin drink-ing at an early age face enormous risks of becoming alcoholics: 47 percent of people who begin drinking alcohol before age 14 become alcohol dependent at some time in their lives, com-pared with 9 percent of those who wait until at least age 21.[17]

Cardiovascular Effects Alcohol affects the cardiovascular system in a number of ways. Numerous studies have associated light to moderate alcohol consumption (no more than 2 drinks a day) with a reduced risk of coronary artery disease. Several mechanisms have been proposed to explain how this might happen. The strongest evidence points to an increase in high-density lipoprotein (HDL) cholesterol, which is known as "good" cholesterol. Studies have shown that moderate drinkers have higher levels of HDL.

However, alcohol consumption is not a preventive measure against heart disease—it causes many more cardiovascular health hazards than benefits. Alcohol contributes to high blood pressure and slightly increased heart rate and cardiac output. People who report drinking three to five drinks a day, regardless of race or sex, have higher blood pressure than those who drink less.

Liver Disease One of the most common diseases related to alcohol abuse is **cirrhosis** of the liver (Figure 8.6). It is among the leading 12 causes of death in the United States. One result of heavy drinking is that the liver begins to store fat—a condition known as *fatty liver*. If there is insufficient time between drinking episodes, this fat cannot be transported to storage sites, and the fat-filled liver cells stop functioning. Continued drinking can cause a further stage of liver deterioration called *fibrosis,* in which the damaged area of the liver develops fibrous scar tissue. Cell function can be partially restored at this stage with proper nutrition and abstinence from alcohol. If the person continues to drink, however, cirrhosis results. At this point, the liver cells die, and the damage becomes permanent. **Alcoholic hepatitis** is a serious condition resulting from prolonged use of alcohol. A chronic inflammation of the liver develops, which may be fatal in itself or progress to cirrhosis.

Cancer Alcohol is considered a carcinogen. The repeated irritation caused by long-term use of alcohol has been linked to cancers of the esophagus, stomach, mouth, tongue, and liver. There is substantial evidence that women consuming high levels of alcohol (more than three drinks per day) have a higher risk of breast cancer compared with abstainers.[18]

Other Effects Alcohol abuse is a major cause of chronic inflammation of the pancreas, the organ that produces digestive enzymes and insulin. Chronic abuse of alcohol inhibits enzyme production, which further inhibits the absorption of nutrients. Drinking alcohol can block the absorption of calcium, a nutrient that strengthens bones. This should be of particular concern to women because of their risk for osteoporosis; bone thinning and calcium loss increase with age (see Chapter 14). Heavy consumption of alcohol worsens this condition.

Evidence also suggests that alcohol impairs the body's ability to recognize and fight foreign bodies, such as bacteria and viruses. The relationship between alcohol and AIDS is unclear, especially because some of the populations at risk for AIDS are also at risk for alcohol abuse. But any stressor, including alcohol, with a known effect on the immune system would probably contribute to the development of the disease.

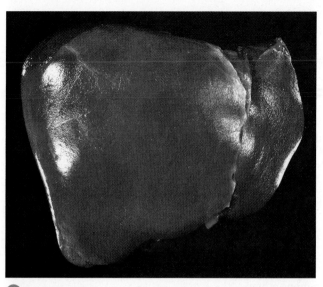

a A normal liver

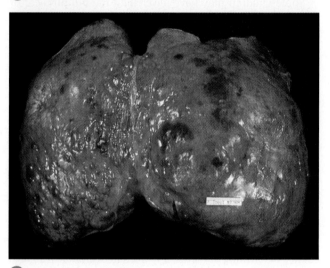

b A liver with cirrhosis

FIGURE 8.6 **Comparison of a Healthy Liver with a Cirrhotic Liver** In cirrhosis, healthy liver cells are replaced with scar tissue that interferes with the liver's ability to perform its many vital functions.

Alcohol and Pregnancy

Recall from Chapter 6 that *teratogenic* substances cause birth defects. Of the 30 known teratogens in the environment, alcohol is one of the most dangerous and common. If a woman ingests alcohol while pregnant, it will pass through the placenta and enter the growing fetus's bloodstream. More than 10 percent of all children have been exposed to high levels of alcohol in utero. All will suffer varying degrees of effects, ranging from mild learning disabilities to major physical, mental, and intellectual impairment. Alcohol consumed during the first trimester

cirrhosis The last stage of liver disease associated with chronic heavy use of alcohol, during which liver cells die and damage becomes permanent.
alcoholic hepatitis Condition resulting from prolonged use of alcohol, in which the liver is inflamed; can be fatal.

poses the greatest threat to organ development; exposure during the last trimester, when the brain is developing rapidly, is most likely to affect CNS development.

A disorder called **fetal alcohol syndrome (FAS)** is associated with alcohol consumption during pregnancy. FAS is the third most common birth defect and the second leading cause of mental retardation in the United States, with an estimated incidence of 1 to 2 in every 1,000 live births. It is the most common preventable cause of mental impairment in the Western world. Among the symptoms of FAS are mental retardation, small head, tremors, and abnormalities of the face, limbs, heart, and brain. Children with FAS may experience problems such as poor memory and impaired learning, reduced attention span, impulsive behavior, and poor problem-solving abilities, among others.

fetal alcohol syndrome (FAS) A disorder involving physical and mental impairment that may affect the fetus when the mother consumes alcohol during pregnancy.

Some children may have fewer than the full physical or behavioral symptoms of FAS, and may be diagnosed with disorders such as partial fetal alcohol syndrome (PFAS) or alcohol-related neurodevelopmental disorder (ARND); all of these disorders (including FAS) fall under the umbrella term *fetal alcohol spectrum disorders* (FASD). An estimated 40,000 infants in the United States are affected by FASD each year—more than those affected by spina bifida, Down syndrome, and muscular dystrophy combined.[19] Infants whose mothers habitually consumed more than 3 ounces of alcohol (approximately six drinks) in a short time period when pregnant are at high risk for FASD. Risk levels for babies whose mothers consume smaller amounts are uncertain. To avoid any chance of harming her fetus, any woman of childbearing age who is or may become pregnant is advised to refrain from consuming any amount of alcohol.

Drinking and Driving

Traffic accidents are the leading cause of death for all age groups from 5 to 45 years old (including college students). Approximately 32 percent of all traffic fatalities in 2008 involved at least one alcohol-impaired driver (having a BAC of 0.08 percent or higher).[20] Unfortunately, college students are overrepresented in alcohol-related crashes. Surveys report more than 2.8 million college students, or 31.4 percent, have driven under the influence of alcohol.

In the United States in 2008, there were 11,773 alcohol-impaired driving fatalities. This number represents an average of one alcohol-related fatality approximately every 45 minutes.[21] Over the past 20 years, the percentage of drivers involved in fatal crashes who were intoxicated decreased for all age groups (Figure 8.7). Several factors probably contributed to these reductions in fatalities: laws that raised the drinking age to 21; stricter law enforcement; increased

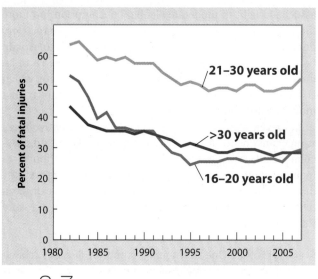

FIGURE 8.7 **Percentage of Fatally Injured Passenger Vehicle Drivers with BACs > 0.08 Percent, by Driver Age**

Source: Insurance Institute for Highway Safety, "Fatality Facts 2007: Alcohol," 2009, www.iihs.org/research/fatality_facts_2007/alcohol.html.

emphasis on zero tolerance (laws prohibiting anyone under 21 from driving with any detectable BAC); and educational programs designed to discourage drinking and driving. Furthermore, all states have zero-tolerance laws for driving while intoxicated, and the penalty is usually suspension of the driver's license.

Despite all these measures, the risk of being involved in an alcohol-related automobile crash remains substantial. Laboratory and test track research shows that the vast majority of drivers are impaired even at 0.08 BAC with regard to critical driving tasks. Braking, steering, lane changing, judgment, and ability to divide attention, among other measures, are all affected significantly at 0.08 percent BAC. Researchers have shown a direct relationship between the amount of alcohol in a driver's bloodstream and the likelihood of a crash. A driver with a BAC of 0.10 percent is approximately ten times more likely to be involved in a car accident than a driver who has not been drinking.

Driving after drinking can lead to disaster.

Alcohol-related fatal crashes occur more often at night than during the day; the hours between midnight and 3:00 AM are the most dangerous. Seventy-five percent of fatally injured drivers involved in nighttime single-vehicle crashes had detectable levels of alcohol in their

3 in 10

Americans will be involved in an alcohol-related accident at some time in their lives.

blood.[22] The risk of being involved in an alcohol-related crash also increases with the day of the week. In 2008, 25 percent of all fatal crashes during the week were alcohol related, compared with 49 percent on weekends.[23] For a driver with a BAC of 0.15 percent on weekend nights, the likelihood of dying in a single-vehicle crash is more than 382 times higher than for a nondrinker.

what do you think?

What do you think the legal BAC for drivers should be? ● What should the penalty be for people arrested for driving under the influence of alcohol (DUI) for the first offense? The second offense?

Alcohol Abuse and Alcoholism

Alcohol use becomes **alcohol abuse** when it interferes with work, school, or social and family relationships, or when it entails any violation of the law, including driving under the influence (DUI). **Alcoholism,** or **alcohol dependence,** results when personal and health problems related to alcohol use are severe, and stopping alcohol use results in withdrawal symptoms. Approximately 8 million Americans can be described as alcohol dependent.

Identifying a Problem Drinker

As with other drug addictions, tolerance, psychological dependence, and withdrawal symptoms must be present to qualify a drinker as an addict (see Chapter 7). Irresponsible and problem drinkers, such as people who get into fights or embarrass themselves or others when they drink, are not necessarily alcoholics. Alcoholics can be found at all socioeconomic levels and in all professions, ethnic groups, geographical locations, religions, and races. Studies suggest that the lifetime risk of alcoholism in the United States is about 10 percent for men and 3 percent for women.[24]

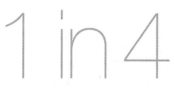

1 in 4 Americans is affected by the alcoholism of a friend or family member.

Recognizing and admitting the existence of an alcohol problem is often extremely difficult. Alcoholics themselves deny their problem, often making statements such as, "I can stop any time I want to. I just don't want to right now." Their families also tend to deny the problem, saying things like, "He really has been under a lot of stress lately. Besides, he only drinks beer." The fear of being labeled a "problem drinker" often prevents people from seeking help.

Alcoholism is characterized by several symptoms, including craving, loss of control, physical dependence, and tolerance. People who recognize one or more of these behaviors in themselves may wish to seek professional help to determine whether alcohol has become a controlling factor in their lives. (The **Skills for Behavior Change** box on page 234 gives tips for cutting down on drinking.)

One study has shown that 6 percent of college students meet the criteria for a diagnosis of alcohol dependence, and 31 percent meet the criteria for alcohol abuse. Students who attend colleges with heavy drinking environments are more likely to be diagnosed with abuse or dependence. Despite the prevalence of alcohol disorders on campus, very few students seek treatment.

Alcohol and Prescription Drug Abuse

Recent studies have shown that men and women with alcohol use disorders are 18 times more likely to report nonmedical use of prescription drugs than people who do not drink at all. Young adults aged 18 to 24 are at most risk for concurrent or simultaneous abuse of both alcohol and drugs. In a study of college students, it was revealed that in the past year, 12 percent had used both alcohol and prescription drugs nonmedically but at different times, and 7 percent had taken them simultaneously.[25] When alcohol and prescription drugs are taken together, severe medical problems can result, including alcohol poisoning, unconsciousness, respiratory depression, and death. The study reported that college students who took prescription drugs while drinking were more likely than those who drank without taking drugs to black out, vomit, and engage in other risky behaviors such as drunk driving and unplanned sex. The prescription drugs that are most commonly combined with alcohol include opioids (e.g., Vicodin, OxyContin, Percocet), stimulants (e.g., Ritalin, Adderall, Concerta), sedative/anxiety medications (e.g., Ativan, Xanax), and sleeping medications (e.g., Ambien, Halcion).

alcohol abuse Use of alcohol that interferes with work, school, or personal relationships or that entails violations of the law.

alcoholism (alcohol dependence) Condition in which personal and health problems related to alcohol use are severe and stopping alcohol use results in withdrawal symptoms.

The Causes of Alcohol Abuse and Alcoholism

We know that alcoholism is a disease with biological and social/environmental components, but we do not know what role each component plays in the disease.

Biological and Family Factors Research into the hereditary and environmental causes of alcoholism has found higher rates of alcoholism among children of alcoholics than in the general population. In fact, alcoholism is four to five times more common among children of alcoholics. These children may be strongly influenced by their parents' behavior.[26]

Despite evidence of heredity's role in alcoholism, scientists do not yet understand the precise role of genes and

Cut Down on Your Drinking

If you suspect that you drink too much, talk with a counselor or a clinician at your student health center. Your counselor or clinician will advise you about what is right for you. If you have a severe drinking problem, alcoholism in your family, or other medical problems, you should stop drinking completely; if you need to cut down on your drinking, these steps can help you:

✳ *Write your reasons for cutting down or stopping.* You may want to improve your health, sleep better, or get along better with your family or friends.

✳ *Set a drinking goal.* Determine a limit for how much you will drink. If you aren't sure what goal is right for you, talk with your counselor. Once you determine your goal, write it down and put it where you can see it, such as on your refrigerator or bathroom mirror.

✳ *Keep a diary of your drinking.* Write down every time you have a drink. Try to keep your diary for 3 or 4 weeks. This will show you how much you drink and when.

✳ *Keep little or no alcohol at home.* You don't need the temptation.

✳ *Drink slowly.* When you drink, sip slowly. Take a break of 1 hour between drinks. Drink a nonalcoholic beverage after every alcoholic drink you consume.

✳ *Learn how to say no.* You do not have to drink when other people are, or take a drink when offered one. Practice ways to say no politely. Stay away from people who give you a hard time about not drinking.

✳ *Stay active.* Use the time and money once spent on drinking to do something fun with your family or friends.

✳ *Get support.* Ask your family and friends for support to help you reach your goal. Talk to your counselor if you are having trouble cutting down.

✳ *Avoid temptations.* Watch out for people, places, or times that make you drink, even if you do not want to. Plan ahead of time what you will do to avoid drinking when you are tempted.

✳ *Remember, don't give up!* Most people don't cut down or give up drinking all at once. If you don't reach your goal the first time, try again. Remember, get support from people who care about you and want to help.

increased risk for alcoholism, nor have they identified a specific "alcoholism" gene. Studies of identical twins (twins who share the same genes) and fraternal twins (who share about half of their genes, like other siblings) suggest that heredity, in both men and women, accounts for two-thirds of the risk for becoming alcoholic.[27]

Social and Cultural Factors Social and cultural factors may trigger the affliction for many people who are not genetically predisposed to alcoholism. Some people begin drinking as a way to dull the pain of an acute loss or an emotional or social problem. For example, college students may drink to escape the stress of college life; disappointment over unfulfilled expectations; difficulties in forming relationships; or loss of the security of home, loved ones, and close friends. Involvement in a painful relationship, death of a family member, and other problems may trigger a search for an anesthetic. Unfortunately, the emotional discomfort that causes many people to turn to alcohol also ultimately causes them to become even more uncomfortable as the depressant effect of the drug begins to take its toll. Thus, the person who is already depressed may become even more depressed, antagonizing friends and other social supports. Eventually, the drinker becomes physically dependent on the drug.

Family attitudes toward alcohol also seem to influence whether a person will develop a drinking problem. It has been clearly demonstrated that people who are raised in cultures in which drinking is a part of religious or ceremonial activities or in which alcohol is a traditional part of the family meal are less prone to alcohol dependence. In contrast, in societies in which alcohol purchase is carefully controlled and drinking is regarded as a rite of passage to adulthood, the tendency for abuse appears to be greater.

Apparently, then, some combination of heredity and environment plays a decisive role in the development of alcoholism. The **Health in a Diverse World** box on the next page discusses some of the patterns of alcohol use and abuse among different racial and ethnic groups.

Costs to Society

Alcohol-related costs to society are estimated to be well over $185 billion when health insurance, criminal justice costs, treatment costs, and lost productivity are factored in. Reportedly, alcoholism is directly or indirectly responsible for over 25 percent of the nation's medical expenses and lost earnings.[28] A recent study estimated that underage drinking alone costs society $61.9 billion annually. These costs take into consideration vehicle crashes, violence, property crime, suicide, burns, drowning, fetal alcohol syndrome, high-risk sex, poisoning, psychosis, and treatments for alcohol dependence. The largest costs were related to violence ($34.7 billion) and drunken driving accidents ($13.5 billion), followed by high-risk sex (nearly $5 billion), property crime ($3 billion), and addiction treatment programs (nearly $2 billion). By dividing the cost of underage drinking by the estimated number of underage drinkers, the study estimated that every underage drinker costs society an average of $4,680 a year.[29]

Women and Alcoholism

Studies indicate that there are now almost as many female as male alcoholics. Women tend to become alcoholic at a later age and after fewer years of heavy drinking than do male alcoholics. Women get addicted faster with less alcohol use and then suffer the consequences more profoundly. Women

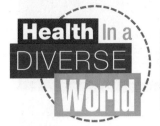

Health In a DIVERSE World

Alcohol and Ethnic or Racial Differences

Different ethnic and racial minority groups have their own patterns of alcohol consumption and abuse. Social or cultural factors, such as drinking norms and attitudes and, in some cases, genetic factors, may account for those differences. Better understanding of ethnic and racial differences in alcohol use patterns and factors that influence alcohol use can help guide the development of culturally appropriate prevention and treatment programs.

Among Native American populations, alcohol is the most widely used drug; the rate of alcoholism in this population is two to three times higher than the national average, and the death rate from alcohol-related causes is eight times higher than the national average. Poor economic conditions and the cultural belief that alcoholism is a spiritual problem, not a physical disease may partially account for high rates of alcoholism in this group.

African American and Latino populations also exhibit distinct patterns of abuse. On average, African Americans drink less than white Americans; however, those who do drink tend to be heavy drinkers. Among Latinos, men have a higher than average rate of alcohol abuse and alcohol-related health problems.

In contrast, many Latino women abstain. Many researchers agree that a major factor for alcohol problems in this ethnic group is the key role that drinking plays in Latino culture.

Asian Americans have a very low rate of alcoholism. Social and cultural influences, such as strong kinship ties, are thought to discourage heavy drinking in Asian groups. Asians also have a genetic predisposition that might influence their low risk for alcohol abuse: Many possess a variant of the gene coding the enzyme aldehyde dehydrogenase, which plays a key role in the metabolism of alcohol. People with this variant gene experience unpleasant side effects from

consuming alcohol, making drinking a less pleasurable experience. Because of the presence of this gene, Asian populations tend to consume less alcohol and have lower rates of alcoholism than do other ethnic groups.

Sources: Substance Abuse and Mental Health Services Administration, "Results from the 2007 National Survey on Drug Use and Health: National Findings," NSDUH Series H-34, DHHS Publication no. SMA 08-4343 (Rockville, MD: Office of Applied Studies, U.S. Department of Health and Human Services, 2008); F. H. Galvan et al., "Alcohol Use and Related Problems among Ethnic Minorities in the United States," *Alcohol and Health Research* 27, no. 1 (2003): 87–94; T. Wall and C. Ehlers, "Genetic Influences Affecting Alcohol Use among Asians," *Alcohol Health and Research World* 19, no. 3 (1995): 184–89.

Prevalence of Alcohol Abuse or Dependence by Ethnicity

Ethnic Group	Percent of Total Population
Whites	9.4
African Americans	8.5
Native Americans/Alaska Natives	13.4
Native Hawaiians/other Pacific Islanders	9.9
Asian Americans	4.7
Persons reporting two or more races	10.8

alcoholics have death rates 50 to 100 percent higher than male alcoholics, including deaths from suicide, alcohol-related accidents, heart disease and stroke, and cirrhosis.[30]

Women at highest risk are those who are unmarried but living with a partner, are in their twenties or early thirties, or have a husband or partner who drinks heavily. Other risk factors for drinking problems among *all women* include a family history of drinking problems, pressure to drink from a peer or spouse, depression, and stress.

It is estimated that only 14 percent of women who need treatment get it. In one study, women cited the following reasons for not seeking treatment: potential loss of income, not wanting others to know they may have a problem, inability to pay for treatment, and fear that treatment would not be confidential.[31]

Recovery

Despite growing recognition of our national alcohol problem, fewer than 10 percent of alcoholics in the United States receive any care. Factors contributing to this low figure include inability or unwillingness to admit to an alcohol problem; the social stigma attached to alcoholism; breakdowns in referral and delivery systems (failure of physicians or psychotherapists to follow up on referrals, failure of clients to follow through with recommended treatments, or failure of rehabilitation facilities to give quality care); and failure of

what do you think?

Why do you think women appear to be drinking more heavily today than they did in the past? ● Does society look at men's and women's drinking habits in the same way? ● Can you think of ways to increase support for women in their recovery process?

the professional medical establishment to recognize and diagnose alcoholic symptoms among patients.

Most problem drinkers who seek help have experienced a turning point: A spouse walks out, taking children and possessions; the boss issues an ultimatum to dry out or ship out. Devoid of hope, physically depleted, and spiritually despairing, the alcoholic finally recognizes that alcohol controls his or her life. The first steps on the road to recovery are to regain that control and to assume responsibility for personal actions.

The Family's Role in Recovery

Members of an alcoholic's family sometimes take action before the alcoholic does. They may go to an organization or a treatment facility to seek help for themselves and their relative. An effective method of helping an alcoholic to confront the disease is a process called **intervention.** Essentially, an intervention is a planned confrontation with the alcoholic that involves several family members and friends plus professional counselors. Family members express their love and concern, telling the alcoholic that they will no longer refrain from acknowledging the problem and affirming their support for appropriate treatment.

Treatment Programs

The alcoholic who is ready for help has several avenues of treatment: psychologists and psychiatrists specializing in the treatment of alcoholism, private treatment centers, hospitals specifically designed to treat alcoholics, community mental health facilities, and support groups such as **Alcoholics Anonymous (AA).**

Private Treatment Facilities Upon admission to a private treatment facility, the patient receives a complete physical exam to determine whether underlying medical problems will interfere with treatment.

Alcoholics who decide to quit drinking will experience *detoxification,* the process by which addicts end their dependence on a drug. Withdrawal symptoms include hyperexcitability, confusion and agitation, sleep disorders, convulsions, tremors of the hands, depression, headache, and seizures. For a small percentage of people, alcohol withdrawal results in a severe syndrome known as **delirium tremens (DTs),** characterized by confusion, delusions, agitated behavior, and hallucinations.

Shortly after detoxification, alcoholics begin their treatment for psychological addiction. Most treatment facilities keep their patients from 3 to 6 weeks. Treatment at private treatment centers costs several thousand dollars, but some insurance programs or employers will assume most of this expense.

intervention A planned confrontation with an alcoholic in which family members, friends, and professional counselors express their concern about the alcoholic's drinking.

Alcoholics Anonymous (AA) An organization whose goal is to help alcoholics stop drinking; includes auxiliary branches such as Al-Anon and Alateen.

delirium tremens (DTs) A state of confusion and delusions brought on by withdrawal from alcohol.

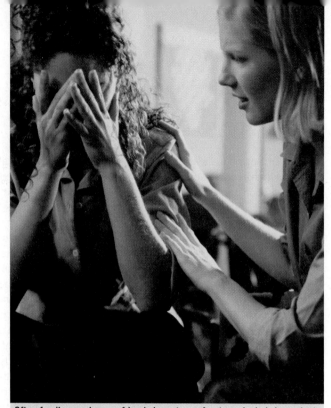

Often family members or friends have to confront an alcohol-dependent person to help him or her take the first steps toward recovery.

Therapy Several types of therapy, including family therapy, individual therapy, and group therapy, are commonly used in alcoholism recovery programs. In family therapy, the person and family members gradually examine the psychological reasons underlying the addiction. In individual and group therapy with fellow addicts, alcoholics learn positive coping skills for situations that have regularly caused them to turn to alcohol.

On some college campuses, the problems associated with alcohol abuse are so great that student health centers are opening their own treatment programs. For example, the University of Texas offers a support service called Complete Recovery 101, and at other schools students in recovery live together in special housing. Because it can be difficult to recover from an alcohol abuse problem in college, support programs such as these hope to offer the support and comfortable environment recovering students need.

Relapse

Success in recovery varies with the individual. Roughly 60 percent of alcoholics relapse (resume drinking) within the first 3 months of treatment. Why is the relapse rate so high? Treating an addiction requires more than getting the addict to stop using a substance; it also requires getting the person to break a pattern of behavior that has dominated his or her life. Many alcoholics refer to themselves as "recovering" throughout their lifetime; they never use the word *cured.*

People who are seeking to regain a healthy lifestyle must not only confront their addiction, but also guard against the tendency to relapse. Drinkers with compulsive personalities need to learn to understand themselves and take control. To be effective, a recovery program must offer the alcoholic ways to increase self-esteem and resume personal growth.

Tobacco Use in the United States

Tobacco use is the single most preventable cause of death in the United States: Nearly 438,000 Americans die each year of tobacco-related diseases.[32] This is 50 times as many that will die from all illegal drugs combined. Moreover, another 10 million people will suffer from health disorders caused by tobacco. To date, tobacco is known to cause about 25 diseases, and about half of all regular smokers die of smoking-related diseases.

In 1991, the Youth Risk Assessment Survey, which includes students in grades 9 through 12, indicated that 27.5 percent of teenagers smoked; by 2005, 23 percent were current smokers, indicating a downward trend among adolescent smokers.[33] Every day, another 3,600 teens under the age of 18 smoke their first cigarette, and more than 1,100 others become daily smokers.[34] Cigarette use among teens is attributed to the ready availability of tobacco products through vending machines and the aggressive drive by tobacco companies to entice young people to smoke.

Tobacco and Social Issues

The production and distribution of tobacco products involve many political and economic issues. Tobacco-growing states derive substantial income from tobacco production, and federal, state, and local governments benefit enormously from cigarette taxes. More recently, nationwide health awareness has led to a decrease in the use of tobacco products among U.S. adults. Table 8.1 shows the percentages of Americans who smoke, by demographic group.

Advertising The tobacco industry spends an estimated $36 million per day on advertising and promotional material.[35] Campaigns are directed at all age, social, and ethnic groups, but because children and teenagers constitute 90 percent of all new smokers, much of the advertising has been directed toward them. Evidence of product recognition among underage smokers is clear: 86 percent of underage smokers prefer one of the three most heavily advertised brands—Marlboro, Newport, or Camel.

Advertisements in women's magazines imply that smoking is the key to financial success, independence, and social acceptance. These ads have apparently been working. From the mid-1970s through the early 2000s, cigarette sales to women increased dramatically. Not coincidentally, by 1987 cigarette-induced lung cancer had surpassed breast cancer as the leading cancer killer among women.

Women are not the only targets of gender-based cigarette advertisements. Men are depicted in locker rooms, charging over rugged terrain in off-road vehicles, or riding stallions into the sunset in blatant appeals to a need to feel and appear masculine. Minorities are also often targeted. Recent studies have shown a higher concentration of tobacco advertising in magazines aimed at African Americans, such as *Jet* and *Ebony*, than in similar magazines aimed at broader audiences, such as *Time* and *People*. Billboards and posters aiming the cigarette message at Hispanics have dotted the landscape and store windows in Hispanic communities for many years, especially in low-income areas. Recent innovations by tobacco companies have included sponsorship of community-based events such as festivals and annual fairs.

Financial Costs to Society The use of tobacco products is costly to all of us in terms of lost productivity and lost lives. Estimates show that tobacco use causes more than $193 billion in annual health-related economic losses. The economic burden of tobacco use totals more than $96 billion in medical expenditures (costs include hospital, physician, and nursing home expenses; prescription drugs; and home health care

TABLE 8.1	Percentage of Population That Smokes (Age 18 and Older) among Select Groups in the United States

	Percent
United States overall	19.8
Race	
Native American	36.4
Asian	9.6
Black, non-Hispanic	19.8
Hispanic	13.3
White, non-Hispanic	21.4
Age	
18–24	22.2
25–44	22.8
45–64	21.0
65+	8.3
Sex	
Male	22.3
Female	17.5
Education	
Undergraduate	11.4
Some college	20.9
High school	23.7
9–11 years	33.3
Income Level	
Below poverty level	28.2
At or above poverty level	20.3

Source: Centers for Disease Control, and Prevention, "Cigarette Smoking among Adults—United States, 2007," *Morbidity and Mortality Weekly Report* 57, no. 45 (2008): 1221–26.

expenditures) and $97 billion in indirect costs (absenteeism, added cost of fire insurance, training costs to replace employees who die prematurely, disability payments, and so on).[36]

College Students and Tobacco Use

College students are the targets of heavy tobacco marketing and advertising campaigns. The tobacco industry has set up aggressive marketing promotions at bars, music festivals, and the like, specifically targeted at the 18-to-24-year-old age group. Being placed in a new, often stressful, social and academic environment makes college students especially vulnerable to outside influences. For many, the college years are their initial taste of freedom from parental supervision. Peer influence can prompt students to start smoking, and many colleges and universities still sell tobacco products in campus stores.

However, cigarette smoking among U.S. college students has decreased slightly in recent years. In a 2007 study, about 19 percent of college students reported having smoked cigarettes in the past 30 days, down from about 30 percent in 1999 (see Figure 8.8). About 11 percent of college students meet the criteria for tobacco dependence. Many who report smoking in college (80%) started doing so before the age of 18. Those who began smoking before the age of 18 report smoking four times as many cigarettes in the past month and on twice as many days as those who began smoking after the age of 18.[37] College men and women have nearly identical rates of cigarette smoking, but men use more cigars and smokeless tobacco.

Why Do College Students Smoke?

In a recent survey, the main reason students gave for their smoking was to relax or to reduce stress (38%). According to this study, smokers are more likely to have higher levels of perceived stress than nonsmokers. Other key reasons provided by students were to fit in/social pressure (16%) and because they cannot stop/are addicted (12%).[38]

Other studies confirm that many students smoke to feel more accepted by their peers. Some research also shows that weight control is an important motivator for smoking among young people. For many students, the fear of weight gain is a common reason for smoking relapse among those who quit.

Students who have reported being depressed in the past year are much more likely to smoke than those who were not (35.3% vs. 20.4%). Other research finds that students diagnosed or treated for depression are 7.5 times more likely to use tobacco compared to students who were never diagnosed or treated for depression.[39]

Social Smoking Many college smokers identify themselves as "social smokers"—those who smoke only when they are with people, rather than alone. Among college students who smoked within the past 30 days, 51 percent were identified as social smokers. What differentiates a social smoker from a smoker? Social smokers smoke less often and less intensely, and they are less dependent on nicotine. They also do not view themselves as being addicted to cigarettes but are less likely to quit or have any intention to quit.[40] However, even occasional smoking is not without risks of damaging health effects. Social smoking in college can lead to a complete dependence on nicotine and, thus, to all the same health risks as smoking regularly.

> ## what do you think?
> Have you noticed a change in the number of your friends who are regular smokers or occasional smokers? ● How many of them smoked prior to coming to college, and how many picked up the habit at college? ● What are their reasons for smoking?
> ● What barriers keep your friends from quitting?

Tobacco and Its Effects

Smoking, the most common form of tobacco use, delivers directly to the lungs a strong dose of nicotine, as well as 4,700 other chemical substances, including arsenic,

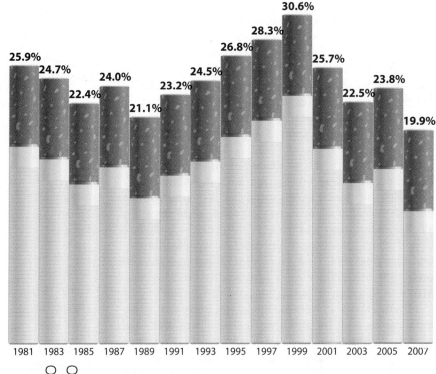

FIGURE 8.8 **Trends in Prevalence of Cigarette Smoking in the Past Month among College Students**

Source: Data are from L. D. Johnston, P. M. O'Malley, J. G. Bachman, and J. E. Schulenberg, *Monitoring the Future National Survey Results on Drug Use, 1975–2007: Volume II, College Students and Adults Ages 19–45,* NIH Publication no. 08-6418B (Bethesda, MD: National Institute on Drug Abuse, 2008).

Tar and Carbon Monoxide

Particulate matter condenses in the lungs to form a thick, brownish sludge called **tar,** which contains various carcinogenic (cancer-causing) agents such as benzo[*a*]pyrene and chemical irritants, such as phenol. In healthy lungs, millions of tiny hairlike projections *(cilia)* on the surfaces lining the upper-respiratory passages sweep away foreign matter, which is expelled from the lungs by coughing. However, the cilia's cleansing function is impaired in smokers' lungs by nicotine, which paralyzes the cilia for up to 1 hour following a single cigarette. This allows tars and other solids in tobacco smoke to accumulate and irritate sensitive lung tissue.

Tar accounts for about 8 percent of tobacco smoke. The remaining 92 percent consists of various gases, the most dangerous of which is **carbon monoxide.** The concentration of carbon monoxide in tobacco smoke is 800 times higher than the level considered safe by the U.S. Environmental Protection Agency (EPA). In the human body, carbon monoxide reduces the oxygen-carrying capacity of the red blood cells by binding with the receptor sites for oxygen; this causes oxygen deprivation in many body tissues.

nicotine The primary stimulant chemical in tobacco products; nicotine is highly addictive.
tar A thick, brownish substance condensed from particulate matter in smoked tobacco.
carbon monoxide A gas found in tobacco smoke that binds at oxygen receptor sites in the blood.
nicotine poisoning Symptoms often experienced by beginning smokers, including dizziness, diarrhea, light-headedness, rapid and erratic pulse, clammy skin, nausea, and vomiting.
pairings Associations (such as coffee and a cigarette) that trigger cravings.

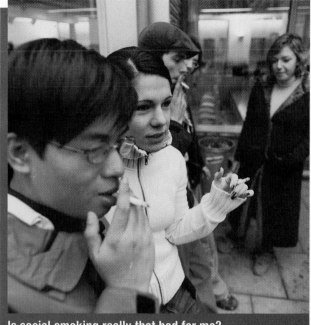

Is social smoking really that bad for me?

An occasional puff once in a while when you are out with friends can't hurt, right? Wrong! There is no "safe" amount of tobacco use—any smoking or exposure to smoke increases your risks for negative health effects such as heart disease and lung cancer. And even if you only smoke once or twice a week and consider yourself a "social smoker," chances are you're on the road to dependence and a more frequent smoking habit.

formaldehyde, and ammonia. Among these chemicals are more than 60 known or suspected carcinogens.[41] The heat from tobacco smoke, which can reach 1,616°F, is also harmful. Inhaling hot toxic gases exposes sensitive mucous membranes to irritating chemicals that weaken the tissues and contribute to cancers of the mouth, larynx, and throat.

Nicotine

The highly addictive chemical stimulant **nicotine** is the major psychoactive substance in all tobacco products. In its natural form, nicotine is a colorless liquid that turns brown upon exposure to air. When tobacco leaves are burned in a cigarette, pipe, or cigar, nicotine is released and inhaled into the lungs. Sucking or chewing tobacco releases nicotine into the saliva, and the nicotine is then absorbed through the mucous membranes in the mouth.

Nicotine is a powerful CNS stimulant that produces a variety of physiological effects. In the cerebral cortex, it produces an aroused, alert mental state. Nicotine stimulates the adrenal glands, which increases the production of adrenaline. It also increases heart and respiratory rates, constricts blood vessels, and, in turn, increases blood pressure because the heart must work harder to pump blood through the narrowed vessels.

Tobacco Addiction

Smoking is a complicated behavior. Somewhere between 60 and 80 percent of people have tried a cigarette. Why do some walk away from cigarettes while others get hooked? For one thing, smoking is a very efficient drug-delivery system. It gets the drug to the brain in just a few seconds, much faster than it would travel if injected.

Beginning smokers usually feel the effects of nicotine with their first puff. These symptoms, called **nicotine poisoning,** include dizziness, light-headedness, rapid and erratic pulse, clammy skin, nausea, vomiting, and diarrhea. These symptoms cease as tolerance to the chemical develops, which happens almost immediately in new users, perhaps after the second or third cigarette. In contrast, tolerance to most other drugs, such as alcohol, develops over a period of months or years. Regular smokers often no longer experience the "buzz" of smoking. They continue to smoke simply because stopping is too difficult.

A pack-a-day smoker experiences 300 "hits," or **pairings,** a day—that's 109,500 pairings per year. In pairing, an environmental cue triggers a craving

what do you think?
Because nicotine is highly addictive, should it be regulated as a controlled substance? ● How could tobacco be regulated effectively? ● Should more resources be used for research into nicotine addiction? Why or why not?

for nicotine.[42] Simple pairings, such as drinking a cup of coffee, sitting in a car, finishing a meal, or sipping a beer, induce nicotine craving. The brain gets used to these pairings and cries out in displeasure when the association is missing. It is easy to see how stopping even occasional use can be very difficult.

Tobacco Products

Tobacco comes in several forms. Cigarettes, cigars, and bidis are used for burning and inhaling tobacco. Smokeless tobacco is inhaled or placed in the mouth.

Cigarettes *Filtered cigarettes,* which are designed to reduce levels of gases such as hydrogen cyanide and carbon monoxide, may actually deliver more hazardous gases to the user than nonfiltered brands. Some smokers use low-tar and low-nicotine products as an excuse to smoke more cigarettes. This practice is self-defeating because they wind up exposing themselves to more harmful substances than they would with regular-strength cigarettes.

Clove cigarettes contain about 40 percent ground cloves (a spice) and about 60 percent tobacco. Many users mistakenly believe that these products are made entirely of ground cloves and that smoking them eliminates the risks associated with tobacco. In fact, clove cigarettes contain higher levels of tar, nicotine, and carbon monoxide than do regular cigarettes—and the numbing effect of eugenol, the active ingredient in cloves, allows smokers to inhale the smoke more deeply.

Cigars Since 1991, cigar sales in the United States have increased dramatically. The fad, especially popular among young men and women, is fueled in part by the willingness of celebrities to be photographed puffing on one. Among some women, cigar smoking symbolizes an impulse to be slightly outrageous and liberated.

Many people believe that cigars are safer than cigarettes, when in fact nothing could be further from the truth. Cigar smoke contains 23 poisons and 43 carcinogens. Most cigars contain as much nicotine as several cigarettes, and when cigar smokers inhale, nicotine is absorbed as rapidly as it is with cigarettes. For those who don't inhale, nicotine is still absorbed through the mucous membranes in the mouth.

Bidis Generally made in India or Southeast Asia, **bidis** are small, hand-rolled cigarettes that come in a variety of flavors, such as vanilla, chocolate, and cherry, and resemble a marijuana joint or a clove cigarette. They have become increasingly popular with college students, because they are viewed to be safer and cheaper than cigarettes. However, they are far more toxic than cigarettes. A study by the Massachusetts Department of Health found that bidis produced three times more carbon monoxide and nicotine

bidis Hand-rolled flavored cigarettes.
chewing tobacco A stringy type of tobacco that is placed in the mouth and then sucked or chewed.
dipping Placing a small amount of chewing tobacco between the front lip and teeth for rapid nicotine absorption.
snuff A powdered form of tobacco that is sniffed and absorbed through the mucous membranes in the nose or placed inside the cheek and sucked.

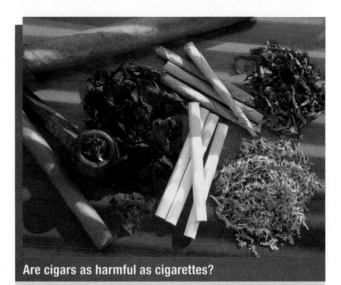

Are cigars as harmful as cigarettes?

No matter what form you use—cigar, pipe, bidi, dip, snuff, or cigarette—tobacco is hazardous to your health. Because they are usually "puffed" rather than inhaled, you may think cigars are safer, but actually they have two or three times the nicotine of a cigarette, which is quickly absorbed through the mucous membranes of the mouth, and their smoke contains just as many toxic chemicals and carcinogens as cigarette smoke.

and five times more tar than cigarettes. The leaf wrappers are nonporous, which means that smokers have to pull harder to inhale and inhale more to keep the bidi lit. During testing, it took an average of 28 puffs to smoke a bidi, compared to only 9 puffs for a regular cigarette. This results in much more exposure to the higher amounts of tar, nicotine, and carbon monoxide, and bidis lack any sort of filter to lower these levels.

Smokeless Tobacco Approximately 5 million U.S. teenagers and adults use smokeless tobacco. Most of them are teenaged (20% of male high school students) and young adult men, many of whom take up the habit to emulate a professional sports figure or family member. There are two types of smokeless tobacco: chewing tobacco and snuff.

Chewing tobacco comes in three forms—loose leaf, plug, or in a pouch—and contains tobacco leaves treated with molasses and other flavorings. The user dips the tobacco by placing a small amount between the lower lip and teeth to stimulate the flow of saliva and release the nicotine. **Dipping** rapidly releases nicotine into the bloodstream.

Snuff is a finely ground form of tobacco that can be inhaled, chewed, or placed against the gums. It comes in dry or moist powdered form or sachets (tea bag–like pouches). In 2009, "snus" became the latest form of smokeless tobacco to hit the market in the United States. Popular for more than 100 years in Sweden, these small sachets of tobacco are placed inside the cheek and sucked. Some people prefer snus to chewing tobacco because it doesn't require the user to spit frequently.

Smokeless tobacco is just as addictive as cigarettes and actually contains more nicotine—holding an average-sized dip or chew in the mouth for 30 minutes delivers as much nicotine as smoking four cigarettes. A two-can-a-week snuff user gets as much nicotine as a ten-pack-a-week smoker. Smokeless tobacco contains 10 times the amount of cancer-producing substances found in cigarettes and 100 times more than the U.S. Food and Drug Administration (FDA) allows in foods and other substances used by the public.

Dental problems are common among users of smokeless tobacco. Contact with tobacco juice causes receding gums, tooth decay, bad breath, and discolored teeth. Damage to both the teeth and jawbone can contribute to early loss of teeth.

Health Hazards of Tobacco Products

Cigarette smoking adversely affects the health of every person who smokes, as well as the health of everyone nearby. Each day, cigarettes contribute to more than 1,000 deaths from cancer, cardiovascular disease, and respiratory disorders. In addition, tobacco use can negatively impact the health of almost every system in your body. **Figure 8.9** summarizes some of the physiological and health effects of smoking.

Cancer

Lung cancer is the leading cause of cancer deaths in the United States. The American Cancer Society estimates that tobacco smoking causes 85 to 90 percent of all cases of lung cancer; fewer than 10 percent of cases occur among non-smokers. There were an estimated 219,440 *new* cases of lung cancer in the United States in 2009 alone, and an estimated 159,390 Americans died from the disease in 2009.[43] **Figure 8.10** on the next page illustrates how tobacco smoke damages the lungs.

Lung cancer can take 10 to 30 years to develop, and the outlook for its victims is poor. Most lung cancer is not diagnosed until it is fairly widespread in the body; at that point, the 5-year survival rate is only 13 percent. When a malignancy is diagnosed and recognized while still localized, the 5-year survival rate rises to 47 percent.

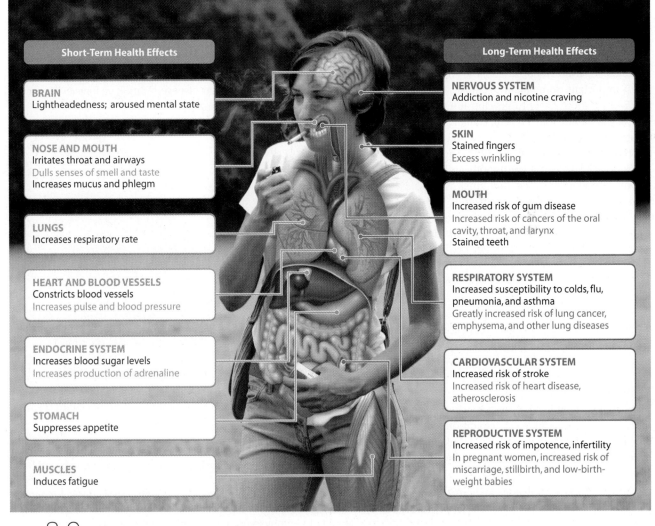

Short-Term Health Effects

BRAIN
Lightheadedness; aroused mental state

NOSE AND MOUTH
Irritates throat and airways
Dulls senses of smell and taste
Increases mucus and phlegm

LUNGS
Increases respiratory rate

HEART AND BLOOD VESSELS
Constricts blood vessels
Increases pulse and blood pressure

ENDOCRINE SYSTEM
Increases blood sugar levels
Increases production of adrenaline

STOMACH
Suppresses appetite

MUSCLES
Induces fatigue

Long-Term Health Effects

NERVOUS SYSTEM
Addiction and nicotine craving

SKIN
Stained fingers
Excess wrinkling

MOUTH
Increased risk of gum disease
Increased risk of cancers of the oral cavity, throat, and larynx
Stained teeth

RESPIRATORY SYSTEM
Increased susceptibility to colds, flu, pneumonia, and asthma
Greatly increased risk of lung cancer, emphysema, and other lung diseases

CARDIOVASCULAR SYSTEM
Increased risk of stroke
Increased risk of heart disease, atherosclerosis

REPRODUCTIVE SYSTEM
Increased risk of impotence, infertility
In pregnant women, increased risk of miscarriage, stillbirth, and low-birth-weight babies

FIGURE 8.9 **Effects of Smoking on the Body and Health**

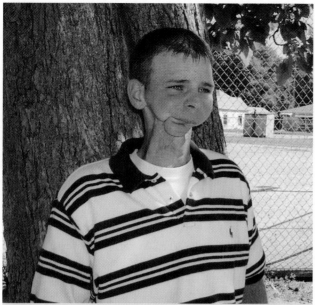
This young cancer survivor has undergone surgery to remove neck muscles, lymph nodes, and his tongue. He began using smokeless tobacco at age 13; by age 17, he was diagnosed with squamous cell carcinoma. He now educates others about the dangers of chewing tobacco.

either smokeless tobacco or cigarettes.[44] Users of smokeless tobacco are 50 times more likely to develop oral cancers than are nonusers. Warning signs include lumps in the jaw or neck; color changes or lumps inside the lips; white, smooth, or scaly patches in the mouth or on the neck, lips, or tongue; a red spot or sore on the lips or gums or inside the mouth that does not heal in 2 weeks; repeated bleeding in the mouth; and difficulty or abnormality in speaking or swallowing.

The lag time between first use and contracting cancer is shorter for smokeless tobacco users than for smokers, because absorption through the gums is the most efficient route of nicotine administration. Many smokeless tobacco users eventually "graduate" to cigarettes and further increase their risk for developing additional problems.

Tobacco is linked to other cancers as well. The rate of pancreatic cancer is more than twice as high for smokers as nonsmokers. Typically, people diagnosed with pancreatic cancer live only about 3 months after their diagnosis. Cancers of the lip, tongue, salivary glands, and esophagus are five times more likely to occur among smokers than among nonsmokers. Smokers are also more likely to develop kidney, bladder, and larynx cancers. A growing body of evidence suggests that long-term use of smokeless tobacco also increases the risk of cancer of the larynx, esophagus, nasal cavity, pancreas, kidney, and bladder.

Cardiovascular Disease

Over a third of all tobacco-related deaths occur from some form of cardiovascular disease.[45] Smokers have a 70 percent

If you are a smoker, your risk of developing lung cancer depends on several factors. First, the amount you smoke per day is important. Someone who smokes two packs a day is 15 to 25 times more likely to develop lung cancer than a nonsmoker. Also, smoking as little as one cigar per day can double the risk of several cancers, including that of the oral cavity (lip, tongue, mouth, and throat), esophagus, larynx, and lungs. A second factor is when you started smoking; if you started in your teens, you have a greater chance of developing lung cancer than people who start later. And a third risk factor is if you inhale deeply when you smoke. Smokers are also more susceptible to the cancer-causing effects of exposure to other irritants, such as asbestos and radon, than are nonsmokers.

A major health risk of chewing tobacco is **leukoplakia,** a condition characterized by leathery white patches inside the mouth that are produced by contact with irritants in tobacco juice. Three to 17 percent of diagnosed leukoplakia cases develop into oral cancer. An estimated 75 percent of the 35,720 new oral cancer cases in 2009 resulted from

leukoplakia A condition characterized by leathery white patches inside the mouth; produced by contact with irritants in tobacco juice.

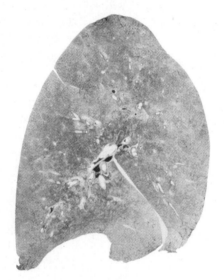
a A healthy lung

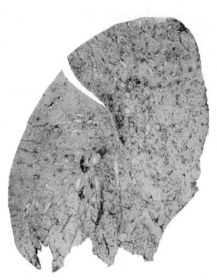
b A smoker's lung permeated with deposits of tar

FIGURE 8.10 **Comparison of Cross Sections of a Healthy Lung with the Lung of a Smoker** Smoke particles irritate lung pathways, causing extra mucus production, and nicotine paralyzes the cilia that normally function to keep the lungs clear of excess mucus. The result is difficulty breathing, "smoker's cough," and chronic bronchitis. At the same time, tar collects within the alveoli (air sacs), ultimately causing their walls to break, leading to emphysema. Tar and other carcinogens in tobacco smoke also cause cellular mutations that lead to cancer.

higher death rate from heart disease than nonsmokers do, and heavy smokers have a 200 percent higher death rate than moderate smokers do. In fact, smoking cigarettes poses as great a risk for developing heart disease as high blood pressure and high cholesterol levels do (see Chapter 12). Daily cigar smoking, especially for people who inhale, also increases the risk of heart disease (cigar smokers double their risk of heart attack and stroke). Bidi smokers are at the same, if not higher, risk for coronary heart disease and cancer.

Smoking contributes to heart disease by adding the equivalent of 10 years of aging to the arteries.[46] One explanation for the mechanism behind this is that smoking and exposure to environmental tobacco smoke (ETS) encourage and accelerate the buildup of fatty deposits (plaque) in the heart and major blood vessels (*atherosclerosis*). Smokers can experience a 50 percent increase in plaque accumulation in the arteries, compared with ex-smokers, and a 20 percent increase in plaque buildup for people regularly exposed to ETS. For unknown reasons, smoking decreases blood levels of HDLs, the "good cholesterol" that helps protect against heart attacks.

Smoking also contributes to **platelet adhesiveness,** the sticking together of red blood cells that is associated with blood clots. The oxygen deprivation associated with smoking decreases the oxygen supplied to the heart and can weaken tissues. Smoking also contributes to irregular heart rhythms, which can trigger a heart attack. Both carbon monoxide and nicotine in cigarette smoke can precipitate angina attacks (pain spasms in the chest when the heart muscle does not get the blood supply it needs).

Smokers are twice as likely to suffer strokes as nonsmokers.[47] A stroke occurs when a small blood vessel in the brain bursts or is blocked by a blood clot, denying oxygen and nourishment to vital portions of the brain. Depending on the area of the brain affected, stroke can result in paralysis, loss of mental functioning, or death. Smoking contributes to strokes by raising blood pressure, which increases the stress on vessel walls. Platelet adhesiveness contributes to blood clot formation.

If a person quits smoking, the risk of dying from a heart attack falls by half after only 1 year without smoking and declines steadily thereafter. After about 15 years without smoking, the ex-smoker's risk of coronary heart disease is similar to that of people who have never smoked.[48]

Respiratory Disorders

Smoking quickly impairs the respiratory system. Smokers can feel its impact in a relatively short period of time—they are more prone to breathlessness, chronic cough, and excess phlegm production than are nonsmokers their age. Over time, cumulative lung damage can lead to chronic obstructive pulmonary disease (COPD) including chronic bronchitis and emphysema (see Chapter 13). Ultimately, smokers are up to 18 times more likely to die of lung disease than are nonsmokers.[49]

Chronic bronchitis may develop in smokers because their inflamed lungs produce more mucus, which they constantly try to expel along with foreign particles. This results in the persistent cough known as "smoker's hack." Smokers are also more prone than nonsmokers to respiratory ailments such as influenza, pneumonia, and colds.

Emphysema is a chronic disease in which the alveoli (the tiny air sacs in the lungs) are destroyed, impairing the lungs' ability to obtain oxygen and remove carbon dioxide. As a result, breathing becomes difficult. Whereas healthy people expend only about 5 percent of their energy in breathing, people with advanced emphysema expend nearly 80 percent. Because the heart has to work harder to do even the simplest tasks, it may become enlarged and death from heart damage may result. There is no known cure for emphysema, and the damage is irreversible. Approximately 80 percent of all cases are related to cigarette smoking.

platelet adhesiveness Stickiness of red blood cells associated with blood clots.

emphysema A chronic lung disease in which the tiny air sacs in the lungs are destroyed, making breathing difficult.

Sexual Dysfunction and Fertility Problems

Despite attempts by tobacco advertisers to make smoking appear sexy, research shows just the opposite: It can cause impotence in men. Several studies have found that male smokers are about two times more likely than are nonsmokers to suffer from some form of impotence. Toxins in cigarette smoke damage blood vessels, reducing blood flow to the penis and leading to an inadequate erection. It is thought that impotence may indicate oncoming cardiovascular disease.

In women, smoking can lead to infertility and problems with pregnancy. Women who smoke increase their risk for infertility, ectopic pregnancy, spontaneous abortion, and stillbirth. Smoking during pregnancy accounts for 20 to 30 percent of low-birth-weight babies, up to 14 percent of preterm deliveries, and about 10 percent of all infant deaths.

Other Health Effects

Gum disease is three times more common among smokers than among nonsmokers, and smokers lose significantly more teeth.[50] In addition, smoking increases risk of macular degeneration, one of the most common causes of blindness in older adults. It also causes premature skin wrinkling, staining of the teeth, yellowing of the fingernails, and bad breath. Nicotine and other ingredients in tobacco smoke can interfere with the body's metabolism of certain drugs. In particular, nicotine speeds

what do you think?
Most smokers are very aware of the long-term hazards of tobacco use yet continue to smoke. Why do you think this is? ● What strategies might be effective to reduce the number of people who begin smoking?

Catching Up to the Men: Women and Smoking

Cigarette smoking was rare among women in the early twentieth century; however, by the end of the century, the number of women smokers had almost caught up to that of men. What led to this increase? Part of the answer lies in the marketing efforts of the tobacco industry. Themes of social desirability, independence, and weight control in ads with slim, attractive models dominate tobacco marketing programs that target women.

Today, more than 1 in 6 women in America smoke, and men's and women's smoking rates are nearly equal: 17.4 percent for women, 22.3 percent for men. Accordingly, women have assumed a much larger burden of smoking-related diseases than they did in the past. However, not all women are equally likely to smoke. For example:

✳ Smoking among women differs by race and ethnicity: non-Hispanic white women—19.8 percent; African American women—15.8 percent; Hispanic women—8.3 percent; Asian American women—4 percent; and Native American/Alaskan Native women—36 percent.
✳ Smoking among women varies with education level. Among U.S. women who earned a general equivalency diploma (GED), 38.9 percent are smokers. Among college graduates, 9.4 percent are smokers, whereas only 6 percent of those who completed graduate work smoke.

✳ Affluent women are less likely to smoke than women are who are poor. Twenty-six percent of women with incomes below the poverty line smoke.

Despite recent declines in smoking overall, the prevalence of tobacco-related disease continues to increase, especially among women. Consider the following:

✳ Every year, tobacco-related disease kills an estimated 174,000 women, making it the largest preventable cause of death among women in the United States.
✳ Women who die of a smoking-related disease lose, on average, 14.5 years of potential life. Men who die of a smoking-related disease lose 13 years of life, on average.
✳ Women who begin smoking at an early age (within 5 years of their first menstrual period) are at higher risk of developing breast cancer.
✳ Evidence suggests that breast cancer is more likely to spread to the lungs in women who smoke than it is in women who do not smoke.
✳ Recent Centers for Disease Control and Prevention (CDC) data indicate that smoking-related cancer deaths are decreasing among men but are increasing among women.
✳ Some studies suggest that smoking cigarettes dramatically increases the risk

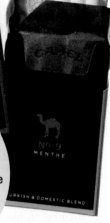

Cigarette companies have become adept at marketing to women with "glamorous" packaging and ad campaigns borrowed from cosmetics, perfume (such as the famous Chanel scents evoked by this Camel No. 9 brand), and the fashion industry.

of heart disease among younger women who are also taking birth control pills.
✳ Postmenopausal women who smoke have lower bone density than do women who never smoked, putting these women at increased risk for osteoporosis.

Sources: American Cancer Society, "Women and Smoking: An Epidemic," www.cancer.org/docroot/PED/content/PED_10_2X_Women_and_Smoking.asp Revised May 2009; American Heart Association, "Women, Heart Disease, and Stroke," 2009, www.americanheart.org/presenter.jhtml?identifier=4786; Office on Smoking and Health, Centers for Disease Control and Prevention, "Cigarette Smoking among Adults—United States, 2007," *Morbidity and Mortality Weekly Report* 57, no. 45 (2008): 1221–1226; Centers for Disease Control and Prevention, "Smoking-Attributable Mortality, Years of Potential Life Lost, and Productivity Losses—United States, 2000–2004," *Morbidity and Mortality Weekly Report* 57, no. 45 (2008): 1226–28.

up the process by which the body uses and eliminates drugs, making medications less effective. In addition, recent research suggests that heavy smokers might be accelerating damage to the brain, which could lead to Alzheimer's disease. It was found that Alzheimer's patients who smoked at least a pack a day developed the disease 2.3 years sooner, and those with a genetic risk for Alzheimer's and who were pack-a-day smokers developed the disease 3 years sooner than those who don't have the gene.[51] There are also

environmental tobacco smoke (ETS) Smoke from tobacco products, including secondhand and mainstream smoke.

health effects of special concern to women (see the **Gender & Health** box above).

Environmental Tobacco Smoke

Although fewer than 30 percent of Americans smoke, air pollution from smoking in public places continues to be a problem. **Environmental tobacco smoke (ETS)** is divided into two categories: mainstream and sidestream smoke. **Mainstream smoke** refers to smoke drawn through tobacco while inhaling; **sidestream smoke** (commonly called *secondhand smoke*) refers to smoke from the burning end of a cigarette or smoke exhaled by a smoker. People who breathe smoke from someone else's smoking product are said to be *involuntary* or *passive* smokers. Since the 1986 Surgeon General's *Report on the Health Consequences of Involuntary Smoking,* detectable levels of nicotine exposure in nonsmoking Americans has decreased, from 88 percent to 43 percent.[52]

Children are more heavily exposed to ETS than adults. Almost 60 percent of U.S. children aged 3 to 11 years—or 22 million children—are exposed to ETS. Disparities in ETS also occur among ethnic and racial lines and among income levels. African Americans have been found to have higher levels of exposure to ETS than whites and Hispanics. ETS exposure is also higher among low-income persons.[53]

46 **states have sued tobacco companies to recover health care costs related to treating smokers.**

Risks from Environmental Tobacco Smoke

Although involuntary smokers breathe less tobacco than active smokers do, they still face risks from exposure to tobacco smoke. Secondhand smoke actually contains more carcinogenic substances than the smoke that a smoker inhales. According to the American Lung Association, secondhand smoke has about 2 times more tar and nicotine, 5 times more carbon monoxide, and 50 times more ammonia than mainstream smoke. Every year, ETS is estimated to be responsible for approximately 3,000 lung cancer deaths, 46,000 coronary and heart disease deaths, and 430 deaths in newborns from sudden infant death sydrome.[54]

The Environmental Protection Agency has designated secondhand smoke as a known carcinogen (group A carcinogen). According to the Surgeon General's report titled *The Health Consequences of Involuntary Exposure to Tobacco Smoke,* there are more than 50 cancer-causing agents found in secondhand smoke.[55] There is also strong evidence that secondhand smoke interferes with normal functioning of the heart, blood, and vascular systems, significantly increasing the risk for heart disease and having immediate effects on the cardiovascular system. Studies indicate that nonsmokers exposed to secondhand smoke were 20 to 30 percent more likely to have coronary heart disease than nonsmokers who are not exposed to smoke.[56] The **Green Guide** on page 246 discusses some of the measures being taken to address the problem

what do you think?

What rights, if any, should smokers have with regard to smoking in public places? ● Does your campus allow smoking in residence halls? ● Do you think your community would support nonsmoking restaurants and bars? Why or why not?

of ETS, as well as steps you can take to protect yourself and others from its hazards.

Tobacco Use and Prevention Policies

It has been more than 40 years since the government began warning that tobacco use is hazardous to the health of the nation. Despite all the education on the health hazards of tobacco use, health care spending associated with smoking still exceeds $96 billion each year.[57]

In 1998, the tobacco industry reached a Master's Settlement Agreement with 40 states. This agreement requires tobacco companies to pay approximately $206 billion over 25 years nationwide. The agreement also included a variety of measures to support antismoking education and advertising and to fund research to determine effective smoking cessation strategies.

Unfortunately, most of the money designated for tobacco control and prevention at the state level has not been used for this purpose. Facing budget woes, many states have drastically cut spending on antismoking programs. In the few states that have spent the settlement money on smoking cessation programs, there has been some reported success in decreasing cigarette use.

Quitting

Quitting smoking isn't easy. Smokers must break both the physical addiction to nicotine and the habit of lighting up at certain times of day. Approximately 70 percent of adult smokers in the United States want to quit smoking, and up to 40 percent make a serious attempt to quit each year. However, fewer than 5 percent succeed.[58] Quitting is often a lengthy process involving several unsuccessful attempts before success is finally achieved. Stopping smoking is a dynamic process that occurs over time; even successful quitters suffer occasional slips.

The person who wishes to quit smoking has several options. Most people who are successful quit "cold turkey"— that is, they decide simply not to smoke again. Others resort to short-term programs, such as those offered by the American Cancer Society, which are based on behavior modification and a system of self-rewards. Still others turn to treatment centers that are part of large franchises, to a community outreach plan sponsored by a local medical clinic, or to a telephone quit line. Finally, some people work privately with their physicians to reach their goal. Programs that combine several approaches have shown the most promise.

mainstream smoke Smoke that is drawn through tobacco while inhaling. **sidestream smoke** The cigarette, pipe, or cigar smoke breathed by nonsmokers; commonly called *secondhand smoke.*

GREEN GUIDE

Clear the Air!

What's the primary cause of indoor air pollution? The answer is secondhand tobacco smoke. From irritating allergies to contributing to heart disease, tobacco smoke in the environment poses a health risk to all who encounter it. Efforts to reduce the hazards associated with secondhand smoke have gained momentum in recent years. The Surgeon General has concluded that smoke-free policies are the only effective way to eliminate secondhand smoke exposure in the workplace—separating smokers from nonsmokers, cleaning the air, and ventilating buildings are not enough to eliminate exposure. Groups such as Action on Smoking and Health (ASH), and Americans for Nonsmokers' Rights (ANR) have been working since the early 1970s to reduce smoking in public places, both indoors and out. As a result of their efforts, 17,059 municipalities across the United States are covered by a 100 percent smoke-free provision in workplaces, and/or restaurants, and/or bars, by either a state, commonwealth, or local law, representing 70.8 percent of the U.S. population. To break this down further:

✳ 37 states and the District of Columbia have local laws in effect that require 100 percent smoke-free workplaces *and/or* restaurants *and/or* bars.

✳ 31 states, along with Puerto Rico and the District of Columbia, have laws in effect that require 100 percent smoke-free workplaces *and/or* restaurants *and/or* bars.

✳ 23 states, along with Puerto Rico and the District of Columbia, have a state law in effect that requires restaurants *and* bars to be 100 percent smoke free. These state laws, along with local laws, protect 53.6 percent of the U.S. population.

✳ 17 states, along with Puerto Rico and the District of Columbia, have a state law in effect that requires workplaces, restaurants, *and* bars to be 100 percent smoke free. These state laws, along with local laws, protect 40.3 percent of the U.S. population.

In addition to government bans on smoking, the hospitality industry has also taken steps to protect the health of nonsmokers. Hotels and motels set aside rooms for nonsmokers, and many hotels are now 100 percent smoke free. Car rental agencies designate certain vehicles for nonsmokers. Smoking is banned on all U.S. airlines, and many other countries ban smoking on their airlines as well. Many other organizations and facilities, including colleges and universities have rules in effect banning smoking in all public places.

Do you know the smoke-free policies of your school, your town, and your state? You can take steps to protect yourself and your loved ones from secondhand smoke by finding out about these policies and advocating for change. The ANR provides information about smoking-free communities across the United States on its website, www.no-smoke.org, as well as tips for taking action to ban smoking in your home, workplace, or in other public places you frequent.

If you are a smoker, the single best way to protect your family and others from secondhand smoke is to quit smoking. In the meantime, you can protect your family and friends by making your home and vehicles smoke free and smoking only outside. A smoke-free home rule can also help you quit smoking.

If you live in a multiunit building and you are encountering secondhand smoke in your home, speak to the management about enacting smoke-free policies. Property owners, be they landlords, corporations, or educational institutions, have the right to ban smoking on their property. Smokers are not a protected class: It is not discrimination to prohibit smoking, there is no legal "right to smoke."

Business owners have the right to ban smoking on their premises as well, so talk to your boss about enacting a smoke-free policy if you are encountering secondhand smoke in your workplace. Make sure that your children's day care center or school

is also smoke free and teach your children to avoid secondhand smoke in general. Let business owners who allow smoking know that secondhand smoke is harmful to your health and the health of others, and that the presence of smoke on their premises is preventing you from patronizing them. Even if you are uncomfortable approaching business owners about their policies, you can encourage change simply by choosing to patronize only smoke-free businesses, and by thanking them for being smoke free.

Sources: American Nonsmokers' Rights Foundation, "Overview List: How Many Smokefree Laws?" 2009, www.no-smoke.org/pdf/mediaordlist .pdf; Office on Smoking and Health, *The Health Consequences of Involuntary Exposure to Tobacco Smoke: A Report of the Surgeon General— Executive Summary.* (Washington, DC: U.S. Department of Health and Human Services, 2006).

No Smoking in the Bar Thank You

Many state and local lawmakers have taken action to protect individuals' health by banning smoking in public places.

Breaking the Nicotine Addiction

Nicotine addiction may be one of the toughest addictions to overcome. Symptoms of **nicotine withdrawal** include irritability, restlessness, nausea, vomiting, and intense cravings for tobacco. The evidence is strong that consistent pharmacological treatments can help a smoker quit: An estimated 17 to 30 percent of people who have used nicotine replacement therapy or smoking-cessation medications continue to abstain from cigarettes.[59]

Nicotine Replacement Products Nontobacco products that replace depleted levels of nicotine in the bloodstream have helped some people stop using tobacco. The two most common are nicotine chewing gum and the nicotine patch, both of which are available over the counter. The FDA has also approved a nicotine nasal spray, a nicotine inhaler, and nicotine lozenges.

Nicotine gum is available without a prescription. The user chews up to 20 pieces of gum a day for 1 to 3 months. Nicotine gum delivers about as much nicotine as a cigarette does, but because it is absorbed through the mucous membrane of the mouth, it doesn't produce the same rush. Users experience no withdrawal symptoms and fewer cravings for nicotine as the dosage is reduced until they are completely weaned.

The nicotine patch is generally used in conjunction with a comprehensive smoking-behavior cessation program. A small, thin, patch placed on the smoker's upper body delivers a continuous flow of nicotine through the skin, helping to relieve cravings. Patches can be bought with or without a prescription and are available in different dosages. The FDA recommends using the patch for a total of 3 to 5 months. During this time, the dose of nicotine is gradually reduced until the smoker is fully weaned from the drug. Occasional side effects include mild skin irritation, insomnia, dry mouth, and nervousness. The patch costs less than a pack of cigarettes—about $4—and some insurance plans will pay for it.

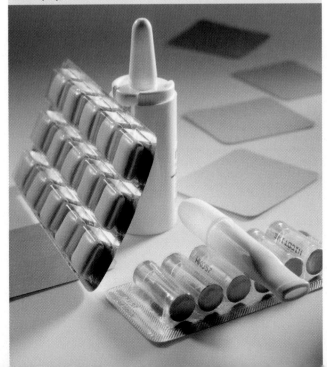

The FDA has approved five types of nicotine replacement therapy: nicotine gum, nicotine patches (transdermal nicotine systems), nicotine nasal spray, nicotine inhalers, and nicotine lozenges (not shown).

The nasal spray, which requires a prescription, is much more powerful and delivers nicotine to the bloodstream faster than gum or the patch. Patients are warned to be careful not to overdose; as little as 40 mg nicotine taken at once could be lethal. The FDA has advised that it should be used for no more than 3 months and never for more than 6 months, so that smokers don't find themselves as dependent on nicotine in spray form as they were on cigarettes. The FDA also advises that no one who experiences nasal or sinus problems, allergies, or asthma should use it.

The nicotine inhaler, which also requires a prescription, consists of a mouthpiece and cartridge. By puffing on the mouthpiece, the smoker inhales air saturated with nicotine, which is absorbed through the lining of the mouth, not the lungs. This nicotine enters the body much more slowly than the nicotine in cigarettes does. Using the inhaler mimics the hand-to-mouth actions used in smoking and causes the back of the throat to feel as it would when inhaling tobacco smoke.

nicotine withdrawal Symptoms, including nausea, headaches, irritability, and intense tobacco cravings, suffered by nicotine-addicted individuals who cease using tobacco.

Nicotine-containing lozenges are the newest form of nicotine-replacement therapy on the market. Lozenges are available over the counter and, as with nicotine gum, come in two strengths: 2 mg and 4 mg. The manufacturer recommends a 12-week program of lozenge use that allows the user to taper off the drug.

Smoking Cessation Medications Although the gum, patch, nasal spray, inhaler, and lozenges all serve to replace nicotine in the system, some smoking-cessation aids are aimed at reducing withdrawal symptoms and decreasing craving for nicotine. In 1997, the FDA approved buproprion, an antidepressant, for use as a smoking-cessation aid. The drug, sold under the brand name Zyban, is thought to work on dopamine and norepinephrine receptors in the brain to decrease craving and withdrawal symptoms.

Chantix (varinicline), approved by the FDA in March 2006, works in two ways: It reduces nicotine cravings and the urge to smoke, and it blocks the effects of nicotine at nicotine receptor sites in the brain. In July 2009, the FDA issued an advisory that the use of both Chantix and Zyban had been associated with changes in behavior such as hostility, agitation, depressed mood, and suicidal thoughts or actions. People taking one of these drugs who experience any unusual changes in mood or behavior or who feel like hurting themselves or others are advised to stop taking the drug immediately and contact their health care professional.[60]

A radical new way to help smokers quit is NicVAX, an anti-smoking vaccine due out on the market soon. The vaccination is intended to prevent nicotine from reaching the brain, making smoking less pleasurable and therefore easier to give up. A small amount that may reach the brain eases the discomfort of withdrawal. One of the advantages of the vaccine over other cessation methods is that it will reduce relapses by making the cigarette much less enjoyable when the quitter tries one again. Early clinical trial results report that twice as many people given the vaccine had quit smoking as those given the placebo.[61]

Breaking the Smoking Habit

For some smokers, the road to quitting includes antismoking therapy. Two common techniques are operant conditioning and self-control therapy. Pairing the act of smoking with an external stimulus is a typical example of an operant strategy. For example, one technique requires smokers to carry a timer that sounds a buzzer at different intervals. When the buzzer sounds, the patient is required to smoke a cigarette. Once the smoker is conditioned to associate the buzzer with smoking, the buzzer is eliminated, and, one hopes, so is the smoking. Self-control strategies view smoking as a learned habit associated with specific situations. Therapy is aimed at identifying these situations and teaching smokers the skills necessary to resist smoking. The **Skills for Behavior Change** box at right presents one of the American Cancer Society's approaches for quitting smoking.

Benefits of Quitting

According to the American Cancer Society, many tissues damaged by smoking can repair themselves. As soon as a smoker stops, the body begins the repair process (Figure 8.11). Within 8 hours, carbon monoxide and oxygen levels return to normal, and "smoker's breath" disappears. Often, within a month of quitting, the mucus that clogs airways is broken up and eliminated. Circulation and the senses of taste and smell improve within weeks. Many ex-smokers say they have more energy, sleep better, and feel more alert. Women are less likely to bear babies with low birth weight. At the end of 10 smoke-free years, the ex-smoker can expect to live out his or her normal life span.

Another significant benefit of quitting smoking is the money saved. A pack of cigarettes averages $4.87 including taxes. Using this number, a pack-a-day smoker burns through about $34.09 per week, or $1,772.68 per year saved. It is estimated that a 40-year-old who quits smoking and puts the savings into a 401(k) earning 9 percent a year would have nearly $250,000 by age 70.

Tips for Quitting

If you're a smoker and you're ready to quit, try these tips to help kick the habit:

* Use the four Ds to fight the urge to smoke:
  Delay—put off smoking for 10 minutes; when the 10 minutes are up, put it off for another 10 minutes.
  Deep breathing
  Drink water
  Do something else
* Keep "mouth toys" handy: hard candy, gum, toothpicks, and carrot sticks can help.
* If you've had trouble stopping before, ask your doctor about nicotine chewing gum, patches, nasal sprays, inhalers, or lozenges.
* Tell your family and friends that you've stopped smoking so they won't offer you a cigarette.
* Aim to spend your time in places that don't allow smoking.
* Take up a new sport, exercise program, hobby, or organizational commitment. This will help shake up your routine and distract you from smoking.
* Throw out your cigarettes or keep them in a place that's harder to access or that makes smoking inconvenient, such as the freezer, in your car's glove compartment, or at a friend's house.

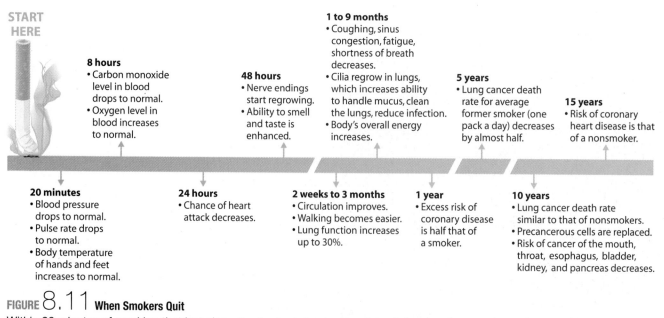

START HERE

8 hours
• Carbon monoxide level in blood drops to normal.
• Oxygen level in blood increases to normal.

48 hours
• Nerve endings start regrowing.
• Ability to smell and taste is enhanced.

1 to 9 months
• Coughing, sinus congestion, fatigue, shortness of breath decreases.
• Cilia regrow in lungs, which increases ability to handle mucus, clean the lungs, reduce infection.
• Body's overall energy increases.

5 years
• Lung cancer death rate for average former smoker (one pack a day) decreases by almost half.

15 years
• Risk of coronary heart disease is that of a nonsmoker.

20 minutes
• Blood pressure drops to normal.
• Pulse rate drops to normal.
• Body temperature of hands and feet increases to normal.

24 hours
• Chance of heart attack decreases.

2 weeks to 3 months
• Circulation improves.
• Walking becomes easier.
• Lung function increases up to 30%.

1 year
• Excess risk of coronary disease is half that of a smoker.

10 years
• Lung cancer death rate similar to that of nonsmokers.
• Precancerous cells are replaced.
• Risk of cancer of the mouth, throat, esophagus, bladder, kidney, and pancreas decreases.

FIGURE 8.11 **When Smokers Quit**
Within 20 minutes of smoking that last cigarette, the body begins a series of changes that continues for years. However, by smoking just one cigarette a day, the smoker loses all these benefits, according to the American Cancer Society.

Alcohol and Tobacco: Are Your Habits Placing You at Risk?

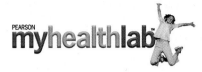

Fill out this assessment online at www.pearsonhighered.com/myhealthlab or www.pearsonhighered.com/donatelle.

1 Are You Nicotine Dependent?

Most college students don't smoke; however, many social smokers (who often consider themselves nonsmokers) may be more addicted to nicotine than they think. Do you have a dependence on nicotine? Take the following quiz to see.

1. **How soon after you wake up do you smoke your first cigarette?**
   - ⓪ After 60 minutes ① 31–60 minutes
   - ② 6–30 minutes ③ Within 5 minutes

2. **Do you find it difficult to refrain from smoking in places where it is not allowed?**
   - ⓪ No ① Yes

3. **Which cigarette would you hate most to give up?**
   - ⓪ The first one in the morning
   - ① Any other

4. **How many cigarettes a day do you smoke?**
   - ⓪ 10 or less ① 11–20
   - ② 21–30 ③ 31 or more

5. **Do you smoke more frequently during the first hours after awakening than during the rest of the day?**
   - ⓪ No ① Yes

6. **Do you smoke even if you are so ill that you are in bed most of the day?**
   - ⓪ No ① Yes

Interpreting Part 1

If you scored 7 or 8 points, your level of nicotine dependence is high. You should consider discussing smoking-cessation methods with your health care provider, or research smoking-cessation therapies in your area. If you scored under 4 points, you can probably stop smoking without nicotine-replacement techniques or medication.

Source: T. F. Heatherton, L. T. Kozlowski, R. C. Frecker, and K. O. Fagerstrom, "The Fagerstrom Test for Nicotine Dependence: A Revision of the Fagerstrom Tolerance Questionnaire," *British Journal of Addictions* 86 (1991): 1119–27. Reprinted by permission of Dr. Karl Fagerstrom.

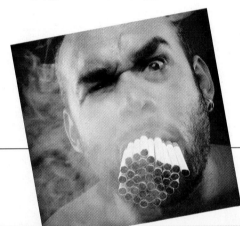

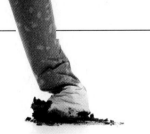

YOUR PLAN FOR CHANGE

This **Assess yourself** activity gave you the chance to evaluate your current smoking habits. Regardless of your current level of nicotine addiction, if you smoke at all, now is the time to take steps toward kicking the habit.

Today, you can:

◯ Develop a plan to kick the tobacco habit. The first step in quitting smoking is to identify why you want to quit. Write your reasons down and carry a copy of it with you. Every time you are tempted to smoke, go over your reasons for stopping.

◯ Think about the times and places you usually smoke. What could you do instead of smoking at those times? Make a list of positive tobacco alternatives.

Within the next 2 weeks, you can:

◯ Pick a day to stop smoking, fill out the Behavior Change Contract (available in the front of this text and online), and have a family member or friend sign it.

◯ Throw away all your cigarettes, lighters, and ashtrays.

By the end of the semester, you can:

◯ Focus on the positives. Now that you have stopped smoking, your mind and your body will begin to feel better. Make a list of the good things about not smoking. Carry a copy with you, and look at it whenever you have the urge to smoke.

◯ Reward yourself for stopping. Go to a movie, go out to dinner, or buy yourself a gift.

2 What's Your Risk of Alcohol Abuse?

Many college students engage in potentially dangerous drinking behaviors. Do you have a problem with alcohol use? Take the following quiz to see.

1. How often do you have a drink containing alcohol?
- ⓪ Never
- ① Monthly or less
- ② 2 to 4 times a month
- ③ 2 to 3 times a week
- ④ 4 or more times a week

2. How many alcoholic drinks do you have on a typical day when you are drinking?
- ⓪ 1 or 2
- ① 3 or 4
- ② 5 or 6
- ③ 7 to 9
- ④ 10 or more

3. How often do you have six drinks or more on one occasion?
- ⓪ Never
- ① Less than monthly
- ② Monthly
- ③ Weekly
- ④ Daily or almost daily

4. How often during the past year have you been unable to stop drinking once you had started?
- ⓪ Never
- ① Less than monthly
- ② Monthly
- ③ Weekly
- ④ Daily or almost daily

5. How often during the past year have you failed to do what was normally expected from you because of drinking?
- ⓪ Never
- ① Less than monthly
- ② Monthly
- ③ Weekly
- ④ Daily or almost daily

6. How often during the past year have you needed a first drink in the morning to get yourself going after a heavy drinking session?
- ⓪ Never
- ① Less than monthly
- ② Monthly
- ③ Weekly
- ④ Daily or almost daily

7. How often during the past year have you had a feeling of guilt or remorse after drinking?
- ⓪ Never
- ① Less than monthly
- ② Monthly
- ③ Weekly
- ④ Daily or almost daily

8. How often during the past year have you been unable to remember what happened the night before because you had been drinking?
- ⓪ Never
- ① Less than monthly
- ② Monthly
- ③ Weekly
- ④ Daily or almost daily

9. Have you or someone else been injured as a result of your drinking?
- ⓪ No
- ① Yes, but not in the past year
- ② Yes, during the past year

10. Has a relative, friend, or a doctor or other health care professional been concerned about your drinking or suggested you cut down?
- ⓪ No
- ① Yes, but not in the past year
- ② Yes, during the past year

Interpreting Part 2

Scores below 6: Congratulations! You are in control of your drinking behaviors and do a good job of consuming alcohol responsibly and in moderation.

Scores between 6 and 8: Your alcohol consumption is possibly risky. Try taking steps to change your drinking behavior and make some positive changes for your health and safety.

Scores above 8: Your drinking patterns are putting you at high risk for illness, unsafe sexual situations, or alcohol-related injuries, and may even affect your academic performance.

Source: Taken from the AUDIT Manual, box 4, p. 17, World Health Organization, Division of Mental Health and Prevention of Substance Abuse. http://whqlibdoc.who.int/hq/2001/WHO_MSD_MSB_01.6a.pdf. Copyright © 2001 World Health Organization. Used with permission.

YOUR PLAN FOR CHANGE

This **Assessyourself** activity gave you the chance to evaluate your alcohol consumption. If some of your answers surprised you or if you were unsure how to answer some of the questions, consider taking steps to change your behavior.

Today, you can:

◯ Start a diary of your drinking habits. Keeping track of how much you drink—as well as how much money you spend on drinks and how you feel when you are drinking—will make you more aware of your true drinking habits.

◯ Spend some time thinking about the ways your family members use alcohol. Is there a family history of alcohol abuse or addiction? Did your family's alcohol consumption have any effect on you while you were growing up? Consider whether your current alcohol use is healthy, or whether it is likely to create problems for you in the future.

Within the next 2 weeks, you can:

◯ Make your first drink a glass of water or another nonalcoholic beverage the next time you go to a party. Intersperse alcoholic drinks with nonalcoholic beverages to help you pace your consumption.

◯ Challenge yourself and a few close friends to get together at least once a week for a non-alcoholic social occasion, such as a sports event or movie night.

By the end of the semester, you can:

◯ Commit yourself to limiting your alcohol intake at every social function you attend. Decide ahead of time whether you want to drink and, if so, what your limit will be; then stick to it.

◯ Cultivate friendships and explore activities that do not center on alcohol. If your current group of friends drinks heavily, and it is becoming a problem for you, you may need to step back from the group for a while.

Summary

* Alcohol is a central nervous system (CNS) depressant used by 61 percent of all Americans, about 10 percent of whom are heavy drinkers. Over 44 percent of all college students are binge drinkers.
* Negative consequences associated with alcohol use among college students are lower grade point averages, academic problems, traffic accidents, dropping out of school, unplanned sex, hangovers, alcohol poisoning, and injury.
* Alcohol's effect is measured by the blood alcohol concentration (BAC), the ratio of alcohol to total blood volume. The higher the BAC, the greater drowsiness and impaired judgment and coordination will be.
* Long-term alcohol overuse can cause damage to the nervous system, cardiovascular damage, liver disease, and increased risk for cancer. Drinking during pregnancy can cause fetal alcohol spectrum disorders (FASDs).
* Alcohol use becomes alcoholism when it interferes with school, work, or social and family relationships or entails violations of the law. Causes of alcoholism include biological, family, social, and cultural factors.
* Most alcoholics do not admit to a problem until reaching a major life crisis or having their families intervene. Treatment options include detoxification at private medical facilities, therapy, and self-help programs. Most alcoholics relapse because alcoholism is a behavioral addiction as well as a chemical addiction.
* Tobacco use involves many social and political issues, including advertising targeted at youth and women, the fastest growing populations of smokers. Health care and lost productivity resulting from smoking costs the nation as much as $193 billion per year.
* Tobacco is available in smoking and smokeless forms. Both contain nicotine, an addictive psychoactive substance. Smoking also delivers 4,700 other chemicals to the lungs of smokers.
* Health hazards of smoking include markedly higher rates of cancer, heart and circulatory disorders, respiratory diseases, and gum diseases. Smoking during pregnancy increases risk of miscarriage and low birth weight. Smokeless tobacco increases risks for oral cancer and other oral problems. Environmental tobacco smoke puts nonsmokers at risk for cancer and heart disease.
* To quit, smokers must kick a chemical addiction and a behavioral habit. Nicotine-replacement products or drugs such as Zyban and Chantix can help wean smokers off nicotine. Therapy methods can also help.

Pop Quiz

1. If a man and a woman drink the same amount of alcohol, the woman's blood alcohol concentration (BAC) will be approximately
   a. the same as the man's BAC.
   b. 60% higher than the man's BAC.
   c. 30% higher than the man's BAC.
   d. 30% lower than the man's BAC.

2. Blood alcohol concentration (BAC) is the
   a. concentration of plant sugars in the bloodstream.
   b. percentage of alcohol in a beverage.
   c. level of alcohol content in the blood.
   d. ratio of alcohol to the total blood volume.

3. Which of the following is false?
   a. College students under 21 drink less often than older students but drink more heavily.
   b. College students tend to underestimate the amount that their peers drink.
   c. In the past 10 years, the number of college-aged women who report being drunk ten or more times has increased.
   d. Alcohol is involved in at least two-thirds of campus suicides.

4. When Amanda goes out on the weekends, she usually has four to five beers in a row. This type of high-risk drinking is called
   a. tolerance.
   b. alcoholic addiction.
   c. alcohol overconsumption.
   d. binge drinking.

5. Which of the following is *not* a potential long-term effect of alcohol abuse?
   a. increased risk of some cancers
   b. increased risk of liver damage
   c. increased risk of hangover
   d. increased risk of infertility

6. What effect does carbon monoxide have on a smoker's body?
   a. It accumulates on the alveoli in the lungs, making breathing difficult.
   b. It increases heart rate.
   c. It interferes with the ability of hemoglobin in the blood to carry oxygen.
   d. It dulls the senses of taste and smell.

7. What age group is most targeted by tobacco advertisers?
   a. teenagers aged 14 to 17
   b. college students aged 18 to 24
   c. young adults aged 25 to 30
   d. married men aged 31 to 35

8. What is the major psychoactive ingredient in tobacco products?
   a. carbon monoxide
   b. tar
   c. formaldehyde
   d. nicotine

9. What does nicotine do to the cilia hairs found in the lungs?
   a. instantly destroys them
   b. thickens them

c. paralyzes them

d. accumulates on them

10. How quickly will an individual begin to see health benefits after quitting smoking?

a. within a day

b. within a month

c. within a year

d. never

Answers to these questions can be found on page A-1.

Think about It!

1. When it comes to drinking alcohol, how much is too much? How can you avoid drinking amounts that will affect your judgment? If you see a friend having too many drinks at a party, what actions could you take?

2. What are some of the most common negative consequences college students experience as a result of drinking? What are secondhand effects of binge drinking?

3. Describe the difference between a problem drinker and an alcoholic. What factors can cause someone to become an alcoholic? What effect does alcoholism have on an alcoholic's family?

4. Discuss health hazards associated with tobacco. Who should be responsible for the medical expenses of smokers? Insurance companies? Smokers themselves?

5. Do you think restrictions on smokers are fair? Do they infringe on people's rights? Are the restrictions too strict or not strict enough?

6. Describe the various methods of tobacco cessation. Which would be most effective for you? Why?

Accessing Your Health on the Internet

The following websites explore further topics and issues related to personal health. For links to the websites below, visit the Companion Website for *Health: The Basics,* Green Edition at www.pearsonhighered.com/donatelle.

1. *Alcoholics Anonymous.* Provides general information about AA and the 12-step program. www.aa.org

2. *American Lung Association.* This site offers a wealth of information regarding smoking trends, environmental smoke, and advice on smoking cessation. www.lungusa.org

3. *ASH (Action on Smoking and Health).* The nation's oldest and largest antismoking organization, ASH takes legal actions and does other work to fight smoking and protect nonsmokers' rights. www.ash.org

4. *College Drinking: Changing the Culture.* This online resource center targets three audiences: the student population as a whole, the college and its surrounding environment, and the individual at-risk or alcohol-dependent drinker. www.collegedrinkingprevention.gov

5. *Had Enough.* This site is designed for college students who have suffered the secondhand effects (babysitting a roommate who has been drinking, having sleep interrupted, and so on) of other students' drinking. http://gbgm-umc.org/mission_programs/cim/hadenough/home

6. *The Tobacco Atlas.* This book and website, a joint production of the World Lung Foundation and the American Cancer Society, cover a range of topics including the history of tobacco use, prevalence of use, youth smoking, secondhand smoke, quitting, and more. www.tobaccoatlas.com

References

1. Centers for Disease Control and Prevention, National Center for Health Statistics, *Health, United States, 2008, with Special Feature on the Health of Young Adults* (Hyattsville, MD: National Center for Health Statistics, 2009).

2. American College Health Association, *American College Health Association—National College Health Assessment: Reference Group Data Report Fall 2008* (Baltimore: American College Health Association, 2009).

3. U.S. Department of Health and Human Services, National Institute on Alcohol Abuse and Alcoholism, "What Colleges Need to Know: An Update on College Drinking Research," NIH Publication no. 07-5010, November 2007, www.collegedrinkingprevention.gov.

4. American College Health Association, *American College Health Association—National College Health Assessment: Reference Group Data Report Fall 2008,* 2009.

5. Ibid.

6. U.S. Department of Health and Human Services, National Institute on Alcohol Abuse and Alcoholism, "What Colleges Need to Know," 2007.

7. National Social Norms Institute, "Case Studies: Alcohol," Accessed 2009, www.socialnorms.org/CaseStudies/alcohol.php.

8. R. Hingson et al., "Magnitude of Alcohol-Related Mortality and Morbidity among U.S. College Students Ages 18–24: Changes from 1998 to 2001," *Annual Review of Public Health* 26 (2005): 259–79.

9. H. Wechsler et al., "Trends in College Binge Drinking during a Period of Increased Prevention Efforts: Findings from Four Harvard School of Public Health College Study Surveys: 1993–2001," *Journal of American College Health* 50, no. 5 (2002): 207.

10. H. Wechsler et al., "College Binge Drinking in the 1990s: A Continuing Problem, Results of the Harvard School of Public Health 1999 College Alcohol Study," *Journal of American College Health* 48, no. 10 (2000): 199–210.

11. R. Hingson et al., "Magnitude of Alcohol-Related Mortality and Morbidity," 2005.

12. M. Mohler-Kuo et al., "Correlates of Rape While Intoxicated in a National Sample of College Women," *Journal of Studies on Alcohol* 65, no. 1 (2004): 37.

13. R. LaVallee et al., "Apparent Per Capita Alcohol Consumption: National, State, and Regional Trends, 1977–2007" "Surveillance Report #87" (National Institute on Alcohol Abuse and Alcoholism, 2009), http://pubs.niaaa.nih.gov/publications/survelliance87/CONS07.htm.

14. S. MacDonald, "The Criteria for Causation of Alcohol in Violent Injuries in Six Countries," *Addictive Behaviors* 30, no. 1 (2005): 103–13.

15. J. Turner et al., "Serious Health Consequences Associated with Alcohol Use among College Students: Demographic and Clinical Characteristics of Patients

Seen in the Emergency Department," *Journal of Studies on Alcohol* 65, no. 2 (2004): 179.

16. K. Butler, "The Grim Neurology of Teenage Drinking," *New York Times*, July 4, 2006.

17. R. W. Hingson et al., "Age at Drinking Onset and Alcohol Dependence," *Archives of Pediatric and Adolescent Medicine* 160 (2006): 739–46.

18. National Institute on Alcohol Abuse and Alcoholism, "Alcohol: A Women's Health Issue," NIH Publication No. 03-4956, (Bethesda, MD: National Institutes of Health, revised 2008), http://pubs.niaaa .nih.gov/publications/brochurewomen/ women.htm.

19. National Organization on Fetal Alcohol Syndrome, "FASD: What Everyone Should Know," 2006, www.nofas.org/MediaFiles/ PDFs/factsheets/everyone.pdf.

20. National Highway Traffic Safety Administration, "Traffic Safety Facts Research Note: 2008 Traffic Safety Annual Assessment—Highlights," DOT HS 811 172, 2009, www-nrd.nhtsa.dot.gov/Pubs/ 811172.PDF.

21. Ibid.

22. Insurance Institute for Highway Safety, "Fatality Facts 2008: Alcohol," 2009, www .iihs.org/research/fatality_facts_2008/ alcohol.html.

23. Ibid.

24. Substance Abuse and Mental Health Services Administration, "Results from the 2007 National Survey on Drug Use and Health: National Findings" NHSDA Series H-34, DHHS Publication no. SMA 08-4343 (Rockville, MD, Office of Applied Studies; U.S. Department of Health and Human Services, 2008).

25. National Institute on Drug Abuse, "Alcohol Abuse Makes Prescription Drug Abuse More Likely," *NIDA Notes* 21, no. 5 (March 2008).

26. C. Wilson and J. Knight, "When Parents Have a Drinking Problem," *Contemporary Pediatrics* 18, no. 1 (January 2001): 67.

27. Ibid.

28. Ensuring Solutions to Alcohol Problems, *Workplace Screening & Brief Intervention: What Employers Can and Should Do about Excessive Alcohol Use*, (Washington, DC: The George Washington University Medical Center, March 2008).

29. T. R. Miller et al., "Societal Costs of Underage Drinking," *Journal of Studies on Alcohol* 67, no. 4 (2006): 519–28.

30. National Institute on Alcohol Abuse and Alcoholism, "Alcohol: A Women's Health Issue," 2008.

31. National Institute on Drug Abuse, "Info Facts: Treatment Methods for Women," Updated 2009, www.nida.nih.gov/Infofax/ treatwomen.html.

32. Centers for Disease Control and Prevention, "Smoking & Tobacco Use: Fast Facts," Updated May 2009, www.cdc.gov/tobacco/ data_statistics/fact_sheets/fast_facts.

33. Substance Abuse and Mental Health Services Administration, "Results from the 2007 National Survey on Drug Use and Health: National Findings," 2008.

34. Ibid.

35. Campaign for Tobacco-Free Kids, "Toll of Tobacco in the United States of America," 2009, www.tobaccofreekids.org/research/ factsheets/pdf/0072.pdf.

36. Centers for Disease Control and Prevention, "Smoking-Attributable Mortality, Years of Potential Life Lost, and Productivity Losses—United States, 2000–2004," *Morbidity and Mortality Weekly Report* 57, no. 45 (2008): 1226–28.

37. National Center on Addiction and Substance Abuse at Columbia University, *Wasting the Best and the Brightest: Substance Abuse at America's Colleges and Universities* (New York: National Center on Addiction and Substance Abuse at Columbia University, March 2007).

38. National Center on Addiction and Substance Abuse at Columbia University, *Wasting the Best and the Brightest*, 2007.

39. Ibid.

40. S. Moran et al., "Social Smoking among U.S. College Students," *Pediatrics* 114 (2004): 1028–34.

41. American Cancer Society, "Secondhand Smoke," www.cancer.org/docroot/PED/ content/PED_10_2X_Secondhand _Smoke-Clean_Indoor_Air.asp. Revised 2009.

42. National Institute on Drug Abuse Research Report Series, *Tobacco Addiction*, NIH Publication no. 09-4342 (Bethesda, MD: National Institute on Drug Abuse, 2009).

43. American Cancer Society, *Cancer Facts & Figures, 2009*. (Atlanta: American Cancer Society, 2009).

44. Ibid.

45. American Heart Association, *Heart Disease and Stroke Statistics—2009 Update At-A-Glance* (Dallas: American Heart Association, 2009).

46. Ibid.

47. American Heart Association, "Stroke Risk Factors," 2009. www.americanheart.org/ presenter.jhtml?identifier=4716.

48. Office on Smoking and Health, "The Benefits of Quitting," Poster, www.cdc.gov/ tobacco/data_statistics/sgr/2004/posters/ benefits/index.htm. Updated 2009.

49. American Cancer Society, *Cancer Facts & Figures, 2008*, 2008.

50. American Academy of Periodontology, "Tobacco Use and Periodontal Disease," Updated 2008, www.perio.org/consumer/ smoking.htm.

51. American Academy of Neurology, "Alzheimer's Starts Earlier for Heavy Drinkers, Smokers," Press Release, April 16, 2008.

52. Centers for Disease Control and Prevention, "Smoking and Tobacco Use Fact Sheet: Secondhand Smoke," Updated May 2009, www.cdc.gov/tobacco/data _statistics/fact_sheets/secondhand _smoke/general_facts/index.htm.

53. U.S. Department of Health and Human Services, *The Health Consequences of Involuntary Exposure to Tobacco Smoke: A Report of the Surgeon General* (Atlanta: U.S. Department of Health and Human Services, Centers for Disease Control and Prevention, Coordinating Center for Health Promotion, National Center for Chronic Disease Prevention and Health Promotion, Office on Smoking and Health, 2006).

54. Ibid.

55. Ibid.

56. Ibid.

57. Centers for Disease Control and Prevention, "Smoking-Attributable Mortality, Years of Potential Life Lost, and Productivity Losses—United States, 2000–2004," *Morbidity and Mortality Weekly Report* 57, no. 45 (2008): 1226–28. Available at www .cdc.gov/mmwr/preview/mmwrhtml/ mm5745a3.htm.

58. U.S. Department of Health and Human Services, "Effective Strategies for Tobacco Cessation Underused, Panel Says" *National Institutes of Health News*, June 2006.

59. American Cancer Society, *Cancer Facts & Figures, 2008*, 2008.

60. U.S. Food and Drug Administration, "Public Health Advisory: FDA Requires New Boxed Warnings for the Smoking Cessation Drugs Chantix and Zyban," July 1, 2009, www.fda.gov/Drugs/DrugSafety/ PublicHealthAdvisories/ucm169988.htm.

61. J. Interlandi, "Are Vaccines the Answer to Addiction?" *Newsweek* CLI, no. 2 (January 14, 2008): 17.

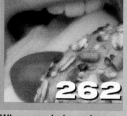
262
Why are whole grains better than refined ones?

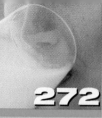
272
Do teenagers really need to drink milk?

278
Is vegetarianism healthy?

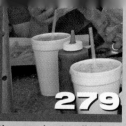
279
How can I eat well when I'm in a hurry?

9 Nutrition and You

Objectives

✳ List the six classes of nutrients, and explain the primary functions of each and their roles in maintaining long-term health.

✳ Understand the factors that influence dietary choices.

✳ Discuss how to change old eating habits, improve dietary behaviors, and use the USDA MyPyramid Plan to make the best nutritional choices.

✳ Distinguish fact from fiction about trends in nutrition, potential risks versus benefits of food supplements, and the role of nutrition in fighting various diseases.

✳ Discuss issues surrounding gender, culture, and other factors that influence decision making about healthy nutrition.

✳ Discuss the unique challenges that college students face when trying to eat healthy foods and the actions they can take to eat healthfully.

✳ Explain food safety concerns facing Americans and people in other regions of the world.

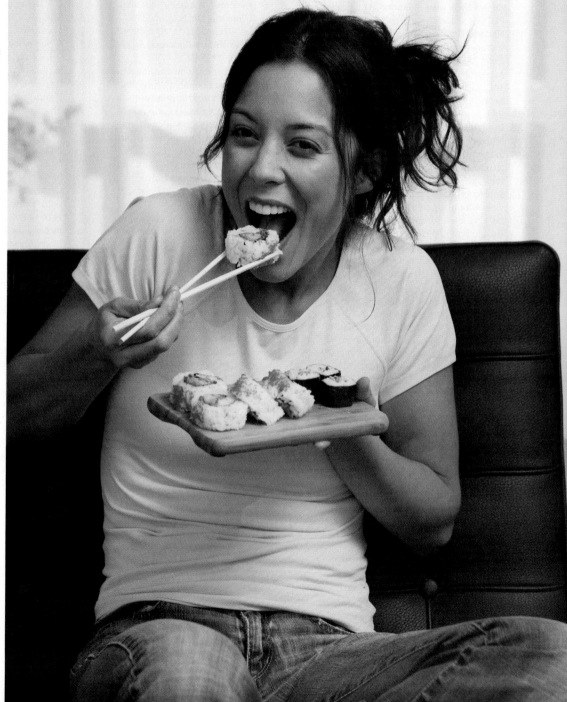

When was the last time you ate something without regard for its fat or calorie content? Can you remember when you last went out to dinner with friends and didn't think twice before ordering the fried foods or high-calorie desserts? Do you eat differently around your health-conscious friends than when by yourself? If so, you are not alone. Clearly, Americans are trying to heed expert advice and the multiple pressures to eat low-fat, high-fiber foods, and to consume fewer calories overall. However, knowing what to eat, how much to eat, and how to choose from a media-driven array of foods and nutrition advice can be mind-boggling.

The good news is that in survey after survey, 60 to 80 percent of food shoppers say they read food labels before selecting products; they consume more vegetables, fruits, and lower-fat foods; and they are cutting down on portion sizes and total calories.[1] Diet-book sales are at an all-time high as millions of people make the leap toward what they think is healthy eating. But we still have a long way to go. In fact, although reports indicate that increasing numbers of us read labels and are trying to eat more healthfully, nearly 78 percent of all adults indicate that they are not eating the recommended servings of fruits and vegetables and that they are still eating too many refined carbohydrates and high-fat foods.

Just how important is sound nutrition? Thousands of individual studies have shown associations between what we eat and a wide range of chronic diseases, such as diabetes, heart disease, hypertension, stroke, and many types of cancer.[2] A landmark review of over 4,500 research studies concluded that widespread consumption of five to six servings of fruits and vegetables daily would lower cancer rates by more than 20 percent in the global population.[3] Newer reviews have focused on specific chronic diseases, and all have shown an important link between diet and risks for certain diseases.[4]

Many documented studies indicate that undernutrition and overnutrition play major roles in global population health (See the **Health in a Diverse World** box on page 256). Indeed, undernutrition, overnutrition, and diet-related chronic diseases account for more than half of the world's diseases and

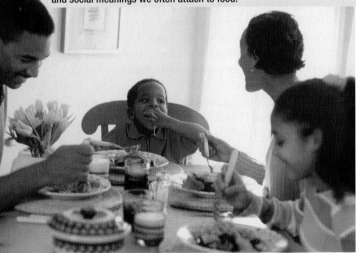

Family mealtimes and the traditions they involve can reinforce the cultural and social meanings we often attach to food.

hundreds of millions of dollars in public expenditures.[5] The evidence is compelling and clear. Your health depends largely on what you eat, how much you eat, and the amount of exercise that you get throughout your life.

Assessing Eating Behaviors: Are You What You Eat?

True **hunger** occurs when there is a lack or shortage of basic foods needed to provide the energy and nutrients that support health.[6] When we are hungry, chemical messages in the brain, especially in the hypothalamus, initiate a physiological response that prompts us to seek food. Few Americans have experienced the type of hunger that continues for days and threatens survival. Most of us eat because of our **appetite,** a learned psychological desire to eat that may or may not have anything to do with feeling hungry. Appetite can be triggered by smells, tastes, and other triggers such as certain times of day, special occasions, or proximity to a favorite food.

hunger The physiological impulse to seek food, prompted by the lack or shortage of basic foods needed to provide the energy and nutrients that support health.
appetite The desire to eat; normally accompanies hunger but is more psychological than physiological.
nutrition The science that investigates the relationship between physiological function and the essential elements of foods eaten.

Hunger and appetite are not the only forces involved in our physiological drive to eat. Other factors that influence when, how, and what we eat include the following:

● **Cultural and social meanings attached to food.** Cultural traditions and food choices give us many of our *food preferences.* We learn to like the tastes of certain foods, especially the foods we grew up eating. A yearning for sweet, salty, or high-fat foods can evolve from our earliest days.
● **Convenience and advertising.** That juicy burger on TV looked really good. You've got to have it.
● **Habit or custom.** Often we select foods because they are familiar and fit religious, political, or spiritual views.
● **Emotional comfort.** Eating makes you feel better—a form of reward and security. We derive pleasure or sensory delight from eating specific foods and reward ourselves with foods.
● **Nutritional value.** You think the food is good or bad for you, or it may help you maintain your weight.
● **Social interaction.** Eating out or having company over for a meal is an enjoyable social event.
● **Regional/seasonal trends.** Some foods may be favored in your area by season or overall climate.

With all the factors that influence our dietary choices and the wide array of foods available, the challenge of eating for health increases daily. Fortunately, we have a wealth of solid information that serves as a foundation for our decisions.

Eating for Health

Nutrition is the science that investigates the relationship between physiological function and the essential elements

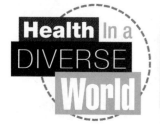
Global Nutrition: Threats to World Populations

Although it's widely accepted that in general good nutrition means stronger immune systems, better productivity, fewer illnesses, and better health, millions of people in the developed and developing world suffer from food scarcity, food insecurity, and malnutrition. Just how much of an impact does poor nutrition have on the health of global populations? Consider this:

✱ Poor nutrition contributes to one out of two deaths (53 percent) associated with infectious diseases among children under age 5 in developing countries.
✱ One out of four preschool children suffers from undernutrition in the global population.
✱ One in three people in developing countries are affected by vitamin and mineral deficiencies and therefore are more at risk for infection, birth defects, and impaired physical and intellectual development.
✱ In the United States, nearly 12 percent of the population suffers from *food insecurity,* meaning that they are unable to provide sufficient food for themselves or their families.

Ironically, at the same time that food insecurity and insufficient food levels plague the world, the global population is also seeing a dramatic increase in other

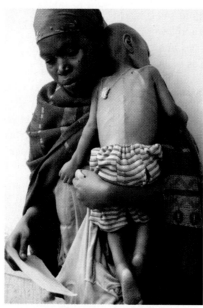

Drought, high food prices, and political unrest all contribute to the severe malnutrition experienced by millions of people worldwide.

forms of malnutrition. These are characterized by obesity and the long-term implications of unbalanced dietary and lifestyle practices that result in chronic diseases such as cardiovascular disease, cancer, and diabetes. Although we often think that obesity is a problem of excess and affluence, this isn't always the case. In fact, obesity flourishes in populations where acute hunger also persists.

✱ Two out of three overweight and obese people now live in developing countries, the vast majority in emerging markets and transition economies.
✱ Under- and overnutrition problems and diet-related chronic diseases (including obesity-related diseases) account for more than half of the world's diseases and hundreds of millions of dollars in public expenditure to combat them.

Sources: World Health Organization, "Nutrition for Health and Development: Challenges," 2009, www.who.int/nutrition/challenges/en/index.html; M. Nord, M. Andrews, and S. Carlson, *Household Food Security in the United States, 2007,* Economic Research Report no. 66, U.S. Department of Agriculture, Economic Research Service, November 2008, www.ers.usda.gov/Publications/ERR66.

of the foods we eat. Generally, a healthful diet provides the proper combination of energy and **nutrients,** the compounds in food that your body requires to sustain proper functioning. A healthful diet should be

● **Adequate.** It provides enough of the energy, nutrients, and fiber to maintain health and essential body functions. A **calorie** is the unit of measurement used to quantify the amount of energy we obtain from a particular food. Everyone's energy needs differ (Table 9.1). For example, a small woman who has a sedentary lifestyle may need only 1,700 calories of energy to support her body's functions, whereas a professional biker may need several thousand calories of energy to be up for his competition.
● **Moderate.** The quantity of food you consume can cause you to gain weight. Moderate caloric consumption, portion

nutrients The constituents of food that sustain humans physiologically: proteins, carbohydrates, fats, vitamins, minerals, and water.
calorie A unit of measure that indicates the amount of energy obtained from a particular food.

control, and awareness of the total amount of nutrients in the foods you eat are key aspects of dietary health.
● **Balanced.** Your diet should contain the proper combination of foods from different groups. Following the recommendations for the MyPyramid plan, discussed later in the chapter, should help you achieve balance.
● **Varied.** Eat a lot of different foods each day. Variety helps you avoid boredom and can make it easier to keep your diet interesting and in control.
● **Nutrient dense.** Nutrient density refers to the proportion of nutrients compared to the number of calories. In short, the foods you eat should have the biggest nutritional bang for the calories consumed. Making each bite count and not wasting calories on foods that give you little nutritional value are key to healthful eating.

Trends indicate that Americans today overall eat more food than ever before (see Figure 9.1). In a 30-year study of changes in consumption, women's overall caloric intake

GREEN GUIDE

Bottled Water Boom: Who Pays the Price?

Globally, factories are churning out bottled water at unprecedented rates. Conservative estimates are that bottled water is now our second most popular drink, right behind soda, with over $100 billion in sales each year. The consumption of bottled water in the United States rose 20 times, or 2,000 percent, between 1978 and 2006. People all over the world have developed a love affair with their special brands of water, many thinking that bottled water is better, safer, and more pure than tap water. It isn't enough that we are spending between 500 to 4,000 times more for bottled than we do for tap water. Most experts argue that all that money is being spent on a product that doesn't really deliver any benefits.

We may imagine that bottled water comes from medicinal mountain streams or aquifers that ensure purity, but the fact is that most of the water sold in bottles comes from municipal water supplies, sometimes with extra minerals being added, or with an extra step in purification. If it was just your money going down the drain and you could afford it, it wouldn't be so worrisome. However, the environmental consequences of bottled water are significant. Consider the following:

✳ Around the world, factories are using more than 18 million barrels of oil and up to 130 billion gallons of fresh water to quench our bottled water thirst. When you include the resource cost of transporting bottled water, it is estimated that the total amount of energy required to create and transport every bottle is the equivalent of filling the bottle one-quarter full of oil.

✳ In general, systems such as reverse osmosis purifiers use about 2 liters of fresh water running through a system to realize 1 liter of bottled water.

✳ In 2006, more than 900,000 tons of plastic were used to package 8 billion gallons of bottled water.

✳ There is a growing concern about negative health risks from certain chemicals found in plastic bottles that can leach into the water, particularly *bisphenol-A (BPA)*. Research has suggested links between BPA and negative estrogen-related effects, including breast enlargement in young boys, some forms of cancer, early onset of puberty, and increased risk for type 2 diabetes.

✳ Tap water in the United States is among the safest in the world, largely because community water supplies are subject to strict and constant monitoring required by the Safe Drinking Act, while bottled water is considered a "food" and requires much less frequent monitoring for safety and quality by the Food and Drug Administration (FDA) or individual state oversight.

✳ Nationwide, less than 15 percent of discarded bottles are recycled.

✳ Companies taking part in the bottled water boom are buying water supplies throughout the world for financial gain, leaving entire populations vulnerable to water shortages.

You can help to curb the personal and global environmental threats caused by bottled water use:

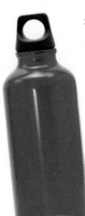

Purchasing a stainless steel bottle that you can reuse is a better choice than buying plastic bottles every day.

✳ Don't buy bottled water unless it's absolutely necessary. Instead, purchase a stainless steel or glass container and use it again and again. Look for a container with a wide mouth so that you can wash and dry it regularly.

✳ When you have parties, use covered pitchers of ice water and recyclable paper cups, rather than serving bottles or using plastic cups.

✳ Buy an inexpensive water filter to help remove the taste of chlorine from tap water. Refrigerate your water jug as a means of improving taste and clarity.

✳ Recycle any plastic bottles you use or come across. Many states offer 5 cent deposits on beverage bottles and cans as an incentive to increase recycling efforts.

✳ Become involved in initiatives to ensure quality tap water in your community. Ask questions about the filters being used, the chemicals and minerals that are removed, and the chemicals and minerals that remain.

Sources: Sierra Club, "Bottled Water: Learning the Facts and Taking Action," 2008, www.sierraclub.org/committees/cac/water/bottled_water/bottled_water.pdf; Oregon State University, "Bottled Water Boom Has Environmental Drawbacks," Media Release, 2007, http://oregonstate.edu/dept/ncs/newsarch/2007/May07/bottledwater.html.

water isn't going to help clear more toxins from your body, cure your headaches, or improve your skin or health. That's not to say that water isn't important to cell functioning and overall health, but we usually get all the fluids that we need per day through the food we eat. In fact, fruits and vegetables are 80 to 95 percent water, meats are more than 50 percent water, and even dry bread and cheese are about 35 percent water. Contrary to popular opinion, caffeinated drinks, including coffee, tea, and soda, also count toward total fluid intake for those who regularly consume them. Caffeinated beverages have not been found to dehydrate people whose bodies are used to caffeine.

Researchers have looked at climates around the world and have concluded that people who live in hot, desertlike places or those who engage in activities where they sweat profusely, such as heavy laborers or athletes, probably need to replenish their lost fluids regularly.[11] In addition, certain diseases, such as diabetes and cystic fibrosis, cause people to lose fluids at a rate necessitating a higher volume of fluid intake. However, for the typical person, if you are thirsty, drink; if you are sweating profusely, drink; and if you have a fever or other illness where there is vomiting and diarrhea, drink even more. Remember that no two people are alike when it comes to water consumption needs. If you are an athlete or are just wondering about general water recommendations, check the guidelines at the American College of Sports Medicine website, www.acsm.org.[12]

Proteins

Next to water, **proteins** are the most abundant substances in the human body. Proteins are major components of nearly every cell and have been called the "body builders" because of their role in developing and repairing bone, muscle, skin, and blood cells. They are the key elements of the antibodies that protect us from disease, of enzymes that control chemical activities in the body, and of hormones that regulate body functions. Proteins help transport iron, oxygen, and nutrients to all body cells and supply another source of energy to cells when fats and carbohydrates are not readily available. In short, adequate amounts of protein in the diet are vital to many body functions and ultimately to survival.

Whenever you consume proteins, your body breaks them down into smaller molecules known as **amino acids,** the building blocks of protein. Nine of the 20 different amino acids are termed **essential amino acids,** which means the body must obtain them from the diet; the other 11 can be produced by the body. Dietary protein that supplies all the essential amino acids is called **complete (high-quality) protein.** Typically, protein from animal products is complete. When we consume foods that are deficient in some of the essential amino acids, the total amount of protein that can be synthesized from the other amino acids is decreased. For proteins to be complete, they also must be present in digestible form and in amounts proportional to body requirements.

What about plant sources of protein? Proteins from plant sources are often **incomplete proteins** in that they may lack one or two of the essential amino acids. Nevertheless, it is relatively easy for the nonmeat eater to combine plant foods effectively and eat complementary sources of plant protein (Figure 9.3).

Plant sources of protein fall into three general categories: *legumes* (beans, peas, peanuts, and soy products), *grains* (e.g., wheat, corn, rice, and oats), and *nuts and seeds.* Certain vegetables, such as leafy green vegetables and broccoli, also

proteins The essential constituents of nearly all body cells; necessary for the development and repair of bone, muscle, skin, and blood; the key elements of antibodies, enzymes, and hormones.
amino acids The nitrogen-containing building blocks of protein.
essential amino acids Nine of the basic nitrogen-containing building blocks of protein, which must be obtained from foods to ensure health.
complete (high-quality) proteins Proteins that contain all nine of the essential amino acids.
incomplete proteins Proteins that lack one or more of the essential amino acids.

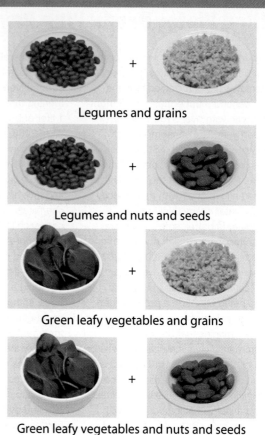

Eaten in the right combinations, plant-based foods can provide complementary proteins and all essential amino acids.

Legumes and grains

Legumes and nuts and seeds

Green leafy vegetables and grains

Green leafy vegetables and nuts and seeds

FIGURE 9.3 Complementary Proteins

contribute valuable plant proteins. Mixing two or more foods from each of these categories during the same meal will provide all the essential amino acids necessary to ensure adequate protein absorption.

Although protein deficiency continues to pose a threat to the global population, few Americans suffer from protein deficiencies. In fact, the average American consumes more than 100 grams of protein daily, and about 70 percent of this comes from high-fat animal flesh and dairy products.[13] The recommended protein intake for adults is only 0.8 gram (g) per kilogram (kg) of body weight per day. The typical recommendation is that in a 2,000-calorie diet, 10 to 35 percent of calories should come from protein, for a total average of 50 to 175 grams per day (a 6-ounce steak contains 53 grams of protein—more than the daily needs of an average-sized woman!).

A person might need to eat extra protein if fighting off a serious infection, recovering from surgery or blood loss, or recovering from burns. In these instances, proteins that are lost to cellular repair need to be replaced. There is considerable controversy over whether someone in high-level physical training needs additional protein to build and repair muscle fibers or whether normal daily requirements should suffice.

Carbohydrates

Although we should not underestimate the importance of water and proteins in the body, it is **carbohydrates** that supply us with the energy needed to sustain normal daily activity. Carbohydrates can actually be metabolized more quickly and efficiently than proteins and are a quick source of energy for the body, being easily converted to glucose, the fuel for the body's cells. These foods also play an important role in the functioning of internal organs, the nervous system, and the muscles. They are the best fuel for endurance athletics because they provide both an immediate and a time-released energy source; they are digested easily and then consistently metabolized in the bloodstream. There are two major types of carbohydrates: **simple carbohydrates** or *simple sugars,* which are found primarily in fruits and many vegetables, and **complex carbohydrates,** which are found in grains, cereals, and vegetables.

Simple Carbohydrates

A typical American diet contains large amounts of simple carbohydrates. The most common form is *glucose.* Eventually, the human body converts all types of simple sugars to glucose to provide energy to cells. *Fructose* (commonly called *fruit sugar*) is another simple sugar found in fruits and berries. Glucose and fructose are **monosaccharides.**

Disaccharides are combinations of two monosaccharides. Perhaps the best-known example is *sucrose* (granulated table sugar). *Lactose* (milk sugar), found in milk and milk products, and *maltose* (malt sugar) are other examples of common disaccharides. These must be broken down into monosaccharides before the body can use them.

Sugar is found in high amounts in a wide range of food products that many people never even think about. Items such as ketchup, barbecue sauce, and flavored coffee creamers derive 30 to 65 percent of their calories from sugar. Read food labels carefully before purchasing. If *sugar* or one of its aliases (including *high fructose corn syrup*) appears near the top of the ingredients list, then that product contains a lot of sugar and is probably not your best nutritional bet. Also, most labels provide the amount of sugar as a percentage of total calories.

Complex Carbohydrates: Starches and Glycogen

Complex carbohydrates, or **polysaccharides,** are formed by long chains of monosaccharides. They must be broken down into simple sugars before the body can use them. *Starches, glycogen,* and *fiber* are the main types of complex carbohydrates.

Starches make up the majority of the complex carbohydrate group and come from flours, breads, pasta, rice, corn, oats, barley, potatoes, and related foods. The body breaks down these complex carbohydrates into glucose, which can be easily absorbed by cells and used as energy. Polysaccharides can also be stored in body muscles and the liver as **glycogen.** When the body requires a sudden burst of energy, it breaks down glycogen into glucose.

Glycemic Index and Glycemic Load

Americans consume far too many refined carbohydrates, which have few health benefits and are a major factor in our growing epidemic of overweight and obesity. Many of these simple sugars come from *added sugars,* sweeteners that are put in during processing to flavor foods, make sodas taste good, and ease our cravings for sweets. A classic example is the amount of added sugar in one can of soda: over 10 teaspoons per can! All that refined sugar can cause tooth decay and put on pounds; however, the greater threats may come from the sudden spike in blood glucose that comes from eating them. In response to an overload of blood glucose, insulin levels also may surge in order to drive blood glucose levels down. Through a typical day, these surges of sugar, bursts of insulin, and resultant dips in blood glucose may cause a cascade of ill health effects.

The **glycemic index (GI)** is a system for rating the potential of foods to raise blood glucose levels. Foods that break down quickly and result in that fast blood glucose surge have a high glycemic index rating. Those that digest slowly and release glucose slowly into the blood tend to have low glycemic index ratings. **Glycemic load (GL)** refers to the amount of carbohydrates in the food you eat multiplied by the glycemic index of that food. In other words, if you eat a tiny amount of a high glycemic index food, the net effect won't be as severe as if you ate a huge serving.

Combining carbohydrates with fats and proteins can lower the overall GI. If, instead of just drinking a glass of orange juice in the morning, you also ate a piece of whole-grain bread with peanut butter, the level of blood glucose surging in your blood would be substantially lower than without that protein and fat combination. Diabetics and others can benefit from eating such combinations of whole grains, proteins, and fats throughout the day as a means of controlling blood glucose levels.[14]

Complex Carbohydrates: Fiber

Fiber, often referred to as "bulk" or "roughage," is the indigestible portion of plant foods that helps move foods through the

---

carbohydrates Basic nutrients that supply the body with glucose, the energy form most commonly used to sustain normal activity.

simple carbohydrates A major type of carbohydrate, which provides short-term energy; also called simple sugars.

complex carbohydrates A major type of carbohydrate, which provides sustained energy.

monosaccharides Simple sugars that contain only one molecule of sugar.

disaccharides Combinations of two monosaccharides.

polysaccharides Complex carbohydrates formed by the combination of long chains of monosaccharides.

starch Polysaccharide that is the storage form of glucose in plants.

glycogen The polysaccharide form in which glucose is stored in the liver and, to a lesser extent, in muscles.

glycemic index (GI) A measure of the effect of particular carbohydrates on blood glucose levels.

glycemic load (GL) A measure of the carbohydrate content of a portion of food multiplied by its glycemic index.

fiber The indigestible portion of plant foods that helps move food through the digestive system and softens stools by absorbing water.

digestive system, delays absorption of cholesterol and other nutrients, and softens stools by absorbing water. Dietary fiber is found only in plant foods, such as fruits, vegetables, nuts, and grains. The Food and Nutrition Board of the Institute of Medicine proposed three fiber distinctions: dietary fiber, functional fiber, and total fiber.[15] *Dietary fiber* is the nondigestible parts of plants that form the structure of leaves, stems, and seeds— the plant's "skeleton." *Functional fiber* consists of nondigestible forms of carbohydrates that may come from plants or are manufactured in the laboratory and have known health benefits. *Total fiber* is the sum of dietary fiber and functional fiber in a person's diet.

A more user-friendly classification of fiber types is either *soluble* or *insoluble*. Soluble fibers, such as pectins, gums, and mucilages, dissolve in water, form gel-like substances, and can be easily digested by bacteria in the colon. Major food sources of soluble fiber include citrus fruits, berries, oat bran, dried beans (such as kidney, garbanzo, pinto, and navy beans), and some vegetables. Insoluble fibers, such as lignins and cellulose, are those that typically do not dissolve in water and that cannot be fermented by bacteria in the colon. They are found in whole grains, such as brown rice, wheat, bran, whole-grain breads and cereals, and most fruits and vegetables.

Research supports many benefits of fiber:

- **Protection against colon and rectal cancer.** One of the leading causes of cancer deaths in the United States, colorectal cancer is much rarer in countries with diets high in fiber and low in animal fat. Several studies have contributed to the theory that fiber-rich diets, particularly those including insoluble fiber, prevent the development of precancerous growths.[16]
- **Protection against constipation.** Insoluble fiber, consumed with adequate fluids, acts like a sponge, absorbing moisture and producing softer, bulkier stools that are easily passed.
- **Protection against diverticulosis.** Diverticulosis is a condition in which tiny bulges or pouches form on the large intestinal wall. These bulges can become irritated and cause chronic pain if under strain from constipation. Insoluble fiber helps to reduce constipation and discomfort.
- **Protection against breast cancer.** Research into the effects of fiber

fats Basic nutrients composed of carbon and hydrogen atoms; needed for the proper functioning of cells, insulation of body organs against shock, maintenance of body temperature, and healthy skin and hair.

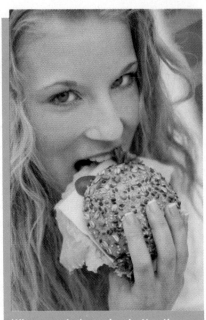

Why are whole grains better than refined ones?

Whole grain foods contain fiber, a crucial form of carbohydrate that protects against some gastrointestinal disorders and reduces risk for certain cancers. Fiber is also associated with lowered blood cholesterol levels; studies have shown that eating 2.5 servings of whole grains per day can reduce cardiovascular disease risk by as much as 21%. But are people getting the message? One nutrition survey showed that only 8% of U.S. adults consume three or more servings of whole grains each day, and 42% ate no whole grains at all on a given day.

on breast cancer risk is inconclusive. However, some studies indicate that wheat bran (rich in insoluble fiber) reduces blood estrogen levels, which may affect the risk for breast cancer.
- **Protection against heart disease.** Many studies have indicated that soluble fiber helps reduce blood cholesterol, primarily by lowering low-density lipoprotein (LDL: "bad") cholesterol.
- **Protection against type 2 diabetes.** Some studies suggest that soluble fiber improves control of blood sugar and can reduce the need for insulin or medication in people with type 2 diabetes.[17]
- **Protection against obesity.** Because most high-fiber foods are high in carbohydrates and low in fat, they help control caloric intake. Many take longer to chew, which slows you down at the table, and fiber stays in the digestive tract longer than other nutrients, making you feel full sooner.

In spite of growing evidence supporting the benefits of whole grains and high-fiber diets, intake among the general public remains low. Most experts believe that Americans should double their current consumption of dietary fiber—to 20 to 35 grams per day for most people and perhaps to 40 to 50 grams for others. What's the best way to increase your intake of dietary fiber? Eat more foods high in complex carbohydrates, such as whole grains, fruits, vegetables, legumes (peas and beans), nuts, and seeds. See the **Skills for Behavior Change** box on the next page for more tips to increase your fiber intake. As with most nutritional advice, however, too much of a good thing can pose problems. Sudden increases in dietary fiber may cause flatulence (intestinal gas), cramping, or bloating. Consume plenty of water or other liquids to reduce such side effects.

Fats

Fats, another group of basic nutrients, are perhaps the most misunderstood of the body's required energy sources. Fats play a vital role in maintaining healthy skin and hair, insulating body organs against shock, maintaining body temperature, and promoting healthy cell function. Fats make foods taste better and carry the fat-soluble vitamins A, D, E, and K to the cells. They also provide a concentrated form of energy in the absence of sufficient amounts of carbohydrates and make you feel full after eating.

If fats perform all these functions, why are we constantly urged to cut back on them? Although moderate consumption

Bulk Up Your Fiber Intake!

✳ Whenever possible, select whole-grain breads, especially those that are low in fat and sugars. Choose breads with three or more grams of fiber per serving. Read labels—just because bread is brown doesn't mean it is better for you.

✳ Eat whole, unpeeled fruits and vegetables rather than drinking their juices. The fiber in the whole fruit tends to slow blood sugar increases and helps you feel full longer.

✳ Substitute whole-grain pastas, bagels, and pizza crust for the refined, white flour versions.

✳ Add wheat crumbs or grains to meat loaf and burgers to increase fiber intake.

✳ Toast grains to bring out their nutty flavor and make foods more appealing.

✳ Sprinkle ground flaxseed on cereals, yogurt, and salads, or add to casseroles, burgers, and baked goods. Flaxseeds have a mild flavor and are also high in beneficial fatty acids.

of fats is essential to health, overconsumption can be dangerous. **Triglycerides,** which make up about 95 percent of total body fat, are the most common form of fat circulating in the blood. When we consume too many calories, the liver converts the excess into triglycerides, which are stored throughout our bodies.

The remaining 5 percent of body fat is composed of substances such as **cholesterol,** which can accumulate on the inner walls of arteries and narrow the channels through which blood flows. This buildup, called **plaque,** is a major cause of *atherosclerosis*, a component of cardiovascular disease (see Chapter 12).

The ratio of total cholesterol to a group of compounds called **high-density lipoproteins (HDLs)** is important to determining risk for heart disease. Lipoproteins facilitate the transport of cholesterol in the blood. High-density lipoproteins are capable of transporting more cholesterol than are **low-density lipoproteins (LDLs).** Whereas LDLs transport cholesterol to the body's cells, HDLs apparently transport circulating cholesterol to the liver for metabolism and elimination from the body. People with a high percentage of HDLs therefore appear to be at lower risk for developing cholesterol-clogged arteries. Regular vigorous exercise plays a part in reducing cholesterol by increasing high-density lipoproteins.

Types of Dietary Fats
Fat molecules consist of chains of carbon and hydrogen atoms. Those that are unable to hold any more hydrogen in their chemical structure are labeled **saturated fats.** They generally come from animal sources, such as meat, poultry, and dairy products, and are solid at room temperature. **Unsaturated fats,** which come from plants and include most vegetable oils, are generally liquid at

room temperature and have room for additional hydrogen atoms in their chemical structure.

The terms *monounsaturated fat* (MUFA) and *polyunsaturated fat* (PUFA) refer to the relative number of hydrogen atoms that are missing in an unsaturated fat. Peanut and olive oils are high in monounsaturated fats, whereas corn, sunflower, and safflower oils are high in polyunsaturated fats. There is currently a great deal of controversy about which type of unsaturated fat is most beneficial. Many nutritional researchers believe that PUFAs may decrease levels of beneficial HDLs as well as those of harmful LDLs. PUFAs come in two forms: omega-3 fatty acids and omega-6 fatty acids. MUFAs, such as olive oil, seem to lower LDL levels and increase HDL levels and thus are currently the preferred fats. MUFAs are also resistant to oxidation, a process that leads to cell and tissue damage. For a breakdown of the types of fats in common vegetable oils, see **Figure 9.4** on page 264.

triglycerides The most common form of fat in the body; excess calories consumed are converted into triglycerides and stored as body fat.

cholesterol A form of fat circulating in the blood that can accumulate on the inner walls of arteries, causing a narrowing of the channel through which blood flows.

plaque Cholesterol buildup on the inner walls of arteries; a major cause of atherosclerosis.

high-density lipoproteins (HDLs) Compounds that facilitate the transport of cholesterol in the blood to the liver for metabolism and elimination from the body.

low-density lipoproteins (LDLs) Compounds that facilitate the transport of cholesterol in the blood to the body's cells.

saturated fats Fats that are unable to hold any more hydrogen in their chemical structure; derived mostly from animal sources; solid at room temperature.

unsaturated fats Fats that do have room for more hydrogen in their chemical structure; derived mostly from plants; liquid at room temperature.

trans fats (trans fatty acids) Fatty acids that are produced when polyunsaturated oils are hydrogenated to make them more solid.

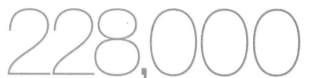

228,000

deaths related to coronary heart disease could be averted each year by reducing Americans' consumption of *trans* fats, according to some estimates.

Avoiding *Trans* Fatty Acids For decades, Americans shunned saturated fats found in butter, certain cuts of red meat, and a host of other foods. What they didn't know is that foods low in saturated fat, such as margarine, could be just as bad for us. As early as the 1990s Dutch researchers reported that a form of fat known as *trans* fats increased LDL cholesterol levels while decreasing HDL cholesterol levels. In a more recent study, researchers concluded that just a 2 percent caloric intake of *trans* fats was associated with an increased risk for heart disease of 23 percent and a 47 percent increased chance of sudden cardiac death.[18]

What are **trans** fats (***trans* fatty acids**)? *Trans* fats are fatty acids that are produced by adding hydrogen molecules to liquid oil to make the oil into a solid. Unlike regular fats and oils, these "partially hydrogenated" fats stay solid or semisolid at room temperature. They change into irregular shapes at the molecular level, priming them to clog up arteries. *Trans* fats

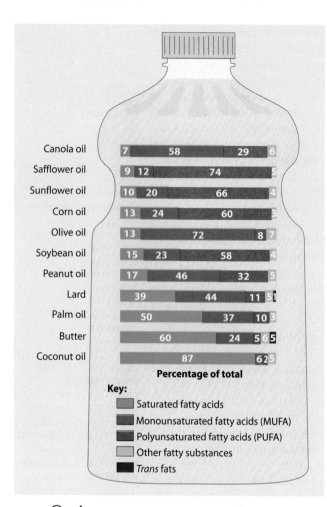

FIGURE 9.4 Percentages of Saturated, Monounsaturated, Polyunsaturated, and *Trans* Fats in Common Vegetable Oils

Canola oil: 7 | 58 | 29 | 6
Safflower oil: 9 | 12 | 74 | 5
Sunflower oil: 10 | 20 | 66 | 4
Corn oil: 13 | 24 | 60 | 3
Olive oil: 13 | 72 | 8 | 7
Soybean oil: 15 | 23 | 58 | 4
Peanut oil: 17 | 46 | 32 | 5
Lard: 39 | 44 | 11 | 5 | 1
Palm oil: 50 | 37 | 10 | 3
Butter: 60 | 24 | 5 | 6 | 5
Coconut oil: 87 | 6 | 2 | 5

Percentage of total

Key:
- Saturated fatty acids
- Monounsaturated fatty acids (MUFA)
- Polyunsaturated fatty acids (PUFA)
- Other fatty substances
- *Trans* fats

have been used in margarines, many commercial baked goods, and restaurant deep-fried foods.

In 2006, the Food and Drug Administration began to require labeling that tells consumers how much *trans* fat is in that cookie they are putting in their mouths. In July 2008, California took bold steps toward health by becoming the first state to ban *trans* fats from restaurant food. The American Medical Association (AMA) promptly followed suit in November 2008 by saying that banning *trans* fats would save up to 100,000 lives a year. Today, *trans* fats are being removed from most foods, and, if they *are* present, they must be clearly indicated. If you see the words *partially hydrogenated oils, fractionated oils, shortening, lard,* or *hydrogenation,* then *trans* fats are present.

New Fat Advice: Is More Fat Ever Better?
Although most of this section has promoted the long-term recommendation to reduce saturated fat, avoid *trans* fatty acids, and eat more monounsaturated fats, some researchers worry that we have gone too far in our anti-fat frenzy. In fact, according to some experts, our zeal to eat no-fat or low-fat foods may be one of the greatest causes of obesity in America today. According to the American Heart Association, eating fewer than 15 percent of our calories as fat (fewer than 34 g a day on a 2,000-calorie diet) can actually

Trimming the Fat for a Healthier You!

Enjoying a healthy intake of dietary fat doesn't have to be difficult or confusing. Follow these guidelines to add more healthy fats to your diet:

✳ Eat fatty fish (bluefish, herring, mackerel, salmon, sardines, or tuna) at least twice weekly.
✳ Substitute soy and canola oils for corn, safflower, and sunflower oils. Keep using olive oil, too.
✳ Add healthy doses of green leafy vegetables, walnuts, walnut oil, and ground flaxseed to your diet.

Follow these guidelines to help reduce your overall intake of less healthy fats:

✳ Read the Nutrition Facts Panel on foods to find out how much fat is in your food. Remember that no more than 10 percent of your total calories should come from saturated fat, and no more than 30 percent should come from all forms of fat.
✳ Use olive oil for baking and sautéing.
✳ Chill soups and stews and scrape off any fat that hardens on top, then reheat to serve.
✳ Fill up on fruits and vegetables.
✳ Hold the creams and sauces.
✳ Avoid margarine products with *trans* fatty acids. Whenever possible, opt for other condiments on your bread, such as fresh vegetable spreads, sugar-free jams, fat-free cheese, and other healthy toppings.
✳ Choose lean meats, fish, or skinless poultry. Broil or bake whenever possible. Drain off fat after cooking.
✳ Experiment with eating whole wheat pastas, brown rice, beans, or vegetables as the main dish.
✳ Choose fewer cold cuts, bacon, sausages, hot dogs, and organ meats.
✳ Select nonfat and low-fat dairy products.
✳ When cooking, use substitutes for butter, margarine, oils, sour cream, mayonnaise, and salad dressings. Chicken or beef broth, fresh herbs, wine, vinegar, and low-calorie dressings provide flavor with less fat.

increase blood triglycerides to levels that promote heart disease while lowering levels of protective HDLs.

The bottom line for fat intake is that moderation is the key. Remember that no more than 7 to 10 percent of your total calories should come from saturated fat and that no more than 30 percent should come from all forms of fat. In general, switching to beneficial fats without increasing total fat intake is a good idea. See the **Skills for Behavior Change** box above for tips on how to include more healthy fats, including the essential fatty acids, in your diet, while reducing your overall fat intake. The **Green Guide** at right provides tips for making healthy and sustainable seafood choices to fulfill your need for omega-3 fatty acids.

GREEN GUIDE

Toward Sustainable Seafood

The USDA recommends consuming fish two or three times per week to reduce saturated fat and cholesterol levels, and to increase omega-3 fatty acid levels. However, there are many environmental concerns surrounding the seafood industry today that call into question the sustainability and safety of such consumption. More than 70 percent of the world's natural fishing grounds have been overfished, and whole stretches of the oceans are, in fact, dead zones, where fish and shellfish can no longer live.

In an effort to counteract the loss of wild fish populations, increasing numbers of fish are being farmed, which poses additional health risks and environmental concerns. Some farmed fish are laden with antibiotics, while highly concentrated levels of parasites and bacteria from fish farm runoff may enter the ocean and river fish populations through adjacent

waterways. There are other reasons to think carefully about your farmed fish alternatives. Farmed salmon, for example, are often fed wild fish, resulting in a net loss of fish from the sea.

At the same time that fish populations are threatened, high levels of chemicals, parasites, bacteria, and toxins are also being found in many of the fish available on the market. Mercury, a waste product of many industries, binds to proteins and stays in an animal's body, accumulating as it moves up the food chain; in humans mercury can cause damage to the nervous system and kidneys, and birth defects and developmental problems in fetuses and children. Polychlorinated biphenyls (PCBs), chemicals that can build up in the fatty tissue of fish, are another cause of major concern.

So what is a savvy fish consumer to do? Knowing where your fish are caught

and the methods by which they are caught is important. Several major environmental groups have developed guides to inform consumers of safe and sustainable seafood choices. The guide shown here provides general national guidelines for seafood available for purchase in the United States. This guide is also available as a free iPhone application, or can be accessed on other mobile devices at http://mobile.seafoodwatch.org. Another great resource is the FishPhone service offered by the Blue Ocean Institute. Simply send a text message to 30644 with the word FISH and the type of fish you want to know about, and it will send you information about whether it is safe to eat. Remember: Your consumer choices make a difference. Purchasing seafood from environmentally responsible sources will support fisheries and fish farms that are healthier for you and the environment.

BEST CHOICES	GOOD ALTERNATIVES	AVOID	Support Ocean-Friendly Seafood
Arctic Char (farmed) Barramundi (US farmed) Catfish (US farmed) Clams (farmed) Cobia (US farmed) Cod: Pacific (Alaska longline)✦ Crab: Dungeness, Stone Halibut: Pacific✦ Lobster: Spiny (US) Mussels (farmed) Oysters (farmed) Pollock (Alaska wild)✦ Salmon (Alaska wild)✦ Scallops: Bay (farmed) Striped Bass (farmed or wild✳) Tilapia (US farmed) Trout: Rainbow (farmed) Tuna: Albacore (troll/pole, US✦ or British Columbia) Tuna: Skipjack (troll/pole)	Caviar, Sturgeon (US farmed) Clams (wild) Cod: Pacific (US trawled) Crab: Blue✳, King (US), Snow Crab: Imitation/Surimi Flounders, Soles (Pacific) Herring: Atlantic Lobster: American/Maine Mahi mahi/Dolphinfish (US) Oysters (wild)✳ Scallops: Sea (wild) Shrimp (US, Canada) Squid Swai, Basa (farmed) Swordfish (US)✳ Tilapia (Central America, farmed) Tuna: Bigeye, Yellowfin (troll/pole) Tuna: Canned Skipjack and Albacore✳ Yellowtail (US farmed)	Caviar, Sturgeon✳ (imported wild) Chilean Seabass/Toothfish✳ Cobia (imported farmed) Cod: Atlantic, imported Pacific Flounders, Halibut, Soles (Atlantic) Groupers✳ Lobster: Spiny (Caribbean) Mahi mahi/Dolphinfish (imported) Marlin: Blue✳, Striped✳ Monkfish Orange Roughy✳ Salmon (farmed, including Atlantic)✳ Sharks✳ Shrimp (imported) Snapper: Red Swordfish (imported)✳ Tilapia (Asia farmed) Tuna: Albacore, Bigeye, Yellowfin (longline)✳ Tuna: Bluefin✳, Tongol, Canned (except Albacore and Skipjack) Yellowtail (imported, farmed)	**Best Choices** are abundant, well-managed and caught or farmed in environmentally friendly ways. **Good Alternatives** are an option, but there are concerns with how they're caught or farmed — or with the health of their habitat due to other human impacts. **Avoid** for now as these items are caught or farmed in ways that harm other marine life or the environment. **Key** ✳ Limit consumption due to concerns about mercury or other contaminants. Visit www.edf.org/seafood ✦ Some or all of this fishery is certified as sustainable to the Marine Stewardship Council standard. Visit www.msc.org Seafood may appear in more than one column

Sustainable Seafood Guide

Source: Monterey Bay Aquarium Seafood Watch, *National Sustainable Seafood Guide, July 2009* Copyright © 2009, Monterey Bay Aquarium Foundation. Used with permission.

Vitamins

Vitamins are potent and essential organic compounds that promote growth and help maintain life and health. Every minute of every day, vitamins help maintain nerves and skin, produce blood cells, build bones and teeth, heal wounds, and convert food energy to body energy—and they do all this without adding any calories to your diet.

Vitamins can be classified as either *fat soluble,* which means they are absorbed through the intestinal tract with the help of fats, or *water soluble,* which means they are dissolved easily in water. Vitamins A, D, E, and K are fat soluble; B-complex vitamins and vitamin C are water soluble. Fat-soluble vitamins tend to be stored in the body, and toxic accumulations in the liver may cause cirrhosis-like symptoms. Water-soluble vitamins generally are excreted and cause few toxicity problems. See Tables 9.2 and 9.3 on pages 267 and 268 for more information on the benefits and dangers of specific vitamins.

Antioxidants The old adage "you are what you eat" is indeed a motto to live by. Beneficial foods are termed **functional foods** based on the ancient belief that eating the right foods not only may prevent disease, but also may actually cure some diseases. This perspective is gaining credibility among the scientific community. Some of the most popular functional foods today are items containing **antioxidants** or other phytochemicals (from the Greek word meaning "plant"). Among the more commonly cited nutrients touted as providing a protective antioxidant effect are vitamin C, vitamin E, and beta-carotene. Although these substances do appear to protect people from the ravages of oxidative stress and resultant tissue damage at the cellular level, you may want to consider all the evidence. First, it is important to understand what damage from *oxidative stress* really is. This damage occurs in a complex process in which *free radicals* (molecules with unpaired electrons that are produced in excess when the body is overly stressed) either damage or kill healthy cells, cell proteins, or genetic material in the cells. Antioxidants produce enzymes that scavenge free radicals, slow their formation, or actually repair oxidative stress damage.

To date, many claims about the benefits of antioxidants in reducing the risk of heart disease, improving vision, and slowing the aging process have not been fully investigated, and conclusive statements about their true benefits are difficult to find (see the **Health Headlines** box on soy on page 269). Large, longitudinal epidemiological studies support the hypothesis that antioxidants in foods, mostly fruits and vegetables, help protect against cognitive decline and risk of Parkinson's disease.[19] Other studies indicate that these vitamins, particularly when taken as supplements, have no effect on atherosclerosis.[20]

Some studies indicate that when people's diets include foods rich in vitamin C, they seem to develop fewer cancers, but other studies detect no effect from dietary vitamin C.[21] Recent studies indicate that high-dose vitamin C given intravenously, rather than orally, may be effective in treating cancer and protecting from diseases affecting the central nervous system.[22]

Possible effects of vitamin E intake are even more controversial. Researchers have long theorized that because many cancers result from DNA damage, and because vitamin E appears to protect against DNA damage, vitamin E would also reduce cancer risk. Surprisingly, the great majority of studies have demonstrated no effect or, in some cases, a negative effect.[23]

Carotenoids are part of the red, orange, and yellow pigments found in fruits and vegetables. They are fat soluble, transported in the blood by lipoproteins, and stored in the fatty tissues of the body. Beta-carotene, the most researched carotenoid, is a precursor of vitamin A. This means that vitamin A can be produced in the body from beta-carotene; like vitamin A, beta-carotene has antioxidant properties.[24] Although there are over 600 carotenoids in nature, two that have received a great deal of attention are *lycopene* (found in tomatoes, papaya, pink grapefruit, and guava) and *lutein* (found in green leafy vegetables such as spinach, broccoli, kale, and brussels sprouts). Both are believed to be more beneficial than beta-carotene in preventing disease.

The National Cancer Institute and the American Cancer Society have endorsed lycopene as a possible factor in reducing the risk of cancer. A landmark study assessing the effects of tomato-based foods reported that men who ate ten or more servings of lycopene-rich foods per week had a 45 percent lower risk of prostate cancer.[25] However, subsequent research has questioned the benefits of lycopene, and some professional groups are modifying their endorsements of tomato-based products.

Lutein is most often touted as a means of protecting the eyes, particularly from age-related macular degeneration (ARMD), a leading cause of blindness for people aged 65 and older. Although there is considerable controversy over many of the benefits of these nutrients in protecting against selected illnesses, experts generally agree that the best way to obtain these nutrients is through foods, rather than pills.

Folate A form of vitamin B that is needed for DNA production in body cells, folate, is particularly important during fetal development; folate deficiencies during

> Blueberries are a great source of antioxidants.

vitamins Essential organic compounds that promote growth and reproduction and help maintain life and health.

functional foods Foods believed to have specific health benefits and/or to prevent disease.

antioxidants Substances believed to protect against oxidative stress and resultant tissue damage at the cellular level.

carotenoids Fat-soluble plant pigments with antioxidant properties.

TABLE

9.2   A Guide to Water-Soluble Vitamins

Vitamin Name and Recommended Intake	Reliable Food Sources	Primary Functions	Toxicity/Deficiency Symptoms
Thiamin (vitamin B$_1$) RDA: Men = 1.2 mg/day Women = 1.1 mg/day	Pork, fortified cereals, enriched rice and pasta, peas, tuna, legumes	Required as enzyme cofactor for carbohydrate and amino acid metabolism	*Toxicity:* none known *Deficiency:* beriberi, fatigue, apathy, decreased memory, confusion, irritability, muscle weakness
Riboflavin (vitamin B$_2$) RDA: Men = 1.3 mg/day Women = 1.1 mg/day	Beef liver, shrimp, milk and dairy foods, fortified cereals, enriched breads and grains	Required as enzyme cofactor for carbohydrate and fat metabolism	*Toxicity:* none known *Deficiency:* ariboflavinosis, swollen mouth and throat, seborrheic dermatitis, anemia
Niacin, nicotinamide, nicotinic acid RDA: Men = 16 mg/day Women = 14 mg/day UL = 35 mg/day	Beef liver, most cuts of meat/fish/poultry, fortified cereals, enriched breads and grains, canned tomato products	Required for carbohydrate and fat metabolism; plays role in DNA replication and repair and cell differentiation	*Toxicity:* flushing, liver damage, glucose intolerance, blurred vision differentiation *Deficiency:* pellagra; vomiting, constipation, or diarrhea; apathy
Vitamin B$_6$ (pyridoxine, pyridoxal, pyridoxamine) RDA: Men and women 19–50 = 1.3 mg/day Men > 50 = 1.7 mg/day Women > 50 = 1.5 mg/day UL = 100 mg/day	Chickpeas (garbanzo beans), most cuts of meat/fish/ poultry, fortified cereals, white potatoes	Required as enzyme cofactor for carbohydrate and amino acid metabolism; assists synthesis of blood cells	*Toxicity:* nerve damage, skin lesions *Deficiency:* anemia; seborrheic dermatitis; depression, confusion, and convulsions
Folate (folic acid) RDA: Men = 400 µg/day Women = 400 µg/day UL = 1,000 µg/day	Fortified cereals, enriched breads and grains, spinach, legumes (lentils, chickpeas, pinto beans), greens (spinach, romaine lettuce), liver	Required as enzyme cofactor for amino acid metabolism; required for DNA synthesis; involved in metabolism of homocysteine	*Toxicity:* masks symptoms of vitamin B$_{12}$ deficiency, specifically signs of nerve damage *Deficiency:* macrocytic anemia; neural tube defects in a developing fetus; elevated homocysteine levels
Vitamin B$_{12}$ (cobalamin) RDA: Men = 2.4 µg/day Women = 2.4 µg/day	Shellfish, all cuts of meat/fish/poultry, milk and dairy foods, fortified cereals	Assists with formation of blood; required for healthy nervous system function; involved as enzyme cofactor in metabolism of homocysteine	*Toxicity:* none known *Deficiency:* pernicious anemia; tingling and numbness of extremities; nerve damage; memory loss, disorientation, and dementia
Pantothenic acid AI: Men = 5 mg/day Women = 5 mg/day	Meat/fish/poultry, shiitake mushrooms, fortified cereals, egg yolk	Assists with fat metabolism	*Toxicity:* none known *Deficiency:* rare
Biotin RDA: Men = 30 µg/day Women = 30 µg/day	Nuts, egg yolk	Involved as enzyme cofactor in carbohydrate, fat, and protein metabolism	*Toxicity:* none known *Deficiency:* rare
Vitamin C (ascorbic acid) RDA: Men = 90 mg/day Women = 75 mg/day Smokers = 35 mg more per day than RDA UL = 2,000 mg	Sweet peppers, citrus fruits and juices, broccoli, strawberries, kiwi	Antioxidant in extracellular fluid and lungs; regenerates oxidized vitamin E; assists with collagen synthesis; enhances immune function; assists in synthesis of hormones, neurotransmitters, and DNA; enhances iron absorption	*Toxicity:* nausea and diarrhea, nosebleeds, increased oxidative damage, increased formation of kidney stones in people with kidney disease *Deficiency:* scurvy, bone pain and fractures, depression, and anemia

Note: RDA = Recommended Daily Allowance; AI = Adequate Intakes; UL = Tolerable Upper Level Intakes. Values are for all adults aged 19 and older, except as noted. Values increase among women who are pregnant or lactating.

Source: From J. Thompson and M. Manore, *Nutrition: An Applied Approach.* 2d ed. (San Francisco: Benjamin Cummings, 2009). Reprinted by permission of Pearson Education.

Vitamin Name and Recommended Intake	Reliable Food Sources	Primary Functions	Toxicity/Deficiency Symptoms
Vitamin A (retinol, retinal, retinoic acid) RDA: Men = 900 µg Women = 700 µg UL = 3,000 µg/day	Preformed retinol: beef and chicken liver, egg yolks, milk Carotenoid precursors: spinach, carrots, mango, apricots, cantaloupe, pumpkin, yams	Required for ability of eyes to adjust to changes in light; protects color vision; assists cell differentiation; required for sperm production in men and fertilization in women; contributes to healthy bone and healthy immune system	*Toxicity:* fatigue; bone and joint pain; spontaneous abortion and birth defects of fetuses in pregnant women; nausea and diarrhea; liver damage; nervous system damage; blurred vision; hair loss; skin disorders *Deficiency:* night blindness, xerophthalmia; impaired growth, immunity, and reproductive function
Vitamin D (cholecalciferol) AI (assumes that person does not get adequate sun exposure): Adult 19–50 = 5 µg/day Adult 50–70 = 10 µg/day Adult > 70 = 15 µg/day UL = 50 µg/day	Canned salmon and mackerel, milk, fortified cereals	Regulates blood calcium levels; maintains bone health; assists cell differentiation	*Toxicity:* hypercalcemia *Deficiency:* rickets in children; osteomalacia and/or osteoporosis in adults
Vitamin E (tocopherol) RDA: Men = 15 mg/day Women = 15 mg/day UL = 1,000 mg/day	Sunflower seeds, almonds, vegetable oils, fortified cereals	As a powerful antioxidant, protects cell membranes, polyunsaturated fatty acids, and vitamin A from oxidation; protects white blood cells; enhances immune function; improves absorption of vitamin A	*Toxicity:* rare *Deficiency:* hemolytic anemia; impairment of nerve, muscle, and immune function
Vitamin K (phylloquinone, menaquinone, menadione) AI: Men = 120 µg/day Women = 90 µg/day	Kale, spinach, turnip greens, brussels sprouts	Serves as a coenzyme during production of specific proteins that assist in blood coagulation and bone metabolism	*Toxicity:* none known *Deficiency:* impaired blood clotting; possible effect on bone health

Note: RDA = Recommended Daily Allowance; AI = Adequate Intakes; UL = Tolerable Upper Level Intakes. Values are for all adults aged 19 and older, except as noted. Values increase among women who are pregnant or lactating.

Source: From J. Thompson and M. Manore, *Nutrition: An Applied Approach.* 2d ed. (San Francisco: Benjamin Cummings, 2009). Reprinted by permission of Pearson Education.

pregnancy can result in spina bifida, a birth defect in which a baby's spine and spinal cord are not fully developed. In 1998, the FDA began requiring that all bread, cereal, rice, and pasta products sold in the United States be fortified with folic acid, the synthetic form of folate. This practice, which boosts folate intake by an average of 100 micrograms daily, is intended to decrease the number of infants born with spina bifida and other neural tube defects.

Folate was widely studied in the late 1990s for its potential to decrease blood levels of *homocysteine* (an amino acid that has been linked to vascular diseases) and to protect against cardiovascular disease (CVD).[26] More recent research has raised questions about the benefits of the B vitamins in

minerals Inorganic, indestructible elements that aid physiological processes.

macrominerals Minerals that the body needs in fairly large amounts.

trace minerals Minerals that the body needs in only very small amounts.

reducing the risks of CVD or stroke, leading researchers to question these earlier results.[27]

Minerals

Minerals are the inorganic, indestructible elements that aid physiological processes within the body. Without minerals, vitamins could not be absorbed. Minerals are readily excreted and are usually not toxic. **Macrominerals** (also called *major minerals*) are those minerals that the body needs in fairly large amounts: sodium, calcium, phosphorus, magnesium, potassium, sulfur, and chloride. **Trace minerals** include iron, zinc, manganese, copper, and iodine. Only very small amounts of trace minerals are needed, and serious problems may result if excesses or deficiencies occur (see Tables 9.4 and 9.5 on pages 270 and 271).

Health Headlines

SOY WONDER?

Vegetarians and health enthusiasts have long known that foods made from soybeans offer a great alternative to meat, poultry, and other animal-based products. Soy protein is generally lower in calories and fat than animal protein. The FDA, American Heart Association, and others have provided endorsements or support for soy as a staple in the diet, suggesting it is associated with a host of health benefits, including reductions in heart disease, breast cancer, high cholesterol levels, and hot flashes during menopause. But is it all too good to be true?

An increasing number of new studies have failed to support such health claims, and have raised concern over certain components of soy products, particularly specific phytochemicals. In plants, mainly soybeans and other legumes, phytochemicals are biologically active, naturally occurring chemical components that are believed to act as natural defenses for the plant, protecting them from oxidative damage, infection, and microbial invasions. One type of phytochemical, *flavonoids* (a group of over 800 blue, red, and violet plant pigments found in foods ranging from teas and apples to grapes and red wine), have been shown to reduce the risk of heart disease by acting as antioxidants. While

soy may have a small effect on reducing lipids, other potential CVD effects need more research. In particular, researchers are looking at the way in which soy is processed, which may reduce its potential effects.

Another phyto-chemical group, the *isoflavones*, are among those soy components most intensely scrutinized in recent years, particularly in studies focused on their role in reducing cancer. Why the scrutiny? Because some isoflavones are phytoestrogens, that is, plant steroidal versions of estrogens. The simplified theory, based on early research, was that they may be cancer protective and may decrease the hormone-related effects of estrogen-positive breast cancer by blocking carcinogens or suppressing tumors. Newer research calls into question the effect of soy in reducing cancer risk or on survival, particularly at the lower consumption levels typically seen in Western populations. Additional research is needed to assess whether soy consumption that begins during the adult years or earlier affects subsequent risk of cancer development.

The bottom line is that soy foods don't seem to lower cholesterol and triglyceride levels as much as previously thought. If you're supplementing your diet with soy as

an alternative to high-fat, high-cholesterol, high-calorie foods or for humane or environmental reasons, you're probably doing the right thing. Most soy products also contain higher fiber and omega-3 fatty acids, which may reduce inflammation and certain health risks. If you are mega-dosing on soy to protect against heart disease, breast cancer, hot flashes, or other chronic diseases, you should take a close look at the research, as more is needed to prove the effectiveness of such actions.

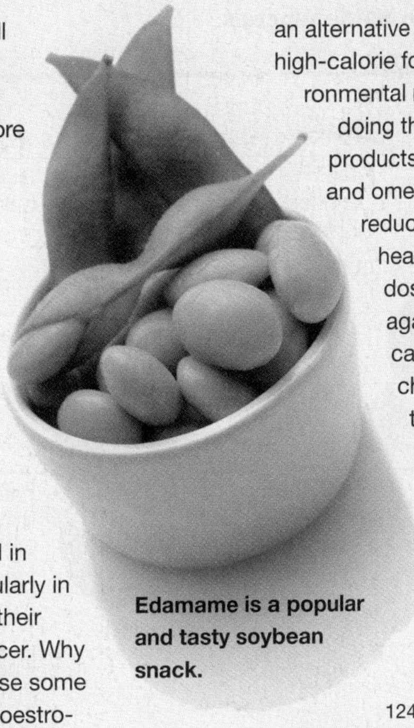

Edamame is a popular and tasty soybean snack.

Sources: C. W. Xiao, "Health Effects of Soy Protein and Isoflavones in Humans," *Journal of Nutrition* 138 (2008): 1244S–49S; E. Balk et al., *Effects of Soy on Health Outcomes,* Evidence Report/Technology Assessment Number 126, AHRQ Publication Number 05-E024-1 (Rockville, MD: Agency for Healthcare Research and Quality, 2005); F. Sacks et al., "Soy Proteins, Isoflavones and Cardiovascular Health: An American Heart Association Science Advisory for Professionals from the Nutrition Committee," *Circulation* 113 (2006): 1034–44; A.C. Yh et al., "Isoflavone Intake in Persons at High Risk of Cardiovascular Events: Implications for Vascular Endothelial Function and the Carotid Atherosclerotic Burden," *American Journal of Clinical Nutrition* 86, no. 4 (2007): 938–44; M. Gammons, B. Fink, S. Steck, and M. Wolff, "Soy Intake and Breast Cancer: An Elucidation of an Unanswered Question," *British Journal of Cancer* 98 (2008): 2–3; S. Boyapati et al., "Soyfood Intake and Breast Cancer Survival: A Followup of the Shanghai Breast Cancer Study," *Breast Cancer Research and Treatment* 92, no. 1 (2005): 11–17; B. Fink et al., "Dietary Flavonoid Intake and Breast Cancer Risk among Women on Long Island," *American Journal of Epidemiology* 165, no. 5 (2007): 514–23.

Sodium Sodium is necessary for the regulation of blood and body fluids, transmission of nerve impulses, heart activity, and certain metabolic functions. It enhances flavors, balances the bitterness of certain foods, acts as a preservative, and tenderizes meats, so it's often present in high quantities in many of the foods we eat. As a result, most of us consume far too much sodium. Today, the Institute of Medicine, the American Heart Association, the FDA, and the USDA are among the many professional organizations that recommend that healthy people consume fewer than 2,300 milligrams of sodium each day. What does that really mean?

For most of us, that means consuming less than 1 teaspoon of table salt per day! Recent studies indicate that, on average, we eat nearly twice that amount each day.[28]

A common misconception is that salt and sodium are the same thing. However, table salt accounts for only 15 percent of sodium intake. The majority of sodium in our diet comes from highly processed foods that are infused with sodium to enhance flavor and preservation. Pickles, salty snack foods, processed cheeses, canned soups, frozen dinners, many breads and bakery products, and smoked meats and sausages often contain several hundred milligrams of sodium per serving.

TABLE
9.4 | **A Guide to Major Minerals**

Mineral Name and Recommended Intake	Reliable Food Sources	Primary Functions	Toxicity/Deficiency Symptoms
Sodium AI: Adults = 1.5 g/day (1,500 mg/day)	Table salt, pickles, most canned soups, snack foods, cured luncheon meats, canned tomato products	Fluid balance; acid–base balance; transmission of nerve impulses; muscle contraction	*Toxicity:* water retention, high blood pressure, loss of calcium *Deficiency:* muscle cramps, dizziness, fatigue, nausea, vomiting, mental confusion
Potassium AI: Adults = 4.7 g/day (4,700 mg/day)	Most fresh fruits and vegetables: potato, banana, tomato juice, orange juice, melon	Fluid balance; transmission of nerve impulses; muscle contraction	*Toxicity:* muscle weakness, vomiting, irregular heartbeat *Deficiency:* muscle weakness, paralysis, mental confusion, irregular heartbeat
Phosphorus RDA: Adults = 700 mg/day	Milk/cheese/yogurt, soy milk and tofu, legumes (lentils, black beans), nuts (almonds, peanuts), poultry	Fluid balance; bone formation; component of ATP, which provides energy for our bodies	*Toxicity:* muscle spasms, convulsions, low blood calcium *Deficiency:* muscle weakness, muscle damage, bone pain, dizziness
Chloride AI: Adults = 2.3 g/day (2,300 mg/day)	Table salt	Fluid balance; transmission of nerve impulses; component of stomach acid (HCL); antibacterial	*Toxicity:* none known *Deficiency:* dangerous blood acid–base imbalances, irregular heartbeat
Calcium AI: Adults 19–50 = 1,000 mg/day Adults > 50 = 1,200 mg/day UL = 2,500 mg	Milk/yogurt/cheese (best absorbed form of calcium), sardines, collard greens and spinach, calcium-fortified juices	Primary component of bone; acid–base balance; transmission of nerve impulses; muscle contraction	*Toxicity:* mineral imbalances, shock, kidney failure, fatigue, mental confusion *Deficiency:* osteoporosis, convulsions, heart failure
Magnesium RDA: Men 19–30 = 400 mg/day Men > 30 = 420 mg/day Women 19–30 = 310 mg/day Women > 30 = 320 mg/day UL = 350 mg/day	Greens (spinach, kale, collards), whole grains, seeds, nuts, legumes (navy and black beans)	Component of bone; muscle contraction; assists more than 300 enzyme systems	*Toxicity:* none known *Deficiency:* low blood calcium; muscle spasms or seizures; nausea; weakness; increased risk of chronic diseases such as heart disease, hypertension, osteoporosis, and type 2 diabetes
Sulfur No DRI	Protein-rich foods	Component of certain B vitamins and amino acids; acid–base balance; detoxification in liver	*Toxicity:* none known *Deficiency:* none known

Note: RDA = Recommended Daily Allowance; AI = Adequate Intakes; UL = Tolerable Upper Level Intake. Values are for all adults aged 19 and older, except as noted.

Source: From J. Thompson and M. Manore, *Nutrition: An Applied Approach.* 2d ed. (San Francisco: Benjamin Cummings, 2009). Reprinted by permission of Pearson Education.

Why is high sodium intake a concern? Many experts believe that there is a link between excessive sodium intake and hypertension (high blood pressure). Although this theory is controversial, it is recommended that hypertensive Americans cut back on sodium to reduce their risk for cardiovascular disorders including stroke, debilitating bone fractures, and other health problems.[29]

Calcium The issue of calcium consumption has gained national attention with the rising incidence of osteoporosis among older adults. Although calcium plays a vital role in building strong bones and teeth, muscle contraction, blood clotting, nerve impulse transmission, regulating heartbeat, and fluid balance within cells, most Americans do not consume the recommended 1,000–1,200 milligrams of calcium per day.[30]

It is critical to consume the minimum required amount each day. Milk is one of the richest sources of dietary calcium. Calcium-fortified orange juice and soy milk are good alternatives if you do not drink dairy milk. Many green leafy vegetables are good sources of calcium, but some contain oxalic acid,

Mineral Name and Recommended Intake	Reliable Food Sources	Primary Functions	Toxicity/Deficiency Symptoms
Selenium RDA: Adults = 55 µg/day UL = 400 µg/day	Nuts, shellfish, meat/fish/poultry, whole grains	Required for carbohydrate and fat metabolism	*Toxicity:* brittle hair and nails, skin rashes, nausea and vomiting, weakness, liver disease *Deficiency:* specific forms of heart disease and arthritis, impaired immune function, muscle pain and wasting, depression, hostility
Fluoride AI: Men = 4 mg/day Women = 3 mg/day UL = 2.2 mg/day for children 4–8 years; children > 8 years = 10 mg/day	Fluoridated water and other beverages made with this water	Development and maintenance of healthy teeth and bones	*Toxicity:* fluorosis of teeth and bones *Deficiency:* dental caries, low bone density
Iodine RDA: Adults = 150 µg/day UL = 1,100 µg/day	Iodized salt and foods processed with iodized salt	Synthesis of thyroid hormones; temperature regulation; reproduction and growth	*Toxicity:* goiter *Deficiency:* goiter, hypothyroidism, cretinism in infant of mother who is iodine deficient
Chromium AI: Men 19–50 = 35 µg/day Men > 50 = 30 µg/day Women 19–50 = 25 µg/day Women > 50 = 20 µg/day	Grains, meat/fish/poultry, some fruits and vegetables	Glucose transport; metabolism of DNA and RNA; immune function and growth	*Toxicity:* none known *Deficiency:* elevated blood glucose and blood lipids, damage to brain and nervous system
Manganese AI: Men = 2.3 mg/day Women = 1.8 mg/day UL = 11 mg/day for adults	Whole grains, nuts, legumes, some fruits and vegetables	Assists many enzyme systems; synthesis of protein found in bone and cartilage	*Toxicity:* impairment of neuromuscular system *Deficiency:* impaired growth and reproductive function, reduced bone density, impaired glucose and lipid metabolism, skin rash
Iron RDA: Men = 8 mg/day Women 19–50 = 18 mg/day Women > 50 = 8 mg/day	Meat/fish/poultry (best absorbed form of iron), fortified cereals, legumes, spinach	Component of hemoglobin in blood cells; component of myoglobin in muscle cells; assists many enzyme systems	*Toxicity:* nausea, vomiting, and diarrhea; dizziness, confusion; rapid heartbeat; organ damage; death *Deficiency:* iron-deficiency microcytic anemia, hypochromic anemia
Zinc RDA: Men 11 mg/day Women = 8 mg/day UL = 40 mg/day	Meat/fish/poultry (best absorbed form of zinc), fortified cereals, legumes	Assists more than 100 enzyme systems; immune system function; growth and sexual maturation; gene regulation	*Toxicity:* nausea, vomiting, and diarrhea; headaches; depressed immune function; reduced absorption of copper *Deficiency:* growth retardation, delayed sexual maturation, eye and skin lesions, hair loss, increased incidence of illness and infection
Copper RDA: Adults = 900 µg/day UL = 10 mg/day	Shellfish, organ meats, nuts, legumes	Assists many enzyme systems; iron transport	*Toxicity:* nausea, vomiting, and diarrhea; liver damage *Deficiency:* anemia, reduced levels of white blood cells, osteoporosis in infants and growing children

Note: RDA = Recommended Daily Allowance; AI = Adequate Intakes; UL = Tolerable Upper Intake Level. Values are for all adults aged 19 and older, except as noted.

Source: Adapted from J. Thompson and M. Manore, *Nutrition: An Applied Approach.* 2d ed. (San Francisco: Benjamin Cummings, 2009). Reprinted by permission of Pearson Education.

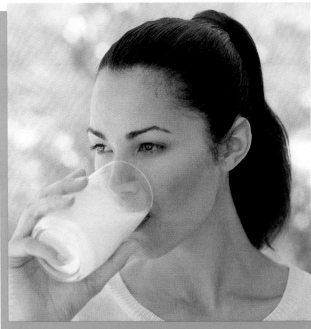

Do teenagers really need to drink milk?

Consumption of calcium, one of the many nutrients in milk, is important for people of all ages. To build healthy bones and teeth, and to prevent bone loss later in life, you need to get enough calcium while you are young; women, in particular, should be sure to obtain adequate amounts. Yet, 85% of adolescent girls do not consume enough calcium, and during the last 25 years, consumption of milk has decreased 36% among teenage girls. If you are one of those who do not drink milk, be sure you are getting enough calcium—at least 1,200 milligrams per day—through other sources.

which makes their calcium harder to absorb. Spinach, chard, and beet greens are not particularly good sources of calcium, whereas broccoli, cauliflower, and many peas and beans offer good supplies.

It is generally best to take calcium throughout the day, consuming it with foods containing protein, vitamin D, and vitamin C for optimal absorption. Many dairy products are fortified with vitamin D, which is known to improve calcium absorption. We also know that sunlight increases the manufacture of vitamin D in the body and is therefore like an extra calcium source.

Do you consume carbonated soft drinks? Be aware that the added phosphoric acid (phosphate) in these drinks can cause you to excrete extra calcium, which may result in calcium loss from your bones. A recent study of 2,500 men and women found that in women who consumed at least three cans of cola per week, even diet cola, bone density of the hip was 4 to 5 percent lower than in women who drank fewer than one cola per month. Colas did not seem to have the same effect on men.[31]

anemia Condition that results from the body's inability to produce hemoglobin.

Recommended Dietary Allowances (RDAs) The average daily intakes of energy and nutrients considered adequate to meet the needs of most healthy people in the United States under usual conditions.

Iron Worldwide, iron deficiency is the most common nutrient deficiency, affecting more than 2 billion people, nearly 30 percent of the world's population. In the United States iron deficiency is less prevalent, but it is still the most common micronutrient deficiency.[32] How much iron do we need? Women aged 19 to 50 need about 18 milligrams per day, and men aged 19 to 50 need about 8 milligrams.

Iron deficiency frequently leads to *iron-deficiency anemia.* **Anemia** is a problem resulting from the body's inability to produce hemoglobin (the bright red oxygen-carrying component of the blood). When iron-deficiency anemia occurs, body cells receive less oxygen, and carbon dioxide wastes are removed less efficiently. As a result, the iron-deficient person feels tired and run down. Iron deficiency in the diet is a common cause, but not the only cause, of anemia; anemia can also result from blood loss, cancer, ulcers, and other conditions.

Iron overload or iron toxicity due to ingesting too many iron-containing supplements remains the leading cause of accidental poisoning in small children in the United States. Symptoms of toxicity include nausea, vomiting, diarrhea, rapid heartbeat, weak pulse, dizziness, shock, and confusion. Excess iron intake has also been associated with other problems: a recent study of over 45,000 men indicated that those who consumed excess heme iron—the kind found in meat, seafood, and poultry—had a 20 percent higher risk of gallstones than those who consumed low-iron foods or got their iron from supplements.[33]

Determining Your Nutritional Needs

Historically, various government and scientific organizations developed dietary guidelines to reduce the public's risk of diseases from nutrient deficiency. Known as the **Recommended Dietary Allowances (RDAs),** these guidelines have provided Americans and Canadians with recommended intake levels that meet the nutritional needs of about 97 percent of healthy individuals. In 1997, the U.S. Food and Nutrition Board replaced and expanded upon the RDAs by creating new *Dietary Reference Intakes (DRIs),* a list of 26 nutrients essential to maintaining health. The DRIs identify recommended and maximum safe intake levels for healthy people and establish the amount of a nutrient needed to prevent deficiencies or to reduce the risk of chronic disease. DRIs are considered the umbrella guidelines under which the following categories fall:

- *U.S. Recommended Dietary Allowances (USRDAs):* The reference standard for intake levels necessary to meet the nutritional needs of 97 to 98 percent of healthy individuals
- *Adequate Intake (AI):* The recommended average daily nutrient intake level by healthy people when there is not enough research to determine the full RDA
- *Tolerable Upper Intake Level (UL):* The highest amount of a nutrient an individual can consume daily without the risk of adverse health effects

Reading Labels for Health

To help consumers determine the nutritional values of foods, the FDA and the USDA developed the *Reference Daily Intakes (RDIs)* and the *Daily Reference Values (DRVs)*. RDIs are the recommended daily amounts of 19 vitamins and minerals, also known as *micronutrients,* and DRVs are the recommended amounts for macronutrients, such as total fat, saturated fat, cholesterol, total carbohydrates, dietary fiber, sodium, potassium, and protein.

Confused by all of these values? Don't despair—many people are confused by all the numbers, percentages, and serving sizes that make up today's labels. Just remember this: Together, RDIs and DRVs make up the **Daily Values (DVs).** These are the percentages that you will find listed as "% Daily Value" on food and supplement labels (see Figure 9.5). In addition to the percentage of nutrients found in a serving of food, labels include information on the serving size, calories, calories from fat per serving, and percentage of *trans* fats in a food.

Supplements: Research on the Daily Dose

Dietary supplements are products—usually vitamins and minerals—taken by mouth and intended to supplement existing diets. Ingredients range from vitamins, minerals, and herbs to enzymes, amino acids, fatty acids, and organ tissues. They can come in tablet, capsule, liquid, powder, and other forms. Because of dietary supplements' potential for influencing health, their sales have skyrocketed in the past decades.

It is important to note that all dietary supplements are not regulated like other food and drug products. The FDA does not evaluate the safety and efficacy of supplements prior to their marketing; it can take action to remove a supplement from the market only after it has been proven harmful. Currently, the United States has no formal

Daily Values (DVs) Percentages listed as "% DV" on food and supplement labels; made up of the RDIs and DRVs together.

dietary supplements Vitamins and minerals taken by mouth that are intended to supplement existing diets.

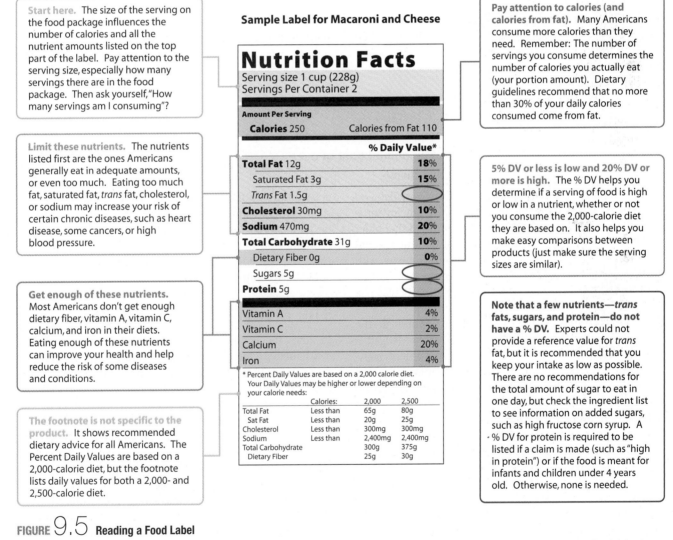

Start here. The size of the serving on the food package influences the number of calories and all the nutrient amounts listed on the top part of the label. Pay attention to the serving size, especially how many servings there are in the food package. Then ask yourself, "How many servings am I consuming"?

Limit these nutrients. The nutrients listed first are the ones Americans generally eat in adequate amounts, or even too much. Eating too much fat, saturated fat, *trans* fat, cholesterol, or sodium may increase your risk of certain chronic diseases, such as heart disease, some cancers, or high blood pressure.

Get enough of these nutrients. Most Americans don't get enough dietary fiber, vitamin A, vitamin C, calcium, and iron in their diets. Eating enough of these nutrients can improve your health and help reduce the risk of some diseases and conditions.

The footnote is not specific to the product. It shows recommended dietary advice for all Americans. The Percent Daily Values are based on a 2,000-calorie diet, but the footnote lists daily values for both a 2,000- and 2,500-calorie diet.

Pay attention to calories (and calories from fat). Many Americans consume more calories than they need. Remember: The number of servings you consume determines the number of calories you actually eat (your portion amount). Dietary guidelines recommend that no more than 30% of your daily calories consumed come from fat.

5% DV or less is low and 20% DV or more is high. The % DV helps you determine if a serving of food is high or low in a nutrient, whether or not you consume the 2,000-calorie diet they are based on. It also helps you make easy comparisons between products (just make sure the serving sizes are similar).

Note that a few nutrients—*trans* fats, sugars, and protein—do not have a % DV. Experts could not provide a reference value for *trans* fat, but it is recommended that you keep your intake as low as possible. There are no recommendations for the total amount of sugar to eat in one day, but check the ingredient list to see information on added sugars, such as high fructose corn syrup. A % DV for protein is required to be listed if a claim is made (such as "high in protein") or if the food is meant for infants and children under 4 years old. Otherwise, none is needed.

Sample Label for Macaroni and Cheese

Nutrition Facts
Serving size 1 cup (228g)
Servings Per Container 2

Amount Per Serving

Calories 250 — Calories from Fat 110

% Daily Value*

Total Fat 12g	**18%**
Saturated Fat 3g	**15%**
Trans Fat 1.5g	
Cholesterol 30mg	**10%**
Sodium 470mg	**20%**
Total Carbohydrate 31g	**10%**
Dietary Fiber 0g	**0%**
Sugars 5g	
Protein 5g	
Vitamin A	4%
Vitamin C	2%
Calcium	20%
Iron	4%

* Percent Daily Values are based on a 2,000 calorie diet. Your Daily Values may be higher or lower depending on your calorie needs:

	Calories:	2,000	2,500
Total Fat	Less than	65g	80g
Sat Fat	Less than	20g	25g
Cholesterol	Less than	300mg	300mg
Sodium	Less than	2,400mg	2,400mg
Total Carbohydrate		300g	375g
Dietary Fiber		25g	30g

FIGURE 9.5 **Reading a Food Label**

Source: Center for Food Safety and Applied Nutrition, "How to Understand and Use the Nutrition Facts Label," 2004, www.cfsan.fda.gov/~dms/foodlab.html.

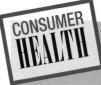

CONSUMER HEALTH: MAKING SENSE OF NUTRITION HYPE

Frustrated by health food discoveries that seem to fizzle as fast as they burst onto the scene? You're not alone. In the past few decades, we've been bombarded with a wide variety of conflicting scientific evidence and claims about dietary choices we can make to reduce the risk of certain diseases and promote health. The good news is that there are positive outcomes in all this research, and positive health effects can be gained from proper nutrition.

The bad news? This plethora of studies produces conflicting reports that leave many of us scratching our heads. Here is what you need to consider about reports you hear and read about in the media:

1. Remember that any single study must be viewed with caution. Often there are other, equally reputable, studies that may prove opposite findings.
2. Many of these studies are meta-analyses. This means they summarize the results of many studies, often without regard to population, study design, age of the population studied, confounders (things that could influence effects), dosage, underlying bias of the population, and many other factors.
3. Information gained from studies like the Women's Health Initiative about diet and exercise is largely based on self-reporting. Many people question the validity of some responses. Even randomized, controlled trials have limitations, and results should be viewed in light of potential limitations and the results of previous studies.
4. The best studies will conclude that more research must be done. Though this may seem frustrating and may not give the definitive answers we are looking for, this is the most current and accurate response that researchers can give.

---

guidelines for supplement sale and safety, and supplement manufacturers are responsible for self-monitoring their activities. (See the **Consumer Health** box above for tips on how to evaluate nutritional claims and hype.)

For years, health experts had touted the benefits of eating a balanced diet over popping a vitamin or mineral supplement, so it came as a surprise when a 2001 article in the *Journal of the American Medical Association (JAMA)* recommended that "a vitamin/mineral supplement a day just might be important in keeping the doctor away, particularly for some groups of people."[34] The article indicated that older adults, vegans, alcohol-dependent individuals, and patients with malabsorption problems may be at particular risk for deficiency of several vitamins. Although the article acknowledged a possible risk of overdosing on fat-soluble vitamins, it noted that preliminary research has linked inadequate amounts of vitamins B_6, B_{12}, D, and E and lycopene to chronic diseases, including coronary heart disease, cancer, and osteoporosis.

Yet, the scientific debate doesn't stop there. In a 2006 report issued by the National Institutes of Health, a 13-member panel of experts concluded that "the present evidence is insufficient to recommend either for or against the use of multivitamins and minerals by the American public to prevent

52%
of U.S. adults take multivitamins, at an annual cost of over $23 billion.

chronic diseases."[35] The committee concluded that much more research must be done to evaluate the huge amount of seemingly contradictory studies about using supplements individually or in combination.

Probiotics Probiotics—live microorganisms found in, or added to, fermented foods that optimize the bacterial environment in our intestines—are currently receiving much attention as natural healers. Commonly, they are found in fermented milk products such as yogurt, and you will see them labeled as *Lactobacillus* or *Bifidobacterium* in a product's list of ingredients. Probiotics do not typically pose harm to healthy humans. However, someone with a compromised immune system could have complications over time.

The MyPyramid Food Guide

In 2005, the Food Guide Pyramid underwent a landmark overhaul to account more completely for the variety of nutritional needs throughout the U.S. population (Figure 9.6). This new pyramid, called the MyPyramid Plan, replaced the former Food Guide Pyramid promoted since 1993 by the USDA and incorporated the *2005 Dietary Guidelines for Americans*.[36] These guidelines are updated every 5 years; the *2010 Guidelines* are currently being developed, and will be released in the fall of 2010.[37] Although the former pyramid emphasized variety in daily intake, it did not reflect what we now know about restricting fats, eating more fruits and vegetables, and consuming whole grains. The MyPyramid Plan also takes into consideration the various dietary and caloric needs for a variety of individuals (such as people over age 65,

---

probiotics Live microorganisms found in or added to fermented foods; they are intended to optimize the bacterial environment in our intestines.

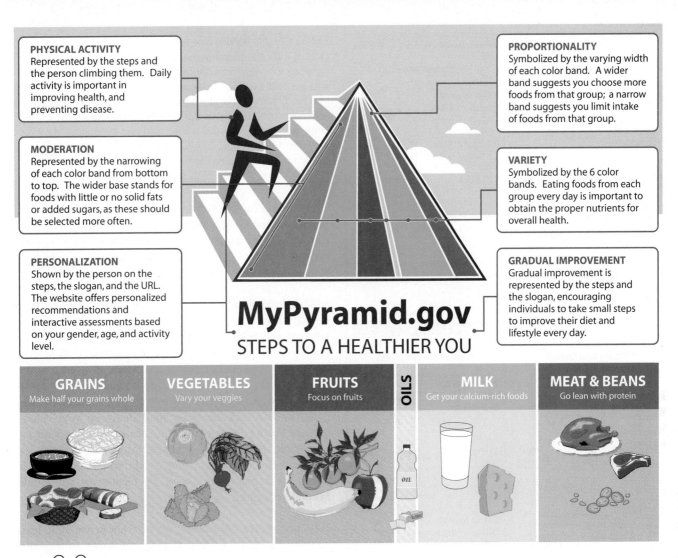

PHYSICAL ACTIVITY
Represented by the steps and the person climbing them. Daily activity is important in improving health, and preventing disease.

MODERATION
Represented by the narrowing of each color band from bottom to top. The wider base stands for foods with little or no solid fats or added sugars, as these should be selected more often.

PERSONALIZATION
Shown by the person on the steps, the slogan, and the URL. The website offers personalized recommendations and interactive assessments based on your gender, age, and activity level.

PROPORTIONALITY
Symbolized by the varying width of each color band. A wider band suggests you choose more foods from that group; a narrow band suggests you limit intake of foods from that group.

VARIETY
Symbolized by the 6 color bands. Eating foods from each group every day is important to obtain the proper nutrients for overall health.

GRADUAL IMPROVEMENT
Gradual improvement is represented by the steps and the slogan, encouraging individuals to take small steps to improve their diet and lifestyle every day.

MyPyramid.gov
STEPS TO A HEALTHIER YOU

GRAINS Make half your grains whole
VEGETABLES Vary your veggies
FRUITS Focus on fruits
OILS
MILK Get your calcium-rich foods
MEAT & BEANS Go lean with protein

FIGURE 9.6 **MyPyramid Plan**
The USDA MyPyramid Plan takes a new approach to dietary and exercise recommendations. Each colored section of the pyramid represents a food group, with the specific needs of individuals in mind.
Source: U.S. Department of Agriculture, 2005, www.MyPyramid.gov.

children, and active adults) as well as activity levels. (See the **Gender & Health** box on page 277 for a discussion of men's and women's different nutritional needs.) The MyPyramid Plan promotes personalizing dietary and exercise recommendations based on individual needs.[38]

Using the MyPyramid Plan

Understanding serving sizes, incorporating daily physical activity, and eating a nutritionally balanced diet are key components to using the MyPyramid Plan recommendations successfully. Though these elements are not new to the 2005 pyramid, they have been updated to reflect the latest in nutritional science.

Understanding Serving Sizes How much is one serving? Is it different from a portion? Although these two terms are often used interchangeably, they actually mean very

different things. A *serving* is the recommended amount you should consume, whereas a *portion* is the amount you choose to eat at any one time. Most of us select portions that are much bigger than servings. According to a survey conducted by the American Institute for Cancer Research (AICR), respondents were asked to estimate the standard servings defined by the old USDA Food Guide Pyramid for eight different foods. Only 1 percent of those surveyed correctly answered all serving size questions, and nearly 65 percent answered five or more of them incorrectly.[39] See **Figure 9.7** on page 276 for a handy pocket guide with tips on recognizing serving sizes.

Unfortunately, we don't always get a clear picture from food producers and advertisers about what a serving really is. Consider a bottle of soda: The food label may list one serving size as 8 fluid ounces and 100 calories. However, note the size of the entire bottle; the bottle may hold 20 ounces, and drinking the entire bottle serves up a whopping 250 calories.

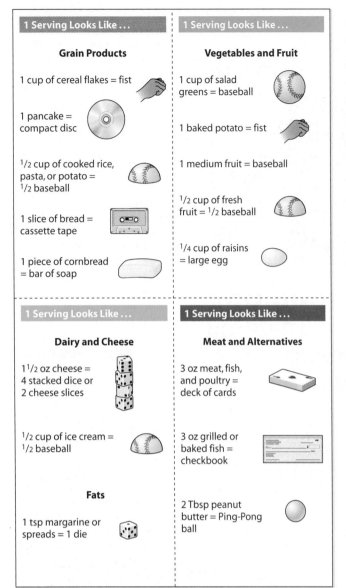

1 Serving Looks Like ...	1 Serving Looks Like ...
Grain Products	**Vegetables and Fruit**
1 cup of cereal flakes = fist	1 cup of salad greens = baseball
1 pancake = compact disc	1 baked potato = fist
1/2 cup of cooked rice, pasta, or potato = 1/2 baseball	1 medium fruit = baseball
1 slice of bread = cassette tape	1/2 cup of fresh fruit = 1/2 baseball
1 piece of cornbread = bar of soap	1/4 cup of raisins = large egg

1 Serving Looks Like ...	1 Serving Looks Like ...
Dairy and Cheese	**Meat and Alternatives**
1 1/2 oz cheese = 4 stacked dice or 2 cheese slices	3 oz meat, fish, and poultry = deck of cards
1/2 cup of ice cream = 1/2 baseball	3 oz grilled or baked fish = checkbook
Fats	
1 tsp margarine or spreads = 1 die	2 Tbsp peanut butter = Ping-Pong ball

FIGURE 9.7 Serving Size Card

One of the challenges of following a healthy diet is judging how big a portion size should be and how many servings you are really eating. The comparisons on this card can help you recall what a standard food serving looks like. For easy reference, photocopy or cut out this card, fold on the dotted lines, and keep it in your wallet. You can even laminate it for long-term use.

Source: National Heart, Lung and Blood Institute, "Portion Distortion," 2007, http://hp2010.nhlbihin.net/portion.

Be sure to eat at least the lowest number of servings from the major food groups; you need them for the nutrients they provide. If you eat a large portion, count it as more than one serving. **Figure 9.8** lists the suggested daily amount of food from each group for a variety of calorie intake levels.

Discretionary Calories Every day you must consume a certain number of nutrient-rich foods to maintain health. *Discretionary calories* are those obtained from foods that do not provide a significant amount of nutritional value. Most of us have a very small discretionary caloric allowance at the end of the day. For example, suppose you are on a 2,000-calorie diet and have eaten wisely all day, choosing whole-grain, low-fat, and low-sugar food items, so your calorie balance for the day is 1,800. This means you can spend the remaining 200 calories on what might be considered indulgences. This might include a soda, a small serving of ice cream, or a higher fat cheese or meat than you would normally consume.

Physical Activity Strive to be physically active for at least 30 minutes daily, preferably with moderate to vigorous activity levels on most days. Physical activity does not mean you have to go to the gym, jog 3 miles a day, or hire a personal trainer. Any activity that gets your heart pumping (such as

	1,200	1,400	1,600	1,800	2,000	2,200	2,400	2,600	2,800	3,000
Fruits	1 cup	1.5 cups	1.5 cups	1.5 cups	2 cups	2 cups	2 cups	2 cups	2.5 cups	2.5 cups
Vegetables	1.5 cups	1.5 cups	2 cups	2.5 cups	2.5 cups	3 cups	3 cups	3.5 cups	3.5 cups	4 cups
Grains	4 oz-eq.	5 oz-eq.	5 oz-eq.	6 oz-eq.	6 oz-eq.	7 oz-eq.	8 oz-eq.	9 oz-eq.	10 oz-eq.	10 oz-eq.
Meat and Beans	3 oz-eq.	4 oz-eq.	5 oz-eq.	5 oz-eq.	5.5 oz-eq.	6 oz-eq.	6.5 oz-eq.	6.5 oz-eq.	7 oz-eq.	7 oz-eq.
Milk	2 cups	2 cups	3 cups	3 cups	3 cups	3 cups	3 cups	3 cups	3 cups	3 cups
Oils	4 tsp	4 tsp	5 tsp	5 tsp	6 tsp	6 tsp	7 tsp	8 tsp	8 tsp	10 tsp
Discretionary calories	171	171	132	195	267	290	362	410	426	512

FIGURE 9.8 Nutritional Needs for People with Different Energy Requirements

Once you've determined your daily caloric requirements (Table 9.1), use this chart to determine how many servings of each food group you need per day to maintain good health.

Source: U.S. Department of Agriculture, 2005, www.MyPyramid.gov.

Different Bodies, Different Needs

Men and women differ in body size, body composition, and overall metabolic rates. They therefore have differing needs for most nutrients throughout their lives (see Tables 9.2–9.5 for specifics on vitamin and mineral requirements) and face unique difficulties in keeping on track with their dietary goals. Have you ever wondered why men can eat more than women without gaining weight? Although there are many possible reasons, one factor is that women have a lower ratio of lean body mass to adipose (fatty) tissue at all ages and stages of life. Also, after sexual maturation, men's metabolic rate is higher, meaning that they will burn more calories doing the same activities.

In addition, women have many "milestone" times in the life when their nutritional needs vary significantly. From menarche to menopause, women undergo cyclical physiological changes that can have dramatic effects on metabolism and nutritional needs. For example, during pregnancy and lactation, women's nutritional requirements increase substantially. Those who are unable to follow their doctor's strict dietary recommendations may gain too much weight during pregnancy and retain it afterward. During the menstrual cycle, many women report significant food cravings. Those who experience very heavy menstrual cycles may benefit from increased iron in their diet or by taking a supplement. Later in life, with the advent of menopause, nutritional needs again change rather dramatically. With depletion of the hormone estrogen, the body's need for calcium to ward off bone deterioration becomes pronounced. Women must pay closer attention to exercising and getting enough calcium through diet or dietary supplements, or they run the risk of osteoporosis.

Men and women also tend to have different eating habits. For example, women tend to enjoy more fruits and vegetables than men. The average American male eats fewer than three servings of fruits and vegetables per day although five to nine servings are recommended. Women average three to seven servings per day. Men also tend to consume more red meat than women.

---

gardening, playing basketball, heavy yard work, and dancing) are all examples of ways to get moving. For more on physical fitness, see Chapter 11.

Eating Nutrient-Dense Foods Although eating the proper number of servings from MyPyramid is important, it is also important to recognize that there are large caloric, fat, and energy differences among foods within a given food group. For example, fish and hot dogs provide vastly different fat and energy levels per ounce, with fish providing better energy and caloric value per serving. It is important to eat foods that have a high nutritional value for their caloric content. Avoid "empty calories," that is, high-calorie foods that have little nutritional value.

Vegetarianism

According to a new, representative study of over 5,500 U.S. adults, 7.3 million (3.2% of all American adults) are vegetarians and another 22.8 million are "vegetarian inclined" meaning that they are actively choosing to reduce meat consumption in favor of other "faceless" forms of protein.[40] Millions more report being very curious about or contemplating a vegetarian lifestyle. The majority of those who describe themselves as vegetarians are females (59%). Why are so many moving toward meat/dairy reduction and/or elimination in their diets? Of those surveyed, the most common reasons for pursuing a vegetarian lifestyle were:

- Animal welfare (54%)
- Improving health (53%)
- Environmental concerns (47%)
- Natural approaches to wellness (39%)
- Food safety (31%)
- Weight loss (25%)
- Weight maintenance (24%)

Normally, vegetarianism provides a superb alternative to our high-fat, high-calorie, meat-based cuisine. But without proper information and food choices, vegetarians can develop serious dietary problems in much the same way as their meat-eating counterparts.

The term **vegetarian** means different things to different people. Strict vegetarians, or *vegans,* avoid all foods of animal origin, including dairy products and eggs. Far more common are *lacto-vegetarians,* who eat dairy products but avoid flesh foods. *Ovo-vegetarians* add eggs to a vegan diet, and *lacto-ovo-vegetarians* eat both dairy products and eggs. *Pesco-vegetarians* eat fish, dairy products, and eggs, and *semivegetarians* eat chicken, fish, dairy products, and eggs. Some people in the semivegetarian category prefer to call themselves "non-red meat eaters."

Generally, people who follow a balanced vegetarian diet weigh less and have better cholesterol levels, fewer problems with irregular bowel movements (constipation and diarrhea), and a lower risk of heart disease than do nonvegetarians. The benefits of vegetarianism also include a reduced risk of some cancers, particularly colon cancer, and a reduced risk of kidney disease.[41]

Although in the past vegetarians often suffered from vitamin deficiencies, most vegetarians today are adept at

vegetarian A person who follows a diet that excludes some or all animal products.

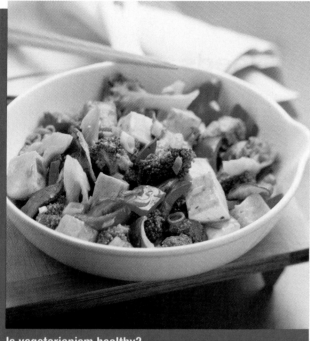

Is vegetarianism healthy?

Adopting a vegan or vegetarian diet can be a very healthy way to eat, as long as you take care to prepare your food healthfully by limiting the use of oils and avoiding added sugars and sodium. Vegetarians also need to ensure that they are getting all the essential amino acids. Meals like this tofu and vegetable stir-fry provide the vegetarian with essential vitamins and protein; adding a whole grain, such as brown rice, would further enhance it by making use of complementary plant proteins.

combining the right types of foods and eating a variety of different foods to ensure proper nutrient intake. Vegan diets may be deficient in vitamins B_2 (riboflavin), B_{12}, and D. Vegans are also at risk for deficiencies of calcium, iron, zinc, and other minerals but can obtain these nutrients from supplements. Strict vegans have to pay much more attention to what they eat than the average person does, but by eating complementary combinations of plant products, they can receive adequate amounts of essential amino acids. In fact, whereas vegans typically get 50 to 60 grams of protein per day, lacto-ovo-vegetarians normally consume between 70 and 90 grams per day, well beyond the RDA. Eating a full variety of grains, legumes, fruits, vegetables, and seeds each day will keep even the strictest vegetarian in excellent health. Pregnant women, older adults, sick people, and children who are vegans need to take special care to ensure that their diets are adequate. In all cases, seek advice from a health care professional if you have questions.

what do you think?

Why are so many people today becoming vegetarians? ● How easy is it to be a vegetarian on your campus? ● What concerns about vegetarianism would you be likely to have, if any?

Improved Eating for the College Student

College students often face a challenge when trying to eat healthy foods. Some students live in dorms and do not have their own cooking or refrigeration facilities. Others live in crowded apartments where everyone forages in the refrigerator for everyone else's food. Still others eat at university food services where food choices may be overwhelming. Nearly all have financial and time constraints that make buying, preparing, and eating healthy food a difficult task. What's a student to do?

When Time and Money Are Short

Many college students may find it hard to fit a well-balanced meal into the day, but eating breakfast and lunch are important to keep energy levels up and get the most out of your classes. If your campus is like many others, you've probably noticed a distinct move toward fast-food restaurants in your student unions. Eating a complete breakfast that includes complex carbohydrates and protein and bringing a small healthy snack (such as carrots, an apple, or even a small sandwich on whole-grain bread) to class are ways to ensure you fit meals into your day. If you must eat fast food, follow the tips below to get more nutritional bang for your buck:

- Ask for nutritional analyses of items. Most fast-food chains now have them.
- Order salads, but be careful about what you add to them. Taco salads and Cobb salads are often high in fat, calories, and sodium. Ask for dressing on the side, and use sparingly. Try the vinaigrette or low-fat alternative dressings. Stay away from eggs and other high-fat add-ons, such as bacon bits, croutons, and crispy noodles.
- If you must have fries, check to see what type of oil is used to cook them. Avoid lard-based or other saturated-fat products and *trans* fats. Some fast-food restaurants offer baked "fries," which may be lower in fat.
- Avoid giant sizes, and refrain from ordering extra sauce, bacon, cheese, dressings, and other extras that add additional calories, sodium, carboydrates, and fat.
- Limit beverages and foods high in added sugars. Common forms of added sugars include sucrose, glucose, fructose, maltose, dextrose, corn syrups, concentrated fruit juices, and honey.
- At least once per week, substitute a vegetable-based meat substitute into your fast-food choices. Most places now offer Gardenburgers, Boca burgers, and similar products, which provide excellent sources of protein and often have considerably less fat and fewer calories.

Maintaining a nutritious diet within the confines of student life can be challenging. However, if you take the time to plan healthy meals, you will find that you are eating better, enjoying it more, and actually saving money. Follow the steps in the **Skills for Behavior Change** box at right for a healthy, affordable diet.

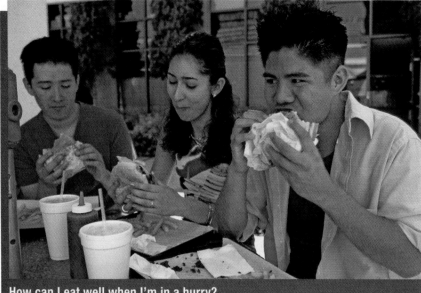

How can I eat well when I'm in a hurry?

Meals like this one may be convenient, but they are high in fat and calories. Even when you are short on time and money, it is possible—and worthwhile—to make healthier choices. Most fast-food restaurants make nutritional analyses of their offerings available to the public. If you are ordering fast food, opt for foods prepared by baking, roasting, or steaming; ask for the leanest meat option; request that sauces, dressings, and gravies be served on the side; and substitute a healthier option for a high-fat one, such as a baked potato or fresh vegetables instead of French fries.

over 76 million people and cause some 400,000 hospitalizations and 5,000 deaths in the United States annually. These numbers have remained fairly constant since 2004, in spite of increased attention to prevention in the United States.[42] Because most of us don't go to the doctor every time we feel ill, we may not make a connection between what we eat and later symptoms.

Signs of foodborne illnesses vary and usually include one or several symptoms: diarrhea, nausea, cramping, and vomiting. Depending on the amount and virulence of the pathogen, symptoms may appear as early as 30 minutes after eating contaminated food or as long as several days or weeks later. Most of the time, symptoms occur 5 to 8 hours after eating and last only a day or two. For certain populations, however, including the very young, older adults, and people with severe illnesses such as cancer, diabetes, kidney disease, or AIDS, foodborne diseases can be fatal.

Several factors may be contributing to the increase in foodborne illnesses. The movement away from a traditional meat-and-potato American diet to "heart-healthy" eating—increased consumption of fruits, vegetables, and grains—has spurred

Food Safety: A Growing Concern

Eating unhealthy food is one thing. Eating food that has been contaminated with a pathogen, toxin, or other harmful substance is quite another. You may be surprised to know that more than 200 diseases are transmitted through food. As outbreaks of salmonella in chicken, peanut butter, and vegetables or *Escherichia coli* (a potentially lethal bacterial pathogen) in spinach or beef continue to periodically make the news, the food industry has come under fire. To convince us that their products are safe, some manufacturers have come up with "new and improved" ways of protecting our foods. What are the dangers of contaminated foods, and how well do food manufacturers' new strategies work? Let's find out.

Foodborne Illnesses

Are you concerned that the chicken you are buying doesn't look pleasingly pink or that your "fresh" fish smells a little *too* fishy? You may have good reason to be worried. In increasing numbers, Americans are becoming sick from what they eat, and many of these illnesses are life-threatening. Based on several studies conducted over the past 10 years, scientists estimate that foodborne pathogens sicken

Budget Nutrition Tips

* Buy fruits and vegetables in season whenever possible for their lower cost, higher nutrient quality, and greater variety.
* Use coupons and specials to get price reductions. Plan your menu for the week, make a list, and stick to it so you can avoid impulse shopping. No food is cheap if you don't eat it.
* Shop at discount warehouse food chains; capitalize on volume discounts and no-frills products. However, don't buy more than you can reasonably use before the products expire.
* Purchase meats and other products in volume, freeze portions in vacuum-packed bags or freezer bags, put dates on them, and save for future needs. Or purchase small amounts of meat and other expensive proteins and combine them with beans and plant proteins for lower cost, calories, and fat.
* Invest in storage containers that hold up well to microwaving and dishwashing. Cook larger quantities at a time, and freeze leftovers.

demand for fresh foods that are not in season most of the year. This means that we must import fresh fruits and vegetables, thus putting ourselves at risk for ingesting exotic pathogens or even pesticides that have been banned in the United States for safety reasons. Depending on the season, up to 70 percent of the fruits and vegetables consumed in the United States come from Mexico alone. Although we are told when we travel to developing countries, "boil it, peel it, or don't eat it," we bring these foods into our kitchens and eat them, often without even washing them. Food can become contaminated by being watered with contaminated water, being fertilized with animal manure, being picked by people who have not washed their hands properly, or by being exposed to pesticides. To give you an idea of the implications, studies have shown that *E. coli* can survive in cow manure for up to 70 days and can multiply in foods grown with manure unless heat or additives such as salt or preservatives are used to kill the microbes.[43] There are no regulations that prohibit farmers from using animal manure to fertilize crops. Additionally, *E. coli* actually increases in summer months as cows await slaughter in crowded, overheated pens. This increases the chances of meat's coming to market already contaminated.[44]

Other key factors associated with the increasing spread of foodborne diseases include inadvertent introduction of pathogens into new geographic regions and insufficient education about food safety.

Avoiding Risks in the Home

Part of the responsibility for preventing foodborne illness lies with consumers—more than 30 percent of all such illnesses result from unsafe handling of food at home. Fortunately, consumers can take several steps to reduce the likelihood of contaminating their food. Among the most basic precautions are to wash your hands and to wash all produce before eating it. Also, avoid cross-contamination in the kitchen by using separate cutting boards and utensils for meats and produce. Temperature control is also important, and refrigerators must be set at 40 degrees Fahrenheit or less. Hot foods must be kept hot and cold foods kept cold in order to avoid unchecked bacterial growth. Leftovers need to be eaten within 3 days, and if you're unsure how long something has been sitting in the fridge, don't take chances. When in doubt, throw it out. See the **Skills for Behavior Change** box at

food irradiation Treating foods with gamma radiation from radioactive cobalt, cesium, or other sources of X rays to kill microorganisms.

U.S. FDA label for irradiated foods

Many people worldwide enjoy sushi. Use caution when eating it, however, as raw fish can be a breeding ground for dangerous microbes.

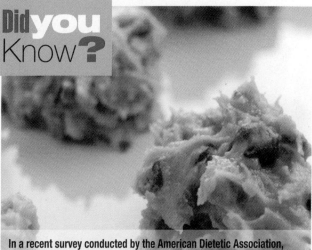

right for more tips about reducing risk of foodborne illness when shopping for and preparing food.

Food Irradiation: How Safe Is It?

Food irradiation is a process that involves treating foods with invisible waves of energy that damage microorganisms. These energy waves are actually low doses of radiation, or ionizing energy, which breaks chemical bonds in the DNA of harmful bacteria, destroying the pathogens and keeping them from replicating. The rays essentially pass through the food without leaving any radioactive residue.[45]

Irradiation lengthens food products' shelf life and prevents the spread of deadly microorganisms, particularly in high-risk foods such as ground beef and pork. Thus, the minimal costs of irradiation should result in lower overall costs to consumers and reduce the need for toxic chemicals now used to preserve foods and prevent contamination from external pathogens. Some environmentalists and consumer groups have raised concerns; however, food irradiation is now common in more than 40 countries. In the United States, foods that have been irradiated are marked with the "radura" logo.

Food Additives

Additives are substances added to food to reduce the risk of foodborne illness, prevent spoilage, and enhance the look and taste of foods. Additives can also enhance nutrient value, especially to benefit the general public. Good examples include the fortification of milk with vitamin D and of grain products with folate. Although the FDA regulates additives according to effectiveness, safety, and ability to detect them in foods, ques-

Reduce Your Risk For Foodborne Illness

✻ When shopping for fish, buy from markets that get their supplies from state-approved sources.

✻ Check for cleanliness at the salad bar and at the meat and fish counters.

✻ Keep most cuts of meat, fish, and poultry in the refrigerator no more than 1 or 2 days. Check the shelf life of all products before buying. Use the sniff test—if fish smells really fishy, don't eat it.

✻ Use a meat thermometer to ensure that meats are completely cooked. Beef and lamb steaks and roasts should be cooked to at least 145°F; ground meat, pork chops, ribs, and egg dishes to 160°F; ground poultry and hot dogs to 165°F; chicken and turkey breasts to 170°F; and chicken and turkey legs, thighs, and whole birds to 180°F. Fish is done when the thickest part becomes opaque and the fish flakes easily when poked with a fork.

✻ Never leave cooked food standing on the stove or table for more than 2 hours.

✻ Never thaw frozen foods at room temperature. Put them in the refrigerator for a day to thaw or thaw in cold water, changing the water every 30 minutes.

✻ Wash your hands and countertop with soap and water when preparing food, particularly after handling meat, fish, or poultry.

✻ When freezing chicken or other raw foods, make sure juices can't spill over into ice cubes or into other areas of the refrigerator.

tions have been raised about those additives put into foods intentionally and those that get in unintentionally before or after processing. Whenever these substances are added, consumers should take the time to determine what they are and whether there are alternatives. As a general rule, the fewer chemicals, colorants, and preservatives there are, the better. Examples of common additives include the following:

- **Antimicrobial agents.** Substances such as salt, sugar, nitrates, and others that tend to make foods less hospitable for microbes.
- **Antioxidants.** Substances that preserve color and flavor by reducing loss due to exposure to oxygen. Vitamins C and E are among the antioxidants believed to reduce the risk of cancer and cardiovascular disease. The additives BHA and BHT are also antioxidants.
- **Artificial colors, nutrient additives, and flavor enhancers such as MSG (monosodium glutamate).**
- **Sulfites.** Used to preserve vegetable color; some people have severe allergic reactions to them.

Food Allergy or Food Intolerance?

One out of every three people today *think* they have an allergy or avoid a certain food because they think they are allergic to it; however, only 4 percent of the population has a true food allergy. Still, that 4 percent accounts for more than 12 million Americans, and the number may increase in coming years, as rates are on the rise among children under the age of 3.[46]

A **food allergy,** or hypersensitivity, is an abnormal response to a food that is triggered by the immune system. Symptoms of an allergic reaction vary in severity and may include a tingling sensation in the mouth; swelling of the lips, tongue, and throat; difficulty breathing; hives; vomiting; abdominal cramps; diarrhea; drop in blood pressure; loss of consciousness; and death. Approximately 200 deaths per year occur from the anaphylaxis (the acute systemic immune and inflammatory response) that occurs with allergic reactions. These symptoms may appear within seconds to hours after eating the foods to which one is allergic.[47]

Peanuts are among the 8 most common food allergens: 0.6% of the general population are allergic to them, with slightly higher rates in children.

In 2004, Congress passed the Food Allergen Labeling and Consumer Protection Act (FALCPA), which requires food manufacturers to clearly label foods indicating the presence of (or possible contamination by) any of the 8 major food allergens: milk, eggs, peanuts, wheat, soy, tree nuts (walnuts, pecans, etc.), fish, and shellfish. Although over 160 foods have been identified as allergy triggers, these 8 foods account for 90 percent of all food allergies in the United States.[48]

In contrast to allergies, **food intolerance** can cause you to have symptoms of gastric upset, but it is not the result of an immune system response. Probably the best example of a food intolerance is *lactose intolerance,* a problem that affects about one in every ten adults. Lactase is an enzyme in the lining of the gut that degrades lactose, which is in dairy products. If you don't have enough lactase, you cannot digest lactose, and it remains in the gut to be used by bacteria. Gas is formed, and you experience bloating, abdominal pain, and sometimes diarrhea. Food intolerance also occurs in response to some food additives, such as the flavor enhancer MSG, certain dyes, sulfites, gluten, and other substances. In some cases, the food intolerance may have psychological triggers.

food allergy Overreaction by the body to normally harmless proteins, which are perceived as allergens. In response, the body produces antibodies, triggering allergic symptoms.

food intolerance Adverse effects resulting when people who lack the digestive chemicals needed to break down certain substances eat those substances.

If you suspect that you have an actual allergic reaction to food, see an allergist to be tested to determine the source of the problem. Because there are several diseases that share symptoms with food allergies (ulcers and cancers of the gastrointestinal tract can cause vomiting, bloating, diarrhea, nausea, and pain), you should have persistent symptoms checked out as soon as possible. If particular foods seem to bother you consistently, look for alternatives or modify your diet. In true allergic instances, you may not be able to consume even the smallest amount safely.

Is Organic for You?

Mounting concerns about food safety and the health impacts of chemicals used in the growth and production of food have led many people to refuse to buy processed foods and mass-produced agricultural products. Instead, they purchase foods that are **organic**—foods and beverages developed, grown, or raised without the use of synthetic pesticides, chemicals, or hormones.

As of 2002, any food sold in the United States as organic has to meet criteria set by the USDA under the National Organic Rule and can carry a USDA seal verifying products as "certified organic." Under this rule, a product that is certified may carry one of the following terms: "100 percent Organic" (100% compliance with organic criteria), "Organic" (must contain at least 95% organic materials), "Made with Organic Ingredients" (must contain at least 70% organic ingredients), or "Some Organic Ingredients" (contains less than 70% organic ingredients—usually listed individually). To be labeled with any of the above terms, the foods must be produced without hormones, antibiotics, herbicides, insecticides, chemical fertilizers, genetic modification, or germ-killing radiation. However, reliable monitoring systems to ensure credibility are still under development.

Is buying organic really better for you? Perhaps if we could put a group of people in a pristine environment and

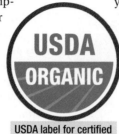

USDA label for certified organic foods

organic Grown without use of pesticides, chemicals, or hormones.
locavore A person who primarily eats food grown or produced locally.

ensure that they never ate, drank, or were exposed to chemicals, we could test this hypothesis. In real life, however, it is almost impossible to assess the health impact of organic versus nonorganic foods. Nevertheless, the market for organics has been increasing by more than 20 percent per year—five times faster than food sales in general. Nearly 40 percent of U.S. consumers now reach occasionally for something labeled organic; as of 2010, annual organic food sales are estimated to be about $23.8 billion.[49]

In 2007, several reports by consumer groups questioned the nutrient value of organic foods. Some sources have actually indicated that smaller organic farmers may have more trouble getting their produce to market in the proper climate-controlled vehicles. As such, their foods might lose valuable nutrients while sitting in warm trucks or at a roadside stand as compared to the refrigerated section of a local supermarket; or, more important, increased bacterial growth may be noted. In general, the closer to the field you can purchase produce and the faster you can get it home and into the refrigerator, the more nutritious foods will be.

Today, the new word **locavore** has been coined to describe people who eat only food grown or produced locally, usually within close proximity to their homes. Farmers' markets or home-grown foods or those grown by independent farmers are thought to be fresher, more environmentally friendly, and requiring far fewer resources to get them to market and keep them fresh for longer periods of time. Locavores believe that locally grown organic food is preferable to large corporation or supermarket-based organic foods, as they have a smaller impact on the environment. Although there are many reasons why organic farming is better for the environment, the fact that pesticides, herbicides, and other products are not used is perhaps the greatest benefit. Other benefits of locally grown organic products include the fact that they can often be harvested and brought to market with minimal fossil-fuel usage and are more likely to be grown on independent, small farms rather than on huge corporate farms.

Assess yourself

How Healthy Are Your Eating Habits?

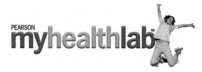

1 Keep Track of Your Food Intake

Keep a food diary for 5 days, writing down everything you eat or drink. Be sure to include the approximate amount or portion size. Add up the number of servings from each of the major food groups on each day and enter them into the chart below.

Number of Servings of:						
	Day 1	Day 2	Day 3	Day 4	Day 5	Average
Fruits						
Vegetables						
Grains						
Protein Foods						
Dairy						
Fats and Oils						
Sweets						

Fill out this assessment online at www.pearsonhighered.com/myhealthlab or www.pearsonhighered.com/donatelle.

2A Does your diet have proportionality?

	Yes	No
1. Are grains the main food choice at all your meals?	◯	◯
2. Do you often forget to eat vegetables?	◯	◯
3. Do you typically eat fewer than three pieces of fruit daily?	◯	◯
4. Do you often have fewer than 3 cups of milk daily?	◯	◯
5. Is the portion of meat, chicken, or fish the largest item on your dinner plate?	◯	◯

Scoring 2A

If you answered yes to three or more of these questions, your diet probably lacks proportionality. Review the recommendations in this chapter, particularly the MyPyramid guidelines, to learn how to balance your diet.

2 Evaluate Your Food Intake

Now compare your consumption patterns to the MyPyramid recommendations. Look at Table 9.1 (page 257) and Figure 9.8 (page 276) or visit www.mypyramid.gov/mypyramid/index.aspx to evaluate your daily caloric needs and the recommended consumption rates for the different food groups. How does your diet match up?

	Less than the recommended amount	About equal to the recommended amount	More than the recommended amount
1. How does your daily fruit consumption compare to the recommendation for your age and activity level?	◯	◯	◯
2. How does your daily vegetable consumption compare to the recommendation for your age and activity level?	◯	◯	◯
3. How does your daily grain consumption compare to the recommendation for your age and activity level?	◯	◯	◯
4. How does your daily protein food consumption compare to the recommendation for your age and activity level?	◯	◯	◯
5. How does your daily fats and oils consumption compare to the recommendation for your age and activity level?	◯	◯	◯
6. How does your daily consumption of discretionary calories compare to the recommendation for your age and activity level?	◯	◯	◯

Scoring

If you found that your food intake is consistent with the MyPyramid recommendations, congratulations! If, on the other hand, you are falling short in a major food group or are overdoing it in certain categories, consider taking steps to adopt healthier eating habits. There are some additional assessments at left and on the next page to help you figure out where your diet is lacking.

2B Are you getting enough fat-soluble vitamins in your diet?

	Yes	No
1. Do you eat at least 1 cup of deep yellow or orange vegetables, such as carrots and sweet potatoes, or dark green vegetables, such as spinach, every day?	○	○
2. Do you consume at least two glasses (8 ounces each) of milk daily?	○	○
3. Do you eat a tablespoon of vegetable oil, such as corn or olive oil, daily (tip: salad dressings, unless they are fat free, count!)?	○	○
4. Do you eat at least 1 cup of leafy green vegetables in your salad and/or put lettuce in your sandwich every day?	○	○

Scoring 2B

If you answered yes to all four questions, you are on your way to acing your fat-soluble vitamin needs! If you answered no to any of the questions, your diet needs some fine-tuning. Deep orange and dark green vegetables are excellent sources of vitamin A, and milk is an excellent choice for vitamin D. Vegetable oils provide vitamin E, and if you put them on top of your vitamin K-rich leafy green salad, you'll hit the vitamin jackpot.

2C Are you getting enough water-soluble vitamins in your diet?

	Yes	No
1. Do you consume at least 1/2 cup of rice or pasta daily?	○	○
2. Do you eat at least 1 cup of a ready-to-eat cereal or hot cereal every day?	○	○
3. Do you have at least one slice of bread, a bagel, or a muffin daily?	○	○
4. Do you enjoy a citrus fruit or fruit juice, such as an orange, a grapefruit, or orange juice every day?	○	○
5. Do you have at least 1 cup of vegetables throughout your day?	○	○

Scoring 2C

If you answered yes to all of these questions, you are a vitamin B and C superstar! If you answered no to any of the questions, your diet could use some refinement. Rice, pasta, cereals, bread, and bread products are all excellent sources of B vitamins. Citrus fruits are a ringer for vitamin C. In fact, all vegetables can contribute to meeting your vitamin C needs daily.

Source: Adapted from J. Blake, *Nutrition and You* (San Francisco: Benjamin Cummings, 2008).

YOUR PLAN FOR CHANGE

The **Assess**yourself activity gave you the chance to evaluate your current nutritional habits. Now that you have considered these results, you can decide whether you need to make changes in your daily eating for long-term health.

Today, you can:

○ Start keeping a more detailed food log. Take note of the nutritional information of the various foods you eat and write down particulars about the number of calories, grams of fat, grams of sugar, milligrams of sodium, and so on of each food. Try to find specific weak spots: Are you consuming too many calories or too much salt or sugar? Do you eat too little calcium or iron?

○ Take a field trip to the grocery store. Forgo your fast-food dinner and instead spend some time in the produce section of the supermarket. Purchase your favorite fruits and vegetables, and try something new to expand your tastes.

Within the next 2 weeks, you can:

○ Plan at least three meals that you can make at home or in your dorm room, and purchase the ingredients you'll need ahead of time. Something as simple as a chicken sandwich on whole-grain bread will be more nutritious, and probably cheaper, than heading out for a fast-food meal.

○ Start reading labels. Be aware of the amounts of calories, sodium, sugars, and fats in prepared foods; aim to buy and consume those that are lower in all of these and are higher in calcium and fiber.

By the end of the semester, you can:

○ Get in the habit of eating a healthy breakfast every morning. Combine whole grains, proteins, and fruit in your breakfast—for example, eat a bowl of cereal with milk and bananas or a cup of yogurt combined with granola and berries. Eating a healthy breakfast will jump-start your metabolism, prevent drops in blood glucose levels, and keep your brain and body performing at their best through those morning classes.

○ Commit to one or two healthful changes to your eating patterns for the rest of the semester. You might resolve to eat five servings of fruits and vegetables every day, to switch to low-fat or nonfat dairy products, to stop drinking soft drinks, or to use only olive oil in your cooking. Use your food diary to help you spot places where you can make healthier choices on a daily basis.

Summary

* Recognizing that we eat for more reasons than just survival is the first step toward changing our nutritional habits.
* The essential nutrients include water, proteins, carbohydrates, fats, vitamins, and minerals. Water makes up 50 to 60 percent of our body weight and is necessary for nearly all life processes. Proteins are major components of our cells and are key elements of antibodies, enzymes, and hormones. Carbohydrates are our primary sources of energy. Fats play important roles in maintaining body temperature and cushioning and protecting organs. Vitamins are organic compounds, and minerals are inorganic compounds. We need both in relatively small amounts to maintain healthy body function.
* Food labels provide information on the serving size, number of calories in a food, as well as the amounts of various nutrients and the percentage of recommended daily values those amounts represent.
* MyPyramid provides guidelines for healthy eating. These recommendations, developed by the USDA, place emphasis on personalization, proportionality, moderation, variety, physical activity, and gradual improvement.
* Vegetarianism can provide a healthy alternative for people wishing to reduce animal consumption from their diets.
* College students face unique challenges in eating healthfully. Learning to make better choices at fast-food restaurants, to eat healthfully when funds are short, and to eat nutritionally in the dorm are all possible when you use the information in this chapter.
* Foodborne illnesses, food irradiation, food allergies, and other food safety and health concerns are becoming increasingly important to health-wise consumers. Recognizing potential risks and taking steps to prevent problems are part of a sound nutritional plan.
* Organic foods are grown and produced without the use of synthetic pesticides, chemicals, or hormones. The USDA offers certification of organics. These foods have become increasingly available and popular, as people take a greater interest in eating healthfully and sustainably.

Pop Quiz

1. What type of carbohydrates is found primarily in fruits?
   a. glucose
   b. dextrose
   c. simple carbohydrates
   d. complex carbohydrates

2. Which of the following foods would be considered a healthy, *nutrient-dense* food?
   a. nonfat milk
   b. cheddar cheese
   c. soft drink
   d. potato chips

3. What is the most crucial nutrient?
   a. water
   b. fiber
   c. minerals
   d. starch

4. Which of the following nutrients moves food through the digestive tract?
   a. water
   b. fiber
   c. minerals
   d. starch

5. Which of the following nutrients are required for the repair and growth of body tissue?
   a. carbohydrates
   b. proteins
   c. vitamins
   d. fats

6. What substance plays a vital role in maintaining healthy skin and hair, insulating body organs against shock, maintaining body temperature, and promoting healthy cell function?
   a. fats
   b. fibers
   c. proteins
   d. carbohydrates

7. What substance supplies us with the energy needed to sustain normal daily activity?
   a. fats
   b. fibers
   c. proteins
   d. carbohydrates

8. What is the most common nutrient deficiency worldwide?
   a. fat deficiency
   b. iron deficiency
   c. fiber deficiency
   d. calcium deficiency

9. Carrie eats fish, dairy products, and eggs, but she does not eat red meat. Carrie is considered a(n)
   a. vegan.
   b. lacto-vegetarian.
   c. ovo-vegetarian.
   d. pesco-vegetarian.

10. Which of the following fats is a healthier fat to include in the diet?
   a. *trans* fats
   b. saturated fats
   c. unsaturated fats
   d. hydrogenated fats

Answers to these questions can be found on page A-1.

Think about It!

1. Which factors influence a person's dietary patterns and behaviors? What factors have been the greatest influences on your eating behaviors?
2. What are the six major food groups in MyPyramid? From which groups do you eat too few servings? What can you do to increase or decrease your intake of selected food groups?

3. What are the major types of nutrients that you need to obtain from the foods you eat? What happens if you fail to get enough of some of them? Are there significant differences between men and women in particular areas of nutrition?

4. Distinguish between the different types of vegetarianism. Which types are most likely to lead to nutrient deficiencies? What can be done to ensure that even the most strict vegetarian receives enough of the major nutrients?

5. What are the major problems that many college students face when trying to eat the right foods? List five actions that you and your classmates could take immediately to improve your eating.

6. What are the major risks for foodborne illnesses, and what can you do to protect yourself? How do food illnesses differ from food allergies?

Accessing Your Health on the Internet

The following websites explore further topics and issues related to personal health. For links to the websites below, visit the Companion Website for *Health: The Basics,* Green Edition at www.pearsonhighered.com/donatelle.

1. *American Dietetic Association (ADA).* Provides information on a full range of dietary topics, including sports nutrition, healthful cooking, and nutritional eating. Links to scientific publications and information on scholarships and public meetings. www.eatright.org

2. *U.S. Food and Drug Administration (FDA).* Provides information for consumers and professionals in the areas of food safety, supplements, and medical devices. Links to other sources of information about nutrition and food. www.fda.gov

3. *Food and Nutrition Information Center.* Offers a wide variety of information related to food and nutrition. http://fnic.nal.usda.gov

4. *National Institutes of Health: Office of Dietary Supplements.* Site of the International Bibliographic Information on Dietary Supplements (IBIDS), updated quarterly. http://dietary-supplements.info.nih.gov

5. *U.S. Department of Agriculture (USDA).* Offers a full discussion of the USDA Dietary Guidelines for Americans. www.usda.gov

6. *Linus Pauling Institute.* Key U.S. research center for studies on macro- and micronutrients; leaders in antioxidant research. http://lpi.oregonstate.edu

References

1. D. Mackinson, A. Anderson, and W. Wriden, "A Review of Consumers' Use and Understanding of Nutrition Information on Food Labels," *Proceedings of the Nutrition Society* 67 (2008): E215; G. Cowburn and L. Stockly, "Consumer Understanding and Use of Consumer Labeling: A Systematic Review," *Public Health Nutrition* 8 (2007): 21–28; R. Eckel et al., "Americans' Awareness, Knowledge, and Behaviors Regarding Fats: 2006–2007," *Journal of the American Dietetic Association* 109, no. 2 (2009): 288–96.

2. K. Flegal et al., "Cause-Specific Excess Deaths Associated with Underweight, Overweight, and Obesity," *Journal of the American Medical Association* 298 (2007): 2020–37.

3. American Institute of Cancer Research, *Food, Nutrition and the Prevention of Cancer: A Global Perspective* (Washington, DC: American Institute of Cancer Research, 1997).

4. F. Sofi et al., "Adherence to Mediterranean Diet and Health Status: Meta-Analysis," *BMJ* 337 (2008): a1344; M. Streppel et al., "Dietary Fiber Intake in Relation to Coronary Heart Disease and All Cause Mortality over 40," *American Journal of Clinical Nutrition* 88, no. 4 (2008): 1119–25; D. A. Timm and J. Slavin, "Dietary Fiber and the Relationship to Chronic Diseases," *American Journal of Lifestyle Medicine* 2, no. 3 (2008): 233–40.

5. World Health Organization, "Nutrition for Health and Development: Challenges," 2009, www.who.int/nutrition/challenges/en/index.html.

6. J. Thompson, M. Manore, and L. Vaughn, *The Science of Nutrition* (San Francisco: Benjamin Cummings, 2008).

7. U.S. Department of Agriculture, "Food Consumption Patterns: How We've Changed, 1970–2005," December 2005, www.usda.gov.

8. U.S. Department of Agriculture, "Economic Research Services," March 2008, www.ers.usda.gov.

9. J. Thompson and M. Manore, *Nutrition: An Applied Approach.* 2d ed. (San Francisco: Benjamin Cummings, 2009).

10. G. Block, "Foods Contributing to Energy Intake in the U.S.: Data from NHANES III and NHANES 1999–2000," *Journal of Food Composition and Analysis* 17, nos. 3–4 (2004): 439–47.

11. S. Goldfarb and D. Negoianu, "Just Add Water," *Journal of the American Society of Nephrology* 19 (2008): 1–3.

12. American College of Sports Medicine, "Exercise and Fluid Replacement," *Medicine and Science in Sports and Exercise* 39, no. 2 (2007): 377–90.

13. U.S. Department of Agriculture, Center for Nutrition Policy and Promotion. "Food Availability (Per Capita) Data System," 2009, www.ers.usda.gov.

14. J. E. Miltonal et al., "Relationship of Glycemic Index with Cardiovascular Risk Factors: Analysis of the National Diet and Nutrition Survey for People Aged 65 and Older," *Public Health Nutrition* 10, no. 11 (2007): 1321–35.

15. Institute of Medicine of the National Academies, "Dietary, Functional, and Total Fiber," in *Dietary Reference Intakes for Energy, Carbohydrate, Fiber, Fat, Fatty Acids, Cholesterol, Protein, and Amino Acids* (Washington, DC: The National Academies Press, 2002) pp. 7-1–7-2.

16. E. T. Jacobs et al., "Fiber, Sex, and Colorectal Adenoma: Results of a Pooled Analysis," *American Journal of Clinical Nutrition* 83 (2006): 343–49; American Institute for Cancer Research, "Colorectal Cancer Called 'Most Preventable,'" News Release, March 10, 2008, www.aicr.org; A. Millen et al., "Fruit and Vegetable Intake and Prevalence of Colorectal Adenoma in Cancer Screening Trial," *American Journal of Clinical Nutrition* 86, no. 6 (2007) 1754–64; P. "Newby et al., "Intake of Whole Grains, Refined Grains and Cereal Fiber Measured with 7-d Diet Records and Associations with Risk Factors for Chronic Disease," *American Journal of Clinical Nutrition* 86, no. 6 (2007): 1745–53.

17. E. J. Brunner et al., "Dietary Patterns and 15 Year Risks of Major Coronary Events, Diabetes and Mortality," *American Journal of Clinical Nutrition* 87, no. 5 (2008): 1414–21; P. Newby et al., "Intake of

Whole Grains, Refined Grains and Cereal Fiber," 2007.

18. D. Mozaffarian et al., "Trans Fatty Acids and Cardiovascular Disease," *New England Journal of Medicine* 354 (2006): 1601–13.

19. G. Bjelakovic et al., "Mortality in Randomized Trials of Antioxidant Supplements for Primary and Secondary Prevention: Systematic Review and Meta-Analysis," *Journal of the American Medical Association* 297, no. 8 (2007): 842–57; J. H. Kang and F. Grodstein, "Plasma Carotenoids and Tocopherols and Cognitive Function: A Prospective Study," *Neurobiological Aging* 29, no. 9 (2008): 1394–1403.

20. J. May, "Ascorbic Acid Transporters in Health and Disease," Paper presented at the Linus Pauling Diet and Optimum Health Annual Conference (Portland, OR: May 2007).

21. D. Albanes, "Vitamin Supplements and Cancer Prevention: Where Do Randomized Controlled Trials Stand?" *Journal of the National Cancer Institute* 101, no. 1 (2009): 2–4; J. Lin, et al., "Vitamins C and E and Beta Carotene Supplementation and Cancer Risk: A Randomized Controlled Trial," *Journal of the National Cancer Institute* 101, no. 1 (2009): 14–23.

22. M. Levine, "Pharmacologic Ascorbate Concentrations Selectively Kill Cancer Cells: Ascorbic Acid as a Pro-Drug for Ascorbate Radical and/or H_2O_2 Delivery to Tissues," Paper presented at the Linus Pauling Diet and Optimum Health Annual Conference (Portland, OR: May 2007); J. May, "Ascorbic Acid Transporters in Health and Disease," 2007.

23. C. M. Hasler et al., "Position Statement of the American Dietetic Association: Functional Foods," *Journal of the American Dietetic Association* 104, no. 5 (2004): 814–18; Linus Pauling Institute, Oregon State University, 2009, http://lpi.oregonstate.edu/infocenter.

24. M. Manore and J. Thompson, *Sport Nutrition for Health and Performance* (Champaign, IL: Human Kinetics, 2000), 283.

25. J. Chan and E. Giovannucci, "Vegetables, Fruits, Associated Micronutrients and Risk of Prostate Cancer," *Epidemiology Review* 23, no. 1 (2001): 82–86.

26. A. Chait et al., "Increased Dietary Micronutrients Decrease Serum Homocysteine Concentrations in Patients at High Risk of Cardiovascular Disease," *American Journal of Clinical Nutrition* 70, no. 5 (1999): 881–87.

27. J. Manson et al., "A Randomized Trial of Folic Acid and B-Vitamins in the Secondary Prevention of Cardiovascular Events in Women: Results from the Women's Antioxidant and Folic Acid Cardiovascular Study (WAFACS)," *Circulation* 114, no. 22 (2006): 2424; J. Manson et al., "A Randomized Factorial Trial of Vitamins C, E, and Beta-Carotene in the Secondary Prevention of Cardiovascular Events in Women: Results from the Women's Antioxidant Cardiovascular Study (WACS)," *Circulation* 114, no. 22 (2006): 2424.

28. Institute of Medicine, *Dietary Reference Intake for Water, Potassium, Sodium, Chloride, and Sulfate* (Washington, DC: The National Academies Press, 2004); H. Cohen et al., "Sodium Intake and Mortality in the NHANES II Follow-Up Study," *American Journal of Medicine* 119, no. 275 (2006): e7–e14.

29. H. Cohen et al., "Sodium Intake," (2006); J. Feng et al., "Salt Intake and Cardiovascular Mortality," *American Journal of Medicine* 120, no. 1 (2007): e5–e7; H. Harpannen and E. Mervaala, "Sodium Intake and Hypertension," *Progress in Cardiovascular Diseases* 49, no. 2 (2006): 59–75.

30. J. Ma, R. Johns, and R. Stafford, "Americans Are Not Meeting Current Calcium Recommendations," *American Journal of Clinical Nutrition* 85 (2007): 1361–66.

31. K. Tucker et al., "Colas, but Not Other Carbonated Beverages, Are Associated with Low Bone Mineral Density in Older Women: The Framingham Osteoporosis Study," *American Journal of Clinical Nutrition* 84 (2006): 936–42.

32. World Health Organization, "Micronutrient Deficiencies," www.who.int/nutrition/topics/ida/en/index.html. Accessed June 2008.

33. C. Tsai et al., "Heme and Non-Heme Iron Consumption and Risk of Gallstone Disease in Men," *American Journal of Clinical Nutrition* 85 (2007): 518–22.

34. K. M. Fairfield and R. H. Fletcher, "Vitamins for Chronic Disease Prevention in Adults: Scientific Review," *Journal of the American Medical Association* 287, no. 23 (2001): 3116–26.

35. "NIH State-of-the-Science Conference Statement on Multivitamin/Mineral Supplements and Chronic Disease Prevention," *Annals of Internal Medicine* 145 (2006): 364–71.

36. U.S. Department of Health and Human Services and U.S. Department of Agriculture, *Dietary Guidelines for Americans, 2005* (Washington, DC: Government Printing Office, 2005).

37. U.S. Department of Agriculture, Center for Nutrition Policy and Promotion, 2009, www.cnpp.usda.gov/DietaryGuidelines.htm.

38. U.S. Department of Agriculture, "Johanns Reveals USDA's Steps to a Healthier You," Press Release, April 19, 2005.

39. B. Black, "Health Library: Just How Much Food Is on That Plate? Understanding Portion Control," Last reviewed February 2009, EBSCO Publishing, www.ebscohost.com/healthLibrary.

40. "*Vegetarian Times* Study Shows 7.3 Million Americans Are Vegetarians" *Vegetarian Times*, Press Release, April 15, 2008, www.vegetariantimes.com/features/667.

41. J. Thompson and M. Manore, *Nutrition: An Applied Approach* (San Francisco: Benjamin Cummings, 2005).

42. Centers for Disease Control and Prevention, "Preliminary FoodNet Data on the Incidence of Infection with Pathogens Transmitted Commonly Through Food—10 States, 2007," *Morbidity and Mortality Weekly Report* 57, no. 14 (April 11, 2008): 366–70.

43. National Center for Infectious Diseases, Division of Bacterial and Mycotic Diseases, "*E. Coli,*" Updated 2007, www.cdc.gov/ecoli; Centers for Disease Control and Prevention, "Preliminary FoodNet Data," April, 11, 2008.

44. Ibid.

45. Iowa State University, "Food Irradiation: What Is It?" *Iowa State University Extension Newsletter,* www.extension.iastate.edu/foodsafety/irradiation. Revised August 2006.

46. Food Allergy and Anaphylaxis Network, "Food Allergy Facts and Statistics," 2008, www.foodallergy.org.

47. Ibid.

48. Food Allergy and Anaphylaxis Network, "Advocacy: Food Labeling," 2008, www.foodallergy.org.

49. U.S. Department of Agriculture, Economic Research Services, "Diet Quality and Food Consumption," 2006, www.ers.usda.gov/briefing/DietQuality.

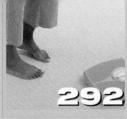

292

How can I tell if I am overweight?

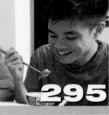

295

Do my genes have any effect on my weight?

296

Why don't most diets succeed?

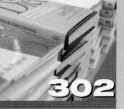

302

Is there a best way to lose weight?

10 Managing Your Weight

Objectives

✻ Define *overweight* and *obesity*, describe the current epidemic of overweight/obesity in the United States and globally, and understand risk factors associated with these weight problems.

✻ Explain why so many people are obsessed with thinness.

✻ Discuss reliable options for determining body fat content and the right weight for you.

✻ Describe factors that place people at risk for problems with obesity. Distinguish factors that can and cannot be controlled.

✻ Discuss the roles of exercise, dieting, nutrition, lifestyle modification, fad diets, and other strategies of weight control, and evaluate which methods are most effective.

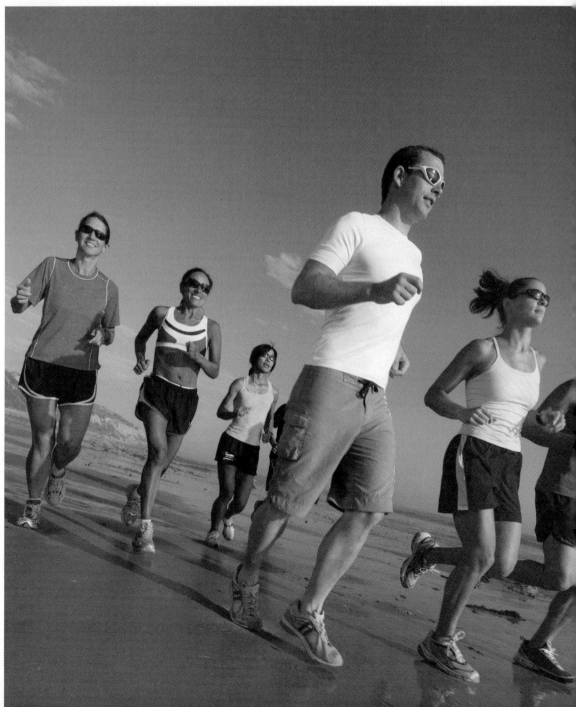

During the past 20 years, the world's population has grown progressively heavier. Globally, there are more than 1.6 billion overweight adults, at least 400 million of them obese.[1] Since 1980, rates have risen threefold or more in some areas of North America, the United Kingdom, eastern Europe, the Middle East, the Pacific Islands, Australasia, and China. Many developing regions of the world are demonstrating even faster rates of obesity.[2] The **Health in a Diverse World** box on page 291 looks more closely at the different rates of obesity across the globe.

The United States has the dubious distinction of being among the fattest nations on Earth. Young and old, rich and poor, rural and urban, educated and noneducated Americans share one thing in common—they are fatter than virtually all previous generations. The U.S. maps in Figure 10.1 illustrate the increasing levels of obesity that have occurred in the last two decades. Research indicates that the rate of increase in obesity began to slow in the past few years.[3] However, although the rate of increase has slowed down, obesity is still very much on the rise, and current rates are still extremely high, with more than 66 percent of U.S. adults considered to be overweight or obese. That translates into a whopping 72 million people—33.3 percent of men and 35.3 percent of women—who are classified as obese. Some researchers predict that by 2015, 41 percent of all Americans will be obese and 34 percent will be overweight—a possibility that holds staggering implications for health and health care costs.[4]

Research suggests that the prospect is even more bleak for certain populations within the United States. A recent study of American preschool children showed obesity rates of nearly 19 percent among children under age 4. Rates are even more troubling when broken down by ethnicity: In the under-4 age group, nearly 32 percent of Native Americans/Native Alaskans, 22 percent of Hispanics, and nearly 21 percent of non-Hispanic blacks were found to be obese. Rates among non-Hispanic whites and Asian Americans were 16 percent and 13 percent, respectively.[5] Other research points to higher obesity risks among adults of different ethnicities—most notably African American women, who have been found to have rates of overweight/obesity as high as 80 percent.[6]

Obesity is one of the top underlying preventable causes of death in the United States. Obesity and inactivity increase the risks from three of our leading killers: heart disease, cancer, and cerebrovascular ailments, including strokes.[7] Other associated health risks include diabetes, gallstones, sleep apnea, osteoarthritis, and several cancers. Figure 10.2 on the next page summarizes these and other potential health consequences of obesity. Some experts predict that the number of Americans diagnosed with diabetes, a major obesity-associated problem, will increase by 165 percent, from 15 million in 2005 to well over 30 million in 2030.[8]

Short- and long-term health consequences of obesity are not our only concern: The estimated annual cost of obesity in the United States exceeds $152 billion in medical expenses and lost productivity.[9] Of course, it is impossible to place a dollar value on a life lost prematurely due to diabetes, stroke, or heart attack or to assess the cost of the social isolation of and discrimination against overweight individuals. Of growing importance is the recognition that obese individuals suffer significant disability during their lives, in terms of both mobility and activities of daily living.[10]

This chapter will help you understand why we have such a weight problem in America today and provide simple strategies to help you manage your own weight. It will also help you understand what *underweight, normal weight, overweight,* and *obesity* really mean and why managing your weight is essential to overall health and well-being.

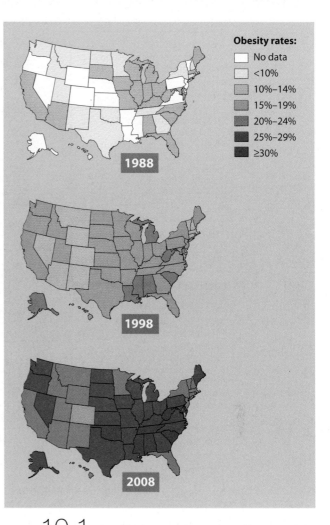

FIGURE 10.1 **Obesity Trends among U.S. Adults, 1988, 1998, and 2008**

These maps indicate the percentage of population in each state that is considered obese, based on a body mass index of 30 or higher, or about 30 pounds overweight for a person 5 feet 4 inches tall.

Source: Centers for Disease Control and Prevention, "U.S. Obesity Trends: 1985–2008," 2009, www.cdc.gov/obesity/data/trends.html#State.

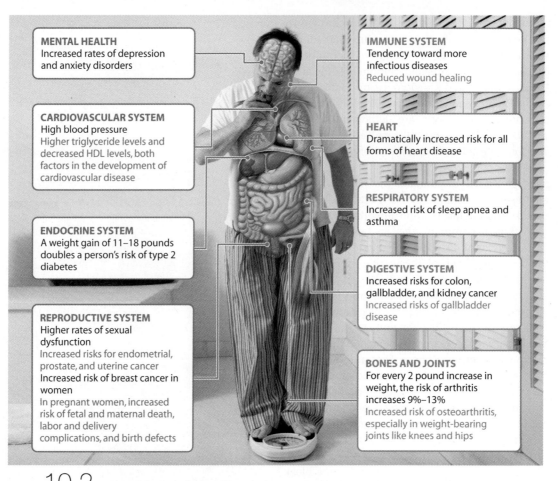

MENTAL HEALTH
Increased rates of depression and anxiety disorders

IMMUNE SYSTEM
Tendency toward more infectious diseases
Reduced wound healing

CARDIOVASCULAR SYSTEM
High blood pressure
Higher triglyceride levels and decreased HDL levels, both factors in the development of cardiovascular disease

HEART
Dramatically increased risk for all forms of heart disease

ENDOCRINE SYSTEM
A weight gain of 11–18 pounds doubles a person's risk of type 2 diabetes

RESPIRATORY SYSTEM
Increased risk of sleep apnea and asthma

DIGESTIVE SYSTEM
Increased risks for colon, gallbladder, and kidney cancer
Increased risks of gallbladder disease

REPRODUCTIVE SYSTEM
Higher rates of sexual dysfunction
Increased risks for endometrial, prostate, and uterine cancer
Increased risk of breast cancer in women
In pregnant women, increased risk of fetal and maternal death, labor and delivery complications, and birth defects

BONES AND JOINTS
For every 2 pound increase in weight, the risk of arthritis increases 9%–13%
Increased risk of osteoarthritis, especially in weight-bearing joints like knees and hips

FIGURE 10.2 **Potential Negative Health Effects of Overweight and Obesity**

Assessing Body Weight and Body Composition

What weight is right for you? Everyone has their own ideal weight, based on individual variables such as body structure, height, and fat distribution. Traditionally, experts used measurement techniques such as height–weight charts to determine whether an individual fell into the ideal weight, overweight, or obese category. However, these charts can be misleading because they don't take body composition—that is, a person's ratio of fat to lean muscle—or fat distribution into account. In fact, weight can be a deceptive indicator. Many extremely muscular athletes would be considered overweight based on traditional height–weight charts, whereas many young women might think their weight is normal based on charts, only to be shocked to discover that 35 to 40 percent of their weight is body fat! More accurate measures of evaluating healthy weight and disease risk focus on a person's percent body fat, and how that fat is distributed in his or her body.

overweight Having a body weight more than 10 percent above healthy recommended levels; in an adult, having a BMI of 25 to 29.
obesity A body weight more than 20 percent above healthy recommended levels; in an adult, a BMI of 30 or more.
morbidly obese Having a body weight 100 percent or more above healthy recommended levels; in an adult, having a BMI of 40 or more.

Overweight and Obesity

Most of us cringe at the thought of having one of the big O words attached to us: overweight and obesity. But what's the difference between these two words? *Overweight* and *obese* both refer to ranges of weight that are higher than what is considered to be healthy for a given height and body size. In general, **overweight** is increased body weight due to excess fat that exceeds healthy recommendations, whereas **obesity** refers to body weight that greatly exceeds health recommendations. Traditionally, *overweight* was defined as 1 to 19 percent above one's ideal weight, based on a standard height–weight chart, and *obesity* was defined as 20 percent of more above one's ideal weight. **Morbidly obese** people are 100 percent or more above their ideal weight. Experts now usually define *overweight* and *obesity* in terms of body mass index, a measure discussed below, or percentage of body fat, as determined by some of the methods we'll discuss shortly. Although opinion varies somewhat, most experts agree that men's bodies should contain between 8 and 20 percent total body fat, and women should be within the range of 20 to 30 percent. At various ages and stages of life, these ranges also vary, but generally, men who exceed 22 percent body fat and women who exceed 35 percent are considered overweight (see Table 10.1 on page 292).

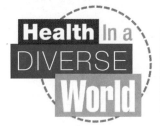

COMBATING GLOBESITY

The United States is not alone in being a "fat" country. During the past decade, epidemic rates of obesity and diabetes have joined underweight, malnutrition, and infectious diseases as major problems threatening the developing world. In fact, a higher body weight is associated with up to 16 percent of the global burden of all diseases. The global epidemic of obesity has been attributed to increased consumption of energy-dense foods, nutrient-poor foods, high levels of sugar and saturated fats; reduced physical activity; and the ready availability of fast foods.

In the past 20 years, rates of obesity have tripled in westernized developing countries. Arab, migrant Asian, Indian, Chinese, and U.S. Hispanic communities that are becoming westernized have diabetes rates that approach 20 percent.

Today, more than 1.6 billion adults worldwide are overweight, and 400 million of them are obese. Add to that the 155 million children worldwide—20 million under age 5—who are overweight or obese and the vastness of the problem is clear. The World Health Organization (WHO) projects that by 2015 approximately 2.3 billion adults will be overweight and more than 700 million will be obese.

As the problems of obesity and overweight capture international attention, there appears to be a growing public backlash against those who are too fat. Some people argue that obese patients raise health care costs by taxing an already overburdened health care system. The implication is that being overweight is a negative health behavior—a "choice"—that ultimately affects all of society. Such an attitude toward obesity has resulted in legislation banning *trans* fats and requiring restaurants to post nutritional information about menu items. It has also led to discussion of taxes on foods considered to contribute to obesity.

To a certain extent, such legislation may seem sensible, but once you begin taxing or removing unhealthy foods from the marketplace, where would you stop? A myriad of factors contribute to overweight and obesity—not just a person's choice in food purchases—so will singling out any one food item make a difference? And does a government have a right to restrict the foods available to its citizens?

At the same time this debate is raging in the United States, countries around the world are beginning to establish their own sets of policies and procedures. Consider these:

✳ In Great Britain, residents of some cities are being recruited to wear accelerometers that track movement and calories burned. Daily exercise is rewarded with coupons and even days off from work. Britain's National Health Service is paying for more than 30,000 people to take weight-loss classes.

✳ A 2006 British Medical Association (BMA) survey found that four in ten doctors were in favor of refusing joint surgery for obese patients if resources were limited. The study raised the idea of obesity being grouped alongside smoking and alcoholism as a self-inflicted risk.

✳ New Zealand has rules barring people who weigh too much from immigrating to the country, because such individuals would pose a potential burden to the health care system.

✳ In Japan, health officials check the waistlines of citizens over age 40, and those who are considered too fat undergo diet counseling. Failure to slim down can lead to fines.

✳ Ten female Air India flight attendants were fired in 2008 for failing to meet company weight restrictions. This action came after a June 2008 ruling by India's High Court that employees' physiques may be deemed integral to their "personality."

✳ In Germany, the equivalent of nearly $50 million is being spent on healthier school lunches and sports programs, as well as new, tougher nutritional standards.

In some states and cities, new legislation is being passed requiring restaurants to post nutritional information, leading to advertisements like this one at a New York City Dunkin' Donuts, listing the calorie range for a six-donut special.

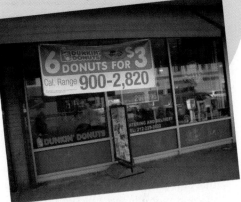

✳ And in the United States, 20 states have passed legislation requiring schools to perform weight screenings of children and adolescents.

How do you feel about policies such as those listed above? What are the potential pros and cons of some of these actions? How is the regulation of overweight and obesity similar to or different from that of other health-related behaviors such as smoking or drinking alcohol?

Sources: World Health Organization, *The World Health Report 2006: Working Together for Health* (Geneva: World Health Organization, 2006); P. Hossain, K. Bisher, and M. El Nahas, "Obesity and Diabetes in the Developing World—A Growing Challenge," *New England Journal of Medicine* 356, no. 3 (2007): 312–15; R. Blakely, "Air India Fires Air Hostesses for Being Too Fat to Fly," TimesOnline, January 6, 2009, www .timesonline.co.uk/tol/travel/news/article5452570 .ece?print=yes&randnum=12; J. Levi et al., *F as in FAT: How Obesity Policies Are Failing in America 2009* (Washington, DC: Robert Wood Johnson Foundation and Trust for America's Health, 2009); P. Rowland, "Today: Too Fat for Surgery Tomorrow: Where Do We Draw the Line?" RedOrbit, 2006, www.redorbit.com/news/health/ 381336/today_too_fat_for_surgery_tomorrow _where_do_we_draw/index.html; New Zealand Press Association, "135kg Woman Refused NZ Residency Over Size," *New Zealand Herald,* February 16, 2009, www.nzherald.co.nz/nz/news/ article.cfm?c_id= 1&objectid=10557061.

TABLE
10.1
Body Fat Percentage Recommendations for Men and Women*

	Recommended	Overweight	Obese
Men	≤34 years old: 8%–22%	≤34 years old: 23%–25%	≤34 years old: >25%
	35–55 years old: 10%–25%	>35 years old: 26%–28%	>35 years old: >28%
	>55 years old: 10%–25%		
Women	≤34 years old: 20%–35%	≤34 years old: 36%–38%	≤34 years old: >38%
	35–55 years old: 23%–38%	>35 years old: 39%–40%	>35 years old: >40%
	>55 years old: 25%–38%		

*Assumes nonathletes. For athletes, recommended body fat is 5 to 15 percent for men and 12 to 22 percent for women. Please note that there are no agreed-upon national standards for recommended body fat percentage.

Source: American College of Sports Medicine, *ACSM's Resource Manual for Guidelines for Exercise Testing and Prescription.* 5th ed. (Baltimore, MD: Lippincott Williams & Wilkins, 2006). Copyright © 2006 ACSM. Reprinted by permission of Wolters/Kluwer.

Underweight

Although many people are concerned about becoming fat, a certain amount of fat is essential for healthy body functioning. Body fat is composed of two types: essential fat and storage fat. *Essential fat* is that amount necessary for maintenance of life and reproductive functions. Fat regulates body temperature, cushions and insulates organs and tissues, and is the body's main source of stored energy. As such, there are percentages of body fat below which a person is considered **underweight,** and health is compromised. In men, this lower limit is approximately 3 to 7 percent of total body weight and in women it is approximately 8 to 15 percent. *Storage fat,* the nonessential fat that many of us try to shed, makes up the remainder of our fat reserves. Excessively low body fat in females, as seen in those with eating disorders or other rigid diet and exercise regimens, may result in amenorrhea, a disruption of the normal menstrual cycle, skin problems, hair loss, visual disturbances, a tendency to fracture bones easily, digestive system disturbances, heart irregularities, gastrointestinal problems, difficulties in maintaining body temperature, and a host of other problems. Problems with being underweight and having too low body fat are on the increase today, particularly as our obsession with appearance

underweight Having a body weight more than 10 percent below healthy recommended levels; in an adult, having a BMI below 18.5.
body mass index (BMI) A number calculated from a person's weight and height that is used to assess risk for possible present or future health problems.

grows. Pressure to conform to societal views of ideal weight and pressure to succeed in athletic endeavors and other competitive physical activities have caused increasing numbers of men and women to become dangerously thin. Some studies indicate that between 20 to 40 percent of female college students may suffer from some form of eating disorder.[11] See **Focus On: Your Body Image** beginning on page 314 for an in-depth discussion of eating disorders and body image issues.

Body Mass Index

Body mass index (BMI) is a useful index of the relationship of height and weight and is a standard measurement used by obesity researchers and health professionals. It is not gender specific. Although it does not directly measure percentage of body fat, it does provide a more accurate measure of overweight and obesity than does weight alone.[12] We calculate BMI by dividing a person's weight in kilograms by height in meters squared. The mathematical formula is

$$\text{BMI} = \text{weight (kg)} / \text{height squared (m}^2)$$

Figure 10.3 shows BMI as calculated for various heights in inches and weights in pounds. A BMI calculator is also available at the National Heart, Lung, and Blood Institute's website at http://nhlbisupport.com/bmi/bmicalc.htm.

Desirable BMI levels may vary with age and by sex; however, most BMI tables for adults do not account for such variables. *Healthy weights* are defined as those with BMIs of 18.5 to 25, the range

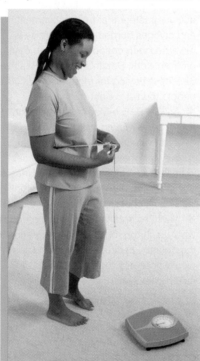

How can I tell if I am overweight?

Observing the way you look and how your clothes fit can give you a general idea of whether you weigh more or less than in the past. But for evaluating your weight and body fat levels in terms of potential health risks, it's best to use more scientific measures, such as BMI, waist circumference, waist-to-hip ratio, or a technician-administered body composition test.

BMI	19	20	21	22	23	24	25	26	27	28	29	30	31	32	33	34	35	36	37	38	39	40	41	42
Height												Weight in pounds												
4'10"	91	96	100	105	110	115	119	124	129	134	138	143	148	153	158	162	167	172	177	181	186	191	196	201
4'11"	94	99	104	109	114	119	124	128	133	138	143	148	153	158	163	168	173	178	183	188	193	198	203	208
5'	97	102	107	112	118	123	128	133	138	143	148	153	158	163	168	174	179	184	189	194	199	204	209	215
5'1"	100	106	111	116	122	127	132	137	143	148	153	158	164	169	174	180	185	190	195	201	206	211	217	222
5'2"	104	109	115	120	126	131	136	142	147	153	158	164	169	175	180	186	191	196	202	207	213	218	224	229
5'3"	107	113	118	124	130	135	141	146	152	158	163	169	175	180	186	191	197	203	208	214	220	225	231	237
5'4"	110	116	122	128	134	140	145	151	157	163	169	175	180	186	192	197	204	209	215	221	227	232	238	244
5'5"	114	120	126	132	138	144	150	156	162	168	174	180	186	192	198	204	210	216	222	228	234	240	246	252
5'6"	118	124	130	136	142	148	155	161	167	173	179	186	192	198	204	210	216	223	229	235	241	247	253	260
5'7"	121	127	134	140	146	153	159	166	172	178	185	191	198	204	211	217	223	230	236	242	249	255	261	268
5'8"	125	131	138	144	151	158	164	171	177	184	190	197	204	210	216	223	230	236	243	249	256	262	269	276
5'9"	128	135	142	149	155	162	169	176	182	189	196	203	210	216	223	230	236	243	250	257	263	270	277	284
5'10"	132	139	146	153	160	167	174	181	188	195	202	209	216	222	229	236	243	250	257	264	271	278	285	292
5'11"	136	143	150	157	165	172	179	186	193	200	208	215	222	229	236	243	250	257	265	272	279	286	293	301
6'	140	147	154	162	169	177	184	191	199	206	213	221	228	235	242	250	258	265	272	279	287	294	302	309
6'1"	144	151	159	166	174	182	189	197	204	212	219	227	235	242	250	257	265	275	280	288	295	302	310	318
6'2"	148	155	163	171	179	186	194	202	210	218	225	233	241	249	256	264	272	280	287	295	303	311	319	326
6'3"	152	160	168	176	184	193	200	208	216	224	232	240	248	256	264	272	279	287	295	303	311	319	327	335
6'4"	156	164	172	180	189	197	205	213	221	230	238	246	254	263	271	279	287	295	304	312	320	328	336	344

Healthy weight BMI 18.5–24.9	Overweight BMI 25–29.9	Obese BMI 30–39.9	Morbidly obese BMI ≥40

FIGURE 10.3 **Body Mass Index (BMI)**

Locate your height, read across to find your weight, then read up to determine your BMI. Any weight less than those listed for a given height would yield a BMI of less than 18.5, classified as underweight.

Source: NIH/National Heart, Lung, and Blood Institute (NHLBI). *Evidence Report of Clinical Guidelines on the Identification, Evaluation, and Treatment of Overweight and Obesity in Adults,* 1998, www.nhlbi.nih.gov/guidelines/obesity/ob_gdlns.htm.

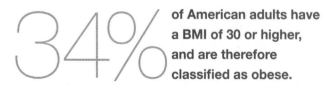

34% of American adults have a BMI of 30 or higher, and are therefore classified as obese.

of lowest statistical health risk.[13] The desirable range for women falls between 21 and 23; for men, it is between 22 and 24.[14] A BMI of 25 to 29.9 indicates overweight and potentially significant health risks. A BMI of 30 or above is classified as obese, while a BMI of 40 or higher is morbidly obese.[15] Nearly 3 percent of obese men and almost 7 percent of obese women are morbidly obese.[16]

Although useful, BMI levels don't really account for the fact that muscle weighs more than fat and a well-muscled person could weigh enough to be classified as obese according to his or her BMI, nor are bone mass and water weight considered in BMI calculations. For people who are under

5 feet tall, are highly muscled, or are older and have little muscle mass, BMI levels can be highly inaccurate. More precise methods of determining body fat, described below, should be used for these individuals.

Youth and BMI Although the labels *obese* and *morbidly obese* have been used for years for adults, there is growing concern about what the long-term consequences are of pinning these potentially stigmatizing labels on children.[17] Often, for children and teens BMI ranges above a normal weight are labeled differently, as "at risk of overweight" and "overweight," to avoid the sense of shame such words may cause. In addition, BMI ranges for children and teens are defined so that they take into account normal differences in body fat between boys and girls and the differences in body fat that occur at various ages. After BMI is calculated, the BMI number is plotted on the Centers for Disease Control and Prevention (CDC) BMI-for-age growth charts (for either girls or boys) to obtain a percentile ranking. Percentiles are the most commonly used indicator to assess the size and growth patterns of individual children in the United States. The percentile indicates the relative position of the child's BMI number among children of the same sex and age.[18]

Waist Circumference and Ratio Measurements

Waist circumference measurement is a useful tool to assess abdominal fat, which is considered more health threatening than fat in other regions of the body. Research indicates that a waistline greater than 40 inches (102 centimeters) in men and 35 inches (88 centimeters) in women may indicate greater health risk.[19] If a person is less than 5 feet tall or has a BMI of 35 or above, waist circumference standards used for the general population might not apply.

The **waist-to-hip ratio** measures regional fat distribution. A waist-to-hip ratio greater than 1 in men and 0.8 in women indicates increased health risks.[20] Therefore, knowing where your fat is carried may be more important than knowing how much you carry. Men and postmenopausal women tend to store fat in the upper regions of the body, particularly in the abdominal area. Premenopausal women usually store fat in the lower regions of their bodies, particularly the hips, buttocks, and thighs.

waist-to-hip ratio Waist circumference divided by hip circumference; a high ratio indicates increased health risks due to unhealthy fat distribution.

Measures of Body Fat

There are numerous ways besides BMI calculations and waist measurements to assess whether your body fat levels are too high. One low-tech way is simply to look in the mirror or consider how your clothes fit now compared with how they fit the last season you wore them. Of course, we've all seen people who appear to have a disconnect between how they look and the size of their clothes or between how

Underwater (hydrostatic) weighing:
Measures the amount of water a person displaces when completely submerged. Because fat tissue is less dense than muscle or bone tissue, body fat can be computed by comparing underwater and out-of-water weights.

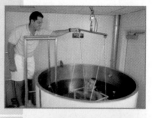

Skinfolds:
Involves "pinching" a person's fold of skin (with its underlying layer of fat) at various locations of the body. The fold is measured using a specially designed caliper. When performed by a skilled technician, it can estimate body fat with an error of 3%–4%.

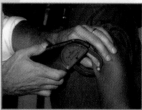

Bioelectrical impedance analysis (BIA):
Involves sending a very low level of electrical current through a person's body. As lean body mass is made up of mostly water, the rate at which the electricity is conducted gives an indication of a person's lean body mass and body fat. Under the best circumstances, BIA can estimate body fat with an error of 3%–4%.

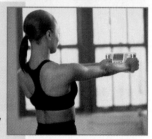

Dual-energy X-ray absorptiometry (DXA):
The technology is based on using very-low-level X-ray to differentiate between bone tissue, soft (or lean) tissue, and fat (or adipose) tissue. The margin of error for predicting body fat is 2%–4%.

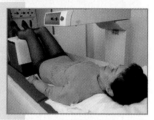

Bod Pod:
Uses air displacement to measure body composition. This machine is a large, egg-shaped chamber made from fiberglass. The person being measured sits in the machine wearing a swimsuit. The door is closed and the machine measures how much air is displaced.

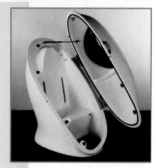

FIGURE 10.4 **Overview of Various Body Composition Assessment Methods**

Source: Adapted from J. Thompson and M. Manore, *Nutrition: An Applied Approach.* 2d ed. (San Francisco: Benjamin Cummings, 2009), Figure 11.3.

they really look and how they perceive themselves. For those who wish to take a more precise measurement of their percentage of body fat, more accurate techniques are available, several of which are described and depicted in Figure 10.4. These methods usually involve the help of a skilled professional and typically must be done in a lab or clinical setting. Before undergoing any procedure, make sure you understand the expense, potential for inaccuracy, risks, and the tester's training and background.

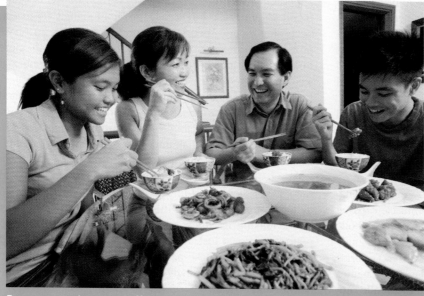

Do my genes have any effect on my weight?

Many factors help determine weight and body type, including heredity and genetic makeup, environment, and learned eating patterns, which are often connected to family habits.

Factors Contributing to Overweight and Obesity

In a major 2005 report, the U.S. Surgeon General stated it quite simply: Overweight and obesity result from an energy imbalance. If you eat too many calories and don't exercise, you'll gain weight.[21] However, since this landmark report, many have criticized such a simplistic view of a multifaceted problem. If all it took was the willpower to eat less and exercise more, Americans would merely reevaluate their diets; cut calories; and exercise, exercise, exercise. Unfortunately, it's not that easy.

What factors predispose us to excess weight? Although diet and exercise are clearly two of the major contributors, other factors, including genetics and physiology, are also important. In addition, the environment you live in, eat in, exercise in, and play and work in has a significant influence on what you eat, how much you eat, and when you eat.[22]

Genetic and Physiological Factors

Are some people born to be fat? Several factors appear to influence why one person becomes obese and another remains thin; genes, hormones, and other aspects of a person's physiology seem to interact with many of these factors.

Body Type and Genes Many scientists have explored the role of heredity in determining human body shape. Children whose parents are obese also tend to be overweight. In fact, a family history of obesity has long been thought to increase one's chances of becoming obese. Researchers have found that adopted individuals tend to be similar in weight to their biological parents and that identical twins are twice as likely

to weigh the same as are fraternal twins, even if they are raised separately.[23]

Over 250 gene markers have shown positive association to obesity in over 400 separate studies.[24] Genes play a significant role in how the body balances calories and energy. Although the exact mechanism remains unknown, it is believed that genes set metabolic rates, influencing how the body handles calories. Some genes, such as the *CD36* gene, may influence our cravings for fatty foods.[25] Also, by influencing the amount of body fat and fat distribution, genes can make a person more susceptible to gaining weight.[26]

In the past decade, more and more research has pointed to the existence of a "fat gene." Rather than inheriting a particular body type that predisposes us to overweight, it may be that our genes predispose us toward certain satiety and feeding behaviors. This "I need to eat" gene may account for up to one-third of our risk for obesity.[27] The most promising candidate is the *GAD2* gene. For some individuals, a variation in this gene increases the production of a chemical that boosts appetite and signals a person to eat.[28]

Another gene getting a lot of attention is an *Ob* gene (for obesity), which is believed to disrupt the body's "I've had enough to eat" signaling system and may prompt individuals to keep eating past the point of being comfortably full. Research on Pima Indians, who have an estimated 75 percent obesity rate (nine out of ten are overweight), points to an *Ob* gene that is a "thrifty gene." It is theorized that because their ancestors struggled through centuries of famine, during which the *Ob* gene prompted them to eat as much as possible whenever food was available, their metabolic rates slowed, allowing them to store precious fat for survival. Survivors may have passed these genes on to their children, which would explain the lower metabolic rates found in Pimas today and their tendency toward obesity.[29] If this thrifty-gene hypothesis is true, certain people may be genetically programmed to burn fewer calories.

Metabolic Rates Although the number of calories you consume as a part of your daily energy supply is important in the weight-gain equation, several aspects of your metabolism also help determine whether you gain, maintain, or lose weight. Each of us seems to have an innate energy-burning capacity that hums along even when we are in the deepest levels of sleep. This **basal metabolic rate (BMR),** is the minimum rate at which the body uses energy when at complete rest in a neutrally temperate environment when activities such as digestion are not occurring and the body is simply working to maintain basic vital functions. Technically,

> **basal metabolic rate (BMR)** The rate of energy expenditure by a body at complete rest in a neutral environment.

to measure BMR, a person would be awake, but all major stimuli, including stressors to the sympathetic nervous system, would be at rest. Usually, the best time to measure BMR is after 8 hours of sleep and after a 12-hour fast. A BMR for the average, healthy adult is usually between 1,200 and 1,800 calories per day. If you consume more than that and don't find other ways to burn energy, you will gain weight.

A more commonly used, less restrictive, and more practical way of assessing your energy expenditure levels is the **resting metabolic rate (RMR).** Slightly higher than the BMR, the RMR includes the BMR plus any additional energy expended through daily sedentary activities such as food digestion, sitting, studying, or standing. Because lean muscle tissue appears to influence metabolic rates, increasing muscle mass may be a factor in burning calories throughout the day (see Chapter 11).[30] The **exercise metabolic rate (EMR)** accounts for the remaining percentage of all daily calorie expenditures. It refers to the energy expenditure that occurs during physical exercise. For most of us, these calories come from light daily activities, such as walking, climbing stairs, and mowing the lawn. If we increase the level of physical activity to moderate or heavy, however, our EMR may be 10 to 20 times greater and can contribute substantially to weight loss.

resting metabolic rate (RMR) The energy expenditure of the body under BMR conditions plus other daily sedentary activities.

exercise metabolic rate (EMR) The energy expenditure that occurs during exercise.

thermic effect of food An estimate of how much energy is required to digest, absorb, and process food.

adaptive thermogenesis Theoretical mechanism by which the brain regulates metabolic activity according to caloric intake.

yo-yo diets Cycles in which people diet and regain weight.

satiety The feeling of fullness or satisfaction at the end of a meal.

Your BMR (and RMR) can fluctuate considerably, with several factors influencing whether it slows down or speeds up. In general, the younger you are, the higher your BMR will be, partly because cells undergo rapid subdivision during periods of growth, an activity that consumes a good deal of energy. The BMR is highest during infancy, puberty, and pregnancy, when bodily changes are most rapid. After age 30, a person's BMR slows down by about 1 to 2 percent a year. Therefore, people over age 30 commonly find that they must work harder to burn off an extra helping of ice cream than they did in their teens. A slower BMR, coupled with less activity, shifting priorities (family and career become more important than fitness), and loss in muscle mass, puts the weight of many middle-aged people in jeopardy.

Not surprisingly, the type and amount of food you actually consume may influence how you burn calories for energy. The **thermic effect of food** is an estimate of how much energy is necessary to burn food calories. Actions such as chewing, digesting, peristaltic action of the stomach and intestines, and production of digestive enzymes require energy from calories. It may take more energy per unit to burn certain foods than others and the amount of food you eat also is a factor.

Theories abound concerning the mechanisms that regulate metabolism and food intake. Some sources indicate that the hypothalamus (the part of the brain that regulates appetite) closely monitors levels of certain nutrients in the blood. When these levels fall, the brain signals us to eat. According to one theory, the monitoring system in obese people does not work properly, and the cues to eat are more frequent and intense than they are in people of normal weight. Another theory is that thin people send more effective messages to the hypothalamus. This concept, called **adaptive thermogenesis,** states that thin people can consume large amounts of food without gaining weight because the appetite center of their brains speeds up metabolic activity to compensate for the increased consumption.

Yo-yo diets, in which people repeatedly gain weight and then starve themselves to lose it, are doomed to fail. When dieters resume eating after their weight loss, their BMR is set lower, making it almost certain that they will regain the pounds they just lost. After repeated cycles of dieting and regaining weight, these people find it increasingly hard to lose weight and increasingly easy to regain it, so they become heavier and heavier.

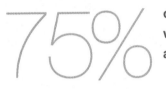

75% of dieters regain lost weight within 2 years of a major diet.

Endocrine Influence: The Hungry Hormones Over the years, many people have attributed obesity to problems with their thyroid gland and resultant hormone imbalances.

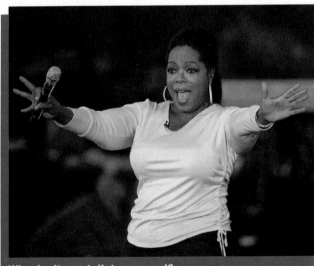

Why don't most diets succeed?

Just about any calorie-cutting diet can produce weight loss in the short term, often through water-weight loss. However, without improved nutrition and sustained exercise and activity, lost weight will return and the overall dieting process will have failed. Talk show host and media personality Oprah Winfrey has been candid about her struggles with this pattern of weight cycling, or yo-yo dieting. Such a pattern disrupts the body's metabolism and makes future weight loss more difficult and permanent changes even harder to maintain.

They believed that an underactive thyroid impeded their ability to burn calories. Today, most authorities agree that less than 2 percent of the obese population have a thyroid problem and can trace their weight problems to a metabolic or hormone imbalance.[31] However, researchers are investigating the impact of various hormones on a person's ability to lose weight, control appetite, and sense fullness.

Scientists distinguish *hunger,* an inborn physiological response to nutritional needs, from *appetite,* a learned response to food that is tied to an emotional or psychological craving and is often unrelated to nutritional need. Obese people may be more likely than thin people to satisfy their appetite and eat for reasons other than nutrition.[32] In some instances, the problem with overconsumption may be related more to **satiety** than it is to appetite or hunger. People generally feel satiated, or full, when they have satisfied their nutritional needs and their stomach signals "no more."

One hormone that researchers suspect may influence satiety and play a role in our ability to keep weight off is *ghrelin,* sometimes referred to as "the hunger hormone," which is produced in the stomach. Researchers at the University of Washington studied a small group of obese people who had lost weight over a 6-month period.[33] They noted that ghrelin levels rose before every meal and fell drastically shortly afterward, suggesting that the hormone plays a role in appetite stimulation. New attention is also being paid by researchers to the hormone *obestatin,* a genetic relative of gherlin. Animal studies show significant effects of obestatin on food intake, leading scientists to see potential for developing it for use in humans.[34]

Another hormone gaining increased attention and research is *leptin,* which scientists believe serves as a form of satiety signal, telling the brain when you are full.[35] When levels of leptin in the blood rise, appetite levels drop. Although obese people have adequate amounts of leptin and leptin receptors, they do not seem to work properly. Other scientists have isolated a hormone called *GLP-1,* which is known to slow down the passage of food through the intestines to allow the absorption of nutrients. Research suggests that the GLP-1 hormone may stimulate insulin production and may eventually be a key factor in preventing and controlling diabetes and obesity.[36] Researchers speculate that leptin and GLP-1 might play complementary roles in weight control. Leptin and its receptors may regulate body weight over the long term, calling on fast-acting appetite suppressants such as GLP-1 when necessary.

Environmental Factors

With all our twenty-first-century conveniences, environmental factors have come to play a large role in weight maintenance. Automobiles, remote controls, "desk" jobs, and long sessions on the Internet all cause us to sit more and move less, and this lack of physical activity causes a decrease

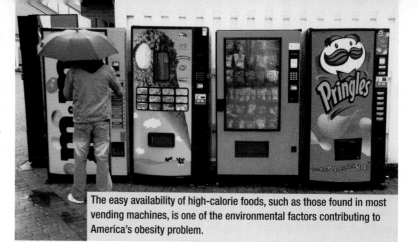

The easy availability of high-calorie foods, such as those found in most vending machines, is one of the environmental factors contributing to America's obesity problem.

in energy expenditure. Time our grandparents spent going for a walk after dinner we now spend watching our favorite television shows. Our culture also urges us to eat more. There is a long list of environmental factors that encourage us to increase our consumption:[37]

what do you think?

In addition to those listed, can you think of other environmental factors that contribute to obesity? ● What actions could you take to reduce your risk for each of these factors?

● Bombardment with advertising designed to increase energy intake—ads for high-calorie foods at a low price, marketing super-sized portions (see the **Consumer Health** box on page 298). Prepackaged meals, fast food, and soft drinks are all increasingly widespread. High-calorie drinks such as coffee lattes and energy drinks add to daily caloric intake.

● Changes in the number of working women, leading to greater consumption of restaurant meals, fast foods, and convenience foods. As society eats out more, higher-calorie, high-fat foods become the norm, and increased weight is the result.

● Bottle-feeding of infants, which may increase energy intake relative to breast-feeding.

● Misleading food labels that confuse consumers about portion and serving sizes.

● Increased opportunities for eating. Fast-food restaurants, cafes, vending machines, and quick-stop markets are everywhere, offering easy access to high-calorie foods and beverages. Meals, mini-meals, and snacks have become common diversions for many of us.

Early Sabotage: A Youthful Start on Obesity Children have always loved junk food, from sugary sweets and beverages to fat-laden chips and salty french fries. However, today's youth tend to eat larger portions and, from their earliest years, exercise less than any previous generation.[38] Video games, television, cell phones, and the Internet often keep them exercising their fingers more than any other part of their bodies, and children are subject to the same environmental, social, and cultural factors that influence obesity in their elders.

Portion Inflation

When you go out to your local restaurant, do you think your dinner looks the same as one your grandmother might have ordered 50 years ago? Would you be surprised to learn that today's serving portions are significantly larger than those of past decades? From burgers and fries to meat-and-potato or pasta meals, today's popular restaurant foods dwarf their earlier counterparts. A 25-ounce prime-rib dinner served at one local steak chain, for example, contains nearly 3,000 calories and 150 grams of fat in the meat alone. Add a baked potato with sour cream or butter, a salad loaded with creamy dressing, and fresh bread with real butter, and the meal may surpass the 5,000-calorie mark and ring in at close to 300 grams of fat. In other words, it exceeds what most adults should eat in 2 days!

And that is just the beginning. Soft drinks, once commonly served in 12-ounce sizes, now come in "big gulps" and 1-liter bottles. Cinnamon buns used to be the size of a dinner roll; now one chain sells them in giant, butter-laden, 700-calorie portions.

What accounts for the increased portion sizes of today? Restaurant owners might say that they are only giving customers what they want. While there may be some merit to this claim, it's also true that bigger portions can justify higher prices, which help increase an owner's bottom line.

A quick glance at the fattening of Americans provides growing evidence of a significant health problem. Many researchers believe that the main reason Americans are gaining weight is that people no longer recognize a normal serving size. The National Heart, Lung, and Blood Institute has developed a pair of "Portion Distortion" quizzes that show how today's portions compare with those of 20 years ago. Test yourself online at http://hp2010.nhlbihin.net/portion to see whether you can guess the differences between today's meals and those previously considered normal. Just one example is the difference between an average cheeseburger 20 years ago and the typical cheeseburger of today (see figure at left). According to the "Portion Distortion" quiz, today's cheeseburger has 590 calories—257 more calories than the cheeseburger of 20 years ago!

Carrie Wiatt, a Los Angeles dietitian and author of *Portion Savvy*, explains that a telling marker of the big-food trend is that restaurant plates have grown from an average of 9 inches to 13 inches in the past decade. Studies show that people eat 40 to 50 percent more than they normally would when larger portions are made available.

To make sure you're not overeating when you dine out, follow these strategies:

✳ Order the smallest size available. Focus on taste, not quantity. Get used to eating less and enjoy what you eat.
✳ Take your time, and let your fullness indicator have a chance to kick in while there is still time to quit.
✳ Always order dressings, gravies, and sauces on the side, and use these added calories sparingly.
✳ Order an appetizer as your main meal.
✳ Split your main entrée with a friend, and order a side salad for each of you. Alternatively, eat only half your dinner and save the rest to take home and eat another day.
✳ Avoid buffets and all-you-can-eat establishments. Most of us can eat two to three times what we need—or more.
✳ Skip dessert or split one among several people.

Sources: E. J. Fried, "The Potential for Policy Initiatives to Address the Obesity Epidemic in the United States," in *Obesity Prevention and Public Health*, eds. D. Crawford and R. W. Jeffrey (New York: Oxford University Press, 2005); K. D. Brownell et al., "Does a Toxic Environment Make Obesity Inevitable?" *Obesity Management* (2005): 52–55.

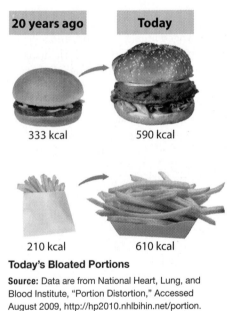

20 years ago	Today
333 kcal	590 kcal
210 kcal	610 kcal

Today's Bloated Portions

Source: Data are from National Heart, Lung, and Blood Institute, "Portion Distortion," Accessed August 2009, http://hp2010.nhlbihin.net/portion.

In addition, youth are at risk because of factors that are only beginning to be understood. Epidemiological studies suggest that maternal undernutrition, obesity, and diabetes during gestation and lactation are strong predictors of obesity in children.[39] Research also shows that race and ethnicity seem to be intricately interwoven with environmental factors in increasing risks to young people by as much as three times in selected populations, most notably among Native Americans/Alaska Natives, Hispanics, and African Americans.[40]

Obese kids not only suffer from the potential physical problems of obesity, but they also often face weight-related stigma, and are subjected to insults, slurs, and hateful comments about their size from their peers.[41] As a result, overweight and obese children may suffer lasting blows to their self-esteem, feelings of social acceptance, and emotional health, affecting personal identity and fostering mistrust and fear of others.

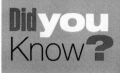
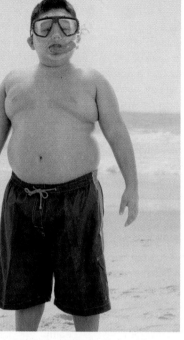

Psychosocial and Economic Factors

The relationship of weight problems to deeply rooted emotional insecurities, needs, and wants remains uncertain. Food often is used as a reward for good behavior in childhood. As adults face unemployment, broken relationships, financial uncertainty, fears about health, and other problems, the bright spot in the day is often "what's on the table for dinner" or "we're going to that restaurant tonight." Again, the research underlying this theory is controversial. What is certain is that eating tends to be a focal point of people's lives; it has become a social ritual associated with companionship, celebration, and enjoyment. For many people, the psychosocial aspect of the eating experience is a major obstacle to successful weight control.

Socioeconomic factors can provide obstacles or aids to weight control, as well. When economic times are tough, people tend to eat more inexpensive, high-calorie processed foods.[42] Unsafe neighborhoods and poor infrastructure (lack of, recreational areas, for example) make it difficult for less-affluent people to exercise.[43] New research suggests that the more educated you are, the lower your BMI and overall obesity profile is likely to be. In a study of comparative international data, highly educated men and particularly highly educated women in the United States have a lower average BMI than their less-educated counterparts. Conversely, highly educated men and women in poor countries where malnutrition is prevalent tend to have a higher BMI than less-educated people. Essentially, education appears to confer a buffer against obesity or malnutrition, depending on the country

you live in. Other studies have shown that the more you know about nutrition, the more likely you are to have a lower BMI.[44]

Lifestyle Factors

Athough heredity, metabolism, and environment all have an impact on weight management, the increasingly high rate of overweight and obesity in the past decades is largely due to the way we live our lives. In general, Americans are eating more and moving less than ever before, and the result shows up on our bathroom scales.

Of all the factors affecting obesity, perhaps the most critical is the relationship between activity level and calorie intake. Obesity rates are rising, but aren't more people exercising than ever before?

Although the many advertisements for sports equipment and the popularity of athletes may give the impression that Americans love a good workout, the facts are not so positive. Data from the National Health Interview Survey show that four in ten adults in the United States *never* engage in any exercise, sports, or physically active hobbies in their leisure time.[45] Nor are most of these adults particularly active during their nonleisure time. See the **Health Headlines** box on page 300 for an exploration of the idea of "sitting behavior" and its impact on health.

Do you know people who seemingly can eat whatever they want without gaining weight? With few exceptions, if you were to follow them around for a typical day and monitor the level and intensity of their activity, you would discover the reason. Even if their schedule does not include jogging

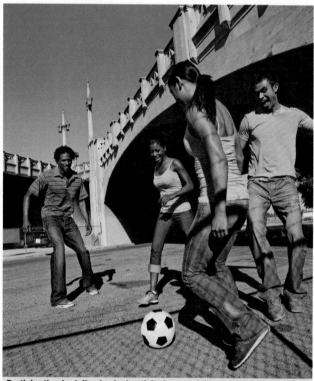

Participating in daily physical activity is one of the most important things you can do to manage your weight.

IS SITTING MAKING YOU FAT?

For many years, diet and exercise professionals have urged us all to exercise. The latest guidelines say that the way to health and fitness as well as prevention of chronic diseases in healthy adults is to engage in moderate-intensity aerobic physical activity for a minimum of 30 minutes, 5 days a week, or vigorous activity for 20 minutes, 3 days a week, adding muscle-strengthening activity to your workouts and, in general, picking up the pace of all of your exercise. As a part of these recommendations, experts acknowledge that routine daily activities such as vacuuming, shopping, and walking to the parking lot are all important in helping ensure health and fitness.

Not until recently have health and fitness experts begun to turn their attention to the level of activity that people engage in when they are not exercising. Although, say, 60 minutes of exercise is surely important, what about the other 23 hours of the day? If a person takes a 30-minute walk in the morning, but then lounges on the couch the rest of the day watching television and snacking, wouldn't that sedentary behavior affect his or her health negatively—in spite of the morning exercise? What about the woman or man who sits at a desk all day, busily answering the phone, pushing papers, and typing away on a computer keyboard?

Surprisingly, it is only recently that experts have begun to focus on "sitting behavior," a term used to describe sedentary activities. Recent studies point out the troubling amount of time that adults spend sitting. For about 15 hours or more each day, the only body parts that many of us move are our hands on computer keyboards or cell phones. New research indicates that there is a dose-response association between sitting time and mortality from all causes and from cardiovascular disease (CVD), independent of leisure-time activity. In fact, some people are so prone to sitting that they spend large parts of their day subconsciously seeking their next place to sit down.

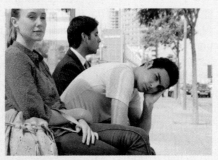

Americans today spend 15 or more hours each day sitting—and many of us have the weight problems to prove it!

Recent research suggests that we should make an effort to balance light-intensity activities and sedentary behaviors throughout our days. The implications of this "upside-down" way of looking at the obesity epidemic are staggering. What if instead of spending all of our effort on getting in 30 minutes of exercise each day, we focused more on the little things we can do to burn calories 24/7? What if workplaces were designed to get people up and moving and using larger muscle groups at various intervals throughout the day? How about standing to use your computer, or riding a stationary bike at a comfortable speed while watching TV? These little extra bouts of movement may make a big difference in daily calories burned, weight management, and overall health.

Sources: W. Haskell et al., "Physical Activity and Public Health: Updated Recommendation for Adults from the American College of Sports Medicine and the American Heart Association. 2007," *Medicine and Science in Sports and Exercise* 39, no. 8 (2007): 1423–34; N. Owen, A. Bauman, and W. Brown, "Too Much Sitting: A Novel and Important Predictor of Chronic Disease Risk?" *British Journal of Sports Medicine* 43, no. 2 (2009): 81–83; S. A. Anderssen et al., "Changes in Physical Activity Behavior and the Development of Body Mass Index during the Last 30 Years in Norway," *Scandinavian Journal of Medicine and Science in Sports* 18, no. 3 (2008): 309–17; P. Katzmarzyk, P. T. Church, C. L. Craig, and C. Bouchard, "Sitting Time and Mortality from All Causes, Cardiovascular Diseases, and Cancer," *Medicine and Science in Sports and Exercise* 41, no. 5 (2009): 998–1005; M. T. Hamilton, D. G. Hamilton, and T. W. Zderic, "The Role of Low Energy Expenditure and Sitting in Obesity, Metabolic Syndrome, Type 2 Diabetes and Cardiovascular Disease," *Diabetes* 56, no. 11 (2007): 2655–67.

or intense exercise, it probably includes a high level of activity. Walking up a flight of stairs rather than taking the elevator, speeding up the pace while mowing the lawn, getting up to change the TV channel rather than using the remote, and doing housework all burn extra calories.

Managing Your Weight

At some point in our lives, almost all of us will decide to lose weight or modify our diet to reduce risks from chronic diseases. Many will have mixed success. The problem is probably related to us thinking about losing weight in terms of short-term "dieting" rather than carefully analyzing our individual risks for obesity and adjusting our long-term lifestyle and eating behaviors. Research has consistently shown that low-calorie diets produce only temporary weight losses and may actually lead to disordered binge eating or related problems.[46] Repeated bouts of restrictive dieting may be physiologically harmful; moreover, the sense of failure we experience each time we don't meet our goal can exact far-reaching psychological costs. Drugs and intensive counseling can contribute to positive weight loss, but even then, many people regain weight after treatment. Maintaining a healthful body takes constant attention and nurturing over the course of your lifetime.

Keeping Weight Control in Perspective

Weight loss is difficult for many people and may require supportive friends, relatives, and community resources, plus extraordinary efforts to prime the body for burning extra calories. Although experts say that losing weight simply requires burning more calories than are consumed, putting this principle into practice is far from simple (Figure 10.5). People of the same age, sex, height, and weight can have differences of as much as 1,000 calories a day in RMR—this may explain why one person's gluttony is another's starvation. Other factors such as depression, stress, culture, and available foods can also affect a person's ability to lose weight. Being overweight does not mean people are weak willed or lazy.

To reach and maintain the weight at which you will be healthy and feel your best, you must develop a program of exercise and healthy eating behaviors that will work for you now and in the long term. See the **Skills for Behavior Change** box at right for strategies to make your weight management program succeed. To become a wise weight manager, you also need to become familiar with important concepts in weight control.

Understanding Calories

A *calorie* is a unit of measure that indicates the amount of energy gained from food or expended through activity.

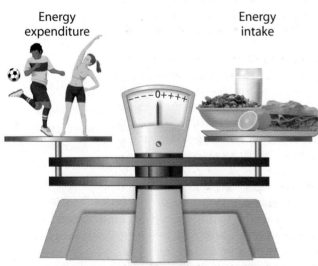

Energy expenditure = Energy intake

FIGURE 10.5 **The Concept of Energy Balance**
If you consume more calories than you burn, you will gain weight. If you burn more than you consume, you will lose weight. If both are equal, your weight will not change, according to this concept.

Sensible and Safe Weight Management

The key to successful weight management is finding a sustainable way to control food: one that will work for you. Remember, this is not a short-term diet that will end in a few weeks. You are making long-term behavior changes that will result in weight loss and better health.

BEFORE YOU BEGIN

✻ Talk with your health care provider. Be sure to discuss any medical conditions you have or medicines you take.
✻ Ask yourself some key questions. Why do you want to make this change? What are your weight-loss goals? Are you ready to change your eating habits and incorporate physical activity into your lifestyle?
✻ Assess where you are by keeping a food and exercise log for 2 or 3 days, taking careful note of the good things you are doing, the things that need improvement, and the triggers you need to address.

MAKE A PLAN

✻ Set realistic short- and long-term goals.
✻ Establish a plan. What are the diet and exercise changes you can make this week? Once you do 1 week, plot a course for 2 weeks, and so on.
✻ Look for balance. Remember that it is calories taken in and burned over time that make the difference.
✻ Be patient and persistent. Don't expect instant results.

CHANGE YOUR DIET

✻ Be adventurous. Expand your usual meals and snacks to enjoy a wide variety of different options.
✻ Do not constantly deprive yourself or set unrealistic guidelines.
✻ Eat only when you are hungry, and do not skip meals or let yourself get too hungry.
✻ Eat breakfast. This will prevent you from being too hungry and overeating at lunch.
✻ Plan ahead and always have healthy food options available for when and where you get hungry.

INCORPORATE EXERCISE

✻ Be active and slowly increase activity by increasing time, speed, distance, or resistance levels.
✻ Be creative with your physical activity. Find activities that you really love and try things you haven't tried before.
✻ Find an exercise partner to help you stay motivated.

Each time you consume 3,500 calories more than your body needs to maintain weight, you gain a pound of storage fat. Conversely, each time your body expends an extra 3,500 calories, you lose a pound of fat. If you consume 140 calories (the amount in one can of regular soda) more than you need every single day and make no other changes in diet or activity, you would gain 1 pound in 25 days (3,500 calories ÷ 140 calories/day = 25 days). Even when you think you are being good by ordering your Starbucks vanilla latte with skim milk, you are consuming a whopping 230 calories with every 16 ounces. Assuming you have the same drink every day and do nothing else differently, you'll gain 1 pound every 15 days! Conversely, if you walk for 30 minutes each day at a pace of 15 minutes per mile (172 calories burned) in addition to your regular activities, you would lose 1 pound in 20 days (3,500 calories ÷ 172 calories/day = 20.3 days).

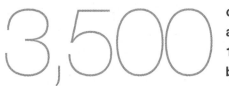 **calories equal approximately 1 pound of body fat.**

Of course, these are generic formulas. If you weigh more, moving your body through the same exercise routine will burn more calories than someone who is much thinner. Unfortunately, moving a bigger body is harder, and thus, people who are overweight or obese rarely enjoy this advantage.

Including Exercise

Increasing BMR, RMR, or EMR levels will help burn calories. Any increase in the intensity, frequency, and duration of daily exercise levels can have a significant impact on total calorie expenditure.

Physical activity makes a greater contribution to metabolic rate when large muscle groups are used. The energy spent on physical activity is the energy used to move the body's muscles and the extra energy used to speed up heartbeat and respiration rate. The number of calories spent depends on three factors:

1. The amount of muscle mass moved
2. The amount of weight moved
3. The amount of time the activity takes

An activity involving both the arms and legs burns more calories than one involving only the legs. An activity performed by a heavy person burns more calories than the same activity performed by a lighter person. And an activity performed for 40 minutes requires twice as much energy as the same activity performed for only 20 minutes. Thus, an obese person walking for 1 mile burns more calories than does a slim person walking the same distance. It also may take overweight people longer to walk the mile, which means that they are burning energy for a longer time and therefore expending more overall calories than the thin walkers.

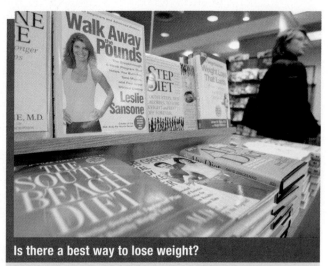

Is there a best way to lose weight?

There are hundreds of weight-loss plans currently being commercially marketed, but no one plan is a miracle fix. Ultimately, the best way to lose weight is by evaluating and modifying your own eating and exercising behaviors. Enlisting the aid of a registered dietician or other reliable health professional can help you craft a healthy plan that will work for you.

Improving Your Eating Habits

Before you can change a behavior, you must first determine what causes (or "triggers") it. Many people find it helpful to keep a chart of their eating patterns: when they feel like eating, where they are when they decide to eat, the amount of time they spend eating, other activities they engage in during the meal (watching television or reading), whether they eat alone or with others, what and how much they consume, and how they felt before they took their first bite. If you keep a detailed daily log of eating triggers for at least a week, you will discover useful clues about what in your environment or your emotional makeup causes you to want food. Typically, these dietary triggers center on problems in everyday living rather than on real hunger pangs. Many people eat compulsively when stressed; however, for other people, the same circumstances diminish their appetite, causing them to lose weight. See **Figure 10.6** and the **Skills for Behavior Change** box on page 304 for ways you can adjust your eating triggers and snack more healthfully in order to manage your weight.

what do you think?
If you wanted to lose weight, what strategies would you most likely choose? ● Which strategies, if any, have worked for you before? ● Which strategies offer the lowest health risk and the greatest chance for success? ● What factors might serve to help or hinder your weight-loss efforts?

Once you have evaluated your behaviors and determined your triggers, you can begin to devise a plan for improved eating. If you are unsure of where to start, seek assistance from reputable sources in selecting a dietary plan that is nutritious and easy to follow, such as the MyPyramid Plan discussed in Chapter 9. Registered dietitians, some

If your trigger is ...	then	try this strategy ...
A stressful situation		Acknowledge and address feelings of anxiety or stress, and develop stress management techniques to practice daily.
Feeling angry or upset		Analyze your emotions and look for a noneating activity to deal with them, such as taking a quick walk or calling a friend.
A certain time of day		Change your eating schedule to avoid skipping or delaying meals and overeating later; make a plan of what you'll eat ahead of time to avoid impulse or emotional eating.
Pressure from friends and family		Have a response ready to help you refuse food you do not want, or look for healthy alternatives you can eat instead when in social settings.
Being in an environment where food is available		Avoid the environment that causes you to want to eat: Sit far away from the food at meetings, take a different route to class to avoid passing the vending machines, shop from a list and only when you aren't hungry, arrange nonfood outings with your friends.
Feeling bored and tired		Identify the times when you feel low energy and fill them with activities other than eating, such as exercise breaks; cultivate a new interest or hobby that keeps your mind and hands busy.
The sight and smell of food		Stop buying high-calorie foods that tempt you to snack, or store them in an inconvenient place, out of sight; avoid walking past or sitting or standing near the table of tempting treats at a meeting, party, or other gathering.
Eating mindlessly or inattentively		Turn off all distractions, including phones, computers, television, and radio, and eat more slowly, savoring your food and putting your fork down between bites so you can become aware of when your hunger is satisfied.
Feeling deprived		Allow yourself to eat "indulgences" in moderation, so you won't crave them; focus on balancing your calorie input to calorie output.
Eating out of habit		Establish a new routine to circumvent the old, such as taking a new route to class so you don't feel compelled to stop at your favorite fast-food restaurant on the way.
Watching television		Look for something else to occupy your hands and body while your mind is engaged with the screen: Ride an exercise bike, do stretching exercises, doodle on a pad of paper, or learn to knit.

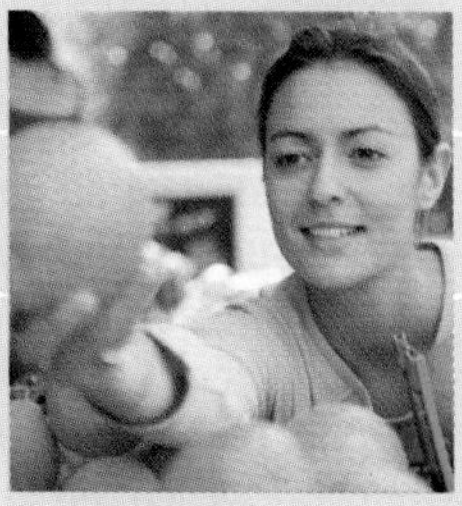

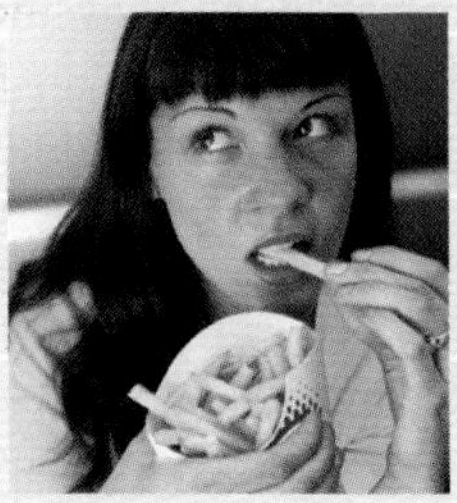

FIGURE 10.6 **Avoid Trigger-Happy Eating**
Learn what triggers your "eat" response—and what stops it—by keeping a daily log.

physicians (not all doctors have a strong background in nutrition), health educators and exercise physiologists with nutritional training, and other health professionals can provide reliable information. Beware of people who call themselves nutritionists. There is no such official designation. Avoid weight-loss programs that promise quick, "miracle" results or that are run by "trainees," often people with short courses on nutrition and exercise that are designed to sell products or services.

Before engaging in any weight-loss program, ask about the credentials of the adviser; assess the nutrient value of the prescribed diet; verify that dietary guidelines are consistent with reliable nutrition research; and analyze the suitability of the diet to your tastes, budget, and lifestyle. Any diet that requires radical behavior changes or sets up artificial dietary programs through prepackaged products that don't teach you how to eat healthfully is likely to fail. Supplements and fad diets that claim fast weight loss will invariably

mean fast weight regain. The most successful plans allow you to make food choices in real-world settings and do not ask you to sacrifice everything you enjoy. See Table 10.2 on page 305 for an analysis of some of the popular diets books being marketed today. For information on other books, check out the regularly updated list of the diet book reviews on the American Dietetic Association website at www.eatright .org/cps/rde/xchg/ada/hs.xsl/nutrition_8815_ENU_HTML.htm.

Reward yourself when you lose pounds. If you binge and go off your nutrition plan, get right back on it the next day. Remember that you didn't gain your weight in 1 week, so you're not likely to lose it all in the week or two before spring break. It is unrealistic and potentially dangerous to punish your body by trying to lose weight in a short period of time. Instead, try to lose a healthy 1 to 2 pounds during the first week, and stay with this slow and easy regimen. Making permanent changes to your lifestyle by adding exercise and cutting back on calories to expend about 500 calories more

Tips for Sensible Snacking

✳ **Keep healthy munchies around.** Buy whole-wheat breads, and if you need something to spice that up, use low-fat or soy cheese, low-fat cream cheese, or other healthy favorites.

✳ **Keep "crunchies" on hand.** Apples, pears, green-pepper sticks, popcorn, carrots, and celery all are good choices. Wash the fruits and vegetables and cut them up to carry with you; eat them when a snack attack comes on.

✳ **Quench your thirst with hot drinks.** Hot tea, heated milk, decaffeinated coffee, hot chocolate made with nonfat milk or water, or soup broths will help keep you satisfied.

✳ **Choose natural beverages.** Drink plain water, 100 percent juice, or other low-sugar choices to satisfy your thirst. Avoid soft drinks or other sugary, calorie-laden beverages.

✳ **Eat nuts instead of candy.** Although nuts are relatively high in calories, they are also loaded with healthy fats and make a healthy snack when consumed in moderation.

✳ **If you must have a piece of chocolate, keep it small.** Note that dark chocolate is better than milk chocolate or white chocolate because of its antioxidant content.

✳ **Avoid high-calorie energy bars.** Eat these only if you are exercising hard and don't have an opportunity to eat a regular meal. If you buy energy bars, look for those with a good mixture of fiber and protein and that are low in fat and calories.

than you consume each day will help you lose weight at a rate of 1 pound per week.

Considering Drastic Weight-Loss Measures

When nothing seems to work, people often become willing to take significant risks to lose weight. Dramatic weight loss may be recommended in cases of extreme health risk. However, even in such situations, drastic dietary, pharmacological, or surgical measures should be considered carefully and discussed with several knowledgeable health professionals.

very-low-calorie diets (VLCDs) Diets with a daily caloric value of 400 to 700 calories.

ketosis The body's process of converting body fat into ketones that can be used as fuel.

Very-Low-Calorie Diets In severe cases of obesity that are not responsive to traditional dietary strategies, medically supervised, powdered formulas with daily values of 400 to 700 calories plus vitamin and mineral supplements may be given to patients. Such **very-low-calorie diets (VLCDs)** should never be undertaken without strict medical supervision. These severe diets do not teach healthy eating and persons who manage to lose weight on them may experience significant weight regain. More important, fasting, starvation diets, and other forms of VLCDs have been shown to cause significant health risks and can, in fact, be deadly. Problems associated with any form of severe caloric restriction include blood sugar imbalance, cold intolerance, constipation, decreased BMR, dehydration, diarrhea, emotional problems, fatigue, headaches, heart irregularity, kidney infections and failure, loss of lean body tissue, weakness, and the potential for coma and death.

One particularly dangerous potential complication of VLCDs or starvation diets is *ketoacidosis*. After a prolonged period of inadequate carbohydrate or food intake, the body will have depleted its immediate energy stores and will begin metabolizing fat stores through **ketosis** in order to supply the brain and nervous system with an alternative fuel known as *ketones*. Ketosis is the body's normal process for metabolizing fat and may help provide energy to the brain during times of fasting, low carbohydrate intake, or vigorous exercise. However, ketones may also suppress appetite and cause dehydration at a time when a person should feel hungry and seek out food. As ketones increase in the body, the blood may become more acidic, and ketoacidosis may occur.[47] People with untreated type 1 diabetes and individuals with anorexia nervosa or bulimia nervosa are at risk of developing ketoacidotic symptoms as damage to body tissues begins.

If fasting continues, the body will turn to its last resort—protein—for energy, breaking down muscle and organ tissue to stay alive. As this occurs, the body loses weight rapidly. At the same time, it also loses significant water stores. Eventually, the body begins to run out of liver tissue, heart muscle,

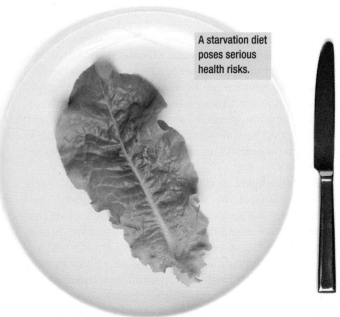

A starvation diet poses serious health risks.

TABLE

10.2 | Analyzing Popular Diet Books

Name	Claim	What You Eat	Is the Science Solid?	Is the Diet Healthy?	Worst Feature	Most Preposterous Claim
The South Beach Diet by Arthur Agatson	Switching to good carbs stops insulin resistance, cures cravings, and causes weight loss. Good fats protect the heart and prevent hunger.	**Yes:** Seafood, chicken breast, lean meat, low-fat cheese, most veggies, nuts, oils; (*later*) whole grains, most fruits, low-fat milk or yogurt, beans **Less:** Fatty meats, full-fat cheese, refined grains, sweets, juice, potatoes	Healthy version of Atkins diet that's backed by solid evidence on fats and heart disease.	↑Mostly healthy foods	Restricts carrots, bananas, pineapple, and watermelon.	You won't ever be hungry (despite menus that average just 1,200 calories a day).
The Ultimate Weight Solution by Phil McGraw	Foods that take time to prepare and chew lead to weight loss. Other "Keys to Weight Freedom" include "no-fail environment," "right thinking," "healing feelings," and "circle of support."	**Yes:** Seafood, poultry, meat, low-fat dairy, whole grains, most veggies, fruits, (*limited*) oils **Less:** Fatty meats, refined grains, full-fat dairy, microwave-able entrées, fried foods	Tough-love manual that relies more on Dr. Phil's opinion than science.	↑Mostly healthy foods. ↓ Gives no menus, recipes, or advice on how much of what to eat.	Readers may buy Dr. Phil's expensive, questionable supplements, bars, and shakes.	"Each of these nutrients [in his supplements] has solid clinical evidence (and a record of safety) behind it."
Dr. Atkins' New Diet Revolution by Robert C. Atkins	A low-carb diet is the key to weight loss (and good health) because carbs cause high insulin levels.	**Yes:** Seafood, poultry, meat, eggs, cheese, salad veggies, oils, butter, cream; (*later*) limited amounts of nuts, fruits, wine, beans, veggies, whole grains **Less:** Sweets, refined grains, milk, yogurt	Low-carb "bible" overstates the results of weak studies and the evidence on supplements. (However, in recent small studies, people lost more weight after 6—but not 12—months on Atkins than on a typical diet.)	↓ Too much red meat may raise risk of colon or prostate cancer. ↓ Lack of fiber, vegetables, and fruits may raise risk of heart disease, stroke, cancer, diverticulosis, and constipation.	Long-term safety not established.	"Only by doing Atkins can you lose weight eating the same number of calories on which you used to gain weight."
Eat More, Weigh Less by Dean Ornish	Slashing fat is the key to weight loss.	**Yes:** Beans, fruits, veggies, grains, (*limited*) nonfat dairy **Less:** Meat, seafood, poultry, oils, nuts, butter, dairy (except nonfat), sweets, alcohol	Diet worked (when combined with exercise and stress reduction) in a small-but-long-term study.	↑Mostly healthy foods. ↓ Too many carbs may raise triglycerides and lower HDL ("good") cholesterol if people don't exercise, lose weight, and reduce stress.	Unnecessarily restricts seafood, turkey, and chicken breast, oils, nuts, and fat-free dairy.	Eating a very-low-fat vegetarian diet is easy.

Source: D. Schardt, adapted from "Battle of the Diet Books," *Nutrition Action Healthletter* (January/February 2004): 6–7. Copyright © 2004 Center for Science in the Public Interest.

and so on. Within about 10 days after the typical adult begins a complete fast, the body will have depleted its energy stores, and death may occur.

Drug Treatment Individuals looking for help in losing weight often turn to thousands of commercially marketed weight-loss supplements, which are available on the Internet and at drug and health food stores. Food and Drug Administration (FDA) approval is not required for over-the-counter "diet aids" or supplements, and many manufacturers simply feed off people's frustrations. Want to lose weight and eat whatever you want? Try diet pill X. Most of these supplements contain stimulants such as caffeine or diuretics, and their effectiveness in promoting weight loss has been largely untested and unproved by any scientific studies. In many cases, the only thing that users lose is money they might have put to better use.

In contrast, FDA-approved diet pills have historically been available only by prescription. These lines were blurred in 2007 when the FDA approved the first over-the-counter weight-loss pill—a half-strength version of the prescription drug orlistat (brand name Xenical), marketed as Alli. This drug inhibits the action of lipase, an enzyme that helps digest fats, causing about 30 percent of consumed fat to pass through the digestive system undigested, leading to reduced overall caloric intake. Known side effects of orlistat include gas with watery fecal discharge; fecal urgency; oily stools and spotting; frequent, often unexpected, bowel movements; and possible deficiencies of fat-soluble vitamins.

When used as part of a long-term, comprehensive weight-loss program, drugs can help people who are severely obese lose up to 10 percent of their weight and maintain the loss. The challenge is to develop an effective drug that can be used over time without adverse effects or risks of abuse, and no such drug currently exists. A classic example of supposedly safe drugs that later were found to have dangerous side effects were Pondimen and Redux, known as *fen-phen* (from their chemical names, fenfluramine and phentermine), two of the most widely prescribed diet drugs in U.S. history.[48] When they were found to damage heart valves and contribute to pulmonary hypertension, a massive recall and lawsuit occurred.

In general, diet pills have not proved to be all that effective when used alone. A recent meta-analysis involving long-term diet-pill use showed that a few of these pills may result in modest weight loss and may have differing effects on the cardiovascular system and varying degrees of adverse side effects. However, virtually all persons who used these pills in the review studies regained their weight once they stopped taking them.[49]

Surgery When all else fails, particularly for people who are severely overweight and have weight-related diseases such as diabetes or hypertension, a person may be a candidate for weight-loss surgery. Generally, these surgeries fall into one of two major categories: *restrictive surgeries* that limit food intake, and *malabsorption surgeries* that decrease the absorption of food into the body, such as *gastric bypass*.

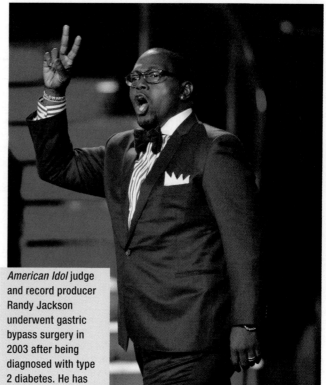

American Idol judge and record producer Randy Jackson underwent gastric bypass surgery in 2003 after being diagnosed with type 2 diabetes. He has since lost 110 pounds.

Common types of operations performed in the United States include laparoscopic adjustable gastric banding (Lap-Band, LAGB), Roux-en-Y gastric bypass (RYGB), vertical banded gastroplasty (VBG), gastric sleeve (GS), and biliopancreatic bypass with a duodenal switch (BPD). Each has its own benefits and risks. To select the best option, a physician will consider that operation's benefits and risks along with many other factors, including the patient's BMI, eating behaviors, obesity-related health conditions, and previous operations.

In gastric banding and other restrictive surgeries, the surgeon uses an inflatable band to partition off part of the stomach. The band is wrapped around that part of the stomach and is pulled tight, like a belt, leaving only a small opening between the two parts of the stomach. The upper part of the stomach is smaller, so the person feels full more quickly, and food digestion slows so that the person also feels full longer. Although the bands are designed to stay in place, they can be removed surgically. They can also be inflated to different levels to adjust the amount of restriction. This procedure is usually done using laparoscopy—that is, by making several small incisions through which the surgical instruments and a camera (laparoscope) connected to a video monitor can be passed. The surgical team operates using the images from the laparoscope as guidance, rather than having to open up a large portion of the patient's abdomen.

In contrast to the restrictive surgeries, gastric bypass is designed to drastically decrease the amount of food a person can eat and absorb. It is done with general anesthesia, hospitalization is required, and it is irreversible. Results are fast and dramatic, but there are many risks, including blood clots in the legs, a leak in a staple line in the stomach, pneumonia, infection, and death. Because the stomach pouch that remains after surgery is so small (about the size of a lime), the person can drink only a few tablespoons of liquid and consume only a very small amount of food at a time. For this reason, possible side effects include nausea and vomiting (if the person consumes too much), vitamin and mineral deficiencies, and dehydration (if the patient cannot eat or drink enough).

Aftercare for gastric surgery patients often includes counseling to help them cope with the urge to eat after the ability to eat normal portions has been removed, as well as other adjustment problems. Recent research has shown that gastric bypass may help prevent certain types of cancer and both prevent and treat type 2 diabetes mellitus.[50] In one study, nearly 99 percent of the morbidly obese who had gastric bypass and had a previous history of type 2 diabetes were free of the disease after surgery, even before they began to lose weight. This finding has caused much excitement in the scientific community as researchers explore surgical options for prevention of diabetes in other populations.[51] For those at high risk from these diseases, these benefits may factor into surgical decisions in the future.

Keep in mind that it is always best to lose weight through a healthy diet and regular physical activity. Ironically, even after going through surgery, people must learn to eat healthy foods and exercise. Otherwise, they can continue to gain weight, even returning to their original weight.

Unlike restrictive and malabsorption surgeries, which facilitate overall weight loss, *liposuction* is a surgical procedure in which fat cells are removed from specific areas of the body. Generally, liposuction is considered cosmetic surgery rather than weight-loss surgery and is used for spot reducing and body contouring. Although this technique has garnered much attention, it too is not without risk: Infections, severe scarring, and even death have resulted. In many cases, people who have liposuction regain fat in those areas or require multiple surgeries to repair lumpy, irregular surfaces from which the fat was removed.

Trying to Gain Weight

For some people, trying to gain weight is a challenge for a variety of metabolic, hereditary, psychological, and other reasons. If you are one of these individuals, the first priority is

Tips for Gaining Weight

✳ Eat at regularly scheduled times, whether you're hungry or not.

✳ Eat more frequently, spend more time eating, eat high-calorie foods first if you fill up fast, and always start with the main course.

✳ Take time to shop, to cook, and to eat slowly.

✳ Put extra spreads such as peanut butter, cream cheese, or cheese on your foods. Make your sandwiches with extra-thick slices of bread and add more filling.

✳ Take seconds whenever possible, and eat high-calorie, nutrient-dense snacks such as nuts, cheese, whole-grain tortilla chips, and guacamole during the day.

✳ Supplement your diet. Add high-calorie drinks that have a healthy balance of nutrients, such as whole milk.

✳ Try to eat with people you are comfortable with. Avoid people who you feel are analyzing what you eat or make you feel like you should eat less.

✳ If you are sedentary, be aware that exercise can increase appetite. If you are exercising, or exercising to extremes, moderate your activities until you've gained some weight.

✳ Avoid diuretics, laxatives, and other medications that cause you to lose body fluids and nutrients.

✳ Relax. Many people who are underweight operate at high gear most of the time. Slow down, get more rest, and control stress.

to determine why you cannot gain weight. For example, among older adults, the senses of taste and smell may decline, which makes food taste different and be less pleasurable. Visual problems and other disabilities may make meals more difficult to prepare, and dental problems may make eating more difficult. People who engage in sports that require extreme nutritional supplementation may be at risk for nutritional deficiencies, which can lead to immune system problems and organ dysfunction, weakness that leads to falls and fractures, slower recovery from diseases, and a host of other problems. See the **Skills for Behavior Change** box above for several weight-gaining strategies.

Are You Ready for Weight Loss?

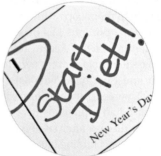

PEARSON
myhealthlab

How well do your attitudes equip you for a weight-loss program? For each question, circle the answer that best describes your attitude. As you complete sections 2–5, tally your score and analyze it according to the scoring guide.

Fill out this assessment online at www.pearsonhighered.com/myhealthlab or www.pearsonhighered.com/donatelle.

1 Diet History

A. How many times have you been on a diet?

| 0 times | 1–3 times | 4–10 times | 11–20 times | More than 20 |

B. How much weight did you lose?

| 0 lb | 1–5 lb | 6–10 lb | 11–20 lb | More than 20 lb |

C. How long did you stay at the new lower weight?

| Less than 1 mo | 2–3 mo | 4–6 mo | 6 to 12 mo | Over 1 yr |

D. Put a check mark by each dieting method you have tried:

____ skipping breakfast   ____ skipping lunch or dinner   ____ taking over-the-counter appetite suppressants

____ counting calories   ____ cutting out most fats   ____ cutting out most carbohydrates

____ increasing regular exercise   ____ taking weight-loss supplements   ____ cutting out all snacks

____ using meal replacements such as Slim Fast   ____ taking prescription appetite suppressants   ____ taking laxatives

____ inducing vomiting   ____ other _____

2 Readiness to Start a Weight-Loss Program

If you are thinking about starting a weight-loss program, answer questions A–F.

A. How motivated are you to lose weight?

1	2	3	4	5
Not at all motivated	Slightly motivated	Somewhat motivated	Quite motivated	Extremely motivated

B. How certain are you that you will stay committed to a weight-loss program long enough to reach your goal?

1	2	3	4	5
Not at all certain	Slightly certain	Somewhat certain	Quite certain	Extremely certain

C. Taking into account other stresses in your life (school, work, and relationships), to what extent can you tolerate the effort required to stick to your diet plan?

1	2	3	4	5
Cannot tolerate	Can tolerate somewhat	Uncertain	Can tolerate well	Can tolerate easily

D. Assuming you should lose no more than 1 to 2 pounds per week, have you allotted a realistic amount of time for weight loss?

1	2	3	4	5
Very unrealistic	Somewhat unrealistic	Moderately realistic	Somewhat realistic	Realistic

E. While dieting, do you fantasize about eating your favorite foods?

1	2	3	4	5
Always	Frequently	Occasionally	Rarely	Never

F. While dieting, do you feel deprived, angry, upset?

1	2	3	4	5
Always	Frequently	Occasionally	Rarely	Never

Total your scores

from questions A–F and circle your score category.

6 to 16: This may not be a good time for you to start a diet. Inadequate motivation and commitment and unrealistic goals could block your progress. Think about what contributes to your unreadiness. What are some of the factors? Consider changing these factors before undertaking a diet.

17 to 23: You may be nearly ready to begin a program but should think about ways to boost your readiness.

24 to 30: The path is clear—you can decide how to lose weight in a safe, effective way.

3 Hunger, Appetite, and Eating

Think about your hunger and the cues that stimulate your appetite or eating, and then answer questions A–C.

A. When food comes up in conversation or in something you read, do you want to eat, even if you are not hungry?

1	2	3	4	5
Never	Rarely	Occasionally	Frequently	Always

B. How often do you eat for a reason other than physical hunger?

1	2	3	4	5
Never	Rarely	Occasionally	Frequently	Always

C. When your favorite foods are around the house, do you succumb to eating them between meals?

1	2	3	4	5
Never	Rarely	Occasionally	Frequently	Always

> **Total your scores**
> from questions A–C and circle your score category.
>
> **3 to 6:** You might occasionally eat more than you should, but it is due more to your own attitudes than to temptation and other environmental cues. Controlling your own attitudes toward hunger and eating may help you.
>
> **7 to 9:** You may have a moderate tendency to eat just because food is available. Losing weight may be easier for you if you try to resist external cues and eat only when you are physically hungry.
>
> **10 to 15:** Some or much of your eating may be in response to thinking about food or exposing yourself to temptations to eat. Think of ways to minimize your exposure to temptations so you eat only in response to physical hunger.

4 Controlling Overeating

How good are you at controlling overeating when you are on a diet? Answer questions A–C.

A. A friend talks you into going out to a restaurant for a midday meal instead of eating a brown-bag lunch. As a result, you:

1	2	3	4	5
Would eat much less	Would eat somewhat less	Would make no difference	Would eat somewhat more	Would eat much more

B. You "break" your diet by eating a fattening, "forbidden" food. As a result, for the day, you:

1	2	3	4	5
Would eat much less	Would eat somewhat less	Would make no difference	Would eat somewhat more	Would eat much more

C. You have been following your diet faithfully and decide to test yourself by taking a bite of something you consider a treat. As a result, for the day, you:

1	2	3	4	5
Would eat much less	Would eat somewhat less	Would make no difference	Would eat somewhat more	Would eat much more

> **Total your scores**
> from questions A–C and circle your score category.
>
> **3 to 7:** You recover rapidly from mistakes. However, if you frequently alternate between out-of-control eating and very strict dieting, you may have a serious eating problem and should get professional help.
>
> **8 to 11:** You do not seem to let unplanned eating disrupt your program. This is a flexible, balanced approach.
>
> **12 to 15:** You may be prone to overeating after an event breaks your control or throws you off track. Your reaction to these problem-causing events could use improvement.

5 Emotional Eating

Consider the effects of your emotions on your eating behaviors, and answer questions A–C.

A. Do you eat more than you would like to when you have negative feelings such as anxiety, depression, anger, or loneliness?

1	2	3	4	5
Never	Rarely	Occasionally	Frequently	Always

B. Do you have trouble controlling your eating when you have a positive feelings (i.e., do you celebrate feeling good by eating)?

1	2	3	4	5
Never	Rarely	Occasionally	Frequently	Always

C. When you have unpleasant interactions with others in your life or after a difficult day at work, do you eat more than you'd like?

1	2	3	4	5
Never	Rarely	Occasionally	Frequently	Always

> **Total your scores**
> from questions A–C and circle your score category.
>
> **3 to 8:** You do not appear to let your emotions affect your eating.
>
> **9 to 11:** You sometimes eat in response to emotional highs and lows. Monitor this behavior to learn when and why it occurs, and be prepared to find alternative activities to respond to your emotions.
>
> **12 to 15:** Emotional ups and downs can stimulate your eating. Try to deal with the feelings that trigger the eating and find other ways to express them.

6 Exercise Patterns and Attitudes

Exercise is key for weight loss. Think about your attitudes toward it, and answer questions A–D.

A. How often do you exercise?

1	2	3	4	5
Never	Rarely	Occasionally	Somewhat frequently	Frequently

B. How confident are you that you can exercise regularly?

1	2	3	4	5
Not at all confident	Slightly confident	Somewhat confident	Highly confident	Completely confident

C. When you think about exercise, do you develop a positive or negative picture in your mind?

1	2	3	4	5
Completely negative	Somewhat negative	Neutral	Somewhat positive	Completely positive

D. How certain are you that you can work regular exercise into your daily schedule?

1	2	3	4	5
Not at all certain	Slightly certain	Somewhat certain	Quite certain	Extremely certain

Total your scores

from questions A–D and circle your score category.

4 to 10: You're probably not exercising as regularly as you should. Determine whether it is your attitude about exercise or your lifestyle that is blocking your way, then change what you must and put on those walking shoes!

11 to 16: You need to feel more positive about exercise so you can do it more often. Think of ways to be more active that are fun and fit your lifestyle.

17 to 20: The path is clear for you to be active. Now think of ways to get motivated.

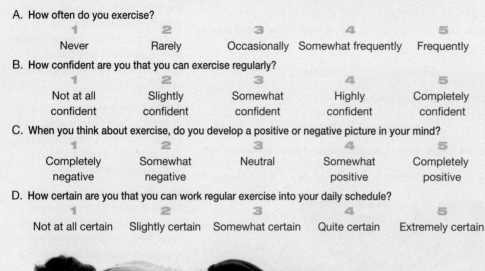

Source: Adapted from "The Diet Readiness Test," in Kelly D. Brownell, "When and How to Diet," *Psychology Today* (June 1989) 41–46. Copyright © 1989 Sussex Publishers, Inc. Reprinted with permission from *Psychology Today Magazine.*

YOUR PLAN FOR CHANGE

The **Assessyourself** activity identifies six areas of importance in determining your readiness for weight loss. If you wish to lose weight to improve your health, understanding your attitudes about food and exercise will help you succeed in your plan.

Today, you can:

○ Set "SMART" goals for weight loss and give them a reality check: Are they **s**pecific, **m**easurable, **a**chievable, **r**elevant, and **t**ime-oriented? For example, rather than aiming to lose 15 pounds this month (which probably wouldn't be healthy or achievable), set a comfortable goal to lose 5 pounds. Realistic goals will encourage weight-loss success by boosting your confidence in your ability to make lifelong healthy changes.

○ Begin keeping a food log and identifying the triggers that influence your eating habits. Think about what you can do to eliminate or reduce the influence of your two most common food triggers.

Within the next 2 weeks, you can:

○ Get in the habit of incorporating more fruits, vegetables, and whole grains in your diet and eating less fat. The next time you make dinner, look at the proportions on your plate. If veggies and whole grains do not take up most of the space, substitute 1 cup of the meat, pasta, or cheese in your meal with 1 cup of legumes, salad greens, or a favorite vegetable. You'll reduce the number of calories while eating the same amount of food!

○ Aim to incorporate more exercise into your daily routine. Visit your campus rec center or a local gym, and familiarize yourself with the equipment and facilities that are available. Try a new machine or sports activity, and experiment until you find a form of exercise you really enjoy.

By the end of the semester, you can:

○ Get in the habit of grocery shopping every week and buying healthy, nutritious foods while avoiding high-fat, high-sugar, or overly processed foods. As you make healthy foods more available and unhealthy foods less available, you'll find it easier to eat better.

○ Chart your progress and reward yourself as you meet your goals. If your goal is to lose weight and you successfully take off 10 pounds, reward yourself with a new pair of jeans or other article of clothing (which will likely fit better than before!).

Summary

* Overweight, obesity, and weight-related health problems appear to be on the rise globally, with the population of the United States being among the fattest of the world's developed nations. *Overweight* is most commonly defined as a body mass index of 25 to 29, and *obesity* is most commonly defined as a body mass index of 30 or greater.

* Societal costs from obesity, including increased health care costs, lowered worker productivity, low self-esteem, increased depression, discrimination, and other factors, exact a considerable toll on the entire population. Individual health risks include a variety of disabling and deadly chronic diseases and increased risks for certain infectious diseases.

* New methods for assessing whether you are overweight or obese no longer rely on height–weight charts or on weight alone. Percentage of body fat is a more reliable indicator for levels of overweight and obesity. There are many different methods of assessing body fat. Body mass index (BMI) is one of the most commonly accepted measures of weight based on height. Waist circumference, or the amount of fat in the belly region, is believed to be related to the risk for several chronic diseases, particularly type 2 diabetes.

* Many factors contribute to one's risk for obesity, including environmental factors, poverty, education level, genetics, developmental factors, endocrine influences, psychosocial factors, eating cues, lack of awareness, metabolic changes, and lifestyle.

* Exercise, dieting, diet pills, surgery, and other strategies are used to maintain or lose weight. However, sensible eating behavior and aerobic exercise and exercise that builds muscle mass offer the best options for weight loss and maintenance.

Pop Quiz

1. The proportion of your total weight made up of fat is called
   a. body composition.
   b. lean mass.
   c. percent body fat.
   d. BMI.

2. *Storage fat* is
   a. fat that is absolutely essential to normal functioning.
   b. nonessential fat.
   c. completely unaffected by genetics.
   d. fat that cannot be altered in any way.

3. All of the following statements about BMI are true EXCEPT,
   a. BMI is based on height and weight measurements.
   b. BMI is accurate for everyone, including those individuals, such as athletes, with high amounts of muscle mass.
   c. very low and very high BMI scores are associated with greater risk of mortality.
   d. BMI stands for "body mass index."

4. Which of the following BMI ratings is considered overweight?
   a. 20
   b. 25
   c. 30
   d. 35

5. Which of the following body circumferences is most strongly associated with risk of heart disease and diabetes?
   a. hip circumference
   b. chest circumference
   c. waist circumference
   d. thigh circumference

6. One pound of body fat contains
   a. 1,500 calories.
   b. 3,500 calories.
   c. 5,000 calories.
   d. 7,000 calories.

7. To lose weight, you must establish a(n)
   a. negative caloric balance.
   b. isocaloric balance.
   c. positive caloric balance.
   d. set point.

8. The rate at which your body consumes food energy to sustain basic functions is your
   a. basal metabolic rate.
   b. resting metabolic rate.
   c. body mass index.
   d. set point.

9. Successful weight maintainers are most likely to do which of the following?
   a. indulge in junk food on weekends.
   b. skip meals.
   c. drink diet sodas.
   d. eat high-volume but low-calorie density foods.

10. Yo-yo dieting is
    a. a pattern of repeatedly losing and regaining weight.
    b. characterized by rigid diets.
    c. characterized by flexible diets.
    d. uncommon.

Answers to these questions can be found on page A-1.

Think about It!

1. Discuss the pressures, if any, you feel to change the shape of your body. Do these pressures come from media, family, friends, and other external sources, or from concern for your personal health?

2. What type of measurement would you choose to assess your fat levels? Why?

3. List the risk factors for obesity. Evaluate which seem to be most important in determining whether you will be obese in middle age.

4. Create a plan to help someone lose the "freshman 15" over the summer vacation. Assume that the person is

male, weighs 180 pounds, and has 15 weeks to lose the excess weight.

5. Why do you think that obesity rates are rising in both developed and less-developed regions of the world? What could be done to help reduce the threat of obesity in these areas?

6. How does your state rank in terms of the percentage of people who are overweight or obese? Why do you think this is the case?

7. What are some factors that increase risks of obesity in a society and among individuals? What strategies can we take collectively and individually to reduce risks of obesity in our society?

Accessing Your Health on the Internet

The following websites explore further topics and issues related to personal health. For links to the websites below, visit the Companion Website for *Health: The Basics,* Green Edition at www.pearsonhighered.com/donatelle.

1. *American Dietetic Association.* Includes recommended dietary guidelines and other current information about weight control.
www.eatright.org

2. *Duke University Diet and Fitness Center.* Includes information about one of the best weight-loss treatment programs in the country; focuses on helping people live healthier, fuller lives through weight control and lifestyle change.
www.dukedietcenter.org

3. *F as in Fat: How Obesity Policies Are Failing in America.* This report by the Robert Wood Johnson Foundation and the Trust for America's Health provides an excellent summary of the current status of obesity, obesity policies, and programs in the United States, as well as suggestions for new strategies and policies to reduce

risks. http://healthyamericans.org/reports/obesity2009

4. *Weight-Control Information Network.* Excellent resource for diet and weight control information. Offers practical strategies and current information on research.
http://win.niddk.nih.gov

5. *The Rudd Center for Foods Policy and Obesity.* Website for the research center at Yale University. Provides excellent information on the latest in obesity research, public policy, and ways we can put a stop to the obesity epidemic at the community level.
www.yaleruddcenter.org

References

1. World Health Organization, "Global Strategy on Diet, Physical Activity and Health," 2009, www.who.int/dietphysicalactivity/publications/facts/obesity/en.

2. Ibid.

3. Centers for Disease Control and Prevention, "Obesity among Adults in the United States–No Statistically Significant Change since 2003–2004," *National Health and Nutrition Examination Survey (NHANES) 2005–2006,* Data brief, number 1, November 2007.

4. Y. Wang and M. A. Beydoun, "The Obesity Epidemic in the United States–Gender, Age, Socioeconomic, Racial/Ethnic, and Geographic Characteristics: A Systematic Review and Meta-Regression Analysis," *Epidemiologic Reviews* 29, no. 1 (2007): 6–28; Centers for Disease Control and Prevention, "Obesity among Adults in the United States," 2007.

5. S. Anderson and R. Whitaker, "Prevalence of Obesity among U.S. Preschool Children in Different Racial and Ethnic Groups," *Archives of Pediatrics and Adolescent Medicine* 163, no. 4 (2009): 344–48.

6. C. Ogden, "Disparities in Obesity Prevalence in the United States: Black Women at Risk," *American Journal of Clinical Nutrition* 89, no. 4 (2009): 1001–02.

7. K. Flegal et al., "Excess Deaths Associated with Underweight, Overweight and Obesity," *Journal of the American Medical Association* 293 (2005): 1861–67.

8. N. Pandey and V. Gupta, "Trends in Diabetes," *Lancet* 369, no. 14 (2007): 1256–57.

9. E. Finkelstein et al., "Economic Causes and Consequences of Obesity," *Annual Reviews of Public Health* 26 (2005): 239–57.

10. K. Butcher and K. Park, "Obesity, Disability, and the Labor Force," *Economic Perspectives* 32, no. 1 (2008); H. Chen and X. Guo, "Obesity and Functional Disability in Elderly Americans," *Journal of the American Geriatrics Society* 56, no. 4 (2008): 689–94; A. Peeters et al., "Adult Obesity and the Burden of Disability throughout Life," *Obesity Research* 12 (2004): 1145–51.

11. J. I. Hudson, E. Hiripi, H. G. Pope, and R. C. Kessler, "The Prevalence and Correlates of Eating Disorders in the National Comorbidity Survey Replication," *Biological Psychiatry* 61, no. 3 (2007): 348–58; National Institute of Mental Health, "Eating Disorders," 2009, www.nimh.nih.gov/health/topics/eating-disorders/index.shtml; K. Berg, P. Frazier, and L. Sherr, "Change in Eating Disorder Attitudes and Behavior in College Women: Prevalence and Predictors," *Eating Behaviors* 10, no. 3 (2009): 137–42; C. Greenleaf, T. Petrie, J. Carter, and J. Reel, "Female Collegiate Athletes: Prevalence of Eating Disorders and Disordered Eating Behaviors," *Journal of American College Health* 57, no. 5 (2009): 489–95.

12. C. Ogden et al., "Prevalence of Overweight and Obesity in the United States, 1999–2004," *Journal of the American Medical Association* 295, no. 13 (April 2006): 1549–55.

13. Obesity Society, "What Is Obesity?" Accessed November 2009, www.obesity.org/information/what_is_obesity.asp.

14. National Center for Health Statistics (NCHS), *Prevalence of Overweight and Obesity among Adults: United States, 1999–2002* (Hyattsville, MD: NCHS, 2004).

15. Centers for Disease Control and Prevention, "Defining Overweight and Obesity," 2008, www.cdc.gov/obesity/defining.html.

16. C. Ogden et al., "Prevalence of Overweight and Obesity in the United States, 1999–2004," 2006.

17. J. Hill and H. Wyatt, "Is it OK to Call Children Obese?" *Obesity Management* 2, no. 4 (2006): 131–32.

18. Centers for Disease Control and Prevention, "About BMI for Children and Teens," Updated 2009, www.cdc.gov/healthyweight/assessing/bmi/childrens_BMI/about_childrens_BMI.html.

19. National Heart, Lung, and Blood Institute, "Classification of Overweight and Obesity by BMI, Waist Circumference and Associated Disease Risks," 2009, www.nhlbi.nih.gov/health/public/heart/obesity/lose_wt/bmi_dis.htm.

20. Rush University, "Waist to Hip Ratio Calculator," Accessed August 2009, www.rush.edu/itools/hip/hipcalc.html.

21. U.S. Department of Health and Human Services (USDHHS), *Surgeon General's Call to Action to Prevent and Decrease Overweight and Obesity* (Washington, DC: USDHHS, 2005).

22. J. Spence, N. Cutumisu, J. Edwards, K. Raine, and K. Smoyer-Tomic, "Relation between Local Food Environments and Obesity among Adults," *BMC Public Health* 9, no. 1 (2009): 192.

23. D. Cummings and M. Schwartz, "Genetics and Pathophysiology of Human Obesity," *Annual Review of Medicine* 54 (2003): 453–71.

24. T. Rankinen et al., "The Human Obesity Gene Map: 2005 Update," *Obesity* 14 (2006): 529–644.

25. N. Abumad, "CD36 May Determine Our Desire for Dietary Fats," *Journal of Clinical Nutrition* 115 (2005): 2965–67.

26. C. Bell et al., "The Genetics of Obesity," *Nature Reviews Genetics* 6 (2005): 221–34.

27. T. Rankinen et al., "The Human Obesity Gene Map," 2006.

28. Ibid.

29. C. Bouchard, "Thrifty Gene Hypothesis: Maybe Everyone Is Right?" *International Journal of Obesity* 32, no. 4 (2008): 25–27; R. Stoger, "The Thrifty Epigenotype: An Acquired and Heritable Predisposition for Obesity and Diabetes?" *Bioessays* 30, no. 2 (2008): 156–66.

30. Centers for Disease Control and Prevention, "Growing Stronger: Strength Training for Older Adults: Why Strength Training?" Updated December 2008, www.cdc.gov/physicalactivity/growingstronger/why/index.html.

31. T. Reinehr et al., "Thyroid Hormones and Their Relation to Weight Status," *Hormone Research* 70, no. 1 (2008): 51–57; Mayo Clinic, "Special Report: Weight Control," 2005, www.mayoclinic.com.

32. E. Schuer et al., "Activation in Brain Energy Regulation and Reward Centers by Food Cues Varies with Choice of Visual Stimulation," *International Journal of Obesity* 33, no. 6 (2009): 653–61.

33. D. E. Cummings et al., "Plasma Ghrelin Levels after Diet-Induced Weight Loss or Gastric Bypass Surgery," *New England Journal of Medicine* 346, no. 21 (2002): 1623–30.

34. J. Beasley et al., "Characteristics Associated with Fasting Appetite Hormones (Obestatin, Ghrelin, and Leptin)," *Obesity* 17, no. 2 (2009): 349–54.

35. T. Reinehr et al., "Thyroid Hormones and Their Relation to Weight Status," 2008; V. Paracchini, P. Pedotti, and E. Taioli, "Genetics of Leptin and Obesity: A HuGE Review," *American Journal of Epidemiology* 162, no. 2 (2005): 101–14; Y. Friedlander et al., "Leptin, Insulin, and Obesity-Related Phenotypes: Genetic Influences on Levels and Longitudinal Changes," *Obesity* 17, no. 7 (2009): 1458–60.

36. D. Williams, D. Baskin, and M. Schwartz, "Leptin Regulation of Anorexic Responses to Glucagon-Like Peptide-1 Receptor Stimulation," *Diabetes* 55, no. 12 (2006): 3387–93.

37. J. Spence, N. Cutumisu, J. Edwards, K. Raine, and K. Smoyer-Tomic, "Relation between Local Food Environments and Obesity among Adults," 2009; T. Harder et al., "Duration of Breast Feeding and Risk of Overweight," *American Journal of Epidemiology* 162, no. 5 (2005): 397–403; M. Wang, C. Cubbin, D. Ahn, and M. Winkelby, "Changes in Neighbourhood Food Store Environment, Food Behaviour, and Body Mass Index, 1981–1990," *Public Health Nutrition* 11, no. 9 (2008): 963–70; R. P. Lopez, "Neighborhood Risk Factors for Obesity," *Obesity* 15, no. 8 (2007): 2111–19.

38. M. Treuth et al., "A Longitudinal Study of Sedentary Behavior and Overweight in Adolescent Girls," *Obesity* 17, no. 5 (2009): 1003–08.

39. B. Levin, "Synergy of Nurture and Nature in the Development of Childhood Obesity," *International Journal of Obesity* 33, Supplement 1 (2009): S53–S56.

40. S. Anderson and R. Whitaker, "Prevalence of Obesity among U.S. Preschool Children in Different Racial and Ethnic Groups," 2009.

41. K. Doheny, "Stigma of Obesity Not Easy to Shed," WebMD Health News, June 19, 2008, www.webmd.com/balance/news/20080619/stigma-of-obesity-not-easy-to-shed.

42. M. Beydoun, L. Powell, and Y. Yang, "The Association of Fast Food, Fruit, and Vegetable Prices with Dietary Intakes among U.S. Adults: Is There Modification by Family Income?" *Social Science and Medicine* 66, no. 11 (2008): 2218–29.

43. F. Li et al., "Built Environment, Adiposity, and Physical Activity in Adults Aged 50–75," *American Journal of Preventive Medicine* 35, no. 1 (2008): 38–46.

44. G. O'Brian and M. Davis, "Nutrition Knowledge and BMI," *Health Education Research* 22, no. 4 (2007): 571–75.

45. Centers for Disease Control and Prevention, "U.S. Physical Activity Statistics," Updated June 2008, www.cdc.gov/nccdphp/dnpa/physical/stats/index.htm; National Center for Health Statistics, "Prevalence of Sedentary Leisure Time Behavior among Adults in the United States," Reviewed January 2007, www.cdc.gov/nchs/data/hestat/3and4/sedentary.htm.

46. F. Fernandez-Aranda et al., "Individual and Family Eating Patterns during Childhood and Early Adolescence: An Analysis of Associated Eating Disorder Factors," *Appetite* 49, no. 2 (2007): 476–85.

47. J. Thompson and M. Manore, *Nutrition: An Applied Approach.* 2d ed. (San Francisco: Benjamin Cummings, 2009), 126.

48. U.S. Food and Drug Administration, "Fen-Phen Safety Update Information," Updated September 2009, www.fda.gov/Drugs/DrugSafety/PostmarketDrugSafetyInformationforPatientsandProviders/ucm072820.htm.

49. D. Rucker et al., "Long-Term Pharmacotherapy for Obesity and Overweight: Updated Meta-Analysis," *British Medical Journal* 335, no. 7631 (2007): 1194–99.

50. D. Van der Worde et al., "Bariatric Surgery and Mortality," *New England Journal of Medicine* 357, no. 8 (2007): 741–52.

51. C. Mottin et. al., "Behavior of Type 2 Diabetes Mellitus in Morbid Obese Patients Submitted to Gastric Bypass," *Obesity Surgery* 18, no. 2 (2008): 179–82.

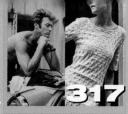
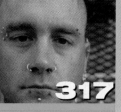
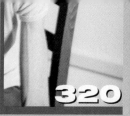
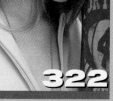
FOCUS ON Your Body Image

As he began his arm curls, Ali checked his form in the full-length mirror on the weight-room wall. His biceps were bulking up, but after 6 months, he expected more. His pecs, too, still lacked definition, and his abdomen wasn't the washboard he envisioned. So after a 45-minute upper-body workout, he added 200 sit-ups. Then he left the gym to shower back at his apartment: No way was he going to risk any of the gym regulars seeing his flabby torso unclothed. But by the time Ali got home and looked in the mirror, frustration had turned to anger. He was just too fat! To punish himself for his slow progress, instead of taking a shower, he put on his Nikes and went for a 4-mile run.

When you look in the mirror, do you like what you see? If you feel disappointed, frustrated, or even angry like Ali, you're not alone. A spate of recent studies is revealing that a majority of adults are dissatisfied with their bodies. For instance, a study of men in the United States, Austria, and France found that the ideal bodies they envisioned for themselves were an average of 28 pounds more muscular than their actual bodies. Most adult women—80 percent in one study—are also dissatisfied with their appearance, but for a different reason: Most want to lose

80%

of adult American women report dissatisfaction with their appearance.

weight.[1] Tragically, negative feelings about one's body can contribute to disordered eating, excessive exercise, and other behaviors that can threaten your health—and your life. Having a healthy body image is a key indicator of self-esteem, and can contribute to reduced stress, an increased sense of personal empowerment, and more joyful living.

Dissatisfaction with one's appearance and shape is an all-to-common feeling in today's society that can foster unhealthy attitudes and thought patterns, as well as disordered eating and exercising behaviors.

What Is Body Image?

This chapter focuses on body image because it's so fundamental to our sense of who we are. Consider the fact that mirrors made from polished stone have been found at archaeological sites dating from before 6000 BCE; humans have been viewing themselves for millennia.[2] But the term **body image** refers to more than just what you see when you look in a mirror. The National Eating Disorders Association (NEDA) identifies several additional components of body image:[3]

● How you see yourself in your mind
● What you believe about your own appearance (including your memories, assumptions, and generalizations)
● How you feel about your body, including your height, shape, and weight
● How you sense and control your body as you move

NEDA identifies a *negative body image* as either a distorted perception of your shape, or feelings of discomfort, shame, or anxiety about your body. You may be convinced that only other people are attractive, whereas your own body is a sign of personal failure. Does this attitude remind you of Ali? It should, because he clearly exhibits signs of a negative body image. In contrast, NEDA describes a *positive body image* as a true perception of your appearance: You see yourself as you really are. You understand that everyone is different, and you celebrate your uniqueness—including your "flaws," which you know have nothing to do with your value as a person.

Is your body image negative or positive—or is it somewhere in between? Researchers at the University of Arizona have developed a body image continuum that may help you decide (see **Figure 1** on page 316). Like a spectrum of light, a continuum represents a series of stages that aren't entirely distinct. Notice that the continuum identifies behaviors associated with particular states, from total dissociation with one's body to body acceptance and body ownership.

Many Factors Influence Body Image

You're not born with a body image, but you do begin to develop one at an early age as you compare yourself against images you see in the world around you, and interpret the responses of family members and peers to your appearance. Let's look more closely at the factors that probably played a role in the development of your body image.

The Media and Popular Culture

Although photos of bulked-up actors such as Brad Pitt and Tobey Maguire sell fitness magazines, snapshots of emaciated celebrities such as Lindsay Lohan and Paris Hilton dominate the tabloids. The images and celebrities in the media set the standard for what we find attractive, leading some people to go to dangerous extremes to have the biggest biceps or fit into size 2 jeans. Most of us think of this obsession with appearance as a recent phenomenon. The truth is, it has long been part of American culture. During the early twentieth century, while men idolized the hearty outdoorsman President Teddy Roosevelt, women pulled their corsets ever tighter to achieve unrealistically tiny waists. In the 1920s and 1930s, men emulated the burly cops and robbers in gangster films, while women dieted and bound their breasts to achieve the boyish "flapper" look. After World War II, both men and women strove for a healthy, wholesome appearance, but by the 1960s, tough-guys like Clint Eastwood and Marlon Brando were the male ideal, whereas rail-thin supermodel Twiggy embodied the nation's standard of female beauty.

Today, more than 66 percent of Americans are overweight or obese;[4] thus, a significant disconnect exists between the media's idealized images of male and female bodies and the typical American body. At the same time, the media—in the form of television, the Internet,

body image Most fundamentally, how you see yourself when you look in a mirror or picture yourself in your mind and how you feel about your body.

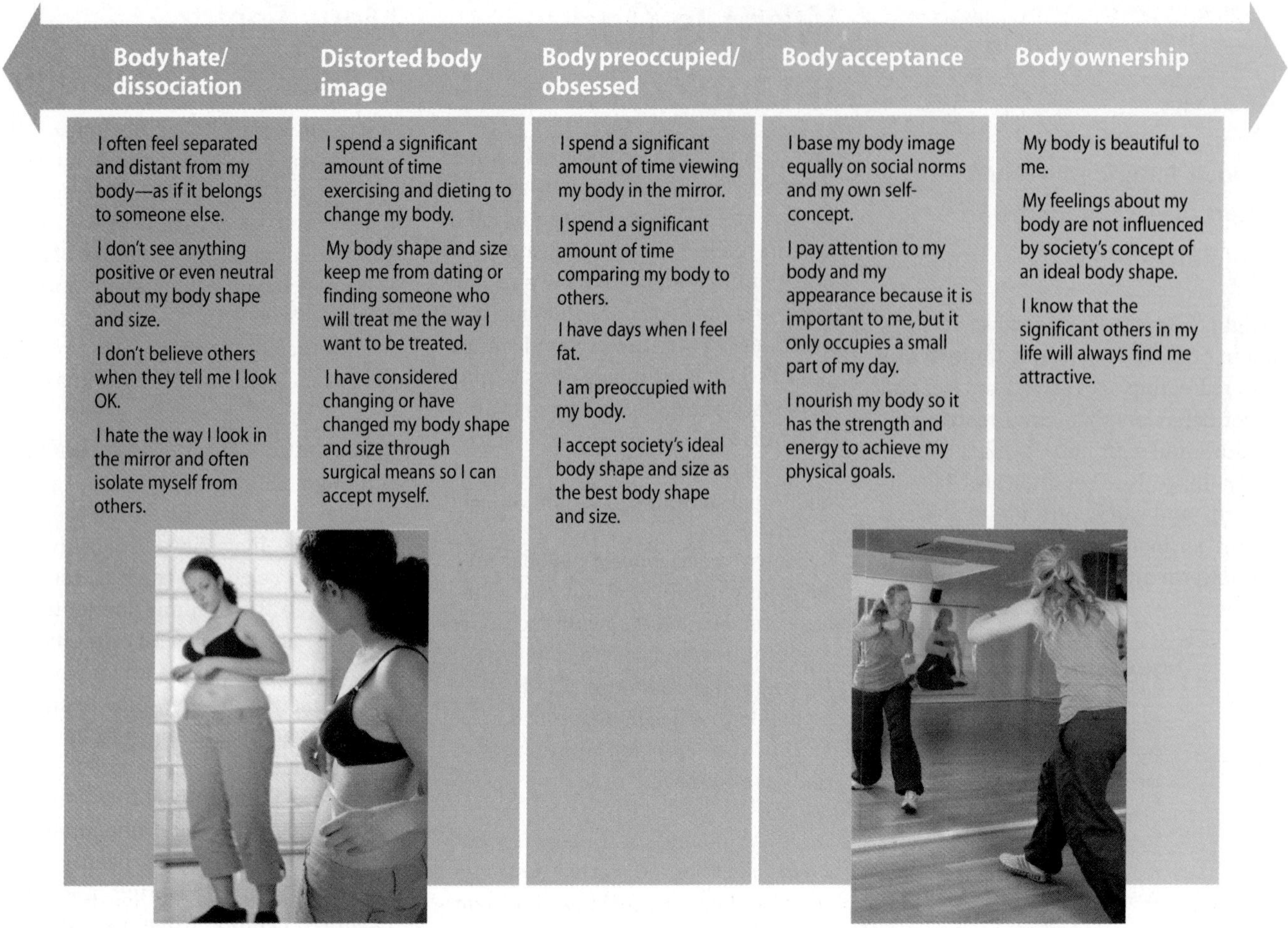

Body hate/ dissociation	Distorted body image	Body preoccupied/ obsessed	Body acceptance	Body ownership
I often feel separated and distant from my body—as if it belongs to someone else.	I spend a significant amount of time exercising and dieting to change my body.	I spend a significant amount of time viewing my body in the mirror.	I base my body image equally on social norms and my own self-concept.	My body is beautiful to me.
I don't see anything positive or even neutral about my body shape and size.	My body shape and size keep me from dating or finding someone who will treat me the way I want to be treated.	I spend a significant amount of time comparing my body to others.	I pay attention to my body and my appearance because it is important to me, but it only occupies a small part of my day.	My feelings about my body are not influenced by society's concept of an ideal body shape.
I don't believe others when they tell me I look OK.	I have considered changing or have changed my body shape and size through surgical means so I can accept myself.	I have days when I feel fat.	I nourish my body so it has the strength and energy to achieve my physical goals.	I know that the significant others in my life will always find me attractive.
I hate the way I look in the mirror and often isolate myself from others.		I am preoccupied with my body.		
		I accept society's ideal body shape and size as the best body shape and size.		

FIGURE 1 | **Body Image Continuum**

This is part of a two-part continuum, the second part of which is shown in Figure 2. Individuals whose responses fall to the far left side of the continuum have a highly negative body image, whereas responses to the right indicate a positive body image.

Source: Adapted from Smiley/King/Avery, Campus Health Service. Original continuum, C. Schislak, *Preventive Medicine and Public Health.* Copyright © 1997 Arizona Board of Regents. Used with permission.

movies, and print publications—is a more powerful and pervasive presence than ever before. In fact, one study of more than 4,000 television commercials revealed that more than one out of every four sends some sort of "attractiveness message."[5] Thus, Americans are daily bombarded with messages telling us that we just don't measure up.

Family, Community, and Cultural Groups The members of society with whom we most often interact—our family members, friends, and others—strongly influence the way we see ourselves. Parents are especially influential in body image development. For instance, it's common and natural for fathers of adolescent girls to experience feelings of discomfort related to their daughters' changing bodies. If they are

able to successfully navigate these feelings, and validate the acceptability of their daughters' appearance throughout puberty, they'll help their daughters maintain a positive body image. In contrast, if they make even subtle judgments about their daughters' changing bodies, girls can interpret these as revealing how their bodies are perceived by members of the opposite sex in general. In addition, mothers who model body acceptance or body ownership foster a similar positive body image in their daughters, whereas mothers who are frustrated with or ashamed of their bodies foster these attitudes in their daughters.

Interactions with siblings and other relatives, peers, teachers, coworkers, and other community members can also influence body image development. For

instance, peer harassment (teasing and bullying) is widely acknowledged to contribute to a negative body image. Moreover, associations within one's cultural group appear to influence body image. For example, studies have found that European American females experience the highest rates of body dissatisfaction, but as acculturation of a minority group increases, the body dissatisfaction levels of women in that group increase.[6]

Physiological and Psychological Factors Recent neurological research has suggested that people who have been diagnosed with a body image disorder show differences in the brain's ability to regulate chemicals called *neurotransmitters,* which are linked to mood.[7] Poor regulation of neurotransmitters is also involved in depression

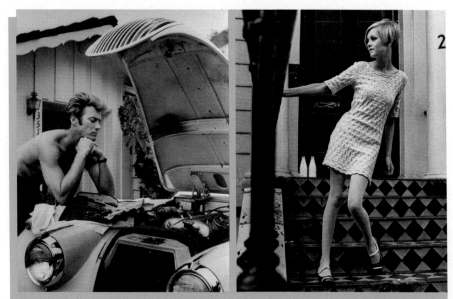

Is the media's mania for burly men and scrawny women a new phenomenon?

Although the exact nature of the "in" look may change from generation to generation, unrealistic images of both male and female celebrities are nothing new. In the 1960s, images of brawny film stars such as Clint Eastwood and ultrathin models such as Twiggy dominated the media.

with BDD are obsessively concerned with their appearance, and have a distorted view of their own body shape, body size, weight, perceived lack of muscles, facial blemishes, size of body parts, and so on. Although the precise cause of the disorder isn't known, an anxiety disorder such as obsessive-compulsive disorder is often present as well. Contributing factors may include genetic susceptibility, childhood teasing, physical or sexual abuse, low self-esteem, and rigid sociocultural expectations of beauty.[12] People with BDD may try to fix their perceived flaws through abuse of steroids, excessive

and in anxiety disorders, including obsessive-compulsive disorder (see Chapter 2). One study linked distortions in body image to a malfunctioning in the brain's visual processing region that was revealed by MRI scanning.[8]

How Can I Build a More Positive Body Image?

If you want to develop a more positive body image, your first step might be to bust some toxic myths pervasive in contemporary society. Have you been accepting these four myths as facts?[9]

Myth 1: How you look is more important than who you are.

Myth 2: Anyone can be slender and attractive if they work at it.

Myth 3: Extreme dieting is an effective weight-loss strategy.

Myth 4: Appearance is more important than health.

To learn ways to bust these toxic myths and build a more positive body image, check out the **Skills for Behavior Change** box on page 318.

Some People Develop Body Image Disorders

Although most Americans are dissatisfied with some aspect of their appearance, very few have a true body image disorder. However, several diagnosable body image disorders affect a small percentage of the population. Let's look at two of the most common.

An emerging problem, seen in both young men and women, is **social physique anxiety (SPA).** Consider this a concern about your appearance taken to the extreme: The desire to "look good" is so strong that it has a destructive and sometimes disabling effect on the person's ability to function effectively in relationships and interactions with others. People suffering from SPA may spend a disproportionate amount of time fixating on their bodies, working out, and performing tasks that are ego centered and self-directed, rather than focusing on interpersonal relationships and general tasks.[10] Experts speculate that this anxiety may contribute to disordered eating behaviors (discussed shortly).

Approximately 1 percent of people in the United States suffer from **body dysmorphic disorder (BDD).**[11] Persons

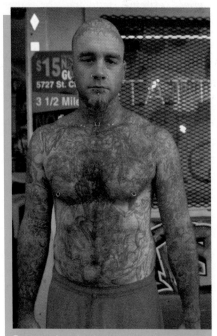

Do people who keep changing their looks really hate their bodies?

It's not always easy to spot people who are highly dissatisfied with their bodies, as they don't necessarily stick out in a crowd. For instance, people who cover their bodies with tattoos may have a strong sense of self-esteem. On the other hand, extreme tattooing can be an outward sign of a severe body image disturbance known as *body dysmorphic disorder.*

The average "female" store mannequin is 6 feet tall and has a 23-inch waist, whereas the average woman is 5 feet, 4 inches tall and has a 30-inch waist.

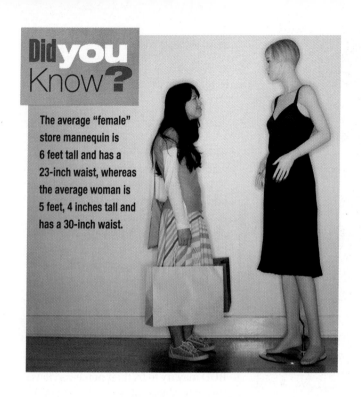

bodybuilding, repeated cosmetic surgeries, extreme tattooing, or other appearance-changing behaviors. Not only do such actions fail to address the underlying problem, they are actually considered diagnostic signs of BDD. In contrast, psychiatric treatment, including psychotherapy and/or antidepressant medications, is often successful.

What Are Eating Disorders?

As we've seen, people with a negative body image can fixate on a wide range of physical "flaws," from thinning hair to flat feet. Still, the "flaw" that causes distress to the majority of people with negative body image is overweight.

Some people channel their anxiety about their weight into self-defeating thoughts and harmful behaviors. Check out the eating issues continuum in **Figure 2**: the far left identifies a pattern of thoughts and behaviors associated with **disordered eating.** These behaviors can include chronic dieting,

abuse of diet pills and laxatives, self-induced vomiting, and many others.

Only some people who exhibit disordered eating patterns progress to a clinical **eating disorder.** The diagnosis of an eating disorder can be applied only by a physician to a patient who exhibits severe disturbances in thoughts, behavior, and body functioning—disturbances that can prove fatal. These diagnostic criteria are defined by the American Psychiatric Association (APA). The three APA-defined eating disorders are *anorexia nervosa, bulimia nervosa,* and a cluster of less distinct conditions collectively referred to as *eating disorders not otherwise specified (EDNOS).*

disordered eating A pattern of atypical eating behaviors that are used to achieve or maintain a lower body weight.

eating disorder A psychiatric disorder characterized by severe disturbances in body image and eating behaviors.

Ten Steps to a Positive Body Image

One list cannot automatically tell you how to turn negative body thoughts into a positive body image, but it can help you think about new ways of looking more healthfully and happily at yourself and your body. The more you do that, the more likely you are to feel good about who you are and the body you naturally have.

✳ **Step 1.** Appreciate all that your body can do. Every day your body carries you closer to your dreams. Celebrate all of the amazing things your body does for you—running, dancing, breathing, laughing, dreaming.

✳ **Step 2.** Keep a list of things you like about yourself—things that aren't related to how much you weigh or how you look. Read your list often. Add to it as you become aware of more things to like about yourself.

✳ **Step 3.** Remind yourself that true beauty is not simply skin deep. When you feel good about yourself and who you are, you carry yourself with a sense of confidence, self-acceptance, and openness that makes you beautiful. Beauty is a state of mind, not a state of your body.

✳ **Step 4.** Look at yourself as a whole person. When you see yourself in a mirror or in your mind, choose not to focus on specific body parts. See yourself as you want others to see you—as a whole person.

✳ **Step 5.** Surround yourself with positive people. It is easier to feel good about yourself and your body when you are around others who are supportive and who recognize the importance of liking yourself just as you naturally are.

✳ **Step 6.** Shut down those voices in your head that tell you your body is not "right" or that you are a "bad" person. You can overpower those negative thoughts with positive ones.

✳ **Step 7.** Wear clothes that are comfortable and that make you feel good about your body. Work with your body, not against it.

✳ **Step 8.** Become a critical viewer of social and media messages. Pay attention to images, slogans, or attitudes that make you feel bad about yourself or your body. Protest these messages: Write a letter to the advertiser or talk back to the image or message.

✳ **Step 9.** Do something nice for yourself—something that lets your body know you appreciate it. Take a bubble bath, make time for a nap, or find a peaceful place outside to relax.

✳ **Step 10.** Use the time and energy that you might have spent worrying about food, calories, and your weight to do something to help others. Sometimes reaching out to other people can help you feel better about yourself and can make a positive change in our world.

Eating disordered	Disruptive eating patterns	Food preoccupied/ obsessed	Concerned well	Food is not an issue
I regularly stuff myself and then exercise, vomit, use diet pills or laxatives to get rid of the food or calories. My friends/family tell me I am too thin. I am terrified of eating fat. When I let myself eat, I have a hard time controlling the amount of food I eat. I am afraid to eat in front of others.	I have tried diet pills, laxatives, vomiting, or extra time exercising in order to lose or maintain my weight. I have fasted or avoided eating for long periods of time in order to lose or maintain my weight. I feel strong when I can restrict how much I eat. Eating more than I wanted to makes me feel out of control.	I think about food a lot. I feel I don't eat well most of the time. It's hard for me to enjoy eating with others. I feel ashamed when I eat more than others or more than what I feel I should be eating. I am afraid of getting fat. I wish I could change how much I want to eat and what I am hungry for.	I pay attention to what I eat in order to maintain a healthy body. I may weigh more than what I like, but I enjoy eating and balance my pleasure with eating with my concern for a healthy body. I am moderate and flexible in goals for eating well. I try to follow Dietary Guidelines for healthy eating.	I am not concerned about what others think regarding what and how much I eat. When I am upset or depressed I eat whatever I am hungry for without any guilt or shame. Food is an important part of my life but only occupies a small part of my time.

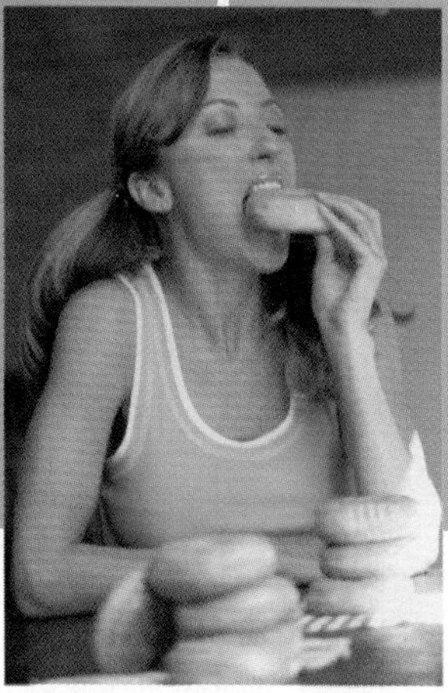

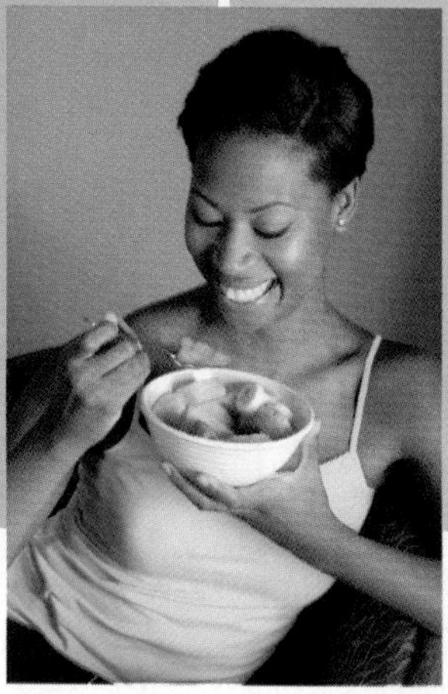

FIGURE 2 Eating Issues Continuum

This second part of the continuum shown in Figure 1 suggests that the progression from normal eating to eating disorders occurs on a continuum.

Source: Adapted from Smiley/King/Avery: Campus Health Service. Original continuum, C. Schislak, *Preventive Medicine and Public Health*. Copyright © 1997 Arizona Board of Regents. Used with permission.

Who's at Risk?

In the United States, as many as 24 million people of all ages meet the established criteria for an eating disorder.[13] Although anorexia nervosa and bulimia nervosa affect people primarily in their teens and twenties, increasing numbers of children as young as 6 have been diagnosed, as have women as old as 76. In 2007, 3.8 percent of college students reported that they were dealing with either anorexia or bulimia. In addition, 1.3 percent of college students said that their eating disorder had affected their academic performance.[14]

Eating disorders are on the rise among men, who currently represent up to 25 percent of anorexia and

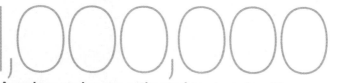

American males are estimated to struggle with some form of eating disorder.

bulimia patients and almost 40 percent of binge eaters (a category within EDNOS).[15] Many men suffering from eating disorders fail to seek treatment, because these illnesses are traditionally thought of as being a woman's problem, and treatment centers are often geared toward women. Disordered eating and eating disorders are also common among athletes, affecting up to 62 percent of college athletes in sports such as gymnastics, wrestling, swimming, and figure skating.[16]

What factors put individuals at risk? Eating disorders are very complex, and despite scientific research to try to understand them, their biological, behavioral, and social underpinnings remain elusive. Many people with these disorders feel disempowered in other aspects of their lives, and try to

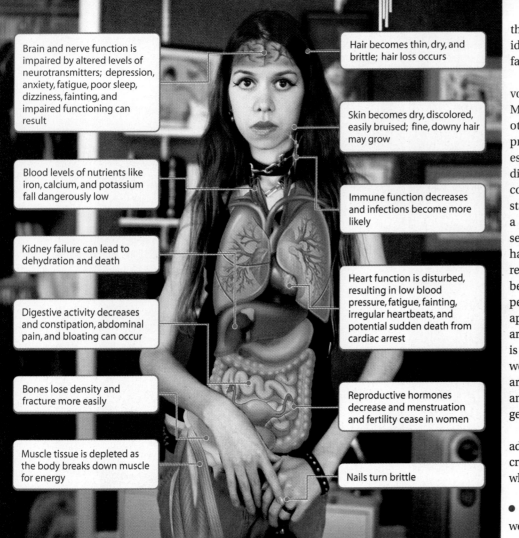

Brain and nerve function is impaired by altered levels of neurotransmitters; depression, anxiety, fatigue, poor sleep, dizziness, fainting, and impaired functioning can result

Hair becomes thin, dry, and brittle; hair loss occurs

Blood levels of nutrients like iron, calcium, and potassium fall dangerously low

Skin becomes dry, discolored, easily bruised; fine, downy hair may grow

Kidney failure can lead to dehydration and death

Immune function decreases and infections become more likely

Digestive activity decreases and constipation, abdominal pain, and bloating can occur

Heart function is disturbed, resulting in low blood pressure, fatigue, fainting, irregular heartbeats, and potential sudden death from cardiac arrest

Bones lose density and fracture more easily

Reproductive hormones decrease and menstruation and fertility cease in women

Muscle tissue is depleted as the body breaks down muscle for energy

Nails turn brittle

FIGURE 3 What Anorexia Nervosa Can Do to the Body

thin enough and constantly identify body parts that are "too fat."

The causes of anorexia nervosa are complex and variable. Many people with anorexia have other coexisting psychiatric problems, including low self-esteem, depression, an anxiety disorder such as obsessive-compulsive disorder, and substance abuse. Some people have a history of being physically or sexually abused, and others have troubled interpersonal relationships with family members. Cultural norms that value people on the basis of their appearance and glorify thinness are of course a factor, as is weight-based teasing and weight bias.[18] Physical factors are thought to include an imbalance of neurotransmitters and genetic susceptibility.[19]

Nearly 1 percent of girls in late adolescence meet the full APA criteria for anorexia nervosa, which are as follows:[20]

● Refusal to maintain body weight at or above a minimally normal weight for age and height

gain a sense of control through food. Many are clinically depressed, suffer from obsessive-compulsive disorder, or have other psychiatric problems. In addition, studies have shown that individuals with low self-esteem, negative body image, and a high tendency for perfectionism are at risk.[17]

Anorexia Nervosa Involves Severe Food Restriction

Anorexia nervosa is a persistent, chronic eating disorder characterized by delib-

anorexia nervosa Eating disorder characterized by excessive preoccupation with food, self-starvation, or extreme exercising to achieve weight loss.

erate food restriction and severe, life-threatening weight loss. It involves self-starvation motivated by an intense fear of gaining weight along with an extremely distorted body image. Initially, most people with anorexia nervosa lose weight by reducing total food intake, particularly of high-calorie foods. Eventually, they come to restrict their intake of almost all foods. The little they do eat, they may purge through vomiting or using laxatives. Although they lose weight, people with anorexia nervosa never seem to feel

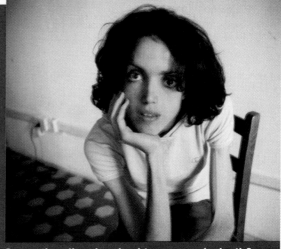

Can eating disorders lead to a person's death?

People with anorexia nervosa put themselves at risk for starving to death. In addition, they may die from sudden cardiac arrest caused by electrolyte imbalances; this is also a risk for people with bulimia nervosa. About 20% to 25% of people with a serious eating disorder die from it.

- Intense fear of gaining weight or becoming fat, even though considered underweight by all medical criteria
- Disturbance in the way in which one's body weight or shape is experienced, undue influence of body weight or shape on self-evaluation, or denial of the seriousness of the current low body weight
- Amenorrhea (the absence of at least three menstrual periods in a row) in females who are past puberty

The physical symptoms and consequences of anorexia nervosa are illustrated in Figure 3. Because it involves starvation and can lead to heart attacks and seizures, anorexia nervosa has the highest death rate (20%) of any psychological illness.

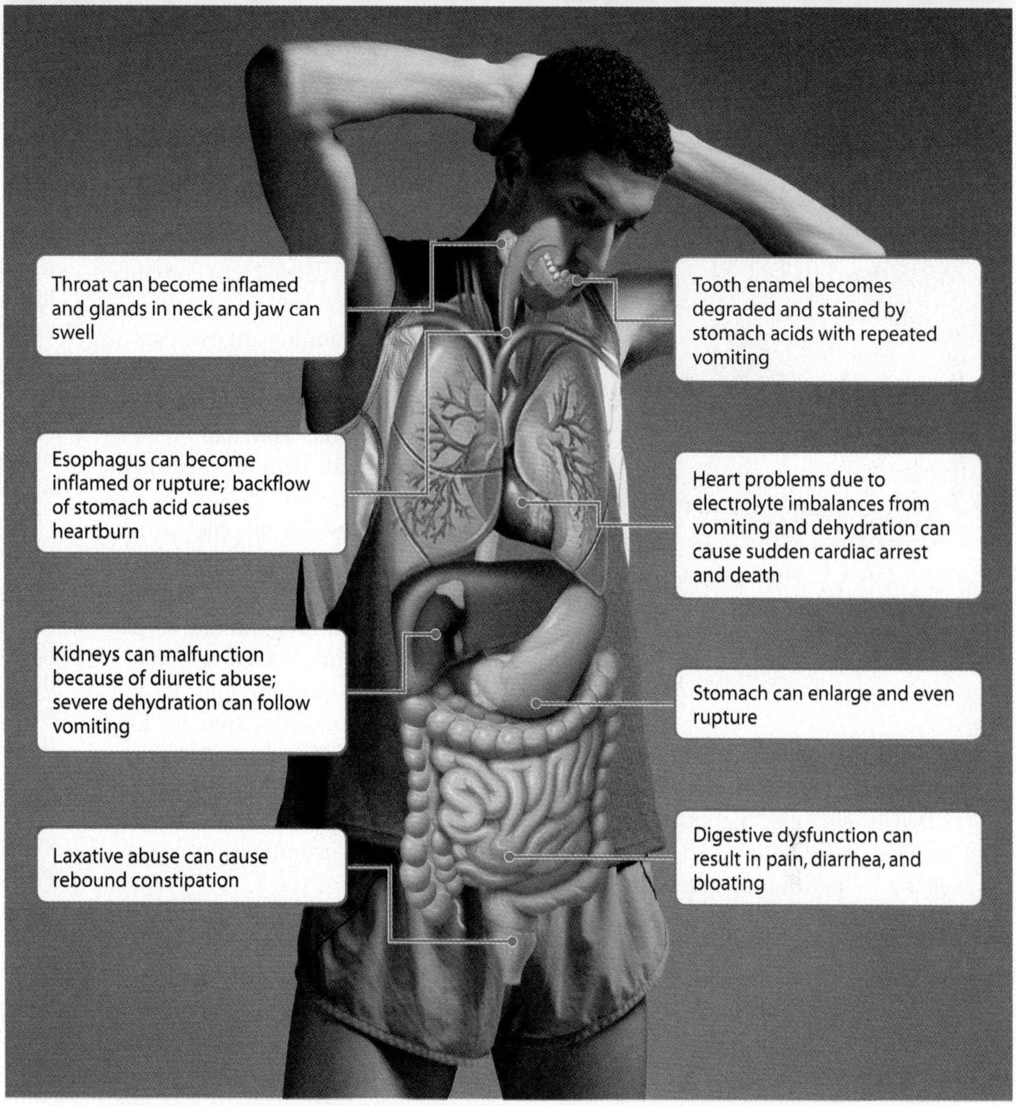

Bulimia Nervosa Involves Bingeing and Purging

People with **bulimia nervosa** often binge on huge amounts of food and then engage in some kind of purging, or "compensatory behavior," such as vomiting, taking laxatives, or exercising excessively, to lose the calories they have just consumed. Up to 3 percent of adolescents and young women are bulimic; rates among men are about 10 percent of the rate among women. People with bulimia are obsessed with their bodies, weight gain, and appearance, but unlike those with anorexia, their problem is often "hidden" from the public eye because their weight may fall within a normal range or they may be overweight.

A combination of genetic and environmental factors is thought to cause bulimia nervosa.[21] A family history of obesity, an underlying anxiety disorder, and an imbalance in neurotransmitters are all possible contributing factors. In support of the role of neurotransmitters, a recent study showed that brain circuitry involved in regulating impulsive behavior seems to be less active in

Throat can become inflamed and glands in neck and jaw can swell

Esophagus can become inflamed or rupture; backflow of stomach acid causes heartburn

Kidneys can malfunction because of diuretic abuse; severe dehydration can follow vomiting

Laxative abuse can cause rebound constipation

Tooth enamel becomes degraded and stained by stomach acids with repeated vomiting

Heart problems due to electrolyte imbalances from vomiting and dehydration can cause sudden cardiac arrest and death

Stomach can enlarge and even rupture

Digestive dysfunction can result in pain, diarrhea, and bloating

FIGURE 4 **What Bulimia Nervosa Can Do to the Body**

women with bulimia than in normal women.[22] However, it is impossible at this point to determine whether such differences exist before bulimia develops or arise as a consequence of the disorder.

The APA diagnostic criteria for bulimia nervosa are as follows:[23]

- Recurrent episodes of binge eating
- Recurrent inappropriate compensatory behavior
- Binge eating occurs on average at least twice a week for 3 months
- Body shape and weight unduly influence self-evaluation
- The disturbance does not occur exclusively during episodes of anorexia nervosa

The physical symptoms and consequences of bulimia nervosa are shown in Figure 4. One of the more common

symptoms of bulimia is tooth erosion, which results from the excessive vomiting associated with this disorder. Bulimics who vomit are also at risk for electrolyte imbalances and dehydration, both of which can contribute to a heart attack and sudden death.

Some Eating Disorders Are Not Easily Classified

The APA recognizes that some patterns of disordered eating qualify as a legitimate psychiatric illness but don't fit into the strict diagnostic criteria for either anorexia or bulimia. These are

bulimia nervosa Eating disorder characterized by binge eating followed by inappropriate measures, such as vomiting, to prevent weight gain.

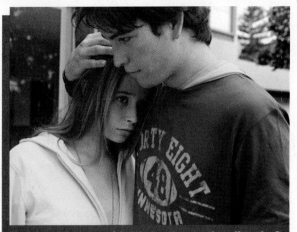

How can I talk to a friend about an eating disorder?

When talking to a friend about an eating disorder, avoid casting blame, preaching, or offering unsolicited advice. Instead, be a good listener, let the person know that you care, and offer your support.

the **eating disorders not otherwise specified (EDNOS).** Patients with EDNOS are the highest treatment-seeking population, and represent 40 to 75 percent of individuals with eating disorders.[24]

A form of EDNOS that has recently received considerable research attention is binge-eating disorder. Individuals with **binge-eating disorder** gorge like their bulimic counterparts but do not take excessive measures to lose the weight that they gain. Thus, they are often clinically obese. As in bulimia, binge-eating episodes are typically characterized by eating large amounts of food rapidly, even when not feeling hungry, and feeling guilty or depressed after overeating.[25]

A national survey on eating disorders conducted by Harvard-affiliated McLean Hospital reported that binge-eating disorder is more prevalent than either anorexia nervosa or bulimia nervosa. The survey showed that 3.5 percent of women and 2 percent of men experience binge-eating disorder at some point in their lives.[26]

eating disorder not otherwise specified (EDNOS) An eating disorder that is a true psychiatric illness but does not fit the strict diagnostic criteria for either anorexia nervosa or bulimia nervosa.
binge-eating disorder A type of EDNOS characterized by binge eating twice a week or more, but not typically followed by a compensatory behavior.

Eating Disorders Can Be Treated

Because eating disorders are caused by a combination of many factors, spanning many years of development, there are no quick or simple solutions. The bad news is that without treatment, between 20 and 25 percent of people with a serious eating disorder will die from it. With treatment, about 60 percent will recover, whereas 20 percent improve but remain focused on food and weight and often engage in excessive exercise. The remaining 20 percent do not improve and spend considerable time and resources in various treatments.[27]

Treatment often focuses first on reducing the threat to life; once the patient is stabilized, long-term therapy focuses on the psychological, social, environmental, and physiological factors that have led to the problem. Therapy allows the patient to work on adopting new eating behaviors, building self-confidence, and finding other ways to deal with life's problems. Support groups can help the family and the individual learn to foster positive actions and interactions. Treatment of an underlying anxiety disorder or depression may also be a focus.

How Can You Help Someone You Suspect Has an Eating Disorder?

Although every situation is different, there are several things you can do if you suspect someone you know is struggling with an eating disorder:[28]

● Learn as much as possible about eating disorders before talking to the

person. Check out resources on your campus and in your local community. Have a list of therapeutic referrals ready to give to the person.

● Set up a time to meet and share your concerns openly, honestly, and in a caring and supportive way. Be a good listener, and don't give advice unless asked.

● Provide examples of why you think there might be a problem. Talk about health, relationships, and changes in behaviors.

● Avoid conflicts or a battle of wills with this person. If he or she denies that there is a problem or minimizes it, repeat your concerns in a nonjudgmental way. You want the person to feel comfortable talking to you—you don't want to drive him or her away.

● Never nag, plead, beg, bribe, threaten, or manipulate. Be straightforward and acknowledge it will be hard but that you know the person can work through this.

● Don't talk about how thin the person is or focus on weight, diets, or exercise. Remember that people with these disorders want to hear they are thin; if you say it's good they are gaining weight, they will try to lose it.

● If the person is nervous about counseling, offer to go along as support.

● Avoid placing shame, guilt, or accusations. Use "I" words (such as "I am worried that you won't be able to do such and such if you don't eat") rather than "you" statements (such as "you need to eat or you are going to make yourself really sick").

● Stay calm and realize your own limitations. Be patient, supportive, and there if the person asks for your help.

What Are Exercise Disorders?

While exercise is generally beneficial to health, in excess it can be a problem. In addition to being a common compensatory behavior used by people with anorexia or bulimia, exercise can become a compulsion, or contribute to either of two more complex disorders.

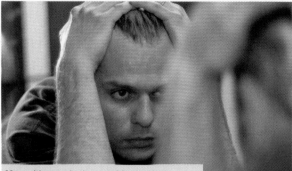
Men with muscle dysmorphia may have unusually muscular bodies but suffer from very low self-esteem.

Exercise Can Become a Compulsion

A recent study of almost 600 college students revealed that 18 percent met the criteria for **compulsive exercise.**[29] Also called *anorexia athletica*, compulsive exercise is characterized not by a *desire* to exercise but a *compulsion* to do so. That is, the person struggles with guilt and anxiety if he or she doesn't work out. Compulsive exercisers, like people with eating disorders, often define their self-worth externally. They overexercise in order to feel more in control of their lives. Disordered eating or a true eating disorder is often part of the picture.

Compulsive exercise can contribute to a variety of other problems, including injuries to joints and broken bones. It can also put significant stress on the heart, especially if combined with disordered eating. Psychologically, people who engage in compulsive exercise are often plagued by anxiety and/or depression. Their social life and academic success can suffer as they fixate more and more on exercise.

Muscle Dysmorphia Is a Body Image and Exercise Disorder

Muscle dysmorphia appears to be a relatively new form of body image disturbance among men in which a man believes that his body is insufficiently lean or muscular.[30] Men with muscle dysmorphia believe that they look "puny," when in reality they look normal or may even be unusually muscular. As a result of their adherence to a meticulous diet, their time-consuming workout schedule, and their shame over their perceived appearance flaws, they may neglect important social or occupational activities. Other behaviors characteristic of muscle dysmorphia include comparing oneself unfavorably to others, checking one's appearance in the mirror, and camouflaging one's appearance. Men with muscle dysmorphia also have higher rates of substance abuse and suicide than men without the disorder.[31]

The Female Athlete Triad Involves Three Interrelated Disorders

Female athletes in competitive sports often strive for perfection. In an effort to be the best, they may do more damage than good, and put themselves at risk for developing a syndrome called the **female athlete triad**. *Triad* means "three," and the three interrelated problems are as follows (Figure 5):[32]

● Low energy intake, typically prompted by disordered eating behaviors
● Menstrual dysfunction such as amenorrhea
● Poor bone density

How does the female athlete triad develop, and what makes it so dangerous? Through a chronic pattern of low energy intake and intensive exercise an athlete can deplete her body stores of nutrients essential to health. At the same time, her body will begin to burn its stores of fat tissue for energy. Adequate body fat is essential to maintaining healthy levels of the female reproductive hormone *estrogen*; when an athlete isn't getting enough food, estrogen levels decline. This can manifest as amenorrhea. In addition, fat-soluble vitamins, calcium, and estrogen are all essential for dense, healthy bones, so their depletion weakens the athlete's bones, leaving her at high risk for fracture.

Not all athletes are equally prone to the female athlete triad: It is particularly prevalent in women who participate in highly competitive individual sports or activities that emphasize leanness and require the wearing of body-contouring clothing. Gymnasts, figure skaters, cross-country runners, and ballet dancers are among those at highest risk for the female athlete triad.

Menstrual dysfunction

Low bone density

Energy deficit (e.g., from disordered eating)

FIGURE 5 **The Female Athlete Triad**
The female athlete triad is a cluster of three interrelated health problems.

Assess yourself

Are Your Efforts to Be Thin Sensible— Or Spinning Out of Control?

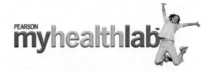

Fill out this assessment online at www.pearsonhighered.com/myhealthlab or www.pearsonhighered.com/donatelle.

On one hand, just because you weigh yourself, count calories, or work out every day, don't jump to the conclusion that you have any of the health concerns discussed in this chapter. On the other hand, efforts to lose a few pounds can spiral out of control. To find out whether your efforts to be thin are harmful to you, take the following quiz from the National Eating Disorders Association (NEDA).

1. I constantly calculate numbers of fat grams and calories. **T   F**

2. I weigh myself often and find myself obsessed with the number on the scale. **T   F**

3. I exercise to burn calories and not for health or enjoyment. **T   F**

4. I sometimes feel out of control while eating. **T   F**

5. I often go on extreme diets. **T   F**

6. I engage in rituals to get me through meal-times and/or secretively binge. **T   F**

7. Weight loss, dieting, and controlling my food intake have become my major concerns. **T   F**

8. I feel ashamed, disgusted, or guilty after eating. **T   F**

9. I constantly worry about the weight, shape, and/or size of my body. **T   F**

10. I feel my identity and value are based on how I look or how much I weigh. **T   F**

If you marked True to any of these questions, you could be dealing with disordered eating. If so, talk about it! Tell a friend, parent, teacher, coach, youth group leader, doctor, counselor, or nutritionist what you're going through. Check out the NEDA's Sharing with EEEase handout at www.nationaleatingdisorders .org/nedaDir/files/documents/handouts/ShEEEase.pdf for help planning what to say the first time you talk to someone about your eating and exercise habits.

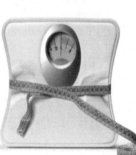

Source: Copyright © 2005 by National Eating Disorders Association. All rights reserved. Available at www.nationaleatingdisorders.org.

YOUR PLAN FOR CHANGE

The **Assess yourself** activity gave you the chance to evaluate your feelings about your body, and to determine whether or not you might be engaging in eating or exercise behaviors that could undermine your health and happiness. Below are some steps you can take to improve your body image, starting today.

Today, you can:

○ Talk back to the media. Write letters to advertisers and magazines who depict unhealthy and unrealistic body types. Boycott their products or start a blog commenting on harmful body image messages in the media.

○ Visit www.mypyramid.gov and print out your personalized food plan. Just for today, eat the recommended number of servings from every food group at every meal, and don't count calories!

Within the next 2 weeks, you can:

○ Find a photograph of a person you admire *not* for his or her appearance, but for his or her contribution to humanity. Paste it up next to your mirror to remind yourself that true beauty comes from within and benefits others.

○ Start a diary. Each day, record one thing you are grateful for that has nothing to do with your appearance. At the end of each day, record one small thing you did to make someone's world a little brighter.

By the end of the semester, you can:

○ Establish a group of friends who support you for who you are, not what you look like, and who get the same support from you. Form a group on a favorite social-networking site, and keep in touch, especially when you start to feel troubled by self-defeating thoughts or have the urge to engage in unhealthy eating or exercise behaviors.

○ Borrow from the library or purchase one of the many books on body image now available, and read it!

References

1. H. G. Pope Jr, A. J. Gruber, B. Mangweth et al., "Body Image Perception among Men in Three Countries," *American Journal of Psychiatry* 157 (2000): 1297–1301; National Eating Disorders Association, "Statistics: Eating Disorders and Their Precursors," 2008, www.nationaleatingdisorders.org/p.asp?WebPage_ID=286&Profile_ID=41138.

2. J. M. Enoch, "History of Mirrors Dating Back 8000 Years," *Optometry and Vision Science* 83, no. 10 (2006): 775–81.

3. National Eating Disorders Association, "Body Image," 2008, www.nationaleatingdisorders.org/p.asp?WebPage_ID=286&Profile_ID=41157.

4. Centers for Disease Control and Prevention, "U.S. Obesity Trends 1985 to 2008," 2009, www.cdc.gov/nccdphp/dnpa/obesity/trends.html.

5. National Eating Disorders Association, "The Media, Body Image, and Eating Disorders," 2008, www.nationaleatingdisorders.org/p.asp?WebPage_ID=286&Profile_ID=41166.

6. S. Grogan, *Body Image: Understanding Body Dissatisfaction in Men, Women, and Children*, 2d ed. (New York: Psychology Press, 2008), 159–61.

7. Mayo Clinic Staff, "Body Dysmorphic Disorder," 2008, www.mayoclinic.com/health/body-dysmorphic-disorder/DS00559; KidsHealth, "Body Dysmorphic Disorder," 2007, http://kidshealth.org/parent/emotions/feelings/bdd.html.

8. University of California—Los Angeles, "Distorted Self-Image in Body Image Disorder Due to Visual Brain Glitch, Study Suggests," *ScienceDaily*, 2007, www.sciencedaily.com/releases/2007/12/071203103409.htm.

9. K. Kater, "Building Healthy Body Esteem," *Healthy Body Image: Teaching Kids to Eat and Love Their Bodies Too* (Seattle: National Eating Disorders Association, 2005). Available at www.bodyimagehealth.org.

10. G. Flett and P. Hewitt, "The Perils of Perfectionism in Sports and Exercise," *Current Directions in Psychological Science* 14, no. 1 (2005): 14–22; P. Crocker et al., "Examining Current Ideal Discrepancy Scores and Exercise Motivations as Predictors of Social Physique Anxiety in Exercising Females," *Journal of Sport Behavior* 28 (2005): 63–72.

11. Mayo Clinic Staff, "Body Dysmorphic Disorder," 2008.

12. Mayo Clinic Staff, "Body Dysmorphic Disorder," 2008; KidsHealth, "Body Dysmorphic Disorder," 2007.

13. Disordered Eating, UK, "Eating Disorders Statistics (U.S.)," 2008, www.disordered-eating.co.uk/eating-disorders-statistics/eating-disorders-statistics-us.html; National Eating Disorder Association, "Statistics: Eating Disorders and Their Precursors," 2008, www.nationaleatingdisorders.org.

14. American College Health Association, *National College Health Assessment Reference Group Executive Summary,* Fall 2007, www.achancha.org/pubs_rpts.html.

15. E. Bernstein, "Men, Boys Lack Options to Treat Eating Disorders," *Wall Street Journal* (April 17, 2007): D1–D2.

16. K. Beals and A. Hill, "The Prevalence of Disordered Eating, Menstrual Dysfunction, and Low Bone Mineral Density among U.S. Collegiate Athletes," *International Journal of Sport Nutrition and Exercise Metabolism* 16, no. 3 (2006): 1–23; American College of Sports Medicine, "Female Athlete Health Challenges Prevalent but Misunderstood: Study Shows Too Few Coaches Aware of Conditions, Implications," June 2006, www.acsm.org; L. Ronco, "The Female Athlete Triad: When Women Push Their Limits in High-Performance Sports," *American Fitness* 25, no. 2 (2007): 22–24.

17. S. Forsberg and J. Lock, "The Relationship between Perfectionism, Eating Disorders and Athletes: A Review," *Minerva Pediatrica* 58, no. 6 (2006): 525–34.

18. A. L. Ahern, K. M. Bennett, and M. M. Hetherington, "Internalization of the Ultra-Thin Ideal: Positive Implicit Associations with Underweight Fashion Models Are Associated with Drive for Thinness in Young Women," *Eating Disorders* 16, no. 4 (2008): 294–307; M. Eisenberg, and D Neumark-Sztainer, "Peer Harassment and Disordered Eating," *International Journal of Adolescent Medicine and Health* 20, no. 2 (2008): 155–64.

19. National Eating Disorders Association, "Causes of Eating Disorders," 2006, www.nationaleatingdisorders.org/p.asp?WebPage_ID=286&Profile_ID=41144.

20. American Psychiatric Association, *Diagnostic and Statistical Manual of Mental Disorders.* 4th ed., *Text Revision (DSM-IV-TR).* (Washington, DC: American Psychiatric Association, 2004).

21. National Alliance on Mental Illness, "Bulimia Nervosa," 2009, www.nami.org/template.cfm?Section=by_illness&template=/ContentManagement/ContentDisplay.cfm&ContentID=65839.

22. R. Marsh, J. E. Steinglass, A. J. Gerber, K. Graziano O'Leary, Z. Wang, D. Murphy, B. T. Walsh, and B. S. Peterson, "Deficient Activity in the Neural Systems That Mediate Self-Regulatory Control in Bulimia Nervosa," *Archives of General Psychiatry* 66, no. 1 (2009): 51–63.

23. American Psychiatric Association, *Diagnostic and Statistical Manual of Mental Disorders,* 2004.

24. D. Satir, "EDNOS: The Meaning of 'Eating Disorder Not Otherwise Specified' and Its Implications," *National Eating Disorders Association Newsletter* 21 (2009): 4.

25. J. Manwaring et al., "Risk Factors and Patterns of Onset in Binge Eating Disorder," *International Journal of Eating Disorders* 39, no. 2 (2005): 101–7.

26. J. Hudson et al., "The Prevalence and Correlates of Eating Disorders in the National Comorbidity Survey Replication," *Biological Psychiatry* 61, no. 3 (2007): 348–58.

27. National Association of Anorexia Nervosa and Associated Eating Disorders, 2009, www.anad.org.

28. National Eating Disorders Association, "What Should I Say? Tips for Talking to a Friend Who May Be Struggling with an Eating Disorder," 2006, www.nationaleatingdisorders.org.

29. J. Guidi, M. Pender, S. D. Hollon, S. Zisook, F. H. Schwartz, P. Pedrelli, A. Farabaugh, M. Fava, and T. J. Petersen, "The Prevalence of Compulsive Eating and Exercise among College Students: An Exploratory Study," *Psychiatry Research* 165, nos. 1–2 (2009): 154–62.

30. C. G. Pope, H. G. Pope, W. Menard, C. Fay, R. Olivardia, and K. A. Phillips, "Clinical Features of Muscle Dysmorphia among Males with Body Dysmorphic Disorder," *Body Image* 2, no. 4 (2005): 395–400.

31. Ibid.

32. A. Nattiv, A. B. Loucks, M. M. Manore, C. F. Sanborn, J. Sundgot-Borgen, and M. P. Warren, "American College of Sports Medicine Position Stand: The Female Athlete Triad," *Medicine and Science in Sports and Exercise* 39, no. 10 (2007): 1867–82.

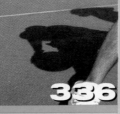
331
Can exercise really reduce stress?

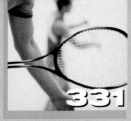
336
Why is core strength training important?

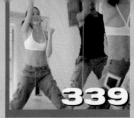
339
How can I motivate myself to exercise more?

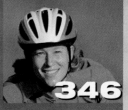
346
What can I do to avoid injury while I'm exercising?

11

Personal Fitness

Objectives

✴ Distinguish among physical activity for health, for fitness, and for performance.

✴ Describe the benefits of regular physical activity, including improvements in physical health, mental health, stress management, and life span.

✴ Explain the components of an aerobic exercise program, a strength-training program, and a stretching program.

✴ Summarize ways to prevent and treat common fitness injuries.

✴ Summarize the key components of a personal fitness program, and design a program that works for you.

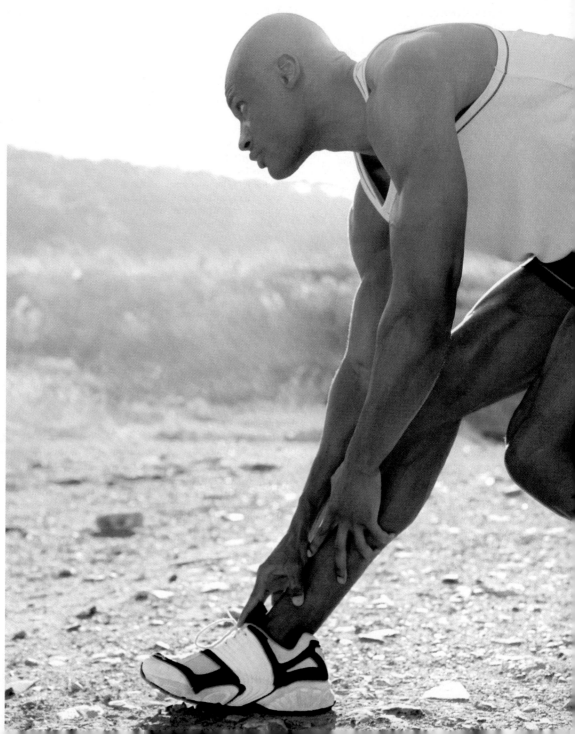

A century ago in the United States, just to survive meant you had to perform physical labor on a daily basis. However, science and technology have transformed our lives. Today most adults in our country lead sedentary lifestyles and perform little physical labor or exercise. Students are no different; a recent survey indicated that 57 percent of college women and 47 percent of college men do not meet recommended health guidelines for engaging in moderate or vigorous physical activities.[1] The growing percentage of Americans who live sedentary lives has been linked to dramatic increases in the incidence of obesity, diabetes, and other chronic diseases.[2] More than 145 million Americans are overweight or obese, 73.6 million have high blood pressure, 16.8 million have coronary artery disease, 23.6 million have diabetes, and approximately 57 million have pre-diabetes.[3]

Decades of research show that physical activity has tremendous health-promoting and disease-preventing benefits. Now is an excellent time to develop exercise habits that will improve the quality and duration of your own life.

Physical Activity for Health, Fitness, and Performance

Physical activity refers to any bodily movement that involves muscle contractions and an increase in metabolism.[4] Walking, swimming, heavy lifting, and housework are all examples of physical activity. Physical activities also may vary by intensity. For example, walking to class may require little effort, but walking to class up a hill while carrying a heavy backpack makes the activity more intense. There are three general categories of physical activity defined by the purpose for which they are done: physical activity for health, physical activity for fitness, and physical activity for performance.

Physical Activity for Health

Just about everyone can improve general health by increasing overall physical activity. Simply adding more physical movement to your day can benefit your health. A physically active lifestyle might include choices such as parking farther away from your destination, taking walking breaks while studying, or choosing to take the stairs instead of the elevator. In addition to these incidental ways to increase activity, there are lots of ways you can enjoy being physically active in recreation. Going dancing, playing Frisbee, or walking your dog are all good examples of recreational physical activity. The good thing about lifestyle physical activity is that you don't necessarily have to sustain your activity for an extended period of time to get a health benefit. Research shows that accumulating activity throughout the day can contribute to overall health and well-being. In their 2007 updated recommendations for adults, the American College of Sports Medicine (ACSM) and the American Heart Association (AHA) stated that to promote and maintain

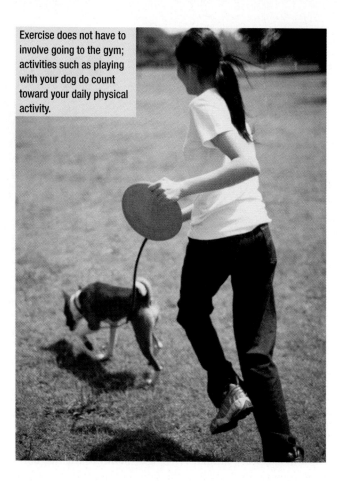

Exercise does not have to involve going to the gym; activities such as playing with your dog do count toward your daily physical activity.

good health, adults under age 65 should perform 30 minutes of moderate-intensity activity 5 days a week. This activity is in addition to the light-intensity activities of daily life and can be accumulated in bouts of at least 10 minutes.[5] In their 2008 physical activity guidelines, the U.S. Department of Health and Human Services made a similar recommendation of 150 minutes of moderate physical activity per week, preferably spread throughout the week and performed in episodes of at least 10 minutes.[6]

Physical Activity for Fitness

The word **exercise** is a bit more specific than the term *physical activity*. Although all exercise is physical activity, not all physical activity may be exercise. For example, walking from your car to class is physical activity, but going for a brisk 30-minute walk is considered exercise. *Exercise* is defined as planned, structured, and repetitive bodily movement done to improve or maintain one or more components of physical fitness, such as endurance, flexibility, and strength. **Physical fitness** is the ability to perform moderate to vigorous physical activity on a regular basis

physical activity Any bodily movement that involves muscle contractions and an increase in metabolism.

exercise Planned, structured, and repetitive bodily movement done to improve or maintain one or more components of physical fitness.

physical fitness The ability to perform regular moderate to vigorous levels of physical activity without excessive fatigue.

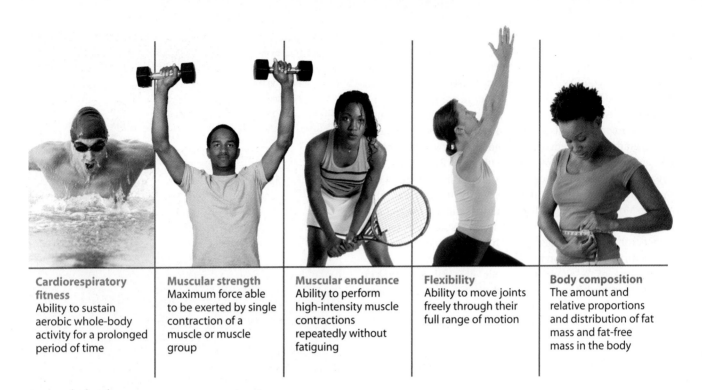

Cardiorespiratory fitness	Muscular strength	Muscular endurance	Flexibility	Body composition
Ability to sustain aerobic whole-body activity for a prolonged period of time	Maximum force able to be exerted by single contraction of a muscle or muscle group	Ability to perform high-intensity muscle contractions repeatedly without fatiguing	Ability to move joints freely through their full range of motion	The amount and relative proportions and distribution of fat mass and fat-free mass in the body

FIGURE 11.1 **Components of Physical Fitness**

without excessive fatigue. **Figure 11.1** identifies the five core components that make up the foundation of fitness. Each of these elements makes a unique contribution to overall fitness. For example, a person who jogs regularly has well-developed cardiorespiratory fitness, but also needs flexibility to avoid injury, muscle strength to make it up hills, muscle endurance to be able to jog without lower body fatigue, and a normal body composition for effective body movement.

Both the Centers for Disease Control and Prevention (CDC) and the ACSM recommend that adults engage in moderate-intensity physical activities for at least 30 minutes on most days of the week or vigorous-intensity exercise for at least 20 minutes three times a week (or some combination of the two).[7] This amount of physical activity can improve your overall health and can result in some cardiovascular improvements. If you want to improve your cardiorespiratory fitness even more, the ACSM and CDC recommend you perform vigorous physical activities (e.g., jogging or running, circuit weight training, singles tennis) at least 3 days per week for at least 20 minutes at a time; if losing weight is your goal, you need to add 60 to 90 minutes of moderate to vigorous exercise to your daily routine.

Some people have physical limitations that make achieving these recommendations difficult, but they can still be physically active and reap the benefits of a regular exercise program. For example, a woman with arthritis in the knee and hip joints might not be able to jog without extreme pain, but she can engage in water exercise in a swimming pool. The water will help relieve much of the stress on her joints, and she can improve her range of motion. Similarly, a man who uses a wheelchair may be unable to walk or run, but he can stay physically fit by playing wheelchair basketball.

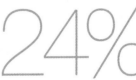 **of American women report getting recommended amounts of vigorous physical activity, compared with 33% of American men.**

Physical Activity for Performance

People who want to take their fitness level one step further can add exercise to improve performance. Programs can be designed to increase speed, strength, endurance, or specific muscle strength. Examples include plyometrics to improve control and speed in changing directions, and interval training to improve power and cardiovascular fitness.

Performance training is meant for people who already have a high level of physical fitness and are training to enhance some aspect of their ability. Those who engage in this level of activity will achieve a high level of fitness but are also more prone to risk of injury and overtraining.

what do you think?

Which of the three categories of physical activity best describes your motivation for being physically active: health, fitness, or performance? ● What physical activities could you do to improve your health, fitness, or performance?

Benefits of Regular Physical Activity

Regular physical activity has been shown to improve more than 50 different physiological, metabolic, and psychological aspects of human life. Figure 11.2 summarizes some of the major health-related benefits of regular physical activity and exercise.

Improved Cardiorespiratory Fitness

Exercise is good for the heart and lungs. It can reduce the risk for heart-related diseases, and it can improve blood flow and make performing everyday tasks much easier. Something as mundane as carrying a bag of groceries up a flight of stairs can leave someone with poor cardiorespiratory fitness winded and fatigued, while someone who's in better shape could make several trips without breaking a sweat.

Cardiorespiratory fitness is the ability to perform exercise using large-muscle groups at moderate to high intensity for prolonged periods.[8] Because it requires the cardiovascular and respiratory systems to supply oxygen to the body during sustained physical activity, it is a good indicator of overall health. Low levels of cardiorespiratory fitness are associated with increased risk of premature death and disease.[9]

Regular exercise makes the circulatory and respiratory systems more efficient by enlarging the heart muscle, enabling more blood to be pumped with each stroke and increasing the number of *capillaries* (small blood vessels that allow gas exchange between blood and surrounding tissues) in trained skeletal muscles, which supply more blood to working muscles. Exercise also improves the respiratory system by increasing the amount of oxygen that is inhaled and distributed to body tissues.[10]

cardiorespiratory fitness The ability of the heart, lungs, and blood vessels to supply oxygen to skeletal muscles during sustained physical activity.

Reduced Risk of Heart Disease Exercise significantly lowers the risk of coronary heart disease.[11] Your heart is a muscular organ made up of highly specialized tissue. Because muscles become stronger and more efficient with use, regular exercise strengthens the heart, which enables it

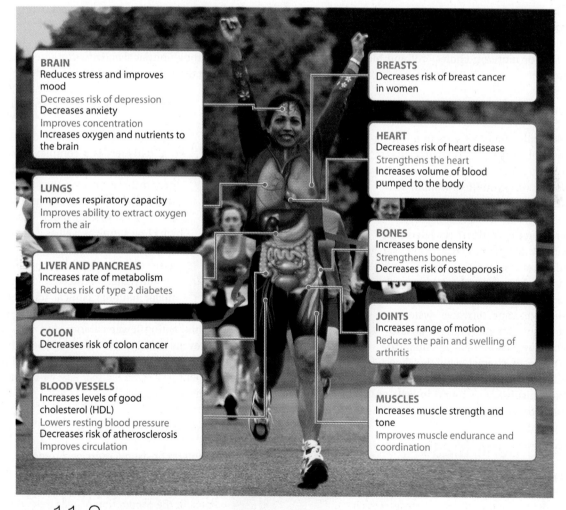

BRAIN
Reduces stress and improves mood
Decreases risk of depression
Decreases anxiety
Improves concentration
Increases oxygen and nutrients to the brain

LUNGS
Improves respiratory capacity
Improves ability to extract oxygen from the air

LIVER AND PANCREAS
Increases rate of metabolism
Reduces risk of type 2 diabetes

COLON
Decreases risk of colon cancer

BLOOD VESSELS
Increases levels of good cholesterol (HDL)
Lowers resting blood pressure
Decreases risk of atherosclerosis
Improves circulation

BREASTS
Decreases risk of breast cancer in women

HEART
Decreases risk of heart disease
Strengthens the heart
Increases volume of blood pumped to the body

BONES
Increases bone density
Strengthens bones
Decreases risk of osteoporosis

JOINTS
Increases range of motion
Reduces the pain and swelling of arthritis

MUSCLES
Increases muscle strength and tone
Improves muscle endurance and coordination

FIGURE 11.2 **Some Health Benefits of Regular Exercise**

to pump more blood with each beat. This increased efficiency means that the heart requires fewer beats per minute to circulate blood throughout the body. A stronger, more efficient heart is better able to meet the ordinary demands of life.

Prevention of Hypertension *Blood pressure* refers to the force exerted by blood against blood vessel walls, generated by the pumping action of the heart. *Hypertension*, the medical term for abnormally high blood pressure, is a significant risk factor for cardiovascular disease and stroke. People with consistently elevated blood pressure are more susceptible to heart disease and die at a younger age than people with normal blood pressure. Studies report that moderate exercise can reduce both diastolic and systolic blood pressure by 7 mm Hg.[12]

Improved Blood Lipid and Lipoprotein Profile Regular exercise is known to increase the number of high-density lipoproteins (HDLs, or "good" cholesterol) and decrease the number of low-density lipoproteins (LDLs, or "bad" cholesterol) in the blood.[13] Higher HDL levels are associated with lower risk for artery disease, because they remove some of the "bad" cholesterol from artery walls and hence reduce clogging. Similarly, high levels of LDLs are associated with higher risk for artery disease, because they carry cholesterol in the blood and deposit it along blood vessel walls. For more on cholesterol and blood pressure, see Chapter 12.

Reduced Cancer Risk

Regular physical activity appears to lower the risk for some types of cancer, particularly breast cancer. Research on exercise and breast cancer risk has found that the earlier in life a woman starts to exercise, the lower her breast cancer risk will be.[14]

Regular exercise is also associated with lower risk for colon cancer. One theory is that exercise decreases intestinal transit time. Experts say that because physical activity makes food move more quickly through your digestive system, there is less time for the body to absorb potential carcinogens and for potential carcinogens to be in contact with the digestive tract. Physical activity also decreases the levels of prostaglandins, substances found in cells of the large intestine that are implicated in cancer.[15]

Improved Bone Mass

A common affliction among older adults is *osteoporosis*, a disease characterized by low bone mass and deterioration of bone tissue, which increase fracture risk. Bone, like other human tissues, responds to the demands placed upon it. Women (and men) have much to gain by remaining physically active as they age—bone mass levels are significantly higher among active than among sedentary women.[16] Regular weight-bearing exercise, when combined with a balanced diet containing adequate calcium, helps keep bones healthy.

Improved Weight Control

Many people start exercising because they want to lose weight. Level of physical activity has a direct effect on metabolic rate and can raise it for several hours following a vigorous workout. This increase in metabolic rate can reduce body fat and increase lean muscle mass. An effective method for losing weight combines regular endurance-type exercises with a moderate decrease in food intake. In addition to helping you lose weight, increased physical activity also improves your chances of keeping the weight off.[17]

For healthy weight loss, the ACSM recommends 30 minutes of moderate physical activity daily with an intake of between 1,500 and 2,000 calories per day.[18] Although exercise and dietary changes work best for weight loss, research shows that exercise alone can reduce obesity. For example, in a study of obese men, those who exercised at a moderate intensity for 60 minutes five times a week with no dietary changes significantly decreased their body fat and increased muscle mass.[19] However, remember that if you want to lose weight only through physical activity, you must spend more time exercising than if you also reduce your caloric intake.

If you want to lose weight, you have to work it off!

Prevention of Diabetes

Noninsulin-dependent diabetes (type 2 diabetes) is a complex disorder that affects millions of Americans, many of whom have no idea that they have the disease. Risk factors for this type of diabetes include obesity, high blood pressure, and high cholesterol, as well as a family history of the disease.[20] Physicians suggest exercise combined with weight loss and healthy diet to prevent diabetes. In a major national clinical trial, researchers found that exercising 150 minutes per week while eating fewer calories and less fat could prevent or delay the onset of type 2 diabetes.[21] For more on diabetes prevention and management, see **Focus On: Your Risk for Diabetes** beginning on page 386.

Improved Immunity

Regular, consistent exercise promotes a healthy immune system. Research shows that moderate exercise gives the immune system a temporary boost in the production of cells that attack bacteria.[22] But whereas moderate amounts of exercise can be beneficial, extreme exercise may actually be detrimental. For example, athletes engaging in marathon-type events or very intense physical training have an increased risk of colds and flu.[23]

Just how exercise alters immunity is not well understood. We do know that brisk exercise temporarily increases the number of white blood cells (WBCs), which are responsible for fighting infection.[24] The largest changes in immunity are seen in people who are sedentary and begin a moderately energetic program. Because their fitness level is low when they embark on an exercise program, they gain a large number of WBCs.

Improved Mental Health and Stress Management

People who engage in regular physical activity also notice psychological benefits. Regular vigorous exercise has been shown to "burn off" the chemical by-products of the stress response and increase endorphins, giving your mood a natural boost. Regular exercise improves a person's physical appearance by toning and developing muscles and reducing body fat. Feeling good about personal appearance boosts self-esteem. At the same time, as exercisers come to appreciate the improved strength, skills, and flexibility that accompany fitness, they often become less obsessed with physical appearance.[25]

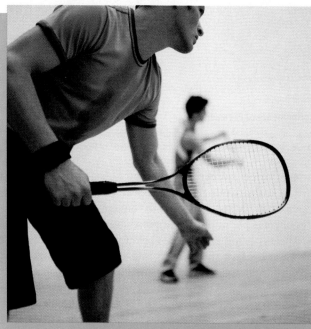

Can exercise really reduce stress?

You bet it can! Improving your overall level of fitness may be the most helpful thing you can do to combat stress. Exercise actually stimulates the stress response, but a well-exercised body adapts to the *eustress* of exercise, and as a result is able to tolerate greater levels of *distress* of all kinds. Of course, some activities involving competition or physical risk may add to your overall stress load. The trick is to balance exercise, fun, and recreational activities in your free time so that you can stay fit and reduce chronic stress.

Longer Life Span

Several large studies that followed groups of people over time found that those who exercised or were more fit lived longer. In a study of over 5,000 middle-aged and older Americans, researchers found that those who had moderate to high levels of activity lived 1.3 to 3.7 years longer than those who got little exercise. Study subjects who exercised at a more intense level outlived sedentary subjects by 3.5 to 3.7 years.[26]

Cardiorespiratory Fitness

There are many options for improving cardiorespiratory fitness. Swimming, cycling, jogging, and in-line skating are just a few options for **aerobic exercise.** The term *aerobic* means "with oxygen" and describes any type of exercise, typically performed at moderate levels of intensity for extended periods of time, that increases your heart rate. A person said to be in good shape has an above-average **aerobic capacity**—a term used to describe the functional status of the cardiorespiratory system (heart, lungs, and blood vessels). Aerobic capacity (commonly written as $\dot{V}O_{2max}$) is defined as the maximum volume of oxygen consumed by the muscles during exercise.

There are three main dimensions to an aerobic exercise program: frequency, intensity, and duration. The characteristics of these dimensions vary by individual exercise goal and beginning fitness level. These same dimensions also apply to the other components of fitness: muscular strength, muscular endurance, and flexibility. You can remember them with the acronym FITT, which stands for *frequency, intensity, time (duration),* and *type* of activity. **Figure 11.3** on the next page shows how the FITT principle can be applied to the different fitness components.

aerobic exercise Any type of exercise that increases heart rate.
aerobic capacity The current functional status of a person's cardiovascular system; measured as $\dot{V}O_{2max}$.
target heart rate Percentage of maximum heart rate; heart rate is taken during aerobic exercise to check whether exercise intensity is at the desired level.

Determining Exercise Frequency

To best improve your cardiovascular endurance, you will need to exercise vigorously at least three times a week. If you are a newcomer to exercise, you can still make improvements by doing less intense exercise but doing it more days a week, following the recommendations from the CDC and the ACSM for moderate physical activity at least 5 days a week.

Determining Exercise Intensity

There are several ways to measure exercise intensity. One of the main ways is using your **target heart rate** zone. To calculate target heart rate zone, start by subtracting your age from 220 to find your maximum heart rate. Your target heart rate zone is a certain range of this maximum heart rate. For moderate-intensity physical activity, you should work out at 50 to

	Cardiorespiratory endurance	Strength	Flexibility
Frequency	3–5 days a week	2–3 nonconsecutive days a week	Minimum of 2–3 days a week
Intensity	55/65–90% of maximum heart rate	70–85% of maximal resistance. Sufficient resistance to enhance strength and endurance	Sufficient to develop and maintain full range of motion
Time	20–60 minutes continuous aerobic activity	1 or more sets (8–12 repetitions) of 8–10 exercises conditioning all the major muscle groups	2–4 repetitions of each stretch held for 15–30 seconds
Type	Continuous aerobic activity that uses large-muscle groups	Resistance exercises in a full range of motion for all major muscle groups	Stretching for all major joints and muscle groups

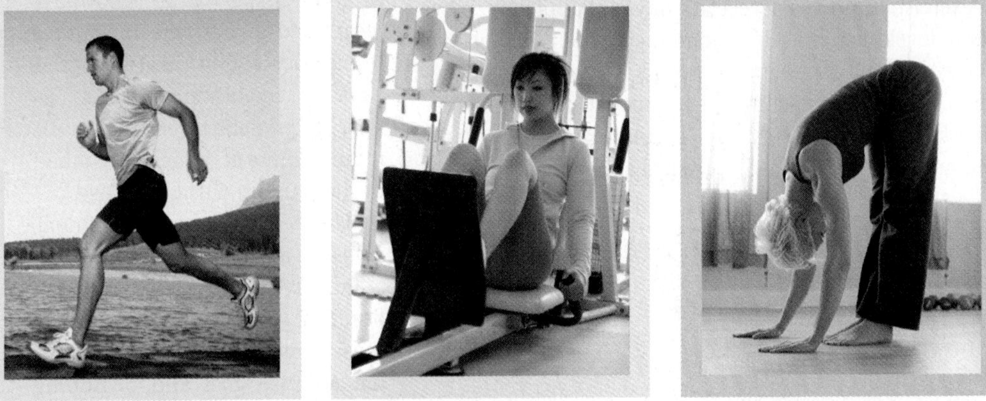

FIGURE 11.3 **The FITT Principle Applied to the Health-Related Components of Fitness**

Source: Adapted from "Position Stand on the Recommended Quantity and Quality of Exercise for Developing and Maintaining Cardiorespiratory and Muscular Fitness and Flexibility in Adults," *Medicine and Science in Sports and Exercise* 30 (1998): 975–91. Copyright © 1998 American College of Sports Medicine.

70 percent of your maximum heart rate. Thus, if you are 20 years old, your 50 percent target heart rate zone would be

$$(220 - 20) \times 0.50, \text{ or } 100 \text{ beats per minute (bpm)}$$

To determine 70 percent of a 20-year-old's maximum heart rate, you would use the following calculations:

$$(220 - 20) \times 0.70, \text{ or } 140 \text{ bpm}$$

Thus, for a moderately intense cardiovascular workout, a 20-year-old would try to maintain aerobic exercise at an intensity of 100 to 140 beats per minute, or 50 to 70 percent of his or her maximum heart rate. For more vigorous activities (e.g., running), aim for 70 to 85 percent of your maximum heart rate. People in poor physical condition should set a target heart rate between 40 and 50 percent of maximum and gradually increase the target rate in 5 percent increments.

Once you know your target heart rate zone, you can take your pulse to determine how close you are to this value during your workout. As you exercise, lightly place your index and middle fingers (don't use your thumb) on your radial artery (inside your wrist, on the thumb side). Using a watch or clock, take your pulse for 6 seconds, and multiply this number by 10 (just add a zero to your count) to get the number of beats per minute. Your pulse should be within a range of 5 beats per minute above or below your target heart rate. If necessary, adjust the pace or intensity of your workout to achieve your target heart rate.

Another way of determining intensity is to use the Borg rating of perceived exertion (RPE) scale (Figure 11.4). Perceived exertion is how hard you feel you are working, based on your heart rate, increased breathing rate, sweating, and muscle fatigue. This scale uses a rating from 6 (no exertion at all) to 20 (maximal exertion). This method corresponds to heart rate for most people, that is, if a person's RPE is 12, then the person's heart rate will be approximately 120 beats per minute. (This is just an estimation of heart rate, as the actual rate can vary depending on age and physical condition.) Experts agree that RPE ratings of 12 to 14 correspond to moderate-intensity activity and ratings of 15 to 17 to vigorous activity.

6	No exertion at all
7	Extremely light
8	
9	Very light
10	
11	Light
12	
13	Somewhat hard
14	
15	Hard (heavy)
16	
17	Very hard
18	
19	Extremely hard
20	Maximal exertion

Target heart rate for most people — 13, 14, 15, 16

FIGURE 11.4 Borg's Rating of Perceived Exertion (RPE) Scale

Source: Borg-RPE-scale ® from G. Borg, *Borg's Perceived Exertion and Pain Scales* (Champaign, IL: Human Kinetics, 1998). © Gunnar Borg, 1970, 1985, 1994, 1998. Used with permission of Dr. G. Borg.

The easiest, but least scientific, method of measuring exercise intensity is the "talk test." If you are exercising moderately, you should be able to carry on a conversation comfortably. If you are too out of breath to carry on a conversation, you are exercising vigorously.

Determining Exercise Duration

Duration refers to the number of minutes of activity performed during any one session. To achieve health benefits, the ACSM recommends that vigorous activities be performed for at least 20 minutes at a time, and moderate activities for at least 30 minutes at a time.[27]

The lower the intensity of your activity, the longer the duration you'll need to get the same caloric expenditure. See **Figure 11.5** for approximations of the number of calories burned during different activities. The numbers of calories burned is higher for a person who weighs more than for someone who weighs less.[28] Aim to expend 300 to 500 calories per exercise session, with an eventual weekly goal of 1,500 to 2,000 calories. As you progress, add to your exercise load by increasing duration or intensity, but not both at the same time. From week to week, don't increase duration or intensity by more than 10 percent.

Muscular Strength and Endurance

To get a sense of what resistance training is about, do a resistance exercise. Start by holding your right arm straight down by your side, then turn your hand palm up and bring it up toward your shoulder. That's a resistance exercise: using a muscle, your biceps, to move a resistance, in this case just the weight of your hand—not very much resistance. Resistance training usually involves more weight or tension than this. Free weights, such as dumbbells and barbells, and all sorts of tension-producing machines are usually part of resistance training. It's not just bodybuilding that uses this type of exercise, either: Fitness programs and many sports employ resistance training to improve strength and endurance. Also, resistance exercises are an integral part of rehabilitation programs to help patients recover from muscle and joint injury.

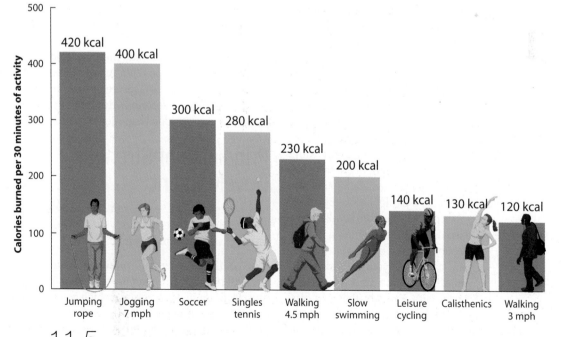

FIGURE 11.5 Calories Burned by Different Activities
The harder you exercise, the more energy you expend. Estimated calories burned for various moderate and vigorous activities are listed for a 30-minute bout of activity.

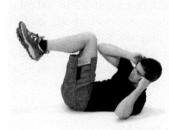

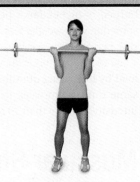

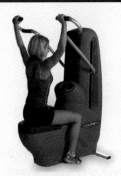

Body Weight Resistance (Calisthenics)	Fixed Resistance	Variable Resistance	Accommodating Resistance
• Using your own body weight to help develop skeletal muscle strength • Can improve general muscle fitness and muscle tone and help maintain muscle strength	• Provides a constant amount of resistance throughout the full range of movement • Requires balance and coordination and may promote development of more joint and stabilizer muscles	• Resistance is altered so that the muscle's effort is more consistent throughout the movement • Provides more controlled motion and isolates certain muscle groups	• Sometimes called isokinetic machines • Maintain a constant speed through the range of motion • Often used for rehabilitation after injury
Examples: Push-ups, pull-ups, sit-ups	**Examples:** Free weights such as barbells, dumbbells, and some machines	**Examples:** Specific machines in gyms, some home models available, such as Nautilus or Bowflex machines	**Examples:** Specific machines in rehab facilities and gyms

Many college students are incorporating strengthening exercises into their physical fitness program. In a 2008 survey, 44 percent of college-aged men and 28 percent of women reported doing exercises to strengthen or tone muscles at least twice a week.[29] See the **Gender & Health** box at right for information about gender differences in weight training. **Table 11.1** presents information about the four most commonly used resistance exercise methods: body weight resistance and fixed, variable, and accommodating resistance devices.

In the field of resistance training, **muscular strength** refers to the amount of force a muscle or group of muscles is capable of exerting. The most common way to assess strength in a resistance exercise program is to measure the **one repetition maximum (1 RM)**, which is the maximum amount of weight a person can move one time (and no more) in a particular exercise. For example, 1 RM for the simple exercise done at the beginning of this section is the maximum weight you can lift to your shoulder one time. To calculate your maximum, begin with a weight that you can lift easily. Rest for 2 to 3 minutes between lifts, and then add 5 to 10 pounds of weight until you can no longer complete a successful lift. This muscle strength assessment is a good way to help create an effective weight-training program and monitor progress.

muscular strength The amount of force that a muscle is capable of exerting.

one repetition maximum (1 RM) The amount of weight or resistance that can be lifted or moved only once.

muscular endurance A muscle's ability to exert force repeatedly without fatiguing.

Muscular endurance is the ability of muscle to exert force repeatedly without fatiguing. If you can perform the exercise described earlier holding a 5-pound weight in your hand and lifting 10 times, you will have greater endurance than someone who attempts that same exercise but is able to lift the weight only seven times. There are two categories of muscle endurance. The first is static muscular endurance, or a force that is held as long as possible. An example of static abdominal endurance would be a measure of how long you can hold a double leg lift. The second is dynamic muscular endurance, or maximum repetitions completed at a determined rate.

Principles of Strength Development

According to the ACSM, an effective resistance exercise program involves these key principles: overload, specificity of training, variation, and reversibility.[30]

Overload The overload principle is the foundation of strength training. *Overload* doesn't mean forcing a muscle or muscle group to do too much, which could result in injuries; rather, it's requiring muscles to do more than they are used to doing. Everyone begins a resistance-training exercise program with an initial level of strength. To become stronger, you must regularly create a greater degree of tension in your muscles than you are accustomed to. Tension is created by

Gender Differences in Exercise

Exercise is good for everyone's health, but research shows that there are differences in the ways men and women choose, participate in, and react to exercise. Overall, men have higher rates of physical activity than women in all age groups. A national survey found that 73 percent of high school–aged boys report regular physical activity, compared with 60 percent of girls. Also, almost 50 percent of girls reported *not* playing on a sports team, compared with 38 percent of boys. Gender differences in participation are also reported in college-aged men and women. According to the American College Health Association (ACHA) National College Health Assessment, fewer women than men report participating in regular exercise 3 or more days per week.

Why such differences? There are several reasons, including socialization, physiology, and access. In the past, women were not encouraged to exercise because it was thought that physical exertion would cause damage to their bodies, especially their reproductive organs. Women were also thought to be physiologically incapable of feats such as weight lifting or endurance running.

Even though it is now known that exercise is beneficial—not detrimental—to the health of women, there are several physiological differences between men and women that account for performance differences, if not participation ones. First, aerobic capacity differs. While there are many women with a significantly higher $\dot{V}O_{2max}$ level than many men, on average, there is a 43 percent difference between the $\dot{V}O_{2max}$ level in a young, untrained man and a young, untrained woman. Part of this difference is explained by the fact that in general, men have larger hearts, which relates to more capacity. Also, men may have higher levels of blood hemoglobin, which affects the oxygen-carrying ability of the blood. Exercise performance can also be affected by percentage of body fat. Overall, women have an average body fat percentage of 25 percent, with men averaging 15 percent.

Muscle strength also can differ between men and women. While studies show that there is no difference in "muscle quality"—a muscle cell in a man is the same as a muscle cell in a woman—there are strength and power differences, which are a function of muscle *quantity.* Flexibility is another area in which men and women differ, with women having greater hip and elbow flexibility.

The results of resistance training in men and women are quite different. Women do not develop muscle to the extent that men do because of differences in testosterone levels in their blood. Before puberty, testosterone levels are similar for both boys and girls. During adolescence, testosterone levels in boys increase dramatically (about tenfold), while testosterone levels in girls remain unchanged. Any individual's muscles will become larger (hypertrophy) as a result of resistance-training exercise, but typically this change is less dramatic in women because of their lower testosterone levels.

Resistance training is beneficial to everyone's health.

Sources: Centers for Disease Control and Prevention, "Behavioral Risk Factor Surveillance System Prevalence Data." Physical Activity, 2007. http://apps.nccd.cdc.gov/BRFSS; American College Health Association, *American College Health Association—National College Health Assessment II (ACHA-NCHA) Reference Group Data Report Fall 2008* (Baltimore: American College Health Association, 2009); S. Seiler, J. J. De Koning, and C. Foster, "The Fall and Rise of the Gender Difference in Elite Anaerobic Performance 1952–2006," *Medicine and Science in Sports and Exercise* 39, no. 3 (2007): 534–40; M. Tarnopolsky, "Sex Differences in Exercise Metabolism and the Role of 17-Beta Estradiol," *Medicine and Science in Sports and Exercise* 40, no. 4 (2008): 648–54.

resistance; progressively overloading your muscles will cause them to adapt to a new level, thus becoming stronger.

Resistance-training exercises cause microscopic damage (tears) to muscle fibers, and the rebuilding process that increases the size and capacity of the muscle takes 24 to 48 hours. Thus, resistance-training exercise programs should include at least 1 day of rest and recovery between workouts before you overload the same muscles again.

Specificity of Training According to the specificity-of-training principle, the effects of resistance exercise training are specific to the muscles being exercised. Only the muscle or muscle group that you exercise responds to the demands placed on it. For example, if you regularly do curls, the muscles involved—your biceps—will become larger and stronger, but the other muscles in your body won't change. It is important to note that if you exercise only certain muscle groups, you may put opposing muscle groups at increased risk for injury. For example, overworking your quadriceps muscles but neglecting your hamstrings can put you at risk for a hamstring muscle pull or strain.

Variation Variation is a fundamental principle in strength training. This principle supports the need for changes in one or more parts of your workout routine over time to allow for the training effects to remain at an optimal level. It has been shown that varying duration and intensity is most effective for long-term results.

Reversibility Another important principle is reversibility. Reversibility means that if you stop putting demands on your body, the body responds by deconditioning. Even after only 4 days without training, muscles begin to revert back to their untrained state. The saying "use it or lose it" is applicable when it comes to strength (or cardiorespiratory) training.

Strength-Training Elements

There are several elements you should consider when developing a strength-training routine, including the following:

- **Exercise selection.** Exercises that work a single joint (e.g., chest presses) are effective for building muscle strength, but multiple-joint exercises (e.g., a squat coupled with an overhead press) are some of the most effective for increasing overall muscle strength. The ACSM recommends that both exercise types be included in a strength-training program, with an emphasis on multiple-joint exercises for maximizing muscle strength.[31]
- **Exercise order.** The sequence of exercises can affect your results. When training all major muscle groups in a workout, complete large-muscle exercises before small-muscle-group exercises, multiple-joint exercises before single-joint exercises, and high-intensity exercises before lower-intensity exercises.
- **Sets and repetitions.** One element that is very important in strength training is how much weight to lift and how many times to lift it to achieve your fitness goals. The SAID principle refers to "**s**pecific **a**daptation to **i**mposed **d**emand." More simply put, the types of demands that you put on your body will result in the kind of adaptation that will follow. For example, if your strength-training goal is to become stronger and increase muscle size, a program with three to six sets of four to eight repetitions at approximately 85 percent of your 1 RM would be effective. If your goal is to tone your muscles without a major increase in muscle size, a program that includes 8 to 12 repetitions would be sufficient. When you can comfortably and correctly complete 12 repetitions, increase the weight load by 10 percent.[32]
- **Rest periods.** The amount of rest between exercises is key to an effective strength-training workout. Resting in between exercises can reduce fatigue and help maintain performance and safety in subsequent sets. A rest period of 2 to 3 minutes is recommended for multiple-joint exercises that use large-muscle groups (squats with overhead presses) and a rest period of 1 to 2 minutes for single-joint exercises or for strength exercises using machines.
- **Exercise frequency.** Performing eight to ten exercises that train the major muscle groups 2 to 3 days a week is recommended.

Increased awareness of the benefits of strength training and muscle development have led to a proliferation of "performance-enhancing" drugs and supplements. In recent years, the use of such drugs has become a major problem on college campuses and among athletes (see the **Health Headlines** box at right).

Core Strength Training

The body's core muscles are the foundation for movement.[33] These muscles are the deep back and abdominal muscles that attach to the spine and pelvis. The contraction of these muscles provides the basis of support for movements of the upper and lower body and powerful movements of the extremities. A weak core increases your chances for poor posture, lower back pain, and muscle injuries. A strong core gives you a more stable center of gravity and a more stable platform for movements, thus reducing the chance of injury.

You can develop core strength by simple calisthenics, using fitness equipment such as a fitness ball, or taking an exercise class such as yoga or Pilates. Holding yourself in a plank, or "up" push-up position and doing abdominal curl-ups are two examples of calisthenic exercises to increase core strength. Experts recommend doing core strengthening activities at least three times per week.[34]

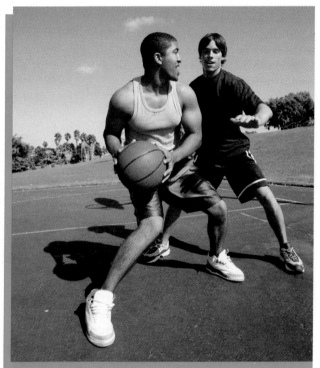

Why is core strength training important?

Your core muscles are essential for supporting your spine in everything you do—from standing to sitting, from dancing to playing basketball. Core muscles work together to effectively transmit forces between your upper and lower body, allowing you to twist, jump, lift, bend, and change directions. While weak core muscles can lead to back pain, strong core muscles can lead to increased performance levels in all of your activities.

PERFORMANCE-ENHANCING DRUGS: THE MAGIC BULLET?

It seems as if every year, newspaper headlines declare that certain elite athletes are being reprimanded for using performance-enhancing drugs. But it is not just professional athletes who turn to performance-enhancing drugs to "step up their game." For some athletes, both amateur and professional alike, gaining the competitive edge by taking performance-enhancing drugs seems like just another training strategy. What these athletes don't realize is that these drugs affect more than performance. Becoming faster or stronger may be a short-term benefit but there are side effects and health risks to taking these drugs. Legal risks also stem from the fact that many of these drugs are illegal without medical prescriptions. Listed below are some of the major types of drugs used for performance enhancement.

ANABOLIC STEROIDS

Athletes take anabolic steroids to increase their muscle mass and strength. The presence of the hormone testosterone—the main anabolic steroid—in the body has two main effects: anabolic effects that promote muscle building, and androgenic effects that promote male traits such as facial hair and a deep voice. Synthetic versions of this hormone do have some medicinal purposes in treating AIDS and rare types of anemia, but athletes often use doses much higher than are medically prescribed. Men who use this steroid can develop prominent breasts, baldness, shrunken testicles, a higher voice, and infertility. Side effects for women include a deeper voice, increased body hair, baldness, and increased appetite. Both sexes can suffer from severe acne, liver abnormalities and tumors, high LDL cholesterol and low HDL cholesterol, aggressive behavior, and drug dependence.

Androstenedione is a hormone produced by the adrenal glands, ovaries, and testes and converted by the body into testosterone in men and estradiol in women. The synthetic version is marketed to increase the body's production of testosterone. The claims have been refuted by scientific studies, and androstenedione is now listed as a controlled substance whose use is banned by most sports associations. Side effects from this drug are similar to those of anabolic steroids.

CREATINE

Creatine monohydrate is a compound produced by the body that helps release energy in muscles. It is marketed as a nutritional supplement and is readily available at many retail stores. Some research shows that creatine can produce small gains in short-term bursts of power. Research does not support any benefits to aerobic or endurance activities. Some side effects of creatine include stomach cramps, muscle cramps, nausea, vomiting, diarrhea, and risk of dehydration. High doses may increase risk of damage to the kidneys, liver, and heart.

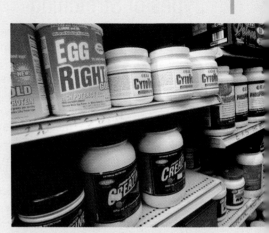

More performance-enhancing supplements hit the shelves all the time, but are they more likely to hurt you than to help?

STIMULANTS

Stimulants are drugs that affect the central nervous system by increasing heart rate, blood pressure, and metabolism. These drugs can reduce fatigue, suppress appetite, and increase alertness. The illegal drugs cocaine and methamphetamine are both stimulants, as are some drugs sold in pharmacies, such as pseudoephedrine, which is found in many cold and allergy remedies. Caffeine, the active ingredient in coffee, tea, and many soft drinks, is also a stimulant. Athletes have been known to use caffeine to decrease fatigue and increase aggressiveness. Side effects of such use of caffeine and over-the-counter stimulants include nervousness and irritability, insomnia, and psychological dependence.

Sources: Mayo Clinic Staff, "Performance-Enhancing Drugs: Are They a Risk to Your Health?," Mayo Clinic, December 23, 2008, http://mayoclinic.com/health/performance-drugs-enhancing/hq01105; A. A. Walter et al., "Effects of Creatine Loading on Electromyographic Fatigue Threshold in Cycle Ergometry in College-Age Men," *International Journal of Sport Nutrition and Exercise Metabolism* 18, no. 2 (2008): 142–51.

Flexibility

Improved **flexibility**—a measure of the range of motion, or the amount of movement possible, at a particular joint—can give you a sense of well-being, help you deal with stress better, and stop your joints from hurting as much as they used to. Stretching exercises are the main way to improve flexibility. Today, stretching exercises are extremely popular, both because they are effective and because people can begin them at virtually any age and enjoy them for a lifetime. Flexibility exercises are effective in reducing the incidence and severity of lower back problems and muscle or tendon injuries that can occur during sports and everyday physical activities.[35] Improved flexibility also means less tension and pressure on joints, resulting in less joint pain and joint deterioration.[36]

flexibility The measure of the range of motion, or the amount of movement possible, at a particular joint.

Types of Stretching

Static stretching techniques involve the slow, gradual stretching of muscles and their tendons, then holding them at a point. During this holding period—the stretch— participants may feel mild discomfort and a warm sensation in the stretched muscles. Static stretching exercises involve specialized tension receptors in our muscles. When done properly, these exercises slightly lessen the sensitivity of tension receptors, which allows the muscle to relax and be stretched to greater length.[37] The stretch is followed by a slow return to the starting position and a rest period of 15 to 30 seconds before stretching again.

To improve flexibility, it is recommended that you stretch major muscles and joints at least 2 or 3 days a week, but daily stretching is optimal. A stretching routine completed after cardiovascular activity is a good strategy to improve flexibility because muscles and joints are already warmed by prior activity, therefore giving a much more efficient stretch.

Three major styles of exercise that include stretching have become widely practiced in the United States and other Western countries: yoga, tai chi, and Pilates. All three emphasize a joining of mind and body as a result of intense concentration on breathing and body position. As mentioned earlier in the section on strength training, these styles are also an excellent way to improve core body strength.

Yoga One of the most popular fitness and static stretching activities, **yoga** originated in India about 5,000 years ago. Yoga blends the mental and physical aspects of exercise, a union of mind and body that participants find relaxing and satisfying. Done regularly, its combination of mental focus and physical effort improves flexibility, vitality, posture, agility, and coordination.

The practice of yoga focuses attention on controlled breathing as well as purely physical exercise. In addition to its mental dimensions, yoga incorporates a complex array of static stretching exercises expressed as postures (*asanas*). During a session, participants move to different asanas and hold them for 30 seconds or more.

Some forms of yoga are more meditative in their practice (see Chapter 3 for a discussion of a few of these forms), while other forms, such as Ashtanga and Bikram, are more athletic.

Ashtanga yoga, also called "power yoga," is an energetic yoga that focuses on a series of poses done in a continuous, repeated flow, with controlled breath. *Bikram yoga*, also known as *hot yoga*, is unique in that classes are held in rooms that are heated to 105°F. While many people extol the virtues of Bikram yoga, there have been reports of heat exhaustion, dehydration, and other problems. This style of yoga is risky for people with hypertension, certain respiratory conditions, and other cardiovascular risks or for people who don't tolerate heat very well.

Tai chi **Tai chi** is an ancient Chinese form of exercise that, like yoga, combines stretching, balance, coordination, and meditation. It is designed to increase range of motion and flexibility while reducing muscular tension. It involves a series of positions called *forms* that are performed continuously. Both yoga and tai chi are excellent for improving flexibility and muscular coordination.

Pilates **Pilates** combines stretching with movement against resistance, which is aided by devices such as tension springs or heavy rubber bands. Pilates differs from yoga and tai chi because it includes a component specifically designed to increase strength. Pilates exercises are carried out on specially designed equipment, whereas others are performed on mats. Each exercise stretches and strengthens the muscles involved and has a specific breathing pattern associated with it.

Body Composition

Body composition is the fifth and final component of a comprehensive fitness program. It describes the relative proportions of lean tissue (muscle, bone, water, organs) and fat tissue in the body. Body composition parameters that can be influenced by regular physical activity include total body mass, fat mass, fat-free mass, and regional fat distribution. Aerobic activities that improve cardiovascular endurance also help improve body composition, because they expend calories and contribute to and help maintain weight loss. There are many ways to assess body composition. These range from simple (e.g., height–weight charts) to complex (e.g., underwater weighing). See the section on assessing fat levels in Chapter 10.

Creating Your Own Fitness Program

Now that you know the benefits of improved physical fitness and the components that make up a physical fitness program, you can begin your own plan to become more physically fit.

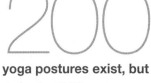

200 yoga postures exist, but only about 50 are commonly practiced.

static stretching Techniques that gradually lengthen a muscle to an elongated position (to the point of discomfort) and hold that position for 10 to 30 seconds.

yoga A variety of Indian traditions geared toward self-discipline and the realization of unity; includes forms that promote balance, coordination, flexibility, and meditation through postures and breathing exercises.

tai chi An ancient Chinese form of exercise, originally developed as a martial art, that promotes balance, coordination, flexibility, and stress reduction through a series of flowing postures and movements.

Pilates Exercise program developed by Joseph Pilates that combines stretching with movement against resistance.

body composition The relative proportions of lean tissue (muscle, bone, water, organs) and fat tissue in the body.

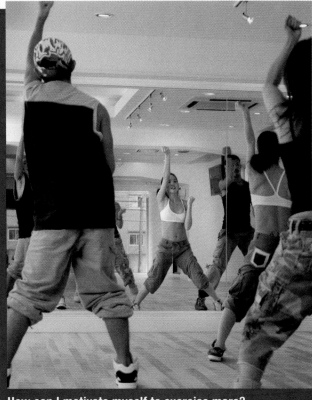

How can I motivate myself to exercise more?

One great way to motivate yourself is to sign up for a class. Find something that interests you—be it dance, yoga, aerobics, martial arts, or acrobatics—and get yourself involved. The structure, regular schedule, social interaction, and challenge of learning a new skill can all be terrific motivators that make exercising exciting and fun.

Overcoming Common Obstacles to Exercise

The first step in forming a fitness program is identifying any hurdles that may keep you from getting started. There are many reasons why people do not exercise, ranging from personal ("I don't have time") to environmental ("I don't have a safe place to exercise"). People may also be reluctant to start exercising if they are overweight or out of shape.

What keeps you from being more active? Is it time? Do you lack a support group? Is the gym inconvenient, or do you lack money for a membership or equipment? Perhaps you're ready to begin but just can't get started. Once you've evaluated why you don't move more, look at Table 11.2 to determine how you can overcome your hurdles.

Identifying Your Fitness Goals

The next step in creating your fitness program is to identify your fitness goals. Do you want to improve your quality of life? Lose weight? Train for an upcoming 5K race? Think about a time line for your goals. Do you want to be able to jog 3 miles before spring break? Hike across campus next semester with a heavy backpack and not be out of breath? Once you develop a specific goal, you can create a plan to help you achieve that goal.

Designing Your Program

There are several factors to consider that will boost your chances of successfully achieving your fitness goal. First,

---

TABLE 11.2 Overcoming Obstacles to Physical Activity

Obstacles	Possible Solutions
Lack of time	• Take a good look at your schedule. Can you find three 30-minute time slots in your week?
	• Multitask. Read while riding an exercise bike or listen to lecture tapes while walking.
	• Exercise during your lunch breaks or between classes.
	• Select activities that require minimal time, such as brisk walking or jogging.
Social influence	• Invite family and friends to exercise with you.
	• Join a class to meet new people who share your exercise interests.
	• Explain the importance of exercise to people who may not support your efforts.
Lack of motivation, willpower, or energy	• Write your planned workout time in your schedule book.
	• Enlist the help of an exercise partner to make you accountable for working out.
	• Give yourself an incentive.
	• Schedule your workouts when you feel most energetic.
	• Remind yourself that exercise can give you more energy.
Lack of resources	• Select an activity that requires minimal equipment, such as walking, jogging, jumping rope, or calisthenics.
	• Identify inexpensive resources on campus or in the community.

Source: Adapted from National Center for Chronic Disease Prevention and Health Promotion, "How Can I Overcome Barriers to Physical Activity?" Updated 2008, www.cdc.gov/nccdphp/dnpa/physical/life/overcome.htm.

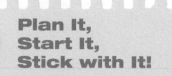
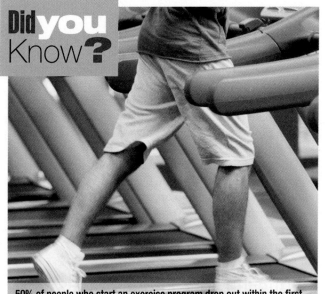

50% of people who start an exercise program drop out within the first 6 months. Pick an activity that you like doing, and you'll have a better chance of sticking to it!

Plan It, Start It, Stick with It!

The most successful exercise program is one that is realistic and appropriate for your skill level and needs.

✽ **Start slow.** For the sedentary, first-time exerciser, any type and amount of physical activity will be a step in the right direction. If you are extremely overweight or are out of condition, you might be able to walk for only 5 minutes at a time. Don't be discouraged; you're on your way!

✽ **Make only one life change at a time.** Success with one major behavioral change will encourage you to make other positive changes.

✽ **Set reasonable expectations** for yourself and your fitness program. Many people become exercise dropouts because their expectations were too high to begin with.

✽ **Choose a specific time to exercise and stick with it.** Learning to establish priorities and keeping to a schedule are vital steps toward improved fitness. Try exercising at different times of the day to learn what schedule works best for you.

✽ **Keep a record of your progress.** Include various facts about your physical activities (duration, intensity) and chronicle your emotions and personal achievements as you progress.

✽ **Take lapses in stride.** Physical deconditioning—a decline in fitness level—occurs at about the same rate as physical conditioning. Renew your commitment to fitness, and restart your exercise program.

choose an activity that is appropriate for you. For example, don't plan on swimming if the pool is difficult to access. Choose activities that you like to do. If you hate to run, don't choose running as your exercise. Be creative in your activity choice; try something new! There are many different classes (e.g., salsa aerobics, boot camp classes) that can keep you motivated—and if you don't like one activity, you can always try another. The **Consumer Health** box on the next page offers suggestions on evaluating and choosing a fitness center and fitness equipment you may want to incorporate into your plan. Table 11.3 on page 342 shows some popular fitness gadgets and equipment you may consider.

Your plan should include very specific ways to incorporate physical activity into your lifestyle. When will you exercise? For how long? At what intensity? How often? As you make specific goals for yourself, keep in mind the FITT principle and the recommendations in Figure 11.3 on page 332.

You may also find that writing out these goals and putting them in your daily planner, as you would any other activity, will help you keep to your schedule. Lack of time is the number one reason given for not exercising. Think about ways you can work more activity into the things you already do—for example, taking stairs rather than an elevator or walking or biking to run errands, rather than using the car. (See the **Green Guide** on page 344 for more on active transportation and how it can benefit the planet's health as well as your own.)

Reevaluate your fitness goal and action plan after 30 days. This time period should give you a good idea of whether or not the program is working for you. Make changes if necessary, and then make a plan to reevaluate after another 30-day period. The **Skills for Behavior Change** box at right offers more tips on starting and maintaining an exercise plan.

Fitness Program Components

Good fitness programs are designed to improve or maintain cardiorespiratory fitness, flexibility, muscular strength and endurance, and body composition. A comprehensive program could include a warm-up period of easy walking, followed by stretching activities to improve flexibility, then selected strength development exercises, followed by an aerobic activity for 20 minutes or more, and concluding with a cool-down period of gentle flexibility exercises.

Warming Up and Stretching Warming up and stretching prepare your body for exercise and provide a transition from rest to physical activity. A 5-minute warm-up may consist of a 5-minute brisk walk to ease your cardiovascular system into the more vigorous activity and to increase blood flow to the exercising muscles. This 5-minute warm-up can increase the temperature and elasticity of muscles and connective tissue,

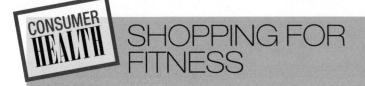

SHOPPING FOR FITNESS

If you have a treadmill that you use as a clothes rack or belong to a gym you haven't visited in months, you are not alone. Many people buy great equipment and don't get motivated to use it, but others buy services and equipment that don't have a ghost's chance of being useful. As with so many other products, consumers need to evaluate advertising claims carefully for fitness products and facilities.

Joining a fitness club can be a great motivator when you are starting a new exercise plan—just be sure that you find one that will work for you. Most college campuses include recreational facilities, so start your search for a workout center there. Visit the facilities, find out when they are open, and consider whether they are convenient for you and offer classes and equipment that interest you.

If you want to join a private health club, shop around at several facilities before making a decision. You should carefully consider the convenience of the clubs and how using them will fit into your schedule. Visit the clubs during the hours you'd be most likely to use them so you can see how crowded they are. Tour the club and observe classes. A good club should offer a complete workout; it should have a variety of aerobic exercising machines and a complete set of strength-training machines, free weights, mats for stretching, and aerobics classes. The club should also have plenty of well-trained and qualified staff. Take note of the staff during your visit to see if they seem friendly and helpful. Ask about the training of the personnel—including training in first aid and CPR—and inquire about the options for working with a personal trainer.

Finally, before you decide on a club, carefully weigh the financial implications. Find out what membership benefits entail and whether there are student rates or other discounts available to you. Steer clear of clubs that pressure you to make a long-term commitment or don't offer a trial membership or a grace period during which you can get your money refunded.

Even if you opt not to join a club, there are many useful exercise products available to help you take your exercise program to the next level—they can provide variety, allowing you to work out at home, or encourage you to monitor your progress. Fitness products are a multimillion-dollar industry, and some may make claims that sound too good to be true. Remember that no equipment is ever a quick fix—in order to see changes in your fitness and health, you must do the work yourself. General tips on evaluating fitness equipment include the following:

✳ Ignore claims that an exercise machine or device can provide lasting "no sweat" results in a short time.
✳ Question claims that a device can "target" or burn fat off a particular part of the body.
✳ Read the fine print. Advertised results may be based on more than just using a machine; they may also be based on caloric restriction.
✳ Be skeptical of testimonials and before-and-after pictures of "satisfied" customers.
✳ Calculate the cost and find out details about any shipping and handling fees, sales tax, delivery and setup charges, or long-term commitments.
✳ Get details on warranties, guarantees, and return policies.
✳ Try before you buy. You may be able to try out items at a gym or borrow one from someone before you invest in it.
✳ Do your research. Check out consumer reports or online resources for the best product ratings and reviews.

---

making stretching more effective. Add 5 to 10 minutes of stretching to your fitness routine, and you'll be ready to go! Figure 11.6 on page 343 shows a selection of exercises that will stretch the major muscle groups of your body and can be used as a warm-up for other physical activities and exercise programs.

Resistance Training When beginning a resistance-exercise program, always consider your age, fitness level, and personal goals. Strength-training exercises are done in a set, or a single series of multiple repetitions using the same resistance. For both men and women under the age of 50, the ACSM recommends working major muscle groups with at least one set of eight to ten different exercises 2 to 3 days per week.[38] Weight loads should be at a level to allow up to 8 to 12 repetitions. Beginners should use lighter weights and complete 10 to 15 repetitions. Remember, experts suggest allowing at least one day of rest and recovery between workouts of any specific muscle group.

Cardiorespiratory Training You should spend the greatest proportion of exercise time developing cardiovascular fitness. Choose an aerobic activity you think you will like. Many people find cross training—alternate-day participation in two or more aerobic activities (such as jogging and swimming)—more enjoyable than long-term participation in only one activity. Cross training is also beneficial because it strengthens a variety of muscles, thus helping you avoid overuse injuries to muscles and joints.

Cooling Down and Stretching Just as you ease into a workout with a warm-up, you should slowly transition from activity to rest. A cool-down is an essential component of a fitness program. Aerobic activity causes an increase in heart rate and the amount of blood pumped to major muscle groups. Stopping without a gradual decrease in the intensity of the activity can cause a dangerous drop in blood pressure. A 5-minute cool-down walk will help heart rate decrease gradually. Be sure to stretch the major muscle groups after

TABLE
11.3 — Some Popular Fitness Gadgets and Equipment

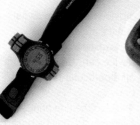
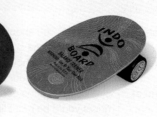

Heart Rate Monitor

A chest strap with a watch device that helps the wearer become aware of heart rate during training.

- Provides instant feedback about the intensity of your workout.
- Needs a good fit for the strap, which may be cumbersome

Cost: $50–$200

Pedometer

A small battery-operated device, usually worn on the belt, that keeps track of number of steps. Some models also monitor calories, distance, and speed.

- Great for motivating to get the recommended 10,000 steps per day
- Needs to be calibrated for your height, weight, and stride length

Cost: $25–$50

Stability Ball

Large ball made of burst-resistant vinyl that can be used for sitting, strengthening core muscles, or stretching.

- Balls must be inflated correctly to be most effective

Cost: $25–$50

Balance Board

A board with a rounded bottom that can be used to improve balance and core muscle strength, and to help stretch muscles.

- Great for improving agility, reaction skills, and ankle strength
- Can be difficult for new users

Cost: $40–$80

Resistance Bands

Rubber or elastic material with handles that can be used to work the muscles without the use of weights.

- Can improve muscle endurance, strength, flexibility, and range of motion
- Lightweight and portable

Cost: $5–$15

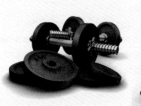
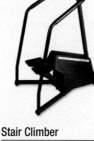

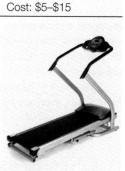

Free Weights

Rubber, plastic, or metal dumbbells or barbells, often with adjustable weight and used with a weight bench.

- Traditional and reliable method for building muscular strength and endurance
- A full set allows you to increase weight load as you train
- Potential for injury if form is incorrect

Cost: $10–$300

Elliptical Trainer

A stationary exercise machine that simulates walking or running without causing impact on the bones and joints. Some machines have arm movements also.

- Nonimpact
- Readout and programs vary

Cost: $300–$4,000

Stair Climber

A stationary exercise machine that provides a low-impact lower-body workout by simulating stair climbing.

- The degree of workout depends on working against your body weight
- Does not provide upper-body workout

Cost: $200–$3,000

Stationary Bike

A lower-body exercise machine designed to simulate bike riding.

- Generally easy to use
- Comes with varied resistance programs
- Recumbent styles offer less strain on back and knees
- Does not provide upper-body workout

Cost: $200–$2,000

Treadmill

Exercise machine for walking or running on a moving platform while remaining in one place.

- Comes with an emergency shutoff
- Different models have varied readouts and programmability
- Lower impact on joints than running on most pavements

Cost: $500–$4,000

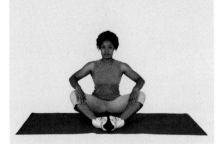

ⓐ Stretching the inside of the thighs

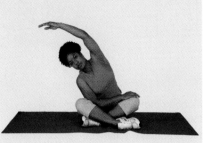

ⓑ Stretching the upper arm and the side of the trunk

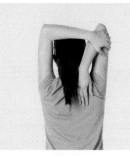

ⓒ Stretching the triceps

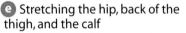

ⓓ Stretching the trunk and the hip

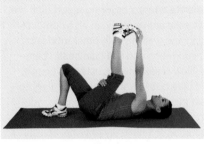

ⓔ Stretching the hip, back of the thigh, and the calf

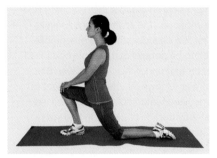

ⓕ Stretching the front of the thigh and the hip flexor

FIGURE 11.6 **Stretching Exercises to Improve Flexibility and Prevent Injury**
Use these stretches as part of your warm-up and cool-down. Hold each stretch for 10 to 30 seconds, and repeat four times for each limb. After only a few weeks of regular stretching, you'll begin to see more flexibility.

cooling down to help reduce the amount of soreness you experience from exercise.

Fitness-Related Injuries

Enthusiastic but out-of-shape beginners often injure themselves by doing too much too soon. Experienced athletes develop *overtraining syndrome* by engaging in systematic and progressive increases in training without getting enough rest and recovery time. Eventually, performance begins to decline, and training sessions become increasingly difficult. Adequate rest, good nutrition, and rehydration are important to sustain or improve fitness levels.

There are two basic types of injuries stemming from fitness-related activities: traumatic injuries and overuse injuries. **Traumatic injuries** occur suddenly and violently, typically by accident. Typical traumatic injuries are broken bones, torn ligaments and muscles, contusions, and lacerations. If your traumatic injury causes a noticeable loss of function and immediate pain or pain that does not go away after 30 minutes, consult a physician.

Doing too much intense exercise, or doing too much exercise without variation, can increase the likelihood of **overuse injuries.** Overuse injuries are those that result from the cumulative effects of day-after-day stresses placed on tendons, muscles, and joints during exercise.

These injuries occur most often in repetitive activities such as swimming, running, bicycling, and step aerobics. The forces that occur normally during physical activity are not enough to cause a ligament sprain or muscle strain, but when these forces are applied daily for weeks or months, they can result in an injury.

The three most common overuse injuries all occur in the lower body: runner's knee, shin splints, and plantar fasciitis. *Runner's knee* is a general term describing a series of problems involving the muscles, tendons, and ligaments around the knee. *Shin splints* is a general term for any pain that occurs below the knee and above the ankle. *Plantar fasciitis* is an inflammation of the plantar fascia, a broad band of dense, inelastic tissue in the foot. For any of these overuse injuries, rest, variation of routine, and stretching are the first lines of treatment. If pain continues, a physician visit is recommended.

traumatic injuries Injuries that are accidental and occur suddenly and violently.
overuse injuries Injuries that result from the cumulative effects of day-after-day stresses placed on tendons, muscles, and joints.
RICE Acronym for the standard first aid treatment for virtually all traumatic and overuse injuries: rest, ice, compression, and elevation.

Treatment of Fitness-Related Injuries

First aid treatment for virtually all personal fitness injuries involves **RICE: r**est, **i**ce, **c**ompression, and **e**levation. *Rest,*

GREEN GUIDE

Transport Yourself!

Before we became a car culture, much of our transportation was human powered. Bicycling and walking historically have been important means of transportation and recreation in the United States. These modes not only helped keep people in good physical shape, but they also had little or no impact on the environment. Even in the first few decades after the automobile started to be popularized, people continued to get around under their own power. Since World War II, however, the development of automobile-oriented communities has led to a steady decline of bicycling and walking. Currently, only about 10 percent of trips are made by foot or bike.

The more we use our cars to get around, the more congested our roads, the more polluted our air, and the more sedentary our lives become. That's why many people are now embracing a movement toward more active transportation. *Active transportation* means getting out of your car and using your own power to get around—whether walking, riding a bike,

skateboarding, or roller skating. The following are just a few of the many reasons to make active transportation a bigger part of your life:

✳ **You will be adding more exercise into your daily routine.** People who walk or bike to complete errands or for transportation are physically active. You can also combine biking and walking with other modes of transportation and still gain health benefits. New research suggests that people who take public transit are more likely to meet the physical activity recommendations. Walking or biking to the bus or train stop adds to total daily physical activity and may curb weight gain.

✳ **Walking or biking can save you money.** With rising gas prices and car maintenance and insurance costs, fewer trips by car per week can add up to considerable savings. For many of our daily trips, bicycling and walking are the most economical choices. During the course of a year, regular bicycle commuters who ride 5 miles to work can save about $500 on fuel and more than $1,000 on other expenses related to driving.

✳ **You will enjoy being outdoors.** Research is emerging on the physical and mental health benefits of nature and being outdoors. So much of what we do is inside, with recirculated air and artificial lighting, that our bodies are deficient in receiving fresh air and sunlight. New studies point to the mental and physical health benefits of being out in nature.

✳ **You will be making a significant contribution to the reduction of air pollution.** Driving less means fewer pollutants being emitted into the air. Leaving your car at home just 2 days a week will reduce greenhouse gas emissions by an average of 1,600 pounds per year.

✳ **You will help reduce traffic.** The average traveler now wastes the equivalent of a full work week stuck in traffic every year. More active commuters mean fewer cars on the roads and less traffic congestion.

✳ **You'll contribute to global health.** Annually, personal transportation accounts for consumption of approximately 136 billion gallons of gasoline, or the production of 1.2 billion tons of carbon dioxide. Reducing vehicle trips will help reduce overall greenhouse gas emissions and reduce the need to source more fossil fuel.

Sources: T. Gotschi and K. Mills, *Active Transportation for America: The Case for Increased Federal Investment in Bicycling and Walking* (Washington, DC: Rails to Trails Conservancy, 2008); D. Shinkle and A. Teigens, *Encouraging Bicycling and Walking: The State Legislative Role* (Washington, DC: National Conference of State Legislatures, 2008); University of British Columbia, "Public Transit Users Three Times More Likely to Meet Fitness Guidelines," *Science Daily* 27, March 2009, www.sciencedaily.com/releases/2009/03/090326134014.htm; U. Lachapelle and L. Frank, "Transit and Health: Mode of Transport, Employer-Sponsored Public Transit Pass Programs, and Physical Activity," *Journal of Public Health Policy* 30 (2009): s73–s94; U.S. Environmental Protection Agency, "Climate Change: What You Can Do—On the Road," Updated April 2009, www.epa.gov/climatechange/wycd/road.html; C. Maller, M. Townsend, A. Pryor, P. Brown, and L. St. Leger, "Healthy Nature Healthy People: 'Contact with Nature' as an Upstream Health Promotion Intervention for Populations," *Health Promotion International* 21, no. 1 (2005): 45–54.

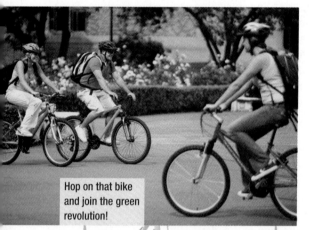

Hop on that bike and join the green revolution!

the first component of this treatment, is required to avoid further irritation of the injured body part. *Ice* is applied to relieve pain and constrict the blood vessels to stop any internal or external bleeding. Never apply ice cubes, reusable gel ice packs, chemical cold packs, or other forms of cold directly to your skin. Instead, place a layer of wet toweling or elastic bandage between the ice and your skin. Ice should be applied to a new injury for approximately 20 minutes every hour for the first 24 to 72 hours. *Compression* of the injured body part can be accomplished with a 4- or 6-inch-wide elastic bandage; this applies indirect pressure to damaged blood vessels to help stop bleeding. Be careful, though, that the compression wrap does not interfere with normal blood flow. Throbbing or pain in the injured part indicates that the compression wrap should be loosened. *Elevation* of an injured extremity above the level of your heart also helps to control internal or external bleeding by making the blood flow upward to reach the injured area.

Preventing Injuries

There are steps that you can take to reduce your risk of overuse or traumatic injuries. Using common sense, identifying and using only the proper gear and equipment, and making sure they're always in fully functional condition, can help you avoid an injury.

Appropriate Footwear Athletic shoes are made to protect the foot from sport-specific movements. Proper footwear can decrease the likelihood of foot, knee, or back injuries.

When you purchase athletic shoes, the two most important factors to consider are (1) how well they fit and (2) the activity for which you'll need them. Feet come in all shapes and sizes. A good fit is essential for comfort and performance. To get the best fit, shop at a sports or fitness specialty store where there are a large selection and salespeople who are trained in properly fitting athletic shoes. Try on shoes later in the day when your feet are largest, and check to make sure there is a little extra room in the toe and that the width is appropriate. Because different activities place different stresses on your feet and joints, you should choose shoes specifically designed for your sport or activity. Shoes of any type should be replaced once they lose their cushioning. Continuing to use a shoe that is worn out will increase your risk of injury.

For individuals looking for quality running shoes, the shoes' ability to absorb shock is critical. Biomechanics research has revealed that running is a collision sport—with each stride, the runner's foot collides with the ground with a force three to five times the runner's body weight.[39] The force not absorbed by the running shoe is transmitted upward into the foot, leg, thigh, and back. Our bodies can absorb forces such as these but may be injured by the cumulative effect of repetitive impacts (such as running 40 miles per week). There are several other key components to a good running shoe as well (see **Figure 11.7**).

Appropriate Protective Equipment Some activities require special protective equipment to reduce chances of injury. Eye injuries can occur in virtually all fitness-related activities, although some are more risky than others. As many as 90 percent of the eye injuries resulting from racquetball and squash could be prevented by wearing appropriate eye protection—for example, goggles with polycarbonate lenses.[40]

Wearing a helmet while bicycle riding is an important safety precaution. An estimated 45 to 88 percent of head

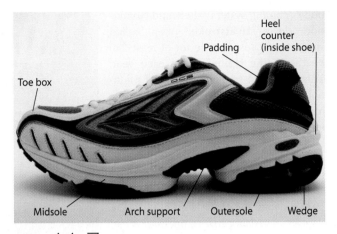

FIGURE 11.7 Anatomy of a Running Shoe
A good running shoe should fit comfortably, allow room for you to wiggle your toes, and provide a firm grip on your heel so it doesn't slip when you are walking or running.

injuries among cyclists can be prevented by wearing a helmet. The direct medical costs from cyclists' failure to wear helmets is $81 million a year.[41] Cyclists aren't the only ones who should be wearing helmets. People who skateboard, use kick-scooters, ski, in-line skate, play contact sports, or snowboard should also wear helmets. Look for helmets that meet the standards established by the American National Standards Institute or the Snell Memorial Foundation.

what do you think?

Given your activity level, what injuries do you risk on a regular basis? ● What changes can you make in your equipment and clothing to reduce your risk?

Exercising in the Heat

Heat stress, which includes several potentially fatal illnesses resulting from excessive core body temperatures, should be a concern whenever you exercise in warm, humid weather. In these conditions, your body's rate of heat production can exceed its ability to cool itself.

The three different heat stress illnesses—heat cramps, heat exhaustion, and heatstroke—are progressive in severity. **Heat cramps** (heat-related muscle cramps), the least serious problem, can usually be prevented by warm-ups, adequate fluid replacement, and a diet that includes the electrolytes lost during sweating (sodium and potassium). **Heat exhaustion** is caused by excessive water loss resulting from prolonged exercise or work. Symptoms of heat exhaustion include nausea, headache, fatigue, dizziness and faintness, and, paradoxically, "goosebumps" and chills. If you are suffering from heat exhaustion, your skin will be cool and moist. Heat exhaustion occurs when the

heat cramps Muscle cramps that occur during or following exercise in warm or hot weather.

heat exhaustion A heat stress illness caused by significant dehydration resulting from exercise in warm or hot conditions.

body's cooling system falters and circulation slows. **Heatstroke,** often called *sunstroke,* is responsible for at least 240 deaths in the United States each year. This condition triggers a series of metabolic events that may result in irreversible injury or death.[42] Heatstroke occurs during vigorous exercise when the body's heat production significantly exceeds its cooling capacities. Body core temperature can rise from normal (98.6°F) to 105°F to 110°F within minutes after the body's cooling mechanism shuts down. Rapidly increasing core temperatures can cause brain damage, permanent disability, and death. Common signs of heatstroke are dry, hot, and usually red skin; very high body temperature; and rapid heart rate.

You can prevent heat stress by following certain precautions. First, proper acclimatization to hot and/or humid climates is essential. The process of heat acclimatization, which increases your body's cooling efficiency, requires about 10 to 14 days of gradually increasing activity in the hot environment. Second, avoid dehydration by replacing the fluids you lose during and after exercise. The ACSM, along with the National Athlete Trainers Association, recommends consuming 14 to 22 ounces of fluid 2 hours prior to exercise. When exercising intensely, you should drink 6 to 12 ounces, every 15 to 20 minutes. The third way to avoid heat stress is to wear clothing appropriate for your activity and the environment. And finally, use common sense—for example, on a day when the temperature is 85°F and the humidity is 80 percent, postpone your usual lunchtime run until the cool of evening. Be aware that heat stress can also result from prolonged immersion in a sauna, hot tub, or steam bath or from performing activity in lots of heavy

heatstroke A deadly heat stress illness resulting from dehydration and overexertion in warm or hot conditions.

hypothermia Potentially fatal condition caused by abnormally low body core temperature.

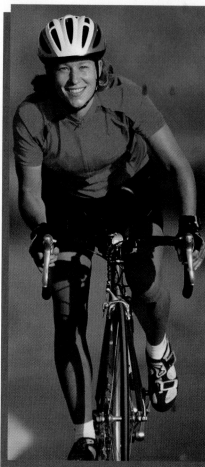

What can I do to avoid injury while I'm exercising?

Avoiding exercise-related injuries simply requires taking proper precautions and being prepared. Wear the protective gear, such as helmets or eyewear, that are appropriate for your activity. Purchase supportive footwear, and vary your activities to avoid overuse injuries. Dress for the weather, try to avoid exercising in extreme conditions, and always stay properly hydrated.

clothing and equipment, such as a football uniform.[43]

Exercising in the Cold

Exercising in cool weather can lead to **hypothermia,** a potentially fatal condition resulting from abnormally low body core temperature, which occurs when body heat is lost faster than it is produced. Temperatures need not be frigid for hypothermia to occur; it can also result from prolonged, vigorous exercise in 40°F to 50°F temperatures, particularly if there is rain, snow, or a strong wind.

In mild cases of hypothermia, as body core temperature drops from the normal 98.6°F to about 93.2°F, you will begin to shiver. Shivering—the involuntary contraction of nearly every muscle in the body—increases body temperature by using the heat given off by muscle activity. You may also experience cold hands and feet, poor judgment, apathy, and amnesia. Shivering ceases in most hypothermia victims as body core temperatures drop to between 87°F and 90°F, a sign that the body has lost its ability to generate heat. Death usually occurs at body core temperatures between 75°F and 80°F.[44]

To prevent hypothermia, analyze weather conditions and your risk of hypothermia before you undertake an outdoor physical activity. Remember that wind and humidity are as significant as temperature. Have a friend join you for cold weather outdoor activities and wear layers of appropriate clothing to prevent excessive heat loss (polypropylene or woolen undergarments, a windproof outer garment, and a wool hat and gloves). Keep your head, hands, and feet warm. Don't allow yourself to become dehydrated. Thirst is suppressed in cold environments, so drink plenty of fluids even if you're not thirsty.[45]

How Physically Fit Are You?

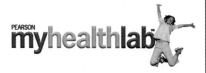

Fill out this assessment online at www.pearsonhighered.com/myhealthlab or www.pearsonhighered.com/donatelle.

1 Evaluating Your Muscular Endurance (the 1-Minute Curl-Up Test)

Your abdominal muscles are important for core stability and back support; this test will assess their muscular endurance.

Description/Procedure

Lie on a mat with your arms by your sides, palms flat on the mat, elbows straight, and fingers extended. Bend your knees at a 90-degree angle. Your instructor or partner will mark your starting finger position with a piece of tape under each hand and your ending position 10 cm or 3 in. away from the first piece of tape—one ending position tape for each hand. Set a metronome to 50 beats per/min and curl up at this slow, controlled pace: one curl-up every 3 sec (25 curl-ups per min). Curl your head and upper back upward, reaching your arms forward along the mat to touch the ending tape. Then curl back down so that your upper back and shoulders touch the floor. During the entire curl-up, your fingers, feet, and buttocks should stay on the mat. Your partner will count the number of correct repetitions you complete. Perform as many curl-ups as you can without pausing, to a maximum of 25.

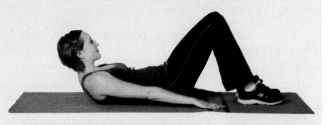

Fitness Categories for 1-Minute Curl-Up Test

Men	Superior	Excellent	Good	Fair	Poor	Very Poor
20–29 yrs	>25	22–25	16–21	13–15	10–12	<10
30–39 yrs	>25	19–25	15–18	13–14	10–12	<10
40–49 yrs	>25	19–25	13–18	8–12	5–7	<5
50–59 yrs	>25	18–25	11–17	9–10	7–8	<7
60–69 yrs	>25	17–25	11–16	8–10	5–7	<5

Women	Superior	Excellent	Good	Fair	Poor	Very Poor
20–29 yrs	>25	19–25	14–18	7–13	4–6	<4
30–39 yrs	>25	20–25	10–19	8–9	5–7	<5
40–49 yrs	>25	20–25	11–19	6–10	3–5	<3
50–59 yrs	>25	20–25	10–19	8–9	5–7	<5
60–69 yrs	>25	18–25	8–17	5–7	2–4	<2

Source: Adapted from Canadian Society for Exercise Physiology, *The Canadian Physical Activity, Fitness & Lifestyle Approach: CSEP-Health & Fitness Program's Health-Related Appraisal & Counseling Strategy,* 3d ed. (Ottawa, ON: Canadian Society for Exercise Physiology, 2003).

2 Evaluating Your Flexibility (the Sit-and-Reach Test)

This test measures the general flexibility of your lower back, hips, and hamstring muscles.

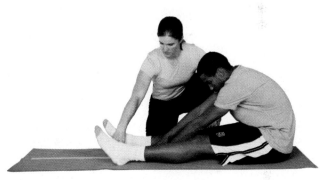

Description/Procedure

Warm up with some light activity and range-of-motion exercises and stretches for the joints and muscles that you will be using. For the test, sit straight-legged on a mat with your shoes removed and your feet about 10 to 12 in. apart. Have a partner place a yardstick on the mat between your feet with the 15-in. mark at the edge of your heels. You can use a preplaced/taped yardstick, tape the yardstick in place at the heels, or just have your partner hold the yardstick. Place your hands on top of the yardstick's end, one hand on top of the other. Keeping your hand on the yardstick and your fingertips together, reach forward as far as you can by slowly bending forward, reaching with your arms, and sliding your fingertips out along the yardstick. Keep your legs straight, drop your head between your arms, and breathe out as you perform the test. Hold your ending position for at least 2 sec. Your *reach distance* is the most distant point reached with both fingertips. If you cannot keep your hands from separating, the most distant point reached by the fingertips of the hand that is farthest back should be considered the reach distance. Record the reach distance in inches, as measured by the yardstick. Perform the test twice. Have your partner point to your reach distance for each trial on the yardstick.

Men	Superior	Excellent	Good	Fair	Poor	Very Poor	Women	Superior	Excellent	Good	Fair	Poor	Very Poor
18–25 yrs	>27	21–27	18–20	15–17	11–14	<11	18–25 yrs	>27	23–27	20–22	17–19	15–16	<15
26–35 yrs	>27	20–27	17–19	14–16	10–13	<10	26–35 yrs	>26	22–26	19–21	16–18	14–15	<14
36–45 yrs	>27	20–27	16–19	13–15	8–12	<8	36–45 yrs	>26	21–26	18–20	15–17	13–14	<13
46–55 yrs	>24	18–24	14–17	11–13	7–10	<7	46–55 yrs	>25	20–25	17–19	14–16	11–13	<11
56–65 yrs	>22	16–22	12–15	9–11	6–8	<6	56–65 yrs	>24	19–24	16–18	13–15	10–12	<10
>65 yrs	>22	16–22	12–15	8–11	5–7	<5	>65 yrs	>24	19–24	16–18	13–15	10–12	<10

Source: Reprinted with permission from Medical Advisory Committee Recommendations: A Resource Guide for YMCAs, February 2007 © 2007 by YMCA of the USA, Chicago. All rights reserved.

3 Evaluating Your Cardiorespiratory Endurance (the 1.5-Mile Run Test)

This test assesses your cardiorespiratory endurance level.

Description/Procedure

Find a local track, typically one-quarter mile per lap, to perform your test. Run 1.5 miles; use a stopwatch to measure how long it takes to reach that distance. If you become extremely fatigued during the test, slow your pace or walk—do not over-stress yourself! If you feel faint or nauseated or experience any unusual pains in your upper body, stop and notify your instructor. Use the chart below to estimate your cardiorespiratory fitness level based on your age and sex. Note that women have lower standards for each fitness category, because they have higher levels of essential fat than men do.

Men	Excellent	Good	Fair	Poor	Women	Excellent	Good	Fair	Poor
20–29 yrs	<10:10	10:10–11:29	11:30–12:38	>12:38	20–29 yrs	<11:59	11:59–13:24	13:25–14:50	>14:50
30–39 yrs	<10:47	10:47–11:54	11:55–12:58	>12:58	30–39 yrs	<12:25	12:25–14:08	14:09–15:43	>15:43
40–49 yrs	<11:16	11:16–12:24	12:25–13:50	>13:50	40–49 yrs	<13:24	13:24–14:53	14:54–16:31	>16:31
50–59 yrs	<12:09	12:09–13:35	13:36–15:06	>15:06	50–59 yrs	<14:35	14:35–16:35	16:36–18:18	>18:18
60–69 yrs	<13:24	13:24–15:04	15:05–16:46	>16:46	60–69 yrs	<16:34	16:34–18:27	18:28–20:16	>20:16

Source: Data are from The Cooper Institute, *Physical Fitness Assessments and Norms for Adults and Law Enforcement* (Dallas, TX: The Cooper Institute, 2009). Reprinted with permission from The Cooper Institute, Dallas, Texas. For more information: www.cooperinstitute.org.

YOUR PLAN FOR CHANGE

The **Assessyourself** activity helped you determine your current fitness levels. Your results may indicate that you should take steps to improve one or more components of your physical fitness.

Today, you can:

◯ Visit your campus fitness facility and familiarize yourself with the equipment and resources. Find out what classes they offer, and take home a copy of the schedule.

◯ Take a stretch break. Spend 5 minutes in between homework projects or just before bed doing some whole-body stretches to release tension.

Within the next 2 weeks, you can:

◯ Shop for comfortable workout clothes or running shoes.

◯ Investigate team sport leagues in your area. Is there an intramural basketball, volleyball, or ultimate Frisbee program on your campus? Look into other group activities you might enjoy.

◯ Ask a friend to join you in your workout once a week. Agree upon a date and time in advance so you'll both be committed to following through.

By the end of the semester, you can:

◯ Establish a regular routine of exercising at least three times a week. Mark your exercise times on your calendar and keep a log to track your progress. After you've been exercising regularly for a month or so, try taking the fitness assessments again.

◯ Take your workouts to the next level. If you have been working out at home, try making a regular habit of going to a gym or participating in an exercise class. If you are walking, perhaps try intermittent jogging or sign up for a fitness event such as a charity 5K.

Summary

* The physiological benefits of regular physical activity include reduced risk of heart attack, some cancers, hypertension, and diabetes; and improved blood profile, skeletal mass, weight control, immunity to disease, mental health and stress management, and physical fitness. Regular physical activity can also increase life span.
* It is recommended that every adult participate in moderate-intensity activities for 30 minutes at least 5 days a week. For improvements in cardiorespiratory fitness, you should work out aerobically for at least 20 minutes, a minimum of 3 days per week. Exercise intensity involves working out at target heart rate. The longer the exercise period, the more calories burned and the greater the improvement in cardiovascular fitness.
* Key principles for developing muscular strength and endurance are overload, specificity-of-training, variation, and reversibility. Resistance-training programs include body weight resistance (calisthenics), fixed resistance, variable resistance, and accommodating resistance devices.
* Flexibility exercises should involve static stretching exercises performed in sets of two to four repetitions held for 15 to 30 seconds, at least 2 to 3 days a week.
* Planning a fitness program involves setting goals and designing a program to achieve these goals. A comprehensive program would include a warm-up period, stretching activities, strength development exercises, an aerobic activity, and a cool-down period.
* Fitness injuries generally are caused by trauma or overuse; the most common ones are runner's knee, shin splints, and plantar fasciitis. Proper footwear and equipment can help prevent injuries. Exercise in the heat or cold requires special precautions.

Pop Quiz

1. The ability to perform regular moderate to vigorous levels of physical activity without excessive fatigue is
   a. physical performance.
   b. plyometrics.
   c. muscular endurance.
   d. cardiorespiratory fitness.

2. Regular exercise is known to increase the number of
   a. high-density lipoproteins.
   b. low-density lipoproteins.
   c. triglycerides.
   d. red blood cells.

3. The sit-and-reach test measures
   a. muscle endurance.
   b. flexibility.
   c. muscle strength.
   d. cardiorespiratory fitness.

4. The foundation of strength training is called the _____ principle.
   a. overload
   b. tension
   c. endurance
   d. contraction

5. Which type of cancer may be prevented by being physically active?
   a. skin
   b. lung
   c. colon
   d. liver

6. Flexibility is the range of motion around
   a. specific bones.
   b. specific joints.
   c. the hips and pelvis.
   d. the muscles

7. An example of aerobic exercise is
   a. brisk walking.
   b. bench pressing weights.
   c. stretching exercises.
   d. yoga breathing.

8. Theresa wants to lower her ratio of fat weight to her total body weight. She wants to work on her
   a. flexibility.
   b. muscular endurance.
   c. muscular strength.
   d. body composition.

9. Miguel is a cross-country runner and is therefore able to sustain moderate-intensity, whole-body activity for an extended time. This ability relates to what component of physical fitness?
   a. flexibility
   b. body composition
   c. cardiorespiratory fitness
   d. muscular strength and endurance

10. Joel enjoys various types of fitness exercises. He alternates his training days with jogging, cycling, and step aerobics. This type of training is called
    a. cardiac fitness training.
    b. static training.
    c. cross training.
    d. multisport training.

Answers to these questions can be found on page A-1.

Think about It!

1. How do you define *physical fitness*? What are the key components of a physical fitness program? What might you need to consider when beginning a fitness program?
2. How would you determine the proper intensity and duration of an exercise program? How often should exercise sessions be scheduled?
3. Why is stretching vital to improving physical flexibility? Why is flexibility important in everyday activities?
4. Identify at least four physiological and psychological benefits of physical fitness. How would you promote these benefits to nonexercisers?
5. What are your core muscles? Why is it important to strengthen them?

6. Your roommate has decided to start running first thing in the morning in an effort to lose weight, tone muscles, and improve cardiorespiratory fitness. What advice would you give to make sure your roommate gets off to a good start and doesn't get injured?

7. What key components are necessary for a personal fitness program?

Accessing Your Health on the Internet

The following websites explore further topics and issues related to personal health. For links to the websites below, visit the Companion Website for *Health: The Basics,* Green Edition at www.pearsonhighered.com/donatelle.

1. *ACSM Online.* A link with the American College of Sports Medicine and all their resources. www.acsm.org

2. *American Council on Exercise.* Information on exercise and disease prevention. www.acefitness.org

3. *Centers for Disease Control and Prevention, National Center for Chronic Disease Prevention and Health Promotion, Division of Nutrition, Physical Activity and Obesity.* A resource for current information on exercise and health. www.cdc.gov/nccdphp/dnpa

4. *National Strength and Conditioning Association.* A resource for personal trainers and others interested in conditioning and fitness. www.nsca-lift.org

5. *President's Council of Physical Fitness and Sports.* Provides information on fitness programs. www.fitness.gov

6. *MyPyramid Tracker.* This tool from the U.S. Department of Agriculture (USDA) is an online dietary and physical activity tracker that provides information on your diet quality and physical activity status, and offers links to nutrient and physical activity information. The Food Calories/Energy Balance feature automatically calculates your energy balance by subtracting the energy you expend from physical activity from your food calories/energy intake. www.mypyramidtracker.gov

References

1. American College Health Association, *American College Health Association— National College Health Assessment II (ACHA-NCHA) Reference Group Executive Summary Fall 2008* (Baltimore: American College Health Association, 2009).

2. National Center for Chronic Disease Prevention and Health Promotion, "Physical Activity for Everyone," Centers for Disease Control and Prevention, Updated 2008, www.cdc.gov/nccdphp/dnpa/physical/everyone/health/index.htm.

3. National Diabetes Information Clearinghouse, National Institute of Diabetes and Digestive and Kidney Diseases (NIDDK), *National Diabetes Statistics, 2007,* NIH Publication no. 08-3892 (Bethesda, MD: National Institutes of Health, 2008), http://diabetes.niddk.nih.gov/dm/pubs/statistics/DM_Statistics.pdf; American Heart Association, *Heart Disease and Stroke Statistics—2009 Update At-a-Glance* (Dallas: American Heart Association, 2009).

4. Harvard Health Publications, *Exercise: A Program You Can Live With* (Cambridge, MA: Harvard Health Publications, 2007).

5. W. L. Haskell et al., "Physical Activity and Public Health: Updated Recommendation for Adults from the American College of Sports Medicine and the American Heart Association," *Medicine and Science in Sports and Exercise* 39, no. 8 (2007): 1423–34.

6. U.S. Department of Health and Human Services, *2008 Physical Activity Guidelines for Americans* ODPHP Publication no. U0036 (Washington, DC: U.S. Department of Health and Human Services, 2008).

7. National Center for Chronic Disease Prevention and Health Promotion, "Physical Activity for Everyone"; W. L. Haskell et al., "Physical Activity and Public Health," 2007.

8. V. H. Heyward, *Advanced Fitness Assessment and Prescription.* 5th ed. (Champaign, IL: Human Kinetics, 2006).

9. X. Sui, M. J. Lamonte, and S. N. Blair, "Cardiorespiratory Fitness and Risk of Nonfatal Cardiovascular Disease in Women and Men with Hypertension," *American Journal of Hypertension* 20, no. 6 (2007): 608–15.

10. S. Plowman and D. Smith *Exercise Physiology for Health, Fitness, and Performance.*

   2d ed. reprint (Philadelphia: Lippincott Williams & Wilkins, 2008): 312–13.

11. G. A. Kelley and K. S. Kelley, "Efficacy of Aerobic Exercise on Coronary Heart Disease Risk Factors," *Preventive Cardiology* 11, no. 2 (2008): 71–75.

12. American Heart Association, "The Number of Adults in the U.S. with High Blood Pressure Rose in the Last Decade," 2004, www.americanheart.org/presenter.jhtml?identifier=3024450#Number; W. Wang et al., "A Longitudinal Study of Hypertension Risk Factors and Their Relation to Cardiovascular Disease," *Hypertension* 47 (2006): 403; American College of Sports Medicine, *ACSM's Certification Review.* 3d ed. (Philadelphia: Lippincott Williams & Wilkins, 2009).

13. American Stroke Association, "Cholesterol," Accessed 2009, www.strokeassociation.org/presenter.jhtml?identifier=4488.

14. C. M. Frienedreich and A. E. Cust, "Physical Activity and Breast Cancer Risk: Impact of Timing, Type, and Dose of Activity and Population Subgroup Effects," *British Journal of Sports Medicine* 42, no. 8 (2008): 636–47.

15. K. Y. Wolin, Y. Yan Y, G. A. Colditz, and I. M. Lee, "Physical Activity and Colon Cancer Prevention: A Meta-Analysis," *British Journal of Cancer* 100, no. 4 (2009): 611–16.

16. K. J. Stewart et al., "Exercise Effects on Bone Mineral Density Relationships to Changes in Fitness and Fatness," *American Journal of Preventive Medicine* 28, no. 5 (2005): 453–60; W. McArdle, F. Katch, and V. Katch, *Exercise Physiology.* 6th ed. (Philadelphia: Lippincott Williams & Wilkins, 2006), 60–65.

17. University of Colorado Health Sciences Center, "National Weight Control Registry," Accessed July 2009, www.uchsc.edu/nutrition/WyattJortberg/nwcr.htm.

18. W. L. Haskell et al., "Physical Activity and Public Health," 2007.

19. P. M. Janiszewski and P. Ross, "Physical Activity in the Treatment of Obesity: Beyond Body Weight Reduction," *Applied Physiology and Nutrition Metabolism* 32, no. 3 (2007): 512–22.

20. American Diabetes Association, "Diabetes Risk Test," Accessed July 2009, www.diabetes.org/risk-test.jsp.

21. National Diabetes Information Clearinghouse, "Diabetes Prevention Program," NIH Publication No. 09–5099, October 2008, http://diabetes.niddk.nih.gov/dm/pubs/preventionprogram.

22. T. Kizaki et al., "Adaptations of Macrophages to Exercise Training Improves Innate Immunity," *Biochemical and Biophysical Research Communications* 372, no. 1 (2008): 152–56.

23. M. Gleeson, "Immune Function in Sport and Exercise," *Journal of Applied Physiology* 103, no. 2 (2007): 693–99.

24. B. F. Burke, "Exercise and Immunity," *MedLine Plus,* National Institutes of Health, Updated May 2008, www.nlm.nih .gov/medlineplus/ency/article/007165 .htm.

25. L. M. Hays, T. M. Damush, and D. O. Clark, "Relationships between Exercise Self-Definitions and Exercise Participation among Urban Women in Primary Care," *Journal of Cardiovascular Nursing* 20, no. 1 (2005): 9–17.

26. O. H. Franco et al., "Effects of Physical Activity on Life Expectancy with Cardio-vascular Disease," *Archives of Internal Medicine* 165, no. 20 (2005): 2355–60.

27. W. L. Haskell et al., "Physical Activity and Public Health," 2007.

28. Centers for Disease Control and Prevention, "Physical Activity for a Healthy Weight," Updated January 2009, www.cdc .gov/healthyweight/physical_activity/ index.html.

29. American College Health Association, *American College Health Association— National College Health Assessment II,* 2009.

30. W. J. Kraemer et al., "Progression Models in Resistance Training for Healthy Adults, American College of Sports Medicine Position Stand," *Medicine and Science in Sports and Exercise* 34, no. 2 (2002): 364–80.

31. Ibid.

32. Ibid.

33. C. Payton and R. Bartlett, eds., *Biomechanical Evaluation of Movement in Sport and Exercise: The British Association of Sport and Exercise Sciences Guide* (New York: Routledge, 2008), 105.

34. Mayo Clinic Staff, "Core Exercises: Beyond Your Average Abs Routine," Mayo Clinic, October 5, 2007, www.mayoclinic.com/ health/core-exercises/SM00071.

35. P. A. Adler and B. L. Roberts, "The Use of Tai Chi to Improve Health in Older Adults," *Orthopedic Nursing* 25, no. 2 (2006): 122–26.

36. Arthritis Foundation, "Exercise and Arthritis," 2009, www.arthritis.org/conditions/ exercise.

37. K. Small, L. McNaughton, and M. Matthews, "A Systematic Review into the Efficacy of Static Stretching as Part of a Warm Up for the Prevention of Exercise Related Injury," *Research in Sports Medicine* 16, no. 3 (2008): 213–31.

38. American College of Sports Medicine, *ACSM's Certification Review.* 3d ed. (Philadelphia: Lippincott Williams & Wilkins, 2009).

39. U. G. Kersting and G. P. Bruggemann, "Midsole Material-Related Force Control During Heel-Toe Running," *Research in Sports Medicine* 14, no. 1 (2006): 1–17.

40. American Academy of Ophthalmology, "Protective Eyewear," Updated February 2009, www.aao.org/eyesmart/injuries/ eyewear.cfm.

41. Bicycle Helmet Safety Institute, "Helmet-Related Statistics," Revised June 2009, www.helmets.org/stats.htm.

42. J. L. Glazer, "Management of Heat Stroke and Heat Exhaustion," *American Family Physician* 71, no. 11 (2005): 2141.

43. International Fitness Association, *Aerobics and Fitness Institute Certification Coursebook* (Orlando, FL: International Fitness Association, 2004).

44. R. Curtis, *Outdoor Action Guide to Hypothermia and Cold Weather Injuries* (Atlanta: Centers for Disease Control and Prevention, 2006).

45. American Council on Exercise, *Exercising in the Cold, 2006* (Indianapolis, IN: American Council on Exercise, 2006).

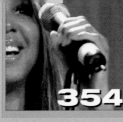
354
Why should I worry about cardiovascular disease?

363
Is heart disease hereditary?

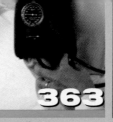
367
What does it mean for a tumor to be malignant?

374
Can having a tan protect me from skin cancer?

12 Cardiovascular Disease and Cancer

Objectives

* Discuss the incidence, prevalence, and outcomes of cardiovascular disease in the United States, including its impact on society.

* Review major types of cardiovascular disease, controllable and uncontrollable risk factors, methods of prevention, and current strategies for diagnosis and treatment.

* Explain what cancer is, and describe the different types of cancer, including the risks they pose to people at different ages and stages of life.

* Discuss cancer's risk factors, and outline strategies and recommendations for prevention, screening, and treatment.

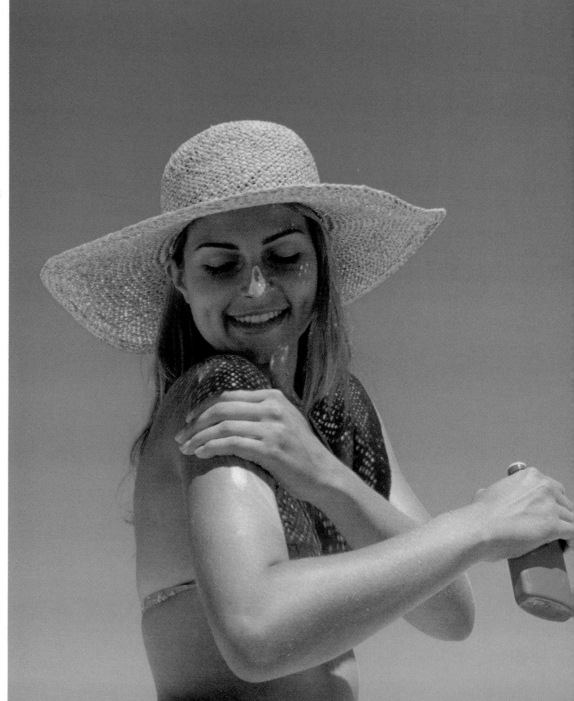

In this chapter, we focus on two groups of chronic diseases that contribute to the greatest global burden of death, illness, and disability of the past century: *cardiovascular diseases* and *cancer*. (Diabetes, another major cause of global health problems, is discussed in **Focus On: Your Risk for Diabetes** beginning on page 386.) Cardiovascular diseases are the number one cause of death globally, with over 17.5 million deaths each year (30% of all deaths). Cancer is another leading cause of death globally, with nearly 7.5 million deaths each year (around 13% of all deaths).[1] More than half of all Americans suffer from one or more chronic diseases, with cardiovascular disease and cancer being the most likely.[2]

What do we mean when we say a disease is chronic? Essentially, **chronic diseases** are defined as illnesses that are prolonged, do not resolve spontaneously, and are rarely cured completely. As such, they are responsible for significant rates of disability, lost productivity, pain, and suffering, not to mention soaring health care costs. Cardiovascular diseases, in particular, and cancer, to a lesser extent, are closely related to lifestyle factors such as obesity, sedentary behavior, poor nutrition, stress, lack of sleep, tobacco use, and excessive alcohol use. The good news is that in many cases, these lifestyle factors can be changed or modified and disease risks will then decrease.

Cardiovascular Disease: An Epidemiological Overview

More than 80 million Americans—one out of every three adults—suffer from one or more types of **cardiovascular disease (CVD),** the broad term used to describe diseases of the heart and blood vessels.[3] Although numbers continue to increase, it's important to note that CVD has been the leading killer of U.S. adults in every year since 1900, with the exception of 1918, when a pandemic flu killed more people. Put into perspective, CVD claims more lives each year than the next four leading causes of death combined (cancer, chronic lower respiratory diseases, accidents, and diabetes), accounting for nearly 37 percent of all deaths in the United States.[4] Although we've made advances in diagnosis and in pharmaceutical and surgical treatments, CVD continues to pose a serious threat to the health of all Americans, no matter their age, socioeconomic status, or gender **(Figure 12.1)**. Consider the following facts: [5]

- Over 150,000 Americans killed by CVD are under age 65, and nearly one third of these deaths are premature (meaning that the person doesn't live to full life expectancy).
- The probability at birth of eventually dying of CVD is 47 percent; of dying from cancer, 22 percent; from accidents, 3 percent; from diabetes, 2 percent; and from HIV, 0.7 percent.

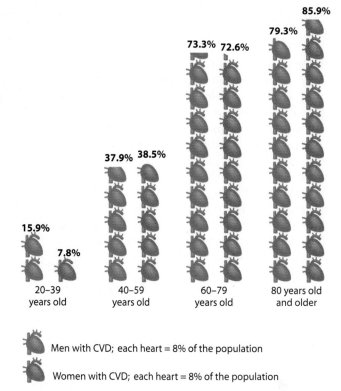

- Lifetime risk for CVD is two in three for men and more than one in two for women at 40 years of age.
- If all forms of major CVD were eliminated, life expectancy would rise by almost 7 years; if all forms of cancer were eliminated, the gain would be 3 years.

The best defense against CVD is to prevent it from developing in the first place. Understanding how your cardiovascular system works and the factors that can impair its functioning will help you understand your risk and how to reduce it.

FIGURE 12.1 **Prevalence of Cardiovascular Diseases (CVDs) in Adults Aged 20 and Older by Age and Sex**
Source: Data are from American Heart Association, *Heart Disease and Stroke Statistics—2009 Update* (Dallas: American Heart Association, 2009).

85.9%
79.3%
73.3% 72.6%
37.9% 38.5%
15.9%
7.8%

20–39 years old
40–59 years old
60–79 years old
80 years old and older

Men with CVD; each heart = 8% of the population

Women with CVD; each heart = 8% of the population

chronic disease An illness that is prolonged, does not resolve spontaneously, and is rarely cured.
cardiovascular disease (CVD) Disease of the heart and blood vessels.
cardiovascular system Organ system, consisting of the heart and blood vessels, that transports nutrients, oxygen, hormones, metabolic wastes, and enzymes throughout the body.

Understanding the Cardiovascular System

The **cardiovascular system** is the network of organs and vessels through which blood flows as it carries oxygen and nutrients to all parts of the body. It includes the *heart, arteries, arterioles* (small arteries), *veins, venules* (small veins), and *capillaries* (minute blood vessels).

The Heart: A Mighty Machine

The heart is a muscular, four-chambered pump, roughly the size of your fist. It is a highly efficient, extremely flexible organ that manages to contract 100,000 times each day and pumps the equivalent of 2,000 gallons of blood to all areas of the body. In a 70-year lifetime, an average human heart beats 2.5 billion times. However, people who are out of shape or overweight have hearts that must work significantly harder, and beat much more often, to keep them moving and functioning throughout the day.

Under normal circumstances, the human body contains approximately 6 quarts of blood, which transports nutrients, oxygen, waste products, hormones, and enzymes throughout the body. Blood also aids in regulating body temperature, cellular water levels, and acidity levels of body components, and it helps defend the body against toxins and harmful microorganisms. An adequate blood supply is essential to health and well-being.

The heart has four chambers that work together to circulate blood constantly throughout the body. The two upper chambers of the heart, called **atria,** are large collecting chambers that receive blood from the rest of the body. The two lower chambers, known as **ventricles,** pump the blood out again. Small valves regulate the steady, rhythmic flow of blood between chambers and prevent leakage or backflow between chambers.

---

atria (singular: *atrium*) The heart's two upper chambers, which receive blood.

ventricles The heart's two lower chambers, which pump blood through the blood vessels.

arteries Vessels that carry blood away from the heart to other regions of the body.

arterioles Branches of the arteries.

capillaries Minute blood vessels that branch out from the arterioles and venules; their thin walls permit exchange of oxygen, carbon dioxide, nutrients, and waste products among body cells.

veins Vessels that carry blood back to the heart from other regions of the body.

venules Branches of the veins.

sinoatrial node (SA node) Cluster of electric pulse–generating cells that serves as a natural pacemaker for the heart.

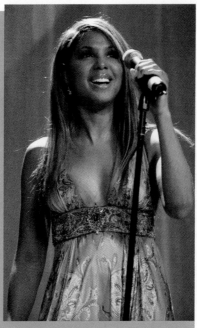

Why should I worry about cardiovascular disease?

Cardiovascular disease can affect even the youngest and most fit people. Grammy-winning singer Toni Braxton was first diagnosed with heart disease in 2003, at the age of 34. At that time she had pericarditis (an inflammation of the lining of the heart) and since then she has been diagnosed with high blood pressure, and briefly hospitalized for microvascular angina. In recent years, Braxton has been a vocal spokesperson for the American Heart Association, urging women not to ignore signs of possible heart disease or to assume that it won't affect them because they are too young and because it is a "men's disease." In fact, heart disease is the number one killer for both men and women.

Heart Function Heart activity depends on a complex interaction of biochemical, physical, and neurological signals. Here are the basic steps involved in heart function (Figure 12.2):

1. Deoxygenated blood enters the right atrium after having been circulated through the body.

2. From the right atrium, blood moves to the right ventricle and is pumped through the pulmonary artery to the lungs, where it receives oxygen.

3. Oxygenated blood from the lungs then returns to the left atrium of the heart.

4. Blood from the left atrium moves into the left ventricle. The left ventricle pumps blood through the aorta to all body parts.

Various types of blood vessels are required for different parts of this process. **Arteries** carry blood away from the heart; all arteries carry oxygenated blood, *except* for pulmonary arteries, which carry deoxygenated blood to the lungs, where the blood picks up oxygen and gives off carbon dioxide. As the arteries branch off from the heart, they branch into smaller blood vessels called **arterioles,** and then into even smaller blood vessels known as **capillaries.** Capillaries have thin walls that permit the exchange of oxygen, carbon dioxide, nutrients, and waste products with body cells. Carbon dioxide and other waste products are transported to the lungs and kidneys through **veins** and **venules** (small veins).

For the heart to function properly, the four chambers must beat in an organized manner. Your heartbeat is governed by an electrical impulse that directs the heart muscle to move when the impulse travels across it, which results in a sequential contraction of the four chambers. This signal starts in a small bundle of highly specialized cells, the **sinoatrial node (SA node),** located in the right atrium. The SA node serves as a natural pacemaker for the heart. People with a damaged SA node must often have a mechanical pacemaker implanted to ensure the smooth passage of blood through the sequential phases of the heartbeat.

The average adult heart at rest beats 70 to 80 times per minute, although a well-conditioned heart may beat only 50 to 60 times per minute to achieve the same results. If your resting heart rate is routinely in the high 80s or 90s, it may indicate that you are out of shape or suffering from some underlying illness. When overly stressed, a heart may beat more than 200 times per minute. A healthy heart functions more efficiently and is less likely to suffer damage from overwork.

Cardiovascular Disease

There are several types of cardiovascular disease, including atherosclerosis, coronary heart disease (CHD), angina pectoris, arrhythmia, congestive heart failure (CHF), and stroke.

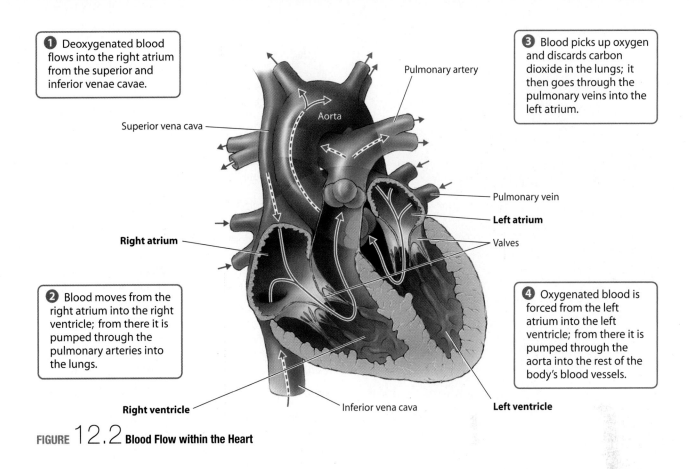

① Deoxygenated blood flows into the right atrium from the superior and inferior venae cavae.

Pulmonary artery

③ Blood picks up oxygen and discards carbon dioxide in the lungs; it then goes through the pulmonary veins into the left atrium.

Superior vena cava

Aorta

Pulmonary vein

Left atrium

Right atrium

Valves

② Blood moves from the right atrium into the right ventricle; from there it is pumped through the pulmonary arteries into the lungs.

④ Oxygenated blood is forced from the left atrium into the left ventricle; from there it is pumped through the aorta into the rest of the body's blood vessels.

Right ventricle

Inferior vena cava

Left ventricle

FIGURE 12.2 **Blood Flow within the Heart**

Many forms of CVD are potentially fatal; Figure 12.3 on page 356 presents the percentage breakdown of deaths from these different diseases in the United States.

Atherosclerosis

Arteriosclerosis, thickening and hardening of arteries, is a condition that underlies many cardiovascular health problems and is believed to be the biggest contributor to disease burden globally. **Atherosclerosis** is a type of arteriosclerosis and is characterized by deposits of fatty substances, cholesterol, cellular waste products, calcium, and fibrin (a clotting material in the blood) in the inner lining of an artery. *Hyperlipidemia* (an abnormally high blood lipid level) is a key factor in this process, and the resulting buildup is referred to as **plaque.**

As plaque accumulates, vessel walls become narrow and may eventually block blood flow or cause vessels to rupture. This is similar to putting your thumb over the end of a hose while water is running through it. Pressure builds within arteries just as pressure builds in the hose. If vessels are weakened and pressure persists, the artery may become weak and eventually burst. Fluctuation in the blood pressure levels within arteries may actually damage their internal walls, making it even more likely that plaque will accumulate.

Atherosclerosis is often called *coronary artery disease (CAD)* because of the resultant damage done to the body's main coronary arteries on the outer surface of the heart. These are the arteries that provide blood supply to the heart

muscle itself. Most heart attacks result from blockage of these arteries.

When atherosclerosis occurs in the lower extremities, such as in the feet, calves, or legs, or in the arms, it is called *peripheral artery disease (PAD)*. In recent years, increased attention has been drawn to PAD's role in subsequent blood clots and resultant heart attacks. In June 2008, when Tim Russert, a well-known NBC news correspondent, died suddenly of a heart attack after a long flight to Italy, there was speculation that he might have had a blood clot form in his legs from sitting for a prolonged period. This theory has not been confirmed; however, people are routinely advised to get up and walk around and flex or extend their legs to keep blood from pooling during long airplane flights or when sitting at a desk for long periods.

arteriosclerosis A general term for thickening and hardening of the arteries.

atherosclerosis Condition characterized by deposits of fatty substances (plaque) on the inner lining of an artery.

plaque Buildup of deposits in the arteries.

Whether from CAD or PAD, damage to vessels and threats to health can be severe. According to current thinking, four factors discussed later in this chapter are responsible for this damage: inflammation, elevated levels of cholesterol and triglycerides in the blood, high blood pressure, and tobacco smoke.

Coronary Heart Disease

Of all the major cardiovascular diseases, coronary heart disease (CHD) is the greatest killer, accounting for nearly one in

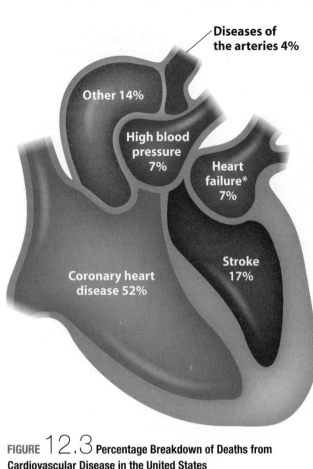

Diseases of
the arteries 4%

Other 14%

High blood
pressure
7%

Heart
failure*
7%

Coronary heart
disease 52%

Stroke
17%

FIGURE 12.3 **Percentage Breakdown of Deaths from Cardiovascular Disease in the United States**
Totals may not add up to 100% due to rounding.
*Not a true underlying cause.
Source: Data are from *Heart Disease and Stroke Statistics—2009 Update.* (Dallas: American Heart Association, 2009).

five deaths in the United States. Of the nearly 785,000 people who suffer a heart attack each year, over 37 percent will die because of it.[6] A **myocardial infarction (MI), or heart attack,** involves an area of the heart that suffers permanent damage because its normal blood supply has been blocked. This condition is often brought on by a blood clot in a coronary artery or an atherosclerotic narrowing that blocks an artery (see **Figure 12.4**). When blood does not flow readily, there is a corresponding decrease in oxygen flow. If the blockage is extremely minor, an otherwise healthy heart will adapt over time by enlarging existing blood vessels and growing new ones to reroute blood through other areas.

myocardial infarction (MI; heart attack) A blockage of normal blood supply to an area in the heart.
ischemia Reduced oxygen supply to a body part or organ.
angina pectoris Chest pain occurring as a result of reduced oxygen flow to the heart.

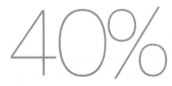

40% of heart attack victims die within the first hour following the heart attack.

When heart blockage is more severe, however, the body is unable to adapt on its own, and outside lifesaving support is critical. See the **Skills for Behavior Change** box above to learn what to do in case of a heart attack.

Angina Pectoris

Atherosclerosis and other circulatory impairments often reduce the heart's blood and oxygen supply, a condition known as **ischemia.** People with ischemia often suffer from varying degrees of **angina pectoris,** or chest pain and pressure. In fact, an estimated 4.3 million men and 5.5 million women suffer

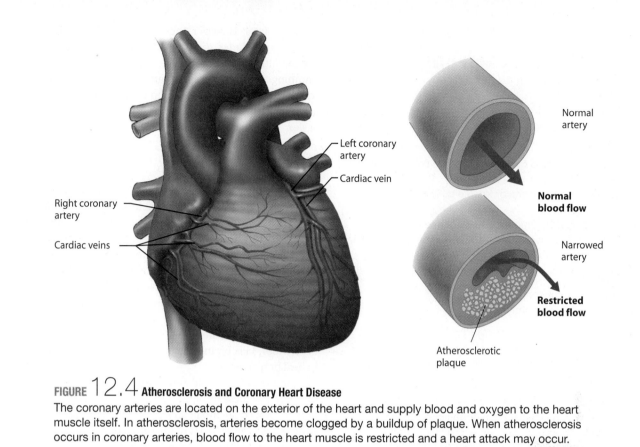

Right coronary artery

Cardiac veins

Left coronary artery

Cardiac vein

Normal artery

Normal blood flow

Narrowed artery

Restricted blood flow

Atherosclerotic plaque

FIGURE 12.4 **Atherosclerosis and Coronary Heart Disease**
The coronary arteries are located on the exterior of the heart and supply blood and oxygen to the heart muscle itself. In atherosclerosis, arteries become clogged by a buildup of plaque. When atherosclerosis occurs in coronary arteries, blood flow to the heart muscle is restricted and a heart attack may occur.
Sources: Adapted from Joan Salge Blake, *Nutrition & You,* p. 152; and Michael D. Johnson, *Human: Biology: Concepts and Current Issues,* 4th ed., p. 172. Both copyright © 2008 Pearson Education, Inc., publishing as Benjamin Cummings. Reprinted by permission.

mild to crushing forms of chest pain each day, many of whom take powerful medications to control their symptoms.[7] Symptoms may range from slight indigestion, to pain upon slight exertion, to a feeling that the heart is being crushed. Generally, the more serious the oxygen deprivation, the more severe the pain. Although angina pectoris is not a heart attack, it does indicate underlying heart disease.

Currently, there are several methods of treating angina. In mild cases, rest is critical. The most common treatments for more severe cases involve drugs that affect either the supply of blood to the heart muscle or the heart's demand for oxygen. Pain and discomfort are often relieved with *nitroglycerin,* a drug used to relax (dilate) veins, thereby reducing the amount of blood returning to the heart and thus lessening its workload. Patients whose angina is caused by spasms of the coronary arteries are often given drugs called *calcium channel blockers,* which prevent calcium atoms from passing through coronary arteries and causing heart contractions. They also appear to reduce blood pressure and slow heart rate. *Beta-blockers,* the other major type of drugs used to treat angina, control potential overactivity of the heart muscle.

Arrhythmias

Over 4 million Americans have experienced some type of **arrhythmia,** an irregularity in heart rhythm.[8] A person who complains of a racing heart in the absence of exercise or anxiety may be experiencing *tachycardia,* the medical term for abnormally fast heartbeat. On the other end of the continuum is *bradycardia,* or abnormally slow heartbeat. When a heart goes into **fibrillation,** it beats in a sporadic, quivering pattern that results in extreme inefficiency in moving blood through the cardiovascular system. If untreated, fibrillation may be fatal.

Not all arrhythmias are life threatening. In many instances, excessive caffeine or nicotine consumption can trigger an arrhythmia episode. However, severe cases may require drug therapy or external electrical stimulus to prevent serious complications.

arrhythmia An irregularity in heartbeat.
fibrillation A sporadic, quivering pattern of heartbeat that results in extreme inefficiency in moving blood through the cardiovascular system.
congestive heart failure (CHF) An abnormal cardiovascular condition that reflects impaired cardiac pumping and blood flow; pooling blood leads to congestion in body tissues.

Congestive Heart Failure

When the heart muscle is damaged or overworked and lacks the strength to keep blood circulating normally through the body, its chambers are often taxed to the limit. **Congestive heart failure (CHF)** affects over 5 million Americans and dramatically increases risk of premature death.[9] The heart muscle may be injured by a number of health conditions, including rheumatic fever, pneumonia, heart attack, or other cardiovascular problems. In some cases, the damage is due to

Stroke Warning Signs

As they do with heart attacks, people often misinterpret the early warning signs of a stroke, or wait too long to seek help. Stroke warning signs include:

* Sudden numbness or weakness of the face, arm, or leg, especially on one side of the body
* Sudden loss of speech or trouble talking or understanding speech
* Sudden dimness or loss of vision in one or both eyes
* Sudden trouble walking, dizziness, or loss of balance or coordination
* Sudden, severe headache with no known cause

If you suspect someone you are with is having a stroke, use the 60-second test:

1. Ask the person to smile.
2. Ask the person to raise both arms.
3. Ask him or her to repeat a simple sentence such as "It is sunny out today."

If you or someone with you has one or more of the signs above or has difficulty performing any of the tasks in the 60-second test, don't delay! Immediately call 9-1-1 or the emergency medical service (EMS) number so an ambulance (ideally with advanced life support) can be dispatched. Also, note the time so that you'll know when the first symptoms appeared. If given within 3 hours of the start of symptoms, a clot-busting drug called *tissue plasminogen activator* (tPA) can reduce long-term disability from ischemic strokes, the most common type of stroke.

Sources: American Heart Association, "Heart Attack, Stroke and Cardiac Arrest Warning Signs," 2009, www.americanheart.org/presenter.jhtml?identifier=3053; American Stroke Foundation, "How to Recognize a Stroke," 2009, www.americanstroke.org/content/view/17/46.

it can be fatal. However, most cases respond well to treatment that includes *diuretics* ("water pills") to relieve fluid accumulation; drugs, such as *digitalis,* that increase the pumping action of the heart; and drugs called *vasodilators,* which expand blood vessels and decrease resistance, allowing blood to flow more freely and making the heart's work easier.

Stroke

Like heart muscle, brain cells must have a continuous adequate supply of oxygen in order to survive. A **stroke** (also called a *cerebrovascular accident*) occurs when the blood supply to the brain is interrupted. Strokes may be either *ischemic* (caused by plaque formation that narrows blood flow or a clot that obstructs a blood vessel) or *hemorrhagic* (due to a weakening of a blood vessel that causes it to bulge or rupture). An **aneurysm** is the most well known of the hemorrhagic strokes, with nearly 40 percent of victims dying within 30 days.[11] When any of these events occurs, oxygen deprivation kills brain cells, which do not have the capacity to heal or regenerate.

Some strokes are mild and cause only temporary dizziness or slight weakness or numbness. More serious interruptions in blood flow may impair speech, memory, or motor control. Other strokes affect parts of the brain that regulate heart and lung function and kill within minutes. According to the American Heart Association's latest statistics, every year more than 6.5 million Americans suffer strokes, 150,000 of whom die as a result. Strokes cause countless levels of disability and suffering, and account for 1 in 15 deaths each year, surpassed only by CHD and cancer.[12]

About 15 percent of all major strokes are preceded days, weeks, or months earlier by **transient ischemic attacks (TIAs),** brief interruptions of the blood supply to the brain that cause only temporary impairment. Symptoms of TIAs include dizziness, particularly when first rising in the morning, weakness, temporary paralysis or numbness in the face or other regions, temporary memory loss, blurred vision, nausea, headache, slurred speech, or other unusual physiological reactions. Some people may actually experience unexpected falls or have blackouts; however, others may have no obvious symptoms. TIAs often indicate an impending major stroke. The earlier a stroke is recognized and treatment started, the more effective that treatment will be. See the **Skills for Behavior Change** box at left for tips on recognizing a stroke.

One of the greatest medical successes in recent years has been the decline in the fatality rate from strokes, which has dropped by one-third in the United States since the 1980s and continues to fall. Improved diagnostic procedures, better surgical options, clot-busting drugs injected soon after a stroke has occurred, and acute care centers specializing in stroke treatment and rehabilitation have all been factors.

Unfortunately, like many victims of other forms of CVD, stroke survivors do not always make a full recovery. Some 50 to 70 percent of stroke survivors regain functional independence, but 15 to 30 percent are permanently disabled and

radiation or chemotherapy treatments for cancer. These weakened muscles respond poorly, impairing blood flow out of the heart through the arteries. The return flow of blood through the veins begins to back up, causing congestion in body tissues. This pooling of blood enlarges the heart, makes it less efficient, and decreases the amount of blood that can be circulated. Fluid begins to accumulate in other body areas, such as the vessels in the legs, ankles, or lungs, where it can leak into surrounding tissues and cause swelling or difficulty in breathing.

Today, CHF is the single most frequent cause of hospitalization in the United States.[10] If untreated,

stroke A condition occurring when the brain is damaged by disrupted blood supply; also called *cerebrovascular accident.*

aneurysm A weakened blood vessel that may bulge under pressure and, in severe cases, burst.

transient ischemic attacks (TIAs) Brief interruption of the blood supply to the brain that causes only temporary impairment; often an indicator of impending major stroke.

require assistance. Today stroke is a leading cause of serious long-term disability and contributes a significant amount to Medicaid and Medicare expenses for older Americans, particularly women.

Reducing Your Risks

Scientific evidence has shown a large cluster of factors related to a person's being at a higher risk for developing cardiovascular diseases over the lifespan. Obesity, lack of physical activity, high cholesterol, and high blood pressure have all shown strong associations with subsequent CVD problems.[13] Interestingly, although selected factors increase risks specific to CVD, the combination of these and other risk factors appears also to increase risks for insulin resistance and type 2 diabetes.[14] The term **cardiometabolic risks** refers to these combined risks that indicate physical and biochemical changes that can lead to these major diseases. Some of these risks result from choices and behaviors, and so are modifiable, whereas others are inherited or are intrinsic to you (such as your age and gender) and therefore cannot be modified.

Metabolic Syndrome: Quick Risk Profile

Over the past decade, different health professionals have attempted to establish diagnostic cutoff points for a cluster of combined cardiometabolic risks, variably labeled as *syndrome X, insulin resistance syndrome,* and, most recently, **metabolic syndrome.** Historically, metabolic syndrome is believed to increase the risk for atherosclerotic heart disease by as much as three times the normal rates. It has captured international attention, as an estimated 50 million people potentially classify as having this syndrome. Typically, for a diagnosis of metabolic syndrome, a person would have three or more of the following risks:

- Abdominal obesity (waist measurement of more than 40 inches in men or 35 inches in women)
- Elevated blood fat (triglycerides greater than 150)
- Low levels of HDL ("good") cholesterol (less than 40 in men and less than 50 in women)
- Elevated blood pressure greater than 130/85
- Elevated fasting glucose greater than 100 mg/dL (a sign of insulin resistance or glucose intolerance)
- High levels of C-reactive proteins, indicating inflammation is present

The use of the metabolic syndrome classification and other, similar terms has been important in highlighting the relationship between the number of risks a person possesses and that person's likelihood of developing CVD and diabetes. Critics have questioned the usefulness of this risk profile, saying that the way data are collected makes it impossible to determine whether additional and compounded risk factors really contribute more to total risk. In addition, these classifications have not been as useful in telling patients and health care providers which risk factors might be more important and which ones should be given the highest priority when taking action to reduce risks.

Modifiable Risks

Although younger adults often think of heart attacks and strokes as something that happens to "old" people, the reality is that you may already be on course to have significant risks. The lifestyle choices you have made and continue making play a significant role in your likelihood for developing CVD well before you hit the golden years. In fact, hypertension, prediabetes, high cholesterol, and other risks have increased significantly among elementary, high school, and college students in the United States and globally. Blacks, Mexican American males, and white females are among the highest risk groups for both obesity and hypertension in children and adolescents, while male college students have higher rates of obesity, hypertension, and triglycerides than do female students.[15] Behaviors you choose today and over the coming decades can actively reduce or promote your risk for CVD. Among the most important behaviors you can adopt are choosing not to smoke, following a healthy diet, staying physically active, controlling blood pressure, and managing stress.

Avoid Tobacco In spite of massive campaigns to educate us about the dangers of smoking, and in spite of increasing numbers of states and municipalities that have enacted policies to go "smoke free," cigarette smoking remains the leading cause of preventable death in the United States, accounting for approximately one of every five deaths. These statistics are particularly surprising given the fact that smoking rates have declined by 49 percent among people aged 18 and older since 1965.[16] The risk for cardiovascular disease is 70 percent greater for smokers than it is for nonsmokers. Smokers who have a heart attack are more likely to die suddenly (within 1 hour) than are nonsmokers. Evidence also indicates that chronic exposure to environmental tobacco smoke (ETS, or secondhand smoke) increases the risk of heart disease by as much as 30 percent, with over 35,000 nonsmokers dying from ETS exposure each year.[17]

How does smoking damage the heart? There are two plausible explanations. One is that nicotine increases heart rate, heart output, blood pressure, and oxygen use by heart muscles. The heart is forced to work harder to obtain sufficient oxygen. The other explanation is that chemicals in smoke damage and inflame the lining of the coronary arteries, allowing cholesterol and plaque to accumulate more easily, increasing blood pressure and forcing the heart to work harder.

When people stop smoking, regardless of how long or how much they've smoked, their risk of heart disease declines rapidly. By 3 years after they quit, the risk of death from heart

cardiometabolic risks Risk factors that impact both the cardiovascular system and the body's biochemical metabolic processes.

metabolic syndrome A group of metabolic conditions occurring together that increases a person's risk of heart disease, stroke, and diabetes.

disease and stroke for people who had smoked a pack a day or less is almost the same as for people who have never smoked.

Cut Back on Saturated Fat and Cholesterol

Cholesterol is a soft, fatty, waxy substance found in the bloodstream and in your body cells. Although we hear only the bad things about it, in truth cholesterol plays an important role in the production of cell membranes and hormones and in other body functions. However, when blood levels of it get too high, risks for CVD escalate. Nearly 36 percent of adults in the United States aged 18 and above have been told they have high cholesterol, and vast numbers of others who have never been tested yet probably have higher than normal levels. Less than half of the people who should be on cholesterol-reducing medications are on them, and many who are on them are unable to reach their cholesterol level goals.

You get cholesterol from two primary sources: from your body (which involves genetic predisposition) and from food. Much of your cholesterol level is predetermined: 75 percent of blood cholesterol is produced by your liver and other cells, and the other 25 percent comes from the foods you eat. The good news is that the 25 percent you get from foods is the part where you can make real improvements in overall cholesterol profiles, even if you have a high genetic risk.

Diets high in saturated fat and *trans* fats are known to raise cholesterol levels, send the body's blood-clotting system into high gear, and make the blood more viscous in just a few hours, increasing the risk of heart attack or stroke. Increased blood levels of cholesterol also contribute to atherosclerosis. Switching to a low-fat diet lowers the risk of clotting; even a 10 percent decrease in total cholesterol levels may result in an estimated 30 percent reduction in the incidence of heart disease.[18]

Total cholesterol level isn't the only level to be concerned about; the type of cholesterol also matters. As discussed in Chapter 9, the two major types of blood cholesterol are *low-density lipoprotein (LDL)* and *high-density lipoprotein (HDL)*. Low-density lipoprotein, often referred to as "bad" cholesterol, is believed to build up on artery walls. In contrast, high-density lipoprotein, or "good" cholesterol, appears to remove cholesterol from artery walls, thus serving as a protector. In theory, if LDL levels get too high or HDL levels too low, cholesterol will accumulate inside arteries and lead to cardiovascular problems. Scientists now believe that there are other blood lipid factors that may also increase CVD risk, such as lipoprotein-associated phospholipase A_2 (Lp-PLA_2), an enzyme that circulates in the blood and attaches to LDL. Lp-PLA_2 plays an important role in plaque accumulation and increased risk for stroke and coronary events, particularly in men. Studies suggest that the higher the Lp-PLA_2 level, the higher the risk of developing CVD.[19] One relatively new consideration in the saturated fat dietary menace is apolipoprotein B (apo B), a primary component of LDL that is essential for cholesterol delivery to cells. Although the mechanism is unclear, some researchers believe that apo B levels may be more important to heart disease risk than total cholesterol or LDL levels.[20]

The most common types of lipids in your body are *triglycerides,* a major energy source that comes from food, and that is manufactured by the body. High levels of blood triglycerides are often found in people who have high cholesterol levels, heart problems or diabetes, or who are overweight. As people get older, heavier, or both, their triglyceride and cholesterol levels tend to rise. It is recommended that a baseline cholesterol test (known as a lipid panel or lipid profile) be taken at age 20, with follow-ups every 5 years. This test, which measures triglyceride levels as well as HDL, LDL, and total cholesterol levels, requires that you fast for 12 hours prior to the test, are well hydrated, and avoid coffee and tea prior to testing. Men over the age of 35 and women over the age of 45 should have their lipid profile checked annually, with more frequent tests for those at high risk. See Table 12.1 for recommended levels of cholesterol and trigylcerides.

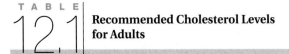

TABLE 12.1	Recommended Cholesterol Levels for Adults

Total Cholesterol Level (lower numbers are better)	
Less than 200 mg/dL	Desirable level that puts you at lower risk for coronary heart disease.
200 to 239 mg/dL	Borderline high
240 mg/dL and above	High blood cholesterol. A person with this level has more than twice the risk of coronary heart disease as someone whose cholesterol is below 200 mg/dL.

HDL Cholesterol Level (higher numbers are better)	
Less than 40 mg/dL (for men) Less than 50 mg/dL (for women)	Low HDL cholesterol. A major risk factor for heart disease.
60 mg/dL and above	High HDL cholesterol. An HDL of 60 mg/dL and above is considered to be protective against heart disease.

LDL Cholesterol Level (lower numbers are better)	
Less than 100 mg/dL	Optimal
100 to 129 mg/dL	Near or above optimal
130 to 159 mg/dL	Borderline high
160 to 189 mg/dL	High
190 mg/dL and above	Very high

Triglyceride Level (lower numbers are better)	
Less than 150 mg/dL	Normal
150–199 mg/dL	Borderline high
200–499 mg/dL	High
500 mg/dL and above	Very high

Source: American Heart Association, "Cholesterol Levels," 2009, www.americanheart.org/presenter.jhtml?identifier=4500.

Health Headlines

HEART-HEALTHY SUPER FOODS

Although there are countless recommendations for reducing your chances of heart disease through exercise, sleep, stress reduction, and so on, the foods you eat also play a major role in your risk by affecting the levels of triglycerides, LDL, and HDL in your bloodstream. Several foods have been shown to reduce the chances that cholesterol will be absorbed in the cells, reduce levels of LDL cholesterol, or enhance the protective effects of HDL cholesterol. To protect your heart, include the following in your diet:

✻ Fish high in omega-3 fatty acids. Consumption of fish such as salmon, sardines, and herring helps reduce blood pressure and the risk associated with blood clots as well as lowering cholesterol.

✻ Olive oil. Using any of a number of monounsaturated fats in cooking, particularly extra virgin olive oil, helps lower total cholesterol and raise your HDL levels. Canola oil; margarine labeled "*trans* fat free"; and cholesterol-lowering margarines such as Benecol, Promise Activ, or Smart Balance are also excellent choices.

✻ Whole grains and fiber. Getting enough fiber each day in the form of 100 percent whole wheat, steel cut oats, oat bran, flaxseed, fruits, and vegetables helps lower LDL or "bad" cholesterol. Soluble fiber, in particular, seems to keep cholesterol from being absorbed in the intestines.

✻ Plant sterols and stanols. Although these sound like substances derived in the lab, they are actually essential components of plant membranes and are found naturally in vegetables, fruits, and legumes. In addition, many food products, including juices and yogurt, are now fortified with them. These compounds are believed to benefit your heart health by blocking cholesterol absorption in the bloodstream, thus reducing LDL levels.

✻ Nuts. Long maligned for being high in calories, walnuts, almonds, and other nuts are naturally high in omega-3 fatty acids, which are important in lowering cholesterol and good for the blood vessels themselves.

✻ Chocolate, red wine, and green tea. Could it really be true? Are dark chocolate, red wine, green tea, and other foods really protecting us from cardiovascular diseases? Over the past decade, several major studies have indicated that dark chocolate appears to significantly reduce blood pressure, whereas green tea seems to reduce LDL cholesterol. The flavonoids in chocolate and green tea act as powerful antioxidants that protect the cells of the heart and blood vessels. Red wine also contains flavonoids and research initially seemed to support beneficial effects; however, newer research has been conflicting. Much more research on all of these foods must be done to say definitively how beneficial they might be, and what dosage is recommended.

Sources: A. Mente, L. deKoning, M. Shannon, and S. Anand, "A Systematic Review of the Evidence Supporting a Causal Link between Dietary Factors and Coronary Heart Disease," *Archives of Internal Medicine* 169, no. 7 (2009): 659–69; L. Hooper, P. Kroon, et al., "Flavonoids, Flavonoid-Rich Foods, and Cardiovascular Risk: A Meta-Analysis of Randomized Controlled Trials," *American Journal of Clinical Nutrition* 88, no. 1 (2008): 38–50; E. Corti et al., "Cocoa and Cardiovascular Health," *Circulation* 119, no. 10 (2009):1433–41; M. Corder, "Red Wine, Chocolate and Vascular Health: Developing the Evidence Base," *Heart* 94, no. 7 (2008): 821–23; N. Tanabe et al., "Consumption of Green and Roasted Teas and the Risk of Stroke Incidence: Results from the Tokamachi-Nakasato Cohort Study in Japan," *International Journal of Epidemiology* 37, no. 5 (2008): 1030–40.

In general, LDL is more closely associated with cardiovascular risk than is total cholesterol. However, most authorities agree that looking only at LDL ignores the positive effects of HDL. Perhaps the best method of evaluating risk is to examine the ratio of HDL to total cholesterol, or the percentage of HDL in total cholesterol. If the level of HDL is lower than 35 Mg/dL, the risk increases dramatically. To reduce risk, the goal is to manage the ratio of HDL to total cholesterol by lowering LDL levels, raising HDL, or both. Regular exercise and a healthy diet low in saturated fat continue to be the best methods for maintaining healthy ratios. See the **Health Headlines** box above for information about foods and dietary practices that can help maintain healthy cholesterol levels.

Of the more than 100 million Americans who have high cholesterol levels, almost half, particularly those at the low to moderate risk levels, should be able to reach their LDL and HDL goals through lifestyle changes alone. People who are at higher risk or those for whom lifestyle modifications are not effective may need to take cholesterol-lowering drugs while they continue modifying their lifestyle.

Maintain a Healthy Weight No question about it—body weight plays a role in CVD. Researchers are not sure whether high-fat, high-sugar, high-calorie diets are a direct risk for CVD or whether they invite risk by causing obesity, which strains the heart, forcing it to push blood through the many miles of capillaries that supply each pound of fat. A heart that has to continuously move blood through an overabundance of vessels may become damaged.

Overweight people are more likely to develop heart disease and stroke even if they have no other risk factors. If you're heavy, losing even 5 to 10 pounds can make a significant difference. This is especially true if you're an "apple" (thicker around your upper body and waist) rather than a "pear" (thicker around your hips and thighs). See Chapter 10 for tips on weight management.

Exercise Regularly
Inactivity is a clear risk factor for CVD.[21] The good news is that you do not have to be an exercise fanatic to reduce your risk. Even modest levels of low-intensity physical activity—walking, gardening, housework, dancing—are beneficial if done regularly and over the long term. Exercise can increase HDL, lower triglycerides, and reduce coronary risks in several ways. For more information on the health benefits of exercise, see Chapter 11.

Control Diabetes
Research underscores the unique CVD risks for people with diabetes.[22] Diabetics who have taken insulin for a number of years have a greater chance of developing CVD. In fact, CVD is the leading cause of death among diabetic patients. Because overweight people have a higher risk for diabetes, distinguishing between the effects of the two conditions is difficult. People with diabetes also tend to have elevated blood fat levels, increased atherosclerosis, and a tendency toward deterioration of small blood vessels, particularly in the eyes and extremities. However, through a prescribed regimen of diet, exercise, and medication, they can control much of their increased risk for CVD. See **Focus On: Your Risk for Diabetes** beginning on page 386 for more on preventing and controlling diabetes.

Control Your Blood Pressure
Hypertension refers to sustained high blood pressure. In general, the higher your blood pressure is, the greater your risk will be for CVD. Hypertension is known as the silent killer because it usually has no symptoms. Its prevalence has increased by over 30 percent in the past 10 years; today one in three adults in the United States has blood pressure above the recommended level.[23] The prevalence of high blood pressure in Blacks in the United States is among the highest in the world and it's increasing. More than 44 percent of Black women have HBP, compared to 28 percent among white women.

Blood pressure is measured in two parts and is expressed as a fraction—for example, 110/80, or "110 over 80." Both values are measured in *millimeters of mercury* (mm Hg). The first number refers to **systolic pressure,** or the pressure being applied to the walls of the arteries when the heart contracts, pumping blood to the rest of the body. The second value is **diastolic pressure,** or the pressure applied to the walls of the arteries during the heart's relaxation phase. During this phase, blood is reentering the chambers of the heart, preparing for the next heartbeat.

Normal blood pressure varies depending on weight; age; physical condition; and for different groups of people, such as women and minorities. Systolic blood pressure tends to increase with age, whereas diastolic blood pressure increases until age 55 and then declines. As a rule, men have a greater risk for high blood pressure than do women until age 55, when their risks become about equal. After age 75, women are more likely to have high blood pressure than men.[24]

For the average person, 110/80 is a healthy blood pressure level. High blood pressure is usually diagnosed when systolic pressure is 140 or above. Diastolic pressure does not have to be high to indicate high blood pressure. When only systolic pressure is high, the condition is known as *isolated systolic hypertension (ISH)*, the most common form of high blood pressure in older Americans. See Table 12.2 for a summary of blood pressure values and what they mean.

Treatment of hypertension can involve dietary changes (reducing sodium and calorie intake), weight loss (when appropriate), the use of diuretics and other medications (only when prescribed by a physician), regular exercise, treatment of sleep disorders such as sleep apnea, and the practice of relaxation techniques and effective coping and communication skills.

Manage Stress
Some scientists have noted a relationship between CVD risk and a person's stress level, behavior habits, and socioeconomic status. These factors may influence established risk factors. For example, people under stress may start smoking or smoke more than they otherwise

hypertension Sustained elevated blood pressure.
systolic pressure The upper number in the fraction that measures blood pressure, indicating pressure on the walls of the arteries when the heart contracts.
diastolic pressure The lower number in the fraction that measures blood pressure, indicating pressure on the walls of the arteries during the relaxation phase of heart activity.

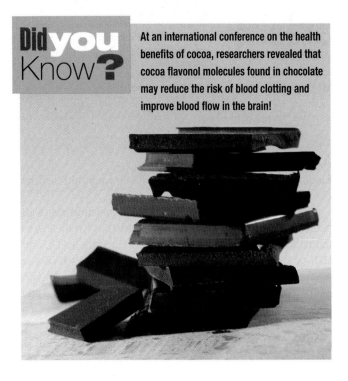

Did you Know?

At an international conference on the health benefits of cocoa, researchers revealed that cocoa flavonol molecules found in chocolate may reduce the risk of blood clotting and improve blood flow in the brain!

TABLE

12.2 | **Blood Pressure Classifications**

Classification	Systolic Reading (mm Hg)		Diastolic Reading (mm Hg)
Normal	<120	and	<80
Prehypertension	120–139	or	80–89
Hypertension			
Stage 1	140–159	or	90–99
Stage 2	≥160	or	≥100

Note: If systolic and diastolic readings fall into different categories, treatment is determined by the highest category. Readings are based on the average of two or more properly measured, seated readings on each of two or more health care provider visits.

Source: National Heart, Lung, and Blood Institute, *The Seventh Report of the Joint National Committee on Prevention, Detection, Evaluation, and Treatment of High Blood Pressure* (NIH Publication no. 03-5233) (Bethesda, MD: National Institutes of Health, revised June 2005).

would. A large study funded by the National Heart, Lung, and Blood Institute found that impatience and hostility, two key components of the Type A behavior pattern, increase young adults' risk of developing high blood pressure. Other related factors, such as competitiveness, depression, and anxiety, did not appear to increase risk. In recent years, scientists have tended to agree that unresolved stress—whether real or perceived, personal, work related, or from a combination of factors—appears to increase risk for hypertension, heart disease, and stroke. Although the exact mechanism is unknown, scientists are closer to discovering why stress can affect us so negatively. Newer studies indicate that chronic stress may result in three times the risk of hypertension, CHD, and sudden cardiac death and that there is a link between anxiety, depression, and negative cardiovascular effects.[25] See Chapter 3 for more on managing stress.

Nonmodifiable Risks

There are, unfortunately, some risk factors for CVD that we cannot prevent or control. The most important are these:

● **Race and ethnicity.** African Americans are at 45 percent greater risk for hypertension and heart disease and tend to have more severe levels of high blood pressure than Caucasians. The rate of high blood pressure in African Americans is among the highest in the world. Heart disease risk is also higher among Mexican Americans, Native Americans, and native Hawaiians (partly due to higher rates of obesity and diabetes).

● **Heredity.** A family history of heart disease appears to increase risk significantly.[26] In fact, as stated previously, the amount of cholesterol you produce, tendencies to form plaque, and a host of other factors seem to have genetic links.

If you have close relatives with CVD, your risk may be double that of others. The younger these relatives are, and the closer their relationship to you (parents or siblings, in particular), the greater your risk will be. The difficulty comes in sorting out genetic influences from the multiple confounders common among family members that may also influence risk, including environment, stress, dietary habits, and so on. Newer research has focused on studying the interactions between nutrition and genes (nutrigenetics) and the role that diet may play in increasing or decreasing risks among certain genetic profiles.[27]

● **Age.** Although cardiovascular disease can affect people of any age, 75 percent of all heart attacks occur in people over age 65. The rate of CVD increases with age for both sexes.

● **Gender.** Men are at greater risk for CVD until about age 60. Women under age 35 have a fairly low risk unless they have high blood pressure, kidney problems, or diabetes. Using oral contraceptives and smoking also increase the risk. Hormonal factors appear to reduce risk for women, although after menopause or after estrogen levels are otherwise reduced (e.g., because of hysterectomy), women's LDL levels tend to go up, which increases their chances for CVD.

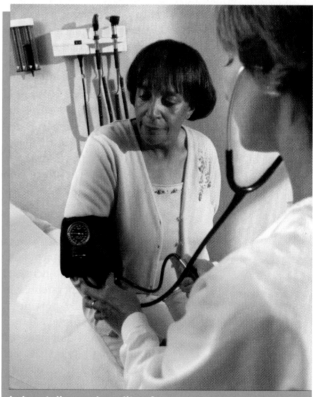

Is heart disease hereditary?

Many behavioral and environmental factors contribute to a person's risk for cardiovascular diseases, but research suggests that there are hereditary aspects as well. If there is a history of CVD in your family or your racial or ethnic background indicates a propensity for CVD, it is all the more important for you to have regular blood pressure and blood cholesterol screenings, and for you to avoid lifestyle risks including tobacco use, physical inactivity, and poor nutrition.

Other Risk Factors Being Studied

Several other factors and indicators have been linked to CVD risk, including inflammation and homocysteine levels.

Inflammation and C-Reactive Protein Recent research has prompted many experts to believe that inflammation may play a major role in atherosclerosis development. Inflammation occurs when tissues are injured by bacteria, trauma, toxins, or heat, among others. Injured vessel walls are more prone to plaque formation. To date, several factors, including cigarette smoke, high blood pressure, high LDL cholesterol, diabetes mellitus, certain forms of arthritis, and exposure to toxic substances, have all been linked to increased risk of inflammation. However, the greatest risk appears to be from certain infectious disease pathogens, most notably *Chlamydia pneumoniae,* a common cause of respiratory infections; *Helicobacter pylori* (a bacterium that causes ulcers); herpes simplex virus (a virus that most of us have been exposed to); and *Cytomegalovirus* (another herpes virus infecting most Americans before the age of 40). During an inflammatory reaction, **C-reactive proteins (CRPs)** tend to be present at high levels. Many scientists believe the presence of these proteins in the blood may signal elevated risk for angina and heart attack. Doctors can test patients using a highly sensitive assay called hs-CRP; if levels are high, action could be taken to prevent progression to a heart attack or other coronary event.[28]

C-reactive protein (CRP) A protein whose blood levels rise in response to inflammation.
homocysteine An amino acid normally present in the blood that, when found at high levels, may be related to higher risk of cardiovascular disease.
electrocardiogram (ECG) A record of the electrical activity of the heart; may be measured during a stress test.
angiography A technique for examining blockages in heart arteries.

Tomatoes, citrus fruit, vegetables, and fortified grain products are good sources of the daily recommended 400 micrograms of folic acid, which is believed to help lower blood levels of homocysteine.

Homocysteine Researchers have discovered another substance that may signal increased risk for CVD: **homocysteine,** an amino acid normally present in the blood. When present at high levels, homocysteine may be related to higher risk of coronary heart disease, stroke, and peripheral vascular disease. Although research is still in its infancy in this area, scientists hypothesize that homocysteine works in much the same way as CRP, inflaming the inner lining of the arterial walls and promoting fat deposits on the damaged walls and development of blood clots.[29] Folic acid and other B vitamins may help break down homocysteine in the body; however, conclusive evidence of risk reduction from folic acid is not available, and authorities such as the American Heart Association do not currently recommend taking folic acid supplements to lower homocysteine levels and prevent CVD.[30] For now, a healthy, balanced diet that includes at least five servings of fruits and vegetables a day is the best preventive action.

Weapons against Cardiovascular Disease

Today, CVD patients have many diagnostic, treatment, prevention, and rehabilitation options that were not available a generation ago. Medications can strengthen heartbeat, control arrhythmias, remove fluids (in the case of congestive heart failure), reduce blood pressure, improve heart function, and reduce pain. Among the most common groups of drugs are the following: *statins*, chemicals used to lower blood cholesterol levels; *ace-inhibitors*, which cause the muscles surrounding blood vessels to contract, thereby lowering blood pressure; and *beta-blockers*, which reduce blood pressure by blocking the effects of the hormone epinephrine. New diagnostic procedures, surgical techniques, and devices are saving countless lives. Even long-standing methods of CPR have been changed recently to focus primarily on chest compressions rather than mouth-to-mouth procedures. The thinking behind this is that people will be more likely to do CPR if the risk for exchange of body fluids is reduced—any effort to save a person in trouble is better than inaction.

Techniques for Diagnosing Cardiovascular Disease

Several techniques are used to diagnose CVD, including electrocardiogram, angiography, and positron emission tomography scans. An **electrocardiogram (ECG)** is a record of the electrical activity of the heart. Patients may undergo a *stress test*—standard exercise on a stationary bike or treadmill with an electrocardiogram and no injections—or a *nuclear stress test*, which involves injecting a radioactive dye and taking images of the heart to reveal problems with blood flow. While these tests provide a good indicator of potential heart blockage or blood flow abnormalities, a more accurate method of testing for heart disease is **angiography** (often referred to as *cardiac catheterization*). In this procedure, a needle-thin tube called a *catheter* is threaded through heart arteries, a dye is injected, and an X-ray image is taken to discover which areas are blocked. A more recent and even more effective method of measuring heart activity is *positron emission tomography (PET)*, which produces three-dimensional images of the heart as blood flows through it. Other tests include the following:

- **Magnetic resonance imaging (MRI).** This test uses powerful magnets to look inside the body. Computer-generated pictures can show the heart muscle and help physicians identify damage from a heart attack and evaluate disease of larger blood vessels such as the aorta.
- **Ultrafast computed tomography (CT).** This is an especially fast form of X-ray imaging of the heart designed to evaluate bypass grafts, diagnose ventricular function, and measure calcium deposits.

One of the newest forms of CT scans is used to assess your *cardiac calcium score*, an indicator of the level of calcium in the plaque in your coronary arteries: The greater amount of calcium, the higher your calcium score and the greater your risk of heart attack. Although some people ask for this as a noninvasive measure of risk (compared to angiograms), recent reports of high radiation levels from some machines have caused many to rethink this procedure.

Bypass Surgery and Angioplasty

Coronary bypass surgery has helped many patients who suffered coronary blockages or heart attacks. In a coronary artery bypass graft (CABG, referred to as a "cabbage"), a blood vessel is taken from another site in the patient's body (usually the saphenous vein in the leg or the internal thoracic artery in the chest) and implanted to "bypass" blocked coronary arteries and transport blood to heart tissue.

Another procedure, **angioplasty** (sometimes called *balloon angioplasty*), carries fewer risks and may be more effective than bypass surgery in selected cases. As in angiography, a thin catheter is threaded through blocked heart arteries. The catheter has a balloon at the tip, which is inflated to flatten fatty deposits against the artery walls, allowing blood to flow more freely. A *stent* (a meshlike tube) may be inserted to prop open the artery. In about 30 percent of patients, the treated arteries become clogged again within 6 months. Some surgeons argue that given this high rate of recurrence, bypass may be a more effective treatment. Today, newer forms of laser angioplasty and *atherectomy*, a procedure that removes plaque, are being done in several clinics.

Can Aspirin Help Heart Disease?

Today, over 50 million people (36% of all adults) pop an aspirin everyday, believing that this will prevent a heart attack.[31] Research indicates that low doses of aspirin (75–81 mg daily or every other day) are beneficial to heart patients because of the drug's blood-thinning properties. Higher levels do not provide significantly more protection. Aspirin has even been advised as a preventive strategy for people with no current heart disease symptoms. Major problems associated with chronic aspirin use are gastrointestinal intolerance and a tendency for some people to have difficulty with blood clotting, and these factors may outweigh aspirin's benefits in some cases.

An Overview of Cancer

Although heart disease is the number one cause of death in the United States, cancer continues to be the second leading cause of death for all age groups, even though cancer-related mortality rates have declined over the past decade.[32] **Five-year survival rates** (the relative rates for survival in persons who are living 5 years after diagnosis) are up dramatically from the virtual death sentences of many cancers in the early 1900s and the 40 to 50 percent survival rates of the 1960s and 1970s. Today, of the approximately 1.5 million people diagnosed each year, about 66 percent will still be alive 5 years from now.[33] Many will be considered "cured," meaning that they have no subsequent cancer in their bodies and can expect to live a long and productive life. Improvements in diagnosis and treatment mean that cancers that used to present a very poor outlook are often cured today.

coronary bypass surgery A surgical technique whereby a blood vessel taken from another part of the body is implanted to bypass a clogged coronary artery.

angioplasty A technique in which a catheter with a balloon at the tip is inserted into a clogged artery; the balloon is inflated to flatten fatty deposits against artery walls and a stent is typically inserted to keep the artery open.

five-year survival rates The percentage of people in a study or treatment group who are alive 5 years after they were diagnosed with or treated for cancer.

cancer A large group of diseases characterized by the uncontrolled growth and spread of abnormal cells.

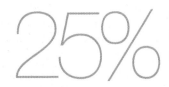 **of all deaths that occur on a given day are from some form of cancer.**

During 2009, approximately 562,340 Americans died of cancer, and nearly 1.5 million new cases were diagnosed.[34] Of these, one-third of the cancers were related to poor nutrition, physical inactivity, and obesity, which means they could have been prevented. Certain other cancers are related to exposure to infectious organisms such as hepatitis B virus (HBV), human papillomavirus (HPV; also the cause of genital warts), HIV (the virus that causes AIDS), *Helicobacter pylori* (the bacterium responsible for most peptic ulcers), and others, and could be prevented through behavioral changes, vaccines, or antibiotics.

What Is Cancer?

Cancer is the name given to a large group of diseases characterized by the uncontrolled growth and spread of abnormal cells. If these cells aren't stopped, they can impair vital functions of the body and lead to death. Think of a healthy cell as a small computer, programmed to operate in a particular fashion. When something interrupts normal cell programming, uncontrolled growth and abnormal cellular development result in a **neoplasm,** a new growth of tissue serving no physiological function. This neoplasmic mass often forms a clumping of cells known as a **tumor.**

Not all tumors are **malignant** (cancerous); in fact, most are **benign** (noncancerous). Benign tumors are generally harmless unless they grow to obstruct or crowd out normal tissues. A benign tumor of the brain, for instance, is life threatening when it grows enough to restrict blood flow and cause a stroke. The only way to determine whether a tumor is malignant is through **biopsy,** or microscopic examination of cell development.

Benign and malignant tumors differ in several key ways. Benign tumors generally consist of ordinary-looking cells enclosed in a fibrous shell or capsule that prevents their spreading to other body areas. Malignant tumors are usually not enclosed in a protective capsule and can therefore spread to other organs (Figure 12.5). This process, known as **metastasis,** makes some forms of cancer particularly aggressive in their ability to overcome bodily defenses. By the time they are diagnosed, malignant tumors have frequently metastasized throughout the body, making treatment extremely difficult. Unlike benign tumors, which merely expand to take over a given space, malignant cells invade surrounding tissue, emitting clawlike protrusions that disturb the RNA and DNA within normal cells. Disrupting these substances, which control cellular metabolism and reproduction, produces **mutant cells** that differ in form, quality, and function from normal cells.

neoplasm A new growth of tissue that serves no physiological function and results from uncontrolled, abnormal cellular development.

tumor A neoplasmic mass that grows more rapidly than surrounding tissue.

malignant Very dangerous or harmful; refers to a cancerous tumor.

benign Harmless; refers to a noncancerous tumor.

biopsy Microscopic examination of tissue to determine whether a cancer is present.

metastasis Process by which cancer spreads from one area to different areas of the body.

mutant cells Cells that differ in form, quality, or function from normal cells.

carcinogens Cancer-causing agents.

What Causes Cancer?

After decades of research, scientists and epidemiologists believe that most cancers are, at least in theory, preventable. Many specific causes of cancer are well documented, the most important of which are represented by two major classes of factors: hereditary risk and acquired (environmental) risk. Heredity factors cannot be modified. Environmental factors are potentially modifiable. In this context they include the macrophysical environment and personal lifestyle factors and situations, such as tobacco use; poor nutrition; physical inactivity; obesity; certain infectious agents; certain medical treatments; drug and alcohol consumption; excessive sun exposure; and exposures to **carcinogens** (cancer-causing agents), such as chemicals in our foods, the air we breathe, the water we drink, and the homes we live in. Several of these hereditary and environmental factors may interact to make cancer more likely, accelerate cancer progression, or increase individual susceptibility during certain periods of life, but the mechanisms are not fully understood. We do not know why some people have malignant cells in their

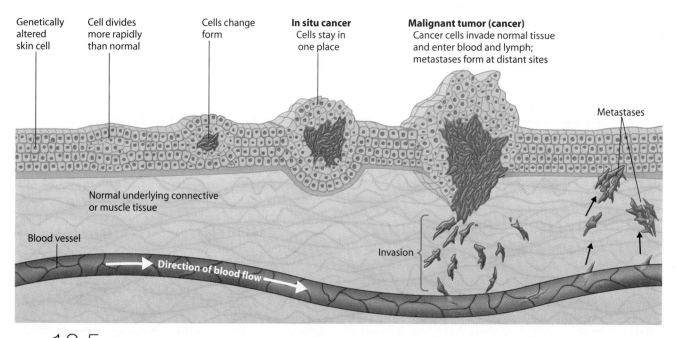

FIGURE 12.5 **Metastasis**
A mutation to the genetic material of a skin cell triggers abnormal cell division and changes cell formation, resulting in a cancerous tumor. If the tumor remains localized, it is considered *in situ* cancer. If the tumor spreads, it is considered a malignant cancer.

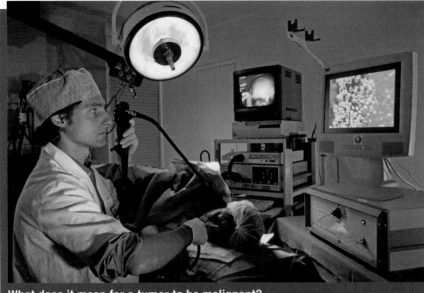

What does it mean for a tumor to be malignant?

A malignant tumor is one whose cells are cancerous. Malignant tumors are generally more dangerous than benign tumors because cancer cells divide quickly and can spread, or metastasize, from the original tumor to other parts of the body. Physicians usually order biopsies of tumors, in which sample cells are taken from the tumor and studied under a microscope to determine whether they are cancerous. Newer techniques, like the minimally invasive "optical biopsy" shown here, allow for the microscopic examination of tissue without doing a physical biopsy.

behaviors. For example, if you are a man and smoke, your relative risk of getting lung cancer is about 23 times greater than that of a male nonsmoker.[36]

Over the years, researchers have found that diet, a sedentary lifestyle (and resultant obesity), overconsumption of alcohol, tobacco use, stress, and other lifestyle factors seem to play a role in the incidence of cancer. Keep in mind that a high relative risk does not guarantee cause and effect. It merely indicates the likelihood of a particular risk factor being related to a particular outcome.

Tobacco Use Of all the potential risk factors for cancer, smoking is among the greatest. In the United States, tobacco is responsible for nearly one in five deaths annually, accounting for at least 30 percent of all cancer deaths and 87 percent of all lung cancer deaths.[37] In fact, by all accounts, smoking is the leading cause of preventable death in the United States and around the world today.[38] Smoking is associated with increased risk of at least 15 different cancers, including those of the nasopharynx, nasal cavity, paranasal sinuses, lip, oral cavity, pharynx, larynx, lung, esophagus, pancreas, uterine cervix, kidney, bladder, and stomach, and acute myeloid leukemia. See Chapter 8 for more on trends in tobacco use.

body and never develop cancer, whereas others may eventually develop the disease.

Lifestyle Risks

Anyone can develop cancer; however, most cases affect adults beginning in middle age. In fact, nearly 76 percent of cancers are diagnosed at age 55 and above. Cancer researchers refer to one's cancer risk when they assess risk factors. *Lifetime risk* refers to the probability that an individual, over the course of a lifetime, will develop cancer or die from it. In the United States, men have a lifetime risk of about one in two; women have a lower risk, at one in three.[35] See Table 12.3 on the next page for an overview of the probability of developing cancer by age and sex.

Relative risk is a measure of the strength of the relationship between risk factors and a particular cancer. Basically, relative risk compares your risk if you engage in certain known risk behaviors with that of someone who does not engage in such

Of the several lifestyle risk factors for cancer, tobacco use is perhaps the most significant and the most preventable.

Poor Nutrition, Physical Inactivity, and Obesity
Mounting scientific evidence suggests that about one-third of the cancer deaths that occur in the United States each year may be due to lifestyle factors such as overweight or obesity, physical inactivity, and poor nutrition—cancers that can be prevented! Dietary choices and physical activity are the most important modifiable determinants of cancer risk (besides not smoking). Several studies indicate a relationship between a high body mass index (BMI) and death rates from cancers of the esophagus, colon, rectum, liver, stomach, kidney, and pancreas. Newer studies point to differences in risks by gender and race.[39]

Women with a high BMI have a higher mortality rate from breast,

TABLE

12.3

Probability of Developing Invasive Cancers during Selected Age Intervals by Sex, United States, 2003–2005*

Site	Sex	Birth to age 39	Ages 40 to 59	Lifetime
All types[†]	Male	1 in 70	1 in 12	1 in 2
	Female	1 in 48	1 in 11	1 in 3
Breast	Female	1 in 208	1 in 26	1 in 8
Colon and rectum	Male	1 in 1,296	1 in 109	1 in 18
	Female	1 in 1,343	1 in 138	1 in 20
Lung and bronchus	Male	1 in 3,398	1 in 101	1 in 13
	Female	1 in 2,997	1 in 124	1 in 16
Melanoma of the skin[§]	Male	1 in 645	1 in 157	1 in 39
	Female	1 in 370	1 in 189	1 in 58
Prostate	Male	1 in 10,002	1 in 41	1 in 6
Uterine cervix	Female	1 in 651	1 in 368	1 in 145
Uterine corpus	Female	1 in 1,499	1 in 140	1 in 40

*For people free of cancer at beginning of age interval.
[†]Excludes basal and squamous cell skin cancers and in situ cancers except in the urinary bladder.
[§]Statistic is for whites only.

Sources: DevCan: Probability of Developing or Dying of Cancer 6.3.0. Statistical Research and Applications Branch, National Cancer Institute, 2008, http://srab.cancer.gov/devcan; American Cancer Society, Surveillance and Health Policy Research, 2009.

Genetic and Physiological Risks

If your parents, aunts and uncles, siblings, or other close family members develop cancer, does it mean that you have a genetic predisposition toward it? Although there is still much uncertainty about this, scientists believe that about 5 percent of all cancers are strongly hereditary, in that some people may be more predisposed to the malfunctioning of genes that ultimately cause cancer.[42]

Cancer development can be affected by suspected cancer-causing genes called **oncogenes.** While these genes are typically dormant, certain conditions such as age, stress, and exposure to carcinogens, viruses, and radiation may activate them. Once activated, they cause cells to grow and reproduce uncontrollably. Scientists are uncertain whether only people who develop cancer have oncogenes, or whether we all have genes that can become oncogenes under certain conditions.

Certain cancers, particularly those of the breast, stomach, colon, prostate, uterus, ovaries, and lungs, appear to run in families. For example, a woman runs a much higher risk of breast cancer if her mother or sisters (primary relatives) have had the disease, particularly at a young age. Hodgkin's disease and certain leukemias show similar familial patterns. Can we attribute these familial patterns to genetic susceptibility or to the fact that people in the same families experience similar environmental risks? To date, the research in this area is inconclusive. It is possible that we can inherit a tendency toward a cancer-prone, weak immune system or, conversely, that we can inherit a cancer-fighting potential. But the complex interaction of hereditary predisposition, lifestyle, and environment on the development of cancer makes it a challenge to determine a single cause. Even among those predisposed to mutations, avoiding risks may decrease chances of cancer development.

Occupational and Environmental Risks

Overall, workplace hazards account for only a small percentage of all cancers. However, various substances are known to cause cancer when exposure levels are high or prolonged. One is asbestos, a fibrous material once widely used in the construction, insulation, and automobile industries. Nickel, chromate, and chemicals such as benzene, arsenic, and vinyl chloride have been shown definitively to be carcinogens for humans. Also, people who routinely work with certain dyes

uterine, cervical, and ovarian cancers; men with a high BMI have higher death rates from prostate and stomach cancers. In a study of over 900,000 U.S. adults, 34 percent of all cancer deaths were attributable to overweight and obesity. The relative risk of breast cancer in postmenopausal women is 50 percent higher for obese women than it is for nonobese women, whereas the relative risk of colon cancer in men is 40 percent higher for obese men than it is for nonobese men. The relative risks of gallbladder and endometrial cancers are five times higher in obese individuals than they are in individuals of healthy weight. Numerous other studies support the link between cancer and obesity.[40]

oncogenes Suspected cancer-causing genes.

Stress and Psychosocial Risks Some researchers claim that social and psychological factors play a major role in determining whether a person gets cancer. Stress has been implicated in increased susceptibility to several types of cancers. Although medical personnel are skeptical of overly simplistic solutions, we cannot rule out the possibility that negative emotional states contribute to illness. People who are under chronic, severe stress or who suffer from depression or other persistent emotional problems show higher rates of cancer than their healthy counterparts. Several newer studies appear to support the premise that stress can play a role in cancer development.[41] Sleep disturbances or an unhealthy diet may weaken the body's immune system, increasing susceptibility to cancer.

GREEN GUIDE

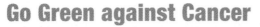

Go Green against Cancer

We live in an environment that is filled with potential cancer-causing agents. Some of them are natural, but many are created by humans, or increased by human activities. There are many things you can do to help reduce the number of carcinogens in the environment and to limit your exposure to those that are there. The following are just a few ideas:

1. Leave the car at home. Try commuting by bicycle or by foot instead of driving a vehicle. This will reduce your daily carbon emissions and your risk for cancer by increasing your physical activity.

2. Choose organic foods when possible. Conventional produce is often sprayed with chemicals and pesticides. When we eat these chemicals, our risk for cancer can be elevated.

3. When shopping for home furnishings, explore ecofriendly furniture, upholstery, and home textiles. Many furnishings are manufactured with toxic chemicals that are released into the air. This can dramatically reduce indoor air quality and increase your risk for cancer. Select products that have not been treated with stain-resistant chemicals and look for ecofriendly flooring, carpets, and other products to ensure the best possible indoor air quality and minimize carcinogenic exposures. Such ecofriendly products include bamboo (which is really a grass and not a wood), recycled glass tiles, recycled metal tiles, cork flooring, and flooring made from reclaimed wood products.

4. Turn off your lights. According to sleep experts and others, artificial light decreases the production of melatonin, a hormone manufactured in the brain that is produced during sleep cycles. This hormone is being shown to have a protective effect against some forms of cancer.

5. Use "green" paper. By purchasing ecofriendly paper products that are bleach free, we reduce the amount of dioxins released into the atmosphere. Dioxins are carcinogenic, and fewer of them in the atmosphere will reduce everyone's risk for cancer.

6. Buy ecofriendly hygiene products. When purchasing personal hygiene products or cosmetics, select items that are environmentally responsible. Many products contain petroleum and plastics, agents that are not good for your skin or the environment. Consider avoiding the following:

* Diethanolamine (DEA), commonly found in shampoos, is thought to be carcinogenic.
* Formaldehyde, commonly found in eye shadows, is well known as a carcinogenic agent.
* Phthalates, found in many hygiene and cosmetic products such as nail polish and perfumes, are thought to be carcinogenic.
* Parabens, used as preservatives in food and cosmetic products such as makeup, lotion, shampoo, and soap, have been found in breast tumors and are being researched as potential carcinogens.

7. Avoid dry cleaning. Try to avoid buying clothes that require dry cleaning. Conventional dry cleaning uses a chemical called *perchloroethylene* (PERC), an agent known to increase the risk for cancer and harm the environment. If dry cleaning is unavoidable, explore local dry cleaners using ecofriendly alternatives such as "wet cleaning," which includes biodegradable soaps or silicone-based solvents and special machinery used to reduce shrinkage.

> **Don't risk your health for beauty! Read the labels on your cosmetics and avoid products containing potentially carcinogenic chemicals such as phthalates and parabens.**

and radioactive substances may have increased risks for cancer. Working with coal tars, as in the mining profession, or with inhalants, as in the auto-painting business, is hazardous. So is working with herbicides and pesticides, although the evidence is inconclusive for low-dose exposures. Several federal and state agencies are responsible for monitoring such exposures and ensuring that businesses comply with standards designed to protect workers.

You don't have to work in one of these industries to come in contact with environmental carcinogens. See the **Green Guide** above to explore some ways you can avoid carcinogens in the products you buy and use every day.

Radiation Ionizing radiation (IR)—radiation from X rays, radon, cosmic rays, and ultraviolet radiation (primarily ultraviolet B, or UVB radiation)—is the only form of radiation proven to cause human cancer. Evidence that high-dose IR causes cancer comes from studies of atomic bomb survivors, patients receiving radiotherapy, and certain occupational groups (e.g., uranium miners). Virtually any part of the body can be affected by IR, but bone marrow and the thyroid are particularly susceptible. Radon exposure in homes can increase lung cancer risk, especially in cigarette smokers. To reduce the risk of harmful effects, diagnostic medical and dental X rays are set at the lowest dose levels possible.

Nonionizing radiation produced by radio waves, cell phones, microwaves, computer screens, televisions, electric blankets, and other products has been a topic of great concern in recent years, but research has not proven excess risk to date. Although highly controversial, some suggest that cell phones beam radio frequency energy that can penetrate the brain, raising concerns about cancers of the head and neck, brain tumors, or leukemia. Most research, including the biggest study of cancer and cell phone risk to date, indicate that having a cell phone glued to your ear for hours causes little more than a sore ear and a hefty bill.[43] See Chapter 15 for more on the potential environmental and health hazards of both ionizing and nonionizing radiation.

Chemicals in Foods

Among the food additives suspected of causing cancer is *sodium nitrate,* a chemical used to preserve and give color to red meat. The actual carcinogen is not sodium nitrate but *nitrosamines,* substances formed when the body digests sodium nitrate. Sodium nitrate has not been banned, primarily because it kills *Clostridium botulinum,* the bacterium that causes the highly virulent foodborne disease botulism. It should also be noted that the bacteria found in the human intestinal tract may contain more nitrates than a person could ever take in from eating cured meats or other nitrate-containing food products. Nonetheless, concern about the carcinogenic properties of nitrates has led to the introduction of meats that are free of nitrates or contain reduced levels of the substance.

Much of the concern about chemicals in foods centers on the possible harm caused by pesticide and herbicide residues. Although some of these chemicals cause cancer at high doses in experimental animals, the very low concentrations found in some foods are well within established government safety levels. Continued research regarding pesticide and herbicide use is essential, and scientists and consumer groups stress the importance of a balance between chemical use and the production of high-quality food products. Prevention efforts should focus on policies to protect consumers, develop low-chemical pesticides and herbicides, and reduce environmental pollution.

Infectious Diseases and Cancer

According to recent estimates, 15 percent of new cancers worldwide in 2007 were attributable to infection. Rates of cancers related to infections are about three times higher in developing countries than in developed countries (26% vs. 8%).[44] Infections are thought to influence cancer development in several ways, most commonly through chronic inflammation, suppression of the immune system, or chronic stimulation.

Hepatitis B, Hepatitis C, and Liver Cancer

Viruses such as hepatitis B (HBV) and C (HCV) are believed to stimulate the growth of cancer cells in the liver because they are chronic diseases that inflame liver tissue. This may prime the liver for cancer or make it more hospitable for cancer development. Global increases in hepatitis B and C rates and concurrent rises in liver cancer rates seem to provide evidence of such an association.

Human Papillomavirus and Cervical Cancer

Nearly 100 percent of women with cervical cancer have evidence of human papillomavirus (HPV) infection, believed to be a major cause of cervical cancer. Fortunately, only a small percentage of HPV cases progress to cervical cancer.[45] Today, a new vaccine is available to help protect young women from becoming infected with HPV and developing cervical cancer. However, as of this writing, preliminary questions have been raised about the safety and potential minor adverse effects of this vaccine. For more on the HPV vaccine, see the discussion in Chapter 13.

what do you think?

How do we determine whether a behavior or substance is a risk factor for a disease? ● Although a direct causal relationship between lung cancer and smoking has not been proved, the evidence supporting such a relationship is strong. Must a clearly established causal link exist before consumers are warned about risk? ● How does the consumer know what to believe?

Types of Cancers

As mentioned earlier, the word *cancer* refers not to a single disease, but to hundreds of different diseases. They are grouped into four broad categories based on the type of tissue from which the cancer arises:

● **Carcinomas.** Epithelial tissues (tissues covering body surfaces and lining most body cavities) are the most common sites for cancers, called *carcinomas.* These cancers affect the outer layer of the skin and mouth as well as the mucous membranes. They metastasize through the circulatory or lymphatic system initially and form solid tumors.
● **Sarcomas.** Sarcomas occur in the mesodermal, or middle, layers of tissue—for example, in bones, muscles, and general connective tissue. They metastasize primarily via the blood in the early stages of disease. These cancers are less common but generally more virulent than carcinomas. They also form solid tumors.
● **Lymphomas.** Lymphomas develop in the lymphatic system—the infection-fighting regions of the body—and metastasize through the lymphatic system. Hodgkin's disease is an example. Lymphomas also form solid tumors.
● **Leukemias.** Cancer of the blood-forming parts of the body, particularly the bone marrow and spleen, is called leukemia. A nonsolid tumor, leukemia is characterized by an abnormal increase in the number of white blood cells.

Figure 12.6 shows the most common sites of cancer and the number of new cases and deaths from each type in 2009. A comprehensive discussion of the many different forms of

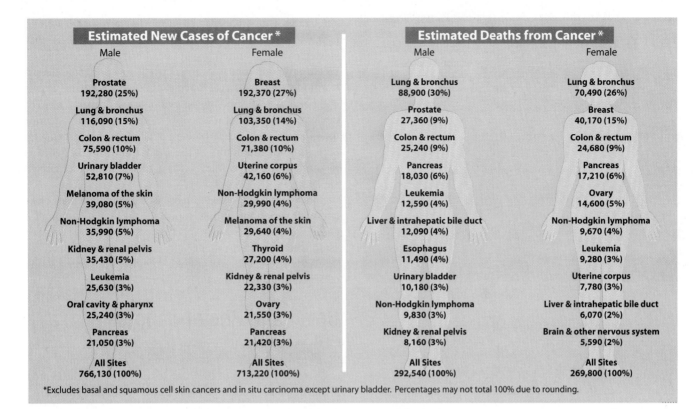

Estimated New Cases of Cancer*		Estimated Deaths from Cancer*	
Male	Female	Male	Female
Prostate 192,280 (25%)	Breast 192,370 (27%)	Lung & bronchus 88,900 (30%)	Lung & bronchus 70,490 (26%)
Lung & bronchus 116,090 (15%)	Lung & bronchus 103,350 (14%)	Prostate 27,360 (9%)	Breast 40,170 (15%)
Colon & rectum 75,590 (10%)	Colon & rectum 71,380 (10%)	Colon & rectum 25,240 (9%)	Colon & rectum 24,680 (9%)
Urinary bladder 52,810 (7%)	Uterine corpus 42,160 (6%)	Pancreas 18,030 (6%)	Pancreas 17,210 (6%)
Melanoma of the skin 39,080 (5%)	Non-Hodgkin lymphoma 29,990 (4%)	Leukemia 12,590 (4%)	Ovary 14,600 (5%)
Non-Hodgkin lymphoma 35,990 (5%)	Melanoma of the skin 29,640 (4%)	Liver & intrahepatic bile duct 12,090 (4%)	Non-Hodgkin lymphoma 9,670 (4%)
Kidney & renal pelvis 35,430 (5%)	Thyroid 27,200 (4%)	Esophagus 11,490 (4%)	Leukemia 9,280 (3%)
Leukemia 25,630 (3%)	Kidney & renal pelvis 22,330 (3%)	Urinary bladder 10,180 (3%)	Uterine corpus 7,780 (3%)
Oral cavity & pharynx 25,240 (3%)	Ovary 21,550 (3%)	Non-Hodgkin lymphoma 9,830 (3%)	Liver & intrahepatic bile duct 6,070 (2%)
Pancreas 21,050 (3%)	Pancreas 21,420 (3%)	Kidney & renal pelvis 8,160 (3%)	Brain & other nervous system 5,590 (2%)
All Sites 766,130 (100%)	All Sites 713,220 (100%)	All Sites 292,540 (100%)	All Sites 269,800 (100%)

*Excludes basal and squamous cell skin cancers and in situ carcinoma except urinary bladder. Percentages may not total 100% due to rounding.

FIGURE 12.6 **Leading Sites of New Cancer Cases and Deaths, 2009 Estimates**

Source: *Cancer Facts and Figures 2009.* Copyright © 2009, American Cancer Society. Used with permission from American Cancer Society, Atlanta, GA.

cancer is beyond the scope of this book, but we will discuss the most common types in the next sections.

Lung Cancer

Lung cancer is the leading cause of cancer deaths for both men and women in the United States, killing an estimated 159,390 Americans in 2009, even as rates for men and women have decreased in recent decades due to declines in smoking and policies that prohibit smoking in public places.[46] Since 1987, more women have died each year from lung cancer than from breast cancer, which over the previous 40 years had been the major cause of cancer deaths in women. Although past reductions in smoking rates have boded well for cancer and CVD statistics, there is growing concern about the number of youth, particularly young women and persons of low income and low educational level, who continue to pick up the habit.

Detection, Symptoms, and Treatment Symptoms of lung cancer include a persistent cough, blood-streaked sputum, chest pain, and recurrent attacks of pneumonia or bronchitis. Treatment depends on the type and stage of the cancer. Surgery, radiation therapy, and chemotherapy are all options. If the cancer is localized, surgery is usually the treatment of choice. If it has spread, surgery is combined

90% of all lung cancers could be avoided if people did not smoke.

with radiation and chemotherapy. Unfortunately, despite advances in medical technology, survival rates 1 year after diagnosis are low, at only 41 percent overall. Newer tests, such as low-dose computerized tomography (CT) scans, molecular markers in sputum, and improved biopsy techniques, have helped improve diagnosis, but we still have a long way to go.

Risk Factors and Prevention Smokers, especially those who have smoked for more than 20 years, and people who have been exposed to industrial substances such as arsenic and asbestos or to radiation are at the highest risk for lung cancer. Exposure to secondhand cigarette smoke increases the risk for nonsmokers. Apparent increases in lung cancer among nonsmokers have caused increasing concern about the hazards of secondhand smoke, leading health advocates to argue vigorously for smoking bans.[47]

Breast Cancer

In 2009, approximately 192,370 women and 1,910 men in the United States were diagnosed with invasive breast cancer for the first time. In addition, 62,280 new cases of in situ breast cancer, a more localized cancer, were diagnosed. About 40,170 women (and 440 men) died, making breast cancer the

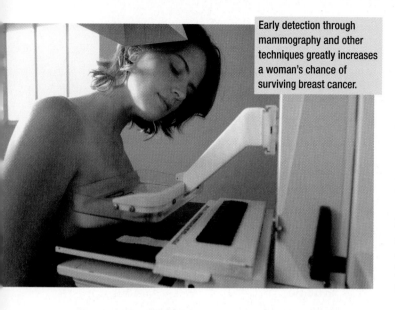

Early detection through mammography and other techniques greatly increases a woman's chance of surviving breast cancer.

second leading cause of cancer death for women, even as rates continue to level off.[48]

Detection, Symptoms, and Treatment The earliest signs of breast cancer are usually observable on mammograms, often before lumps can be felt. However, mammograms are not foolproof. Hence, regular breast self-examination (BSE) is also important (see the **Gender & Health** box on the next page). Although mammograms detect between 80 and 90 percent of breast cancers in women without symptoms, a newer form of magnetic resonance imaging (MRI) appears to be more accurate, particularly in women with genetic risks for tumors.

Once breast cancer has grown enough that it can be felt by palpating the area, many women will recognize the threat and seek medical care. Symptoms may include persistent breast changes, such as a lump in the breast or surrounding lymph nodes, thickening, dimpling, skin irritation, distortion, retraction or scaliness of the nipple, nipple discharge, or tenderness.

Treatments range from a lumpectomy to radical mastectomy to various combinations of radiation or chemotherapy. Among nonsurgical options, promising results have been noted among women using *selective estrogen-receptor modulators (SERMs)* such as tamoxifen and raloxifene, particularly among women whose cancers appear to grow in response to estrogen. These drugs, as well as new *aromatase inhibitors,* work by blocking estrogen. The 5-year survival rate for people with localized breast cancer (which includes all people living 5 years after diagnosis, whether they are in remission, disease free, or under treatment) has risen from 80 percent in the 1950s to 98 percent today. However, these statistics vary dramatically, based on the stage of the cancer when it is first detected and whether it has spread. As with most cancers, the earlier the stage in which it is caught, the greater the chances will be for a full recovery.

Risk Factors and Prevention The incidence of breast cancer increases with age. Although there are many possible

risk factors, those that are well supported by research include family history of breast cancer, menstrual periods that started early and ended late in life, obesity after menopause, recent use of oral contraceptives or postmenopausal hormone therapy, never having children or having a first child after age 30, consuming two or more drinks of alcohol per day, and physical inactivity.[49] Genes appear to account for approximately 5 to 10 percent of all cases of breast cancer. Screening for mutations in the *BRCA1* and *BRCA2* genes is recommended for women with a family history of breast cancer.

International differences in breast cancer incidence correlate with variations in diet, especially fat intake, although a causal role for these dietary factors has not been firmly established. Sudden weight gain has also been implicated. Research also shows that regular exercise, even some forms of recreational exercise, can reduce risk.[50]

Colon and Rectal Cancers

Colorectal cancers (cancers of the colon and rectum) continue to be the third most common cancer in both men and women, with over 146,970 cases diagnosed in the United States in 2009.[51] Although colon cancer rates have increased steadily in recent decades, many people are unaware of their risk.

Detection, Symptoms, and Treatment In its early stages, colorectal cancer has no symptoms. Bleeding from the rectum, blood in the stool, and changes in bowel habits are the major warning signals. Because colorectal cancer tends to spread slowly, the prognosis is quite good if it is caught in the early stages. However, only 21 percent of all Americans over age 50 have had the most basic screening test—the fecal occult blood test—in the past 5 years, and only 33 percent have had a colonoscopy during the same time period. Colonoscopy or barium enemas are recommended screening tests for at-risk populations and everybody over age 50. Treatment often consists of radiation or surgery. Chemotherapy, although not used extensively in the past, is today a possibility.

Risk Factors and Prevention Anyone can get colorectal cancer, but people who are over age 50, who are obese, who have a family history of colon and rectal cancer, a personal or family history of polyps (benign growths) in the colon or rectum, or who have inflammatory bowel problems such as colitis run an increased risk. Other possible risk factors include diets high in fat or low in fiber, smoking, sedentary lifestyle, high alcohol consumption, and low intake of fruits and vegetables. Indeed, approximately 90 percent of all colorectal cancers are preventable.

Regular exercise, a diet with lots of fruits and other plant foods, a healthy weight, and moderation in alcohol consumption appear to be among the most promising prevention strategies. Consumption of milk and calcium appears to decrease risks. New research suggests that aspirin-like drugs,

Breast Awareness and Self-Exam

Women should know how their breasts normally look and feel and report any new breast changes to a health professional as soon as these changes are noted. Finding a breast change does not necessarily mean there is a cancer. A woman can notice changes by being aware of how her breasts normally look and feel and by feeling her breasts for changes (breast awareness), or by choosing to use a step-by-step approach (see below) and using a specific schedule to examine her breasts.

The best time for a woman to examine her breasts is when the breasts are not tender or swollen. Women who examine their breasts should have their technique reviewed during their periodic health exams by their health care professional. Note that the American Cancer Society recommends the use of mammography and clinical breast exam in addition to self-examination.

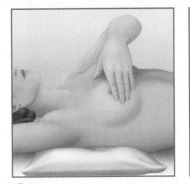

① Perform exam lying down.

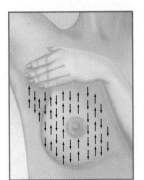

② Use pads of the 3 middle fingers.

③ Follow an up-and-down pattern.

HOW TO EXAMINE YOUR BREASTS

✳ Lie down and place your right arm behind your head (1). When you are lying down, the breast tissue spreads evenly over the chest wall and is as thin as possible, making it much easier to feel all the breast tissue.

✳ Use the finger pads of the three middle fingers on your left hand to feel for lumps in the right breast (2). Use overlapping dime-sized circular motions of the finger pads to feel the tissue.

✳ Use three different levels of pressure to feel all the breast tissue. Light pressure is needed to feel the tissue closest to the skin; medium pressure to feel a little deeper; and firm pressure to feel the tissue closest to the chest and ribs. A firm ridge in the lower curve of each breast is normal. If you're not sure how hard to press, talk with your doctor or nurse. Use each pressure level to feel the breast tissue before moving on to the next spot.

✳ Move around the breast in an up-and-down pattern starting at an imaginary line drawn straight down your side from the underarm and moving across the breast to the middle of the chest bone (sternum or breastbone) (3). Be sure to check the entire breast area going down until you feel only ribs and up to the neck or collarbone (clavicle).

✳ Repeat the exam on your left breast, using the finger pads of the right hand.

✳ While standing in front of a mirror with your hands pressing firmly down on your hips, look at your breasts for any changes of size, shape, contour, or dimpling, or redness or scaliness of the nipple or breast skin. (The pressing down on the hips position contracts the chest wall muscles and enhances any breast changes.)

✳ Examine each underarm while sitting up or standing and with your arm only slightly raised so you can easily feel in this area. Raising your arm straight up tightens the tissue in this area and makes it harder to examine.

Source: American Cancer Society, "Breast Awareness and Self-Examination," Revised May 13, 2009, www.cancer.org/docroot/CRI/content/CRI_2_4_3X _Can_breast_cancer_be_found_early_5.asp. Reprinted by the permission of the American Cancer Society, Inc. from www.cancer.org. All rights reserved.

---

postmenopausal hormones, folic acid, calcium supplements, selenium, and vitamin E may also help.

Skin Cancer

Skin cancer is the most common form of cancer in the United States today, affecting over 1 million people every year (one in five of all adults). In 2009, an estimated 11,590 people died of skin cancer (8,420 from melanoma and 2,940 from other forms of skin cancer).[52] **Malignant melanoma,** the deadliest form of skin cancer, is beginning to occur at a much higher rate in women under age 40. In fact, the highly virulent malignant melanoma has become the most frequent cancer

in women aged 25 to 29 and runs second only to breast cancer in women aged 30 to 34.

Detection, Symptoms, and Treatment Many people do not know what to look for when examining themselves for skin cancer. Fortunately, potentially cancerous growths are often visible as abnormalities on the skin. Basal and squamous cell carcinomas can be a recurrent annoyance, showing up most commonly on the face, ears, neck, arms, hands, and legs as warty bumps, colored spots, or scaly patches. Bleeding, itchiness, pain, or oozing are other symptoms that warrant

malignant melanoma A virulent cancer of the melanocytes (pigment-producing cells) of the skin.

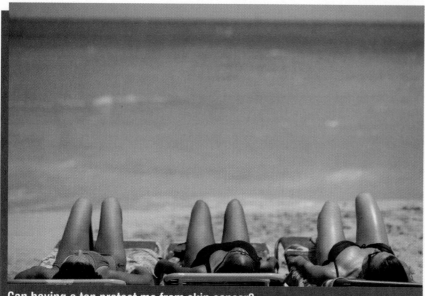

Can having a tan protect me from skin cancer?

It might seem logical that a person's tanned skin would offer protection from the sun's damaging UV rays, but the idea that tanning is healthy and protective has at least three inherent fallacies. First, tanned skin is not healthy but is, by nature, injured skin that has sustained UV-induced damage. Second, a tan isn't protective. According to the American Cancer Society, tanned skin can provide only about the equivalent of sun protection factor (SPF) 4 sunscreen—much too weak to be considered protective. Third, a "base tan" can actually put you at increased risk of sun damage by conferring a false sense of security, leading you to stay out in the sun longer—often without sunscreen.

- **Asymmetry.** One half of the mole or lesion does not match the other half.
- **Border irregularity.** The edges are uneven, notched, or scalloped.
- **Color.** Pigmentation is not uniform. Melanomas may vary in color from tan to deeper brown, reddish black, black, or deep bluish black.
- **Diameter.** Greater than 6 millimeters (about the size of a pea).

Treatment of skin cancer depends on its seriousness. Surgery is performed in 90 percent of all cases. Radiation therapy, *electrodesiccation* (tissue destruction by heat), and *cryosurgery* (tissue destruction by freezing) are also common forms of treatment. For melanoma, treatment may involve surgical removal of the regional lymph nodes, radiation, or chemotherapy.

Risk Factors and Prevention Anyone who overexposes himself or herself to ultraviolet radiation without adequate protection is at risk for skin cancer. The risk is greatest for people who fit the following categories:

attention. Surgery may be necessary to remove them, but they are seldom life threatening.

In striking contrast is melanoma, an invasive killer that may appear as a skin lesion whose size, shape, or color changes and that spreads to regional organs and throughout the body. Malignant melanomas account for over 75 percent of all skin cancer deaths. **Figure 12.7** shows melanoma compared to basal cell and squamous cell carcinomas. A simple *ABCD* rule outlines the warning signs of melanoma:

- Have fair skin; blonde, red, or light brown hair; blue, green, or gray eyes
- Always burn before tanning or burn easily and peel readily
- Don't tan easily but spend lots of time outdoors
- Use no or low–sun protection factor (SPF) sunscreens or old, expired suntan lotions
- Have previously been treated for skin cancer or have a family history of skin cancer
- Have experienced severe sunburns during childhood.

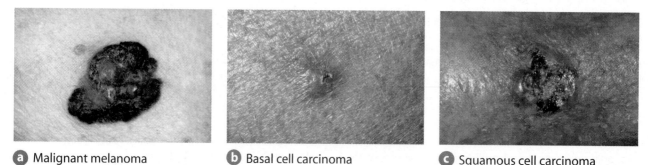

ⓐ Malignant melanoma   ⓑ Basal cell carcinoma   ⓒ Squamous cell carcinoma

FIGURE 12.7 **Types of Skin Cancers**
Preventing skin cancer includes keeping a careful watch for any new pigmented growths and for changes to any moles. The ABCD warning signs of melanoma (a) include *asymmetrical* shapes, irregular *borders, color* variation, and an increase in *diameter.* Basal cell carcinoma (b) and squamous cell carcinoma (c) should be brought to your physician's attention but are not as deadly as melanoma.

Preventing skin cancer is a matter of limiting exposure to harmful UV rays found in sunlight. What happens when you expose yourself to sunlight? Biologically, the skin responds to photodamage by increasing its thickness and the number of pigment cells (melanocytes), which produce the "tan" look. The skin's cells that ward off infection are also prone to photodamage, lowering the normal immune protection of our skin and priming it for cancer. Photodamage also causes wrinkling by impairing the elastic substances (collagens) that keep skin soft and pliable. See the **Skills for Behavior Change** box at right for tips on staying safe in the sun.

Although sun exposure risks have been widely reported, over 60 percent of Americans 25 years old and younger report that they are "working on a tan" at some point during the year. Despite the red flag, why do people continue to tan? Recent research suggests a connection between high levels of ultraviolet light and endorphins. Those who tan in the sun or artificially may experience a short "high" for this reason, and tanning can become a type of addiction. For information on the safety of tanning booths and salons, see the **Consumer Health** box on the next page.

Prostate Cancer

Cancer of the prostate is the most frequently diagnosed cancer in American males today, excluding skin cancer, and is the second leading cause of cancer deaths in men after lung cancer. In 2009, about 192,280 new cases of prostate cancer were diagnosed in the United States. About 1 in 3 men will be diagnosed with prostate cancer during his lifetime, but only 1 in 33 will die of it.[53]

Detection, Symptoms, and Treatment The prostate is a muscular, walnut-sized gland that surrounds part of a man's urethra, the tube that transports urine and sperm out of the body. As part of the male reproductive system, its primary function is to produce seminal fluid. Most symptoms of prostate cancer mimic signs of infection or an enlarged prostate. These may include weak or interrupted urine flow; difficulty starting or stopping urination; feeling the urge to urinate frequently; pain upon urination; blood in the urine; or pain in the low back, pelvis, or thighs. Many men have no symptoms in the early stages.

Men over the age of 40 should have an annual digital rectal prostate examination. The American Cancer Society recommends that men age 50 and over have an annual **prostate-specific antigen (PSA)** test.

Fortunately, 90 percent of all prostate cancers are detected while they are still in the local or regional stages and tend to progress slowly. Over the past 20 years, the 5-year survival rate for all stages combined has increased from 67 percent to almost 99 percent, and the 15-year survival rate is over 76 percent.

Risk Factors and Prevention Chances of developing prostate cancer increase dramatically with age. More than 70 percent of prostate cancers are diagnosed in men over the age of 65. Usually the disease has progressed to the point of

Skills for Behavior Change

Safe Sunning

✳ Avoid the sun or seek shade from 10:00 AM to 2:00 PM, when the sun's rays are strongest. Even on a cloudy day, up to 80 percent of the sun's rays can get through.

✳ Apply an SPF 15 or higher sunscreen evenly to all uncovered skin before going outside. Look for a "broad-spectrum" sunscreen that protects against both UVA and UVB radiation. Check the label for the correct amount of time you should allow between applying the product and going outdoors. If the label does not specify, apply it 30 minutes before going outside.

✳ Check the expiration date on your sunscreen. Sunscreens lose effectiveness over time, just like most other products.

✳ Remember to apply sunscreen to your eyelids, lips, nose, ears, neck, hands, and feet. If you don't have much hair, apply sunscreen to the top of your head, too.

✳ Reapply sunscreen often. The label will tell you how often you need to do this. If it isn't waterproof, reapply it after swimming, or if you are sweating a lot.

✳ Wear loose-fitting, light-colored clothing. You can now purchase clothing that has SPF protection in most sporting goods stores. Wear a wide-brimmed, light-colored hat to protect your head and face.

✳ Use sunglasses with 99 to 100 percent UV protection to protect your eyes. Look for polarization in your shades.

✳ Check your skin regularly for signs of cancer. Remember to look at the backs of your legs, the undersides of your arms, and between your toes. Check parts that are hard to see—your back, neck, scalp, genitals, and buttocks—with a hand mirror. Look for changes in the size, shape, color, or feel of birthmarks, moles, and spots. If you find any changes or find sores that are not healing, see your doctor.

Source: U.S. Food and Drug Administration, "Sun Safety: Save Your Skin!" Updated July 2009, www.fda.gov/ForConsumers/ConsumerUpdates/ucm049090.htm.

displaying symptoms, or, more likely, they are seeing a doctor for other problems and get a screening test or PSA test.

Race is also a risk factor in prostate cancer: African American men are 61 percent more likely to develop prostate cancer than white men and are much more likely to be diagnosed at an advanced stage. Prostate cancer is less common among Asian men and occurs at about the same rates among Hispanic men as it does among white men.

Having a father or brother with prostate cancer more than doubles a man's risk of getting prostate cancer himself (interestingly, the

prostate-specific antigen (PSA) An antigen found in prostate cancer patients.

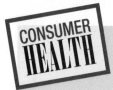

ARTIFICIAL TANS: SACRIFICING HEALTH FOR BEAUTY?

Tanning is a multibillion-dollar industry that draws more than 28 million Americans into over 25,000 salons each year. Being tan is equated with being healthy, chic, and attractive, leading increasing numbers of men and women, particularly adolescent girls, to seek quick tans in packaged visits to tanning beds.

Most tanning salon patrons incorrectly believe that tanning booths are safer than sitting in the sun. However, the truth is that there is no such thing as a safe tan from *any* source! A tan is visible evidence of skin damage. Every time you tan, whether in the sun or in a salon, you are exposing your skin to harmful UV light rays. Such exposure eventually thins the skin, making it less able to heal, as well as contributing to premature aging. The injury accumulated through years of tanning increases your risk for disfiguring forms of skin cancer, eye problems, and possible death from melanoma. Consider the following:

✱ Exposure to tanning beds before age 35 increases melanoma risk by 75 percent.
✱ People who use tanning beds are 2.5 times more likely to develop squamous cell carcinoma and 1.5 times more likely to develop basal cell carcinoma.
✱ New high-pressure sunlamps used in some salons emit doses of UV radiation that can be as much as 15 times that of the sun.
✱ Up to 90 percent of visible skin changes commonly blamed on aging are caused by the sun.

Because of the many salons that are springing up across the country, the artificial tanning industry is difficult to monitor and regulate. Although a growing number of states require UV protective eyewear or have machine operators remain present during a client's session, tanning facilities sometimes fail to enforce regulations.

Dermatologists cite additional factors that make tanning in a salon as bad—or even worse—than sitting in the sun:

✱ Some tanning facilities do not calibrate the ultraviolet output of their tanning bulbs or ensure sufficient rotation of newer and older bulbs, which can lead to more or less exposure than you paid for.
✱ Tanning facility patrons often try for a total body tan. The buttocks and genitalia are particularly sensitive to UV radiation and are prone to developing skin cancer.
✱ Shared tanning booths and beds pose significant hygiene risks. Anytime you come in contact with body secretions from others, you run the risk of an infectious disease. Don't assume that those little colored water sprayers used to "clean" the

The UV light from a tanning bed is just as harmful and damaging to your skin as that from the sun.

inside of the beds are sufficient to kill organisms. The busier the facility, the more likely you are to come into contact with germs that could make you ill.

Sources: S. Danoff-Berg and C. E. Mosher, "Prediction of Tanning Salon Use: Behavioral Alternatives for Enhancing Appearance, Relaxing and Socializing," *Journal of Health Psychology* 11, no. 3 (2006): 511–18; Skin Cancer Foundation, "2008 Skin Cancer Facts," 2008, www .skincancer.org/Skin-Cancer/2008 -Skin-Cancer-Facts.html.

risk is higher for men with an affected brother than it is for those with an affected father). The genes that predispose men to prostate cancer have not been clearly identified; thus, genetic tests like those for breast cancer in women are not yet available.

Eating more fruits and vegetables, particularly those containing lycopene, a pigment found in tomatoes and other red fruits, may lower the risk of prostate cancer. Some studies suggest that taking 50 mg (400 international units, or IU) of vitamin E and adequate amounts of selenium in your diet may reduce risk, whereas consuming high levels of vitamin A may increase risk. The best advice is to follow the dietary recommendations discussed in Chapter 9 and maintain a healthy weight.

Ovarian Cancer

Ovarian cancer is the fifth leading cause of cancer deaths for women, with about 21,550 being diagnosed with it in 2009

and 14,600 dying of it.[54] Ovarian cancer causes more deaths than any other cancer of the reproductive system because its insidious, often silent, course means women tend not to discover it until the cancer is at an advanced stage. Overall, 1-year survival rates are 76 percent, and 5-year suvival rates are 45 percent.

The most common symptom of ovarian cancer is enlargement of the abdomen. Women over 40 may experience persistent digestive disturbances, as well. Other symptoms include fatigue, pain during intercourse, unexplained weight loss, unexplained changes in bowel or bladder habits, and incontinence. However, many women have no early symptoms at all.

Primary relatives (mother, daughter, sister) of a woman who has had ovarian cancer are at increased risk. A family or personal history of breast or colon cancer is also associated with increased risk. Women who have never been pregnant are more likely to develop ovarian cancer than those who have had a child. The use of fertility drugs may also increase a woman's risk.

Research shows that using birth control pills, adhering to a low-fat diet, having multiple children, and breast-feeding can all reduce risk of ovarian cancer. General prevention strategies such as focusing on a healthy diet, exercise, sleep, stress management, and weight control are good ideas to lower your risk for this and any of the diseases discussed in this chapter. To protect yourself, getting thorough annual pelvic examinations is important. Women over the age of 40 should have a cancer-related checkup every year. For those with risk factors or unexplained symptoms, uterine ultrasound or a blood test for the tumor marker CA 125 are often recommended.

Cervical and Endometrial (Uterine) Cancer

Most uterine cancers develop in the body of the uterus, usually in the endometrium (lining). The rest develop in the cervix, located at the base of the uterus. In 2009, an estimated 11,270 new cases of cervical cancer and 42,160 cases of endometrial cancer were diagnosed in the United States.[55] The overall incidence of cervical and uterine cancer has been declining steadily over the past decade. This decline may be due to more regular screenings of younger women using the **Pap test,** a procedure in which cells taken from the cervical region are examined for abnormal cellular activity. Although Pap tests are very effective for detecting early-stage cervical cancer, they are less effective for detecting cancers of the uterine lining. Early warning signs of uterine cancer include bleeding outside the normal menstrual period or after menopause or persistent unusual vaginal discharge. These symptoms should be checked by a physician immediately.

Risk factors for cervical cancer include early age at first intercourse, multiple sex partners, cigarette smoking, and certain sexually transmitted infections, including HPV (the cause of genital warts) and herpes. For endometrial cancer, age is a risk factor; however, estrogen and obesity are also strong risk factors. In addition, risks are increased by treatment with tamoxifen for breast cancer, metabolic syndrome, late menopause, never having children, a history of polyps in the uterus or ovaries, a history of other cancers, and race (white women are at higher risk).[56]

Testicular Cancer

Testicular cancer is one of the most common types of solid tumors found in young adult men, affecting nearly 8,400 young men in 2009. Those between the ages of 15 and 35 are at greatest risk. There has been a steady increase in testicular cancer frequency over the past several years in this age group.[57] However, with a 96 percent 5-year survival rate, it is one of the most curable forms of cancer. Although the cause of testicular cancer is unknown, several risk factors have been identified. Men with undescended testicles appear to be at greatest risk, and some studies indicate a genetic influence.

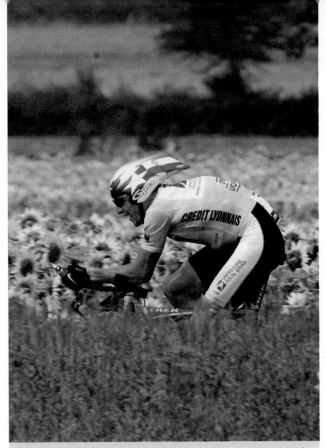

One of the most remarkable testicular cancer stories is the survival of cyclist Lance Armstrong. After recovering from an invasive form of testicular cancer that spread to several parts of his body, including his brain, Armstrong went on to win the Tour de France seven consecutive times and to create a foundation dedicated to cancer education, research, and advocacy.

In general, testicular tumors first appear as an enlargement of the testis or thickening in testicular tissue. Because this enlargement is often painless, it is important that young men practice regular testicular self-examination (see the **Gender & Health** box on the next page).

Facing Cancer

Based on current rates, about 83 million people in the United States will eventually develop cancer. Despite these gloomy predictions, recent advancements in the diagnosis and treatment of many forms of cancer have reduced some of the fear and mystery that once surrounded this disease.

Detecting Cancer

The earlier cancer is diagnosed, the better the prospect that there is for survival. Make a realistic assessment of your own risk factors; avoid those behaviors that put you at risk; and increase healthy behaviors, such as improving your diet and exercise levels,

Pap test A procedure in which cells taken from the cervical region are examined for abnormal activity.

Testicular Self-Exam

Most testicular cancers can be found at an early stage. The American Cancer Society (ACS) advises men to be aware of testicular cancer and to see a doctor right away if they find a lump in a testicle. Because regular testicular self-exams have not been studied enough to show that they reduce the death rate from this cancer, the ACS does not have a recommendation on regular testicular self-exams for all men. If you have certain risk factors that increase your chance of developing testicular cancer (e.g., an undescended testicle, previous germ cell tumor in one testicle, or a family history), you should seriously consider monthly self-exams and talk about it with your doctor.

HOW TO EXAMINE YOUR TESTICLES

The best time for you to examine your testicles is during or after a shower, when the skin of the scrotum is relaxed.

✳ Hold the penis out of the way and examine each testicle separately.

✳ Hold the testicle between your thumbs and fingers with both hands and roll it gently between the fingers.

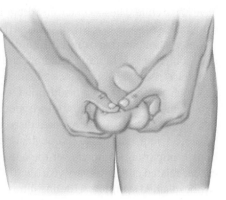

✳ Look and feel for any hard lumps or nodules (smooth, rounded masses) or any change in the size, shape, or consistency of the testes.

You should be aware that each normal testis has an epididymis, which can feel like a small bump on the upper or middle outer side of the testis. Normal testicles also contain blood vessels, supporting tissues, and tubes that conduct sperm. Some men may confuse these with cancer at first. If you have any concerns, ask your doctor. Note that the ACS recommends a testicular exam as part of a routine cancer-related checkup.

Source: American Cancer Society, "Can Testicular Cancer Be Found Early?," Revised August 3, 2009, www.cancer.org/docroot/CRI/content/CRI_2_4_3X _Can_Testicular_Cancer_Be_Found_Early_41.asp?sitearea=. Reprinted by the permission of the American Cancer Society, Inc. from www.cancer.org. All rights reserved.

---

reducing stress, and getting regular checkups. Even if you have significant risks, there are factors you can control. Do you have a family history of cancer? If so, what types? Make sure you know which symptoms to watch for, and follow the recommendations for self-exams and medical checkups outlined in Table 12.4 at right. Avoid known carcinogens—such as tobacco—and other environmental hazards, and eat a nutritious diet.

Several high-tech tools to detect cancer have been developed. In **magnetic resonance imaging (MRI),** a huge electromagnet detects hidden tumors by mapping the vibrations of the various atoms in the body on a computer screen. The **computed tomography scan (CT scan)** uses X rays to examine parts of the body. In both of these painless, noninvasive procedures, cross-sectioned pictures can reveal a tumor's shape and location more accurately than can conventional X-ray images.

magnetic resonance imaging (MRI) A device that uses magnetic fields, radio waves, and computers to generate an image of internal tissues of the body for diagnostic purposes without the use of radiation.

computed tomography scan (CT scan) A scan by a machine that uses radiation to view internal organs not normally visible on X-ray images.

radiotherapy Use of radiation to kill cancerous cells.

chemotherapy Use of drugs to kill cancerous cells.

Cancer Treatments

Cancer treatments vary according to the type of cancer and the stage in which it's detected. Surgery, in which the tumor and surrounding tissue are removed, is one common treatment. **Radiotherapy** (the use of radiation) or **chemotherapy** (the use of drugs) to kill cancerous cells are also used. Radiation works by destroying malignant cells or stopping cell growth. It is most effective in treating localized cancer masses. When cancer has spread throughout the body, it is necessary to use some form of chemotherapy.

Whether used alone or in combination, radiotherapy and chemotherapy have side effects, including nausea, nutritional deficiencies, hair loss, and general fatigue. In the process of killing malignant cells, some healthy cells are also destroyed, and long-term damage to the cardiovascular system and other body systems can be significant.

Although surgery, chemotherapy, and radiation therapy remain the most commonly used treatments for all types of cancer and successfully treat about 50 percent of all cancers, several newer techniques either are in clinical trials or have become available in selected cancer centers throughout the country. Promising areas of research include *immunotherapy,* which enhances the body's own disease-fighting mechanisms, *cancer-fighting vaccines* to combat abnormal cells, *gene therapy* to increase the patient's immune response, and treatment with various substances that block cancer-causing events along the *cancer pathway.* Another promising avenue of potential treatment is *stem cell research,* although controversy around the use of stem cells continues to slow research.

TABLE
12.4
Screening Guidelines for the Early Detection of Cancer in Average-Risk Asymptomatic People

Cancer Site	Population	Test or Procedure	Frequency
Breast	Women, aged 20+	Breast self-examination (BSE)	Beginning in their early 20s, women should be told about the benefits and limitations of BSE. The importance of prompt reporting of any new breast symptoms to a health professional should be emphasized. Women who choose to do BSE should receive instruction and have their technique reviewed on the occasion of a periodic health examination. It is acceptable for women to choose not to do BSE or to do BSE irregularly.
		Clinical breast examination (CBE)	For women in their 20s and 30s, it is recommended that CBE be part of a periodic health examination, preferably at least every 3 years. Asymptomatic women aged 40 and over should continue to receive a CBE as part of a periodic health examination, preferably annually.
		Mammography	Annual, starting at age 40*
Colorectal[†]	Men and women, aged 50+	Fecal occult blood test (FOBT)[‡] with at least 50% test sensitivity for cancer, or fecal immunochemical test (FIT) with at least 50% test sensitivity for cancer, or	Annual, starting at age 50
		Stool DNA test	Interval uncertain, starting at age 50
		Flexible sigmoidoscopy, or	Every 5 years, starting at age 50
		FOBT[‡] and flexible sigmoidoscopy,[§] or	Annual FOBT (or FIT) and flexible sigmoidoscopy every 5 years, starting at age 50
		Double-contrast barium enema (DCBE), or	Every 5 years, starting at age 50
		Colonoscopy	Every 10 years, starting at age 50
		Computerized tomography (CT) colonography	Every 5 years, starting at age 50
Prostate	Men, aged 50+	Digital rectal examination (DRE) and prostate-specific antigen (PSA) test	Health care providers should discuss the potential benefits and limitations of prostate cancer early detection testing with men and offer the PSA blood test and the DRE annually, beginning at age 50, to men who are at average risk of prostate cancer, and who have a life expectancy of at least 10 years.[¶]
Cervix	Women, aged 18+	Pap test	Cervical cancer screening should begin approximately 3 years after a woman begins having vaginal intercourse, but no later than 21 years of age. Screening should be done every year with conventional Pap tests or every 2 years using liquid-based Pap tests. At or after age 30, women who have had three normal test results in a row may get screened every 2 to 3 years with cervical cytology (either conventional or liquid-based Pap test) alone, or every 3 years with a human papillomavirus (HPV) DNA test plus cervical cytology. Women 70 years of age and older who have had three or more normal Pap tests and no abnormal Pap tests in the past 10 years and women who have had a total hysterectomy may choose to stop cervical cancer screening.
Endometrial	Women, at menopause	At the time of menopause, women at average risk should be informed about risks and symptoms of endometrial cancer and strongly encouraged to report any unexpected bleeding or spotting to their physicians.	
Cancer-Related Checkup	Men and women, aged 20+	On the occasion of a periodic health examination, the cancer-related checkup should include examination for cancers of the thyroid, testicles, ovaries, lymph nodes, oral cavity, and skin, as well as health counseling about tobacco, sun exposure, diet and nutrition, risk factors, sexual practices, and environmental and occupational exposures.	

*Beginning at age 40, annual CBE should be performed prior to mammography.

[†]Individuals with a personal or family history of colorectal cancer or adenomas, inflammatory bowel disease, or high-risk genetic syndromes should continue to follow the most recent recommendations for individuals at increased or high risk.

[‡]FOBT as it is sometimes done in physicians' offices, with the single stool sample collected on a fingertip during a DRE, is not an adequate substitute for the recommended at-home procedure of collecting two samples from three consecutive specimens. Toilet bowl FOBT tests also are not recommended. In comparison with guaiac-based tests for the detection of occult blood, immunochemical tests are more patient friendly, and are likely to be equal or better in sensitivity and specificity. There is no justification for repeating FOBT in response to an initial positive finding.

[§]Flexible sigmoidoscopy, together with FOBT, is preferred compared to FOBT or flexible sigmoidoscopy alone.

[¶]Information should be provided to men about the benefits and limitations of testing so that an informed decision about testing can be made with the clinician's assistance.

Source: American Cancer Society, *Cancer Facts & Figures 2009* (Atlanta: American Cancer Society, 2009), www.cancer.org. Used with permission. © 2009, American Cancer Society, Inc.

CVD and Cancer: What's Your Personal Risk?

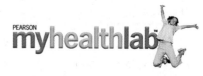

1 Evaluating Your CVD Risk

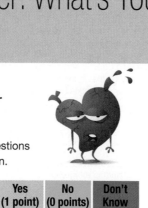

Complete each of the following questions and total your points in each section.

A: Your Family Risk for CVD

	Yes (1 point)	No (0 points)	Don't Know
1. Do any of your primary relatives (parents, grandparents, siblings) have a history of heart disease or stroke?	◯	◯	◯
2. Do any of your primary relatives have diabetes?	◯	◯	◯
3. Do any of your primary relatives have high blood pressure?	◯	◯	◯
4. Do any of your primary relatives have a history of high cholesterol?	◯	◯	◯
5. Would you say that your family consumed a high-fat diet (lots of red meat, whole dairy, butter/margarine) during your time spent at home?	◯	◯	◯

Total points: _____

B: Your Lifestyle Risk for CVD

	Yes (1 point)	No (0 points)	Don't Know
1. Is your total cholesterol level higher than it should be?	◯	◯	◯
2. Do you have high blood pressure?	◯	◯	◯
3. Have you been diagnosed as pre-diabetic or diabetic?	◯	◯	◯
4. Would you describe your life as being highly stressful?	◯	◯	◯
5. Do you smoke?	◯	◯	◯

Total points: _____

C: Your Additional Risks for CVD

1. How would you best describe your current weight?
   a. Lower than what it should be for my height and weight (0 points)
   b. About what it should be for my height and weight (0 points)
   c. Higher than it should be for my height and weight (1 point)

2. How would you describe the level of exercise that you get each day?
   a. Less than what I should be exercising each day (1 point)
   b. About what I should be exercising each day (0 points)
   c. More than what I should be exercising each day (0 points)

3. How would you describe your dietary behaviors?
   a. Eating only the recommended number of calories each day (0 points)
   b. Eating less than the recommended number of calories each day (0 points)
   c. Eating more than the recommended number of calories each day (1 point)

4. Which of the following best describes your typical dietary behavior?
   a. I eat from the major food groups, especially trying to get the recommended fruits and vegetables. (0 points)
   b. I eat too much red meat and consume too much saturated and *trans* fats from meat, dairy products, and processed foods each day. (1 point)
   c. Whenever possible, I try to substitute olive oil or canola oil for other forms of dietary fat. (0 points)

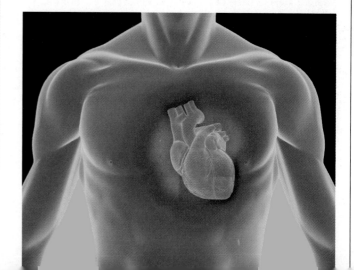

5. Which of the following (if any) describes you?
   a. I watch my sodium intake and try to reduce stress in my life. (0 points)
   b. I have a history of chlamydia infection. (1 point)
   c. I try to eat 5 to 10 mg of soluble fiber each day and try to substitute a soy product for an animal product in my diet at least once each week. (0 points)

Total points: _____

Scoring Part 1

If you scored between 1 and 5 in any section, consider your risk. The higher the number is, the greater your risk will be. If you answered Don't Know for any question, talk to your parents or other family members as soon as possible to find out if you have any unknown risks.

YOUR PLAN FOR CHANGE

The **Assessyourself** activity evaluated your risk of heart disease. Based on your results and the advice of your physician, you may need to take steps to reduce risk of CVD.

Today, you can:

○ Get up and move! Take a walk in the evening, use the stairs instead of the escalator, or ride your bike to class. Start thinking of ways you can incorporate more physical activity into your daily routine.

○ Begin improving your dietary habits by eating a healthier dinner. Replace the meat and processed foods you might normally eat with a serving of fresh fruit or soy-based protein, and green leafy vegetables. Think about the amounts of saturated and *trans* fats you consume—which foods contain them, and how can you reduce consumption of these items?

Within the next 2 weeks, you can:

○ Begin a regular exercise program, even if you start slowly. Set small goals and try to meet them. See Chapter 11 for ideas.

○ Practice a new stress management technique. For example, learn how to meditate. See Chapter 3 for other ideas for managing stress.

○ Get enough rest. Make sure you get at least 8 hours of sleep per night.

By the end of the semester, you can:

○ Find out your hereditary risk for CVD. Call your parents and find out if your grandparents or aunts or uncles developed CVD. Ask if they know their latest cholesterol LDL/HDL levels. Do you have a family history of diabetes?

○ Have your own cholesterol and blood pressure levels checked. Once you know your levels, you'll have a better sense of what risk factors to address. If your levels are high, talk to your doctor about how to reduce them.

2 Evaluating Your Cancer Risk

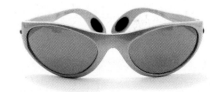

Read each question and circle the number corresponding to each Yes or No. Individual scores for specific questions should not be interpreted as a precise measure of relative risk, but the totals in each section give a general indication.

A: Breast Cancer

	Yes	No
1. Do you check your breasts at least monthly using BSE procedures?	1	2
2. Do you look at your breasts in the mirror regularly, checking for any irregular indentations/lumps, discharge from the nipples, or other noticeable changes?	1	2
3. Has your mother, sister, or daughter been diagnosed with breast cancer?	2	1
4. Have you ever been pregnant?	1	2
5. Have you had a history of lumps or cysts in your breasts or underarm?	2	1

Total points: _____

B: Skin Cancer

	Yes	No
1. Do you spend a lot of time outdoors, either at work or at play?	2	1
2. Do you use sunscreens with an SPF rating of 15 or more when you are in the sun?	1	2
3. Do you use tanning beds or sun booths regularly to maintain a tan?	2	1
4. Do you examine your skin once a month, checking any moles or other irregularities, particularly in hard-to-see areas such as your back, genitals, neck, and under your hair?	1	2
5. Do you purchase and wear sunglasses that adequately filter out harmful sun rays?	1	2

Total points: _____

C: Cancers of the Reproductive System

Men

		Yes	No
1.	Do you examine your penis regularly for unusual bumps or growths?	1	2
2.	Do you perform regular testicular self-examinations?	1	2
3.	Do you have a family history of prostate or testicular cancer?	2	1
4.	Do you practice safe sex and wear condoms during every sexual encounter?	1	2
5.	Do you avoid exposure to harmful environmental hazards such as mercury, coal tars, benzene, chromate, and vinyl chloride?	1	2

Total points: _____

Women

		Yes	No
1.	Do you have regularly scheduled Pap tests?	1	2
2.	Have you been infected with HPV, Epstein-Barr virus, or other viruses believed to increase cancer risk?	2	1
3.	Has your mother, sister, or daughter been diagnosed with breast, cervical, endometrial, or ovarian cancer (particularly at a young age)?	2	1
4.	Do you practice safer sex and use condoms with every sexual encounter?	1	2
5.	Are you obese, taking estrogen, or consuming a diet that is very high in saturated fats?	2	1

Total points: _____

D: Cancers in General

		Yes	No
1.	Do you smoke cigarettes on most days of the week?	2	1
2.	Do you consume a diet that is rich in fruits and vegetables?	1	2
3.	Are you obese, or do you lead a primarily sedentary lifestyle?	2	1
4.	Do you live in an area with high air pollution levels or work in a job where you are exposed to several chemicals on a regular basis?	2	1
5.	Are you careful about the amount of animal fat in your diet, substituting olive oil or canola oil for animal fat whenever possible?	1	2
6.	Do you limit your overall consumption of alcohol?	1	2
7.	Do you eat foods rich in lycopenes (such as tomatoes) and antioxidants?	1	2
8.	Are you "body aware" and alert for changes in your body?	1	2
9.	Do you have a family history of ulcers or of colorectal, stomach, or other digestive system cancers?	2	1
10.	Do you avoid unnecessary exposure to radiation, cell phone emissions, and microwave emissions?	1	2

Total points: _____

Scoring Part 2

Look carefully at each question for which you received a 2. Are there any areas in which you received mostly 2s? Did you receive total points of 6 or higher in A through C? Did you receive total points of 11 or higher in D? If so, you have at least one identifiable risk. The higher the score is, the more risks you may have.

YOUR PLAN FOR CHANGE

The **Assess**yourself activity identified certain factors and behaviors that can contribute to increased cancer risks. If you engage in potentially risky behaviors, consider steps you can take to change these risks and improve your future health.

Today, you can:

○ Perform a breast or testicular self-exam (see pages 373 and 378, respectively, for instructions) and commit to doing one every month.

○ Take advantage of the salad bar in your dining hall for lunch or dinner, and load up on greens, or request veggies such as steamed broccoli or sautéed spinach.

Within the next 2 weeks, you can:

○ Buy a bottle of sunscreen (with SPF 15 or higher) and begin applying it as part of your daily routine. (Be sure to check the expiration date, particularly on sale items!)

○ Find out your family health history. Talk to your parents, grandparents, or an aunt or uncle to find out if family members have developed cancer. This will help you assess your own genetic risk.

By the end of the semester, you can:

○ Work toward achieving a healthy weight. If you aren't already engaged in a regular exercise program, begin one now. Maintaining a healthy body weight and exercising regularly will lower your risk for cancer.

○ Stop smoking, avoid secondhand smoke, and limit your alcohol intake.

Summary

* The cardiovascular system consists of the heart and a network of vessels that supplies the body with nutrients and oxygen. Cardiovascular diseases include atherosclerosis, coronary heart disease, angina pectoris, arrhythmias, congestive heart failure, and stroke.
* *Cardiometabolic risks* refer to combined factors that increase a person's chances of CVD and diabetes. *Metabolic syndrome* is a term for when a person possesses three or more cardiometabolic risk factors.
* Many risk factors for CVD can be controlled, such as cigarette smoking, high blood cholesterol and triglyceride levels, hypertension, lack of exercise, obesity, diabetes, and emotional stress. Some risk factors, such as age, gender, and heredity, cannot be controlled. Other factors being studied include inflammation and homocysteine levels.
* New methods developed for treating heart blockages include coronary bypass surgery and angioplasty. Drugs can reduce high blood pressure and treat other symptoms.
* Cancer is a group of diseases characterized by uncontrolled growth and spread of abnormal cells. These cells may create tumors. Malignant (cancerous) tumors can spread to other parts of the body through metastasis.
* Lifestyle factors for cancer risk include smoking and obesity. Biological factors include inherited genes and gender. Components of the environment that may act as carcinogens include asbestos, radiation, preservatives, and pesticides. Infectious diseases that may lead to cancer include hepatitis and human papillomavirus.
* Common cancers include lung, breast, colon and rectal, skin, prostate, ovarian, uterine, and testicular cancers.
* Early diagnosis improves cancer survival rate. Self-exams aid early diagnosis. New types of cancer treatments include combinations of radiotherapy, chemotherapy, and immunotherapy.

Pop Quiz

1. The function of the aorta is to
   a. return the blood from the lungs.
   b. pump the blood to the arteries in the rest of the body.
   c. pump blood to the lungs.
   d. return blood back to the heart.

2. Severe chest pain due to reduced oxygen flow to the heart is called
   a. angina pectoris.
   b. arrhythmias.
   c. myocardial infarction.
   d. congestive heart failure.

3. Atherosclerosis is referred to as
   a. hardening of the arteries.
   b. heart attack.
   c. high blood pressure.
   d. plaque.

4. A stroke results
   a. when a heart stops beating.
   b. when cardiopulmonary resuscitation has failed to revive the stopped heart.
   c. when blood to the brain has been blocked off.
   d. when the blood pressure rises too high.

5. Which of the following are major causes of cancer?
   a. Sex and socioeconomic status
   b. Environment and genetics
   c. Geographic locations
   d. High-carbohydrate foods

6. The "bad" type of cholesterol found in the bloodstream is known as
   a. high-density lipoprotein.
   b. low-density lipoprotein.
   c. total cholesterol.
   d. triglyceride.

7. The greatest number of cancer deaths for both sexes is caused by
   a. colorectal cancer.
   b. leukemia.
   c. lung cancer.
   d. skin cancer.

8. The more serious, life-threatening type of skin cancer is
   a. basal cell carcinoma.
   b. squamous cell carcinoma.
   c. malignant melanoma.
   d. non-Hodgkin lymphoma.

9. Suspected cancer-causing genes are
   a. epigenes.
   b. oncogenes.
   c. primogenes.
   d. metastogenes.

10. The fecal occult blood test is the most basic screening test used for
    a. lung cancer.
    b. prostate cancer.
    c. cervical cancer.
    d. colorectal cancer.

Answers to these questions can be found on page A-1.

Think about It!

1. List the different types of CVD. Compare and contrast their symptoms, risk factors, prevention, and treatment.
2. Discuss the role that exercise, stress management, dietary changes, medical checkups, and other factors can play in reducing risk for CVD. What role may chronic infections play in CVD risk?
3. Describe some of the diagnostic and treatment alternatives for CVD. If you had a heart attack today, which treatment would you prefer?
4. List the likely causes of cancer. Do any of them put you personally at greater risk? What can you do to reduce your risk? What risk factors do you share with family members? With friends?

5. What are the symptoms of lung, breast, prostate, and testicular cancer? What can you do to reduce your risk of developing these cancers or increase your chances of surviving them?

6. Why are breast and testicular self-exams important for women and men?

Accessing Your Health on the Internet

The following websites explore further topics and issues related to personal health. For links to the websites below, visit the Companion Website for *Health: The Basics*, Green Edition at www.pearsonhighered.com/donatelle.

1. *American Heart Association.* Home page for the leading private organization dedicated to heart health. This site provides information, statistics, and resources regarding cardiovascular care. www.americanheart.org

2. *National Heart, Lung, and Blood Institute.* A valuable resource for information on all aspects of cardiovascular health and wellness. www.nhlbi.nih.gov

3. *American Cancer Society.* Resources from the leading private organization dedicated to cancer prevention. This site provides information, statistics, and resources regarding cancer. www.cancer.org

4. *National Cancer Institute.* Check here for valuable information on clinical trials and the Physician Data Query (PDQ), a comprehensive database of cancer treatment information. www.cancer.gov

5. *Oncolink.* Sponsored by the Abramson Cancer Center of the University of Pennsylvania, this site offers information on cancer support services, cancer causes, screening, and prevention. www.oncolink.com

References

1. Centers for Disease Control and Prevention, "Chronic Disease Overview," Modified October 7, 2009, www.cdc.gov/nccdphp/overview.htm.

2. R. DeVol and A. Bedroussian, *An Unhealthy America: The Economic Burden of Chronic Disease, Charting a New Course to Save Lives and Increase Productivity and Economic Growth* (Santa Monica, CA: Milken Institute, 2007).

3. American Heart Association, *Heart Disease and Stroke Statistics—2009 Update At-A-Glance* (Dallas: American Heart Association, 2009).

4. American Heart Association, *Heart Disease and Stroke Statistics—2009 Update At-A-Glance*, 2009; Centers for Disease Control and Prevention, "Chronic Disease Overview," Updated November 20, 2008, www.cdc.gov/nccdphp/overview.htm.

5. D. Lloyd-Jones et al., "Heart Disease and Stroke Statistics—2009 Update: A Report from the AHA Statistics Committee and the Stroke Statistics Subcommittee." *Circulation* 199, no. 3 (2009): 480–86

6. American Heart Association, *Heart Disease and Stroke Statistics—2009 Update At-A-Glance*, 2009.

7. Ibid.

8. Ibid.

9. Ibid.

10. Ibid.

11. Ibid.

12. Ibid.

13. J. Despres et al., "Abdominal Obesity and Metabolic Syndrome: Contribution to Global Cardiometabolic Risk," *Arteriosclerosis, Thrombosis, and Vascular Biology* 28, no. 6 (2008): 1039–42; S. Haffner, "Epidemiology of Cardiometabolic Diseases," *Mechanisms and Syndromes of Cardiometabolic Disease: Emerging Science in Atherosclerosis Hypertension and Diabetes*, 2009, Medscape CME, http://cme.medscape.com; American Heart Association, *Heart Disease and Stroke Statistics—2009 Update At-A-Glance*, 2009; J. Rosenzwigg, et al., "Primary Prevention of Cardiovascular Disease and Type 2 Diabetes in Patients at Metabolic Risk: An Endocrine Society Clinical Practice Guideline," *Journal of Clinical Endocrinology and Metabolism* 93, no. 10 (2008): 3671–89.

14. S. Haffner, "Epidemiology of Cardiometabolic Diseases," 2009; J. Despres et al., "Abdominal Obesity and Metabolic Syndrome, 2008; A. Gami et al., "Metabolic Syndrome and Risk of Incident Cardiovascular Events and Death: A Systematic Review and Meta-Analysis of Longitudinal Studies," *Journal of the American College of Cardiology* 49, no. 4 (2007): 403–14.

15. U. R. Ximena et al., "High Blood Pressure in Schoolchildren: Prevalence and Risk Factors," *BMC Pediatrics* 6 (2006): 32; R. Din-Dzietham et al., "High Blood Pressure Trends in Children and Adolescents in National Surveys, 1963–2002," *Circulation* 116 (2007): 1488–91; L. Yong, M. Bielo, and F. Shamsa, "Kid's Elevated Blood Pressure Prevalence Linked to Rise in Obesity," *American Heart Association Rapid Access Journal Report*, 2007, www.americanheart.org/presenter.jhtml?identifier=3050261; T. Huang et al., "Metabolic Syndrome and Related Disorders in College Students: Prevalence and Gender Differences," *Metabolic Syndrome and Related Disorders* 5, no. 4 (2007): 365–72.

16. National Center for Health Statistics, *Health, United States, 2008 with Chartbook on Trends in the Health of Americans* (Hyattsville, MD: National Center for Health Statistics, 2009).

17. American Heart Association, *Heart Disease and Stroke Statistics—2009 Update At-A-Glance*, 2009.

18. B. Howard et al., "Low Fat Diet and Risk of Cardiovascular Disease," *JAMA* 295, no. 6 (2006): 655–66; American Heart Association, *Heart Disease and Stroke Statistics—2009 Update At-A-Glance*, 2009.

19. C. A. Garza et al., "The Association between Lipoprotein-Associated Phospholipase A$_2$ and Cardiovascular Disease: A Systematic Review," *Mayo Clinic Proceedings* 82, no. 2 (2007):159–65.

20. P. J. Barter et al., "Apo B versus Cholesterol in Estimating Cardiovascular Risk and in Guiding Therapy: Report of the Thirty-Person/Ten-Country Panel," *Journal of Internal Medicine* 259, no. 3 (2006): 247–58; E. Ingelsson et al., "Clinical Utility of Different Lipid Measures for Prediction of Coronary Heart Disease in Men and Women," *JAMA* 298, no. 7 (2007): 776–85; M. McQueen et al., "Lipids, Lipoproteins and Apolipoproteins as Risk Markers of Myocardial Infarction in 52 Countries (The INTERHEART Study): A Case-Control Study," *Lancet* 372, no. 9634 (2008): 244–33.

21. American Heart Association, *Heart Disease and Stroke Statistics—2009 Update At-A-Glance*, 2009.

22. C. H. Saely, P. Rein, and H. Drexel, "The Metabolic Syndrome and Risk of Cardiovascular Disease and Diabetes: Experiences with the New Diagnostic Criteria from the International Diabetes Federation," *Hormone and Metabolic Research* 39 (2007): 642–50; K. Galassi, K. Reynolds, and J. He, "Metabolic Syndrome and Risk of

Cardiovascular Disease: A Meta-Analysis," *American Journal of Medicine* 119, no. 10 (2007): 812–19.

23. American Heart Association, *Heart Disease and Stroke Statistics—2009 Update At-A-Glance*, 2009.

24. Ibid.

25. M. Esler et al., "Chronic Mental Stress Is a Cause of Essential Hypertension: Presence of Biological Markers of Stress," *Clinical and Experimental Pharmacology and Physiology* 35, no. 4 (2008): 498–502; A. Flaa, I. Eide, S. Kjeldsen, and M. Rostrup, "Sympathoadrenal Stress Reactivity Is a Predictor of Future Blood Pressure. An 18 Year Follow-Up Study," *Hypertension* 52 (2008): 336–41; T. Chadola et al., "Work Stress and Coronary Heart Disease: What Are the Mechanisms," *European Heart Journal* 29, no. 5 (2008): 640–48; J. Yarnell, "Stress at Work—an Independent Risk Factor for Coronary Heart Disease?" *European Heart Journal* 29, no. 5 (2008): 579–81; P. Surtees et al., "Psychological Distress, Major Depressive Disorder, and Risk of Stroke," *Neurology* 70 (2008): 788–94; J. Dimsdale, "Psychological Stress and Cardiovascular Disease," *Journal of the American College of Cardiology* 51 (2008): 1237–46.

26. J. Murabito et al., "Sibling Cardiovascular Disease as a Risk Factor for Cardiovascular Disease in Middle-Aged Adults," *JAMA* 294, no. 24 (2005): 3117–23.

27. J. Ordovas, "Genetic Interactions with Diet Influence the Risk of CVD. Supplement: Living Well to 100: Nutrition, Genetics, Inflammation," *American Journal of Clinical Nutrition* 83, no. 2 (2006): 443S–446S; J. Lovegrove and R. Gitau, "Nutrigenetics and CVD: What Does the Future Hold?" *Proceedings of the Nutrition Society* 67, no. 2 (2008): 206–13.

28. O. Ben-Yehuda, "High-Sensitivity C-Reactive Protein in Every Chart?: The Use of Biomarkers in Individual Patients," *Journal of the American College of Cardiology* 49, no. 21 (2007): 2139–41; D. D. Sin and S. F. P. Man, "Biomarkers in COPD: Are We There Yet?" *Chest* 133, no. 6 (2008): 1296–98; B. Zethelius et al., "Use of Multiple Biomarkers to Improve the Prediction of Death from Cardiovascular Causes," *New England Journal of Medicine* 358, no. 20 (2008): 2107–16; L. Mosca et al., "Narrative Review: Assessment of C-Reactive Protein in Risk Prediction for Cardiovascular Disease," *Annals of Internal Medicine* 145 (2006): 35–42.

29. F. Sofi et al., "Homocysteine-Lowering Therapy and Risk for Venous Thromboem-

bolism: A Randomized Trial," *Annals of Internal Medicine* 146 (2007): 761–67.

30. American Heart Association, "Homocysteine, Folic Acid, and Cardiovascular Disease," 2009, www.americanheart.org/presenter.jhtml?identifier=4677; R. Clarke et al., "Effects of B-Vitamins on Plasma Homocysteine Concentrations and on Risk of Cardiovascular Disease and Dementia," *Current Opinion in Clinical Nutrition and Metabolic Care* 10, no. 1 (2007): 32–39.

31. C. Campbell, S. Smyth, G. Montalescot, and S. Steinhubl, "Aspirin Dose for the Prevention of Cardiovascular Disease: A Systematic Review," *JAMA* 297, no. 18 (2007): 2018–24.

32. American Cancer Society, *Cancer Facts & Figures 2009* (Atlanta: American Cancer Society, 2009).

33. Ibid.

34. Ibid.

35. Ibid.

36. Ibid.

37. Ibid.

38. Centers for Disease Control and Prevention, "Tobacco Use: Targeting The Nation's Leading Killer—at a Glance 2009," 2009, www.cdc.gov/NCCDPHP/publications/aag/osh.htm; World Health Organization, *WHO Report on Global Tobacco Epidemic, 2008: The MPOWER Package* (Geneva, Switzerland: World Health Organization, 2008).

39. K. Flegal et al., "Cause-Specific Excess Deaths Associated with Underweight, Overweight, and Obesity," *Gynecology Obstetrical & Gynecological Survey* 63, no. 3 (2008): 157–59; A. Rehehan, "Body Mass Index and Incidence of Cancer: A Systematic Review and Meta-Analysis of Prospective Observational Studies," *Lancet* 371, no. 9612 (2008): 568–78; G. Reeves et al., "Cancer Incidence and Mortality in Relation to BMI in the Million Women Study: Cohort Study," *BMJ (British Medical Journal)* 1, no. 335 (2007):1134–42; S. Larsson and A. Wolk, "Obesity and Colon and Rectal Cancer Risk: A Meta-Analysis of Prospective Studies," *American Journal of Clinical Nutrition* 86, no. 3 (2008): 556–65.

40. K. Rapp et al., "Obesity and Incidence of Cancer: A Large Cohort Study of over 145,000 Adults in Austria," *British Journal of Cancer* 93 (2005): 1062–67; S. Feedland, "Obesity and Prostate Cancer: A Growing Problem," *Clinical Cancer Research* 11, no. 19 (2005): 6763–66; R. MacInnis et al., "Body Size and Composition and Colon Cancer Risk in Women," *International Cancer Journal* 118 no. 6 (2005): 1496–500; C. Samanic et al., "Relation of Body Mass

Index to Cancer Risk in 362,552 Swedish Men," *Cancer Causes and Control* 17, no. 7 (2005): 10552–600; M. McCullough et al., "Risk Factors for Fatal Breast Cancer in African American Women and White Women in a Large U.S. Prospective Cohort," *American Journal of Epidemiology* 162, no. 8 (2005): 734–42; P. Soliman et al., "Risk Factors for Young Premenopausal Women with Endometrial Cancer," *Obstetrics and Gynecology* 105 (2005): 575–80.

41. E. Reiche, H. Morimoto, and S. Nunes, "Stress and Depression-Induced Immune Dysfunction—Implications for the Development and Progress of Cancer," *International Review of Psychiatry* 17, no. 6 (2005): 515–27; K. Ross, "Mapping Pathways from Stress to Cancer Progression," *Journal of the National Cancer Institute* 100, no. 13 (2008): 914–17; B. Eliyahui, "Stress and Fear Can Affect Cancer's Recurrence," *Science Daily* (February 29, 2008), www.sciencedaily.com/releases/2008/02/080227142656.htm.

42. American Cancer Society, *Cancer Facts & Figures*, 2009.

43. S. Joachim et al., "Cellular Telephone Use and Cancer Risk: Update of a Nationwide Danish Cohort," *Journal of the National Cancer Institute* 98, no. 23 (2006): 1707–13.

44. American Cancer Society, "New Report Estimates 12 Million Cancer Cases Worldwide in 2007," *Science Daily* (December 18, 2008), www.sciencedaily.com/releases/2007/12/071217092929.htm.

45. American Cancer Society, *Cancer Facts & Figures*, 2009.

46. Ibid.

47. H. A. Wakelee et al., "Lung Cancer Incidence in Never Smokers," *Journal of Clinical Oncology* 25, no. 5 (2007): 472–78.

48. American Cancer Society, *Cancer Facts and Figures*, 2009.

49. Ibid.

50. C. M. Dallal et al., "Long-Term Recreational Physical Activity and Risk of Invasive and In Situ Breast Cancer," *Archives of Internal Medicine* 167, no. 4 (2007): 408–15.

51. American Cancer Society, *Cancer Facts & Figures*, 2009.

52. Ibid.

53. Ibid.

54. Ibid.

55. Ibid.

56. National Cancer Institute, "Endometrial Cancer," Accessed August 2009, www.cancer.gov/cancertopics/types/endometrial.

57. National Cancer Institute, "Testicular Cancer," Accessed August 2009, www.cancer.gov/cancertopics/types/testicular.

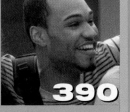
390
Do college students really need to be concerned about diabetes?

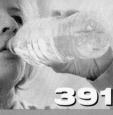
391
What does diabetes feel like?

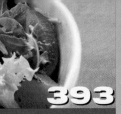
393
People with diabetes can't eat sweets—right?

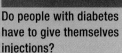
394
Do people with diabetes have to give themselves injections?

FOCUS ON
Your Risk for Diabetes

Like many college students, and a majority of American adults, Nora is overweight. She used to figure it was no big deal, and that she'd put herself on a strict diet and exercise program as soon as she graduated with her engineering degree and started to live "a normal life." But last week, her mom called with some bad news. She told Nora that she'd just found out the results of a routine blood test that her doctor had ordered: Nora's mom has type 2 diabetes. Her voice sounded shaky as she told Nora about her own mother's death from kidney failure—a complication of diabetes—at age 52, a few months before Nora was born. When Nora got off the phone, she searched online for information about diabetes. What she discovered made her feel scared, too: Her Hispanic ethnicity, family history, high stress level, excessive weight, and sedentary lifestyle all increased her own risk for diabetes.

The next morning, Nora stopped off at the campus health center and made an appointment for a diabetes screening. She was instructed to fast the night before, and was scheduled for an appointment first thing in the morning. At her visit, the nurse practitioner took a blood sample. A few days later, she called with the news: Nora has pre-diabetes, and needs to make changes to reduce her risk for developing type 2 diabetes like her mom.

The National Diabetes Information Clearinghouse estimates that 23.6 million Americans of all ages have diabetes.[1] Since 1980, diagnosed diabetes has increased to more than 50 percent of U.S. adults, giving it the dubious distinction of being the fastest growing chronic disease in American history (Figure 1). The rates increase as we age, meaning they aren't as high for college-age adults. The prevalence among Americans aged 20 to 39 is 2.6 percent. Still, one study by the Centers for Disease Control and Pre-

The behaviors you take up in college could lead you on a path to diabetes in the long term—or even in the short term. Do you know whether your lifestyle and family history put you at risk?

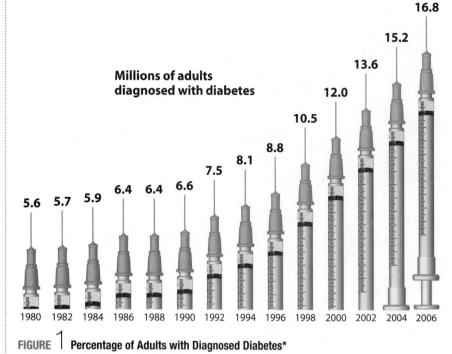

Millions of adults diagnosed with diabetes

5.6 (1980), 5.7 (1982), 5.9 (1984), 6.4 (1986), 6.4 (1988), 6.6 (1990), 7.5 (1992), 8.1 (1994), 8.8 (1996), 10.5 (1998), 12.0 (2000), 13.6 (2002), 15.2 (2004), 16.8 (2006)

FIGURE 1 Percentage of Adults with Diagnosed Diabetes*

*Includes women with gestational diabetes.

Source: Data are from Centers for Disease Control and Prevention, "Diabetes Data and Trends," 2008, http://apps.nccd.cdc.gov/DDTSTRS/default.aspx.

vention (CDC) indicated that diabetes seems to be increasing more dramatically among younger adults than among older Americans—it's up by almost 70 percent among those in their thirties. Approximately 225,000 people die each year of diabetes-related complications, making diabetes the sixth leading cause of death in America today.[2]

7.8%

of the U.S. population has some form of diabetes.

What Is Diabetes?

Diabetes mellitus is a disease characterized by a persistently high level of sugar—technically glucose—in the blood. Its most characteristic sign is the production of an unusually high volume of glucose-laden urine, a fact reflected in its name: *Diabetes* is derived from a Greek word meaning "to

flow through," and *mellitus* is the Latin word for "sweet." The high blood glucose levels—or **hyperglycemia**—seen in diabetes can lead to a variety of serious health problems and even premature death.

Diabetes is actually a group of diseases, each with its own mechanisms. Before we describe what goes wrong to cause the different types of diabetes, let's look at how the body regulates blood glucose in a healthy person.

In Healthy People, Glucose Is Taken Up Efficiently by Body Cells

As you learned in Chapter 9, carbohydrates from the foods you eat are broken down into a monosaccharide called *glucose*. Once the digestive

diabetes mellitus A group of diseases characterized by elevated blood glucose levels.
hyperglycemia Elevated blood glucose level.

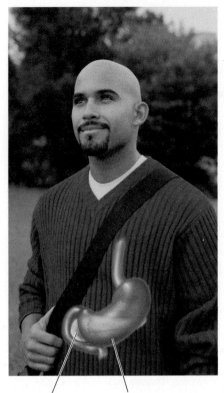

Pancreas   Stomach

FIGURE 2 Diabetes: What It Is and How It Develops

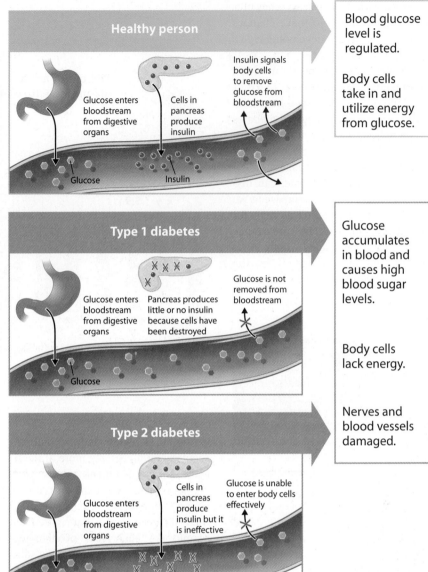

Healthy person

Glucose enters bloodstream from digestive organs

Cells in pancreas produce insulin

Insulin signals body cells to remove glucose from bloodstream

Glucose   Insulin

Blood glucose level is regulated.

Body cells take in and utilize energy from glucose.

Type 1 diabetes

Glucose enters bloodstream from digestive organs

Pancreas produces little or no insulin because cells have been destroyed

Glucose is not removed from bloodstream

Glucose

Glucose accumulates in blood and causes high blood sugar levels.

Body cells lack energy.

Nerves and blood vessels damaged.

Type 2 diabetes

Glucose enters bloodstream from digestive organs

Cells in pancreas produce insulin but it is ineffective

Glucose is unable to enter body cells effectively

system releases it into the bloodstream, glucose becomes available to all body cells. For example, our liver and muscle cells store glucose as glycogen, then use it as needed to fuel metabolism, movement, and other activities. Our red blood cells can use only glucose to fuel their functioning, and brain and other nerve cells prefer glucose over other fuels.

If it's going to power the work of cells, glucose has to be able to get inside them; however, it can't simply cross cell membranes on its own. Instead, cells have structures that transport glucose across in response to a signal. That signal is generated by the **pancreas,** an organ located just beneath the stomach (Figure 2). Whenever a surge of glucose enters the bloodstream, the pancreas secretes a

hormone called **insulin.** Insulin stimulates cells to take up glucose from the bloodstream and carry it into the cell, where it's used for immediate energy or converted to glycogen or fat and stored. Glucose storage is also assisted by insulin. These actions lower the blood level of glucose, and in response, the pancreas stops secreting insulin—until the next influx of glucose arrives.

Type 1 Diabetes Is an Immune Disorder

The more serious and less prevalent form of diabetes, called *type 1 diabetes* (or *insulin-dependent diabetes*), is an

autoimmune disease; that is, the individual's immune system attacks and destroys normal body cells, in this case the insulin-making cells in the pancreas. Destruction of these cells causes a dramatic reduction, or total cessation, of insulin production. Without insulin, cells cannot take up glucose, and blood glucose levels become permanently elevated.

This form of diabetes used to be called *juvenile diabetes* because it most often appears during childhood or adolescence; however, it can begin at any age. European ancestry, a genetic predisposition, and an environmental "insult" such as a viral infection all increase the risk.[3]

pancreas Organ that secretes digestive enzymes into the small intestine, and hormones, including insulin, into the bloodstream.

insulin Hormone secreted by the pancreas and required by body cells for the uptake and storage of glucose.

People with type 1 diabetes require daily insulin injections or infusions and must carefully monitor their diet and exercise levels. Often they face unique challenges as the "lesser known" diabetic type, with fewer funds available for research, fewer community resources, and fewer options for treatment.

Type 2 Diabetes Is a Metabolic Disorder

Type 2 diabetes (non-insulin-dependent diabetes) accounts for 90 to 95 percent of all diabetes cases. In type 2, either the pancreas does not make sufficient insulin, or body cells are resistant to its effects and thus don't efficiently use the insulin that is available (see Figure 2). This latter condition is generally referred to as **insulin resistance.** Unlike type 1 diabetes, which can appear quite suddenly in someone who had previously seemed entirely healthy, type 2 develops slowly.

Development of the Disease In early stages of type 2 diabetes, cells throughout the body begin to resist the effects of insulin. One culprit known to contribute to insulin resistance is the overabundance of free fatty

Singer and pop star Nick Jonas is one of the 5 to 10 percent of diabetics diagnosed with type 1.

acids concentrated in an obese person's fat cells. These free fatty acids directly inhibit glucose uptake by body cells. In addition, they suppress the liver's sensitivity to insulin, so its ability to self-regulate its manufacture of glucose begins to fail. As a consequence of both problems, blood levels of glucose gradually rise. Detecting this elevated blood glucose, the pancreas attempts to compensate by producing more insulin.

The pancreas cannot maintain its hyperproduction of insulin indefinitely. As the progression to type 2 diabetes continues, pancreatic insulin-producing cells become exhausted from overwork. More and more of them sustain physical damage and become nonfunctional. As insulin output declines, blood glucose levels rise high enough to warrant a diagnosis of type 2 diabetes.

Nonmodifiable Risk Factors Type 2 diabetes is associated with a cluster of nonmodifiable risk factors; that is, factors over which you have no control. These include increased age, certain ethnicities, genetic factors, and biological factors.

Type 2 diabetes most often appears after age 40.[4] One in five adults over age 65 has the disease. In fact, type 2 diabetes used to be referred to as *adult-onset diabetes*; now, however, it is being diagnosed at younger ages, even among children and teens. In the United States prior to the year 2000, only 1 to 2 percent of patients below age 18 diagnosed with diabetes had type 2. But recent reports indicate that as many as 45 percent of American youth diagnosed with diabetes have type 2.[5]

In addition, certain ethnic groups have higher rates of type 2 diabetes. Among adults aged 20 and older, 14.2 percent of Native Americans and 11.8 percent of

non-Hispanic blacks have type 2. This makes them about twice as likely as non-Hispanic whites (6.8%) to have the disease. Persons of Hispanic origin have a diabetes rate of 10.4 percent—almost as high as blacks.[6]

Having a close relative with type 2 diabetes is another significant risk factor. Family history suggests a genetic link, and in fact type 2 has a strong genetic component. A small group of "type 2 diabetes genes" has been identified in a variety of studies so far.[7] But even though genetic susceptibility appears to play a role, given the fact that a population's gene pool shifts quite slowly—over centuries—the current epidemic of type 2 diabetes suggests that lifestyle factors, such as increased caloric intake and decreased physical activity, are more to blame.

Modifiable Risk Factors You can't change your age, ethnicity, or genetics, but you can modify lifestyle factors that are considered highly significant in the development of type 2 diabetes. These include your body weight, dietary choices, and your level of physical activity, as well as sleep patterns and your level of stress.

In both children and adults, type 2 diabetes is linked to overweight and obesity. In adults, a body mass index (BMI) of 25 or greater increases the risk. (To determine your BMI, see Chapter 10.) In particular, excess weight carried around the waistline—a condition called *central adiposity*—is risky: A waistline measurement of 40 or more inches in males or 35 or more inches in females is highly correlated to the development of type 2 diabetes.[8]

A sedentary lifestyle also increases the risk, not only because inactivity fails to burn calories, but also because activity itself, and buildup of muscle tissue, improves insulin uptake by cells.[9] People with type 2 diabetes who lose weight and increase their physical

insulin resistance State in which body cells fail to respond to the effects of insulin; obesity increases the risk that cells will become insulin resistant.

activity can significantly improve their blood glucose levels.

Several recent studies suggest that sleep contributes to healthy metabolism, including healthy glucose control. In contrast, inadequate sleep may contribute to the development of type 2 diabetes, as well as obesity.[10] For example, people who routinely fail to get enough sleep have been shown to be at higher risk for *metabolic syndrome* (discussed shortly), a cluster of risk factors that include poor glucose metabolism.[11]

Recent data from large epidemiologic studies have provided evidence of a link between diabetes and psychological or physical stress.[12] When the stress response activates the sympathetic nervous system, it can trigger a combination of increased blood glucose and inadequate production and release of insulin.[13] An occasional stress reaction might not harm you, but chronic stress can contribute to the onset or progression of diabetes. That's why controlling stress (see Chapter 3) is critical for diabetes management.

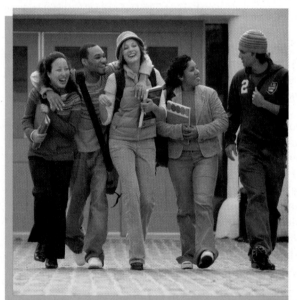

Do college students really need to be concerned about diabetes?

The rate of type 1 and type 2 diabetes among people aged 20 to 39 is 2.6 percent; however, more than 6 percent of college students in one study were found to have pre-diabetes.

Gestational Diabetes Develops during Pregnancy

A third type, *gestational diabetes,* is a state of high blood glucose that is first recognized in a woman during pregnancy. It is thought to be associated with metabolic stresses that occur in response to changing hormonal levels. Gestational diabetes occurs in 3 to 8 percent of all pregnancies. Although experts once considered gestational diabetes a transient event that disappeared after pregnancy, they now realize that women with gestational diabetes have a significantly increased risk of progressing to type 2 diabetes within 5 to 10 years after giving birth.[14] Studies have shown that up to 70 percent of all women with gestational diabetes later develop type 2 diabetes.[15]

In addition, women with gestational diabetes have an increased risk of birth-related complications such as a difficult labor, high blood pressure, high blood acidity, increased infections, and death. The fetus of a woman with gestational diabetes is also endangered: Risks include malformations of the heart, nervous system, and bones; respiratory distress; and excessive growth that can lead to birth trauma. Gestational

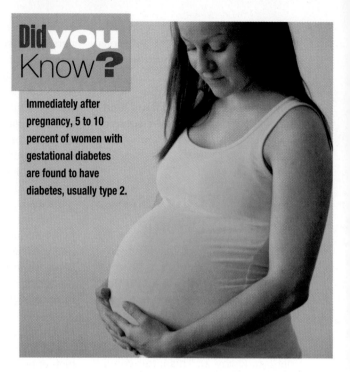

diabetes also increases the risk of fetal death.[16]

Pre-Diabetes Can Lead to Type 2 Diabetes

An estimated 57 million Americans age 20 or older have an ominous set of symptoms known as "pre-diabetes," a condition in which blood glucose levels are higher than normal, but not high enough to be classified as diabetes.[17] This translates into more than 25 percent of the adult population. However, rates of pre-diabetes may not be as high among college students, probably because of the younger age of this population: In one study of college students, just over 6 percent were found to have pre-diabetes.[18]

Although pre-diabetes doesn't cause overt symptoms, the condition is, in a sense, like a ticking time bomb: If it's not "defused," diabetes will eventually strike. On the upside, a diagnosis of pre-diabetes represents a tremendous opportunity to take actions that could prevent diabetes or at least delay its onset. We'll identify these actions shortly.

Pre-Diabetes Plays a Role in Metabolic Syndrome

Often, pre-diabetes is one of the cluster of six conditions linked to overweight and obesity that together constitute a dangerous health risk known as *metabolic syndrome (MetS)*. In fact, of the six conditions, pre-diabetes and central adiposity appear to be the dominant factors for MetS.[19] As we discussed in Chapter 12, MetS dramatically increases an individual's risk for heart disease. In addition, a person with MetS is five times more likely to develop type 2 diabetes than a person without the syndrome.[20]

What Are the Symptoms of Diabetes?

The symptoms of diabetes are similar for both type 1 and type 2. The following are among the most common:

● **Thirst.** It's the job of the kidneys to filter excessive glucose from the blood. When they do, they dilute it with water so that it can be excreted in urine. This pulls too much water from the body, and leaves the person dehydrated and thirsty.

● **Excessive urination.** For the same reason, the person experiences the need to urinate much more frequently than usual. When tested in a lab, a diabetic's urine has a high concentration of glucose.

● **Weight loss.** Because so many calories are lost in the glucose that passes into urine, the person with diabetes often feels unusually hungry. Despite eating more, he or she typically loses weight.

● **Fatigue.** When glucose cannot enter cells, including brain cells and muscle cells, fatigue and weakness become inevitable.

● **Nerve damage.** A high glucose concentration damages the smallest blood vessels of the body, including those supplying nerves in the hands and feet. This can cause numbness and tingling.

● **Blurred vision.** Too much glucose causes body tissues to dry out. When this happens to the lens of the eye, vision deteriorates. In addition, high blood glucose levels can damage microvessels in the eye, leading to vision loss.

● **Poor wound healing and increased infections.** High levels of glucose can affect the body's ability to ward off infection, and may affect overall immune system functioning.

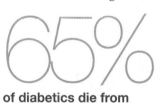

65%
of diabetics die from heart disease or stroke.

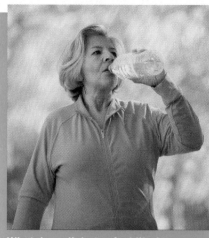

What does diabetes feel like?

People with undiagnosed or uncontrolled diabetes may experience blurred vision, tingling in the hands or feet, and fatigue. One of the most common symptoms is unusual thirst.

Diabetes Can Have Severe Complications

The high blood glucose levels of poorly controlled diabetes can lead to a variety of significant complications. One of the most frightening is a diabetic coma, which results from a state of high blood acidity known as *diabetic ketoacidosis*. It occurs when, in the absence of glucose, body cells break down stored fat for energy. The process produces acidic molecules called *ketones*. Although essential to provide fuel to the brain in the absence of glucose, ketones released in excessive amounts into the blood raise its acid level dangerously high. In a state of ketoacidosis, normal body functions cannot continue. The diabetic slips into a coma and, without prompt medical intervention, will die.

Other complications of poorly controlled diabetes include the following:[21]

● **Cardiovascular disease.** More than 70 percent of diabetics have hypertension. Blood vessels all over the body become damaged as the glucose-laden blood flows more sluggishly and essential nutrients and other substances are not transported as effectively.

● **Kidney disease.** The kidneys become scarred by their extraordinary workload and the high blood pressure in their vessels. Each year, almost 47,000 diabetics develop kidney failure and more than 175,000 are in treatment for this condition.

● **Amputations.** More than 60 percent of nontraumatic amputations of lower limbs are due to diabetes (see **Figure 3a** on page 392). The problem may begin with a minor infection, such as of a toenail; then, an impaired immune response combined with damaged blood vessels enables the infection to spread and resist treatment. Eventually, tissues die and the limb must be amputated.

● **Eye disease and blindness.** Each year, 12,000 to 24,000 people become blind because of diabetic eye disease, making it the leading cause of new blindness in America today (**Figure 3b**).

● **Flu- and pneumonia-related deaths.** Each year, 10,000 to 30,000 people with diabetes die of complications from flu or pneumonia. They are roughly three times more likely to die of these complications than people without diabetes.

● **Tooth and gum diseases.** Diabetics run an increased risk of periodontal disease.

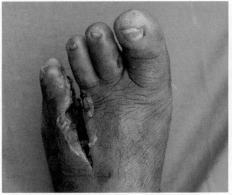

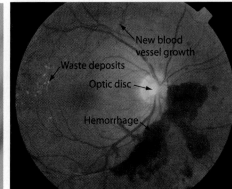

(a) Infections in the feet and legs are common in people with diabetes, and healing is impaired; thus, amputations are often necessary.

(b) Uncontrolled diabetes can damage the eye, causing swelling, leaking, and rupture of blood vessels; growth of new blood vessels; deposits of wastes; and scarring. All of these can progress to blindness.

FIGURE 3 **Complications of Uncontrolled Diabetes: Amputation and Eye Disease**

how to respond when readings are higher or lower than their target level.

How Is Diabetes Treated?

Treatment options for people with pre-diabetes and types 1 and 2 diabetes vary according to the type that they have and how far the disease has progressed.

Blood Tests Are Used to Diagnose and Monitor Diabetes

Diabetes and pre-diabetes are diagnosed when a blood test reveals elevated blood glucose levels. But what tests are used, and exactly what do they show?

Generally, a physician orders either of two blood tests to diagnose pre-diabetes or diabetes:

• The *fasting plasma glucose test (FPG)* requires the patient to fast overnight. Then, a small sample of blood is tested for glucose concentration. As you can see in **Figure 4**, an FPG level greater than or equal to 100 mg/dL indicates pre-diabetes, and a level greater than or equal to 126 mg/dL indicates diabetes.
• The *oral glucose tolerance test (OGTT)* requires the patient to drink a fluid containing a significant level of concentrated glucose. A sample of blood is drawn for testing 2 hours after the patient drinks the solution. As shown in Figure 4, a reading greater than or equal to 140 mg/dL indicates pre-diabetes, whereas a reading greater than or equal to 200 mg/dL indicates diabetes.

If you have any of the risk factors for type 2 diabetes identified earlier, you should talk with your heath care provider about having your blood glucose levels checked. If they're normal, repeat testing should be done every 3 years.[22]

People with diagnosed diabetes typically have their blood glucose levels monitored by their physicians every 3 to 6 months with the *hemoglobin A1C test*. They also need to check their own blood glucose levels several times throughout each day to make sure they stay within their own target range. To check their blood glucose, diabetics must prick their finger to obtain a drop of blood. The blood sample is then evaluated by a handheld glucose meter. Each person has individualized instructions from their heath care provider for

Lifestyle Changes Can Improve Glucose Levels

For people like Nora who have been diagnosed with pre-diabetes, it's important to initiate lifestyle changes immediately to prevent progression of the condition. In fact, studies have shown that people with pre-diabetes can prevent or delay the development of type 2 diabetes by up to 58 percent through

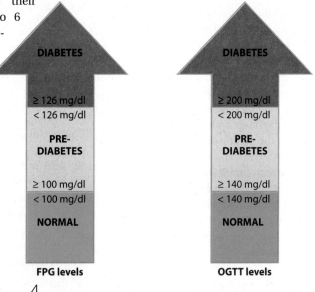

FIGURE 4 **Blood Glucose Levels in Pre-Diabetes and Untreated Diabetes**
The FPG test measures levels of blood glucose after fasting overnight; the OGTT measures levels of blood glucose after consuming a concentrated amount of glucose.

Source: American Diabetes Association, "How to Tell If You Have Pre-Diabetes," www.diabetes.org/diabetes-basics/prevention/pre-diabetes/how-to-tell-if-you -have.html. © 2009 American Diabetes Association. Reprinted with permission.

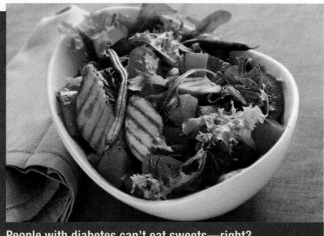

People with diabetes can't eat sweets—right?

People with diabetes can occasionally indulge in sweets, but meals low in saturated and *trans* fats and high in fiber, like this salad of salmon and fresh vegetables, are recommended for helping to control blood glucose and body weight.

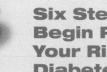

Six Steps to Begin Reducing Your Risk for Diabetes

Step 1. Maintain a healthy weight. For tips on sensible weight loss, see Chapter 10.

Step 2. Eat right. The following tips are from the National Diabetes Education Program's Game Plan to Prevent Type 2 Diabetes:

✳ Eat less fat (especially saturated fats and *trans* fats) than you currently eat.

✳ Eat smaller portions of high-fat and high-calorie foods than you currently eat.

✳ Make fruits, vegetables, and whole grains the focus of your diet.

✳ Choose fat-free or low-fat milk and milk products.

✳ Include lean meats, poultry, fish, beans, eggs, and nuts.

✳ Limit your intake of salt, including the sodium in processed foods.

✳ Limit foods and beverages with added sugars.

Step 3. Get your body moving. Remember that physical activity not only helps you control your weight, but also improves your cells' response to insulin. At least 30 minutes of moderate activity 5 days a week is a minimum recommendation.

Step 4. Quit smoking. You probably know that smoking increases your risk for many types of cancer as well as heart disease, but you might not know that it also increases your blood glucose level. For all these reasons, it's important to quit, and if you don't smoke, don't start.

Step 5. Skip the alcohol, or reduce your intake. Alcohol provides 7 calories per gram, and can keep you from achieving or maintaining weight loss. In addition, alcohol can interfere with blood glucose regulation.

Step 6. Get enough sleep. Inadequate sleep may contribute to the development of type 2 diabetes.

Sources: Adapted from National Diabetes Education Program, *Small Steps, Big Rewards: Your GAME PLAN to Prevent Type 2 Diabetes*, (Bethesda, MD: National Institutes of Health, 2006); American Diabetes Association, "Smoking," 2009, www.diabetes.org/type-1 -diabetes/smoking.jsp.

changes to their lifestyle that include modest weight loss and regular exercise.[23] Even for people who have already been diagnosed with type 2 diabetes, lifestyle changes can sometimes prevent or delay the need for medication or insulin injections. As discussed here, weight loss, exercise, a high-quality diet, stress management, and adequate sleep are all parts of the lifestyle formula. The **Skills for Behavior Change** box at right identifies six steps to get you started!

Weight Loss In people with prediabetes, the key to preventing type 2 diabetes is to lose weight. A Diabetes Prevention Program (DPP) study showed that a loss of as little as 5 to 7 percent of current body weight significantly lowered the risk of progressing to diabetes. Thus, the recommended goal is to lose 5 to 10 percent of current weight.[24] Weight loss is also important for people currently diagnosed with type 2 diabetes.

Adopting a Healthy Diet The DPP recommends that people lose weight by adopting a low-fat, reduced-calorie eating plan. In addition, diabetes researchers have studied a variety of specific foods for their effect on blood glucose levels. Here is a brief summary of some intriguing findings:

● **Whole grains.** A recent review of studies over many years suggests that a diet high in whole grains, especially bran, reduces the risk of developing type 2 diabetes.[25]

● **Coffee.** At least two studies have found that long-term coffee consumption reduces the risk of type 2 diabetes.[26] The findings are controversial, but minerals and antioxidant compounds in coffee are thought to provide the protection.

● **Fatty fish.** An impressive body of evidence links the consumption of fatty fish such as salmon, which is high in omega-3 fatty acids, with decreased progression of insulin resistance.[27]

Eating less overall, and eating fewer animal foods, are two general strategies for weight loss. It is also important to pay attention to the glycemic index (GI) of the foods you eat (see Chapter 9) and to combine carbohydrates with proteins and fats to reduce the overall glycemic load (GL) and prevent surges in blood sugar.

Increasing Physical Fitness The DPP recommends 30 minutes of physical activity 5 days a week to reduce your risk of type 2 diabetes.[28] Brisk walking, swimming, biking, dancing, or any other activity of moderate intensity can be built into your daily schedule. Interestingly, a recent study suggests that improved fitness is even more important than weight loss in improving quality of life for people with diabetes.[29]

Oral Medications and Weight Loss Surgery Can Help

When lifestyle changes fail to provide adequate control of type 2 diabetes, oral medications may be prescribed.[30] These include several types, each of which influences blood glucose in a different way. For example, some medications reduce glucose production by the liver, whereas others slow the absorption of carbohydrates from the small intestine. Other medications increase insulin production by the pancreas, whereas still others work to increase the insulin sensitivity of cells.

Of tremendous interest to the scientific community are recent findings that people who have undergone gastric bypass surgery (discussed in Chapter 10) appear to have high rates of diabetes cure, even before their weight has been lost. This has prompted international focus on the role of various regions of the small intestine in insulin regulation. Although gastric bypass comes with its own set of challenges and risks, other, less drastic methods for achieving these results are under investigation.[31]

Insulin Injections May Be Necessary

Recall that with type 1 diabetes, the pancreas can no longer produce adequate amounts of insulin. Thus, insulin injections are absolutely essential for those with type 1 diabetes. In addition, people with type 2 diabetes whose blood glucose levels cannot be adequately controlled with other treatment options require insulin injections. Incidentally, insulin cannot be taken in pill form because it's a protein, and would be digested in the gastrointestinal tract. It must therefore be injected into the fat layer under the skin, from which it is absorbed into the bloodstream.

People with diabetes used to have to give themselves two or more insulin injections each day. Now, however, many diabetics use an insulin infusion pump. The external portion is only about the size of an MP3 player and can easily be hidden by clothes. It delivers insulin in minute amounts throughout the day through a thin tube and catheter inserted under the patient's skin. This infusion is more effective than delivering a few larger doses of insulin, and obviously less painful. Another form of insulin delivery, insulin inhalers, while available in the past, was taken off the market due to safety concerns. Ongoing research and advances with the technology may lead to their being available again in the future.

Diabetes Care Can Be Expensive

Treatments for diabetes come with a significant price tag. On average, health care costs for diabetics are $15,000 to $25,000 higher per year than for healthy patients. The direct and indirect costs of treating diabetes in the United States total $174 billion per year.[32] However, the full burden of diabetes is hard to measure: Death records often do not reflect the role of diabetes in a person's death, for example, from infection, kidney failure, or a stroke. In addition, the costs related to undiagnosed diabetes are unknown, and the impact of diabetes on quality of life and community resources is difficult to estimate.

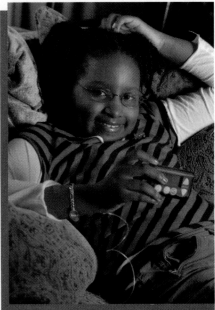

Do people with diabetes have to give themselves injections?

Wearing an insulin infusion pump can help many people with diabetes control their blood glucose levels continuously—and avoid painful injections.

How Can You Prevent Pre-Diabetes?

If you're like Nora, from our chapter-opening story, and have already been diagnosed with pre-diabetes or type 2 diabetes, you can follow the tips in the Skills for Behavior Change box on page 393 to halt or slow the progression of your condition. But what if you've never had your blood glucose tested? Are there any steps you should be taking right now to reduce your risk? Absolutely.

The first step is to consider your risk factors. Use the **Assess Yourself** on the next page to find out whether your risk for diabetes is higher than average. If it is, make an appointment to talk with your heath care provider about diabetes screening.

Assess**yourself**

Are You at Risk for Diabetes?

Certain characteristics place people at greater risk for diabetes. Nevertheless, many people remain unaware of the symptoms of diabetes until after the disease has begun to progress. Take the following quiz to help determine your risk for diabetes. If you answer yes to three or more of these questions, consider seeking medical advice.

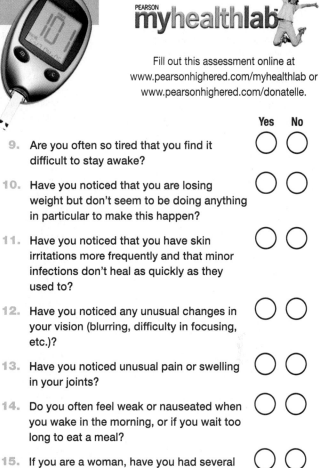

PEARSON myhealthlab

Fill out this assessment online at www.pearsonhighered.com/myhealthlab or www.pearsonhighered.com/donatelle.

		Yes	No
1.	Is there a history of diabetes in your family?	○	○
2.	Do any of your primary relatives (parents, siblings, grandparents) have diabetes?	○	○
3.	Are you overweight or obese?	○	○
4.	Are you typically sedentary (seldom, if ever, engage in vigorous aerobic exercise)?	○	○
5.	Have you noticed an increase in your craving for water or other beverages?	○	○
6.	Have you noticed that you have to urinate more frequently than you used to during a typical day?	○	○
7.	Have you noticed any tingling or numbness in your hands and feet, which might indicate circulatory problems?	○	○
8.	Do you often feel a gnawing hunger during the day, even though you usually eat regular meals?	○	○

		Yes	No
9.	Are you often so tired that you find it difficult to stay awake?	○	○
10.	Have you noticed that you are losing weight but don't seem to be doing anything in particular to make this happen?	○	○
11.	Have you noticed that you have skin irritations more frequently and that minor infections don't heal as quickly as they used to?	○	○
12.	Have you noticed any unusual changes in your vision (blurring, difficulty in focusing, etc.)?	○	○
13.	Have you noticed unusual pain or swelling in your joints?	○	○
14.	Do you often feel weak or nauseated when you wake in the morning, or if you wait too long to eat a meal?	○	○
15.	If you are a woman, have you had several vaginal yeast infections during the past year?	○	○

YOUR PLAN FOR CHANGE

The Assess**yourself** activity asked you to evaluate whether or not you are at risk for diabetes. Now that you have considered your results, you may need to take steps to further understand and address your risks.

Today, you can:

○ Call your parents and ask them if there is a history of diabetes mellitus in your family. If there is, ask which type (type 1, 2, or gestational) the family member(s) had.

○ Take stock of other risk factors you may have for diabetes—do you exercise regularly and watch your weight? Do you eat healthfully? Make a list of small steps you can take in the immediate future to address any of these potential risk factors.

Within the next 2 weeks, you can:

○ If you are at high risk for diabetes, make an appointment with your health care provider to have your blood glucose levels tested.

○ If you smoke, begin devising a plan to quit. Look at the suggestions in Chapter 8 to give you ideas about how to go about this. You may want to consult your doctor about medications or nicotine replacement therapies that could help.

By the end of the semester, you can:

○ Make the lifestyle changes that will reduce your risk. Pay attention to what you eat; increase your intake of whole grains, fruits, and vegetables and decrease your consumption of saturated fats, *trans* fats, and sugar.

○ Make physical activity and exercise part of your daily routine.

References

1. National Diabetes Information Clearinghouse, National Institute of Diabetes and Digestive and Kidney Diseases (NIDDK), *National Diabetes Statistics, 2007* (Bethesda, MD: National Institutes of Health, 2008) NIH Publication no. 08-3892, http://diabetes.niddk.nih.gov/dm/pubs/statistics/DM_Statistics.pdf.

2. Centers for Disease Control and Prevention, "Diabetes Data & Trends," 2008, http://apps.nccd.cdc.gov/ddtstrs.

3. American Diabetes Association, "Type 1 Diabetes," 2009, www.diabetes.org/diabetes-basics/type-1.

4. American Diabetes Association, "Type 2 Diabetes," 2009, www.diabetes.org/diabetes-basics/type-2.

5. H. Rodbard, "Diabetes Screening, Diagnosis, and Therapy in Pediatric Patients with Type 2 Diabetes," *The Medscape Journal of Medicine* 10, no. 8 (2008): 184.

6. American Diabetes Association, "Diabetes Statistics," 2009, www.diabetes .org/diabetes-basics/diabetes-statistics.

7. G. Dedoussis, A. Kaliora, and D. Panagiotakos, "Genes, Diet, and Type 2 Diabetes Mellitus: A Review," *The Review of Diabetic Studies* 4, no. 1 (2007): 13–24; P. Franks, O. Rolandsson, and S. Debenham et al., "Replication of the Association between Variants in the WFS1 Gene and Risk of Type 2 Diabetes in European Populations," *Diabetologia* 51, no. 3 (2008): 458–63; U. Das and A. Rao, "Gene Expression Profile in Obesity and Type 2 Diabetes Mellitus," *Lipids in Health and Disease* 6 (2007): 35; M. van Hoek, A. Dehghan, M. Zillikens, A. Hofman, J. Witteman, and E. Sijbrands, "An RBP4 Promoter Polymorphism Increases Risk of Type 2 Diabetes." *Diabetologia* 51, no. 8 (2008): 1423–28.

8. New Mexico Health Care Takes on Diabetes, "Pre-Diabetes Is a Precursor to Diabetes," *Diabetes Resources* 10, no. 2 (2008), http://nmtod.com/pdfs/precursor.pdf.

9. American Diabetes Association, "Top 10 Benefits of Being Active," 2009, www .diabetes.org/food-nutrition-lifestyle/fitness/fitness-management/top-10-benefits-being-active.jsp.

10. K. Knutson, K. Spiegel, P. Penev, and E. Van Cauter, "The Metabolic Consequences of Sleep Deprivation," *Sleep Medicine Reviews* 11, no. 3 (2007): 163–78;

National Sleep Foundation, "Obesity and Sleep," 2009, www.sleepfoundation.org/article/ask-the-expert/obesity-and-sleep.

11. M. Hall, M. Muldoon, J. Jennings, D. Buysse, J. Flory, and S. Manuck, "Self-Reported Sleep Duration Is Associated with the Metabolic Syndrome in Midlife Adults," *Sleep* 31, no. 5 (2008): 635–43.

12. E. Shiloah and M. Rapoport, "Psychological Stress and New Onset Diabetes," *Pediatric Endocrinology Reviews* 3, no. 3 (2006): 272–75; American Diabetes Association, "Stress," 2008, www.diabetes.org/type-1-diabetes/stress.jsp.

13. R. Rosmond, "Role of Stress in the Pathogenesis of the Metabolic Syndrome," *Pyschoneuroimmunology* 30 (2005): 1–10.

14. American Diabetes Association, "Diabetes Statistics," 2009.

15. C. Kim, K. M. Newton, and R. H. Knopp, "Gestational Diabetes and the Incidence of Type 2 Diabetes," *Diabetes Care* 25, no. 10 (2002): 1862–68; Canadian Medical Association Journal, "Women with Gestational Diabetes at Risk of Type 2 Diabetes," News Release, July 22, 2008, www .cmaj.ca/misc/pr/22jul08_pr_e.shtml.

16. M. Davidson, M. London, and P. Ladewig, *Olds' Maternal-Newborn Nursing & Women's Health across the Lifespan*, 8th ed. (Upper Saddle River, NJ: Pearson Education, 2008), 450–52.

17. American Diabetes Association, "How to Tell If You Have Pre-Diabetes," 2009, www .diabetes.org/diabetes-basics/prevention/pre-diabetes/how-to-tell-if-you-have.html.

18. T. Huang, A. Kempf, M. Strother, C. Li, R. Lee, K. Harris, and H. Kaur, "Overweight and Components of the Metabolic Syndrome in College Students," *Diabetes Care* 27 (2004): 3000–01.

19. American Heart Association, "Metabolic Syndrome," 2009, www.americanheart .org/presenter.jhtml?identifier=4756.

20. National Heart Lung and Blood Institute, "What Is Metabolic Syndrome?" 2007, www.nhlbi.nih.gov/health/dci/Diseases/ms/ms_whatis.html.

21. American Diabetes Association, "Diabetes Statistics," 2008.

22. National Diabetes Education Program, *Small Steps, Big Rewards: Your GAME PLAN to Prevent Type 2 Diabetes* (Bethesda, MD: National Institutes of Health, 2006) NIH Publication no. 06-5334, http://ndep.nih.gov/media/GP_Booklet.pdf.

23. American Diabetes Association, "Frequently Asked Questions about Pre-Diabetes," 2009, www.diabetes.org/diabetes-basics/prevention/pre-diabetes/pre-diabetes-faqs.html.

24. National Diabetes Education Program, *Small Steps, Big Rewards*, 2006.

25. J. de Munter, F. Hu, D. Spiegelman, M. Franz, and R. van Dam, "Whole Grain, Bran, and Germ Intake and Risk of Type 2 Diabetes: A Prospective Cohort Study and Systematic Review," *PLoS Medicine* 4, no. 8 (2007): e261.

26. M. Pereira, E. Parker, and A. Folsom, "Coffee Consumption and Risk of Type 2 Diabetes Mellitus: An 11-Year Prospective Study of 28,812 Postmenopausal Women," *Archives of Internal Medicine* 166, no. 12 (2006): 1311–16; E. Salazar-Martinez, W. Willett, A. Ascherio, J. Manson, M. Leitzmann, M. Stampfer, and F. Hu, "Coffee Consumption and Risk for Type 2 Diabetes Mellitus," *Annals of Internal Medicine* 140, no. 1 (2004): 1–8.

27. M. Lankinen, U. Schwab, and A. Erkkila et al., "Fatty Fish Intake Decreases Lipids Related to Inflammation and Insulin Signaling—A Lipidomics Approach," *PLoS One* 4, no. 4 (2009): e5258; G. Dedoussis, A. Kaliora, and D. Panagiotakos, "Genes, Diet, and Type 2 Diabetes Mellitus: A Review," *The Review of Diabetic Studies* 4, no. 1 (2007): 13–24.

28. National Diabetes Education Program, *Small Steps, Big Rewards*, 2006.

29. W. Bennett, P. Ouyang, A. Wu, B. Barone, and K. Stewart, "Fatness and Fitness: How Do They Influence Health-Related Quality of Life in Type 2 Diabetes Mellitus?" *Health and Quality of Life Outcomes* 6 (2008): 110.

30. G. Gillies et al., "Pharmacological and Lifestyle Interventions to Prevent or Delay Type 2 Diabetes in People with Impaired Glucose Tolerance: Systematic Review and Meta-analysis," *BMJ* 334 (2007): 299.

31. F. Rubino, "Is Type 2 Diabetes an Operable Intestinal Disease? A Provocative yet Reasonable Hypothesis," *Diabetes Care* 31 (2008): S290–96; *60 Minutes*, "Special Report: The Bypass Effect: Stopping Diabetes," April 20, 2008.

32. American Diabetes Association, "Diabetes Statistics," 2008.

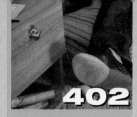
402
Why are vaccinations important?

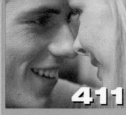
411
How can I tell if someone I'm dating has an STI?

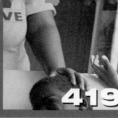
419
Is HIV/AIDS still an epidemic?

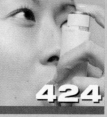
424
What causes asthma?

Infectious and Noninfectious Conditions

13

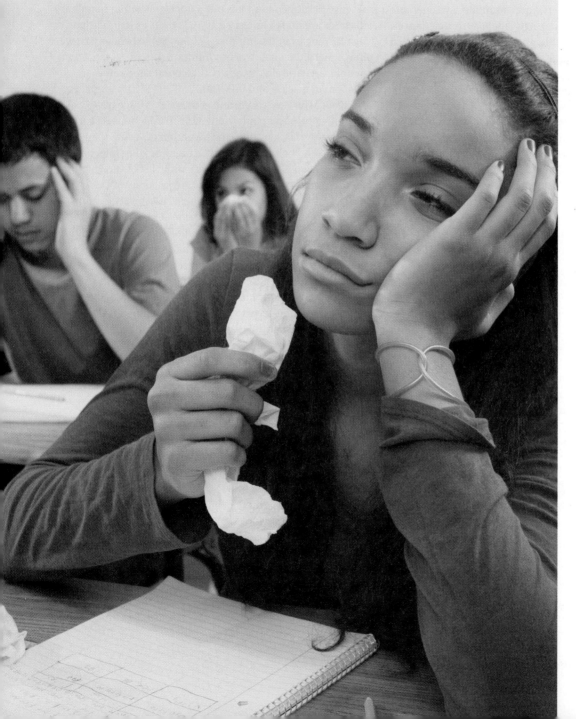

Objectives

✻ Explain how your immune system works to protect you and what you can do to boost its effectiveness.

✻ Describe the most common pathogens infecting humans today and the typical diseases each causes.

✻ Discuss the various sexually transmitted infections, their means of transmission, and actions that can be taken to prevent their spread.

✻ Discuss human immunodeficiency virus (HIV) and acquired immunodeficiency syndrome (AIDS), trends in infection and treatment, and the impact of the disease on special populations.

✻ Discuss common noninfectious conditions, including asthma and low back pain.

Every moment of every day, you are in contact with microscopic organisms that have the ability to cause illness or even death. These disease-causing agents, known as **pathogens,** are found in air and food and on nearly every object and person with whom you come in contact. New varieties of pathogens arise all the time, and scientific evidence indicates that many have existed for as long as there has been life on the planet. Throughout history, infectious diseases have at times wiped out whole groups of people through **epidemics** such as the Black Death, or bubonic plague, which killed up to one-third of the population of Europe in the 1300s. A **pandemic,** or global epidemic, of influenza killed an estimated 30 to 50 million people in 1918, whereas strains of tuberculosis and cholera continue to cause premature death throughout the world.

At times, fear and high levels of anxiety about infectious diseases such as the flu become widespread. However, it's important to remember that in spite of constant bombardment by pathogenic threats, our immune systems are remarkably resilient and amazingly adept at protecting us. Millions of microorganisms live in our bodies all of the time; for example, bacteria inhabit our stomachs, intestines, and mouths without ever triggering our immune systems to fight these invaders. In many cases they are actually beneficial, aiding in digestion and other bodily functions. For people in good health whose immune systems are functioning effectively, these organisms are harmless; however, if the immune system is weakened by other pathogens or chronic diseases, these internal organisms can grow rapidly, overcome the host, and cause serious illness.

When pathogens gain entry to the body, they may produce varying degrees of illness. The more **virulent** the organism, the greater the chance that it can gain entry and sustain itself in the host, and the more likely it is that illness will result. If your immune system is weak, or **immunocompromised,** the greater the chances are that pathogens will be able to overcome your arsenal of immune defenses and make you sick. Keeping your immune system healthy will greatly reduce your chances of developing an infectious disease.

pathogen A disease-causing agent.
epidemic Disease outbreak that affects many people in a community or region at the same time.
pandemic Global epidemic of a disease.
virulent Strong enough to overcome host resistance and cause disease.
immunocompromised Having an immune system that is impaired.

The Process of Infection and Your Body's Defenses

For a disease to occur in a person, or *host,* the host must be *susceptible,* which means that the immune system must be immunocompromised; an *agent* capable of *transmitting* a disease must be present; and the *environment* must be *hospitable* to the pathogen in terms of temperature, light, moisture, and other requirements. Although all pathogens pose a threat if they take hold in your body, the chances that they will do so are actually quite small. First, they must overcome a number of effective barriers, many of which were established in your body before you were born. Figure 13.1 summarizes some of the body's defenses that help protect you against invasion and decrease your susceptibility to disease. Many of these defenses can be improved, meaning that there are actions you can take to make your body's defenses more effective.

Risk Factors You Typically Cannot Control

Unfortunately, some of the factors that make you susceptible to a certain disease are beyond your control. The following are the most common:

- **Heredity.** Perhaps the single greatest factor influencing disease risk is genetics. It is often unclear whether hereditary diseases are due to inherited genetic traits or to inherited insufficiencies in the immune system. Some believe that we may inherit the quality of our immune system, so that some people are naturally "tougher" than others and more resilient to disease and infection.
- **Aging.** The very young and those over the age of 65 tend to be particularly vulnerable to infectious diseases. In the early 1900s, prior to the invention of vaccines, many children died before their fifth birthday as killer infectious diseases swept the country. Today, as the list of vaccinations for the young and for older adults grows, many of these diseases are kept in check. Without access to vaccinations, however, young and old alike become at high risk.
- **Environmental conditions.** Unsanitary conditions and the presence of drugs, chemicals, and hazardous pollutants and wastes in food and water probably have a great effect on our immune systems. A growing body of research points to changes in the environment (like global warming), the potential for long-term exposure to a "melting pot" of toxic chemicals, and natural disasters as significant contributors to increasing numbers of infectious diseases. Add to that the large numbers of displaced refugees in the world population and persons living in squalor and without access to food, clean water, or medical care, and the potential for infectious disease skyrockets.
- **Organism virulence and resistance.** Some organisms, such as the foodborne organism that causes *botulism* (a severe foodborne illness), are particularly virulent, and even tiny amounts may make the most hardy of us ill. Other organisms have mutated and become resistant to the body's defenses and to medical treatments. Multidrug-resistant strains of tuberculosis, *Staphylococcus*, and other organisms are emerging in many parts of the world.

Risk Factors You Can Control

The good news is that we all have some degree of personal control over many risk factors for disease. Too much stress,

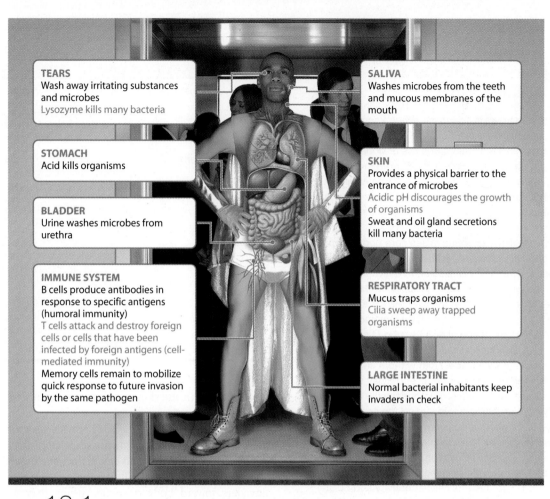

TEARS
Wash away irritating substances and microbes
Lysozyme kills many bacteria

STOMACH
Acid kills organisms

BLADDER
Urine washes microbes from urethra

IMMUNE SYSTEM
B cells produce antibodies in response to specific antigens (humoral immunity)
T cells attack and destroy foreign cells or cells that have been infected by foreign antigens (cell-mediated immunity)
Memory cells remain to mobilize quick response to future invasion by the same pathogen

SALIVA
Washes microbes from the teeth and mucous membranes of the mouth

SKIN
Provides a physical barrier to the entrance of microbes
Acidic pH discourages the growth of organisms
Sweat and oil gland secretions kill many bacteria

RESPIRATORY TRACT
Mucus traps organisms
Cilia sweep away trapped organisms

LARGE INTESTINE
Normal bacterial inhabitants keep invaders in check

FIGURE 13.1 **The Body's Defenses against Disease-Causing Pathogens**
In addition to the defenses listed, many of the body's secretions and fluids, such as earwax, mucus, and blood, contain enzymes and other proteins that can kill some invading pathogens or prevent or slow their reproduction.

inadequate nutrition, a low fitness level, lack of sleep, misuse or abuse of legal and illegal drugs and alcohol, poor personal hygiene, high-risk behaviors, exposure to products and services that increase your risk, and other variables significantly increase the risk for many diseases. Fortunately, there are things you can do to eliminate, reduce, or change your susceptibility to various pathogens. The **Skills for Behavior Change** box on page 400 lists some actions you can take and lifestyle changes you can adopt to keep your body's defenses in top form for warding off infections. There are also changes you can make in your community to clean up toxins, set policies on contaminant levels, and reduce the likelihood of being exposed to pathogens or things that could harm the immune system.

what do you think?
Do you have any risks for infectious disease that may be hereditary? Do you have any that are the result of your lifestyle? ● What actions can you take to reduce your risks? ● Are your risks greater today than before you entered college? Why or why not?

Routes of Transmission

Pathogens enter the body in several ways. They may be transmitted by *direct contact* between infected persons, such as during sexual relations, kissing, or touching, or by *indirect contact,* such as by touching an object the infected person has had contact with. Table 13.1 on the next page lists common routes of transmission. You may also **autoinoculate** yourself, or transmit a pathogen from one part of your body to another. For example, you may touch a sore on your lip that is teeming with viral herpes and then transmit the virus to your eye when you scratch your itchy eyelid.

Your best friend may be the source of *animalborne pathogens.* Dogs, cats, livestock, and wild animals can spread numerous diseases through their bites or feces or by carrying infected insects into living areas and transmitting diseases either directly or indirectly. Although *interspecies transmission* of diseases (diseases passed from humans to animals and vice versa) is rare, it does occur.

autoinoculate Transmit a pathogen from one part of your own body to another part.

Reduce Your Risk of Infectious Disease

✳ **Limit your exposure to pathogens.** When your family, friends, or coworkers are sick, limit your contact with possible germs: Don't share utensils or drinking glasses, keep your toothbrush away from those of other people, and wash your hands often. Remember that your hands are the biggest source of disease transmission. Keep them away from your mouth, nose, eyes, and other body orifices.

✳ **Exercise regularly.** Exercise raises core body temperature, producing a form of "artificial fever" that kills pathogens. Sweat contains salt and enzymes that destroy the cell walls of many bacteria, whereas the oil (sebaceous) glands kick in to lower the pH of the skin, making it a hostile environment for many bacteria.

✳ **Get enough sleep.** Sleep allows the body time to refresh itself, produce necessary cells, and reduce inflammation. Even a single night without sleep can increase inflammatory processes and delay wound healing. Inadequate sleep compromises the ability of every system of the body—including the immune system—to function at peak capacity.

✳ **Stress less.** Stress hormones wreak havoc on immune functioning. Rest and relaxation, stress management practices, laughter, and calming music have all been shown to promote healthy cellular activity and bolster immune functioning.

✳ **Optimize eating.** Enjoy a healthy diet, including adequate amounts of water, protein, and complex carbohydrates. Eat more omega-3 fatty acids to reduce inflammation, and restrict saturated fats, replacing them with good fats such as olive oil. Antioxidants are believed to be important in immune functioning, so make sure you get your daily fruits and vegetables.

TABLE 13.1 Routes of Disease Transmission

Mode of Transmission	Aspects of Transmission
Contact	Either *direct* (e.g., skin or sexual contact) or *indirect* (e.g., infected blood or body fluid)
Food- or waterborne	Eating or coming in contact with contaminated food or water or products passed through them
Airborne	Inhalation; droplet spread as through sneezing, coughing, or talking
Vectorborne	Transmitted by an animal, such as a mosquito, tick, snail, or bird, by means of its secretions, biting, or egg laying
Perinatal	Similar to contact infection; happens in the uterus or as the baby passes through the birth canal or through breast-feeding

breaks occur in the skin can pathogens gain easy access to the body.

The internal linings of the body provide yet another protection. Mucous membranes in the respiratory tract and other linings of the body trap and engulf invading organisms. *Cilia,* hairlike projections in the lungs and respiratory tract, sweep invaders toward body openings, where they are expelled. Tears, nasal secretions, earwax, and other secretions found at body entrances contain enzymes designed to destroy or neutralize pathogens. Finally, any organism that manages to breach these initial lines of defense faces a formidable specialized network of defenses thrown up by the immune system.

The Immune System: Your Body Fights Back

Immunity is a condition of being able to resist a particular disease by counteracting the substance that produces the disease. Any substance capable of triggering an immune response is called an **antigen.** An antigen can be a virus, a bacterium, a fungus, a parasite, a toxin, or a tissue or cell from another organism. When invaded by an antigen, the body responds by forming substances called **antibodies** that are matched to that specific antigen, much as a key is matched to a lock.

Once an antigen breaches the body's initial defenses, the body begins a process of antigen analysis. It considers the size and shape of the invader, verifies that the antigen is not part of the body itself, and then produces a specific antibody to destroy or weaken the antigen. This process, which is much more complex than described here, is part of a system called *humoral immune responses.* **Humoral immunity** is the body's major defense against many bacteria and the poisonous substances, called **toxins,** that they produce.

Physical and Chemical Defenses: Your Body Responds

Our single most critical early defense system is the skin. Layered to provide an intricate web of barriers, the skin allows few pathogens to enter. Enzymes in body secretions such as sweat provide additional protection, destroying microorganisms on skin surfaces by producing inhospitable pH levels. In either case, microorganisms that flourish at a selected pH will be weakened or destroyed as these changes occur. Only when cracks or

antigen Substance capable of triggering an immune response.
antibodies Substances produced by the body that are individually matched to specific antigens.
humoral immunity Aspect of immunity that is mediated by the secretion of antibodies that target cells for destruction.
toxins Poisonous substances produced by certain microorganisms that cause various diseases.

Cell-mediated immunity is characterized by the formation of a population of **lymphocytes** (specialized white blood cells) that can attack and destroy the foreign invader. These lymphocytes constitute the body's main defense against viruses, fungi, parasites, and some bacteria, and they are found in the blood, lymph nodes, bone marrow, and certain glands. Other key players in this immune response are **macrophages** (a type of phagocytic, or cell-eating, white blood cell).

Two forms of lymphocytes in particular, the *B lymphocytes* (B cells) and *T lymphocytes* (T cells), are involved in the immune response. T cells assist the immune system in several ways. *Helper T cells* are essential for activating B cells to produce antibodies. They also activate other T cells, and macrophages. Another form of T cell, known as the *killer T cell* directly attacks infected or malignant cells. Killer T cells enable the body to rid itself of cells that have been infected by viruses or transformed by cancer; they are also responsible for rejecting tissue and organ grafts. *Suppressor T cells* turn off or suppress the activity of B cells, killer T cells, and macrophages. After a successful attack on a pathogen, some of the attacker T and B cells are preserved as *memory T* and *B cells,* enabling the body to recognize and respond quickly to subsequent attacks by the same kind of organism at a later time.

Once people have survived certain infectious diseases, they become immune to those diseases, meaning that in all probability they will not develop them again. Upon subsequent attack by the same disease-causing microorganisms, their memory T and B cells are quickly activated to come to their defense. **Figure 13.2** provides a summary of the cell-mediated immune response.

Autoimmune Diseases

Although white blood cells and the antigen–antibody response generally work in our favor, the body sometimes makes a mistake and targets its own tissue as the enemy, builds up antibodies against that tissue, and attempts to destroy it. This is known as **autoimmune disease** (*auto* means "self"). Common autoimmune disorders include rheumatoid arthritis, systemic lupus erythematosus (SLE), type 1 diabetes, and multiple sclerosis.

Inflammatory Response, Pain, and Fever

If an infection is localized, pus formation, redness, swelling, and irritation often occur. These symptoms are components of the body's inflammatory response, and they indicate that the invading organisms are being fought systematically.

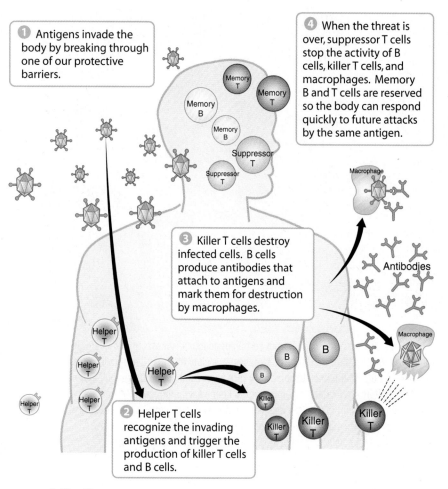

❶ Antigens invade the body by breaking through one of our protective barriers.

❷ Helper T cells recognize the invading antigens and trigger the production of killer T cells and B cells.

❸ Killer T cells destroy infected cells. B cells produce antibodies that attach to antigens and mark them for destruction by macrophages.

❹ When the threat is over, suppressor T cells stop the activity of B cells, killer T cells, and macrophages. Memory B and T cells are reserved so the body can respond quickly to future attacks by the same antigen.

FIGURE 13.2 **The Immune Response**

The four cardinal signs of inflammation are redness, swelling, pain, and heat.

Pain is often one of the earliest signs that an injury or infection has occurred and it can cause the person to avoid activity that may aggravate the injury or site of infection, thereby protecting against further damage. Although pain doesn't feel good, it plays a valuable role in the body's response to injury or invasion. Pathogens can kill or injure tissue at the site of infection, causing swelling that puts pressure on nerve endings in the area, causing pain to occur.

In addition to inflammation, another frequent indicator of infection is the development of a *fever,* or a rise in body temperature above the average norm of 98.6°F. Fever is frequently caused by toxins secreted by pathogens that interfere with the control of body temperature. Although extremely elevated temperatures are harmful to the body, a mild fever is protective: Raising body temperature by one or two degrees provides an environment that destroys some disease-causing organisms. A fever also stimulates the body to produce more white blood cells,

cell-mediated immunity Aspect of immunity that is mediated by specialized white blood cells that attack pathogens and antigens directly.
lymphocyte A type of white blood cell involved in the immune response.
macrophage A type of white blood cell that ingests foreign material.
autoimmune disease Disorders in which the body's tissues are attacked by its own immune system.

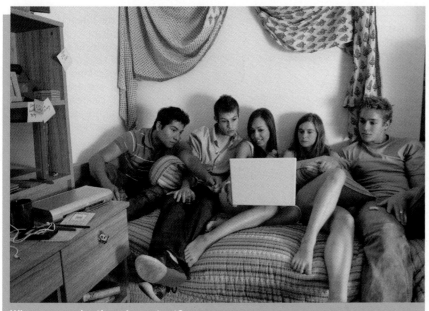

Why are vaccinations important?

Vaccinations can protect an individual from certain infectious diseases, and they are also important in controlling the prevalence of diseases in society at large. Certain diseases such as polio and diphtheria have become very rare as a result of immunizations, but until a disease is completely eradicated, it is important to keep vaccinating people against it. Otherwise, there is nothing to stop the disease from making a comeback and causing an epidemic. People at particular risk, such as college students who often live in close quarters, should be especially certain to stay up to date on their vaccinations.

termed *artificially acquired active immunity,* in contrast to *naturally acquired active immunity* (which is obtained by exposure to antigens in the normal course of daily life) or *naturally acquired passive immunity* (as occurs when a mother passes immunity to her fetus via their shared blood supply or to an infant via breast milk).

Depending on the organism's virulence, vaccines containing live, attenuated (weakened), or dead organisms are given for specific diseases. Regardless of the type of vaccine, specific schedules have been established for optimal vaccine performance in protecting against typical diseases that affect children and adults. **Figure 13.3** shows the recommended schedule for adult vaccinations. Childhood vaccine schedules are available at the Centers for Disease Control and Prevention (CDC) website. Concerns about potential dangers related to vaccines have caused some parents to refuse to vaccinate their children, a potentially dangerous choice that could lead to reemergence of previously eradicated diseases (see the **Health Headlines** box on page 404).

Because of their close living quarters and frequent interaction with people from many different places and backgrounds, college students face higher than average risks of infections from diseases that are largely preventable. Recent increases in some childhood diseases among the general public have prompted campuses across the country to require immunizations against diseases that should no longer plague U.S. citizens, particularly measles, German measles (rubella), and tetanus/diphtheria.

which destroy more invaders. Of course, as fevers increase beyond 101 or 102 degrees Fahrenheit, risks to the patient outweigh any benefits. In these cases, medical treatment should be obtained. Misuse of aspirin in the early stage of (low) fever may inadvertently sabotage the immune system's defenses by keeping temperature ideal for pathogen growth.

Vaccines: Bolstering Your Immunity

Recall that once people have been exposed to a specific pathogen, subsequent attacks will activate their memory T and B cells, thus giving them immunity. This is the principle on which **vaccination** is based.

A vaccine consists of killed or weakened versions of a disease-causing microorganism or an antigen that is similar to but less dangerous than the disease antigen. It is administered to stimulate the person's immune system to produce antibodies against future attacks—without actually causing the disease (or by causing a very minor case of it). Vaccines typically are given orally or by injection, and this form of immunity is

vaccination Inoculation with killed or weakened pathogens or similar, less dangerous antigens to prevent or lessen the effects of some disease.
allergy Hypersensitive reaction to a specific antigen in which the body produces antibodies to a normally harmless substance in the environment.
allergen An antigen that induces a hypersensitive immune response.
histamine Chemical substance that dilates blood vessels, increases mucous secretions, and produces other symptoms of allergies.

Allergies: The Immune System Overreacts

An **allergy** occurs as part of the body's attempt to defend itself against a specific *antigen* or **allergen** by producing specific *antibodies.* Under normal conditions, the production of antibodies is a positive element in the body's defense system. However, for unknown reasons, in some people the body overreacts by developing an overly protective mechanism against relatively harmless substances. The resulting *hypersensitivity reaction* is fairly common, as anyone who has awakened with a runny nose or itchy eyes will testify. Most commonly, these hypersensitivity, or allergic, reactions occur as a response to environmental antigens such as molds, animal dander (hair and dead skin), pollen, ragweed, or dust. Some people are also allergic to certain foods (see Chapter 9). Once excessive antibodies to allergens are produced, they trigger the release of **histamine,** a chemical that dilates blood vessels, increases mucous secretions, causes tissues to swell, and produces rashes, difficulty breathing,

Vaccine	Age group				
	19–26 years	27–49 years	50–59 years	60–64 years	≥ 65 years
Tetanus, diphtheria, pertussis (Td/Tdap)*	Substitute 1-time dose of Tdap for Td booster; then boost with Td every 10 years				Td booster every 10 years
Human papillomavirus (HPV)*	3 doses (females)				
Varicella*	2 doses				
Zoster				1 dose	
Measles, mumps, rubella (MMR)*	1 or 2 doses		1 dose		
Influenza*	1 dose annually				
Pneumococcal (polysaccharide)	1 or 2 doses				1 dose
Hepatitis A*	2 doses				
Hepatitis B*	3 doses				
Meningococcal*	1 or more doses				

*Covered by the Vaccine Injury Compensation Program

For all persons in this category who meet the age requirements and who lack evidence of immunity (e.g., lack documentation of vaccination or have no evidence of prior infection)

Recommended if some other risk factor is present (e.g., on the basis of medical, occupational, lifestyle, or other indications)

No recommendation

FIGURE 13.3 **Recommended Adult Immunization Schedule, by Vaccine and Age Group, 2009**
Note that there are important explanations and additions to these recommendations that should be consulted by checking the latest schedule at www.cdc.gov/vaccines/recs/schedules/adult-schedule.htm.
Source: Centers for Disease Control and Prevention, "Recommended Adult Immunization Schedule—United States, 2009," *MMWR Weekly* 57, no. 53 (2009): 1–4.

and other allergy symptoms. Many people have found that **immunotherapy** treatment, or "allergy shots," somewhat reduce the severity of their symptoms. In most cases, once the offending antigen has disappeared, allergy-prone people suffer few symptoms.

Hay Fever **Hay fever,** or *pollen allergy*, occurs throughout the world and is one of the most common chronic diseases in the United States, affecting over 25 million Americans each year (about 8% of all adults and 10% of children).[1] It is usually considered a seasonal disease, because it is most prevalent when ragweed and flowers are blooming. Symptoms include sneezing and itchy, watery eyes and nose, and they make countless people miserable for weeks at a time every year. As with other allergies, hay fever results from a hypersensitive immune system and an inherited tendency to have this hypersensitivity.

Avoiding the environmental triggers is the best way to prevent hay fever. If you can't prevent it, shots or antihistamines often provide relief. Decongestants can reduce symptoms, as can air-conditioning and air purifiers. Rinsing out your nose can also bring relief. Over-the-counter nose sprays are usually of limited value, and their prolonged use may actually cause symptoms or make them worse. Inhaled steroids are often effective and may be prescribed, as are specific desensitizing injections.[2]

Types of Pathogens and Diseases They Cause

We can categorize pathogenic microorganisms into six major types: bacteria, viruses, fungi, protozoans, parasitic worms, and prions. Each pathogen has a particular route of transmission and characteristic elements that make it unique. In the following pages, we discuss each of these categories and give an overview of some diseases they cause that have a significant impact on public health. Figure 13.4 on page 405 shows examples of several of these pathogens.

Bacteria

Bacteria (singular: *bacterium*) are simple, single-celled microscopic organisms. There are three major types of bacteria, as classified by their shape: cocci, bacilli, and spirilla. Although there are several thousand known species of bacteria (and many thousands more that are unknown), just over 100 cause diseases in humans. In

immunotherapy Treatment strategies based on the concept of regulating the immune system, as by administering antibodies or desensitization shots of allergens.
hay fever A chronic allergy-related respiratory disorder that is most prevalent when ragweed and flowers bloom.
bacteria (singular: *bacterium*) Simple, single-celled microscopic organisms. About 100 known species of bacteria cause disease in humans.

Health Headlines

VACCINE BACKLASH: ARE THEY SAFE? ARE THEY NECESSARY?

Immunizations against widespread infectious diseases are one of the greatest public health success stories of all time—so successful, in fact, that most people have never seen or heard of anyone having the diseases that once wiped out entire populations. As fear of getting these diseases waned, as numbers of vaccines recommended increased, as medical costs increased, and as distrust of all things related to government increased, many people have questioned the ethics, safety, and necessity of these shots. Misinformation and fearmongering about potential hazards of vaccines have prompted more and more people to forgo their shots. How serious a problem is this? In some communities, such as Ashland, Oregon, parents of up to 25 percent of kindergartners opted their children out of at least one vaccine last year. In other U.S. school districts and counties, these rates are even higher, and a general trend of exemptions from vaccinations is growing. Undervaccination rates are particularly high in non-Hispanic, college-educated white families with incomes above $75,000 a year. Religious tenets, fear of vaccine safety, and worry about vaccine overload are among some of the more common reasons for parents' refusal to vaccinate their children. Others object to mandatory vaccinations because they consider them to be a government intrusion into their individual rights.

The vaccine concerns receiving the most attention include fear that the measles, mumps, rubella (MMR) vaccine can lead to autism; fear that the hepatitis B vaccine is related to multiple sclerosis (MS); and fear that the tetanus, diphtheria, pertussis (Td/Tdap vaccine) can cause sudden infant death syndrome (SIDS). Are these concerns valid? While research is ongoing, there is no clear evidence that the MMR vaccine causes autism, that hepatitis B shots are the culprit behind MS, or that the Tdap vaccine leads to SIDS. Virtually all medical and public health organizations support vaccinations, pointing to stringent safety controls in the manufacturing and testing of vaccines, as well as ongoing safety monitoring, the long history of vaccines in wiping out killer diseases across the globe, and the fact that risks from the diseases the themselves are almost always much greater than any risks associated with a vaccine. If large numbers of people were to avoid vaccinations, old killers would be likely to reemerge, and those people who were already sick or weak from other conditions would be extremely vulnerable.

The reasons for vaccination far outweigh any arguments against. That said, it's important to note that, despite extensive testing, no vaccine is completely safe and effective and that there are often risks from temporary, minor side effects from any given vaccine. Local rashes and reactions at injection sites, low-grade fever, discomfort, and even allergic reactions can occur. Major risks from getting vaccinations are extremely rare and studies supporting the "antivaccine" rhetoric are unsubstantiated. The official positions of the international community, the U.S. government, and research groups are in support of vaccine efficacy.

---

many cases, it is not the bacteria themselves that cause disease but rather the toxins that they produce.

Diseases caused by bacteria are often easily treatable with **antibiotics;** penicillin is one of the oldest and historically most well-known antibiotics. However, today's arsenal of antibiotics is becoming less effective, as antibiotic-resistant strains of bacteria become more common. Such "superbugs" can result when successive generations of bacteria mutate to develop **antibiotic resistance,** meaning they are able to withstand the effects of specific drugs. The following are the most common bacterial infections, some of which pose new threats through especially virulent, resistant strains.

antibiotics Medicines used to kill microorganisms, such as bacteria.

antibiotic resistance The ability of bacteria or other microbes to withstand the effects of an antibiotic.

staphylococci A group of round bacteria, usually found in clusters, that cause a variety of diseases in humans and other animals.

colonization The process of bacteria or some other infectious organisms establishing themselves on a host without causing infection.

infection The state of pathogens being established in or on a host and causing disease.

methicillin-resistant staphylococcus aureus (MRSA) Highly resistant form of staph infection that is growing in international prevalence.

Staphylococcal Infections **Staphylococci** are normally present on the skin or in the nostrils of 20 to 30 percent of us at any given time. Usually they cause no problems for otherwise healthy persons. The presence of bacteria on or in a person without infection is called **colonization.** A person can be colonized and spread the infection to others, yet not ever develop the disease. In contrast, when the pathogen is present and there is a cut or break in the *epidermis,* or outer layer of the skin, staphylococci may enter the system and cause an **infection.** If you have ever suffered from acne, boils, styes (infections of the eyelids), or infected wounds, you have probably had a "staph" infection.

Although most of these infections are readily defeated by your immune system, resistant forms of staph bacteria are on the rise. These infections pose serious risks and must be treated with specific antibiotics, of which fewer and fewer remain effective. One of these resistant forms of staph, **methicillin-resistant staphylococcus aureus (MRSA),** has come under intense international scrutiny as numerous cases have arisen around the world, especially in the United States.[3] One form,

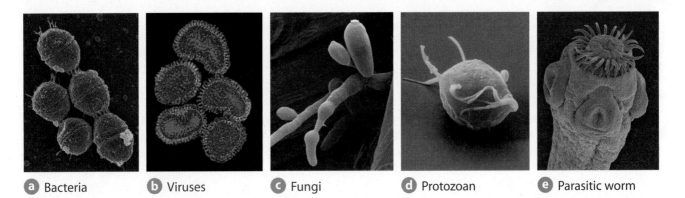

<a> Bacteria   <b> Viruses   <c> Fungi   <d> Protozoan   <e> Parasitic worm

FIGURE 13.4 **Example of 5 Major Types of Pathogens**

(a) Color-enhanced scanning electron micrograph (SEM) of *Streptococcus* bacteria, magnified 40,000×. (b) Colored transmission electron micrograph (TEM) of influenza (flu) viruses, magnified 32,000×. (c) Color SEM of *Candida albicans*, a yeast fungus, magnified 50,000×. (d) Color TEM of *Trichomonas vaginalis*, a protozoan, magnified 9,000×. (e) Color-enhanced SEM of the adult head (scolex) of a mammalian intestinal tapeworm, magnified 20×.

healthcare associated (HA-MRSA), makes up the vast majority of cases and is particularly worrisome in hospitals, nursing homes, and other settings where invasive treatments, persons with weakened immune systems, and other infections are common. A second form, *community acquired (CA-MRSA),* is on the rise in otherwise healthy people who are exposed to the pathogen and can't fight it effectively on their own.

Symptoms of MRSA often start with a rash or pimplelike skin irritation. Within hours, these early symptoms may progress to redness, inflammation, pain, and deeper wounds. If untreated, the MRSA may invade the blood, bones, joints, surgical wounds, heart valves, and lungs and can be fatal. There are only a few antibiotics, such as vancomycin, that are effective—yet even vancomycin is showing signs of weakness against tougher strains of MRSA. For more information on antibiotic-resistant pathogens, including preventive measures, see the **Health Today** box on pages 406–407.

Streptococcal Infections

At least five types of the **streptococcus** microorganism are known to cause bacterial infections. Group A streptococci (GAS) cause the most common diseases, such as streptococcal pharyngitis ("strep throat") and scarlet fever, which is often preceded by a sore throat.[4] One particularly virulent group of GAS can lead to a disease known as *necrotizing faciitis* (often referred to as "flesh-eating strep"), a rare, but serious, disease that leads to death in about 30 percent of all cases, even with vigorous antibiotic treatment.[5] Group B streptococci can cause illness in newborn babies, pregnant women, older adults, and adults with other illnesses such as diabetes or liver disease.

Meningitis

Meningitis is an infection and inflammation of the *meninges,* the membranes that surround the brain and spinal cord. Some forms of bacterial meningitis are contagious and can be spread through contact with saliva, nasal discharge, feces, or respiratory and throat secretions. *Pneumococcal meningitis,* the most common form of meningitis, is the most dangerous form of bacterial meningitis. Approximately

6,000 cases of pneumococcal meningitis are reported in the United States each year. *Meningococcal meningitis,* a virulent form of meningitis, has risen dramatically on college campuses in recent years.[6] College students living in dormitories have a higher risk of contracting this disease than those who live off campus.

The signs of meningitis are sudden fever, severe headache, and a stiff neck, particularly causing difficulty touching your chin to your chest. Persons who are suspected of having meningitis should receive immediate, aggressive medical treatment. Vaccines are available for some types of meningitis.

Pneumonia

In the early twentieth century, **pneumonia** was a leading cause of death in the United States. This lung disease is characterized by chronic cough, chest pain, chills, high fever, fluid accumulation, and eventual respiratory failure. One of the most common forms of pneumonia is caused by bacterial infection and responds readily to antibiotic treatment in the early stages. Other forms are caused by viruses, chemicals, or other substances in the lungs and are more difficult to treat. Although medical advances have reduced the overall incidence of pneumonia, it continues to be a major threat in the United States and throughout the world. Vulnerable populations include the poor, older adults, and people already suffering from other illnesses.

streptococcus A round bacterium, usually found in chain formation.
meningitis An infection of the meninges, the membranes that surround the brain and spinal cord.
pneumonia Disease of the lungs characterized by chronic cough, chest pain, chills, high fever, and fluid accumulation; may be caused by bacteria, viruses, chemicals, or other substances.
tuberculosis (TB) A disease caused by bacterial infiltration of the respiratory system.

Tuberculosis

A major killer in the United States in the early twentieth century, **tuberculosis (TB)** was largely controlled in America by 1950 as a result of improved sanitation, isolation of infected persons, and treatment with drugs such as *rifampin* or *isoniazid.* Though many health professionals assumed that TB had been conquered, that

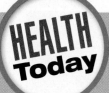

ANTIBIOTIC RESISTANCE: BUGS VERSUS DRUGS

Antibiotics typically wipe out bacteria that are susceptible to them. However, many of our antibiotics are becoming ineffective against resistant strains. Bacteria and other microorganisms that cause infections and diseases are remarkably resilient and continue developing ways to survive drugs that should kill or weaken them. This means that some of the bacteria and microorganisms are becoming "superbugs" that cannot be stopped with medications. Drug resistance is exacerbated by several factors, including over-prescription, underuse, and misuse (poor patient compliance). Consider these examples:

✳ Strains of *Staphylococcus aureus* resistant to most antibiotics, such as methicillin-resistant staphylococcus aureus (MRSA), are endemic in many hospitals today. In some cities, 31 percent of staph infections are resistant to antibiotics, and in nursing homes as many as 71 percent of staph infections defy traditional antibiotic regimens.

✳ The species *Streptococcus pneumoniae* causes thousands of cases of meningitis and pneumonia and 7 million cases of ear infections in the United States each year. Currently, about 30 percent of these cases are resistant to penicillin, the primary drug for treatment. Many penicillin-resistant strains are also resistant to other antibiotics.

✳ An estimated 500 million people worldwide are infected with parasites that cause malaria, and an estimated 700,000 to 2.7 million people die each year from that disease. Resistance to chloroquine,

once a widely used and highly effective treatment, is now found in most regions of the world, and other treatments are losing their effectiveness at alarming rates.

✳ Diarrheal diseases cause almost 3 million deaths per year—mostly in developing countries where resistant forms of *Campylobacter, Shigella, Escherichia coli, Vibrio cholerae,* and *Salmonella* food poisoning have emerged. In some areas, as much as 50 percent of the *Campylobacter* cases are resistant to Cipro, the most effective treatment. A potentially deadly "superbug" called *Salmonella enterica typhimurium* is resistant to most antibiotics and has appeared in Europe, Canada, and the United States.

WHY IS THIS HAPPENING?

In the battle between drugs and bugs, the bugs are clearly scoring some big wins. Why is antibiotic resistance on the rise? Reasons include the following:

1. **Improper use of antibiotics and growth of superbugs.** When used improperly, antibiotics kill only the weak bacteria and leave the strongest versions to thrive and replicate. Because bacteria can swap genes with one another under the right conditions, hardy drug-resistant germs can share their resistance mechanisms with other germs. They adapt, change, and mutate, and eventually an entire colony of resistant bugs grows and passes on its resistance traits to new generations of bacteria. Over time, most pathogens

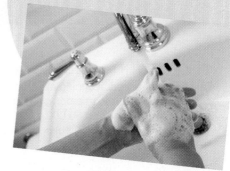

To prevent the spread of infectious disease, wash your hands!

evolve. Human negligence just speeds the healthy ones on their journey.

For example, patients may begin an antibiotic regimen, start to feel better, and stop taking the drug. The surviving bacteria then build immunity to the drugs used to treat them. Also, doctors have overused antibiotics; the Centers for Disease Control and Prevention (CDC) estimates that one-third of the 150 million prescriptions written each year are unnecessary, resulting in bacterial strains that are tougher than the drugs used to fight them.

2. **Overuse of antibiotics in food production.** About 70 percent of antibiotic production today is used to treat sick animals and encourage growth in livestock and poultry. Farmed fish may be given antibiotics to fight off disease in controlled water areas. Although research is only in its infancy, many believe that ingesting meats, animal products, and fish that are rich in antibiotics may contribute to antibiotic resistance in humans. In addition, water runoff from feedlots and sewage

appears not to be the case. During the past 20 years, several factors have led to an epidemic rise in the disease: deteriorating social conditions, including overcrowding and poor sanitation; failure to isolate active cases of TB; a weakening of public health infrastructure, which has led to less funding for screening; and migration of TB to the United States through immigration and international travel. In 2007, the most recent year for which data are available, there were 13,299 active cases of TB in the United States, compared to 85,000 in 1950.[7]

How serious is the TB threat today? The World Health Organization (WHO) reports that almost 2 billion people (a third of the world's entire population) have been exposed to TB, with 9.3 million becoming ill and 2 million dying each year. Some 80 percent of tuberculosis-related deaths occur in developing countries, where it accounts for 26 percent of preventable deaths.[8] TB is the number one infectious killer of women of reproductive age worldwide, as well as the leading cause of death among HIV-positive patients.

can contaminate the water in our rivers and streams with antibiotics.

3. Misuse and overuse of antibacterial soaps and other cleaning products. Preying on the public's fear of germs and disease, the cleaning industry adds antibacterial ingredients to many of their dish soaps, hand cleaners, shower scrubs, surface scrubs, and most household products. Just how much these products contribute to overall resistance is difficult to assess; as with antibiotics, the germs these products do not kill may become stronger than before.

WHO IS AT RISK?

In general, anyone who comes in contact with superbugs such as MRSA can become infected. However, certain groups are at particular risk for these new strains of antibiotic-resistant bugs. Among these are

* Health care workers
* People with weakened immune systems
* Surgical patients and anyone in a hospital with incisions and tissue exposure or persons staying in a health care facility for an extended period of time
* Young children and the elderly
* Diabetics
* People participating in contact sports
* Prisoners or anyone living in confined space with other people

HOW CAN YOU AVOID SUPERBUGS?

Prevention of MRSA and other drug-resistant pathogens involves common infection-control measures in your everyday activities. If someone you know has MRSA or another drug-resistant pathogen, extra precautions may be necessary:

* **Wash your hands often.** Use regular soap and water, wash for at least 10 to 30 seconds, and be sure to scrub the back of the hands and under the fingernails. If you are caring for a patient at home, wash your hands before leaving the house.
* **Keep personal items personal.** Don't share lip balm, makeup, razors, or other personal hygiene implements.
* **Keep wounds clean, sterile, and covered.** Use disposable latex gloves when treating wounds or bandaging. Wash your hands after taking gloves off.
* **Keep surfaces and linens clean.** Any surface that is in frequent contact with an infected person should be washed often with hot, soapy water. Use towels only once and change linens regularly.
* **Take precautions in public athletic facilities.** At the gym, wipe down surfaces you touch with antibiotic washes. Launder your clothes after touching weight machines and other surfaces. Wash hands after touching your dirty clothes. If you are involved in intramural or competitive athletics, shower with hot, soapy water after all contact with individuals, mats, and equipment.
* **Inform others.** If you suspect infection, tell your close friends and health care providers. They can all take precautions to prevent the spread of disease.

WHAT CAN YOU DO ABOUT ANTIBIOTIC RESISTANCE?

To help prevent antibiotic resistance, use antimicrobial drugs only for bacterial, not viral, infections. Take medications as prescribed and finish the full course. Consult with your health care provider if you feel it is necessary to stop your medication. It is also important that you do not keep medication for the next time you are sick. This can lead to an improper dosage, potentially contributing to future antibiotic resistance.

Prescription medications are not the only potential contributors to antibiotic resistance. Next time you go to the grocery store, take note of the multitude of cleaning products that are designed to kill just about any bacterium you face. Some experts say that these antibacterial products do more harm than good. Research suggests that antibacterial agents contained in soaps actually may kill normal bacteria, thus creating an environment for resistant, mutated bacteria that are impervious to antibacterial cleaners and antibiotics.

Sources: Centers for Disease Control and Prevention, National Center for Preparedness, Detection, and Control of Infectious Diseases/Division of Healthcare Quality Promotion, "Antibiotic/Antimicrobial Resistance: Diseases Connected to Antibiotic Resistance," Updated July 2008, www.cdc.gov/drugresistance/diseases.htm; Centers for Disease Control and Prevention, National Center for Immunization and Respiratory Diseases, Division of Bacterial Diseases, "Antibiotic Resistance Questions & Answers," Updated June 2009, www.cdc.gov/getsmart/antibiotic-use/anitbiotic-resistance-faqs.html.

Tuberculosis is caused by bacterial infiltration of the respiratory system that results in a chronic inflammatory reaction in the lungs. Airborne transmission via the respiratory tract is the primary and most efficient mode of transmitting TB. Symptoms include persistent coughing, weight loss, fever, and spitting up blood. Infected people can be contagious without actually showing any symptoms themselves and can transmit the disease while talking, coughing, sneezing, or singing.

Fortunately, TB is fairly difficult to catch, and prolonged exposure, rather than single exposure, is the typical mode of infection. Those at highest risk for TB include the poor, especially children, and the chronically ill. People residing in crowded prisons and homeless shelters with poor ventilation who continuously inhale the same contaminated air are at higher risk. Persons with compromised immune systems are also at high risk, as are those recovering from surgery, cancer therapy, and other situations where comorbidity exists. Treatments are effective for most nonresistant cases and usually include rest, careful infection-control procedures, and anti-TB drug regimens.

As with many bacterial diseases, resistant forms of TB are increasing in the global population. **Multidrug resistant TB (MDR-TB)** is a form of TB that is currently resistant to at least two of the best anti-TB drugs in use today. An even more dangerous form, **extensively drug resistant TB (XDR-TB),** is resistant to nearly all first- and second-line drug defenses against it and is extremely difficult to treat. Fatalities from XDR are increasing globally.

Tickborne Bacterial Diseases In the past few decades, certain tickborne diseases have become major health threats in the United States. Those that are most noteworthy include two bacterially caused diseases, **Lyme disease** and *ehrlichiosis,* each of which spike in the summer months in many states and which can cause significant disability and threats to humans and animals.

Once believed to be closely related to viruses, **rickettsia** are now considered a small form of bacteria. They produce toxins and multiply within small blood vessels, causing vascular blockage and tissue death. Rickettsia require an insect vector (carrier) for transmission to humans. Two common forms of human rickettsial disease are *Rocky Mountain spotted fever* (RMSF), carried by a tick; and *typhus,* carried by a louse, flea, or tick. These diseases produce similar symptoms, including high fever, weakness, rash, and coma, and both can be life threatening.

For all insectborne diseases, the best protection is to stay indoors at dusk and early morning to avoid hours when insects are especially active. If you must go out, wear protective clothing or use bug sprays containing natural oils, pyrethrins, or DEET (diethyl tolumide), all products regarded as generally safe.

multidrug resistant TB (MDR-TB) Form of TB that is resistant to at least two of the best antibiotics available.

extensively drug resistant TB (XDR-TB) Form of TB that is resistant to nearly all existing antibiotics.

Lyme disease A bacterial disease transmitted to humans by the bite of an infected tick.

rickettsia A small form of bacteria that lives inside other living cells.

viruses Microbes consisting of DNA or RNA that invade a host cell and use the cell's resources to reproduce themselves.

incubation period The time between exposure to a disease and the appearance of symptoms.

endemic Describing a disease that is always present to some degree.

influenza A common viral disease of the respiratory tract.

Viruses

Viruses are the smallest known pathogens, approximately 1/500th the size of bacteria. Essentially, a virus consists of a protein structure that contains either *ribonucleic acid (RNA)* or *deoxyribonucleic acid (DNA).* Viruses are incapable of carrying out any life processes on their own. To reproduce, they must invade and inject their own DNA and RNA into the host cell, take it over, and force it to make copies of themselves. The new viruses then erupt out of the host cell and seek other cells to infect.

Viral diseases can be difficult to treat because many viruses can withstand heat, formaldehyde, and large doses of radiation with little effect on their structure. Some viruses have **incubation periods** (the length of time required to develop fully and cause symptoms in their hosts) that last for years, which delays diagnosis. Drug treatment for viral infections is also limited. Drugs powerful enough to kill viruses generally kill the host cells too, although some medications block stages in viral reproduction without damaging host cells.

The Common Cold Colds are responsible for more days lost from work and more uncomfortable days spent at work than any other ailment. Caused by any number of viruses (some experts claim there may be over 200 different viruses responsible), colds are **endemic** (always present to some degree) throughout the world. Current research indicates that otherwise healthy people carry cold viruses in their noses and throats most of the time. These viruses are held in check until the host's resistance is lowered. In the true sense of the word, it is possible to "catch" a cold—from the airborne droplets of another person's sneeze or from skin-to-skin or mucous membrane contact—although the hands are the greatest avenue for transmitting colds and other viruses. Contrary to common thinking, you won't "catch" a cold from getting a chill, but the chill may lower your immune system's resistance to the cold virus or other pathogens.

Influenza In otherwise healthy people, **influenza,** or flu, is usually not life threatening. However, for certain vulnerable populations, such as individuals with respiratory problems or heart disease, older adults (over age 65), or young children (under age 5), the flu can be very serious. Five to 20 percent of Americans get the flu each year, and of these, 200,000 will need hospitalization.[9] Once a person gets the flu, treatment is *palliative,* meaning that it is focused on relief of symptoms, rather than cure.

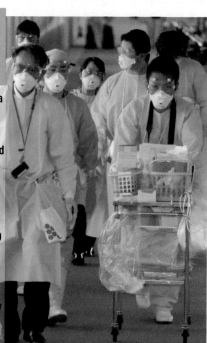

Did you Know?

A pandemic of influenza has the potential to be severe and deadly. The 1918 flu pandemic killed more people than died in World War I: an estimated 30–50 million worldwide, including about 675,000 in the U.S. The 1957 flu pandemic killed 1–2 million worldwide, including approximately 70,000 in the U.S.

What You Can Do to Avoid H1N1 and Other Forms of the Flu

Whether it's the H1N1 flu virus or other strains, there are steps you can take to reduce your risk of contracting the flu, including:

✳ **Stay informed.** Use the Centers for Disease Control and Prevention (CDC) and your state's health division's websites to keep up with the latest information about vaccinations, flu transmission, and ways to protect yourself.

✳ **Take everyday actions to stay healthy.** Influenza is thought to spread mainly person to person through coughing or sneezing.

✳ Cover your nose and mouth with a tissue when you cough or sneeze, or sneeze into your sleeve. Throw the tissue in the trash after you use it.

✳ Wash your hands often with soap and water, especially after you cough or sneeze. Alcohol-based hand cleaners are also effective.

✳ Avoid touching your eyes, nose, or mouth.

✳ Stay home if you get sick, and limit contact with others to keep from infecting them.

✳ Follow public health advice regarding school closures, avoiding crowds, and other social distancing measures.

Source: Centers for Disease Control and Prevention, "2009 H1N1 Flu (Swine Flu)," Updated November 2009, www.cdc.gov/h1n1flu.

To date, three major varieties of flu virus have been discovered, with many different strains existing within each variety. The A form of the virus is generally the most virulent, followed by the B and C varieties. If you contract one form of influenza you may develop immunity to it, but you will not necessarily be immune to other forms of the disease.

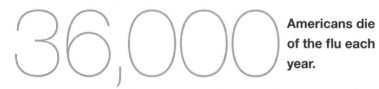

Americans die of the flu each year.

Some vaccines have proven effective against certain strains of flu virus, but they are totally ineffective against others. In spite of minor risks, people over age 65, pregnant women, people with heart or lung disease, and people with certain other illnesses should be vaccinated. Flu shots take 2 to 3 weeks to become effective, so people at risk should get these shots in the fall before the flu season begins.

New strains of influenza are appearing all the time. In 2009, one flu in particular, **H1N1,** the so-called swine flu, captured world attention and rose to pandemic levels. For more about how to avoid H1N1 and other forms of the flu, see the **Skills for Behavior Change** box at left.

Hepatitis One of the most highly publicized viral diseases is **hepatitis,** a virally caused inflammation of the liver. Hepatitis symptoms include fever, headache, nausea, loss of appetite, skin rashes, pain in the upper right abdomen, dark yellow (with brownish tinge) urine, and jaundice. Internationally, viral hepatitis is a major contributor to liver disease and accounts for high morbidity and mortality. Currently, there are seven known forms, with hepatitis A, B, and C having the highest rates of incidence.

Hepatitis A (HAV) is contracted from eating food or drinking water contaminated with human feces. Since vaccinations became available, HAV rates have declined by nearly 90 percent in the United States. However, over 25,000 people per year are still infected.[10] Handlers of infected food, children at day care centers, those who have sexual contact with HAV-positive individuals, or those who travel to international regions where HAV is endemic are at higher risk. In addition, those who ingest seafood from contaminated water, and people who use contaminated needles are also at risk. Fortunately, individuals infected with hepatitis A do not become chronic carriers, and vaccines for the disease are available. Many who contract HAV are asymptomatic.

Hepatitis B (HBV) is spread primarily through body fluids being shared through unprotected sex. However, it is also contracted via sharing needles when injecting drugs; through needlesticks on the job; or, in the case of a newborn baby, from an infected mother. Hepatitis B can lead to chronic liver disease or liver cancer.

H1N1 or "swine flu" A strain of potentially virulent influenza identified in 2009.
hepatitis A viral disease in which the liver becomes inflamed, producing symptoms such as fever, headache, and possibly jaundice.

In spite of vaccine availability since 1982, there are over 43,000 new cases of HBV in the United States each year. Vaccines for HAV and HBV are now available on most college campuses and large numbers of students have been vaccinated. As such, HBV is now one of the only vaccine-preventable forms of sexually transmitted infections. Globally, HBV infections are on the decline, but they continue to be a major health problem, with over 350 million chronic carriers and over 1 million deaths each year. Three-quarters of the world's population live in areas where there are high rates of infection.[11]

Hepatitis C (HCV) infections are on an epidemic rise in many regions of the world as resistant forms of the virus are emerging. Some cases can be traced to blood transfusions or organ transplants. Currently, an estimated 17,000 new cases of HCV are diagnosed in the United States each year, with over 3.2 million people chronically infected.[12] Over 85 percent of those infected develop chronic infections; if the infection is left untreated, the person may develop cirrhosis of the liver, liver cancer, or liver failure. Liver failure resulting from chronic hepatitis C is the leading reason for liver transplants in the United States. Currently, there is no vaccine for HCV, although efforts to develop one have been under way for the past decade.

Other Pathogens

Although bacteria and viruses account for many of the common diseases in both adults and children, they don't account for all of them. Other very small or microscopic organisms can also infect and cause disease symptoms in a host. Among these are fungi, protozoans, parasitic worms, and prions.

Fungi Our environment is inhabited by thousands of species of **fungi,** multicellular or unicellular organisms that obtain their food by infiltrating the bodies of other organisms, both living and dead. Many fungi are useful to humans, such as edible mushrooms, penicillin, and the yeast used in making bread, but some species of fungi can produce infections. *Candidiasis* (a vaginal yeast infection), athlete's foot, ringworm, and jock itch are examples of fungal diseases. With most fungal diseases, keeping the affected area clean and dry plus treating it with appropriate medications will generally bring prompt relief.

Protozoans **Protozoans** are microscopic single-celled organisms that are generally associated with tropical diseases such as African sleeping sickness and malaria. Although these pathogens are prevalent in nonindustrialized countries, they are largely controlled in the United States. The most common protozoan disease in the United States is *trichomoniasis,* which we will discuss later in this chapter's section on sexually transmitted infections. A common waterborne protozoan disease in many regions of the country is *giardiasis.*

Parasitic Worms **Parasitic worms** are the largest of the pathogens. Ranging in size from the small pinworms typically found in children to the relatively large tapeworms that can be found in all warm-blooded animals, most parasitic worms are more a nuisance than a threat. Of special note today are the worm infestations associated with eating raw fish (as in sashimi). Cooking fish and other foods to temperatures sufficient to kill the worms and their eggs can prevent this.

Prions A **prion** is a self-replicating, protein-based agent that can infect humans and other animals. One such prion is believed to be the underlying cause of spongiform diseases such as *bovine spongiform encephalopathy* (BSE, or "mad cow disease"). Evidence indicates that there is a relationship between outbreaks of BSE in Europe and a disease in humans called *variant Creutzfeldt-Jakob disease* (vCJD).[13] Both disorders are invariably fatal brain diseases with unsually long incubation periods measured in years, and both are caused by prions. To date, there have been no known human infections from U.S. beef; however, infected cattle have been found.

fungi A group of multicellular and unicellular organisms that obtain their food by infiltrating the bodies of other organisms, both living and dead; several microscopic varieties are pathogenic.

protozoans Microscopic single-celled organisms that can be pathogenic.

parasitic worms The largest of the pathogens, most of which are more a nuisance than a threat.

prion A recently identified self-replicating, protein-based pathogen.

Emerging and Resurgent Diseases

Although our immune systems are remarkably adept at responding to challenges, microbes and other pathogens appear to be gaining ground. Old scourges are back, and new ones are emerging. Within the past decades, rates for infectious diseases have rapidly increased, particularly for reemerging diseases such as tuberculosis. This trend can be attributed to a combination of overpopulation, inadequate health care systems, increasing poverty, extreme environmental degradation, and drug resistance. As international travel increases (over 1 million people per day cross international boundaries), with germs transported from remote regions to huge urban centers within hours, the likelihood of infection by pathogens previously unknown on U.S. soil increases.

West Nile Virus Until 1999, few Americans had heard of *West Nile virus (WNV),* which is spread by the bite of an infected mosquito. Today, only Alaska and Hawaii remain free of the disease. Several thousand active cases of WNV surface in the United States every year. The elderly and those with impaired immune systems bear the brunt of the disease burden.[14]

Most people who become infected with West Nile virus will have mild symptoms or none at all. Rarely, WNV infection can result in severe and sometimes fatal illness. Symptoms include fever, headache, and body aches, often with skin rash and swollen lymph glands, and a form of encephalitis (inflammation of the brain). There is no vaccine or specific treatment for WNV, but avoiding mosquito bites is the best way to prevent it: using Environmental Protection Agency (EPA)-registered insect repellents such as those with DEET or eucalyptus; wearing long-sleeved clothing and long pants when outdoors; staying indoors during dawn, dusk, and other peak mosquito feeding times; and removing any standing water sources around the home.

Avian (Bird) Flu *Avian influenza* is an infectious disease of birds. There has been considerable media flurry in the past few years over a strain of avian (bird) flu, H5N1, that is highly pathogenic and is capable of crossing the species barrier and causing severe illness in humans. This virulent flu strain began to emerge in bird populations throughout Asia, including domestic birds such as chickens and ducks, as early as 1997. By 2007, H5N1 bird flu had spread to birds in parts of western Europe, eastern Europe, Russia, and northern Africa. Although the virus has yet to mutate into a form highly infectious to humans, outbreaks have occurred in rural areas of the world (where people often live in close proximity to poultry and other animals). As of September 2009, bird flu had caused 262 human deaths worldwide.[15]

Escherichia coli O157:H7 *Escherichia coli* O157:H7 is one of over 170 types of *E. coli* bacteria that can infect humans. Most *E. coli* organisms are harmless and live in the intestines of healthy animals and humans; *E. coli* O157:H7, however, produces a lethal toxin and can cause severe illness or death.

E. coli O157:H7 can live in the intestines of healthy cattle and then contaminate food products at slaughterhouses. Eating ground beef that is rare or undercooked, drinking unpasteurized milk or juice, or swimming in sewage-contaminated water or public pools can cause infection through ingestion of feces that contain *E. coli.*

Although *E. coli* organisms continue to pose threats to public health, strengthened regulations on the cooking of meat and regulation of chlorine levels in pools have helped. However, the 2006 *E. coli* outbreak linked to contaminated spinach and other outbreaks in recent years have caused the U.S. Department of Agriculture (USDA) and others in the agriculture industry to consider new safety measures.

Sexually Transmitted Infections

Sexually transmitted infections (STIs) have been with us since our earliest recorded days on Earth. Today, there are more than 20 known types of STIs. Once referred to as *venereal diseases* and then *sexually transmitted diseases,* the current terminology is more reflective of the number and types of these communicable diseases, and also of the fact that they are caused by infecting pathogens. More virulent strains and antibiotic-resistant forms spell trouble in the days ahead.

65 million people are currently living with an incurable STI.

Sexually transmitted infections affect men and women of all backgrounds and socioeconomic levels. However, they disproportionately affect women, minorities, and infants. In addition, STIs are most prevalent in teens and young adults.[16] In the United States alone, an estimated 19 million new cases of STIs are reported each year.[17]

Early symptoms of an STI are often mild and unrecognizable. Left untreated, some of these infections can have grave consequences, such as sterility, blindness, central nervous system destruction, disfigurement, and even death. Infants born to mothers carrying the organisms for these infections are at risk for a variety of health problems.

As with many communicable diseases, much of the pain, suffering, and anguish associated with STIs can be eliminated through education, responsible action, simple preventive strategies, and prompt treatment. Although STIs can happen to anyone, you can avoid them if you take appropriate precautions when you decide to engage in a sexual relationship.

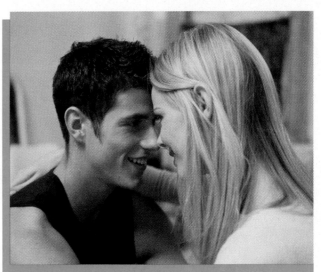

How can I tell if someone I'm dating has an STI?

You can't tell if someone has an STI just by looking at them; it isn't something broadcast on a person's face, and many people with STIs are unaware of the infection because it is asymptomatic. The only way to know for sure is to go to a clinic and get tested. In addition, partners need to be open and honest with each other about their sexual histories, and practice safer sex.

What's Your Risk?

Several reasons have been proposed to explain the present high rates of STIs. The first relates to the moral and social stigma associated with these infections. Shame and embarrassment often keep infected people from seeking treatment. Unfortunately, they usually continue to be sexually active, thereby infecting unsuspecting partners. People who are uncomfortable discussing sexual issues may also be less likely to use and ask their partners to use condoms to protect against STIs and pregnancy.

Another reason proposed for the STI epidemic is our culture's casual attitude about sex. Bombarded by media hype that glamorizes easy sex, many people take sexual partners without considering the consequences. Generally, the more sexual partners a person has, the greater the risk for contracting an STI.

Ignorance—about the infections, their symptoms, and the fact that someone can be asymptomatic but still infected—is also a factor. A person who is infected but asymptomatic can unknowingly spread an STI to an unsuspecting partner, who may, in turn, ignore or misinterpret any symptoms. By the time either partner seeks medical help, he or she may have infected several others. In addition, many people mistakenly believe that certain sexual practices—oral sex, for example—carry no risk for STIs. In fact, oral sex practices among young adults may be

sexually transmitted infections (STIs) Infectious diseases caused by pathogens transmitted through some form of intimate, usually sexual, contact.

High-risk behaviors	Moderate-risk behaviors	Low-risk behaviors	No-risk behaviors
Unprotected vaginal, anal, and oral sex—any activity that involves direct contact with bodily fluids, such as ejaculate, vaginal secretions, or blood—are high-risk behaviors.	Vaginal, anal, or oral sex with a latex or polyurethane condom and a water-based lubricant used properly and consistently can greatly reduce the risk of STI transmission. Dental dams used during oral sex can also greatly reduce the risk of STI transmission.	Mutual masturbation, if there are no cuts on the hand, penis or vagina, is very low risk. Rubbing, kissing, and massaging carry low risk, but herpes can be spread by skin-to-skin contact from an infected partner.	Abstinence, phone sex, talking, and fantasy are all no-risk behaviors.

FIGURE 13.5 Continuum of Risk for Various Sexual Behaviors
There are different levels of risk for various behaviors and various sexually transmitted infections (STIs); however, no matter what, any sexual activity involving direct contact with blood, semen, or vaginal secretions is high risk.

responsible for increases in herpes and other STIs. Figure 13.5 shows the continuum of risk for various sexual behaviors, and the **Skills for Behavior Change** box on the next page offers tips for ways to practice safer sex.

Routes of Transmission

Sexually transmitted infections are generally spread through some form of intimate sexual contact. Sexual intercourse, oral–genital contact, hand–genital contact, and anal intercourse are the most common modes of transmission. Less likely, but still possible, modes of transmission include mouth-to-mouth contact, or contact with fluids from body sores that may be spread by the hands. Although each STI is a different infection caused by a different pathogen, all STI pathogens prefer dark, moist places, especially the mucous membranes lining the reproductive organs. Most of them are susceptible to light, excess heat, cold, and dryness, and many die quickly on exposure to air. Like other communicable infections, STIs have both pathogen-specific incubation periods and periods of time during which transmission is most likely, called *periods of communicability*.

Chlamydia

Chlamydia, an infection caused by the bacterium *Chlamydia trachomatis* that often presents no symptoms, is the most commonly reported STI in the United States. Chlamydia infects about 2.2 million Americans annually, the majority of them women.[18] Public health officials believe that the actual number of cases is probably higher, because these figures represent only those cases reported.

chlamydia Bacterially caused STI of the urogenital tract.
gonorrhea Bacterial infection that is the second most common STI in the United States; if untreated, may cause sterility.

Signs and Symptoms In men, early symptoms may include painful and difficult urination; frequent urination; and a watery, puslike discharge from the penis. Symptoms in women may include a yellowish discharge, spotting between periods, and occasional spotting after intercourse. However, many chlamydia victims display no symptoms and therefore do not seek help until the disease has done secondary damage. Women are especially likely to be asymptomatic; over 70 percent do not realize they have the disease until secondary damage occurs.

Complications The secondary damage resulting from chlamydia is serious in both men and women. Men can suffer injury to the prostate gland, seminal vesicles, and bulbourethral glands, and they can suffer from arthritis-like symptoms and inflammatory damage to the blood vessels and heart. Men can also experience epididymitis, inflammation of the area near the testicles. In women, chlamydia-related inflammation can injure the cervix or fallopian tubes, causing sterility, and it can damage the inner pelvic structure, leading to pelvic inflammatory disease (PID) (see the **Gender & Health** box on page 414). If an infected woman becomes pregnant, she has a high risk for miscarriage and stillbirth. Chlamydia may also be responsible for one type of *conjunctivitis*, an eye infection that affects not only adults but also infants, who can contract the disease from an infected mother during delivery. Untreated conjunctivitis can cause blindness.[19]

Diagnosis and Treatment Diagnosis of chlamydia is determined through a laboratory test. A sample of urine or fluid from the vagina or penis is collected to identify the presence of the bacteria. Unfortunately, chlamydia tests are not a routine part of many health clinics' testing procedures. Usually a person must specifically request it. If detected early, chlamydia is easily treatable with antibiotics such as tetracycline, doxycycline, or erythromycin.

Gonorrhea

Gonorrhea is one of the most common STIs in the United States, surpassed only by chlamydia in number of cases. The CDC estimates that there are over 700,000 cases per year, plus

Safe Is Sexy

Practicing the following behaviors will help you reduce your risk of contracting a sexually transmitted infection (STI):

✳ Avoid casual sexual partners. All sexually active adults who are not in a lifelong monogamous relationship should practice safer sex.

✳ Use latex condoms consistently and correctly. Remember that condoms do not provide 100 percent protection against all STIs.

✳ Postpone sexual involvement with someone until you are assured that your partner is not infected by discussing past sexual history and getting testing.

✳ Avoid injury to body tissue during sexual activity. Some pathogens can enter the bloodstream through microscopic tears in anal or vaginal tissues.

✳ Avoid unprotected oral, anal, or vaginal sexual activity in which semen, blood, or vaginal secretions could penetrate mucous membranes or enter through breaks in the skin.

✳ Always use a condom or a dental dam (a sensitive latex sheet, about the size of a tissue, that can be placed over the female genitals to form a protective layer) during oral sex.

✳ Avoid using drugs and alcohol, which can dull your senses and affect your ability to take responsible precautions with potential sex partners.

✳ Wash your hands before and after sexual encounters. Urinate after sexual relations and, if possible, wash your genitals.

✳ Although total abstinence is the only absolute means of preventing the transmission of STIs, abstinence can be a difficult choice to make. If you have any doubt about the potential risks of having sex, consider other means of intimacy (at least until you can assure your safety)—massage, dry kissing, hugging, holding and touching, and masturbation (alone or with a partner).

✳ If you are worried about your own HIV or STI status, have yourself tested. Don't risk infecting others.

Source: The American College of Obstetricians and Gynecologists, *How to Prevent Sexually Transmitted Diseases* (Atlanta: The American College of Obstetricians and Gynecologists, 2008).

Signs and Symptoms In men, a typical symptom is a white, milky discharge from the penis accompanied by painful, burning urination 2 to 9 days after contact (**Figure 13.6**). Epididymitis can also occur as a symptom of infection. However, about 20 percent of all men with gonorrhea are asymptomatic.

In women, the situation is just the opposite: only 20 percent experience any discharge, and few develop a burning sensation on urinating until much later in the course of the infection (if ever). The organism can remain in the woman's vagina, cervix, uterus, or fallopian tubes for long periods with no apparent symptoms other than an occasional slight fever. Thus a woman can be unaware that she has been infected and that she is infecting her sexual partners.

Complications In a man, untreated gonorrhea may spread to the prostate, testicles, urinary tract, kidney, and bladder. Blockage of the vasa deferentia due to scar tissue may cause sterility. In some cases, the penis develops a painful curvature during erection. If the infection goes undetected in a woman, it can spread to the fallopian tubes and ovaries, causing sterility or, at the very least, severe inflammation and PID. The bacteria can also spread up the reproductive tract or, more rarely, through the blood and infect the joints, heart valves, or brain. If an infected woman becomes pregnant, the infection can be transmitted to her baby during delivery, potentially causing blindness, joint infection, or a life-threatening blood infection.

Diagnosis and Treatment Diagnosis of gonorrhea is similar to that of chlamydia, requiring a sample of either urine or fluid from the vagina or penis to detect the presence of the bacteria. If detected early, gonorrhea is treatable with antibiotics, but the *Neisseria gonorrhoeae* bacterium has

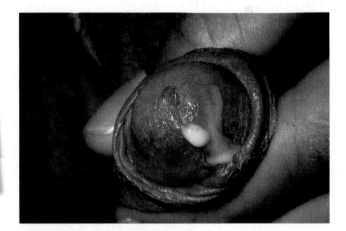

FIGURE 13.6 **Gonorrhea**
One common symptom of gonorrhea in men is a milky discharge from the penis, accompanied by burning sensations during urination. Whereas these symptoms will cause most men to seek diagnosis and treatment, women with gonorrhea are often asymptomatic, so they may not be aware they are infected.

numbers that go unreported.[20] Caused by the bacterial pathogen *Neisseria gonorrhoeae,* gonorrhea primarily infects the linings of the urethra, genital tract, pharynx, and rectum. It may spread to the eyes or other body regions by the hands or through body fluids, typically during vaginal, oral, or anal sex. Most cases occur in individuals between the ages of 20 and 24.[21]

Complications of STIs in Women: PID and UTIs

Women disproportionately experience the long-term consequences of STIs. If not treated, up to 40 percent of women who are infected with *Neisseria gonorrhoeae* or *Chlamydia trachomatis* may develop pelvic inflammatory disease (PID). Pelvic inflammatory disease is a catchall term for a number of infections of the uterus, fallopian tubes, and ovaries that are complications resulting from an untreated STI.

Symptoms of PID vary but generally include lower abdominal pain, fever, unusual vaginal discharge, painful intercourse, painful urination, and irregular menstrual bleeding. The vague symptoms associated with chlamydial and gonococcal PID cause 85 percent of women to delay seeking medical care, thereby increasing the risk of permanent damage and scarring that can lead to infertility and ectopic pregnancy. Among women with PID, ectopic pregnancy (in which an embryo begins to develop outside of the uterus, usually in a fallopian tube) occurs in 9 percent, and chronic pelvic pain in 18 percent.

Women are also at greater risk than men for developing a general urinary tract infection (UTI). Urinary tract infections can be caused by various factors, including untreated STIs. Women are more disproportionately affected by UTIs because a woman's urethra is much shorter than a man's, making it easier for bacteria to enter the bladder. In addition, a woman's urethra is closer to her anus than is a man's, allowing bacteria to spread into her urethra and cause an infection.

Symptoms of a UTI include burning sensation during urination and lower abdominal pain. A UTI can be diagnosed through a urine test and treated by antibiotics. If left untreated, UTIs can cause kidney damage.

These serious complications that can result from untreated STIs in women further illustrate the need for early diagnosis and treatment. Regular screening is particularly important, because women are often asymptomatic, increasing their risk of complications such as PID and UTIs. Therefore, it is recommended that all sexually active women should be screened regularly. Data from a randomized trial of chlamydia screening in a managed care setting suggested that screening programs can reduce the incidence of PID by as much as 60 percent.

Women with undiagnosed and untreated STIs run the risk of developing pelvic inflammatory disease, which may lead to infertility.

Sources: MedlinePlus, "Pelvic Inflammatory Disease (PID)," Updated September 2009, www.nlm.nih.gov/medlineplus/ency/article/000888.htm; Mayo Clinic Staff, "Urinary Tract Infection: Risk Factors," June 2008, Available online: www.mayoclinic.com/health/urinary-tract-infection/DS00286/DSECTION=risk-factors; Centers for Disease Control and Prevention, Division of STD Prevention, National Center for HIV/AIDS, Viral Hepatitis, STD, and TB Prevention, "STDs in Women and Infants," Updated January 2009, www.cdc.gov/std/stats07/womenandinf.htm.

---

begun to develop resistance to some antibiotics. It is also important to recognize that chlamydia and gonorrhea often occur at the same time, but different antibiotics are needed to treat each infection separately.[22]

Syphilis

Syphilis is caused by a bacterium, the spirochete called *Treponema pallidum*. The incidence of syphilis is highest in women aged 20 to 24 and men aged 35 to 39. The incidence of syphilis in newborns has continued to increase in the United States.[23] Because it is extremely delicate and dies readily upon exposure to air, dryness, or cold, the organism is generally transferred only through direct sexual contact or from mother to fetus.

syphilis One of the most widespread STIs; characterized by distinct phases and potentially serious consequences.
chancre Sore often found on the site of primary syphilis infection.

Signs and Symptoms Syphilis is known as the "great imitator," because its symptoms resemble those of several other infections. It should be noted, however, that some people experience no symptoms at all. Syphilis can occur in four distinct stages:[24]

● **Primary syphilis.** The first stage of syphilis, particularly for men, is often characterized by the development of a **chancre** (pronounced "shank-er"), a sore located most frequently at the site of initial infection that usually appears 3 to 4 weeks after initial infection (Figure 13.7). In men, the site of the chancre tends to be the penis or scrotum; in women, the site of infection is often internal, on the vaginal wall or high on the cervix where the chancre is not readily apparent and the likelihood of detection is not great. Whether or not it is detected, the chancre is oozing with bacteria, ready to infect an unsuspecting partner. In both men and women, the chancre will completely disappear in 3 to 6 weeks.

● **Secondary syphilis.** If the infection is left untreated, a month to a year after the chancre disappears, secondary symptoms may appear, including a rash or white patches on the skin or on the mucous membranes of the mouth, throat, or genitals. Hair loss may occur, lymph nodes may enlarge,

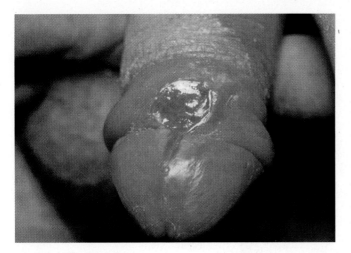

A chancre on the site of the initial infection is a symptom of primary syphilis.

and the victim may develop a slight fever or headache. In rare cases, sores develop around the mouth or genitals. As during the active chancre phase, these sores contain infectious bacteria, and contact with them can spread the infection.

● **Latent syphilis.** After the secondary stage, if the infection is left untreated, the syphilis spirochetes begin to invade body organs, causing lesions called *gummas.* The infection now is rarely transmitted to others, except during pregnancy, when it can be passed to the fetus.

● **Tertiary/late syphilis.** Years after syphilis has entered the body, its effects become all too evident if still untreated. Late-stage syphilis indications include heart and central nervous system damage, blindness, deafness, paralysis, premature senility, and, ultimately, dementia.

Complications Pregnant women with syphilis can experience complications including premature births, miscarriages, and stillbirths. An infected pregnant woman may transmit the syphilis to her unborn child. The infant will then be born with *congenital syphilis,* which can cause death; severe birth defects such as blindness, deafness, or disfigurement; developmental delays; seizures; and other health problems. Because in most cases the fetus does not become infected until after the first trimester, treatment of the mother during this time will usually prevent infection of the fetus.

Diagnosis and Treatment There are two methods that can be used to diagnose syphilis. In the primary stage, a sample from the chancre is collected to identify the bacteria. Another method of diagnosing syphilis is through a blood test. Syphilis can easily be treated with antibiotics, usually penicillin, for all stages except the late stage.

Herpes

Herpes is a general term for a family of infections characterized by sores or eruptions on the skin and caused by herpes simplex virus. The herpes family of diseases is not transmitted exclusively by sexual contact. Kissing or sharing eating utensils can also exchange saliva and transmit the infection. Herpes infections range from mildly uncomfortable to extremely serious. **Genital herpes** affects over 45 million Americans aged 12 and older.[25]

There are two types of herpes simplex virus. Only about one in six Americans currently has HSV-2; however, nearly 58 percent have HSV-1, usually appearing as cold sores on their mouths. Both herpes simplex types 1 and 2 can infect any area of the body, producing lesions (sores) in and around the vaginal area; on the penis; and around the anal opening, buttocks, thighs, or mouth (see **Figure 13.8** on the next page). Whether you contract HSV-1 or HSV-2 on your genitals, the net results may be just as painful, just as long term, and just as infectious for future partners. Herpes simplex virus remains in certain nerve cells for life and can flare up when the body's ability to maintain itself is weakened.

Signs and Symptoms The precursor phase of a herpes infection is characterized by a burning sensation and redness at the site of infection. During this time, prescription medicines such as acyclovir and over-the-counter medications such as Abreva will often keep the disease from spreading. However, this phase of the disease is quickly followed by the second phase, in which a blister filled with a clear fluid containing the virus forms. If you pick at this blister or otherwise touch the site and spread this fluid with fingers, lipstick, lip balm, or other products, you can autoinoculate other body parts. Particularly dangerous is the possibility of spreading the infection to your eyes, for a herpes lesion on the eye can cause blindness.

Over a period of days, the unsightly blister will crust over, dry up, and disappear, and the virus will travel to the base of an affected nerve supplying the area and become dormant. Only when the victim becomes overly stressed, when diet and sleep are inadequate, when the immune system is overworked, or when excessive exposure to sunlight or other stressors occurs will the virus become reactivated (at the same site every time) and begin the blistering cycle all over again. Each time a sore develops, it casts off (sheds) viruses that can be highly infectious. However, it is important to note that a herpes site can shed the virus even when no overt sore is present, particularly during the interval between the earliest symptoms and blistering. People may get genital herpes by having sexual contact with others who don't know they are infected or who are having outbreaks of herpes without any sores. A person with genital herpes can also infect a sexual partner during oral sex. The virus is spread only rarely, if at all, by touching objects such as a toilet seat or hot tub seat.

genital herpes STI caused by the herpes simplex virus.

Complications Genital herpes is especially serious in pregnant women because the baby can be infected as it passes through the vagina during birth. Many physicians

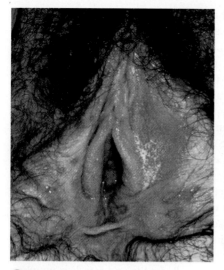

(a) Genital herpes is a highly contagious and incurable STI. It is characterized by recurring cycles of painful blisters on the genitalia.

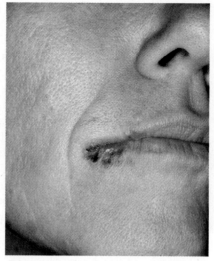

(b) Oral herpes is also extremely contagious and can cause recurrent painful cold sores or fever blisters around the mouth.

FIGURE 13.8 **Herpes**
Herpes can be caused by herpes simplex virus types 1 or 2.

recommend cesarean deliveries for infected women. Additionally, women with a history of genital herpes appear to have a greater risk of developing cervical cancer.

Diagnosis and Treatment Diagnosis of herpes can be determined by collecting a sample from the suspected sore or by performing a blood test to identify an HSV-1 or HSV-2 infection. Although there is no cure for herpes at present, certain drugs can be used to treat symptoms. Unfortunately, they seem to work only if the infection is confirmed during the first few hours after contact. The effectiveness of other treatments, such as L-lysine, is largely unsubstantiated. Over-the-counter medications may reduce the length of time you have sores/symptoms. Other drugs, such as famciclovir (FAMVIR), may reduce viral shedding between outbreaks. This means that if you have outbreaks, you may reduce risks to your sexual partners.[26]

Human Papillomavirus and Genital Warts

Genital warts (also known as *venereal warts* or *condylomas*) are caused by a group of viruses known as **human papillomavirus (HPV)**. There are over 100 different types of HPV; more than 30 types are sexually transmitted and are classified as either low risk or high risk. A person becomes infected when certain types of HPV penetrate the skin and mucous membranes of the genitals or anus. This is among the most common forms of STI,

genital warts Warts that appear in the genital area or the anus; caused by the human papillomavirus (HPV).
human papillomavirus (HPV) A group of viruses, many of which are transmitted sexually; some types of HPV can cause genital warts or cervical cancer.

with 20 million Americans currently infected with genital HPV and approximately 6.2 million new cases each year.[27]

Signs and Symptoms Genital HPV appears to be relatively easy to catch. The typical incubation period is 6 to 8 weeks after contact. People infected with low-risk types of HPV may develop genital warts, a series of bumps or growths on the genitals, ranging in size from small pinheads to large cauliflower-like growths (Figure 13.9).

Complications Infection with high-risk types of HPV poses a significant risk for cervical cancer in women. It may lead to *dysplasia,* or changes in cells that may lead to a precancerous condition. Exactly how high-risk HPV infection leads to cervical cancer is uncertain. It is known that within 5 years after infection, 30 percent of all HPV cases will progress to the precancerous stage. Of those cases that become precancerous and are left untreated, 70 percent will eventually result in actual cancer. In addition, HPV may pose a threat to a fetus that is exposed to the virus during birth. Cesarean deliveries may be considered in serious cases. New research has also implicated HPV as a possible risk factor for coronary artery disease. It is hypothesized that HPV causes an inflammatory response in the artery walls, which leads to cholesterol and plaque buildup (see Chapter 12).

Diagnosis and Treatment Diagnosis of genital warts from low-risk types of HPV is determined through a visual examination by a health care provider. High-risk types can be diagnosed in women through microscopic analysis of cells from a Pap smear or by collecting a sample from the cervix to test for HPV DNA. There is currently no HPV DNA test for men.

Treatment is only available for the low-risk forms of HPV that cause genital warts. The warts can be treated with topical medication or can be frozen with liquid nitrogen and then removed. Large warts may require surgical removal.

HPV Vaccination In 2006, the Food and Drug Administration (FDA) approved a vaccine that protects against four types of HPV. Two of these are low-risk types, 6 and 11, that cause 40 percent of cases of genital warts, and the other two are high-risk types, 16 and 18, that lead to 70 percent of cervical cancer cases. The vaccine is meant primarily for girls and women aged 9 to 26 and is administered as a series of three shots over a 6-month period. See the **Health Headlines** box on page 418 for more information about this vaccine.

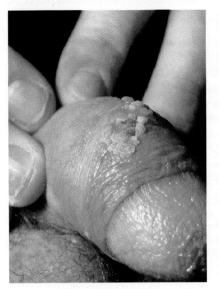
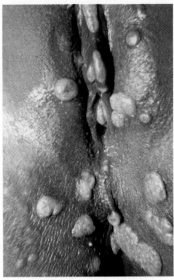

FIGURE 13.9 **Genital Warts**
Genital warts are caused by certain types of human papillomavirus (HPV).

Candidiasis (Moniliasis)

Most STIs are caused by pathogens that come from outside the body; however, the yeastlike fungus *Candida albicans* is a normal inhabitant of the vaginal tract in most women. (See Figure 13.4c on page 405 for a micrograph of this fungus.) Only when the normal chemical balance of the vagina is disturbed will these organisms multiply and cause the fungal disease **candidiasis,** also sometimes called *moniliasis* or a *yeast infection.*

Signs and Symptoms Symptoms of candidiasis include severe itching and burning of the vagina and vulva, and a white, cheesy vaginal discharge.[28] When this microbe infects the mouth, whitish patches form, and the condition is referred to as *thrush.* Thrush infection can also occur in men and is easily transmitted between sexual partners. Symptoms of candidiasis can be aggravated by contact with soaps, douches, perfumed toilet paper, chlorinated water, and spermicides.

Diagnosis and Treatment Diagnosis of candidiasis is usually made by collecting a vaginal sample and analyzing it to identify the pathogen. Antifungal drugs applied on the surface or by suppository usually cure candidiasis in just a few days.

Trichomoniasis

Unlike many STIs, **trichomoniasis** is caused by a protozoan, *Trichomonas vaginalis.* (See Figure 13.4d on page 405 for a micrograph of this organism.) Although as many as half of the men and women in the United States may carry this organism, most remain free of symptoms until their bodily defenses are weakened.

Signs and Symptoms Symptoms among women include a foamy, yellowish, unpleasant-smelling discharge accompanied by a burning sensation, itching, and painful urination. Most men with trichomoniasis do not have any symptoms, though some men experience irritation inside the penis, mild discharge, and a slight burning after urinating.[29] Although usually transmitted by sexual contact, the "trich" organism can also be spread by toilet seats, wet towels, or other items that have discharged fluids on them.

Diagnosis and Treatment Diagnosis of trichomoniasis is determined by collecting fluid samples from the penis or vagina to test for the presence of the protozoan. Treatment includes oral metronidazole, usually given to both sexual partners to avoid the possible "ping-pong" effect of repeated cross-infection typical of STIs.

Pubic Lice

Pubic lice, often called "crabs," are small parasitic insects that are usually transmitted during sexual contact (Figure 13.10). More annoying than dangerous, they move easily from partner to partner during sex. They have an affinity for pubic hair and attach themselves to the base of these hairs, where they deposit their eggs (nits). One to 2 weeks later, these nits develop into adults that lay eggs and migrate to other body parts, thus perpetuating the cycle.

candidiasis Yeastlike fungal infection often transmitted sexually; also called *moniliasis* or *yeast infection.*
trichomoniasis Protozoan STI characterized by foamy, yellowish discharge and unpleasant odor.
pubic lice Parasitic insects that can inhabit various body areas, especially the genitals.

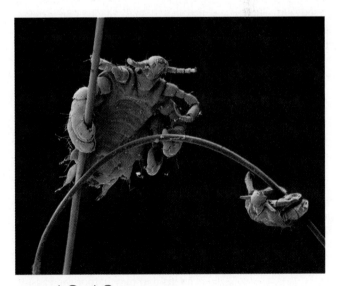

FIGURE 13.10 **Pubic Lice**
Pubic lice, also known as "crabs," are small, parasitic insects that attach themselves to pubic hair.

Q & A ON THE HPV VACCINE

Most sexually active people will contract some form of human papillomarvirus (HPV) at some time in their lives, though they may never even know it. There are about 40 types of sexually transmitted HPV, most of which cause no symptoms and go away on their own. But some high-risk types can cause cervical cancer in women and other less common genital cancers—like cancers of the anus, vagina, and vulva (area around the opening of the vagina). Every year in the United States, about 12,000 women are diagnosed with cervical cancer, and almost 4,000 die from this disease. The new HPV vaccine can help prevent women from becoming infected with HPV and subsequently developing cervical cancer.

✳ **Who should get the HPV vaccine?** The HPV vaccine is recommended for 11- and 12-year-old girls and can also be given to girls 9 or 10 years of age. It is also recommended for girls and women aged 13 through 26 who have not yet been vaccinated or completed the vaccine series. Ideally, females should get the vaccine before they become sexually active. Females who are sexually active may get less benefit from it, because they may have already gotten an HPV type targeted by the vaccine. However they would still get protection from those types they have not yet contracted.

✳ **Why is the HPV vaccine only recommended for girls and women through the age of 26?** The vaccine has been widely tested in girls and women aged 9 through 26 years. New research is being done on the vaccine's safety and efficacy in women older than 26. The FDA will consider licensing the vaccine for these women when there is enough research to show that it is safe and effective for them.

✳ **What about vaccinating boys and men?** Studies are now being done to find out if the vaccine works to prevent HPV infection and disease in males. It is possible that vaccinating men will have health benefits for them by preventing genital warts and rare cancers, such as penile and anal cancer.

✳ **What does the vaccine _not_ protect against?** The vaccine does not protect against all types of HPV—so it will not prevent all cases of cervical cancer. About 30 percent of cervical cancers will not be prevented by the vaccine, so it will be important for women to continue getting screened for cervical cancer (through regular Pap tests). Also, the vaccine does not prevent other sexually transmitted infections (STIs), so it is still important for sexually active persons to lower their risk for other STIs.

✳ **How safe is the HPV vaccine?** This vaccine has been licensed by the FDA and approved by the CDC as safe and effective. It was studied in thousands of females (aged 9 through 26 years) around the world and its safety continues to be monitored by the CDC and the FDA. Studies have found no serious side effects.

Source: Adapted from Centers for Disease Control and Prevention, "HPV Vaccine Information for Young Women," 2008, www.cdc.gov/std/hpv/STDFact-HPV-vaccine-young-women.htm.

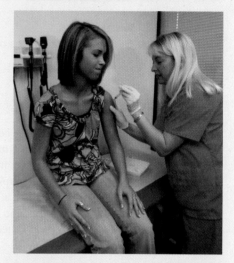

The HPV vaccine is recommended for girls and women aged 9 to 26 as a preventive against cervical cancer. Many state health departments and college campuses offer free or low-cost vaccines for those whose insurance does not cover the cost.

Signs and Symptoms Symptoms of pubic lice infestation include itchiness in the area covered by pubic hair, bluish-gray skin color in the pubic region, and sores in the genital area.

Diagnosis and Treatment Diagnosis of pubic lice involves an examination by a health care provider to identify the eggs in the genital area. Treatment includes washing clothing, furniture, and linens that may harbor the eggs. It usually takes 2 to 3 weeks to kill all larval forms. Although sexual contact is the most common mode of transmission, you can "catch" pubic lice from lying on sheets or sitting on a toilet seat that an infected person has used.

acquired immunodeficiency syndrome (AIDS) A disease caused by a retrovirus, the human immunodeficiency virus (HIV), that attacks the immune system, reducing the number of helper T cells and leaving the victim vulnerable to infections, malignancies, and neurological disorders.

human immunodeficiency virus (HIV) The virus that causes AIDS.

HIV/AIDS

Acquired immunodeficiency syndrome (AIDS) is a significant global health threat. Since 1981, when AIDS was first recognized, approximately 65 million people in the world have become infected with **human immunodeficiency virus (HIV),** the virus that causes AIDS. At the end of 2008, there were approximately 33.4 million people worldwide living with HIV.[30]

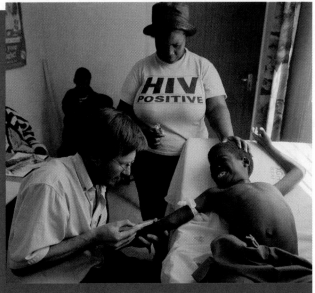

Is HIV/AIDS still an epidemic?

Yes! With swine flu and other emerging diseases dominating the news, it may seem like HIV/AIDS is no longer a problem; however, nothing could be further from the truth. In North America, 1.4 million people are living with HIV, and HIV and AIDS are still at epidemic levels all over the world, especially in developing nations. Sub-Saharan Africa has been hit hardest: 22.4 million people in the region are living with the disease. Another 3.8 million in south/southest Asia are infected and 2 million in Latin America. The epidemic is spreading most rapidly in eastern Europe and central Asia, where 1.5 million people currently have HIV.

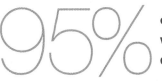

of people with HIV worldwide live in developing nations.

In the United States, there have been approximately 1.1 million people infected with HIV and at least 583,000 have died.[31] In their most recent incidence reports, the CDC estimated that in 2006, there were approximately 56,300 new HIV/AIDS cases diagnosed in the United States.[32]

Initially, people with HIV were diagnosed as having AIDS only when they developed blood infections, the cancer known as Kaposi's sarcoma, or any of 21 other indicator diseases, most of which were common in male AIDS patients. The CDC has expanded the indicator list to include pulmonary tuberculosis, recurrent pneumonia, and invasive cervical cancer. Perhaps the most significant indicator today is a drop in the level of the body's master immune cells, CD4 cells (also called helper T cells), to one-fifth the level in a healthy person.

AIDS cases have been reported state by state throughout the United States since the early 1980s. Today, the CDC recommends that all states report HIV infections as well as AIDS. Because of medical advances in treatment and increasing numbers of HIV-infected persons who do not progress to AIDS, it is believed that AIDS incidence statistics may not provide a true picture of the epidemic, the long-term costs of treating HIV-infected individuals, and other key information.

How HIV Is Transmitted

HIV typically enters one person's body when another person's infected body fluids (e.g., semen, vaginal secretions, blood) gain entry through a breach in body defenses. Mucous membranes of the genital organs and the anus provide the easiest route of entry. If there is a break in the mucous membranes (as can occur during sexual intercourse, particularly anal intercourse), the virus enters and begins to multiply. After initial infection, HIV multiplies rapidly, invading the bloodstream and cerebrospinal fluid. It progressively destroys helper T cells (recall that these cells call the rest of the immune response to action), weakening the body's resistance to disease.

Despite some myths, HIV is not highly contagious. Studies of people living in households with an AIDS patient have turned up no documented cases of HIV infection resulting from casual contact.[33] Other investigations provide overwhelming evidence that insect bites do not transmit HIV.

Engaging in High-Risk Behaviors AIDS is not a disease of gay people or minority groups. Although during the early days of the epidemic it appeared that HIV infected only homosexuals, it quickly became apparent that the disease was not confined to groups of people, but rather was related to high-risk behaviors such as unprotected sexual intercourse and sharing needles (see the **Gender & Health** box on page 421). People who engage in high-risk behaviors increase their risk for the disease; people who do not engage in these behaviors have minimal risk. **Figure 13.11** on page 420 shows the breakdown of sources of HIV infection among U.S. men and women. The majority of HIV infections arise from the following high-risk behaviors:

● **Exchange of body fluids.** The greatest risk factor is the exchange of HIV-infected body fluids during vaginal or anal intercourse. Substantial research indicates that blood, semen, and vaginal secretions are the major fluids of concern. In rare instances, the virus has been found in saliva, but most health officials state that saliva is a less significant risk than other shared body fluids.

● **Injecting drugs.** A significant percentage of AIDS cases in the United States result from sharing or using HIV-contaminated needles and syringes. Though users of illegal drugs are commonly considered the only members of this category, others may also share needles—for example, people with diabetes who inject insulin or athletes who inject steroids. People who share needles and also engage in sexual activities with members of high-risk groups, such as those who exchange sex for drugs, increase their risks dramatically. Tattooing and piercing can also be risky (see the **Consumer Health** box on page 422).

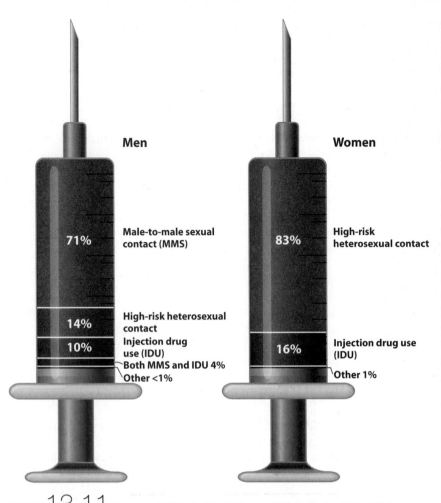

Men

71% — Male-to-male sexual contact (MMS)

14% — High-risk heterosexual contact

10% — Injection drug use (IDU)

Both MMS and IDU 4%

Other <1%

Women

83% — High-risk heterosexual contact

16% — Injection drug use (IDU)

Other 1%

FIGURE 13.11 **Sources of HIV Infection in Men and Women in the United States**

Source: Data are from AVERT, "United States—Statistics by Transmission Route and Gender," Updated August 2009, www.avert.org/usa-transmission-gender.htm.

Blood Transfusion Prior to 1985 A small group of people have become infected after receiving blood transfusions. In 1985, the Red Cross and other blood donation programs implemented a stringent testing program for all donated blood. Today, because of these massive screening efforts, the risk of receiving HIV-infected blood is almost nonexistent in developed countries, including the United States.

Mother-to-Child (Perinatal) Transmission Mother-to-child transmission occurs when an HIV-positive woman passes the virus to her baby. This can occur during pregnancy, during labor and delivery, or through breast-feeding. Without antiretroviral treatment, approximately 25 percent of HIV-positive pregnant women will transmit the virus to their infant.[34]

Symptoms of HIV/AIDS

A person may go for months or years after infection by HIV before any significant symptoms appear. The incubation time varies greatly from person to person. For adults who receive no medical treatment, it takes an average of 8 to 10 years for the virus to cause the slow, degenerative changes in the immune system that are characteristic of AIDS. During this time, the person may experience *opportunistic infections* (infections that gain a foothold when the immune system is not functioning effectively). Colds, sore throats, fever, tiredness, nausea, night sweats, and other generally non–life-threatening conditions commonly appear and are described as pre-AIDS symptoms. Other symptoms of progressing HIV infection include wasting syndrome, swollen lymph nodes, and neurological problems. As the immune system continues to decline, the body becomes more vulnerable to infection. A diagnosis of AIDS, the final stage of HIV infection, is made when the infected person has either a dangerously low CD4 (helper T) cell count (below 200 cells per cubic milliliter of blood) or has contracted one or more opportunistic infections characteristic of the disease (such as Kaposi's sarcoma or *Pneumocystis carinii* pneumonia).

Testing for HIV Antibodies

Once antibodies have formed in reaction to HIV, a blood test known as the *ELISA* (enzyme-linked immunosorbent assay) may detect their presence. It can take 3 to 6 months after initial infection for sufficient antibodies to develop in the body to show a positive test result. Therefore, individuals with negative test results should be retested within 6 months. If sufficient antibodies are present, the test will be positive. When a person who previously tested *negative* (no HIV antibodies present) has a subsequent test that is *positive*, seroconversion is said to have occurred. In such a situation, the person would typically take another ELISA test, followed by a more precise test known as the *Western blot*, to confirm the presence of HIV antibodies.

It should be noted that these tests are not AIDS tests per se. Rather, they detect antibodies for HIV, indicating the presence of the virus in the person's system. Whether the person will develop AIDS depends to some extent on the strength of the immune system. Although we have made remarkable progress in prolonging the relatively symptom-free period between infection, HIV-positive status, and progression to symptomatic AIDS, it is important to

what do you think?

Do you favor mandatory reporting of HIV and AIDS cases? ● On the one hand, if you knew that your name and vital statistics would be "on file" if you tested positive for HIV, would you be less likely to take the HIV test? ● On the other hand, do people who carry this contagious fatal disease have a responsibility to inform the general public and the health professionals who provide their care?

Women and HIV/AIDS

Women are four to ten times more likely than men to contract HIV through unprotected heterosexual intercourse with an infected partner, because the vaginal area is more susceptible to microtears. Also, during intercourse, a woman is exposed to more semen than a man is to vaginal fluids. Women who have sexually transmitted infections (STIs) are more likely to be asymptomatic and therefore unaware they have an infection; preexisting STIs increase the risk of HIV transmission.

Women have been underrepresented in clinical trials for HIV treatment and prevention and may be less likely to seek medical treatment because of caregiving burdens, transportation problems, and lack of money. In some countries, women have few rights regarding sexual relationships and the family. Instead, men are in charge of making the majority of decisions, such as whom they will marry and whether the man will have more than one sexual partner. This power imbalance means that it can be especially difficult for women to protect themselves from getting infected with HIV/AIDS. A woman may not be able to negotiate the use of a condom if her husband makes the decisions. Efforts must be initiated to help women take control of their sexual health and participate actively in sexual decisions with their partners.

In addition, millions of women have been indirectly affected by the HIV/AIDS pandemic. Women's childbearing role means that they have to contend with issues such as mother-to-child transmission of HIV. The responsibility of caring for AIDS patients and orphans is also an issue that has a greater effect on women.

As more and more women become infected with HIV/AIDS, global efforts of aid and prevention need to increase. These efforts should include the promotion and protection of women's human rights; an increase in education and awareness among women; and the development of new, preventive technologies such as microbicides, gels, or creams that could be applied vaginally without a partner even knowing it, to prevent HIV infection. Research has been underway for a number of years, but there is still no microbicide that is currently available.

Sources: Centers for Disease Control and Prevention, Divisions of HIV/AIDS Prevention National Center for HIV/AIDS, Viral Hepatitis, STD, and TB Prevention, "HIV/AIDS among Women," Revised August 2008, www.cdc.gov/hiv/topics/women/resources/factsheets/women.htm; AVERT, "Women, HIV and AIDS," Updated August 2009, www.avert.org/women.htm.

---

note that a cure does not yet exist. The vast majority of infected people eventually develop some form of the disease.

Health officials distinguish between *reported* and *actual* cases of HIV infection because it is believed that many HIV-positive people avoid being tested. One reason is fear of knowing the truth. Another is the fear of recrimination from employers, insurance companies, and medical staff. However, early detection and reporting are important, because immediate treatment for someone in the early stages of HIV disease is critical.

New Hope and Treatments

New drugs have slowed the progression from HIV to AIDS and have prolonged life expectancies for most AIDS patients. Current treatments combine selected drugs, especially protease inhibitors and reverse transcriptase inhibitors. *Protease inhibitors* (e.g., amprenavir, ritonavir, and saquinavir) act to prevent the production of the virus in chronically infected cells that HIV has already invaded. Other drugs, such as AZT, ddI, ddC, d4T, and 3TC, inhibit the HIV enzyme *reverse transcriptase* before the virus has invaded the cell, thereby preventing the virus from infecting new cells. All of the protease drugs seem to work best in combination with other therapies. These combination treatments are still quite experimental, and no combination has proven to be absolute for all people.

Although these drugs provide new hope and longer survival rates for people living with HIV, it is important to

maintain caution. We are still a long way from a cure. Apathy and carelessness may abound if too much confidence is placed in these treatments. Newer drugs that held much promise are becoming less effective as HIV develops resistance to them. Costs of taking multiple drugs are prohibitive, and side effects common. Furthermore, the number of people becoming HIV-infected each year has increased in some communities, meaning that we are still a long way from beating this disease.

Preventing HIV Infection

Although scientists have been working on a variety of HIV vaccine trials, none is currently available. The only way to prevent HIV infection is through the choices you make in sexual behaviors and drug use and by taking responsibility for your own health and the health of your loved ones.

Unfortunately, the message has not gotten through to many Americans. They assume that because they are heterosexual, do not inject illegal drugs, and do not have sex with sex workers, they are not at risk. They couldn't be more wrong. Anyone who engages in unprotected sex is at risk, especially if they have sex with a partner who has engaged in other high-risk behaviors. Sex with multiple partners is the greatest threat. You can't determine the presence of HIV by looking at a person; you can't tell by questioning the person, unless he or she has been tested recently, is HIV-negative, and is giving an honest answer. So what should you do?

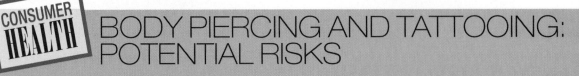
BODY PIERCING AND TATTOOING: POTENTIAL RISKS

A look around any college campus reveals many examples of "body art," the widespread trend of using body piercing and tattoos as a form of self-expression. Although the practice can be done safely, health professionals cite several health concerns. The most common problems include skin reactions,

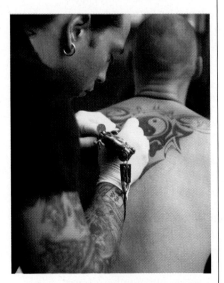

Like any activity that involves bodily fluids, tattooing carries some risk of disease transmission.

infections, allergic reactions, and scarring. Of even greater concern is the potential transmission of dangerous pathogens that can occur with any puncture of the skin. The use of unsterile needles—which can cause serious infections and can transmit staph, HIV, hepatitis B and C, tetanus, and a host of other diseases—poses a very real risk.

Laws and policies regulating body piercing and tattooing vary greatly by state. Standards for safety usually include minimum age of clientele, standards of sanitation, use of aseptic techniques, sterilization of equipment, record keeping, informed risks, instructions for skin care, and recommendations for dealing with adverse reactions. Because of the lack of universal regulatory standards and the potential for transmission of dangerous pathogens, anyone who receives a tattoo, body piercing, or permanent makeup tattoo cannot donate blood for 1 year.

Before deciding on a body artist to do your tattoo or piercing, you may want to watch the artist working on another client to evaluate the person's safety and skill. If you opt for tattooing or body piercing, remember to take the following safety precautions:

✳ Look for clean, well-lighted work areas, and inquire about sterilization procedures. Ask to see the autoclave used for sterilizing the instruments. Be wary of establishments that are reluctant to show you their autoclave or to discuss their sterilization procedures.
✳ Packaged, sterilized needles should be used only once and then discarded. A piercing gun should not be used, because it cannot be sterilized properly. Watch that the artist uses new needles and tubes from a sterile package before your procedure begins. Ask to see the sterile confirmation logo on the bag itself.
✳ Immediately before piercing or tattooing, the body area should be carefully sterilized.

The artist should wash his or her hands and put on new latex gloves for each procedure. Make sure the artist changes those gloves if he or she needs to touch anything else, such as the telephone, while working.
✳ Leftover tattoo ink should be discarded after each procedure. Do not allow the artist to reuse ink that has been used for other customers. Used needles should be disposed of in a "sharps" container, a plastic container with the biohazard symbol clearly marked on it.
✳ If any signs of pus, swelling, redness, or discoloration persist after a piercing, remove the piercing object, and contact a physician.

Sources: Mayo Clinic Staff, "Tattoos: Risks and Precautions to Know First," February 2008, www.mayoclinic.com/health/tattoos-and-piercings/MC00020; Center for Food Safety and Applied Nutrition, "Tattoos and Permanent Makeup," *Office of Cosmetics Fact Sheet*, Updated June 2008, www.fda.gov/Cosmetics/ProductandIngredientSafety/ProductInformation/ucm108530.htm.

Of course, the simplest answer is abstinence. If you don't exchange body fluids, you won't get the disease. As a second line of defense, if you decide to be intimate, the next best option is to use a condom. However, in spite of all the educational campaigns, surveys consistently indicate that most college students throw caution to the wind if they think they "know" someone—and they have unprotected sex. The **Skills for Behavior Change** box at right presents ways to talk to your sexual partner about protecting yourselves from HIV and other STIs.

Noninfectious Conditions

Typically, when we think of major noninfectious ailments, we think of "killer" diseases such as cancer and heart disease. Clearly, these diseases make up the major portion of life-threatening diseases—accounting for nearly two-thirds of all

deaths (see Chapter 12). Although these diseases capture much media attention, other chronic conditions can also cause pain, suffering, and disability.

Generally, noninfectious diseases are not transmitted by a pathogen or by any form of personal contact. Lifestyle and personal health habits are often implicated as underlying causes. Healthy changes in lifestyle and public health efforts aimed at research, prevention, and control can minimize the effects of these diseases.

Chronic Lung Diseases

Lung disease is the number three killer in the United States, right behind heart disease and cancer, and is responsible for one in six deaths, or nearly 400,000 people per year. Today, more than 35 million Americans are living with chronic lung disease such as asthma and chronic obstructive pulmonary disease (COPD), otherwise known as emphysema and chronic bronchitis.[35]

Any disease or disorder in which lung function is impaired is considered a lung disease. The lungs can be damaged by a single exposure to a toxic chemical or severe heat, or they can be impaired from years of inhaling the tar and chemicals in tobacco smoke. Occupational or home exposure to asbestos, silica dust, paint fumes and lacquers, pesticides, and a host of other environmental substances can cause lung deterioration. Of course, cancers, infections, and degenerative changes can also wreak havoc with lung function. When the lungs are impaired, a condition known as **dyspnea,** or a choking type of breathlessness can occur, even with mild exertion. As the lungs are oxygen deprived, the heart is forced to work harder and, over time, cardiovascular problems, suffocation, and death can occur.

Chronic Obstructive Pulmonary Diseases

Chronic obstructive pulmonary diseases (COPDs) include chronic bronchitis and emphysema. Since these conditions often occur together, the abbreviation *COPD* is often preferred by health professionals; COPD does not include other obstructive diseases such as asthma. Currently, about 24 million U.S. adults have impaired lung function, with over 12 million believed to have COPD. Eighty to 90 percent of persons with COPD have a history of smoking.[36] Occupational exposure to certain industrial fumes or gases and exposure to dusts and other lung irritants increases risks, whether this exposure comes in one big dose or over months and years.

Bronchitis Bronchitis refers to an inflammation of the lining of the bronchial tubes. These tubes, the bronchi, connect the windpipe with the lungs. When the bronchi become inflamed or infected, less air is able to flow from the lungs, and heavy mucus begins to form. *Acute bronchitis* is the most common of the bronchial diseases, and symptoms often improve in a week or two.

When the symptoms of bronchitis last for at least 3 months of the year for 2 consecutive years, the condition is considered *chronic bronchitis.* In some cases, this chronic inflammation and irritation goes undiagnosed for years, particularly in smokers who feel it's a normal part of their lives. By the time these individuals receive medical care, the damage to their lungs is severe and may lead to heart and respiratory failure or to a chronic need to carry oxygen to aid in breathing. Nearly 10 million Americans suffer from chronic bronchitis.[37]

Emphysema Emphysema involves the gradual, irreversible destruction of the **alveoli** (tiny air sacs through which gas exchange occurs) of the lungs. Over 4.1 million Americans suffer from emphysema, with nearly 70 percent of cases occurring in men.[38] As the alveoli are destroyed, the affected person finds it more and more difficult to exhale, struggling to take in a fresh supply of air before the air held in the lungs has been expended. The chest cavity gradually begins to expand, producing a barrel-shaped chest. For more on emphysema and smoking, see Chapter 8.

Asthma

Asthma is a long-term, chronic inflammatory disorder that blocks air flow into and out of the lungs. Asthma causes tiny airways in the lung to overreact with spasms in response to certain triggers. Symptoms include wheezing, difficulty breathing, shortness of breath,

dyspnea Shortness of breath, usually associated with disease of the heart or lungs.

chronic obstructive pulmonary diseases (COPDs) A collection of chronic lung diseases including emphysema and chronic bronchitis.

bronchitis Inflammation of the lining of the bronchial tubes.

emphysema A respiratory disease in which the alveoli become distended or ruptured and are no longer functional.

alveoli Tiny air sacs of the lungs where gas exchange occurs (oxygen enters the blood and carbon dioxide is removed).

asthma A chronic respiratory disease characterized by attacks of wheezing, shortness of breath, and coughing spasms.

and coughing spasms. Although most asthma attacks are mild and non–life-threatening, severe attacks can trigger bronchospasms (contractions of the bronchial tubes in the lungs) that are so severe that, without rapid treatment, death may occur. Between attacks, most people have few symptoms.

Asthma falls into two distinctly different types. The more common form of asthma, known as *extrinsic* or *allergic asthma*, is typically associated with allergic triggers; it tends to run in families and develop in childhood. Often by adulthood, a person has few episodes, or the disorder completely goes away. *Intrinsic* or *nonallergic asthma* may be triggered by anything except an allergy.

Several factors can increase your risk of developing asthma: living in a large urban area; being exposed to secondhand smoke during childhood; or having respiratory infections in childhood, low birth weight, obesity, gastroesophageal reflux disease, or one or both parents with asthma.[39] Asthma attacks can be triggered by exposure to irritants or allergens such as tobacco smoke, occupational chemicals, pollen, cockroaches, feathers, foods, molds, dust, or pet dander. In some individuals, stress, exercise, certain medications, cold air, and sulfites are also potential triggers. Interestingly, one in five asthmatics can suffer an attack from taking aspirin.[40]

Approximately 23 million people in the United States currently have asthma, making it one of the most prevalent respiratory diseases.[41] Asthma can occur at any age but is most likely to appear in children between infancy and age 5 and in adults before age 40. In childhood, asthma strikes more boys than girls; in adulthood, it strikes more women than men. The asthma rate is 50 percent higher among African Americans than whites, and four times as many African Americans die of asthma as do whites.[42]

In the past few decades, asthma rates have risen dramatically, increasing by more than 65 percent since the 1980s.[43] Asthma has become the most common chronic disease of childhood, affecting more than 1 child in 20. Among adults, asthma is the fourth leading cause of work absence, resulting in over 10 million lost workdays per year. The annual direct costs of asthma are nearly $20 billion.

Determining whether a specific allergen provokes asthma attacks, taking steps to reduce exposure, and avoiding triggers such as certain types of exercise or stress are important steps in asthma prevention. The **Green Guide**

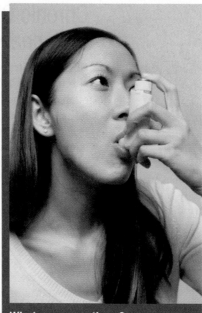

What causes asthma?

Asthma is caused by inflammation of the airways in the lungs, restricting them and leading to wheezing, chest tightness, shortness of breath, and coughing. In most people, asthma is brought on by contact with allergens or irritants in the air; some people also have exercise-induced asthma. People with asthma can generally control their symptoms through the use of inhaled medications, and most asthmatics keep a "rescue" inhaler of bronchodilating medication on hand to use in case of a flare-up.

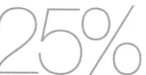

25%

of all school absences are due to asthma.

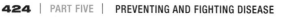

migraine A condition characterized by localized headaches that possibly result from alternating dilation and constriction of blood vessels.

at right offers suggestions for ways to green your home and reduce potential asthma and allergy triggers. In addition to avoiding triggers, finding the most effective medications can help asthmatics control their condition and avoid severe attacks.

Headaches

Almost all of us have experienced at least one major headache. In fact, more than 80 percent of women and 65 percent of men experience headaches on a regular basis.[44] Over 90 percent of all headaches are of three major types: tension headaches, migraines, and cluster headaches.

Tension Headaches

Tension headaches are generally caused by muscle contractions or tension in the neck or head. This tension may be caused by actual strain placed on neck or head muscles due to overuse, to holding static positions for long periods, or to tension triggered by stress. Other possible triggers include red wine, lack of sleep, fasting, and menstruation. Relaxation, hot water treatment, and massage are holistic treatments. Aspirin, ibuprofen, acetaminophen, and naproxen sodium remain the old standby medicinal treatments for pain relief.

Migraine Headaches

Nearly 30 million Americans—three times more women than men—suffer from **migraines,** a type of headache that often has severe, debilitating symptoms. One out of 4 households has a migraine sufferer.[45] If one parent has migraines, his or her children have a 50 percent chance of having them. If both parents have them, there is a 75 percent chance their children will have them. Usually migraine incidence peaks in young adulthood, people aged 20 to 45.

Symptoms vary greatly by individual, and attacks typically last anywhere from 4 to 72 hours, with distinct phases of symptoms. In about 15 percent of cases, migraines are preceded by a sensory warning sign known as an *aura,* such as flashes of light, flickering vision, blind spots, tingling in arms or legs, or sensation of odor or taste. Sometimes nausea, vomiting, and extreme sensitivity to light and sound are present. Symptoms of migraine include excruciating pain behind or around one eye and usually on the same side of the head. In some people, there is sinus pain, neck pain, or an aura without headache.

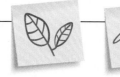

GREEN GUIDE

Be Eco-Clean and Allergen Free

Exposure to household chemicals, dust, and pet dander may exacerbate asthma, allergies, and other respiratory problems. You can reduce exposure to noxious household chemicals and create a clean, comfortable home by practicing green cleaning. This involves using cleaning supplies and household products that are less toxic to one's home environment and less of a burden on water resources. Because some companies may want you to believe their product is greener than it actually is, read the labels carefully and look for independent certifications such as Green Seal and the EPA's Design for the Environment program.

Making your own cleaners is often less expensive than purchasing them at the store, and it is the best way to ensure a cleaner will not harm your health or the environment. Here are a few practical recipes:

✳ For a handy glass and surface cleaner, mix one-half cup white vinegar to 4 cups water. Pour the solution into a spray bottle and keep the remainder for a quick and cheap refill.
✳ Use 2 tablespoons lemon juice to 4 cups water for a surface cleaner.
✳ Baking soda works as a great deodorizer and cleaner. Use it to remove carpet odors and to scour sinks, toilets, and bathtubs.
✳ Because chlorine can damage lungs, skin, and eyes, and chlorine production adds toxic chemicals such as carcinogenic dioxins to our environment, use a chlorine bleach alternative. For example, use one-half cup of hydrogen peroxide in your laundry or use oxygen-based bleaches that can be found in most grocery stores.

✳ An all-purpose cleaner can be made of one-half cup borax (a natural mineral you can find in the laundry aisle) to 1 gallon of hot water.
✳ For green air fresheners, use essential oils, such as lemon or lavender. Many store-bought air fresheners contain phthalates, often called "fragrance," that are related to respiratory problems and other noninfectious conditions. Place a few drops of essential oils on a piece of tissue paper, in a bowl of warm water, or in a store-bought diffuser.

As you transition to green cleaning, do not just throw old products in the trash, as these can wind up polluting landfills and leaching into water supplies. Instead, take them to a hazardous chemical recycling facility.

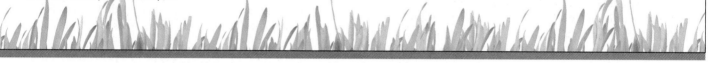

The cause of migraines is unknown, but some research suggests they may occur when blood vessels dilate in the membrane that surrounds the brain. Critics of the blood vessel dilation theory question why only blood vessels of the head dilate in these situations. These researchers suggest that migraines originate in the cortex of the brain, where certain pain sensors are stimulated.

Historically, treatments have centered on reversing or preventing blood vessel dilation, with the most common treatment derived from the rye fungus *ergot*. Today, fast-acting ergot compounds are available by nasal spray, vastly increasing the speed of relief. However, ergot drugs have many side effects, not the least of which may be that they are habit forming. Other drugs that are sometimes prescribed include lidocaine, a new group of drugs called triptans, and Imitrex, a drug tailor-made for migraines.

Cluster Headaches

The pain of a cluster headache is often severe and has been described as "killer" or "suicidal." Usually these headaches cause stabbing pain on one side of the head, behind the eye, or in one defined spot. Other typical cluster headache characteristics include nasal discharge and congestion, tearing of the eye on the same side as the pain, a swollen or drooping eyelid and contracted pupil, flushing of the face

on the affected side, and excessive sweating. Fortunately, cluster headaches are among the more rare forms of headache, affecting less than 1 percent of people, usually men. Young adults in their twenties tend to be particularly susceptible.[46]

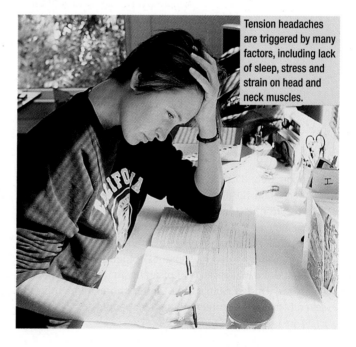

Tension headaches are triggered by many factors, including lack of sleep, stress and strain on head and neck muscles.

Cluster headaches can last for weeks and disappear quickly. However, more commonly they last for 40 to 90 minutes and often occur in the middle of the night, usually during rapid eye movement (REM) sleep. Oxygen therapy, drugs, and even surgery have been used to treat severe cases.

Chronic Fatigue Syndrome

Since the late 1980s, several U.S. clinics have noted a characteristic set of symptoms that include chronic fatigue, headaches, fever, sore throat, enlarged lymph nodes, depression, poor memory, general weakness, and nausea. Researchers initially believed these symptoms were caused by the Epstein-Barr virus, the same one that causes mononucleosis. Since those initial studies, however, researchers have all but ruled out the Epstein-Barr virus. Despite extensive testing, no viral cause has been found.

Today, in the absence of a known pathogen, many researchers believe that the illness, now commonly referred to as **chronic fatigue syndrome (CFS),** may have strong psychosocial roots. Our heightened awareness of health makes some of us scrutinize our bodies so carefully that the slightest deviation becomes amplified. In addition, the growing number of people who suffer from depression seem to be good candidates for chronic fatigue syndrome. Experts worry, however, that too many scientists approach CFS as something that is "in the person's head" and that such an attitude may prevent them from doing the serious research needed to find a cure.

The diagnosis of chronic fatigue syndrome depends on two major criteria and eight or more minor criteria. The major criteria are (1) debilitating fatigue that persists for at least 6 months, and (2) the absence of other illnesses that could cause the symptoms. Minor criteria include headaches, fever, sore throat, painful lymph nodes, weakness, fatigue after exercise, sleep problems, and rapid onset of these symptoms. Because the cause is not apparent, treatment of CFS focuses on improved nutrition, rest, counseling for depression, judicious exercise, and development of a strong support network.

chronic fatigue syndrome (CFS) A condition of unknown cause characterized by extreme fatigue.

repetitive motion disorders (RMDs) A family of painful muscular conditions that result from repeated motions.

carpal tunnel syndrome A common occupational injury in which the median nerve in the wrist becomes irritated, causing numbness, tingling, and pain in the fingers and hands.

Low Back Pain

Approximately 85 percent of all Americans will experience low back pain (LBP) at some point. Some of these episodes result from muscular damage and are short lived and acute; others may involve dislocations, fractures, or other problems with spinal vertebrae or discs, resulting in chronic pain or requiring surgery. Low back pain is epidemic throughout the world and the major cause of disability for people aged 20 to 45 in the United States, who suffer more frequently and severely from this problem than older people do.[47]

Almost 90 percent of all back problems occur in the lumbar spine (lower back). You can avoid many problems by consciously maintaining good posture. Numerous studies have shown that wearing heavy backpacks, particularly among younger, school-aged children, can result in back pain. It is likely that carrying books and computers all day may also be a cause for concern among college students. Although no clear research has pointed this out, common sense suggests you use caution, making sure you purchase a good quality backpack that has straps to off-load some of the weight to your hips, rather than on your shoulders and back. Other things you can do to reduce risks of back pain include the following:

- Purchase a high-quality, supportive mattress, and avoid sleeping on your stomach.
- Avoid high-heeled shoes, which tilt the pelvis forward, and wear shoes with good arch support.
- Control your weight. Extra weight puts increased strain on knees, hips, and your back.
- Warm up and stretch before exercising or lifting heavy objects.
- When lifting something heavy, use your leg muscles and proper form. Do not bend from the waist or take the weight load on your back.
- Buy a chair with good lumbar support for doing your work.
- Move your car seat forward so your knees are elevated slightly.
- Exercise regularly, particularly exercises that strengthen the abdominal muscles and stretch the back muscles.

Repetitive Motion Disorders

It's the end of the term, and you have finished the last of several papers. After hours of nonstop typing, your hands are numb and you feel an intense, burning pain that makes the thought of typing one more word almost unbearable. If this happens, you may be suffering from one of several **repetitive motion disorders (RMDs).** Repetitive motion disorders include carpal tunnel syndrome, bursitis, tendonitis, ganglion cysts, and others.[48] Twisting of the arm or wrist, overexertion, and incorrect posture or position are usually contributors. The areas most likely to be affected are the hands, wrists, elbows, and shoulders, but the neck, back, hips, knees, feet, ankles, and legs can be affected, too. Over time, RMDs can cause permanent damage to nerves, soft tissue, and joints.

One of the most common RMDs is **carpal tunnel syndrome,** a product of spending hours typing at the computer, flipping groceries through computerized scanners, or other jobs requiring repeated hand and wrist movements that can irritate the median nerve in the wrist, causing numbness, tingling, and pain in the fingers and hands. Although carpal tunnel syndrome risk can be reduced by proper placement of the keyboard, mouse, wrist pads, and other techniques, it is often overlooked until significant damage has been done. Better education and ergonomic workplace designs can eliminate many injuries of this nature. Physical and occupational therapy is an important part of treatment and eventual recovery.

Assess yourself

STIs: Do You Really Know What You Think You Know?

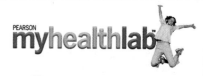

The following quiz will help you evaluate whether your beliefs and attitudes about sexually transmitted infections (STIs) lead you to behaviors that increase your risk of infection. Indicate whether you believe the following items are true or false, then consult the answer key that follows.

1. You can always tell when you've got an STI because the symptoms are so obvious. ○ ○
2. Some STIs can be passed on by skin-to-skin contact in the genital area. ○ ○
3. Herpes can be transmitted only when a person has visible sores on his or her genitals. ○ ○
4. Oral sex is safe sex. ○ ○
5. Condoms reduce your risk of both pregnancy and STIs. ○ ○
6. As long as you don't have anal intercourse, you can't get HIV. ○ ○
7. All sexually active females should have a regular Pap smear. ○ ○
8. Once genital warts have been removed, there is no risk of passing on the virus. ○ ○
9. You can get several STIs at one time. ○ ○
10. If the signs of an STI go away, you are cured. ○ ○
11. People who get an STI have a lot of sex partners. ○ ○
12. All STIs can be cured. ○ ○
13. You can get an STI more than once. ○ ○

TRUE   FALSE

Answer Key

1. **False.** The unfortunate fact is that many STIs show no symptoms. This has serious implications: (1) you can be passing on the infection without knowing it, and (2) the pathogen may be damaging your reproductive organs without you knowing it.

2. **True.** Some viruses are present on the skin around the genital area. Herpes and genital warts are the main culprits.

3. **False.** Herpes is most easily passed on when the sores and blisters are present, because the fluid in the lesions carries the virus. But the virus is also found on the skin around the genital area. Most people contract herpes this way, unaware that the virus is present.

4. **False.** Oral sex is not safe sex. Herpes, genital warts, and chlamydia can all be passed on through oral sex. Condoms should be used on the penis. Dental dams should be placed over the female genitals during oral sex.

5. **True.** Condoms significantly reduce the risk of pregnancy when used correctly. They also reduce the risk of STIs. It is important to point out that abstinence is the only behavior that provides complete protection against pregnancy and STIs.

6. **False.** HIV is present in blood, semen, and vaginal fluid. Any activity that allows for the transfer of these fluids is risky. Anal intercourse is a high-risk activity, especially for the receptive (passive) partner, but other sexual activity is also a risk. When you don't know your partner's sexual history and you're not in a long-term monogamous relationship, condoms are a must.

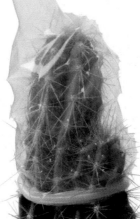

7. **True.** A Pap smear is a simple procedure involving the scraping of a small amount of tissue from the surface of the cervix (at the upper end of the vagina). The sample is tested for abnormal cells that may indicate cancer. All sexually active women should have regular Pap smears.

8. **False.** Genital warts, which may be present on the penis, the anus, and inside and outside the vagina, can be removed. However, the virus that caused the warts will always be present in the body and can be passed on to a sexual partner.

9. **True.** It is possible to have many STIs at one time. In fact, having one STI may make it more likely that a person will acquire more STIs. For example, the open sore from herpes creates a place for HIV to be transmitted.

10. **False.** The symptoms may go away, but your body is still infected. For example, syphilis is characterized by various stages. In the first stage, a painless sore called a *chancre* appears for about a week and then goes away.

11. **False.** If you have sex once with an infected partner, you are at risk for an STI.

12. **False.** Some STIs are viruses and therefore cannot be cured. There is no cure at present for herpes, HIV/AIDS, or genital warts. These STIs are treatable (to lessen the pain and irritation of symptoms), but not curable.

13. **True.** Experiencing one infection with an STI does not mean that you can never be infected again. A person can be reinfected many times with the same STI. This is especially true if a person does not get treated for the STI and thus keeps reinfecting his or her partner with the same STI.

Sources: Adapted from Jefferson County Public Health, "STD Quiz," Modified March 2009, www.co.jefferson.co.us/health/health_T111_R69 .htm; Family Planning Victoria, "Play Safe," Updated July 2005, www.fpv .org.au/1_2_2.html.

YOUR PLAN FOR **CHANGE**

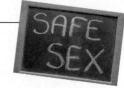

The **Assess**yourself activity let you consider your beliefs and attitudes about STIs and identify possible risks you may be facing. Now that you have considered these results, you can begin to change behaviors that may be putting you at risk for STIs and for infection in general.

Today, you can:

○ Put together an "emergency" supply of condoms. Outside of abstinence, condoms are your best protection against an STI. If you don't have a supply on hand, visit your local drugstore or health clinic. Remember that both men and women are responsible for preventing the transmission of STIs.

○ To prevent infections in general, get in the habit of washing your hands regularly. After you cough, sneeze, blow your nose, use the bathroom, or prepare food, find a sink, wet your hands with warm water, and lather up with soap. Scrub your hands for about 20 seconds (count to 20 or recite the alphabet), rinse well, and dry your hands.

Within the next 2 weeks, you can:

○ Talk with your significant other honestly about your sexual history. Make appointments to get tested if either of you think you may have been exposed to an STI.

○ Adjust your sleep schedule so that you're getting an adequate amount of rest every night. Being well rested is one key aspect of maintaining a healthy immune system.

By the end of the semester, you can:

○ Check your immunization schedule and make sure you're current with all recommended vaccinations. Make an appointment with your health care provider if you need a booster or vaccine.

○ If you are due for an annual pelvic exam, make an appointment. Ask your partner if he or she has had an annual exam and encourage him or her to make an appointment if not.

Summary

* Your body uses a number of defense systems to keep pathogens from invading. The skin is the body's major protection. The immune system creates antibodies to destroy antigens. Fever and pain play a role in defending the body. Vaccines bolster the body's immune system against specific diseases. Allergies are an overreaction of the body's natural defense system.
* The major pathogens are bacteria, viruses, fungi, protozoans, parasitic worms, and prions. Bacterial infections include staphylococcal infections, streptococcal infections, pneumonia, and tuberculosis. Major viral diseases include the common cold, influenza, and hepatitis. Emerging and resurgent diseases pose significant threats for future generations, as do problems related to antibiotic resistance and superbugs.
* Sexually transmitted infections (STIs) are spread through intercourse, oral sex, anal sex, hand–genital contact, and sometimes mouth-to-mouth contact. Major STIs include chlamydia, gonorrhea, syphilis, herpes, human papillomavirus (HPV) and genital warts, candidiasis, trichomoniasis, and pubic lice.
* Acquired immunodeficiency syndrome (AIDS) is caused by the human immunodeficiency virus (HIV). Globally, HIV/AIDS has become a major threat to the world's population. Anyone can get HIV by engaging in high-risk sexual activities that include exchange of body fluids or by injecting drugs with contaminated needles (or having sex with someone who does).
* Chronic lung diseases include chronic bronchitis, emphysema, and asthma. Lung disease is the third leading cause of death in the United States.
* Headaches may be caused by a variety of factors, the most common of which are tension, dilation and/or rapid contraction of blood vessels in the brain, chemical influences on muscles and vessels that cause inflammation and pain, and underlying physiological and psychological disorders.
* Chronic fatigue syndrome is a complex disorder characterized by profound fatigue. Low back pain is a major cause of disability among Americans, but some risks for it can be addressed by proper posture, supportive shoes, and core-strengthening exercises. Repetitive motion disorders are preventable by proper placement and usage of equipment.

Pop Quiz

1. Which of the following is a *viral* disorder?
   a. the common cold
   b. pneumonia
   c. tuberculosis
   d. streptococcal infections

2. Antibiotic resistance is likely caused by
   a. the overuse of antibiotics in food production.
   b. the improper use of antibiotics by patients for whom they are prescribed.
   c. the overuse of antibacterial soaps and other cleaning products.
   d. all of the above.

3. If you are infected, which one of these STIs will remain in your body for life, regardless of treatment?
   a. chlamydia
   b. gonorrhea
   c. syphilis
   d. herpes

4. The term to best describe infections transmitted through some form of intimate contact is
   a. sexually transmitted diseases.
   b. sexually transmitted infections.
   c. venereal disease.
   d. chronic disease.

5. Jennifer touched her viral herpes sore on her lip and then touched her eye. She ended up with herpesvirus in her eye as well. This is an example of
   a. acquired immunity.
   b. passive immunity.
   c. autoinoculation.
   d. self-vaccination.

6. Which of the following is *not* a true statement about HIV/AIDS?
   a. You can tell whether a potential sex partner has the virus by looking at the person.
   b. The virus can be spread through either semen or vaginal fluids.
   c. You cannot get HIV from a public restroom toilet seat.
   d. Unprotected anal sex increases risk of exposure to the HIV virus.

7. Which of the following is true about HPV?
   a. Genital warts are caused by the low-risk types of HPV.
   b. The HPV vaccine is available for men and women.
   c. There are over 100 different types of HPV that are sexually transmitted.
   d. Antibiotics are used to cure HPV.

8. Which of the following is correct?
   a. There is no increased risk for migraines in children born to parents with migraines.
   b. COPDs include low back pain, asthma, and arthritis.
   c. Fever and inflammation are components of the body's immune response and help fight pathogens.
   d. If you have a low fever, taking aspirin is a good idea.

9. The gradual destruction of the alveoli in a smoker's lungs will usually cause which respiratory condition?
   a. dyspnea
   b. bronchitis
   c. emphysema
   d. asthma

10. Which of the following conditions is the leading cause of employee sick time and lost productivity in the United States?
    a. low back pain
    b. the common cold
    c. asthma
    d. on-the-job injuries

Answers to these questions can be found on page A-1.

Think about It!

1. What are the major controllable risk factors for contracting infectious diseases? Using this knowledge, how would you change your current lifestyle to prevent such infection?

2. What is a pathogen? What are the similarities and differences between pathogens and antigens?

3. What are the six types of pathogens? What are the various means by which they can be transmitted?

4. How have social conditions among the poor and homeless increased the risks for certain diseases, such as tuberculosis, influenza, and hepatitis? Why are these conditions a challenge to the efforts of public health officials?

5. Identify five STIs and their symptoms. How do they develop? What are their potential long-term effects?

6. Why are women more susceptible to HIV infection than men? What implications does this have for prevention, treatment, and research?

7. List common respiratory diseases affecting Americans. Which of these diseases has a genetic basis? An environmental basis? An individual basis?

Accessing Your Health on the Internet

The following websites explore further topics and issues related to personal health. For links to the websites below, visit the Companion Website for *Health: The Basics,* Green Edition at www.pearsonhighered.com/donatelle.

1. *American Academy of Allergy, Asthma, and Immunology.* Provides an overview of asthma and allergies. Offers interactive quizzes to test your knowledge and an ask-an-expert section. www.aaaai.org

2. *American Social Health Association.* Provides facts, support, resources, and referrals about sexually transmitted infections and diseases. www.ashastd.org

3. *Centers for Disease Control and Prevention (CDC).* Home page for the government agency dedicated to disease intervention and prevention, with links to all the latest data and publications put out by the CDC, including the *Morbidity and Mortality Weekly Report, HIV/AIDS Surveillance Report,* and the *Journal of Emerging Infectious Diseases.* Also provides access to Wonder, the CDC research database. www.cdc.gov

4. *National Center for Preparedness, Detection, and Control of Infectious Diseases (NCPDCID).* Up-to-date perspectives on infectious diseases of significance to the global community. www.cdc.gov/ncpdcid

5. *San Francisco AIDS Foundation.* This community-based AIDS service organization focuses on ending the HIV/AIDS pandemic through education, services for AIDS patients, advocacy and public policy efforts, and global programs. www.sfaf.org

6. *World Health Organization (WHO).* Provides access to the latest information on world health issues, including infectious disease, and direct access to publications and fact sheets, with keywords to help users find topics of interest. www.who.int

References

1. J. R. Pleis and J. W. Lucas, National Center for Health Statistics, "Summary Health Statistics for U.S. Adults: National Health Interview Survey, 2007," *Vital Health and Statistics* 10, no. 240 (2009).

2. Centers for Disease Control and Prevention, National Center for Health Statistics, "FastStats: Allergies and Hay Fever," Updated April 2009, www.cdc.gov/nchs/fastats/allergies.htm.

3. R. Klevens, "Invasive Methicillin-Resistant Staphylococcus Aureus (MRSA) Infections in the United States," *Journal of the American Medical Association* 298, no. 15 (2007): 1763–71.

4. Centers for Disease Control and Prevention, "Group A Streptococcal Disease (GAS)," Accessed August 2009, www.cdc.gov/ncidod/dbmd/diseaseinfo/groupastreptococcal_g.htm.

5. Ibid.

6. J. Tully et al., "Students May Have Higher Risk for Meningococcal Disease Than Other Adolescents," *British Medical Journal* 332, no. 7539 (2006): 1136–42.

7. Centers for Disease Control and Prevention, *Reported Tuberculosis in the United States, 2007* (Atlanta: U.S. Department of Health and Human Services, CDC, 2008).

8. World Health Organization, *WHO Report 2009—Global Tuberculosis Control: Epidemiology, Strategy, Financing* (Geneva, Switzerland: 2009).

9. Centers for Disease Control and Prevention, "Key Facts about Seasonal Influenza (Flu)," Updated October 2009, www.cdc.gov/flu/keyfacts.htm.

10. Centers for Disease Control and Prevention, "Hepatitis A FAQs for Health Professionals," Updated June 2009, www.cdc.gov/hepatitis/HAV/HAVfaq.htm.

11. World Health Organization, "Global Alert and Response: Hepatitis B," 2009, www.who.int/csr/disease/hepatitis/whocdscsrlyo20022/en/index1.html.

12. Centers for Disease Control and Prevention, Division of Viral Hepatitis, National Center for HIV/AIDS, Viral Hepatitis, STD, and TB Prevention, "Viral Hepatitis," 2009, www.cdc.gov/hepatitis/index.htm.

13. Centers for Disease Control and Prevention, National Center for Infectious Diseases, "vCJD (Variant Creutzfeldt-Jakob Disease)," 2007, www.cdc.gov/ncidod/dvrd/vcjd/index.htm.

14. Centers for Disease Control and Prevention, Division of Vector-Borne Infectious Diseases, National Center for Zoonotic, Vector-Borne, and Enteric Diseases, "West Nile Virus: Statistics, Surveillance and Control,"

2009, www.cdc.gov/ncidod/dvbid/westnile/
surv&controlCaseCount08_detailed.htm.

15. World Health Organization, "Confirmed
Human Cases of Avian Influenza A
(H5N1)," Updated September 2009, www
.who.int/csr/disease/avian_influenza/
country/en.

16. Centers for Disease Control and Preven-
tion, Division of STD Prevention, National
Center for HIV/AIDS, Viral Hepatitis, STD,
and TB Prevention, "Trends in Reportable
Sexually Transmitted Diseases in the
United States, 2008," 2009.

17. Centers for Disease Control and Preven-
tion, Division of STD Prevention, National
Center for HIV/AIDS, Viral Hepatitis, STD,
and TB Prevention, "Trends in Reportable
Sexually Transmitted Diseases in the
United States, 2008: National Surveillance
Data for Chlamydia, Gonorrhea, and
Syphilis," 2009, www.cdc.gov/std/stats08/
trends.htm; American Social Health Asso-
ciation, "STD/STI Statistics: Fast Facts,"
Updated October 2006, www.ashastd.org/
learn/learn_statistics.cfm.

18. Centers for Disease Control and Prevention, Division of STD Prevention, National
Center for HIV/AIDS, Viral Hepatitis, STD,
and TB Prevention, "Chlamydia—CDC
Fact Sheet," Updated December 2007,
www.cdc.gov/std/Chlamydia/STDFact-
Chlamydia.htm.

19. National Institute of Allergy and Infectious
Diseases, "Chlamydia," Updated April
2009, www3.niaid.nih.gov/topics/
chlamydia.

20. Centers for Disease Control and Preven-
tion, Division of STD Prevention, National
Center for HIV/AIDS, Viral Hepatitis, STD,
and TB Prevention, "Gonorrhea—CDC
Fact Sheet," 2008, www.cdc.gov/std/
Gonorrhea/STDFact-gonorrhea.htm.

21. U.S. National Library of Medicine, Medline
Plus, "Gonorrhea," Updated May 2009,
www.nlm.nih.gov/medlineplus/ency/
article/007267.htm.

22. National Institute of Allergy and Infectious
Diseases, "Gonorrhea," Updated March
2009, www3.niaid.nih.gov/topics/
gonorrhea.

23. Centers for Disease Control and Prevention,
Division of STD Prevention, National Center
for HIV/AIDS, Viral Hepatitis, STD, and TB
Prevention, "Syphilis: CDC Fact Sheet,"
2008, www.cdc.gov/std/syphilis/
STDFact-Syphilis.htm.

24. National Institute of Allergy and Infectious
Diseases, "Syphilis," Updated March 2009,
www3.niaid.nih.gov/topics/syphilis.

25. Centers for Disease Control and Preven-
tion, Division of STD Prevention, National
Center for HIV/AIDS, Viral Hepatitis, STD,
and TB Prevention, "Genital Herpes—CDC
Fact Sheet," 2008, www.cdc.gov/std/
Herpes/STDFact-Herpes.htm.

26. American Society for Microbiology, Fourth
Annual Interscience Conference on Antimi-
crobial Agents and Chemotherapy (San
Francisco. September 27–30, 2006); Centers
for Disease Control and Prevention,
"Genital Herpes—CDC Fact Sheet 2008."

27. National Institute of Allergy and Infectious
Diseases, "Human Papillomavirus and
Genital Warts" Updated August 2009,
www3.niaid.nih.gov/topics/genitalWarts.

28. National Institute of Allergy and Infectious
Diseases, "Vaginal Yeast Infection,"
Updated July 2009, www3.niaid.nih.gov/
topics/vaginalYeast.

29. National Institute of Allergy and Infectious
Diseases, "Trichomoniasis," Updated
March 2009, www3.niaid.nih.gov/topics/
trichomoniasis.

30. Joint United Nations Programme on
HIV/AIDS (UNAIDS), *2008 Report on the
Global AIDS Epidemic* (Geneva, Switzerland:
UNAIDS, 2008); AVERT, "Worldwide HIV &
AIDS Statistics," Updated November 2009,
www.avert.org/worldstats.htm.

31. Centers for Disease Control and Prevention,
HIV/AIDS Surveillance Report, 2007 Vol. 19,
(Atlanta: U.S. Department of Health and
Human Services, Centers for Disease
Control and Prevention, 2009) Available at
www.cdc.gov/hiv/topics/surveillance/
resources/reports.

32. Centers for Disease Control and Prevention,
Divisions of HIV/AIDS Prevention, National
Center for HIV/AIDS, Viral Hepatitis, STD,
and TB Prevention, "HIV Incidence,"
Updated September 2008, www.cdc.gov/
hiv/topics/surveillance/incidence.htm;
H. I. Hall et al., "Estimation of HIV
Incidence in the United States," *JAMA:* 300,
no. 5 (2008): 520–29.

33. National Institute of Allergy and Infectious
Diseases, "HIV/AIDS," Updated August
2009, www3.niaid.nih.gov/topics/HIVAIDS.

34. Centers for Disease Control and Preven-
tion, Divisions of HIV/AIDS Prevention,
National Center for HIV/AIDS, Viral
Hepatitis, STD, and TB Prevention,
"Mother-to-Child (Perinatal) HIV
Transmission and Prevention," 2007, www
.cdc.gov/hiv/topics/perinatal/resources/
factsheets/perinatal.htm; Centers for
Disease Control and Prevention, Divisions
of HIV/AIDS Prevention, National Center

for HIV/AIDS, Viral Hepatitis, STD, and
TB Prevention, "HIV/AIDS: Questions
and Answers," Updated February 2009,
www.cdc.gov/hiv/resources/qa; AVERT,
"Preventing Mother to Child Transmission
of HIV," Updated August 2009, www.avert
.org/motherchild.htm.

35. American Lung Association, "Lung Disease," Accessed November 2009, www
.lungusa.org/lung-disease.

36. American Lung Association, "About
COPD," Accessed November 2009,
www.lungusa.org/lung-disease/copd/
about-copd.

37. Ibid.

38. Centers for Disease Control and Preven-
tion, National Center for Health Statistics,
FASTSTATS A to Z, "Chronic Obstructive
Pulmonary Disease (COPD) Includes:
Chronic Bronchitis and Emphysema,"
Updated May 2009, www.cdc.gov/
nchs/fastats/copd.htm.

39. American Lung Association, "About
Asthma," Accessed November 2009, www
.lungusa.org/lung-disease/asthma/
about-asthma.

40. Ibid.

41. Ibid.

42. Ibid.

43. Ibid.

44. National Headache Foundation,
"Headache Topic Sheets," 2009, www
.headaches.org.

45. National Headache Foundation,
"Headache Topic Sheets: Migraine,"
2009, www.headaches.org/education/
Headache_Topic_Sheets/Migraine.

46. National Headache Foundation,
"Headache Topic Sheets: Cluster
Headaches," 2009, www.headaches.org/
education/Headache_Topic_Sheets/
Cluster_Headaches.

47. Centers for Disease Control and Prevention, National Institute of Neurological
Disorders and Stroke, "Low Back Pain Fact
Sheet," Updated August 2009, www.ninds
.nih.gov/disorders/backpain/detail
_backpain.htm.

48. Centers for Disease Control and Prevention, National Institute of Neurological
Disorders, "NINDS Repetitive Motion Disorders Information Page," Updated February 2007, www.ninds.nih.gov/disorders/
repetitive_motion/repetitive_motion.htm
?css=print.

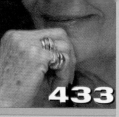
433
Is it really possible to "age gracefully"?

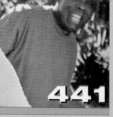
441
Is there any way to slow down the aging process?

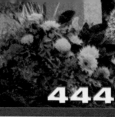
444
How can I help a friend who has just experienced a loss?

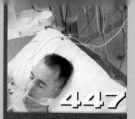
447
Why should I create a living will?

14 Aging, Death, and Dying

Objectives

* Define *aging*.

* Discuss the biological theories of aging, and summarize major physiological changes that occur as a result of the normal aging process.

* Discuss unique health challenges faced by older adults, and describe strategies for successful and healthy aging that can begin during young adulthood.

* Discuss death, the stages of the grieving process, and strategies for coping with death.

* Explain the ethical concerns that arise from the concepts of the right to die and rational suicide.

* Review the decisions that need to be made when someone is dying or has died, including hospice care, funeral arrangements, wills, and organ donations.

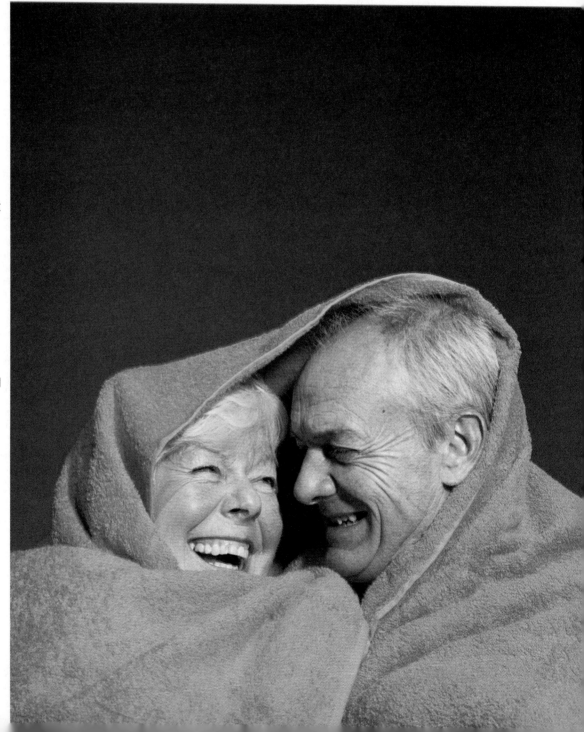

In a society that seems to worship youth, researchers have begun to offer good—even revolutionary—news about the aging process. Growing old doesn't have to mean a slow slide to declining physical and mental health. Health promotion, disease prevention, and wellness-oriented activities can prolong vigor and productivity, even among people who haven't always led model lifestyles or made healthful habits a priority. In fact, getting older can mean getting better in many ways—particularly socially, psychologically, and intellectually.

Aging has traditionally been described as the patterns of life changes that occur in all organisms as they grow older. Some believe that aging begins at the moment of conception. Others contend that it starts at birth. Still others believe that true aging does not begin until we reach our forties. The study of individual and collective aging processes, known as **gerontology,** explores the reasons for aging and the ways in which people cope with and adapt to this process.

aging The patterns of life changes that occur in all organisms as they grow older.

gerontology The study of individual and collective aging processes.

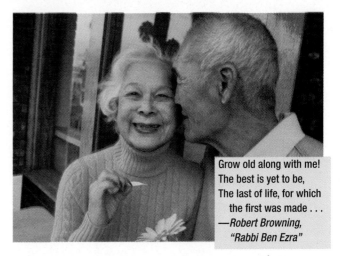

Grow old along with me!
The best is yet to be,
The last of life, for which
the first was made . . .
—*Robert Browning,
"Rabbi Ben Ezra"*

the person has packed into those years. This quality-of-life index, combined with the chronological process, appears to be the best indicator of the phenomenon of "aging gracefully." Most experts agree that the best way to experience a productive, full, and satisfying old age is to lead a productive, full, and satisfying life prior to old age.

What Is Successful Aging?

Many of today's "elderly" individuals lead active, productive lives. For instance, nearly 2.5 million Americans aged 65 or over have completed bachelor's through doctoral or professional degrees. The majority of adults over 65 continue to work, volunteer for humanitarian causes, serve in public office, travel, and remain otherwise active.[1]

Typically, people who have aged successfully have the following characteristics:

● In general, they have managed to avoid serious debilitating diseases and disability.
● They function well physically, live independently, and engage in most normal activities of daily living.
● They have maintained cognitive function and are actively engaged in mentally challenging and stimulating activities and in social and productive pursuits.
● They are resilient and able to cope reasonably well with physical, social, and emotional changes.
● They feel a sense of control over circumstances in their lives.[2]

The question is not how many years someone has lived, but how much life

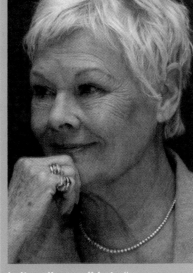

Is it really possible to "age gracefully"?

Growing old will happen to anyone who hangs around long enough, but aging gracefully requires embracing the progress of your years. The people we often think of as aging gracefully—such as actress Dame Judi Dench—are those who continue to be active and productive; who are not frightened or ashamed of growing older; who adapt to the changing circumstances of their lives; and who strive to be healthy, vibrant, and alive at any age.

Older Adults: A Growing Population

The United States and much of the developed world are on the brink of a *longevity revolution,* one that will affect society in ways that we have not even begun to understand. According to the latest statistics, life expectancy for a child born in 2006 is 77.7 years, about 30 years longer than for a child born in 1900.[3] Today there are nearly 38 million people aged 65 or older in the United States, making up over 12 percent of the total population. By 2030, the older population is expected to be twice as large as in 2000, growing to nearly 72 million and representing 20 percent of the population. In comparison, a mere 3 million people were aged 65 and older in 1900 (see Figure 14.1 on the next page).[4] Other nations report a similar trend. The World Health Organization (WHO) predicts that, by 2050, there will be more people over the age of 60 worldwide than those under 60 for the first time in human history.[5]

Within the United States, the population of those over 65 will increase substantially over the next two decades, due to the aging "baby boomer" generation. The baby boomers, born between 1946 and 1964, will start turning 65 in 2011. The needs of this

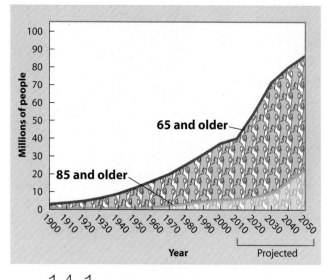

FIGURE 14.1 **Number of Americans 65 and Older (in millions), Years 1900–2006, and Projected 2010–2050**

Note: Data for 2010–2050 are projections of the population.

Source: Data are from Federal Interagency Forum on Aging-Related Statistics, *Older Americans Update 2008: Key Indicators of Well-Being* (Washington, DC: Federal Interagency Forum on Aging-Related Statistics, 2008).

generation of Americans—who are better educated and more racially diverse than past generations—will have a major impact on the economy, housing market, health care system, and Social Security. Because older age is often accompanied by increased risks of disease and disability, there will be a greater need for community resources designed to assist with mental, social, spiritual, psychological, and physical needs.

Recognizing the coming challenges, it is clear that people at all levels of society must take a proactive stance in developing programs and services to promote health and prevent premature disease and disability. In several states, employees are being asked to pay higher health premiums for behaviors that increase health costs. Incentives for screenings, reductions in premiums for improved health, vouchers for participation in health clubs and community-based programs, and other motivational strategies to enhance health throughout the life span are being pushed. More health plans are considering ways to motivate clients to take more initiative and to work harder at health improvements that will save insurers money in the long run. Instead of focusing on negative aspects of aging, more health and social service leaders are focusing on successful aging—what it means and what it will take to ensure that each of us can achieve it.

Health Issues for an Aging Society

Meeting an older population's financial and medical needs, providing health care and adequate housing, and addressing end-of-life ethical considerations are all of

concern in an aging society. No doubt you have heard discussions on the potential bankruptcy of the Social Security system and the large increases in out-of-pocket costs for people on Medicare. Many fear the combination of fewer younger workers paying into the system and more older people drawing for more years than ever before will result in tremendous shortfalls in the future. This is particularly true as the federal government borrows against the existing Social Security revenues and as federal debt continues to soar.

Health Care Costs

Older Americans averaged $4,631 in out-of-pocket medical expenses in 2006, an increase of 62 percent since 1996.[6] These costs included $2,770 (60%) for insurance, $859 (18.5%) for drugs, $844 (18%) for medical services, and $159 (3%) for medical supplies. Actual costs for treatment and aftercare are substantially higher. As people live longer, the chances of developing a costly chronic disease increase, and as technology improves, chronic illnesses that once were quickly fatal may now be treated successfully for years. Projected future costs are staggering. Compared with people aged 18 to 44, people aged 45 to 64 are nearly 3 times more likely to be disabled, 6 times more likely to have high blood pressure, and 15 times more likely to die of cancer. Among people turning 65 today, nearly 70 percent will need some form of long-term care, whether in the community or in a residential care facility.[7]

Housing and Living Arrangements

Most older people live with a spouse, alone, or with relatives or friends. Increasing numbers of people live their later years in communities that offer various levels of assistance for their clients. Some of these communities allow individuals to purchase their own homes and live fairly independently, sometimes with electronically monitored devices that allow some form of supervision. Other communities and facilities can also include 24/7 monitoring of individuals with unique needs, such as Alzheimer's disease or other

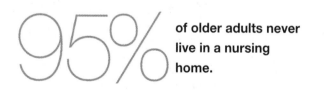

of older adults never live in a nursing home.

disabilities. Newer, technologically advanced housing includes physiological monitoring that actually records heart rate and other life indicators to ensure prompt emergency services in case of problems. Essentially, if you have the means, the sky's the limit in terms of superb care for your later years.

However, tremendous income-based disparities exist in caring for the elderly. Those without means are more likely

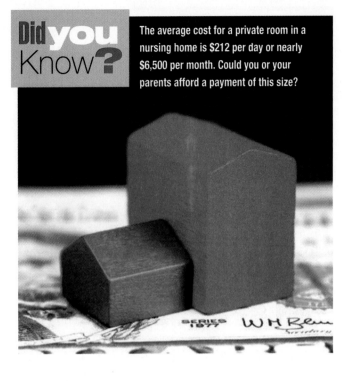

to be homeless or shut out of all but the most meager care situations. Questions arise as to how we as a society will make certain that people will have access not only to health insurance but also to safe and affordable long-term care options.

Ethical and Moral Considerations

Difficult ethical issues arise when we consider the implications for an already overburdened health care system. Given the shortage of donor organs, will we be forced to decide whether a 50-year-old should receive a heart transplant instead of a 75-year-old? Questions have already surfaced regarding the efficacy of hooking up a terminally ill older person to costly machines that prolong life for a few weeks or months but overtax health care resources. Is the prolongation of life at all costs a moral imperative, or will future generations be forced to devise a set of criteria for deciding who will be helped and who will not? The debate over stem cell research asks us to balance scientific achievements with questions of morality (see the **Health Headlines** box on the next page). Understanding the process of aging and knowing what actions each of us can take to prolong our own healthy years are part of our collective responsibility.

Theories of Aging

Social gerontologists, behaviorists, biologists, geneticists, and physiologists continue to explore various potential explanations for why the body breaks down over time.

One explanation for the biological cause of aging is the *wear-and-tear theory,* which states that, like everything else in the world, the human body wears out. Inherent in this theory is the idea that the more you abuse your body, the faster it will wear out. Another theory, the *cellular theory,* proposes that at birth we have only a certain number of usable cells, which are genetically programmed to reproduce a limited number of times. Once cells reach the end of their reproductive cycle, they die, and the organs they make up begin to deteriorate.

According to the *genetic mutation theory,* the number of body cells exhibiting unusual or different characteristics increases with age. Proponents of this theory believe that aging is related to the amount of mutational damage within the genes. The more mutation, the greater the chance that cells will not function properly.

Finally, the *autoimmune theory* attributes aging to the decline of the body's immunological system. Studies indicate that as we age, the ability to produce necessary antibodies declines, and our immune systems become less effective in fighting disease. At the same time, the white blood cells active in immune response become less able to recognize foreign invaders and more likely to mistakenly attack the body's own proteins.

Physical and Mental Changes of Aging

Although the physiological consequences of aging can differ in severity and timing, certain standard changes occur as a result of the aging process. Many of these changes are physical (see **Figure 14.2** on page 437), whereas others are mental or psychosocial.

The Skin

As a normal consequence of aging, the skin becomes thinner and loses elasticity, particularly in the outer surfaces. Fat deposits, which add to the soft lines and shape of the skin, diminish. Starting at about age 30, lines develop on the forehead as a result of smiling, squinting, and other facial expressions. These lines become more pronounced, with added "crow's feet" around the eyes, during the forties. During a person's fifties and sixties, the skin begins to sag and lose color, which leads to pallor in the seventies. Body fat in underlying layers of skin continues to be redistributed away from the limbs and extremities into the trunk region of the body. Age spots become more numerous because of excessive pigment accumulation under the skin, particularly in areas of the skin exposed to heavy sun.

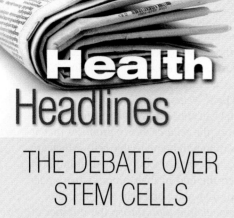

Health Headlines

THE DEBATE OVER STEM CELLS

Stem cells are unique and controversial. Stem cells have two important characteristics: (1) they are capable of renewing themselves by dividing repeatedly; and (2) they are unspecialized, and so can be induced to become specialized cells that perform specific functions, such as muscle cells that make the heart beat or nerve cells that enable the brain to function.

Many scientists believe stem cells have the potential to cure debilitating health conditions that involve the destruction of crucial cells—in the case of type 1 diabetes, for example, the pancreatic cells that secrete insulin. In the laboratory, researchers are working to coax stem cells to develop into these pancreatic cells. The plan is to transplant the new cells into diabetic patients, where they could replace the patients' damaged cells and produce insulin. If successful, this approach could prevent the destructive complications of the disease and free diabetics from the painful burden of injecting insulin for the rest of their lives. Other therapies under investigation involve growing new cells to replace those ravaged by spinal injuries,

Alzheimer's disease, heart disease, and vision and hearing loss.

Generally, stem cells used in research are derived from eggs that were fertilized in vitro. Typically these are "extra" embryos created during fertility treatments at clinics but not used for implantation. Only 4 to 5 days old, embryonic stem cells are *pluripotent* (capable of developing into many different cell types).

Embryonic stem cell research has provoked fierce debate. Opponents believe that an embryo is a human being and that no one has a right to create life and then destroy it, even for humanitarian purposes. Advocates counter that the eggs from which these embryos developed were given freely by donors and would otherwise be discarded.

Are adult stem cells a solution? An adult stem cell is an undifferentiated cell that is found in some body tissues and can specialize to replace certain types of cells. For example, human bone marrow contains at least two kinds of adult stem cells. One kind gives rise to the various types of blood cells, whereas the other can differentiate into bone, cartilage, fat, or fibrous connective tissue. Although research indicates that adult stem cells may be more versatile than previously thought, many scientists think that embryonic stem cells are more medically promising.

In the United States, embryonic stem cell research has been limited by law. In recent years federal funding—a major source of support for universities and labs—has been restricted to experiments on only a small number of stem cell lines (a stem cell line refers to a set of pluripotent, embryonic stem cells that have grown

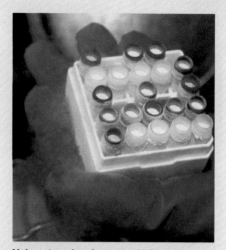

Using stored embryos to derive stem cells for research is a highly controversial matter.

in the laboratory for at least 6 months). In 2009, President Barack Obama expanded federal funding for human embryonic stem cell research, rescinding previous policy. The new policy allows researchers to utilize the many hundreds of lines created since 2001, and relieves them from the challenges of duplicating equipment and other resources in order to separate privately- or state-funded stem cell research from federally funded efforts.

Sources: National Institutes of Health, Stem Cell Information, "Stem Cell Basics," http://stemcells.nih.gov/info/basics/defaultpage, Revised April 2009; Presidential Documents, "Executive Order 13505 of March 9, 2009: Removing Barriers to Responsible Scientific Research Involving Human Stem Cells," *Federal Register* 74, no. 46 (2009), http://edocket.access.gpo.gov/2009/pdf/E9-5441.pdf; International Society for Stem Cell Research (ISSCR), Press Release, "ISSCR Scientists Elated for Future of Human Embryonic Stem Cell Research after Obama Lifts Funding Ban," March 9, 2009, www.isscr.org/press_releases/obama_repeals.html.

Bones and Joints

Throughout the life span, bones are continually changing because of the accumulation and loss of minerals. By the third or fourth decade of life, mineral loss from bones becomes more prevalent than does mineral accumulation, which results in a weakening and porosity (diminishing density) of bone tissue. This loss of minerals (particularly calcium) occurs in both sexes, although it is more common in women. Loss of calcium can contribute to **osteoporosis,** a disease characterized by low

osteoporosis A degenerative bone disorder characterized by increasingly porous bones.

bone density and structural deterioration of bone tissue. These porous, fragile bones are susceptible to fracture and may lead to crippling malformation of the spine characteristic of the dowager's hump seen in stooped individuals.

There are several risk factors for osteoporosis, some of which cannot be controlled (gender, age, body size, ethnicity, and family history). However, there are factors that can be controlled, starting from the early years. In particular, young women should consume adequate nutrients, particularly calcium and vitamin D, to reduce risk of accelerated bone loss that will occur during menopause. See the **Gender & Health** box on page 438 for more information on preventing osteoporosis.

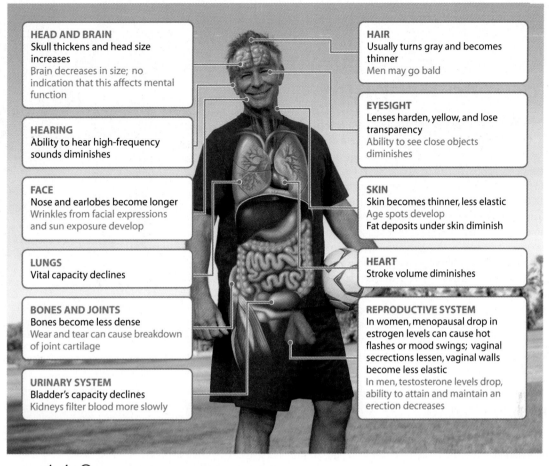

HEAD AND BRAIN
Skull thickens and head size increases
Brain decreases in size; no indication that this affects mental function

HEARING
Ability to hear high-frequency sounds diminishes

FACE
Nose and earlobes become longer
Wrinkles from facial expressions and sun exposure develop

LUNGS
Vital capacity declines

BONES AND JOINTS
Bones become less dense
Wear and tear can cause breakdown of joint cartilage

URINARY SYSTEM
Bladder's capacity declines
Kidneys filter blood more slowly

HAIR
Usually turns gray and becomes thinner
Men may go bald

EYESIGHT
Lenses harden, yellow, and lose transparency
Ability to see close objects diminishes

SKIN
Skin becomes thinner, less elastic
Age spots develop
Fat deposits under skin diminish

HEART
Stroke volume diminishes

REPRODUCTIVE SYSTEM
In women, menopausal drop in estrogen levels can cause hot flashes or mood swings; vaginal secrections lessen, vaginal walls become less elastic
In men, testosterone levels drop, ability to attain and maintain an erection decreases

FIGURE 14.2 **Normal Effects of Aging on the Body**

Another bone condition that afflicts almost 21 million Americans is **osteoarthritis,** a progressive breakdown of joint cartilage that becomes more common with age and is the leading cause of disability in the United States.[8]

The Head and Face

With age, features of the head enlarge and become more noticeable. Increased cartilage and fatty tissue cause the nose to grow a half-inch wider and another half-inch longer. Earlobes get fatter and grow longer. As the skull becomes thicker, the overall head circumference increases one-quarter of an inch per decade, even though the brain itself shrinks.

The Urinary System

At age 70, the kidneys can filter waste from the blood only half as fast as they could at age 30. The need to urinate more frequently occurs because the bladder's capacity declines from 2 cups of urine at age 30 to 1 cup at age 70.

One problem often associated with aging is **urinary incontinence,** which ranges from passing a few drops of urine while laughing or sneezing to having no control over urination. Urinary incontinence affects 15 to 30 percent of the general geriatric population.[9]

Incontinence can pose major social, physical, and emotional problems. Embarrassment and fear of wetting oneself may cause an older person to become isolated and avoid social functions. Caregivers may become frustrated with incontinent patients. Prolonged wetness and the inability to properly care for oneself can lead to irritation, infections, and other problems.

However, incontinence is not an inevitable part of aging. Most cases are caused by medications, highly treatable neurological problems that affect the central nervous system, infections of the pelvic muscles, weakness in the pelvic wall, or other problems. When the problem is treated, the incontinence is usually resolved.

osteoarthritis A progressive breakdown of joint cartilage.
urinary incontinence Inability to control urination.

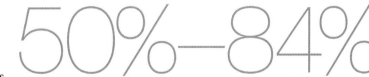

50%–84%
of older adults in long-term care facilities experience urinary incontinence.

Osteoporosis: Preventing an Age-Old Problem

Although many people think osteoporosis is a disease only of older women, it can occur at any age, and it can pose a problem for men, too. In the United States, osteoporosis affects more than 44 million Americans, almost a third of whom (32%) are men. Each year, osteoporosis causes 1.5 million fractures: 300,000 at the hip, 700,000 in the vertebrae, 250,000 in the wrists, and more than 300,000 at other sites. With early detection, steps can be taken to reverse the bone loss and prevent fractures. Bone density scans using dual-energy X-ray absorptiometry can screen for osteoporosis. Although postmenopausal women are often encouraged to have bone-density scans, osteoporosis in men is often underdiagnosed and untreated, leading to increasing numbers of hip fractures and back problems among men.

Although it is most prevalent in older adults, osteoporosis develops over time. Some of the factors that predispose a person to developing osteoporosis are intrinsic and cannot be controlled, including the following:

✱ **Gender.** Women have a higher risk of developing osteoporosis. They have less bone tissue and lose bone more rapidly than men because of the hormonal changes resulting from menopause.

✱ **Age.** Bones become less dense and weaker with age, so the older you are, the greater your risk of osteoporosis.

✱ **Body size.** Small, thin-boned women are at greatest risk.

✱ **Ethnicity.** Caucasian and Asian women are at highest risk; African American and Latina women have a lower but still significant risk.

✱ **Family history.** Susceptibility to fracture may be, in part, hereditary. People whose parents have a history of fractures also seem to have reduced bone mass.

While you cannot modify your age, gender, or ethnicity to prevent osteoporosis, there *are* things you can do to prevent the disease, starting when you are still young. During your lifetime, bone is constantly being added (formation) and being broken down and removed (reabsorption). Through childhood and the young adult years, formation outpaces reabsorption, and bone grows heavier, stronger, and denser. At around 30 years of age, a person reaches what is referred to as "peak

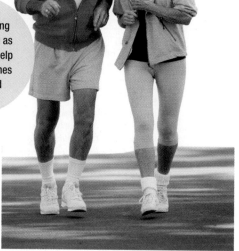

Regular weight-bearing exercise such as walking will help keep your bones healthy and strong.

bone mass." After this peak mass is reached, a slow and steady decline occurs. Individuals who accrue strong, dense, healthy bones through proper diet and exercise begun in young adulthood and continued into middle age and beyond can minimize this decline and reduce their risk for osteoporosis later in life.

In order to create strong healthy bones you need to consume sufficient calcium. Calcium requirements change over the course of a lifetime, with greater needs during childhood and adolescence when the skeleton is growing and during pregnancy and breast-feeding. Postmenopausal women and older men also need more, and medications may deplete calcium reserves as well. Adequate vitamin D, which helps the body absorb and use calcium more efficiently, is also important for creating strong bones. In addition, bone is a living tissue that grows stronger with exercise and weight-bearing activity; therefore, bone loss can be slowed or prevented with regular weight-bearing exercise, such as walking, jogging, dancing, and weight training. To further protect yourself from developing osteoporosis, avoid unhealthy behaviors that contribute to bone loss, including cigarette smoking, excessive alcohol consumption, and anorexia nervosa.

Sources: Osteoporosis and Related Bone Diseases—National Resource Center, "Fast Facts about Osteoporosis," March 2008, www.niams.nih.gov/bone/hi/ff_osteoporosis.htm; National Institute of Arthritis and Musculoskeletal Diseases, "Osteoporosis," Reviewed May 2009, www.niams.nih.gov/Health_Info/Bone/Osteoporosis/default.asp.

The Heart and Lungs

Resting heart rate stays about the same over the course of a person's life, but the stroke volume (the amount of blood the heart pushes out per beat) diminishes as heart muscles deteriorate. Vital capacity, or the amount of air that moves when you inhale and exhale at maximum effort, also declines with age. Exercise can do a great deal to preserve heart and lung function. Not smoking and avoiding smoke-

filled environments are also important to maintain heart and lung health.

The Senses

With aging, the senses (vision, hearing, touch, taste, and smell) become less acute. By the time a person reaches age 30, the lens of the eye begins to harden, which causes problems by the early forties. The lens begins to yellow and loses transparency, and the pupil shrinks, allowing less light to penetrate. By age 60, depth perception declines, and far-sightedness often develops. **Cataracts** (clouding of the lens) and **glaucoma** (elevated pressure within the eyeball) become more likely. Eventually, a tendency toward color blindness may develop, especially for shades of blue and green. **Macular degeneration** is the breakdown of the light-sensitive area of the retina responsible for the sharp, direct vision needed to read or drive. Its effects can be devastating to independent older adults; the causes are still being investigated.

With age, the ear structure also experiences changes and often deteriorates. The eardrum thickens and the inner ear bones are affected. The inner ear is the portion that controls balance (equilibrium). As a result, it often becomes difficult for a person to maintain balance. The ability to hear high-frequency consonants (e.g., *s, t,* and *z*) also diminishes with age. Much of the actual hearing loss lies in the inability to distinguish extreme ranges of sound rather than in the inability to distinguish normal conversational tones.

Many studies have indicated that with age, there is a reduced or changed sensation of pain, vibration, cold, heat, pressure, and touch. It may be that some of these changes are caused by decreased blood flow to the touch receptors or to the brain and spinal cord.[10] It may become difficult, for example, to tell the difference between cool and cold. Decreased temperature sensitivity increases the risk of injuries such as hypothermia and frostbite.

The senses of taste and smell are closely connected. The number of taste buds decreases starting at about age 40 in women and age 50 in men. Each remaining taste bud also begins to atrophy (lose mass). The sense of smell may diminish, especially after age 70. This may be related to loss of nerve endings in the nose. Studies about the cause of decreased sense of taste and smell have conflicting results. Some studies have indicated that normal aging by itself produces very little change in taste and smell.[11] Therefore, changes may be related to chronic diseases, smoking, and environmental exposures over a lifetime.

Sexual Changes

As men age, they experience noticeable alterations in sexual function. Although the degree and rate of change vary greatly from man to man, several changes generally occur, including a slowed ability to obtain an erection, diminished ability to maintain an erection, and a decline in angle of the erection. Men may also experience longer refractory period between orgasms and shortened duration of orgasm.

Women also experience several changes in sexual function as they age. Menopause usually occurs between the ages of 45 and 55. Women may experience hot flashes, mood swings, weight gain, development of facial hair, or other hormone-related symptoms. The walls of the vagina become less elastic,

and the epithelium thins, possibly making intercourse painful. Vaginal secretions, particularly during sexual activity, diminish. The breasts become less firm, and loss of fat in various areas leads to fewer curves, with a decrease in the soft lines of body contours.

Although these physiological changes may sound discouraging, the fact is that sex is an essential component to the lives of people aged 45 and over, and many people remain sexually active throughout their entire adult lives. Indeed, a landmark study by the National Council on Aging refuted long-held beliefs that sexual desire decreases as we age. Results indicated that nearly half of Americans over age 60 engage in sexual activity at least once a month, and four out of ten would like to have sex more frequently than they currently do.[12] With the advent of drugs designed to treat sexual dysfunction, such as Viagra, many older adults may get their wish.

Memory

Is memory loss an inevitable part of aging? No. In fact, all of us have periods in our lives when remembering things seems more difficult than at other times. During times of stress, illness, grief, task overload, injury or trauma, relationship problems, or other life challenges, all of us forget names, can't remember where we were going with a conversation, or have other memory lapses. As we age, drug interactions, vascular deficiencies, hormonal or biochemical imbalances, and other physiological changes can make these lapses occur more frequently.

What can you do to help improve memory and overall mental functioning as you age? Here the research is unclear, but several common themes have emerged. Generally those who maintain their memory have exercised and kept their cardiovascular system and other body systems healthy over the years. Regular physical activity is a key part of this. Another key to maintaining memory is keeping your mind active. Those people who foster their creative side and engage their minds with reading books, solving mental puzzles (e.g., crossword, Sudoku), learning to play musical instruments, becoming involved in volunteer activities, and, in general, sharpening their brains seem to fare much better in the memory department. As with the physical aspects of the body, "use it or lose it" applies to your brain acuity.

> **cataracts** Clouding of the lens that interrupts the focusing of light on the retina, resulting in blurred vision or eventual blindness.
> **glaucoma** Elevation of pressure within the eyeball, leading to hardening of the eyeball, impaired vision, and possible blindness.
> **macular degeneration** Breakdown of the macula, the light-sensitive part of the retina responsible for sharp, direct vision.

For some people, the need for reading glasses is one of the earliest signs of aging.

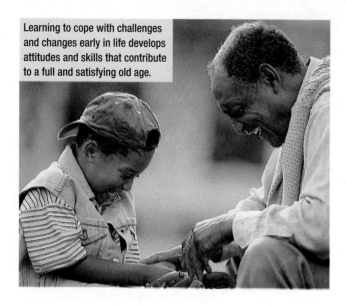

Learning to cope with challenges and changes early in life develops attitudes and skills that contribute to a full and satisfying old age.

Dementias and Alzheimer's Disease

Memory failure, errors in judgment, disorientation, or erratic behavior can occur at any age and for various reasons, including nutrient deficiency (such as vitamin B deficiency), alcohol abuse, medication interactions, vascular problems, tumors, hormonal or metabolic imbalances, or any number of problems. Often, when the underlying issues are corrected, the memory loss and disorientation also improve. The term *dementing diseases,* or **dementias,** are used to describe either reversible symptoms or progressive forms of brain malfunctioning.

Although there are many types of dementia, one of the most common forms is **Alzheimer's disease (AD).** Affecting more than 5.3 million Americans, this disease is one of the most painful and devastating conditions that families can endure.[13] It kills its victims twice: first through a slow loss of personhood (memory loss, disorientation, personality changes, and eventual loss of independent functioning), and then through the deterioration of body systems as they gradually succumb to the powerful impact of neurological problems.

The number of Americans with AD has more than doubled since 1980, and by 2050, a projected 11 to 16 million individuals could suffer from the disease. Eighty-seven percent of current Alzheimer's patients are cared for by relatives, which can take a heavy toll on finances and family dynamics. Patients with AD live for an average of 4 to 6 years after diagnosis, though the disease can last for up to 20 years.[14] Caring for a person with AD can be a heavy financial burden; the

dementias Reversible or progressive brain impairments that interfere with memory and normal intellectual functioning.

Alzheimer's disease (AD) A chronic condition involving changes in nerve fibers of the brain that result in mental deterioration.

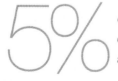

5% of all cases of Alzheimer's disease occur before age 65.

average cost of nursing care is between \$40,000 and \$70,000 each year.[15] Most people associate the disease with the aged, but AD has been diagnosed in people in their late forties.

Alzheimer's disease is a degenerative illness in which areas of the brain develop "tangles" that impair the way nerve cells communicate with one another, eventually causing them to die. This degeneration occurs in the sections of the brain that affect memory, speech, and personality, leaving the parts that control other bodily functions, such as heartbeat and breathing, functioning at near-normal levels. Thus, the mind begins to go while the body lives on.

This disease characteristically progresses in stages, each of which is marked by increasingly impaired memory and judgment. In later stages of the disease these symptoms can be accompanied by agitation and restlessness (especially at night), loss of sensory perceptions, muscle twitching, and repetitive actions. Many patients become depressed, combative, and aggressive. In the final stage of AD, disorientation is often complete. The person becomes dependent on others for eating, dressing, and other activities. Identity loss and speech problems are common. Eventually, control of bodily functions may be lost.

Researchers are investigating several possible causes of the disease, including genetic predisposition, immune system malfunction, a slow-acting virus, chromosomal or genetic defects, chronic inflammation, uncontrolled hypertension, and neurotransmitter imbalance. There is no treatment that can stop the progression of AD, but there are medications that can prevent some symptoms from progressing for a short period of time or relieve symptoms such as sleeplessness, anxiety, and depression. Some researchers are looking at anti-inflammatory drugs, theorizing that AD may develop in response to an inflammatory ailment. Others are focusing on stimulating the brains of AD-prone individuals, believing that as people learn, more connections among cells are formed that may offset those that are lost.[16]

Alcohol and Drug Use and Abuse

A person who is prone to alcoholism during the younger and middle years is more likely to continue during later years. The older alcoholic is probably no more common in American society than the young alcoholic, despite the stereotype of the old, lost soul hiding his or her sorrows in a bottle.

Alcohol abuse is five times more common among older men than among older women. Yet as many as half of all older men and an even higher proportion of older women don't drink at all. Those who do drink do so less than younger persons, consuming only 5 to 6 drinks weekly.

If recent studies are accurate, the reason there aren't many heavy drinkers among older adults may be that very heavy drinkers tend to either die of alcoholic complications before they reach old age, or reform their drinking habits. Some older people reduce their consumption, because they find they cannot process alcohol as readily as they did when they were younger, or because they are afraid of combining it with their prescription drugs.

While older adults rarely use illicit drugs, some do overuse or misuse prescription drugs. *Polypharmacy,* or the use of multiple medications, is common in older adults. Persons aged 65 and older comprise approximately 13 percent of the population of the United States, yet they consume one-third of all prescription medications and more than half of over-the-counter (OTC) medications. Approximately three-quarters of Americans over 65 use prescription medication. For persons aged 65 to 74 years, more than half use two or more prescription drugs, and 12 percent use five or more. The numbers are even higher for persons over 75.[17]

Anyone who combines different drugs runs the risk of dangerous drug interactions. The risks of adverse effects are even greater for people with impaired circulation and declining kidney and liver function. To avoid drug interactions and other problems, older adults should use the same pharmacy consistently, ask questions about medicines and dosages, and read the directions carefully.

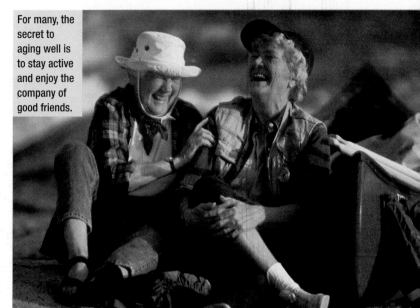
For many, the secret to aging well is to stay active and enjoy the company of good friends.

Strategies for Healthy Aging

As you know from reading this book, you can do many things to prolong and improve the quality of your life. To provide for healthy older years, make each of the following part of your younger years.

Develop and Maintain Healthy Relationships

Social bonds lend vigor and energy to life. Be willing to give to others, and seek variety in your relationships rather than befriending only people who agree with you. By experiencing diverse people and interacting with different points of view, we gain a new perspective on life.

Enrich the Spiritual Side of Life

Although we often take the spiritual side of life for granted, cultivating a relationship

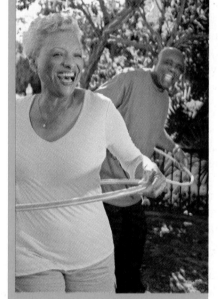
Is there any way to slow down the aging process?

Aging is inevitable, but if you take good care of your body, mind, and spirit, you can prevent disease and delay the deterioration of abilities that can lead to disability or a poor quality of life in old age. Participating in regular physical activity and following a healthy diet are two of the most important things you can do to stay active and thriving throughout all the years of your life.

with nature, the environment, a higher being, and yourself is a key factor in personal growth and development. Take time for thought and quiet contemplation, and enjoy the sunsets, sounds, and energy of life. These moments spent in time you have set aside for yourself will leave you invigorated and fresh—better able to cope with the ups and downs of life. See **Focus On: Your Spiritual Health** beginning on page 474 for more on ways to enhance this aspect of your life.

Improve Fitness

If you're basically sedentary, just about any moderate-intensity exercise that gets your heart beating faster and increases strength and/or flexibility will maximize your physical health and functional years. One of the physical changes that the body undergoes is *sarcopenia,* age-associated loss of muscle mass. The less muscle you have, the less energy you will burn even while resting. The lower your metabolic rate, the more likely you will gain weight. With regular strength training, you can increase your muscle mass, boost your metabolism, strengthen your bones, prevent osteoporosis, and, in general, feel better and function more efficiently.

Both aerobic and muscle-strengthening activities are critical

TABLE 14.1 — Exercise Recommendations for Adults over Age 65

Activity	Duration	Frequency
Moderately intense aerobic exercise	30 minutes	5 days a week
or		
Vigorously intense aerobic exercise	20 minutes	3 days a week
8 to 10 strength-training exercises	10 to 15 repetitions of each exercise	2 to 3 times per week

Source: M. Nelson et al., "Physical Activity and Public Health in Older Adults: Recommendations from the American College of Sports Medicine and the American Heart Association," *Medicine and Science in Sports and Exercise* 39, no. 8 (2007): 1435–45.

for healthy aging. Table 14.1 lists the basic recommendations for aerobic and strength-training exercises in older adults. In addition to these, the American College of Sports Medicine (ACSM) and the American Heart Association (AHA) recommend that people who are at risk of falling perform regular balance exercises. They also recommend that older adults or adults with chronic conditions develop an activity plan with a health professional to manage risks and take therapeutic needs into account.[18] This will maximize the benefits of physical activity and ensure your safety.

death The permanent ending of all vital functions.

brain death The irreversible cessation of all functions of the entire brainstem.

Eat for Health

Although other chapters in this text provide detailed information about nutrition and weight control, certain nutrients are especially essential to healthy aging:

- **Calcium.** During perimenopause and menopause, bone loss accelerates rapidly, with an average of about 3 percent skeletal mass lost per year over a 5-year period. Adequate calcium consumption is necessary to prevent bone loss.
- **Vitamin D.** Vitamin D is necessary for adequate calcium absorption, yet as people age, particularly in their fifties and sixties, they do not absorb vitamin D from foods as readily as they did in their younger years. If vitamin D is unavailable, calcium levels are also likely to be lower.
- **Protein.** As older adults become more concerned about cholesterol and fatty foods, and as their budgets shrink, they often cut back on protein. Because protein is necessary for muscle mass, protein insufficiencies can spell trouble.

Other nutrients, including vitamin E, folic acid (folate), iron, potassium, and vitamin B_{12}, are important to the aging process, and most of these are readily available in any diet that follows the MyPyramid recommendations.

Understanding the Final Transitions: Dying and Death

Death eventually comes to everyone, but if you live life to the fullest and learn as much about end-of-life issues as you can, you will be better able to accept the inevitable. To cope effectively with dying, we must address the needs of people facing life's final transition. Let's begin by investigating what death means, at least in medical terms.

Defining Death

Death can be defined as the "final cessation of the vital functions" and also refers to a state in which these functions are "incapable of being restored."[19] This definition has become more significant as medical advances make it increasingly possible to postpone death.

Legal and ethical issues led to the Uniform Determination of Death Act in 1981. This act, which has been adopted by several states, reads as follows: "An individual who has sustained either (1) irreversible cessation of circulatory and respiratory functions, or (2) irreversible cessation of all functions of the entire brain, including the brainstem, is dead. A determination of death must be made in accordance with accepted medical standards."[20]

The concept of **brain death,** defined as the irreversible cessation of all functions of the entire brainstem, has gained increasing credence. The brainstem is a relay site for sensory and motor pathways and is responsible for such critical body functions as respiration and heart rate. As defined by the Ad Hoc Committee of the Harvard Medical School, brain death occurs when the following criteria are met:[21]

- Unreceptivity and unresponsiveness—that is, no response even to painful stimuli
- No movement for a continuous hour after observation by a physician, and no breathing after 3 minutes off a respirator
- No reflexes, including brainstem reflexes; fixed and dilated pupils
- A "flat" electroencephalogram (EEG, which monitors electrical activity of the brain) for at least 10 minutes
- All of these tests repeated at least 24 hours later with no change
- Certainty that hypothermia (extreme loss of body heat) and depression of the central nervous system caused by use of drugs such as barbiturates are not responsible for these conditions

The Harvard report provides useful guidelines; however, the definition of *death* and all its ramifications continue to concern us.

what do you think?
Why is there so much concern over the definition of death?
● How does modern technology complicate the understanding of when death occurs?

Denying Death

Attitudes toward death tend to fall on a continuum. At one end of the continuum, death is viewed as the mortal enemy of humankind. Both medical science and certain religions have promoted this idea. At the other end of the continuum, death is accepted and even welcomed. For people whose attitudes fall at this end, death is a passage to a better state of being. Most of us, however, perceive ourselves to be in the middle of this continuum. From this perspective, death is a bewildering mystery that elicits fear and apprehension while profoundly influencing beliefs and actions throughout life.

In the United States, a high level of discomfort is associated with death and dying. Those who deny death tend to

- Avoid people who are grieving after the death of a loved one so they won't have to talk about it.
- Fail to validate a dying person's frightening situation by talking to the person as though nothing were wrong.
- Substitute euphemisms for the word *death* (e.g., "passing away," "kicking the bucket," "no longer with us," "going to heaven," or "going to a better place").
- Give false reassurances to dying people by saying things like, "Everything is going to be okay."
- Shut off conversation about death by silencing people who are trying to talk about it.
- Avoid touching people who are dying.

The Process of Dying

Dying is the process of decline in body functions that results in the death of an organism. It is a complex process that includes physical, intellectual, social, spiritual, and emotional dimensions. Now that we have examined the physical indicators of death, we must consider the emotional aspects of dying and "social death."

Coping Emotionally with Death

Science and medicine have enabled us to understand many changes throughout the life span, but they have not fully explained the nature of death. This may explain why the transition from life to death evokes so much mystery and emotion. Although emotional reactions to dying vary, many people share similar experiences during this process.

Kübler-Ross and the Stages of Dying Much of our knowledge about reactions to dying stems from the work of Elisabeth Kübler-Ross, a pioneer in **thanatology,** the study of death and dying. In 1969, Kübler-Ross published *On Death and Dying,* a sensitive analysis of the reactions of terminally ill patients. This pioneering work encouraged the development of death education as a discipline and prompted efforts to improve the care of dying patients. Kübler-Ross identified five psychological stages **(Figure 14.3)** that people coping with death often experience:[22]

> **dying** The process of decline in body functions, resulting in the death of an organism.
> **thanatology** The study of death and dying.

1. **Denial.** ("Not me: there must be a mistake.") A person intellectually accepts the impending death but rejects it emotionally and feels a sense of shock and disbelief. The patient is too confused and stunned to comprehend "not being" and thus rejects the idea.

2. **Anger.** ("Why me?") The person becomes angry at having to face death when others, including loved ones, are healthy and not threatened. The dying person perceives the situation as unfair or senseless and may be hostile to friends, family, physicians, or the world in general.

3. **Bargaining.** ("If I'm allowed to live, I promise . . .") The dying person may resolve to be a better person in return for an extension of life or may secretly pray for a short reprieve from death to experience a special event, such as a family wedding or birth.

4. **Depression.** ("It's really going to happen to me, and I can't do anything about it.") Depression eventually sets in as vitality diminishes and the person begins to experience symptoms with increasing frequency. Common feelings experienced in this stage include doom, loss, worthlessness, and guilt over the emotional suffering of loved ones and the arduous but seemingly futile efforts of caregivers.

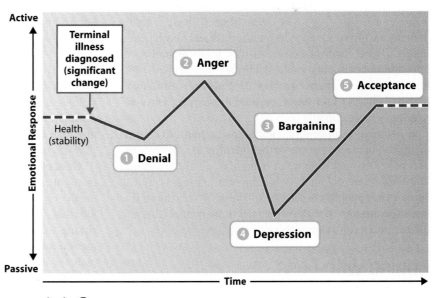

FIGURE 14.3 **Kübler-Ross's Stages of Dying**
Kübler-Ross developed this model while working with terminally ill patients. She later expanded the model to apply to people experiencing grief or significant loss of any kind.

5. **Acceptance.** ("I'm ready.") This is often the final stage. The patient stops battling with emotions and becomes tired and weak. With acceptance, the person does not give up and become sullen or resentfully resigned to death but rather becomes passive.

Some of Kübler-Ross's contemporaries considered her stage theory too neat and orderly. Subsequent research has indicated that the experiences of dying people do not fit easily into specific stages, and patterns vary from person to person. Some people may never go through this process and instead remain emotionally calm; others may pass back and forth between the stages. Even if it is not accurate in all its particulars, however, Kübler-Ross's theory offers valuable insights for those seeking to understand or deal with the process of dying.

Social Death

The need for recognition and appreciation within a social group is nearly universal. Loss of being valued or appreciated by others can lead to **social death,** a situation in which a person is not treated like an active member of society. Dramatic examples of social death include the exile of nonconformists from their native countries or the excommunication of dissident members of religious groups. More often, however, social death is inflicted by denying a person normal social interaction. Numerous studies indicate that people are treated differently when they are dying, leading them to feel more isolated and unable to talk about their feelings: The dying person may be excluded from conversations or referred to as if he or she were already dead.[23] Dying patients are often moved to terminal wards and may be given minimal care; medical personnel may make degrading or impersonal comments about dying patients in their presence. In addition, inadequate pain control may contribute to patient suffering and anger or hostility, making caregiver assistance more difficult.

A decrease in meaningful social interaction often strips dying and bereaved people of their identity as valued members of society at a time when being able to talk, share, and make important decisions or say important things is critical. Some dying people choose not to speak of their inevitable fate in an attempt to make others feel more comfortable and thus preserve vital relationships.

social death A seemingly irreversible situation in which a person is not treated like an active member of society.

bereavement The loss or deprivation experienced by a survivor when a loved one dies.

grief An individual's reaction to significant loss, including one's own impending death, the death of a loved one, or a quasi-death experience; grief can involve mental, physical, social, or emotional responses.

Coping with Loss

The losses resulting from the death of a loved one are extremely difficult to cope with. The dying person, as well as close family and friends, frequently suffers emotionally and physically from the impending loss of critical relationships and roles.

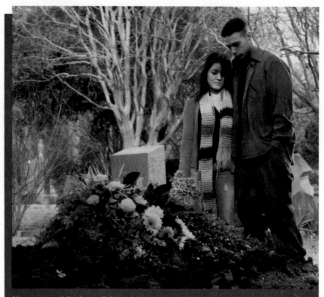

How can I help a friend who has just experienced a loss?

The most important thing you can do for a grieving friend is offer emotional support and a caring presence. Knowing what to say is less important than knowing how to listen. Acknowledge your friend's loss, let them know you care, and be there for them when they need to talk or express their grief.

Bereavement generally is defined as the loss or deprivation that a survivor experiences when a loved one dies. Because relationships vary in type and intensity, reactions to loss also vary. The death of a parent, spouse, sibling, child, friend, or pet will result in different kinds of feelings for different people. We should not make assumptions about the value a person places on his or her relationship with the deceased or the nature of his or her feelings about the loss. For example, often people fail to recognize the importance a pet can have, especially in single people's lives; for some, the loss of a pet may be as significant as the loss of a child. In the lives of the bereaved or of close survivors, the loss of loved ones leaves "holes" and inevitable changes. Loneliness and despair may envelop the survivor. Understanding of these normal reactions, time, patience, and support from loved ones can help the bereaved heal and move on, even though they will not forget.

Grief occurs in reaction to significant loss, including one's own impending death, the death of a loved one, or a *quasi-death* experience (a loss, such as the end of a relationship or job, that resembles death because it involves separation or change in personal identity). Grief may be experienced as a mental, physical, social, or emotional reaction, and often includes changes in patterns of eating, sleeping, working, and even thinking.

When a person experiences a loss that cannot be openly acknowledged, publicly mourned, or socially supported, coping may be much more difficult. This type of grief is referred to as *disenfranchised grief.* It may occur among people who miscarry, are developmentally disabled, or are close friends rather

Talking to Friends When Someone Dies

It's always hard to know just what to say and how to say it when talking with a grieving friend or relative. Here are some do's and don'ts.

DO . . .

✳ Let your genuine concern and caring show; say you are sorry about their loss and about their pain.
✳ Be available to listen, run errands, help with the children, or whatever else seems needed at the time.
✳ Allow them to express as much grief as they are feeling at the moment and are willing to share.
✳ Encourage them to be patient with themselves and not worry about things they should be doing.
✳ Allow them to talk about the person who has died as much and as often as they want to.
✳ Reassure them that they did everything they could, that the medical care given was the best, or whatever else you know to be true and positive about the care given.

DON'T . . .

✳ Let your own sense of helplessness keep you from reaching out to a bereaved person.
✳ Avoid them because you are uncomfortable (this adds pain to an already unbearably painful experience).
✳ Say you know how they feel (unless you've suffered a similar loss, you probably don't).
✳ Say "you ought to be feeling better by now" or anything else that implies judgment about their feelings or what they should be doing.
✳ Change the subject when they mention the person who has died.

than blood relatives of the deceased. It may also include those relationships that are not socially approved, such as those between extramarital lovers or homosexual couples.

Symptoms of grief vary in severity and duration, depending on the situation and the individual. However, the bereaved person can benefit from emotional and social support from family, friends, clergy, employers, and traditional support organizations, including the medical community and the funeral industry. The larger and stronger the support system, the easier readjustment is likely to be. See the **Skills for Behavior Change** box above to learn about how you can best help a grieving friend.

The word *mourning* is often incorrectly equated with the word *grief*. As we have noted, *grief* refers to a wide variety of feelings and actions that occur in response to bereavement. **Mourning,** in contrast, refers to culturally prescribed and accepted time periods and behavior patterns for the expression of grief. In Judaism, for example, *sitting shiva* is a designated mourning period of 7 days that involves prescribed rituals and prayers. Depending on a person's relationship with the deceased, various other rituals may continue for up to a year.

What Is "Typical" Grief?

Grief responses vary widely from person to person but frequently include such symptoms as periodic waves of prolonged physical distress, a feeling of tightness in the throat, choking and shortness of breath, a frequent need to sigh, feelings of emptiness and muscular weakness, or intense anxiety that is described as actually painful.

Other common symptoms of grief include insomnia, memory lapses, loss of appetite, difficulty concentrating, a tendency to engage in repetitive or purposeless behavior, an "observer" sensation or feeling of unreality, difficulty in making decisions, lack of organization, excessive speech, social withdrawal or hostility, guilt feelings, and preoccupation with the image of the deceased. Susceptibility to disease increases with grief and may even be life-threatening in severe and enduring cases.

> **mourning** The culturally prescribed behavior patterns for the expression of grief.
>
> **grief work** The process of accepting the reality of a person's death and coping with memories of the deceased.

A bereaved person may suffer emotional pain and exhibit a variety of grief responses for many months after the death. The rate of the healing process depends on the amount and quality of grief work that a person does. **Grief work** is the process of integrating the reality of the loss into everyday life and learning to feel better. Often, the bereaved person must deliberately and systematically work at reducing denial and coping with the pain that results from memories of the deceased. This process takes time and requires emotional effort.

Worden's Model of Grieving Tasks

William Worden, a researcher into the death process, developed an active grieving model which suggests four developmental tasks to complete in the grief work process:[24]

1. Accept the reality of the loss. This task requires acknowledging and realizing that the person is dead. Traditional rituals, such as the funeral, help many bereaved people move toward acceptance.

2. Work through the pain of grief. It is necessary to acknowledge and work through the pain associated with loss, or it will manifest itself through other symptoms or behaviors.

3. Adjust to an environment in which the deceased is missing. The bereaved may feel lonely and uncertain about a new identity without the person who has died.

4. Emotionally relocate the deceased and move on with life. Individuals never lose memories of a significant relationship. They may need help in letting go of the emotional energy that used to be invested in the person

Skills for Behavior Change

Living with Grief

The reality of death and loss touches everyone. Coping with death is vital to your mental health. The National Mental Health Association offers these suggestions for living with grief and coping effectively with pain:

* **Seek out caring people.** Find relatives and friends who can understand your feelings of loss. Join support groups with others who are experiencing similar losses.
* **Express your feelings.** Tell others how you feel; it will help you to work through the grieving process.
* **Take care of your health.** Maintain regular contact with your family physician and be sure to eat well and get plenty of rest. Be aware of the danger of developing a dependence on medication or alcohol to deal with your grief.
* **Accept that life is for the living.** It takes effort to begin living again in the present and not dwell on the past.
* **Postpone major life decisions.** Try to hold off on making any significant changes, such as moving, remarrying, changing jobs, or having another child. You need time to adjust to your loss.
* **Be patient.** It can take months or even years to absorb a major loss and accept your changed life.

beyond that concept, however, many people today believe that they should be allowed to die if their condition is terminal and their existence depends on mechanical life-support devices or artificial feeding or hydration systems. Artificial life-support techniques that may be legally refused by competent patients include electrical or mechanical heart resuscitation, mechanical respiration by machine, nasogastric tube feedings, intravenous nutrition, gastrostomy (tube feeding directly into the stomach), and medications to treat life-threatening infections.

As long as a person is conscious and competent, he or she has the legal right to refuse treatment, even if this decision will hasten death. However, when a person is in a coma or otherwise incapable of speaking on his or her own behalf, medical personnel, family members, and administrative policy will dictate treatment. This issue has evolved into a battle involving personal freedom, legal rulings, health care administration policy, and physician responsibility. The living will and other **advance directives** were developed to assist in solving these conflicts.

Even young, apparently healthy people need a **living will.** Consider Terri Schiavo, who collapsed at age 26 from heart failure that led to irreversible brain damage. Schiavo, unable to survive without life support, never left any written guidelines about her wishes should she become incapacitated. After a 15-year legal battle between her parents, who wanted her to be kept alive, and her husband, who felt she should be allowed to die, the courts sided with her husband, and she was removed from life support.

Many legal experts suggest that you take the following steps to ensure that your wishes are carried out:[25]

* **Be specific.** Complete an advance directive that permits you to make very specific choices about a variety of procedures, including cardiopulmonary resuscitation (CPR); being placed on a ventilator; being given food, water, or medication through tubes; being given pain medication; and organ donation.
* **Get an agent.** You may want to also appoint a family member or friend to act as your agent, or *proxy,* by making out a form known as either a *durable power of attorney for health care* or a *health care proxy.*
* **Discuss your wishes.** Discuss your preferences in detail with your proxy and your doctor. Going over the situations described in the form will give them a clear idea of just how much you are willing to endure to preserve your life.
* **Deliver the directive.** Distribute several copies, not only to your doctor and your agent, but also to your lawyer and to immediate family members or a close friend. Make sure *someone* knows to bring a copy to the hospital in the event you are hospitalized.

One alternative to the traditional advance directive or living will is a document called *Five Wishes* that meets the legal requirements for advance directive statutes in most states. This document differs from most other living wills because it addresses personal, emotional, and spiritual needs, as well as medical needs.[26] It is available at low cost

what do you think?

If you have experienced death among your family or friends, how did you grieve? ● Did you accomplish Worden's tasks? ● Does the model match your experience?

who has died, finding an appropriate place for the deceased in their emotional lives.

See the **Skills for Behavior Change** box above for more suggestions on coping with grief.

Life-and-Death Decision Making

Many complex—and often expensive—life-and-death decisions must be made during a highly distressing period in people's lives, when a loved one is dying. We will not attempt to present definitive answers to moral and philosophical questions about death; instead, we offer these topics for your consideration.

The Right to Die

Few people would object to the right to a dignified death. Going

advance directive A document that stipulates an individual's wishes about medical care; used to make treatment decisions when and if the individual becomes physically unable to voice his or her preferences.
living will A type of advance directive.

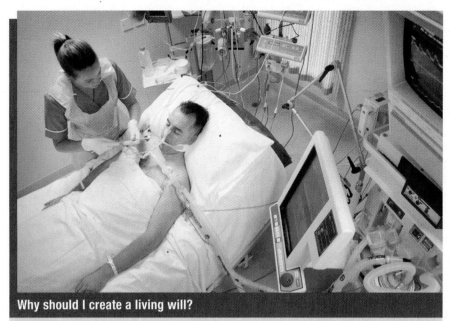

Why should I create a living will?

Unexpected end-of-life situations can happen at any age. Today's sophisticated life-support technology can prolong a patient's life even in cases of terminal illness or mortal injury, yet not everyone would choose to have their life extended by such means. Unfortunately, by the time the situation arises, you may no longer be conscious and able to speak for yourself. Living wills, advance directives, and health care proxies are all legal documents that can protect your wishes and aid your loved ones should you become incapacitated.

online at www.agingwithdignity.org. Written in uncomplicated language, *Five Wishes* allows you to outline the following:

1. Which person you want to make health care decisions for you when you can't make them
2. The kind of medical treatment you want or don't want
3. How comfortable you want to be
4. How you want people to treat you
5. What you want your loved ones to know

Although every state has different guidelines and laws for living wills and advance directives, the above questions are important things to think about now. How would you answer each of the above?

Rational Suicide and Euthanasia

Although exact numbers are not known, medical ethicists and specialists in forensic medicine (the study of legal issues in medicine) estimate that thousands of terminally ill people every year decide to kill themselves rather than endure constant pain and slow decay. This alternative to the extended dying process is known as **rational suicide.** To these people, the prospect of an undignified death is unacceptable. This issue has been complicated by advances in death prevention techniques that allow terminally ill patients to exist in an irreversible disease state for extended periods of time.

According to public opinion polls, most Americans believe that suicide is morally wrong but are divided on whether physician-assisted suicide is morally acceptable. Roughly 70 percent of Americans believe doctors should be allowed to help end an incurably ill patient's life painlessly at the patient's request.[27]

Physician-assisted suicide is not a new phenomenon. It has been practiced in many societies throughout history and currently is legal in some European countries, such as Belgium and the Netherlands. Legalization of assisted suicide has been debated in many states across the nation. Currently, 38 states have enacted statutes explicitly prohibiting assisted suicide and Oregon is the only state that allows physician-assisted suicide under certain circumstances, outlined in Oregon's Death with Dignity Act.[28]

Euthanasia is often referred to as "mercy killing." The term **active euthanasia** refers to ending the life of a person (or animal) who is suffering greatly and has no chance of recovery. An example might be a physician-prescribed lethal injection, as in physician-assisted suicide. **Passive euthanasia** refers to the intentional withholding of treatment that would prolong life. Deciding not to place a person with massive brain trauma on life support is an example of passive euthanasia. Advance directives, such as "do not resuscitate" orders, can provide legal justification for various forms of passive euthanasia.

Making Final Arrangements

Caring for dying people and dealing with the practical and legal questions surrounding death can be difficult and painful. The problems of the dying person and the bereaved loved ones involve a wide variety of psychological, legal, social, spiritual, economic, and interpersonal issues.

Hospice Care: Positive Alternatives

Since the mid-1970s, **hospice** programs have grown from a mere handful to more than 2,500 and are available in nearly every community. These programs are a form of **palliative care** that focus on reducing pain and suffering and attending to the emotional and spiritual needs of dying individuals and their

rational suicide The decision to kill oneself rather than endure constant pain and slow decay.
active euthanasia "Mercy killing," in which a person or organization knowingly acts to end the life of a terminally ill person.
passive euthanasia The intentional withholding of treatment that would prolong life.
hospice A concept of end-of-life care designed to maximize quality of life and help dying people have peace, comfort, and dignity.
palliative care Any form of medical care focused on relieving the pain, symptoms, and stress of serious illness in order to improve the quality of life for patients and their families.

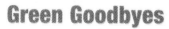

GREEN GUIDE

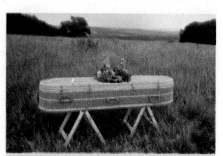

Green Goodbyes

Worldwide, more than 56 million people die each year. Nearly all of those people are given some form of burial, funeral, or cremation, yet traditional burial, funeral, and cremation practices can have significant and negative environmental impacts. With growing awareness of these impacts has come an increased interest in ways to "go green" in funeral, burial, and cremation practices.

Each year, more than 20,000 cemeteries in the United States bury millions of feet of hardwood; tens of thousands of tons of steel, copper, and bronze; and more than a million tons of reinforced concrete. In addition, it is estimated that more than 1 million gallons of embalming fluid are buried in the United States every year. These chemicals (including formaldehyde, glutaraldehyde, phenol, methanol, antibiotics, dyes, and more) eventually make their way into the soil and can potentially contaminate water supplies.

Instead of traditional cemetery and burial sites, you can opt for burial in a green, tomb-free cemetery where chemicals (including chemical lawn treatments) or nonbiodegradable materials are strictly avoided. Green burial sites prohibit the use of formaldehyde-based embalming fluids, metal caskets, and concrete burial vaults. Typically, these sites are located in nature preserves that eschew the manicured expanses of lawn present in modern cemeteries. They have restrictions on the density of burials allowed, as well as strict guidelines aimed at conservation and preservation of the ecosystem. To find global locations of natural cemeteries, start by checking out www.naturalburial.coop or www.greenburialcouncil.org. Woodland burial, a movement started in the United Kingdom, is another natural option available in some areas.

Many green cemeteries and other burial sites choose to plant living markers instead of erecting tombstones. The production of tombstones and burial markers can be wasteful and damaging to the environment. Grave markers are made of stone, a nonrenewable resource, and most leave a carbon footprint, as both the mining and shipping of them produce excess carbon. In contrast, a living marker is a tree, bush, plant, or flowers planted in memory of the deceased loved one. This not only reduces waste and negative environmental impact, but also contributes to the development of green landscape. If you decide on a living marker, consider exploring native plant options for the region in which it will be planted.

Green coffins are also available as an alternative to traditional coffins made of metal, plastic, endangered hardwood, or particleboard with formaldehyde glues. Greener options include coffins made of oak, pine, cardboard, willow, seagrass, wicker, fair-trade bamboo, and other natural materials that are more sustainable, biodegradeable, and renewable. In addition, some burial sites allow one to forgo the coffin altogether and bury loved ones in natural-cloth shrouds.

Cremation has historically been viewed as a more ecofriendly option, because the environmental footprint is much less than that of traditional burials. Although cremation does not involve the land use that burial does, it takes a lot of energy, approximately the same amount required to power an average car for a distance of 4,800 miles, and the burning process releases carbon and particulate emissions into the air. However, these emissions are relatively low in comparison to others in our society. Some fast-food restaurants release 0.46 pound of carbon an hour, whereas the human cremation process emits only 0.08 pound an hour. Environmental monitoring agencies have imposed emission standards on crematoriums that

Ecofriendly burial options include coffins made of biodegradeable materials, such as this wicker model.

help to keep the levels down. Furthermore, some crematoriums are installing additional filters to catch smaller particulate matter.

Another alternative to traditional burial is the controversial and relatively new process of "promession," or freeze-drying. This technique was developed by Swedish biologist Susanne Wiigh-Mäsak as a strategy to reduce the number of corpses buried and as an ecofriendly alternative to cremation. It was patented in 1999 and first introduced to the public in May 2001. Currently, there is only a handful of facilities in Europe that perform promession. The first step in promession involves freezing the body in a vat of liquid nitrogen, a process that makes the body very brittle. Next, the body is gently broken apart with ultrasonic vibration. This creates a damp powder that is then dried and packaged in a small biodegradable coffin. The "promains" can then be easily buried alongside a memorial plant, tree, or garden. As the promains become wet from rain and watering, they will naturally decompose, composting the soil and providing nourishment to the living memorial.

Sources: S. Grover, "How to Go Green: Funerals," Planet Green, 2009, http://planetgreen.discovery.com/go-green/funerals/funerals-basics.html; Green Burial Council, "Frequently Asked Questions," 2009, www.greenburialcouncil.org/faq.php.

caregivers. Hospice programs allow patients to receive end-of-life care at home or at a homelike facility, with family members providing much of the care. Trained volunteers may assist with personal care, medications, and other procedures. In addition, hospice volunteers provide much needed "respite" care for caregivers who often face emotional and physical challenges in caring for dying loved ones.

The primary goals of hospice programs are to relieve the dying person's pain; offer emotional support to the dying person and loved ones; and restore a sense of control to the dying person, family, and friends. Hospice programs usually include the following characteristics.

- The patient and family constitute the unit of care, because the physical, psychological, social, and spiritual problems of dying confront the family as well as the patient.
- Emphasis is placed on symptom control, primarily the alleviation of pain.
- There is overall medical direction of the program, with all health care provided under the direction of a qualified physician.
- Coverage is provided 24 hours a day, 7 days a week, with emphasis on the availability of medical and nursing skills.
- Carefully selected and extensively trained volunteers who augment but do not replace staff service are an integral part of the health care team.
- Care of the family extends through the bereavement period.
- Patients are accepted on the basis of their health needs, not on their ability to pay.

Making Funeral Arrangements

Anthropological evidence indicates that all cultures throughout human history have developed some sort of funeral ritual. For this reason, social scientists agree that funerals assist survivors of the deceased in coping with their loss.

In the United States, with its diversity of religious, regional, and ethnic customs, funeral patterns vary. In some faiths, the deceased may be displayed to formalize last respects and increase social support for the bereaved. This part of the funeral ritual is referred to as a *wake* or *viewing*. The funeral service may be held in a church, in a funeral chapel, or at the burial site. Some people choose to replace the funeral service with a simple memorial service held within a few days of the burial. Social interaction associated with funeral and memorial services is valuable in helping survivors cope with their loss.

Common methods of body disposal include burial in the ground, entombment above ground in a mausoleum, cremation, and anatomical donation. Expenses vary according to the method chosen and the available options. Choosing the container for the remains is only one of many tasks that must be dealt with when a person dies. There are many other decisions concerning the funeral ritual that can also be difficult for survivors. In addition to the method and details of body disposal, the type of memorial service, display of the body, and the site of burial or body disposition, loved ones must also consider the cost of funeral options, organ donation, and floral displays. Then, they usually have to contact friends and relatives, plan for the arrival of guests, choose markers, gather and submit obituary information to newspapers, and print memorial folders, in addition to many other details. Even though funeral directors are available to facilitate decision making, the bereaved may experience undue stress, especially if the death is sudden and unexpected. People who make their own funeral arrangements ahead of time can save their loved ones from having to deal with making many decisions during a time of stress. See the **Green Guide** at left for information on how concern about environmental responsibility is influencing modern funeral, burial, and memorial practices.

Wills

The issue of inheritance is controversial in some families and should be resolved before a person dies to reduce conflict and needless expense. Unfortunately, many people are so intimidated by the thought of making a will that they never do so and die **intestate** (without a will). This is tragic, especially because the procedure for establishing a legal will is relatively simple and inexpensive. In addition, if you don't make a will before you die, the courts (as directed by state laws) will make a will for you. Legal issues, rather than your wishes, will preside. Furthermore, it usually takes longer to settle an estate when the person dies intestate.

intestate Dying without a will.

Organ Donation

In recent years, organ transplant techniques have become so refined, and the demand for transplant tissues and organs so great, that many people are being encouraged to donate these gifts of life upon death. Uniform donor cards are available through the U.S. Department of Health and Human Services, as well as many health care foundations and nonprofit organizations; donor information is printed on the backs of drivers' licenses; and many hospitals include the opportunity for organ donor registration in their admission procedures. Although some people are opposed to organ transplants and tissue donation, others experience personal fulfillment from knowing that their organs may extend and improve someone else's life after their own deaths.

Are You Afraid of Death?

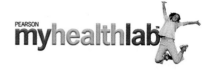

How anxious or accepting are you about the prospect of your death? Indicate how well each statement describes your attitude.

Not True at All = **0**   Mainly Not True = **1**   Not Sure = **2**
Somewhat True = **3**   Very True = **4**

1. I tend not to be very brave in times of crisis situations. **0 1 2 3 4**
2. I am something of a hypochondriac. **0 1 2 3 4**
3. I tend to be unusually frightened in planes at takeoff and landing. **0 1 2 3 4**
4. I would give a lot to be immortal in this body. **0 1 2 3 4**
5. I am superstitious that preparing for dying might hasten my death. **0 1 2 3 4**
6. My experience of friends and family dying has been wholly negative. **0 1 2 3 4**
7. I would feel easier being with a dying relative if he or she had not been told he or she was dying. **0 1 2 3 4**
8. I have fears of dying alone without friends around me. **0 1 2 3 4**
9. I have fears of dying slowly. **0 1 2 3 4**
10. I have fears of dying suddenly. **0 1 2 3 4**
11. I have fears of dying before my time or while my children are still young. **0 1 2 3 4**
12. I have fears of what could happen to my family after my death. **0 1 2 3 4**
13. I have fears of dying in a hospital or an institution. **0 1 2 3 4**

14. I have fears of not getting help with euthanasia. **0 1 2 3 4**
15. I have fears of dying without adequately having expressed my love to those I am close to. **0 1 2 3 4**
16. I have fears of being given unofficial and unwanted euthanasia. **0 1 2 3 4**
17. I have fears of getting insufficient pain control while dying. **0 1 2 3 4**
18. I have fears of being overmedicated and unconscious while dying. **0 1 2 3 4**
19. I have fears of being declared dead when not really dead or being buried alive. **0 1 2 3 4**
20. I have fears of what may happen to my body after death. **0 1 2 3 4**

Total points: _____

Interpreting Your Score

If you are extremely anxious (scoring 38 or more), you might consider counseling or therapy; if you are unusually anxious (scoring between 24 and 37), you might want to find a method of meditation, philosophy, or spiritual practice to help experience, explore, and accept your feelings about death. Average anxiety is a score under 24.

YOUR PLAN FOR **CHANGE**

The **Assess yourself** activity encouraged you to explore your death-related anxiety. Now that you have considered your results, you may want to take steps to lessen your fears about death and dying.

Today, you can:

○ Learn about advance directives. Visit a low-cost legal clinic for information and a sample. You can also locate samples online, including the *Five Wishes* document, which is available at www.agingwithdignity.org.

○ Fill out an organ donation card. Knowing that you may be able to prolong another person's life after your death can help you feel more at peace with your mortality.

Within the next 2 weeks, you can:

○ Write down a list of goals you want to attain by ages 30, 40, and 50. Think about the steps you need to take to attain these goals.

○ Talk to family members about their life goals. What have they achieved, and what do they wish they had done differently? What can you learn from their experiences?

By the end of the semester, you can:

○ Consider how you feel about various medical techniques that might be used in the event you become incapacitated. Do you feel comfortable being kept alive by a machine? Make your wishes on these matters known to family members and friends, and put them in writing.

○ Talk to your parents or grandparents about the arrangements they prefer in the event of their death. Do they want a burial or cremation? A full funeral or a small service? Making these decisions now will save you and your loved ones stress later.

Summary

* *Aging* can be defined as patterns of life changes occurring in individuals as they grow older. The increasing numbers of older adults has a significant impact on society in terms of economy, health care, housing, and ethical considerations.
* Biological explanations of aging include the wear-and-tear theory, the cellular theory, the genetic mutation theory, and the autoimmune theory.
* Aging causes physical changes in skin, bones and joints, head, urinary system, heart and lungs, the senses, and sexual function. Most older people maintain a high level of intelligence and memory. Potential mental problems include Alzheimer's disease.
* Lifestyle choices we make today will affect health status later in life. Choosing to exercise, eat a healthy diet, foster lasting relationships, and avoid tobacco will contribute to healthy aging.
* *Death* can be defined biologically in terms of brain death and/or the final cessation of vital functions. Dying is a multifaceted emotional process, and individuals may experience emotional stages of dying such as denial, anger, bargaining, depression, and acceptance. Social death results when a person is no longer treated as an active member of society. Grief is the state of distress felt after loss.
* The right to die by rational suicide involves ethical, moral, and legal issues. Living wills, health care proxies, and other advance directives allow a person to outline his or her wishes with regard to medical care prior to becoming incapacitated. Choices of care for the terminally ill include hospice care. After death, the need to make funeral arrangements adds to pressures on survivors. Decisions should be made in advance through wills and organ donation cards.

Pop Quiz

1. Which biological theory of aging supports the concept that body cells are able to reproduce only so many times throughout life?
   a. wear-and-tear theory
   b. cellular theory
   c. autoimmune theory
   d. genetic mutation theory

2. The progressive breakdown of joint cartilage is known as
   a. osteoporosis.
   b. osteoarthritis.
   c. calcium loss.
   d. vitamin D deficiency.

3. Walt's ophthalmologist tells him that pressure within his eyeball is elevated. What is this condition?
   a. cataracts
   b. glaucoma
   c. farsightedness
   d. nearsightedness

4. What is the most common form of dementia in older adults?
   a. Alzheimer's disease
   b. incontinence
   c. depression
   d. psychosis

5. The keys to successful aging include
   a. being physically active.
   b. eating a healthy diet.
   c. not smoking.
   d. all of the above.

6. The study of death and dying is called
   a. thanatology.
   b. gerontology.
   c. biology.
   d. living will.

7. Grief work is
   a. the process of integrating the reality of the loss with everyday life and learning to feel better.
   b. the total acceptance that a loved one has died.
   c. assigning feelings to the loss of a loved one.
   d. completing the cultural rituals required to express one's grief.

8. Kerri's elderly grandmother is terminally ill and wants to die without medical intervention. Her family has agreed to withhold treatment that may prolong her life. This is called
   a. rational suicide.
   b. health care proxy.
   c. passive euthanasia.
   d. active euthanasia.

9. When a person dies *intestate*,
   a. the body can be shipped across state boundaries.
   b. burial cannot take place without some authorization.
   c. the person died without a will.
   d. the court will decide what to do about the funeral arrangements.

10. A culturally prescribed and accepted period of grief for someone who has died is known as
    a. bereavement.
    b. grief work.
    c. coping with loss.
    d. mourning.

Answers for these questions can be found on page A-1.

Think about It!

1. Discuss what it means to age successfully. What are some characteristics of successful aging?
2. As the older population grows, how will it affect your life? Would you be willing to pay higher taxes to support government social programs for older adults? Why or why not?
3. List the major physical and mental changes that occur with aging. Which of these, if any, can you change? Discuss actions you can start taking now to ensure a healthier aging process.

4. Discuss why so many of us deny death. How could death become a more acceptable topic to discuss?

5. Debate whether rational suicide should be legalized for the terminally ill. What restrictions would you include in a law?

Accessing Your Health on the Internet

The following websites explore further topics and issues related to personal health. For links to the websites below, visit the Companion Website for *Health: The Basics,* Green Edition at www.pearsonhighered.com/donatelle.

1. *Administration on Aging.* A link to the U.S. Department of Health and Human Services, dedicated to addressing the health needs of older adults. www.aoa.gov

2. *Alzheimer's Association.* Includes media releases, position statements, fact sheets, and research on Alzheimer's disease. www.alz.org

3. *Beyond Indigo.* This site addresses all aspects of grief and loss, including terminal illness, legal issues, and funeral planning. www.beyondindigo.com

4. *Family Caregiver Alliance.* Offers programs at national, state, and local levels to support caregivers. www.caregiver.org

5. *National Hospice and Palliative Care Organization.* Offers information on hospice care, including resources for finding a hospice, end-of-life issues, and advance directives. www.nhpco.org

6. *Organdonor.gov.* This is the official U.S. government site for information on organ and tissue donation and transplantation. www.organdonor.gov

References

1. Centers for Disease Control and Prevention, "Healthy Aging for Older Adults," Modified 2009, www.cdc.gov/aging;
Centers for Disease Control and Prevention and the Merck Company Foundation, *The State of Aging and Health in America 2007* (Whitehouse Station, NJ: The Merck Company Foundation, 2007).

2. M. Lachman, "Aging under Control?" *Psychological Science Agenda* 19, no. 1 (2005): 1–3.

3. M. P. Heron et al., "Deaths: Final Data for 2006," *National Vital Statistics Reports* 57, no. 14 (2009): 1–135; National Center for Health Statistics, *Health, United States, 2008, with Chartbook on Trends in the Health of Americans* (Hyattsville, MD: National Center for Health Statistics, 2009), Table 26.

4. Federal Interagency Forum on Aging-Related Statistics, *Older Americans Update 2008: Key Indicators of Well-Being* (Washington, DC: Federal Interagency Forum on Aging-Related Statistics, 2008); Administration on Aging, "A Profile of Older Americans: 2008," 2009, www.aoa.gov/AoAroot/Aging_Statistics/Profile/index.aspx; Centers for Disease Control and Prevention, "Healthy Aging for Older Adults," 2009.

5. United Nations, Department of Economic and Social Affairs, Population Division, *World Population Prospects: The 2008 Revision, Population Database,* 2009, http://esa.un.org/unpp/index.asp.

6. Administration on Aging, "A Profile of Older Americans: 2008," 2009.

7. American Association of Homes and Services for the Aging, "Aging Services: The Facts," 2009, www.aahsa.org/article.aspx?id=74.

8. Arthritis Foundation, "Disease Center: Osteoarthritis," 2007, www.arthritis.org/disease-center.php?disease_id=32.

9. National Institute of Diabetes and Digestive and Kidney Diseases, "Urinary Tract Infections in Adults," NIH Publication no. 07-2097, 2005, http://kidney.niddk.nih.gov/kudiseases/pubs/utiadult.

10. U.S. National Library of Medicine and National Institutes of Health, Medline Plus, "Aging Changes in the Senses," Updated 2009, www.nlm.nih.gov/medlineplus/ency/article/004013.htm.

11. D. Kemmet and S. Brotherson, "Making Sense of Sensory Losses as We Age— Childhood, Adulthood, Elderhood?" 2008, North Dakota State University, www.ag.ndsu.edu/pubs/yf/famsci/fs1378.html.

12. X. P. Fisher and L. Fisher, *Sexuality at Midlife and Beyond: 2004 Update of Attitudes and Behaviors* (Washington, DC: American Association of Retired Persons, 2005).

13. Alzheimer's Association, *2009 Alzheimer's Disease Facts and Figures* (Chicago: Alzheimer's Association, 2009).

14. B. Kantrowitz and K. Springen, "Confronting Alzheimer's," *Newsweek,* June 15, 2007.

15. Alzheimer's Association, *2009 Alzheimer's Disease Facts and Figures,* 2009.

16. Ibid.

17. J. Wooten and J. Galavis, "Polypharmacy: Keeping the Elderly Safe," *RN* 68, no. 8 (2005): 44–50.

18. M. Nelson et al., "Physical Activity and Public Health in Older Adults: Recommendations from the American College of Sports Medicine and the American Heart Association," *Medicine and Science in Sports and Exercise* 39, no. 8 (2007): 1435–45; National Institute on Aging, *Exercise & Physical Activity: Your Everyday Guide from the National Institute on Aging* (Bethesda, MD: National Institutes of Health, 2009) NIH Publication no. 09-4258, www.nia.nih.gov/HealthInformation/Publications/ExerciseGuide.

19. *The New Shorter Oxford English Dictionary* (Oxford, UK: Oxford University Press, 1993).

20. President's Commission on the Uniform Determination of Death, *Defining Death: Medical, Ethical and Legal Issues in the Determination of Death* (Washington, DC: U.S. Government Printing Office, 1981).

21. Ad Hoc Committee of the Harvard Medical School to Examine the Definition of Brain Death, "A Definition of Irreversible Coma," *Journal of the American Medical Association* 205 (1968): 377.

22. E. Kübler-Ross and D. Kessler, *On Grief and Grieving: Finding the Meaning of Grief through the Five Stages of Loss* (New York: Scribner, 2005).

23. C. Corr, C. Nabe, and D. Corr, *Death and Dying, Life and Living.* 6th ed. (Belmont, CA: Wadsworth, 2008).

24. J. W. Worden, *Grief Counseling and Grief Therapy: A Handbook for the Mental Health Practitioner.* 4th ed. (New York: Springer, 2008).

25. American Bar Association, Commission on Law and Aging, *Consumer's Tool Kit for Health Care Advance Planning.* 2d ed., 2005, www.abanet.org/aging/toolkit/home.html.

26. Aging with Dignity, "Five Wishes," 2009, www.agingwithdignity.org/five-wishes.php.

27. Public Agenda, "Right to Die," 2008, www.publicagenda.org/articles/right-die.

28. Oregon Department of Human Services, "Oregon's Death with Dignity Act," 2008, www.dhs.state.or.us/publichealth/chs/pas/pas.cfm.

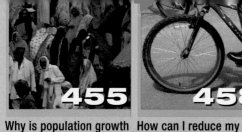
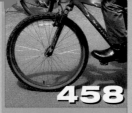
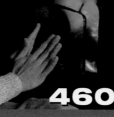
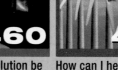

455 Why is population growth an environmental issue?

458 How can I reduce my carbon footprint?

460 How can air pollution be a problem indoors?

463 How can I help prevent global warming?

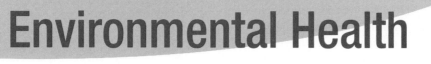

Environmental Health

15

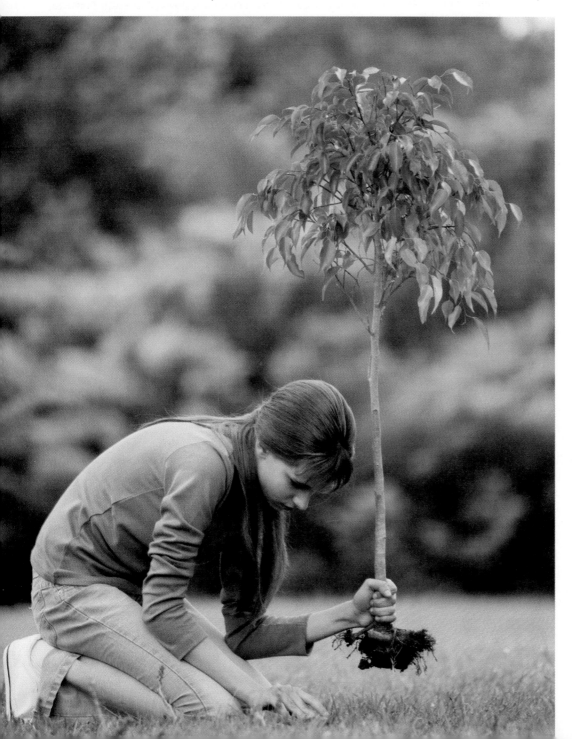

Objectives

* Explain the environmental impact associated with the current global population and its projected growth.

* Discuss major causes of air pollution and the global consequences of the accumulation of greenhouse gases and ozone depletion.

* Identify sources of water pollution and chemical contaminants often found in water.

* Distinguish municipal solid waste from hazardous waste, and list strategies for reducing land pollution.

* Discuss the health concerns associated with ionizing and nonionizing radiation.

* Describe the physiological consequences of noise pollution.

"We have arrived at a moment of decision. Our home—Earth—is in grave danger. What is at risk of being destroyed is not the planet itself, of course, but the conditions that have made it hospitable for human beings."
—Al Gore, opening statement before the Senate Foreign Relations Committee, January 28, 2009

We live in an especially dangerous time—dangerous for us, dangerous for future generations, and dangerous to our very existence. Our global population has grown more in the past 50 years than at any other time in human history. Population growth poses a potentially devastating threat to the water we drink, the air we breathe, the food we eat, and our capacity to survive. Our polar ice caps and glaciers are melting at rates that defy even the most dire predictions of just a decade ago, and threats of rising sea levels loom large. One in four existing mammals in the world is now threatened with extinction as humans destroy habitat, exacerbate drought and flooding due to climate change, and pollute the environment. Clean water is becoming scarce, fossil fuels are being depleted at unprecedented rates, and our solid and hazardous wastes are growing in direct proportion to our global population. In short, we are plundering our natural resources, and greedily consuming and throwing away the future life of all species.

Individuals, communities, and political powers must take action now to make positive change. We must reduce consumption, waste less, be less selfish when it comes to personal comfort and perceived needs, and force governments to enact and enforce environmentally responsible legislation. This chapter provides an overview of the factors contributing to our global environmental crisis. It also provides a blueprint for action—by individuals, communities, policymakers, and governments. Staying informed and becoming involved in the process are key things you can do to help.

Overpopulation

Anthropologist Margaret Mead wrote, "Every human society is faced with not one population problem but two: how to beget and rear enough children and how not to beget and rear too many."[1] As noted health scientist Robert H. Friis has described it, "Every day we share Earth and its resources with 250,000 more people than the day before. Every year, there are another 90 million mouths to feed. This is the equivalent of adding a city the size of Philadelphia to the world population every week, a Los Angeles every 2 weeks, a Mexico every year, and a United States and Canada every 3 years."[2] The United Nations projects that the world population will grow from 7 billion in 2011 to 9.4 billion by 2050 and to 11.5 billion by 2150 (Figure 15.1).[3]

Though our population is expanding exponentially, Earth's resources are not. Fertile land, clean water, and all natural resources are disappearing at a phenomenal rate. There is heavy pressure on the capacity of natural resources to support

ecosystem The collection of physical (nonliving) and biological (living) components of an environment and the relationships between them.

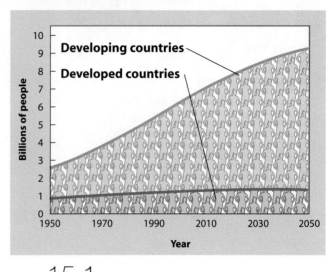

FIGURE 15.1 **World Population Growth, 1950–2050 (Projected)**
Source: Data are from Population Division of the Department of Economic and Social Affairs of the United Nations Secretariat, *World Population Prospects: The 2008 Revision*, 2009, http://esa.un.org/unpp.

human life and world health. According to a recent United Nations Global Environmental Outlook report (GEO-4), the human population is living far beyond its means and is inflicting damage on the environment that may already be irreparable.[4] Population experts believe that the most critical environmental challenge today is to slow the world's population growth.

Bursting with People: Measuring the Impact

While many people question *when* we will reach the "tipping point" at which we will be unable to restore the balance between humans and nature, others argue that it is too late now. Evidence of the effects of unchecked population growth, runaway consumption patterns, and toxic by-products of human use and waste is everywhere:

● **Impact on other species.** Based on current reporting, changes in the **ecosystem** are resulting in mass destruction of many species. We are currently fishing our oceans at rates that are 250 percent more than they can regenerate. At current rates, scientists project a global collapse of all fish species by 2050.

At the same time, 12 percent of birds are threatened with extinction, and 23 percent of mammals and more than 30 percent of amphibians are already gone or nearly gone. Many that survive are sick, have chemically induced ailments, or have genetic disfigurement that will hasten their demise.

● **Impact on our food supply.** In addition to overfishing, aquatic ecosystems continue to be heavily exploited by chemical and human waste. Drought and erosion make growing food increasingly difficult, and food shortages and famine are occurring in many regions of the world with increasing frequency. Faced with decreasing supplies of food products, fish, and the capacity to feed livestock, we may be forced to change the way we think about food. Many experts have long advocated for humans to "eat lower on the food chain" by eating fewer high-resource animal products.

● **Land degradation and contamination of drinking water.** The per capita availability of freshwater is declining rapidly, and contaminated water remains the greatest single environmental cause of human sickness and health. Unsustainable land use and climate change are increasing land degradation, including erosion, nutrient depletion, deforestation, and other problems that will inevitably affect human life.

● **Excessive energy consumption.** "Use it *and* lose it" is an apt saying for our vast greed in using nonrenewable energy sources in the form of **fossil fuels** (oil, coal, natural gas). Although we are seeing a shift toward renewable energy sources, such as hydropower, solar and wind power, and biomass power, the predominant energy sources are still fossil fuels. In many developing regions of the world, demand for limited fossil fuels is growing at unprecedented rates.

● **Impact on our lives.** Imagine waking up in the morning and finding that you have no water for a shower, that your lights can be used only a few hours each day or not at all, that you have to choose between using electricity for your flat-screen TV or your refrigerator. Imagine having very little gas for your car, and going to the grocery store to find half-empty shelves of items you can't afford. Imagine the news filled with stories about long lines at gas stations; natural disasters; and wars over water rights, food, and fuel. Such scenarios are not the imaginings of science fiction. Major difficulties loom unless we take action to change our current rate of population growth and our consumption of natural resources, and unless the global community acts together to enforce policies and programs to check rampant population growth.

Factors That Affect Population Growth

Before we consider how to slow the growing tide of people, we must first understand the factors that have led to the world population's increase. Key among them are changes in fertility and mortality rates.

Fertility rate refers to how many births a woman has by the end of her reproductive life. In the United States today, the fertility rate is just over 2 births per woman, as compared to nearly 3.5 births per woman during the baby boom years after World War II. In other regions of the world, particularly

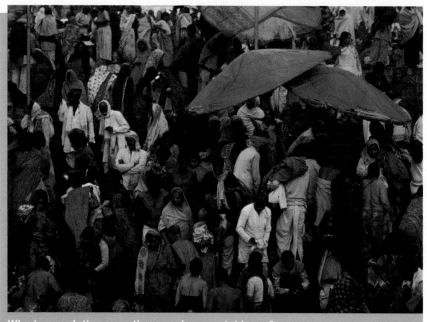

Why is population growth an environmental issue?

Every year the global population grows by 90 million, but Earth's resources are not expanding. Population increases are believed to be responsible for most of the current environmental stress.

in India and in many Asian, Latin American, and African countries, birth rates are about four per woman; this leads to rapid increases in overall population in these poorer countries. In countries where women have little say over reproductive choices, where birth control is either not available or frowned upon, pregnancy rates continue to rise.

Mortality rates from both chronic and infectious diseases have declined in both developed and developing regions of the world as a result of improved public health infrastructure, increased availability of drugs and vaccines, better disaster preparedness, and other factors. Consequently, people are living longer and consuming more over the course of their lifetimes. This, too, contributes to pressure on the environment.

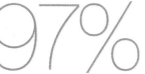

97%

of global growth in the next four decades will happen in Asia, Africa, Latin America, and the Caribbean.

Different Nations, Different Growth Rates

By 2050, India is projected to be the most populous nation at 1.7 billion, overtaking current leader China, which will grow to 1.4 billion.[5] The continued preference for large families in many developing nations is related to several factors: high infant mortality rates; the traditional view of children as "social security" (working from a young age to assist families in daily survival and supporting parents when they grow too old to work); the low educational and economic status of women, which often leaves women with few reproductive

fossil fuels Carbon-based material used for energy; includes oil, coal, and natural gas.

fertility rate The average number of births a female in a certain population has during her reproductive years.

choices; and the traditional desire for sons, which keeps parents of daughters reproducing until they have male offspring.

In contrast to developing nations, the population sizes in wealthier nations are static or declining, with one notable exception—the United States. With a population of 305 million, and an expected 439 million people by 2050, the United States is the only industrialized country in the world currently experiencing significant population growth.[6] Last year, the U.S. growth rate was nearly 1 percent, far greater than that of Canada, England, or other industrialized nations. Each year, the United States adds 3 million more people, or 8,000 per day.[7] This is particularly noteworthy because the United States also has the largest "ecological footprint"—that is, the United States exerts greater impact on many of the planet's resources and ecosystems than any other nation on Earth. Overall, we are the world's largest single emitter of greenhouse gases, the world's largest forest-product consumers, and the generators of the most municipal solid waste per person in the world.[8]

Although the United States makes up only 5 percent of the world's population, it is responsible for nearly 25 percent of total global resource consumption. We consume 2.3 billion metric tons of oil equivalents for energy per year; the rest of the world consumes 10 billion tons per year. Per capita, Americans consume nearly 8,000 kg of oil equivalents for energy, compared to 3,600 kg consumed by Europeans and 900 kg by Asians (see Figure 15.2).[9]

Zero Population Growth

Recognizing that population control will be essential in the decades ahead, many countries have already enacted strict population control measures or have encouraged their citizens to limit the size of their families. Proponents of *zero population growth (ZPG)* believe that each couple should produce only two offspring. When the parents die, these two children are their replacements, allowing the population to stabilize. By 2000, Italy, Spain, Portugal, Greece, and Sweden were among the first to achieve zero population growth.[10] Germany, Russia, Ukraine, Hungary, and Bulgaria had actually achieved negative population growth, causing some people in these countries to worry that they may have gone too far in their population control campaigns.

Education may be the single biggest contributor to ZPG. As education levels of women increase and women achieve equality in pay, job status, and social status with men, fertility rates decline. Access to information about family planning and contraception can also make a big difference.

> ## what do you think?
> Should individuals get tax breaks for having fewer children?
> ● How would such policies compare to our current policies?
> ● Can you think of other policies that might be effective in encouraging population control and resource conservation in the United States?

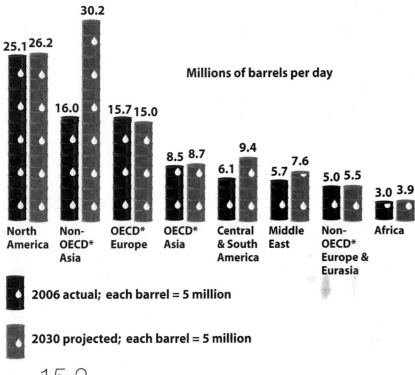

Millions of barrels per day

	2006 actual	2030 projected
North America	25.1	26.2
Non-OECD* Asia	16.0	30.2
OECD* Europe	15.7	15.0
OECD* Asia	8.5	8.7
Central & South America	6.1	9.4
Middle East	5.7	7.6
Non-OECD* Europe & Eurasia	5.0	5.5
Africa	3.0	3.9

■ 2006 actual; each barrel = 5 million

■ 2030 projected; each barrel = 5 million

FIGURE 15.2 World Liquid Fuels Consumption by Region and Country Group, 2006 and 2030 (Projected)
*OECD is the Organization for Economic Cooperation and Development.
Source: Data are from Energy Information Administration (EIA), *International Energy Annual 2006* (June-December 2008), www.eia.doe.gov/iea; and EIA World Energy Projections Plus (2009).

Air Pollution

The term *air pollution* refers to the presence, in varying degrees, of those substances (suspended particles and vapors) not found in perfectly clean air. From the beginning of time, natural events, living creatures, and toxic by-products have been polluting the environment. As such, air pollution is not a new phenomenon. What is new is the vast array of **pollutants** that exist today and the potential interactive effects of many of these substances.

Generally, air pollutants are either *naturally occurring* or *anthropogenic* (human caused). Naturally occurring air pollutants include particulate matter, such as the dust spread from windstorms, smoke and ash from major forest fires, salt spray from the oceans, ash from volcanic eruptions, and others. Anthropogenic sources include those caused by stationary sources (e.g., electric-generating plants, factories, manufacturing complexes, chemical plants, oil and natural gas refineries, coal plants, chemical plants, and incinerators) and mobile sources (e.g., cars, trucks, buses, ATVs, airplanes, ships, and trains). According to Environmental Protection Agency (EPA) estimates, mobile sources produce over half of two major sources of smog—hydrocarbons and nitrogen oxides (NO)—almost 90 percent of carbon monoxide and more than half of hazardous air pollution.[11]

Components of Air Pollution

Concern about air quality prompted Congress to pass the Clean Air Act in 1970 and to amend it in 1977 and again in 1990. The goal was to develop standards for six of the most widespread air pollutants that seriously affect health: sulfur dioxide, particulates, carbon monoxide, nitrogen dioxide, ground-level ozone, and lead. Other common air pollutants include carbon dioxide and hydrocarbons. Today, ozone and particle air pollution are the most widespread and most dangerous of the air pollutants.[12] Table 15.1 ranks the ten best and the ten worst cities in the United States in terms of these two air pollutants.

Sulfur Dioxide Sulfur dioxide (SO_2) is a yellowish brown gas that forms when fuel containing sulfur, particularly coal and oil, is burned; when gasoline is extracted from oil; or when metals are extracted from ore.

Sulfur dioxide is also derived from fertilizers and livestock wastes. More than 65 percent (or more than 13 million tons) of SO_2 released into the air each year comes from electric and coal-fired power plants. Other sources of SO_2 are industrial facilities, locomotives, large ships, and previous-generation diesel engines.

Sulfur dioxide dissolves in water vapor to form acid rain and interacts with other gases and particles in the air to form sulfates and other products. In humans, sulfur dioxide aggravates symptoms of heart and lung disease; obstructs breathing passages; and increases the incidence of respiratory diseases such as colds, asthma, bronchitis, and emphysema. Sulfur dioxide is toxic to plants, destroys some paint pigments, corrodes metals, impairs visibility, and is a precursor to acid deposition (discussed later).

In 2007, a new generation of engines that burn an ultralow sulfur diesel fuel became available in the United States.[13] This new cleaner-burning diesel has been readily available in European countries and has the potential to drastically reduce sulfur-dioxide pollution in the United States, particularly as newer diesel engine technology is developed that will prevent virtually all SO_2 emissions.

Particle Pollution *Particle pollution* refers to a mix of very tiny solid or liquid particles in the air we breathe. **Particulates** vary in size, from coarse to fine to ultrafine; coarse particulates may make you sneeze or cough; fine particles can make your eyes water, or your lungs feel congested. Some of these particles are so small that they can pass through the lungs into the bloodstream. Whether found in solid or liquid form, particle pollution poses one of the greatest health risks to humans today. Depending on the part of the country you live in, the season, or a variety of other factors, you may be exposed to a variety of particle health threats daily. Most particle pollution comes from either mechanical or chemical processes. Dust storms (particularly in drought-ridden areas), construction and demolition, mining, and agriculture are among the most common sources; however, engine exhausts and many industrial and chemical processing releases are also key sources.

How risky is it to breathe particulate pollution? It depends on the size and nature of the particle, the length of and time of exposure, and the concentration in the air. For those prone to asthma, particulate inhalation can be deadly. When combined with SO_2, they can make all respiratory diseases worse.

pollutant A substance that contaminates some aspect of the environment and causes potential harm to living organisms.

sulfur dioxide (SO_2) A yellowish brown gaseous by-product of the burning of fossil fuels.

particulates Nongaseous air pollutants.

TABLE 15.1   The Cleanest and Dirtiest U.S. Cities in Terms of Air Pollution

Top 10 Highest Ozone Pollution	Top 10 Highest Year-Round Particle Pollution	Lowest Ozone Pollution (Not Ranked)	Top 10 Lowest Year-Round Particle Pollution
1. Los Angeles, CA	1. Bakersfield, CA	Billings, MT	1. Cheyenne, WY
2. Bakersfield, CA	2. Pittsburgh, PA	Carson City, NV	2. Santa Fe, NM
3. Visalia, CA	3. Los Angeles, CA	Coeur D'Alene, ID	3. Honolulu, HI
4. Fresno, CA	4. Visalia, CA	Fargo, ND	4. Great Falls, MT
5. Houston, TX	5. Birmingham, AL	Honolulu, HI	5. Farmington, NM
6. Sacramento, CA	6. Hanford, CA	Laredo, TX	6. Anchorage, AK
7. Dallas–Fort Worth, TX	7. Fresno, CA	Lincoln, NE	7. Tucson, AZ
8. Charlotte, NC	8. Cincinnati, OH	Port St. Lucie, FL	8. Bismark, ND
9. Phoenix, AZ	9. Detroit, MI	Sioux Falls, SD	9. Flagstaff, AZ (tie)
10. El Centro, TX	10. Cleveland, OH		10. Salinas, CA (tie)

Source: American Lung Association, "State of the Air," 2009, www.stateoftheair.org/2009/city-rankings.

Symptoms may be similar to those of a long-term smoker. Although risks to the lungs and cardiovascular system are significant, these particles can also corrode metals, damage homes and plant life, and decrease visibility. Short-term spikes in particulate levels can be deadly, particularly for the very young and for older adults who are suffering from chronic illnesses.

carbon monoxide (CO) An odorless, colorless gas that originates primarily from motor vehicle emissions.

nitrogen dioxide An amber-colored gas found in smog; can cause eye and respiratory irritations.

ozone A gas composed of 3 atoms of oxygen; occurs at ground level and in the upper atmosphere.

carbon dioxide (CO_2) Gas created by the combustion of fossil fuels, exhaled by animals, and used by plants for photosynthesis; the primary greenhouse gas in Earth's atmosphere.

greenhouse gases Gases that accumulate in the atmosphere, where they contribute to global warming by trapping heat near Earth's surface.

carbon footprint The amount of greenhouse gases produced, usually expressed in equivalent tons of carbon dioxide emissions.

hydrocarbons Chemical compounds that contain carbon and hydrogen.

Carbon Monoxide

Carbon monoxide (CO) in our atmosphere originates primarily from motor vehicle emissions. Carbon monoxide is an odorless, colorless gas that interferes with the blood's ability to absorb and carry oxygen. It can impair thinking, slow reflexes, and cause drowsiness, unconsciousness, and death. Carbon monoxide poisoning is the third leading cause of death due to unintentional poisoning in the United States, killing nearly 1,400 and injuring 15,000 to 40,000 Americans each year.[14] Carbon monoxide is a major component of both indoor and outdoor air pollution.

Nitrogen Dioxide

Coal-powered electrical utility boilers and motor vehicles emit **nitrogen dioxide,** an amber-colored gas. High concentrations of nitrogen dioxide can be fatal to humans. Lower concentrations increase susceptibility to colds and flu, bronchitis, and pneumonia. Nitrogen dioxide is also toxic to plant life and causes a brown discoloration of the atmosphere.

Ground-Level Ozone

Ground-level **ozone** is a gas and one of the molecular forms of oxygen. When it occurs in nature, ozone has a sharp smell akin to sparks from electrical equipment. Ground-level ozone is produced when nitrogen dioxide reacts with sunlight and oxygen molecules, and it is a main component of smog. (Note, however, that ozone in the upper atmosphere is essential to protecting Earth from the sun's heat and ultraviolet light, as we discuss later.) Ground-level ozone irritates the respiratory system's mucous membranes, causing coughing and choking. It can impair lung function; reduce resistance to colds and pneumonia; and aggravate heart disease, asthma, bronchitis, and pneumonia. Ozone corrodes rubber and paint and can kill vegetation.

Carbon Dioxide

Carbon dioxide (CO_2) is one of the most plentiful gases in Earth's atmosphere, and, as the primary fuel for plant respiration, it is essential to all life. However, CO_2 is also a principal component of emissions from internal combustion engines. Much of the rise in air pollution is directly related to excess CO_2 released from burning carbon-containing fossil fuels. CO_2 is also the most prominent

greenhouse gas and thus the major culprit in global warming (discussed later).

As one of the largest CO_2 emitters in the world, the United States has the largest **carbon footprint**—the measure of impact that human activities have on the environment in terms of greenhouse gases produced, measured in units of CO_2.[15] When you drive your car or heat your house with oil, gas, or coal, the burning of these fossil fuels emits CO_2 into the atmosphere. Each time you turn up your thermostat or leave lights on in your house, the fuel burned adds to your individual carbon footprint. For each gallon of gasoline burned in your car, you emit 8.7 kg of CO_2 into the atmosphere. Multiply that by millions of people driving cars that burn lots of fuel and you can see how the problem escalates. Reducing our individual carbon footprint is a key goal in the struggle to combat air pollution, global warming, and climate change, and has been the purpose of several Green Guide tips throughout this book.

Hydrocarbons

Hydrocarbons are chemical compounds containing different combinations of carbon and hydrogen. They encompass a wide variety of pollutants in the air and play a major part in forming smog. Most automobile engines emit hundreds of different hydrocarbon compounds. By themselves, hydrocarbons seem to cause few problems, but when they combine with sunlight and other pollutants, they form such poisons as formaldehyde, ketones, and peroxyacetyl nitrate, all of which are respiratory irritants. Hydrocarbon combinations such as benzene and benzo[*a*]pyrene are

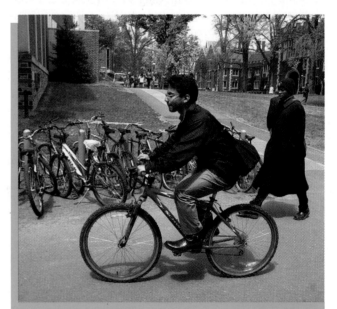

How can I reduce my carbon footprint?

Reducing our individual carbon footprints is a key goal in the struggle to combat air pollution, global warming, and climate change. Making small changes such as driving less, riding your bike more, taking public transportation or carpooling, turning off lights when you leave a room, and recycling and composting can all help reduce your carbon footprint.

When the AQI is in this range:	...air quality conditions are	...as symbolized by this color:
0 to 50	Good	Green
51 to 100	Moderate	Yellow
101 to 150	Unhealthy for sensitive groups	Orange
151 to 200	Unhealthy	Red
201 to 300	Very unhealthy	Purple
301 to 500	Hazardous	Maroon

FIGURE 15.3 Air Quality Index (AQI)
The Environmental Protection Agency (EPA) provides individual AQIs for ground-level ozone, particle pollution, carbon monoxide, sulfur dioxide, and nitrogen dioxide. All of the AQIs are presented using the general values, categories, and colors of this figure.
Source: U.S. Environmental Protection Agency, "Air Quality Index: A Guide to Air Quality and Your Health," Updated April 2009, www.airnow.gov/index.cfm ?action=aqibasics.aqi.

carcinogenic. All of these pollutants are also commonly known as *volatile organic compounds (VOCs)*.

Air Quality Index

A measure of daily air quality, the Air Quality Index (AQI) tells you how clean or polluted your air is and what associated health concerns you should be aware of. The AQI focuses on health effects that can happen within a few hours or days after breathing polluted air.

The AQI runs from 0 to 500: The higher the AQI value, the greater the level of air pollution and associated health risks. An AQI value of 100 generally corresponds to the national air quality standard for the pollutant, which is the level the EPA has set to protect public health. Air Quality Index values below 100 are generally considered satisfactory. When AQI values rise above 100, air quality is considered unhealthy—at first for certain groups of people, then for everyone.

As shown in **Figure 15.3**, the EPA has divided the AQI scale into six categories and color codes. This is the best way for the public to assess the daily quality of the air we breathe.

Indoor Air Pollution

In the past several years, a growing body of scientific evidence has indicated that the air within homes and other buildings can be 10 to 40 times more hazardous than outdoor air, even in the most industrialized cities. Potentially dangerous chemical compounds can increase risks of cancer, contribute to respiratory problems, reduce the immune system's ability to fight disease, and increase problems with allergies and allergic reactions: The higher the dose of these pollutants and the more airtight the house, the greater the risk for individuals.

Shopping to Save the Planet

* Look for products with less packaging or with refillable, reusable, or recyclable containers.
* Bring your own reusable cloth grocery bags to the store.
* Buy foods that are produced with minimal or sustainable energy.
* Purchase organic foods or foods produced with fewer chemicals and pesticides.
* Do not buy plastic bottles of water or other beverages. Purchase a hard plastic or steel, wide-mouth water bottle and fill it from a filtered source.
* Do not use caustic cleansers. Simple vinegar is usually just as effective and less harsh on your home and the environment.
* Buy laundry products that are free of dyes, fragrances, and sulfates.
* Use soap and water to clean surfaces, not disposable cleaning cloths and spray-on shower cleaners.
* Purchase appliances with the Energy Star logo.
* Buy CFLs (compact fluorescent lights) instead of less energy-efficient incandescent bulbs.
* Use reusable mugs, plates, and silverware rather than disposable products.
* Buy recycled paper products.
* Purchase bed linens and bath towels that are made from bamboo, hemp, or organic cotton.

20–100

potentially dangerous chemical compounds can be found in the air of the average American home.

Indoor air pollution comes primarily from these sources: woodstoves, furnaces, passive cigarette smoke exposure (see Chapter 8), asbestos, formaldehyde, radon, and lead. An emerging source of indoor air pollution is mold. In addition, that "new car" smell we like is often related to potentially harmful chemicals found in interior fabrics, upholstery, and glues. Today, more and more manufacturers are offering green building products and furnishings, such as natural fiber fabrics, untreated wood for furniture and floors, low-VOC paints, and many other products in an attempt to reduce potential pollutants. The **Skills for Behavior Change** box above offers ideas for being an environmentally conscious consumer of products for yourself and your home.

Several factors, including age, preexisting medical conditions, individual sensitivity, room temperature and humidity, and functioning of the liver and immune and respiratory systems contribute to one's risk for being affected by indoor air pollution. Those with allergies may be particularly vulnerable. Health effects may develop over years of exposure or may occur in response to toxic levels of pollutants.

Preventing indoor air pollution should focus on three main areas: *source control* (eliminating or reducing individual contaminants), *ventilation improvements* (increasing the amount of outdoor air coming indoors), and *air cleaners* (removing particulates from the air).[16]

Environmental Tobacco Smoke

Perhaps the greatest source of indoor air pollution is *environmental tobacco smoke (ETS),* which contains carbon monoxide and cancer-causing particulates. The level of carbon monoxide in cigarette smoke contained in enclosed places has been found to be 4,000 times higher than that allowed in the clean air standard established by the EPA. Moreover, the Surgeon General has reported that there are more than 50 carcinogens in environmental tobacco smoke. Ten to 15 percent of nonsmokers are extremely sensitive to tobacco smoke. These people experience itchy eyes, difficulty in breathing, painful headaches, nausea, and dizziness in response to minute amounts of smoke. The only truly effective way to eliminate ETS in public places is to enact strict no-smoking policies; ventilation and separate smoking areas are not sufficient. Today, many major U.S. cities have banned smoking in public places, in worksites, and in automobiles where children are present.

asbestos A mineral compound that separates into stringy fibers and lodges in the lungs, where it can cause various diseases.
formaldehyde A colorless, strong-smelling gas released through outgassing; causes respiratory and other health problems.
radon A naturally occurring radioactive gas resulting from the decay of certain radioactive elements.
lead A highly toxic metal found in emissions from lead smelters and processing plants; also sometimes found in pipes or paint in older houses.

Home Heating

Woodstoves emit significant levels of particulates and carbon monoxide in addition to other pollutants, such as sulfur dioxide. If you rely on wood for heating, make sure that your stove is properly installed, vented, and maintained. Burning properly seasoned wood reduces particulates. People who rely on oil- or gas-fired furnaces also need to make sure that these appliances are properly installed, ventilated, and maintained.

Asbestos

Asbestos is a mineral compound that was once commonly used in insulating materials, but it also found its way into vinyl flooring, shingles/roofing materials, heating pipe coverings, and many other products in buildings constructed before 1970. When bonded to other materials, asbestos is relatively harmless, but if its tiny fibers become loosened and airborne, they can embed themselves in the lungs. Their presence leads to cancer of the lungs, stomach, and chest lining, and other life-threatening lung diseases called *mesothelioma* and *asbestosis.* If asbestos is detected in the home, it must be removed or sealed off by a professional.

Formaldehyde

Formaldehyde is a colorless, strong-smelling gas present in some carpets, draperies, furniture, particleboard, plywood, wood paneling, countertops, and many adhesives. It is released into the air in a process called *outgassing.* Outgassing is highest in new products, but the process can continue for many years. Exposure to formaldehyde can cause respiratory problems, dizziness, fatigue, nausea, and rashes. Long-term exposure can lead to central nervous system disorders and cancer.

How can you limit the amount of formaldehyde in your home? Ask about the formaldehyde content of products you purchase, and avoid those that contain it. Some houseplants, such as philodendrons and spider plants, help clean formaldehyde from the air.

Radon

Radon, an odorless, colorless gas, penetrates homes through cracks, pipes, sump pits, and other openings in the basement or foundation. The EPA, National Cancer Institute (NCI), and the American Lung Association estimate that radon causes 7,000 to 30,000 preventable deaths per year.[17] The number of lung cancer deaths per year attributed to radon make it second only to smoking as a cause of lung cancer.[18]

The EPA estimates that as many as 7.7 million homes throughout the country have elevated levels of radon.[19] Short-term testing, taking from 2 to 90 days to complete, is the quickest way to determine whether a potential problem exists. Low-cost radon test kits are available by mail order, in hardware stores, and through other retail outlets. Since 1988, the EPA and the Office of the Surgeon General have recommended that homes below the third floor be tested for radon and that Americans test their homes every 2 years or when they move into a new home.

Lead

Lead is a metal pollutant sometimes found in paint, batteries, drinking water, pipes, dishes with lead-based

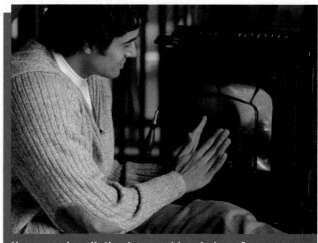

How can air pollution be a problem indoors?

The air within homes can be 10 to 40 times more hazardous than outside air. Indoor air pollution comes from woodstoves, furnaces, cigarette smoke, asbestos, formaldehyde, radon, lead, mold, and household chemicals.

glazes, dirt, soldered cans, and some candies made in Mexico. Recently, toys produced in China and other regions of the world have been recalled due to unsafe levels of lead in their paint.

Lead affects the circulatory, reproductive, urinary, and nervous systems and can accumulate in bone and other tissues. It is particularly detrimental to children and fetuses, and can cause birth defects, learning problems, behavioral abnormalities, and other health problems. By some estimates, as many as 25 percent of U.S. homes still have lead-based paint hazards, and an estimated 250,000 American children aged 1 to 5 have unsafe blood lead levels.[20]

Mold Molds are fungi that live both indoors and outdoors in most regions of the country. Molds produce tiny reproductive spores, which waft through the indoor and outdoor air continually. When they land on a damp spot indoors, they may begin growing and digesting whatever they are on, including wood, paper, carpet, and food. In general, molds are harmless; however, some people are sensitive or allergic to them. In such people, exposure to molds may lead to nasal stuffiness, running nose and eyes, and itchy skin. For those who are really sensitive, molds may cause fever, headache, shortness of breath, nausea, light-headedness, or severe respiratory problems.[21] For ways to reduce your exposure to mold, see the **Skills for Behavior Change** box at right.

Ozone Layer Depletion

As mentioned earlier, the ozone layer forms a protective stratum in Earth's stratosphere—the highest level of our atmosphere, located 12 to 30 miles above Earth's surface. The ozone layer in the stratosphere protects our planet and its inhabitants from ultraviolet B (UVB) radiation, a primary cause of skin cancer. Such radiation damages DNA and weakens immune systems in both humans and animals (radiation in general is discussed later in the chapter).

In the 1970s, scientists began to warn of a breakdown in the ozone layer. Instruments developed to test atmospheric contents indicated that chemicals used on Earth, especially **chlorofluorocarbons (CFCs),** were contributing to the ozone layer's rapid depletion. Chlorofluorocarbons were used as refrigerants, aerosol propellants, and cleaning solvents, and were also used in medical sterilizers, rigid foam insulation, and Styrofoam. When released into the air through spraying or outgassing, CFCs migrate into the ozone layer, where they decompose and release chlorine atoms. These atoms cause ozone molecules to break apart and levels to be depleted.

The U.S. government banned the use of aerosol sprays containing CFCs in the 1970s. The discovery of an ozone "hole" over Antarctica led to the 1987 Montreal Protocol treaty, whereby the United States and other nations agreed to further reduce the use of CFCs and other ozone-depleting chemicals. The treaty was amended in 1995 to ban CFC production in developed countries. Today, over 160 countries have signed the treaty as the international community strives to preserve the ozone layer.[22] Although the ban on CFCs

is believed to be responsible for slowing the depletion of the ozone layer, some CFC replacements may also be damaging because they contribute to the enhanced greenhouse effect.

Global Warming

More than 100 years ago, scientists theorized that carbon dioxide emissions from the burning of fossil fuels would create a buildup of greenhouse gases in Earth's atmosphere that could have a warming effect on Earth's surface.[23] In recent years, these predictions have been supported by reports of leading international scientists in the field and accounts in the popular media, such as the documentary *An Inconvenient Truth,* all detailing startling indicators of a planet in trouble.

The *greenhouse effect* is a natural phenomenon in which greenhouse gases form a gaseous layer in the atmosphere, encircling Earth, allowing solar heat to pass through, and then trapping some of the heat close to Earth's surface, where it warms the planet. Human activities such as burning fossil fuels and land clearing have increased greenhouse gases in the atmosphere, resulting in the **enhanced greenhouse effect,** in which excess solar heat is trapped, raising the planet's temperature (see **Figure 15.4** on the next page). According to data from the National Oceanic and Atmospheric Administration (NOAA) and the National Aeronautics and Space Administration (NASA), Earth's surface temperature has risen about 1.2 to 1.4 degrees

chlorofluorocarbons (CFCs) Chemicals that contribute to the depletion of the atmospheric ozone layer.

enhanced greenhouse effect The warming of Earth's surface as a direct result of human activities that release greenhouse gases into the atmosphere, trapping more of the sun's radiation than is normal.

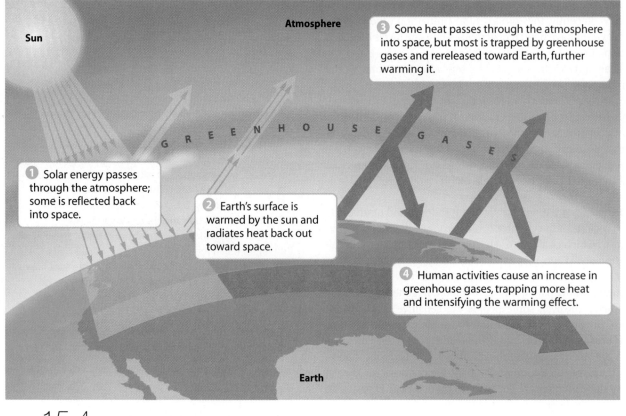

FIGURE 15.4 **The Enhanced Greenhouse Effect**
The natural greenhouse effect is responsible for making Earth habitable; it keeps the planet 33 degrees Celsius (60 degrees Fahrenheit) warmer than it would otherwise be. An increase in greenhouse gases resulting from human activities is creating the enhanced greenhouse effect, trapping more heat and causing dangerous global climate change.

Fahrenheit since 1900, with accelerated warming in the past two decades.[24] Furthermore, the consensus is that temperatures will continue to rise, perhaps by as much as 5 to 10 degrees in the next 100 years, unless immediate steps are taken to reverse the trend. Results of such a temperature increase—which might include rising sea levels (potentially flooding entire countries), glacier retreat, arctic shrinkage at the poles, altered patterns of agriculture (including changes in growing seasons and alterations of climatic zones), deforestation, drought, extreme weather events, increases in tropical diseases, changes in disease trends and patterns, loss of biological species, and economic devastation—would be catastrophic.

The greenhouse gases include carbon dioxide, nitrous oxide, methane, CFCs, and hydrocarbons. The most predominant is carbon dioxide, which accounts for 49 percent of all greenhouse gases. The United States is the greatest producer of greenhouse gases, responsible for over 22 percent of all output, and this output is expected to increase by 43 percent by 2025.[25] Rapid deforestation of the tropical rain forests of Central and South America, Africa, and southeast Asia also contributes to the rapid rise in greenhouse gases. Trees take in carbon dioxide, transform it, store the carbon for food, and release oxygen into the air. As we lose forests, at the rate of hundreds of acres per hour, we lose the capacity to dissipate carbon dioxide.

A United Nations treaty signed in Kyoto in 1997 outlined an international plan to reduce the manmade emissions responsible for climate change. The Kyoto Protocol, which came into effect in 2005, requires participating countries to reduce their emissions between 2008 and 2012 by at least 5 percent below 1990 levels.[26] More than 160 countries signed on to the Kyoto Protocol, including more than 30 industrialized countries.[27] The treaty would require the United States to reduce emissions by 33 percent, but the United States has so far refused to ratify it, stating concerns that major developing nations, including India and China, are not required to reduce emissions under the treaty.

Reducing Air Pollution and the Threat of Global Warming

Air pollution and climate change problems are rooted in our energy, transportation, and industrial practices. Clearly, we must develop comprehensive national strategies that encourage the use of renewable resources such as solar, wind, and water power. Because industrial production is a key contributor to fossil fuel emission, clean energy, green factories, improved technology, and governmental regulation are necessary for preventing climate change.

Most experts agree that reducing consumption of fossil fuels in cars and shifting to alternative fuels, improving gas mileage, and using mass transportation are crucial to air pollution reduction. Many cities have taken steps in this direction by setting high parking fees and road-usage tolls in congested areas and by imposing bans on city driving. Local governments should be encouraged to provide convenient and inexpensive public transportation and to motivate people to use it regularly.

Although stricter laws on vehicular carbon emissions and the development of new cars that operate on electricity, hydrogen, biodiesel, ethanol, or other alternative energy sources are promising, we have a long way to go to reduce fossil-fuel consumption.

Meanwhile, many U.S. communities are creating bicycle lanes and holding "bike to work" days. Scooters and other low-energy modes of transportation are becoming increasingly popular. Some college campuses have enacted new policies allowing increased skateboard and Rollerblade use on campus. Other campuses provide scooter and bike garages to protect students from theft and vandalism and to encourage students to bring energy-efficient vehicles to campus. See the **Green Guide** on page 464 for more ideas about reducing energy use on campus.

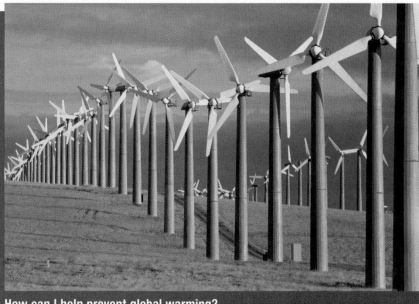

How can I help prevent global warming?

Global warming is a global problem. We need to work with other nations to ensure that everyone does their part. By reducing your use of fossil fuels; using high-efficiency vehicles; and supporting increased use of renewable resources such as solar, wind, and water power, you can help combat global warming.

Water Pollution and Shortages

Seventy-five percent of Earth is covered with water in the form of oceans, seas, lakes, rivers, streams, and wetlands. Beneath the landmass are reservoirs of groundwater. We draw our drinking water from this underground source and from surface freshwater; however, just 1 percent of the world's entire water supply is available for human use. The rest is too salty, too polluted, or locked away in polar ice caps.

We cannot take the safety of our water supply for granted. Over half the global population faces a shortage of clean water. More than 2.6 billion people, about 40 percent of the planet's population, have no access to basic sanitation or adequate toilet facilities. More than 1 billion have no access to clean water, and over 4,000 children die every day from illnesses caused by lack of safe water and sanitation.[28]

Ironically, two regions of the world that have the most severe water shortages also have some of the highest population growth rates—Africa and the Near East, which comprise

99%

of the world's water is unavailable for human use.

20 countries. Estimates suggest that by the year 2025, approximately 2.8 billion people will live in countries with severe water shortages. By 2050, these numbers will increase to 4 billion people in 54 countries.[29]

Considering how little water is available to meet the world's agricultural, manufacturing, community, personal, and sanitation needs, it is no wonder that clean water is a precious commodity that must not be wasted. Each U.S. resident uses an average of 1,500 gallons of water daily for all purposes—domestic consumption, recreation, energy (primarily from cooling at power plants), food production, and industry—about three times the world average.[30] The **Skills for Behavior Change** box on page 465 presents simple conservation measures you can adopt to save water in your home.

Water Contamination

Any substance that gets into the soil can potentially enter the water supply. Industrial pollutants and pesticides eventually work their way into the soil, then into groundwater. Underground storage tanks for gasoline may leak. A recent survey by a group of U.S. Geological Survey researchers discovered the presence of low levels of many chemical compounds in a network of 139 targeted streams across the United States. Steroids, prescription and nonprescription drugs, hormones, insect repellent, and wastewater compounds were all detected.[31]

Tap water in the United States is among the safest in the world. The Safe Drinking Water Act (SDWA) is the main federal

GREEN GUIDE

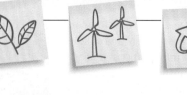

Sustainability on Campus

You are moving into a new dorm room, along with hundreds of other students, and are excited to decorate, meet your new roommate, and make your room the place to be. As a student, this is also your chance to make a positive difference and minimize your ecological footprint. Your actions, and those of your friends, roommates, and school can have a lasting impact on your life and the future of the environment.

More and more universities and colleges are recognizing that students want to attend schools that reflect their values and beliefs around sustainable movements. Several organizations publish annual rankings of the "greenest" schools, including the College Sustainability Report Card and the Sierra Club's "Cool Schools" list (see table below).

The green sustainability movement is picking up steam and turning ideas into realities. You do not need to be an environmental science major or a self-proclaimed "hippie" to make a difference. Going green on campus can be part of the goal for your apartment, your sorority or fraternity, or your residence hall.

Start making a positive impact by turning off lights when you leave a room or bathroom. See if your residence has a way of minimizing the amount of lights used on a floor. Sometimes lights might be connected through several outlets, and turning off a strand might still provide enough light but minimize the amount of energy consumed. Find out whether your administration supports the use of CFLs—compact fluorescent lights—which are typically longer-lasting energy-conserving bulbs that give off the same amount of light as an incandescent bulb at a fraction of the energy used. Next time you go to the store, buy a couple for your new lighting fixtures and start making a positive impact.

When buying a new appliance, look for the Energy Star logo, indicating that the appliance meets energy-efficiency standards set by the EPA and U.S. Department of Energy. Adjust the controls on your new appliances so they do not run at full power all the time. This will help curb unnecessary energy usage and lower the cost of your monthly energy bills. Better yet, consider unplugging items such as iPods, TVs, laptops, desktop computers, hair dryers, and cell phones, all of which still consume energy when not in use.

So what about your computer? While in school, you will probably use it for everything from checking your e-mail to writing your papers. Fortunately, you have many options to help you make better energy-conserving choices when it comes to your computer use. When buying your computer, always look for the Energy Star logo. (Go to www.energystar.gov/index.cfm?c=news.nr_dormroom&Layout=print for more information about creating an Energy Star dorm room.)

Consider buying a laptop rather than a desktop computer, as laptops use less energy. You can also set your computer to sleep or hibernate mode when not in use. When you look for a printer, choose one that prints double-sided, which will help reduce the amount of paper you use. Do not print unnecessary documents, and make sure you recycle used paper—don't just throw it away.

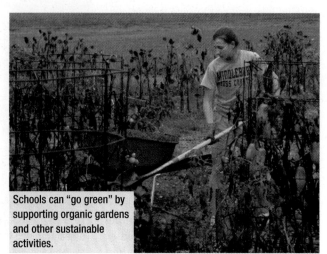

Schools can "go green" by supporting organic gardens and other sustainable activities.

The Ten Most Eco-Enlightened U.S. Colleges and Universities*

1. University of Colorado at Boulder
2. University of Washington at Seattle
3. Middlebury College (VT)
4. University of Vermont
5. College of the Atlantic (ME)
6. Evergreen State College (WA)
7. University of California at Santa Cruz
8. University of California at Berkeley
9. University of California at Los Angeles
10. Oberlin College (OH)

*As ranked by the Sierra Club in their third annual Cool Schools list.

Source: Sierra Club, "Cool Schools: Third Annual List," *Sierra Magazine* September 2009, www.sierraclub.org/sierra/200909/coolschools.

Waste Less Water!

IN THE KITCHEN

* Turn off the tap while washing dishes.
* Check faucets and pipes for leaks. Leaky faucets can waste more than 3,000 gallons of water each year.
* Equip faucets with aerators to reduce water use by 4 percent.
* Run dishwashers only when they are full, and use the energy-saving mode.

IN THE LAUNDRY ROOM

* Wash only full laundry loads.
* Upgrade to a high-efficiency washing machine to use 30 percent less water per load.

IN THE BATHROOM

* Detect and fix leaks. A leaky toilet can waste about 200 gallons of water every day.
* Take showers instead of baths and limit showers to the time it takes to lather up and rinse off.
* Replace old showerheads with new efficient models that use 60 percent less water per minute.
* Turn off the tap while brushing your teeth to save up to 8 gallons of water per day.
* Replace your old toilet with a high-efficiency model that uses 60 percent less water per flush.

law that ensures the quality of Americans' drinking water. Under SDWA, the EPA sets standards for drinking water quality and oversees the states, localities, and water suppliers who implement those standards. Cities and municipalities have strict policies and procedures governing water treatment, filtration, and disinfection to screen out pathogens and microorganisms.

Congress has coined two terms, *point source* and *nonpoint source,* to describe the general sources of water pollution. **Point source pollutants** enter a waterway at a specific location through a pipe, ditch, culvert, or other conduit. The two major sources of point source pollution are sewage treatment plants and industrial facilities. **Nonpoint source pollutants**—commonly known as *runoff* and *sedimentation*—drain or seep into waterways from broad areas of land rather than through a discrete conduit. Nonpoint source pollution results from a variety of human land use practices. It includes soil erosion and sedimentation, construction wastes, pesticide and fertilizer runoff, urban street runoff, acid mine drainage, wastes from engineering projects, leakage from septic tanks, and sewage sludge. Among the pollutants causing the most concern and the greatest potential harm are the following:

- **Gasoline and petroleum products.** There are more than 2 million underground storage tanks for gasoline and petroleum products in the United States, most of which are located at gasoline filling stations. One-quarter of them are thought to be leaking after years of corrosion.

- **Chemical contaminants.** *Organic solvents* are chemicals designed to dissolve grease and oil. These extremely toxic substances are used to clean clothing, painting equipment, plastics, and metal parts. Many household products (e.g., stain and spot removers, degreasers, drain cleaners, septic system cleaners, and paint removers) also contain these toxic chemicals. Organic solvents work their way into the water supply in different ways. Consumers often dump leftover products into the toilet or into street drains. Industries pour leftovers into large barrels, which are then buried. After a while, the chemicals eat through the barrels and leach into groundwater.

- **Polychlorinated biphenyls.** Fire resistant and stable at high temperatures, **polychlorinated biphenyls (PCBs)** were used for many years as insulating materials in high-voltage electrical equipment, such as transformers and older fluorescent lights. The human body does not excrete ingested PCBs but rather stores them in fatty tissues and the liver (i.e., they *bioaccumulate*). Exposure to PCBs is associated with birth defects, cancer, and various skin problems. The manufacture of PCBs was discontinued in the United States in 1977, but approximately 500 million pounds of them have been dumped into landfills and waterways, where they continue to pose an environmental threat.[32]

- **Dioxins. Dioxins** are chlorinated hydrocarbons found in herbicides (chemicals that are used to kill vegetation) and are produced during certain industrial processes. Dioxins have the ability to bioaccumulate and are much more toxic than PCBs. Long-term effects include possible damage to the immune system and increased risk of infections and cancer. Exposure to high concentrations of PCBs or dioxins for a short period of time can also have severe consequences, including nausea, vomiting, diarrhea, painful rashes and sores, and chloracne, an ailment in which the skin develops hard, black, painful pimples that may never go away.

- **Pesticides. Pesticides** are chemicals that are designed to kill insects, rodents, plants, and fungi. There are over 1,055 active ingredients sold as pesticides, marketed as thousands of products sold in stores throughout the world.[33] Americans use more than 1.2 billion pounds of pesticides each year, but only 10 percent actually reach the targeted organisms. The other 90 percent settle on the land and in our air and water. Pesticides evaporate readily, often being dispersed by winds over a large area or carried to the sea. This is particularly true in tropical regions, where many farmers use pesticides heavily and the climate promotes their rapid release into the

point source pollutants Pollutants that enter waterways at a specific point.
nonpoint source pollutants Pollutants that run off or seep into waterways from broad areas of land.
polychlorinated biphenyls (PCBs) Toxic chemicals that were once used as insulating materials in high-voltage electrical equipment.
dioxins Highly toxic chlorinated hydrocarbons contained in herbicides and produced during certain industrial processes.
pesticides Chemicals that kill pests, such as insects or rodents.

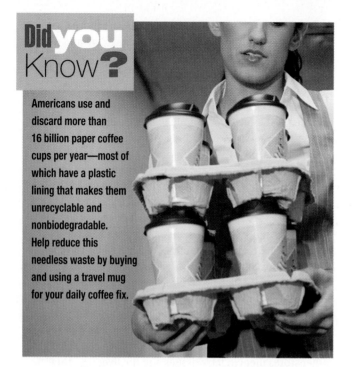

Did you Know?

Americans use and discard more than 16 billion paper coffee cups per year—most of which have a plastic lining that makes them unrecyclable and nonbiodegradable. Help reduce this needless waste by buying and using a travel mug for your daily coffee fix.

atmosphere. Pesticide residues cling to fresh fruits and vegetables and can accumulate in the body when people eat these items. Potential hazards associated with exposure to pesticides include birth defects, liver and kidney damage, and nervous system disorders.

● **Lead.** Lead can sometimes leach into tapwater from lead pipes or water lines, usually in older homes. The EPA has issued new standards to dramatically reduce the levels of lead in drinking water. The new rules stipulate that tap water lead values must not exceed 15 parts per billion (ppb). (The previous standard allowed an average lead level of 50 ppb.) If lead is present in your home's water, you can reduce your risk by running tap water for several minutes before taking a drink or cooking with it. This flushes out water that has been standing overnight in lead-contaminated lines.

municipal solid waste (MSW)
Solid waste such as durable goods; nondurable goods; containers and packaging; food waste; yard waste; and miscellaneous waste from residential, commercial, institutional, and industrial sources.

Land Pollution

Much of the waste that ends up polluting the water starts out polluting the land. The more people there are on the planet, the more waste they create, and the more pressure is put on the land to accommodate increasing amounts of refuse, much of which is nonbiodegradable, and some of which is directly harmful to living organisms.

Solid Waste

Each day, every person in the United States generates more than 4.62 pounds of **municipal solid waste (MSW)** more commonly known as trash or garbage—containers and packaging; discarded food; yard debris; and refuse from residential,

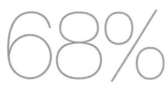 **of all MSW in the United States is burned or buried in landfills.**

commercial, institutional, and industrial sources (Figure 15.5).[34] The total comes to over 254 million tons of MSW each year.[35] Although experts believe that up to 90 percent of our trash is recyclable, we still fall far short of this goal with respect to most types of trash (Figure 15.6). Currently in the United States, 32 percent of all MSW is recovered and recycled or composted, 14 percent is burned at combustion facilities, and the remaining 54 percent is disposed of in landfills.[36]

The number of landfills in the United States has actually decreased in the past decade, but their sheer mass has increased. Many people worry that we are rapidly losing our ability to dispose of all of the waste we create. As communities run out of landfill space, it is becoming more common to haul garbage out to sea to dump, where it contaminates ocean ecosystems, or to ship it to landfills in developing countries, where it becomes someone else's problem. In today's throw-away society, we need to become aware of the amount of waste we generate every day and to look for ways to recycle, reuse, and—most desirable of all—reduce what we consume.

Communities, businesses, and individuals can adopt several strategies to control the growing MSW:

● **Source reduction** (*waste prevention*) involves altering the design, manufacture, or use of products and materials to reduce the amount and toxicity of what gets thrown away.

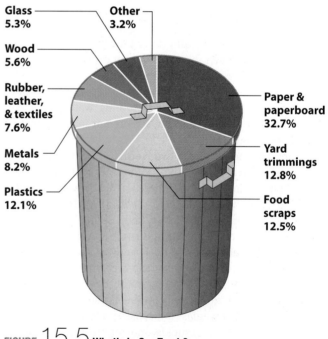

Glass 5.3%
Other 3.2%
Wood 5.6%
Rubber, leather, & textiles 7.6%
Metals 8.2%
Plastics 12.1%
Paper & paperboard 32.7%
Yard trimmings 12.8%
Food scraps 12.5%

FIGURE 15.5 **What's in Our Trash?**

Source: Data are from U.S. Environmental Protection Agency, *Municipal Solid Waste Generation, Recycling, and Disposal in the United States: Facts and Figures for 2007*, EPA-503-F-08-018 (Washington, DC: EPA, 2008), www.epa.gov/epawaste/nonhaz/municipal/msw99.htm.

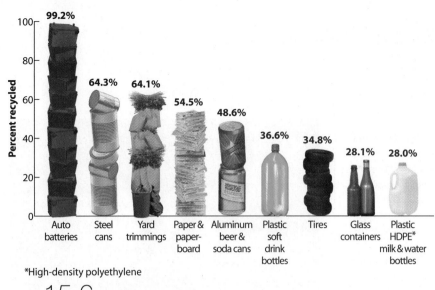

*High-density polyethylene

FIGURE 15.6 **How Much Do We Recycle?**

Source: Data are from U.S. Environmental Protection Agency, *Municipal Solid Waste Generation, Recycling, and Disposal in the United States: Facts and Figures for 2007*, EPA-530-F-08-018 (Washington, DC: EPA, 2008), www.epa.gov/epawaste/nonhaz/municipal/msw99.htm.

The most effective MSW-reducing strategy is to prevent waste from ever being generated in the first place.

● **Recycling** involves sorting, collecting, and processing materials to be reused in manufacturing new products. This process diverts items such as paper, glass, plastic, and metals from the waste stream.

● **Composting** involves collecting organic waste, such as food scraps and yard trimmings, and allowing it to decompose with the help of microorganisms (mainly bacteria and fungi). This process produces a humus-like substance that is suitable for use in gardens and for soil enhancement.

● **Combustion with energy recovery** typically involves the use of boilers and industrial furnaces to generate energy and material recovery or incinerators, which primarily destroy waste but can also recover waste for material use.

what do you think?

Do you know anyone who throws items away rather than recycles them? ● What do you think motivates their behavior? ● What might encourage them to recycle more than they do now?

Hazardous Waste

Hazardous waste is defined as waste with properties that make it capable of harming human health or the environment. In 1980, the *Comprehensive Environmental Response and Liability Act,* known as the **Superfund,** was enacted to provide funds for cleaning up hazardous waste dump sites that endanger public health and land. This fund is financed through taxes on the chemical and petroleum industries (87%) and through general federal tax revenues (13%). To date, 32,500 potentially hazardous waste sites have been identified across the nation, and 90 percent of these have been cleared or "recovered." Currently there are 50 priority sites being actively cleared, with thousands more sites, costing billions of dollars, possible for future clean up.[37] Newer technologies for cleanup are being investigated, including nanotechnologies that could reduce these costs by as much as 75 percent.

The large number of hazardous waste dump sites in the United States indicates the severity of our toxic chemical problem. American manufacturers generate more than 1 ton of chemical waste per person per year (approximately 275 million tons). Many wastes are now banned from land disposal or are being treated to reduce their toxicity before they become part of land disposal sites. The EPA has developed protective requirements for land disposal facilities, such as double liners, detection systems for substances that may leach into groundwater, and groundwater monitoring systems.

Radiation

Radiation is energy that travels in waves or particles. There are many different types of radiation, ranging from radio waves to gamma rays, all making up the electromagnetic spectrum. Exposure to radiation is an inescapable part of life on this planet, and only some of it poses a threat to human health.

Nonionizing Radiation

Nonionizing radiation is radiation at the lower end of the electromagnetic spectrum. This radiation moves in relatively long wavelengths and has enough energy to move atoms around, or cause them to vibrate, but not enough to remove electrons or alter molecular structure. Examples of nonionizing radiation are radio waves, TV signals, microwaves, infrared waves, and visible light.

Concerns have been raised about the safety of the radio frequency waves generated by cell phones, discussed in the **Consumer Health** box on page 468. The potential for exploiting fearful consumers is probably greater than the real hazard to health from this nonionizing form of exposure.

Ionizing Radiation

Ionizing radiation is caused by the release of particles and electromagnetic rays from atomic

hazardous waste Waste that, because of its toxic properties, poses a hazard to humans or to the environment.

Superfund Fund established under the Comprehensive Environmental Response Compensation and Liability Act to be used for cleaning up toxic waste dumps.

nonionizing radiation Electromagnetic waves having relatively long wavelengths and enough energy to move atoms around, or cause them to vibrate.

ionizing radiation Electromagnetic waves and particles having short wavelengths and energy high enough to ionize atoms.

ARE CELL PHONES HAZARDOUS TO YOUR HEALTH?

Although everyone today seems to have a cell phone, most users are unaware that their phone may pose a health risk. Depending on how close the cell phone antenna is to the head, as much as 60 percent of the microwave radiation emitted by the phone may actually penetrate the area around the head, some of it reaching an inch to an inch-and-a-half into the brain.

At high power levels, radio-frequency energy (the energy used in cell phones) can rapidly heat biological tissue and cause damage. However, cell phones operate at power levels well below the level at which such heating occurs. Many countries, including the United States and most European nations, use standards set by the Federal Communications Commission (FCC) for radio-frequency energy based on research by several scientific groups. These groups identified a whole-body *specific absorption rate (SAR)*

value for exposure to radio-frequency energy. Four watts per kilogram was identified as a threshold level of exposure at which harmful biological effects may occur. The FCC requires wireless phones to comply with a safety limit of 1.6 watts per kg.

The U.S. Food and Drug Administration, the World Health Organization, and other major health agencies agree that the research to date has not shown radio-frequency energy emitted from cell phones to be harmful. However, they also point to the need for more research, because cell phones have only been in widespread use for less than two decades, and no long-term studies have been done to determine that cell phones are risk free. Three large studies have compared cell phone use among brain cancer patients and individuals free of brain cancer, finding no correlation between cell phone use and brain tumors. However,

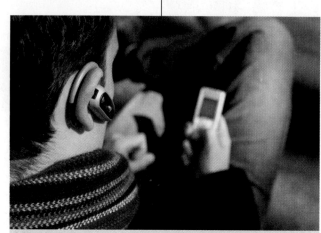

A hands-free device lets you keep your phone—and any radio-frequency energy it may emit—away from your head.

preliminary results from smaller, well-designed studies have continued to raise questions.

To lower any potential risk of problems related to cell phone use, limit your cell phone usage, and purchase a hands-free device that keeps the phone farther from your head. Use landlines whenever possible, or send a text message or e-mail rather than talking on the phone. In addition, check the SAR level of your phone (for

instructions, see www.fcc.gov/cgb/sar). Purchase one with a lower level if yours is near the FCC limit.

Sources: Committee on Identification of Research Needs Relating to Potential Biological or Adverse Health Effects of Wireless Communications Devices, National Research Council (Washington, DC: National Academies Press, 2008); American Cancer Society, "Cellular Phones," 2008, www.cancer.org/docroot/PED/content/PED_1_3X_Cellular_Phones.asp.

nuclei during the normal process of disintegration. This type of radiation has enough energy to remove electrons from the atoms it passes through. Some naturally occurring elements, such as uranium, emit ionizing radiation. The sun is another source of ionizing radiation, in the form of high-frequency ultraviolet rays—those against which the ozone layer protects us.

Reactions to radiation differ from person to person. Exposure is measured in **radiation absorbed doses,** or **rads** (also called *roentgens*). Radiation can cause damage at dosages as low as 100 to 200 rads. At this level, signs of radiation sickness include nausea, diarrhea, fatigue, anemia, sore throat, and hair loss. At 350 to 500 rads, these symptoms become more severe, and death may result because the radiation hinders bone marrow production of the white blood cells we need to protect us from disease. Dosages above 600 to 700 rads are invariably fatal.

radiation absorbed doses (rads)
Units that measure exposure to radioactivity.

Recommended maximum "safe" dosages range from 0.5 to 5 rads per year. Approximately 50 percent of the radiation to which we are exposed comes from natural sources, such as building materials. Another 45 percent comes from medical and dental X rays. The remaining 5 percent is nonionizing radiation that comes from such sources as computer monitors, microwave ovens, television sets, and radar screens. Most of us are exposed to far less radiation than the safe maximum dosage per year. The effects of long-term exposure to relatively low levels of radiation are unknown. Some scientists believe that such exposure can cause lung cancer, leukemia, skin cancer, bone cancer, and skeletal deformities.

Nuclear Power Plants

Although nuclear power plants account for less than 1 percent of the total radiation to which we are exposed, the number of plants may increase in the next decade. Proponents of nuclear energy believe that it is a safe and efficient way to generate electricity. Initial costs of building nuclear power plants are high, but actual power generation is relatively inexpensive. A 1,000-megawatt reactor produces enough energy for 650,000 homes and saves 420 million gallons of fossil fuels each year. In some areas where nuclear power plants were decommissioned, electricity bills tripled when power companies turned to hydroelectric or fossil fuel sources to generate electricity. Nuclear reactors discharge fewer carbon oxides into the air than fossil fuel–powered generators. Advocates believe that converting to nuclear power could help slow global warming.

The advantages of nuclear energy must be weighed against the disadvantages. Currently, disposal of nuclear waste is extremely problematic. In addition, a reactor core meltdown could pose serious threats to a plant's immediate environment and to the world in general. A **nuclear meltdown** occurs when the temperature in the core of a nuclear reactor increases enough to melt both the nuclear fuel and the containment vessel that holds it. Most modern facilities seal their reactors and containment vessels in concrete buildings with pools of cold water on the bottom. If a meltdown occurs, the building and the pool are supposed to prevent the escape of radioactivity.

One serious nuclear accident in particular contributed to a steep decline in public support for nuclear energy: the 1986 reactor core fire and explosion at the Chernobyl nuclear power plant in Russia, which killed 48 people, hospitalized another 200, and led officials to evacuate towns near the plant. Some medical workers estimate that the eventual death toll from radiation-induced cancers related to the Chernobyl incident topped 100,000.

Noise Pollution

Our bodies have definite physiological responses to noise, and it can become a source of physical and mental distress. Sounds are measured in decibels. A sound with a decibel level of 110 is 10 times louder than one at 100 decibels (dB). A jet takeoff from 200 feet has a noise level of approximately 140 dB, whereas the human voice in normal conversation has a level of about 60 dB (Figure 15.7). Short-term exposure to loud noise reduces productivity and concentration and may affect mental and emotional health. Symptoms of noise-related distress include disturbed sleep patterns, headaches, and tension. Prolonged exposure to loud noise can lead to hearing loss; the risks depend on both the decibel level and the length of exposure.

Unfortunately, despite increasing awareness that noise pollution is more than just a nuisance, noise control programs have received low budgetary priority in the United States. According to the National Institute for Occupational Safety and Health, 30 million Americans are exposed to haz-

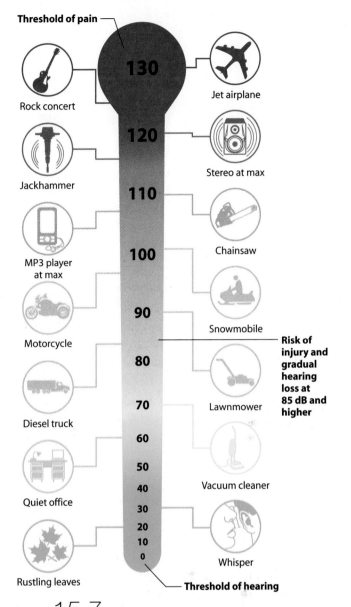

Threshold of pain

130 — Rock concert / Jet airplane

120 — Jackhammer / Stereo at max

110 — Chainsaw

100 — MP3 player at max

90 — Snowmobile

80 — Motorcycle / Lawnmower

70 — Diesel truck

60

50 — Vacuum cleaner

40 — Quiet office

30

20

10

0 — Whisper

Rustling leaves

Threshold of hearing

Risk of injury and gradual hearing loss at 85 dB and higher

FIGURE 15.7 **Noise Levels of Various Sounds (dB)** Decibels increase logarithmically, so each increase of 10 db represents a tenfold increase in loudness.

Source: Adapted from National Institute on Deafness and Other Communication Disorders, "How Loud Is Too Loud? Bookmark," 2006, www.nidcd.nih.gov/health/hearing/ruler.asp.

ardous noise at work, and 10 million suffer from permanent hearing loss.[38] Clearly, to protect your hearing, you must take it upon yourself to avoid voluntary and involuntary exposure to excessive noise. Playing stereos in your car and home at reasonable levels, keeping the volume down on your iPod, wearing earplugs when you use power equipment, and establishing barriers such as closed windows between you and noise will help keep your hearing intact.

nuclear meltdown An accident that results when the temperature in the core of a nuclear reactor increases enough to melt the nuclear fuel and the containment vessel housing it.

Are You Doing All You Can to Protect The Environment?

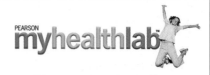

Fill out this assessment online at www.pearsonhighered.com/myhealthlab or www.pearsonhighered.com/donatelle.

Environmental problems often seem too big for one person to make a difference. Each day, though, there are things you can do that contribute to the planet's health. For each statement below, indicate how commonly you follow the described behavior.

		Always	Usually	Sometimes	Never
1.	Whenever possible, I walk or ride my bicycle rather than drive a car.	1	2	3	4
2.	I carpool with others to school or work.	1	2	3	4
3.	I have my car tuned up and inspected every year.	1	2	3	4
4.	When I change the oil in my car, I make sure the oil is properly recycled, rather than dumped on the ground or into a floor drain.	1	2	3	4
5.	I avoid using the air conditioner except in extreme conditions.	1	2	3	4
6.	I turn off the lights when a room is not being used.	1	2	3	4
7.	I take a shower rather than a bath most of the time.	1	2	3	4
8.	I have water-saving devices installed on my shower, toilet, and sinks.	1	2	3	4
9.	I make sure faucets and toilets in my home do not leak.	1	2	3	4
10.	I use my bath towels more than once before putting them in the wash.	1	2	3	4
11.	I wear my clothes more than once between washings when possible.	1	2	3	4
12.	I make sure that the washing machine is full before I wash a load of clothes.	1	2	3	4
13.	I purchase biodegradable soaps and detergents.	1	2	3	4
14.	I use biodegradable trash bags.	1	2	3	4
15.	At home, I use dishes and silverware rather than Styrofoam or plastic.	1	2	3	4
16.	When I buy prepackaged foods, I choose the ones with the least packaging.	1	2	3	4
17.	I do not subscribe to newspapers and magazines that I can view online.	1	2	3	4
18.	I do not use a hair dryer.	1	2	3	4
19.	I recycle plastic bags that I get when I bring something home from the store.	1	2	3	4
20.	I don't run water continuously when washing the dishes, shaving, or brushing my teeth.	1	2	3	4
21.	I use unbleached or recycled paper.	1	2	3	4
22.	I use both sides of printer paper and other paper when possible.	1	2	3	4
23.	If I have items I do not want to use anymore, I donate them to charity so someone else can use them.	1	2	3	4
24.	I carry a reusable mug for my coffee or tea and have it filled rather than using a new paper cup each time I buy a hot beverage.	1	2	3	4
25.	I carry and use a refillable water bottle rather than frequently buying bottled water.	1	2	3	4
26.	I clean up after myself while enjoying the outdoors (picnicking, camping, etc.).	1	2	3	4
27.	I volunteer for cleanup days in the community in which I live.	1	2	3	4
28.	I consider candidates' positions on environmental issues before casting my vote.	1	2	3	4

For Further Thought

Review your scores. Are your responses mostly 1s and 2s? If not, what actions can you take to become more environmentally responsible? Are there ways to help the environment on this list that you had not thought of before? Are there behaviors not on the list that you are already doing?

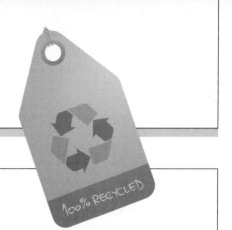

100% RECYCLED

YOUR PLAN FOR CHANGE

The **Assess yourself** activity gave you the chance to look at your behavior and consider ways to conserve energy, save water, reduce waste, and otherwise help protect the planet. Now that you have considered these results, you can take steps to become more environmentally responsible.

Today, you can:

◯ Find out how much energy you are using. Visit www.carbonfund.org, www.carbonoffsets.org, or www.greatest planet.org to find out what your carbon footprint is and to learn about projects you can support to offset your own emissions and energy usage. New carbon offset programs and organizations are popping up all the time, so watch for other opportunities to counter your carbon usage.

◯ Reduce the amount of paper waste in your mailbox. You can stop junk mail, such as credit card offers and unwanted catalogs, by visiting the Direct Marketing Association's Mail Preference Service site at www.dmachoice.org. You can also call 1-888-5 OPT OUT to put an end to unwanted mail. In addition, the website www.catalogchoice.org is a free service that lets you decline paper catalogs you no longer want to receive.

Within the next 2 weeks, you can:

◯ Look into joining an on-campus environmental group, attending an environmental campus event, or taking an environmental science course.

◯ Take part in a local cleanup day or recycling drives. These can be fun opportunities to meet like-minded people while benefiting the planet.

By the end of the semester, you can:

◯ Start a compost pile for all your organic waste. You don't need a yard to do this; the EPA provides information on setting up an indoor compost bin at www.epa.gov/epawaste/conserve/rrr/composting/by_compost.htm.

◯ Make a habit of recycling everything you can rather than adding things to the trash. Find out what items can be recycled in your neighborhood and designate a box or trash can in your apartment or dorm to hold recyclable materials—cans, bottles, newspapers, junk mail, and so on—until you can carry them out to the curbside bins or a drop-off center.

◯ Work to influence the environment on a larger scale. Take part in an environmental activism group on campus or in your community. Listen carefully to what political candidates say about the environment. Let your legislators know how you feel about environmental issues and that you will vote according to their record on the issues.

Summary

* Population growth is the single largest factor affecting the environment. Demand for more food, water, and energy—as well as places to dispose of waste—places great strain on Earth's resources.

* The primary constituents of air pollution are sulfur dioxide, particulate matter, carbon monoxide, nitrogen dioxide, ozone, carbon dioxide, and hydrocarbons. Indoor air pollution is caused primarily by tobacco smoke, woodstove smoke, furnace emissions, asbestos, formaldehyde, radon, lead, and mold. Pollution is depleting Earth's protective ozone layer and contributing to global warming by enhancing the greenhouse effect.

* Water pollution can be caused by either point sources (direct entry) or nonpoint sources (runoff or seepage). Major contributors to water pollution include petroleum products, organic solvents, PCBs, dioxins, pesticides, and lead.

* Solid waste pollution includes household trash, plastics, glass, metal products, and paper. Limited landfill space creates problems. Hazardous waste is toxic; improper disposal creates health hazards for people in surrounding communities.

* Nonionizing radiation comes from electromagnetic fields, such as those around power lines. Ionizing radiation results from the natural erosion of atomic nuclei. The disposal and storage of radioactive waste from nuclear power plants pose potential problems for public health.

* Noise pollution can affect productivity, and lead to physical symptoms including hearing loss.

Pop Quiz

1. The United States is responsible for what percentage of total global resource consumption?
   a. 10 percent
   b. 25 percent
   c. 50 percent
   d. 70 percent

2. The single biggest influence on zero population growth is
   a. income.
   b. gender.
   c. education.
   d. ethnicity.

3. One possible source of indoor air pollution is a gas present in some carpets called
   a. lead.
   b. asbestos.
   c. radon.
   d. formaldehyde.

4. What substance separates into stringy fibers, embeds itself in lungs, and causes mesothelioma?
   a. asbestos
   b. particulate matter
   c. radon
   d. formaldehyde

5. The terms *point source* and *nonpoint source* are used to describe the two general sources of
   a. water pollution.
   b. air pollution.
   c. noise pollution.
   d. ozone depletion.

6. The air pollutant that originates primarily from motor vehicle emissions is
   a. particulates.
   b. nitrogen dioxide.
   c. sulfur dioxide.
   d. carbon monoxide.

7. Which gas is considered radioactive and could become cancer causing when it seeps into a home?
   a. carbon monoxide
   b. radon
   c. hydrogen sulfide
   d. natural gas

8. The phenomenon that creates a barrier to protect us from the sun's harmful ultraviolet radiation rays is
   a. photochemical smog.
   b. ozone layer.
   c. gray air smog.
   d. greenhouse effect.

9. Intensity (exposure) to sound is measured in
   a. foot candles.
   b. noise volume.
   c. hertz.
   d. decibels.

10. Some herbicides contain toxic substances called
    a. THMs.
    b. PCPs.
    c. dioxins.
    d. PCBs.

Answers for these questions can be found on page A-1.

Think about It!

1. How are the rapid increases in global population and consumption of resources related? Is population control the best solution? Why or why not?

2. What are the primary sources of air pollution? What can be done to reduce air pollution?

3. What are the causes and consequences of global warming? What can individuals do to reduce the threat of global warming?

4. What are point and nonpoint sources of water pollution? What can be done to reduce or prevent water pollution?

5. How do you think communities and governments could encourage recycling efforts in the United States?

6. What are the physiological consequences of noise pollution? How can you lessen your exposure to it?

Accessing Your Health on the Internet

The following websites explore further topics and issues related to personal health. For links to the websites below, visit the Companion Website for *Health: The Basics,* Green Edition at www.pearsonhighered.com/donatelle.

1. *Environmental Literacy Council.* This website is an excellent source of information about environmental issues in general. Topics range from how the ozone layer works to why the rain forests are important ecosystems. www.enviroliteracy.org

2. *Environmental Protection Agency (EPA).* The EPA is the government agency responsible for overseeing environmental regulation and protection issues in the United States. www.epa.gov

3. *National Center for Environmental Health (NCEH).* This site provides information on a wide variety of environmental health issues, including a series of helpful fact sheets. www.cdc.gov/nceh

4. *National Environmental Health Association (NEHA).* This organization provides educational resources and opportunities for environmental health professionals. www.neha.org

References

1. R. Caplan, *Our Earth, Ourselves* (New York: Bantam, 1990), 247.
2. R. H. Friis, *Essentials of Environmental Health* (Boston: Jones and Bartlett, 2007), 7.
3. Population Reference Bureau, "2009 World Population Data Sheet," www.prb.org/ Publications/Datasheets/2009/2009wpds .aspx.
4. United Nations, *Global Environment Outlook: Environment for Development (GEO-4)* (United Nations Environment Programme, 2007), www.unep.org/geo/ geo4/media.
5. U.S. Census Bureau, "U.S. and World Population Clocks," 2008, www.census.gov/ main/www/popclock.html.
6. Ibid.
7. V. Markham, "U.S. Population, Energy and Climate Change," 2009, Center for Environment and Population, www.cepnet .org/documents/USPopulationEnergyand ClimateChangeReportCEP.pdf.
8. Ibid.
9. Ibid.
10. Ibid.
11. U.S. Environmental Protection Agency, "Mobile Source Emissions—Past, Present and Future," 2008, www.epa.gov/otaq/ invntory/overview/pollutants/index.htm.
12. American Lung Association, "State of the Air. 2009 Health Risks Overview," www .stateoftheair.org/2009/health-risks/ overview.html.
13. U.S. Environmental Protection Agency, "SO_2—How Sulfur Dioxide Affects the Way We Live and Breathe," 2008, www.epa.gov/ air/sulfurdioxide.
14. E. Lavonas, "Focus On: Carbon Monoxide Poisoning," American College of Emergency Physicians, 2007, www3.acep.org/ publications.aspx?id=26590.
15. V. Markham, "U.S. Population, Energy and Climate Change," 2009.
16. U.S. Environmental Protection Agency, "The Inside Story: A Guide to Indoor Air Quality," 2009, www.epa.gov/iaq/pubs/ insidest.html.
17. Ibid.
18. National Cancer Institute, "Lung Cancer Prevention (PDQ)," 2007, www.cancer.gov/ cancertopics/pdq/prevention/lung/ healthprofessional.
19. Environmental Protection Agency, "U.S. Homes above EPA's Radon Action Level," 2009, http://cfpub.epa.gov/eroe/index .cfm?fuseaction=detail.viewInd&lv=list .listByAlpha&r=201747.
20. Centers for Disease Control Lead Prevention Program, 2009, www.cdc.gov/ nceh/lead.
21. National Center for Environmental Health, "Environmental Hazards and Health Effects: Mold," 2009, www.cdc.gov/mold.
22. U.S. Environmental Protection Agency, *Questions and Answers on Ozone Depletion* (Washington, DC: Stratospheric Protection Division, 2008).
23. S. Arrhenius, "On the Influence of Carbonic Acid in the Air upon the Temperature of the Ground," *Philosophical Magazine and Journal of Science* (fifth series) 41 (1896): 237–75.
24. U.S. Environmental Protection Agency, "Climate Change: Basic Information," 2007, http://epa.gov/climatechange/ basicinfo.html.
25. U.S. General Accounting Office, *Climate Change: Trends in Greenhouse Gas Emissions and Emissions Intensity in the United States and Other High-Emitting Nations,* GAQ04.146R, 2003.
26. United Nations Framework Convention on Climate Change, "Kyoto Protocol," 2007, http://unfccc.int/kyoto_protocol/items/ 2830.php.
27. D. Malakoff and E. M. Williams, "Q & A: An Examination of the Kyoto Protocol," NPR.org (June 6, 2007), www.npr.org/templates/story/story.php ?storyId=5042766.
28. World Health Organization, "World in Danger of Missing Sanitation Target; Drinking-Water Target Also at Risk, New Report Shows," 2006, www.who.int/ mediacentre/news/releases/2006/ pr47/en.
29. R. H. Friis, *Essentials of Environmental Health,* 2007, 204.
30. V. Markham, "U.S. National Report on Population and the Environment," 2006, Center for Environment and Population, www.cepnet.org/documents/ USNatlReptFinal_000.pdf.
31. U.S. Geological Survey, "National Reconnaissance of Pharmaceuticals, Hormones, and Other Organic Wastewater Contaminants in Streams of the U.S., 1999–2000," 2006, http://toxics.usgs.gov/regional/ emc_surfacewater.html.
32. Agency for Toxic Substances and Disease Registry (ATSDR), "Polychlorinated Biphenyls (PCBs)," 2009, www.atsdr .cdc.gov/substances/toxsubstance.asp? toxid=26.
33. U.S. Environmental Protection Agency, "Assessing Health Risks of Pesticides," 2007, www.epa.gov/pesticides/factsheets/ riskassess.htm.
34. U.S. Environmental Protection Agency, "Municipal Solid Waste: Basic Facts," 2007, www.epa.gov/msw/facts.htm.
35. U.S. Environmental Protection Agency, "Municipal Solid Waste in the United States—Facts and Figures," 2007, www .epa.gov/osw/nonhaz/municipal/pubs/ msw07-rpt.pdf.
36. Ibid.
37. U.S. Environmental Protection Agency, "Superfund National Accomplishments Summary, 2008," 2009. www.epa.gov/ superfund/accomp/numbers08.htm.
38. National Institute for Occupational Safety and Health, "Noise and Hearing Loss Prevention: At-Work Solutions for Noise," 2009, www.cdc.gov/niosh/topics/noise/ solutions/atworkSolutions.html.

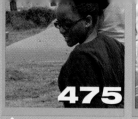

475

How many college students focus on their spiritual health?

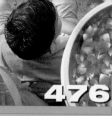

476

Is spirituality the same as religion?

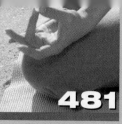

478

Does spirituality influence health?

481

Is meditation boring?

FOCUS ON Your Spiritual Health

Lia's favorite spot on campus is the secluded Japanese garden on the south side of the library. Whether she's feeling stressed about exams or is mulling over an important decision, a few minutes alone in the garden always seem to help. Sometimes she sits quietly and watches the birds come and go. Sometimes she gets out her camera and photographs particularly brilliant blossoms. Often she simply rests, eyes closed, feeling the sun's warmth on her face, and lets her thoughts turn to gratitude for her health, her loving family, and her opportunity to study. However she spends it, her "garden break" leaves Lia feeling refreshed and refocused, with greater confidence in her ability to tackle the challenges of her day.

Lia's desire to cultivate meaning and harmony in her life is shared by a majority of American college students. According to UCLA's Higher Education Research Institute, although undergraduates' religious attendance declines during the college years, they show significant growth in a wide spectrum of spiritual and ethical considerations.[1] Data from nearly 15,000 students at more than 136 colleges and universities (taken as they entered college in the fall of 2004 and again as they prepared for their senior year in 2007) found that interest in the following goals increased by more than 10 percent during the college years, to levels representing more than half of all students surveyed:

● Attaining inner harmony
● Developing a meaningful philosophy of life
● Seeking beauty in life
● Becoming a more loving person

Also, researchers found that, compared with college freshmen, juniors and seniors were more desirous of reducing pain and suffering in the world, were more thankful for all that had happened to them, and expressed higher levels of ecumenical worldviews—that is, views expressing tolerance and respect for other religions and philosophies—and a

A secluded garden can be an ideal spot for quiet contemplation and spiritual renewal.

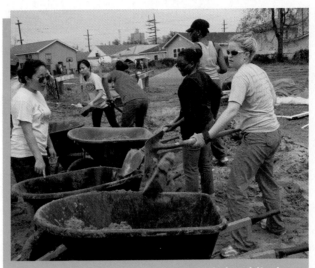

How many college students focus on their spiritual health?

Spiritual and ethical concerns are important to a majority of American college students. For example, more than 80% of college seniors desire to become a more loving person. One of the ways college students express their spirituality is by working to reduce suffering in the world; many contribute their time and skills to volunteer organizations, like these students working to build homes for Habitat for Humanity.

commitment to understanding other countries and cultures.

Back in Chapter 1, we identified spiritual health as one of six key dimensions of health (see Figure 1.4 on page 5). Lia's sense of wonder and respect for the natural world, her gratitude for the good things in her life, and her belief in a "universal spirit" suggest that spiritual health is an important focus of her daily life, bringing her greater self-confidence and serenity. If you're feeling as if you could use a little more of these qualities in your own life, read on: This chapter will help you explore ways to sharpen your spiritual focus.

What Is Spirituality?

From one day to the next, many of us attempt to satisfy our needs for belonging and self-esteem by acquir-

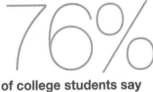

76%

of college students say they are "searching for meaning and purpose in life."

ing material possessions. But at some point we come to realize that new gadgets, clothes, or concert tickets don't necessarily make us happy or improve our sense of self-worth. That's when many of us begin to contemplate another side of ourselves: our spirituality.

But what is spirituality? It isn't easy to define. Although part of the universal human experience, it's highly personal, not to mention intangible, and so it tends to defy the boundaries that strict definitions would impose. Let's begin by exploring its root, *spirit*, which in many cultures refers to *breath*, or the force that animates life. When you're "inspired," your energy flows. You're not held back by doubts about the purpose or meaning of your work and life. Indeed, many definitions of spirituality incorporate this sense of transcendence. For example, the National Center for Complementary and Alternative Medicine (NCCAM) defines **spirituality** as an individual's sense of purpose and meaning in life, beyond material values.[2] Similarly, Harold G. Koenig, MD, one of the foremost researchers of spirituality and health, defines spirituality as the personal quest for understanding answers to ultimate questions about life, about meaning, and about our relationship with the sacred or transcendent.[3]

spirituality An individual's sense of purpose and meaning in life, beyond material values.

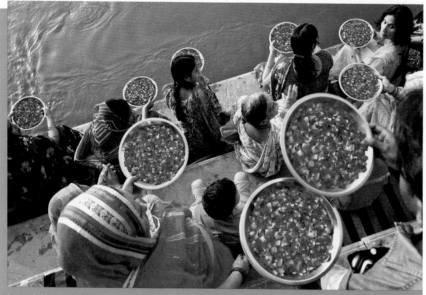

Is spirituality the same as religion?

Spirituality and religion are not the same. Many people find that religious practices, such as attending services or making offerings—like the flowers these Hindus are preparing to place in the sacred Ganges River—help them to focus on their spirituality. However, religion does not have to be part of a spiritual person's life.

Religion and Spirituality Are Distinct Concepts

Spirituality may or may not lead to participation in organized **religion,** that is, a system of beliefs, practices, rituals, and symbols designed to facilitate closeness to the sacred or transcendent.[4] In other words, although spirituality and religion do share some common elements, they are not the same thing. Most Americans consider spirituality to be important in their lives, but not necessarily in the form of religion: A recent national survey of more than 35,000 Americans revealed that 92 percent believe in some kind of "higher power," but not all of these respondents identified themselves as being affiliated with a particular religion.[5] In fact, just over 20 percent of respondents who identified themselves as atheists expressed a belief in a "higher power"! Thus, it's clear that religion does

religion A system of beliefs, practices, rituals, and symbols designed to facilitate closeness to the sacred or transcendent.

perennial philosophy The universal ideas that underlie all spiritual experience.

not have to be part of a spiritual person's life. Table 1 identifies some characteristics that can help you distinguish between religion and spirituality.

Another finding of the same survey was that 70 percent of Americans affiliated with a religious tradition agreed that other religions are also valid.[6] Perhaps this is because all major religions express the **perennial philosophy,** the universal ideas that underlie all spiritual experience. These include, for example, the recognition of a divine Reality and the unity of all beings with

this Reality. As writer and philosopher Aldous Huxley explains, the perennial philosophy has a place in every one of the higher religions.[7] It seems that a majority of Americans recognize and respect this underlying unity of spiritual ideas, expressed in different religious and spiritual practices.

Spirituality Integrates Three Facets

Brian Luke Seaward, a professor at the University of Northern Colorado and author of several books on spirituality and mind–body healing, identifies three facets of human existence that together constitute the core of human spirituality: relationships, values, and purpose in life (Figure 1).[8] Questions arising in these three domains prompt many of us to look for spiritual answers. At the same time, spiritual well-being is characterized by healthy relationships, strong personal values, and a sense that we have a meaningful purpose in life.

Relationships Have you ever wondered if someone you were attracted to is really right for you? Or, conversely, if you should break off a long-term relationship? Have you ever wished you had more friends, or that you were a better friend to yourself? Have you ever tried to make a connection with some sort of Presence or Higher Self? For many people, such questions and yearnings are natural triggers for

TABLE 1	Characteristics Distinguishing Religion and Spirituality	
Religion	**Spirituality**
Community focused	Individualistic
Observable, measurable, objective	Less measurable, more subjective
Formal, orthodox, organized	Less formal, less orthodox, less systematic
Behavior oriented, outward practices	Emotionally oriented, inwardly directed
Authoritarian in terms of behaviors	Not authoritarian, little accountability
Doctrine separating good from evil	Unifying, not doctrine oriented

Source: National Center for Complementary and Alternative Medicine (NCCAM), "Prayer and Spirituality in Health: Ancient Practices, Modern Science," *CAM at the NIH* 12, no. 1 (2005): 1–4.

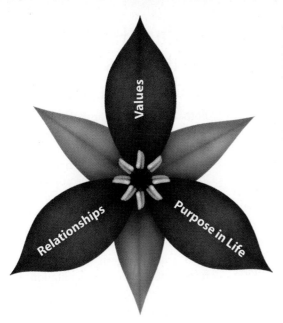

FIGURE 1 Three Facets of Spirituality

Most of us are prompted to explore our spirituality because of questions relating to our relationships, values, and purpose in life. At the same time, these three facets together constitute spiritual well-being.

spiritual growth: As we contemplate whom we should choose as a life partner or how to mend a quarrel with a friend, we begin to foster our own inner wisdom. At the same time, healthy relationships are a sign of spiritual well-being. When we treat ourselves and others with respect, honesty, integrity, and love, we are manifesting our spiritual health.

Values Our personal **values** are our principles—not only the things we say we care about, but also the things that cause us to behave the way we do. For instance, if you value honesty, then you are not likely to call in sick for work when you intend to spend the day at the beach. In other words, our value system is the set of fundamental rules by which we conduct our lives. It's what we stand for. When we attempt to clarify our values, and then to live according to those values, we're engaging in spiritual work. Spiritual health is characterized by a strong personal value system.

Meaningful Purpose in Life What have you chosen as your college major?

What career do you plan to pursue after you graduate? Do you hope to marry? Do you plan to have or adopt children? And how do these choices reflect what you hold as your purpose in life? Contemplating these questions fosters spiritual growth. People who are spiritually healthy are able to articulate their purpose, and to make choices that manifest that purpose. In thinking about your own purpose, avoid the temptation to get too ambitious, as in, "I'm here to eradicate world hunger!" Instead, try to articulate just what you see as your unique contribution to the world—something you can actually do, starting now.

Spiritual Intelligence Is an Inner Wisdom

Our relationships, values, and sense of purpose together contribute to our overall **spiritual intelligence (SI).** This term was introduced by physicist and philosopher Danah Zohar, who defined it as "the intelligence that makes us whole, that gives us our integrity. It is the soul's intelligence, the intelligence of the deep self."[9] Zohar includes qualities such as self-awareness, spontaneity, and compassion in her definition of *spiritual intelligence*, explaining that SI helps us use adversity in a positive way and live according to our values and our vision.

Since Zohar's introduction of SI, dozens of clerics, psychologists, and even business consultants have expanded on the definition. For example, Rabbi Yaacov Kravitz of the Center for Spiritual Intelligence explains that SI helps us find a moral and ethical path to help guide us through life. Similarly, psychologist Robert Emmons emphasizes the ability of people with a high level of SI to solve problems and attain goals.[10] Would you like to find out your own spiritual IQ? See the **Assess Yourself** on page 484.

What Are the Benefits of Focusing on Your Spiritual Health?

The importance of people's spirituality to their wellness and health has been widely acknowledged and is based on hundreds of published studies.[11]

Spiritual Health Contributes to Physical Health

The emerging science of mind–body medicine is a research focus of the NCCAM. One area under study is the association between spiritual health and general health and longevity. The NCCAM cites evidence of a positive influence of spirituality on health, and suggests that the connection may be due to improved immune function, cardiovascular function, and/or other physiological changes.[12] Evidence from a variety of other studies also supports this association. For example, several recent studies have found that Americans who attend religious services regularly live many years longer—on average—than those who do not. Although religious attendance is not the only variable related to spirituality that researchers have found to predict good health and long life, it is currently thought to be the most powerful.[13]

Some researchers believe that a key to understanding the improved health and longer life in spiritually healthy people is their greater self-control. That is, people who are more spiritually healthy may have an increased capacity to restrain themselves from overeating, smoking, and abusing alcohol and other drugs. They may also be

---

values Principles that influence our thoughts and emotions, and guide the choices we make in our lives.
spiritual intelligence (SI) The intelligence of the deep self; a capacity to live in alignment with our inner wisdom, values, and vision.

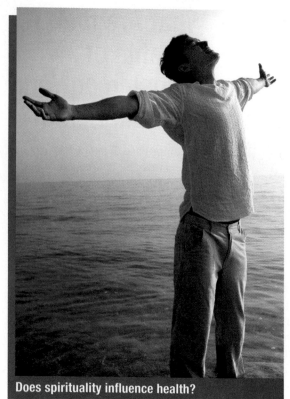

Does spirituality influence health?

Spirituality is widely acknowledged to have a positive impact on health and wellness. The benefits range from reductions in overall morbidity and mortality to improved abilities to cope with illness and stress.

more disciplined about getting adequate exercise and sleep.[14]

When we do get sick, the National Cancer Institute (NCI) contends that spiritual or religious well-being may help restore health and improve quality of life in the following ways:[15]

- By decreasing anxiety, depression, anger, discomfort, and feelings of isolation
- By decreasing alcohol and drug abuse
- By decreasing blood pressure and the risk of heart disease
- By increasing the person's ability to cope with the effects of illness and with medical treatments
- By increasing feelings of hope and optimism, freedom from regret, satisfaction with life, and inner peace

yoga A system of physical and mental training involving controlled breathing, physical postures *(asanas)*, meditation, chanting, and other practices that are believed to cultivate unity with the *Atman*, or Absolute.

Several studies show an association between spiritual health and a person's ability to cope with any of a variety of physical illnesses in addition to cancer.[16] For example, a study of people living with chronic pain and fatigue showed a benefit of spiritual health.[17] Another study of people with HIV showed a slower disease progression over a period of 4 years in people who become more spiritually focused after their diagnosis.[18]

Spiritual Health Contributes to Psychosocial Health

Current research also suggests that spiritual health contributes to psychosocial health. For instance, the NCI and independent studies have found a benefit of spirituality in reducing levels of anxiety and depression.[19] And certain spiritual practices, such as yoga, deep meditation, and prayer, can positively affect brain chemistry in much the same way that conventional antianxiety and antidepressant medications do.[20]

People who have found a spiritual community also benefit from increased social support among members. For instance, participation in religious services, charitable organizations, and social gatherings can help members avoid isolation. At such gatherings, clerics and other members may offer spiritual support on challenges that participants may be facing. Or a community may have retired members who offer child care for harried parents, meals for members with disabilities, or transportation to those needing to get to medical appointments. All such measures can contribute to members' overall feelings of security and belonging.

Spiritual Health Contributes to Reduced Stress

Both the NCCAM and the NCI cite stress reduction as one probable mechanism among spiritually healthy people for improved health and longevity, and for better coping with illness.[21] In addition, several small studies support the contention that positive religious coping supports effective stress management.[22] And a 2009 study suggests that increasing mindfulness through meditation reduces stress levels not only in people with physical and mental disorders, but in healthy people as well.[23]

What Steps Can You Take to Focus on Your Spiritual Health?

Enhancing your spiritual side takes just as much work as becoming physically fit or improving your diet. Here, we introduce some ways to develop your spiritual health by training your body, expanding your mind, tuning in, and reaching out.

Train Your Body

For thousands of years, in regions throughout the world, seekers have cultivated transcendence through physical means. One of the foremost examples is the practice of various forms of **yoga.** The word *yoga* is derived from a verb in Sanskrit, the language of ancient India, meaning "to yoke." Although in the West we think of yoga as involving controlled breathing and physical postures, traditional forms also emphasize meditation, chanting, and other practices that are believed to cultivate unity with the *Atman*, or Absolute. For example, the practices of *kundalini yoga* attempt to awaken the so-called kundalini energy, the divine energy that is said to reside at the base of the spine.

If you are interested in exploring yoga, sign up for a class on campus, at your local YMCA, or at a dedicated yoga center. Make sure you choose a form that seems right to you: Some, such as *hatha yoga*, focus on developing flexibility, deep breathing, and tranquility, whereas others, such as *ashtanga yoga*, are fast-paced and demanding, and thus more appropriate for developing physical fitness than spiritual health. (See Chapter 3 and Chapter 11 for more about individual styles of yoga.) For your first class, dress comfortably in relaxed fabrics that are somewhat close fitting so that, when you bend at the waist or lift your leg, you won't feel constricted or exposed. No shoes or socks are worn. At the beginning of the class, the instructor will likely lead you through some gentle warm-up poses, then add more challenging poses with coordinated inhalations and exhalations to align, stretch, and invigorate each region of your body. Most classes provide yoga mats to cushion your joints as you work through the postures. Your class will probably conclude with several minutes of relaxation and deep breathing.

Training your body to improve your spiritual health doesn't necessarily require you to engage in a formal practice such as yoga. By energizing your body and sharpening your mental focus, jogging, biking, aerobics, or any other exercise you do every day can contribute to your spiritual health. To transform an exercise session into a spiritual workout, begin by acknowledging gratitude for your body's strength and speed, then, throughout the session, try to maintain mindfulness of your breathing. We'll say more about mindful breathing in the discussion of meditation below.

You can also cultivate spirituality through fully engaging your body's senses. In fact, you can think of vision, hearing, taste, smell, and touch as five portals to spiritual health. Viewing an engaging piece of artwork or listening to beautiful music can calm the mind and soothe the spirit. A key reason that Lia, in our opening story, finds sustenance in nature is that she fully engages her senses—smelling the freshly cut grass, listening to the birds, and photographing the flowers.

The flip side of cultivating your senses is depriving them! Closing your eyes and sitting in silence removes the distraction of visual and auditory stimuli, helping you to focus within. To take advantage of silence, turn off your cell phone and take a long, solitary walk.

15.8 million

U.S. adults practice yoga, according to a recent survey by *Yoga Journal*.

You might even spend a weekend at one of the many retreat centers throughout the United States. To find one, see the state-by-state listing at www.SpiritSite.com.

Expand Your Mind

For many people, psychological counseling is a first step toward improving their spiritual health. Therapy helps you let go of the hurts of the past, accept your limitations, manage stress and anger, reduce anxiety and depression, and take control of your life—all of which are also steps toward spiritual growth. If you've never engaged in therapy, making the first appointment can feel daunting. Your campus health department can usually help by providing a referral.

Another practical way to expand your mind is to study the sacred texts of the world's major religions and spiritual practices. Many seekers find guidance in the writings of great spiritual teachers. Libraries and bookstores are filled with volumes that explore the diverse approaches humans take to achieve spiritual fulfillment.

Finally, you can expand your awareness of different spiritual practices by exploring on-campus meditation groups, attending meetings of student religious organizations, going to different churches in your local area, attending public lectures, and checking out the official websites of various spiritual and religious organizations. In addition, many colleges and universities offer courses in spirituality or comparative religions.

Tune In to Yourself and Your Surroundings

Focusing on your spiritual health has been likened to tuning in on a radio: Inner wisdom is perpetually available to us, but if we fail to tune our "receiver," we won't be able to hear it for all the "static" of daily life. Fortunately, four ancient practices still used throughout the world can help you tune in. These are contemplation, mindfulness, meditation, and prayer, which you can think of as studying,

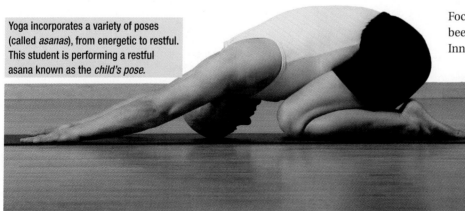

Yoga incorporates a variety of poses (called *asanas*), from energetic to restful. This student is performing a restful asana known as the *child's pose*.

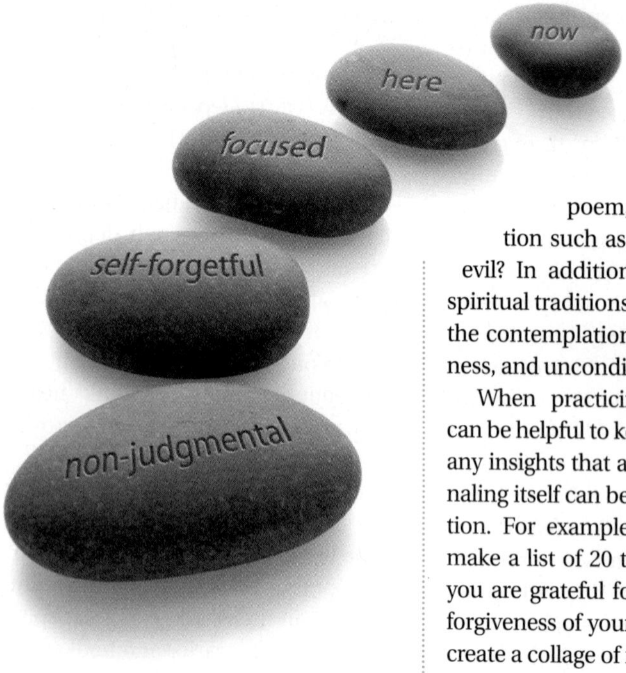

FIGURE 2 Qualities of Mindfulness

contemplation A practice of concentrating the mind on a spiritual or ethical question or subject, a view of the natural world, or an icon or other image representative of divinity.

mindfulness A practice of purposeful, nonjudgmental observation in which we are fully present in the moment.

meditation A practice of emptying the mind of thought.

observing, emptying, and communing with the Divine.

Contemplation If you were to look up the word *contemplation* in a dictionary, you'd find that it means a study of something—whether a candle flame or a theory of quantum mechanics. In the domain of spirituality, **contemplation** usually refers to a practice of concentrating the mind on a spiritual or ethical question or subject, a view of the natural world, or an icon or other image representative of divinity. For instance, a Zen Buddhist might contemplate the solution to a riddle, called a *koan*, such as, what is the sound of one hand clapping? A Sufi might contemplate the 99 names of God. A Roman Catholic might contemplate an image of the Virgin Mary. Spiritual people with no orthodox religious affiliation might contemplate the natural world, a verse from a favorite poem, or an ethical question such as, what is the origin of evil? In addition, most religious and spiritual traditions advocate engaging in the contemplation of gratitude, forgiveness, and unconditional love.

When practicing contemplation, it can be helpful to keep a journal to record any insights that arise. In addition, journaling itself can be a form of contemplation. For example, you might want to make a list of 20 things in your life that you are grateful for, or write a poem of forgiveness of yourself or a loved one, or create a collage of images that symbolize your conception of unconditional love. You might also use your journal to record inspirational quotations that you encounter in your readings.

Mindfulness A practice of focused, nonjudgmental observation, **mindfulness** is the ability to be fully present in the moment (Figure 2). If you have ever "forgotten yourself" while watching the sun set over a mountain, or listening to a great pianist playing Bach, or even while performing a challenging calculation in math, then you have experienced a moment of mindfulness. In other words, mindfulness is an awareness of present-moment reality—a holistic sensation of being totally involved in the moment rather than focused on some past worry or future event.[24]

So how do you practice mindfulness? The range of opportunities is as infinite as the moments of our everyday lives. According to molecular biologist and guru of mindfulness Jon Kabat-Zinn, living mindfully means "making more of your ordinary moments notable and noteworthy by taking note of them."[25] For instance, the next time you get ready to eat an orange, pay attention! What does it feel like to pierce the skin with your thumbnail? Do you smell the fragrance of the orange as you peel it? What does the rind really look like? How do the drops of juice splatter as you separate the orange into segments? And finally, what does it taste like, and how does the taste change from the first bite to the last?

Pursuing almost any endeavor that requires close concentration can help you develop mindfulness. For instance, think of physical and mental challenges, such as a competitive diver leaping from the board, or a physician attempting a difficult diagnosis. Or consider creative and performing arts such as sculpting, painting, writing, dancing, or playing a musical instrument. Even household activities such as cooking or cleaning can foster mindfulness—as long as you pay attention while you do them!

In this era of global environmental concerns, we can also cultivate mindfulness by paying attention to how our choices affect our world. This doesn't only mean mindfulness about recycling our soda cans and taking the subway instead of our car. Those are the easy examples. Instead, mindfulness of our environment calls on us to examine our values and behaviors as we share the Earth every moment of

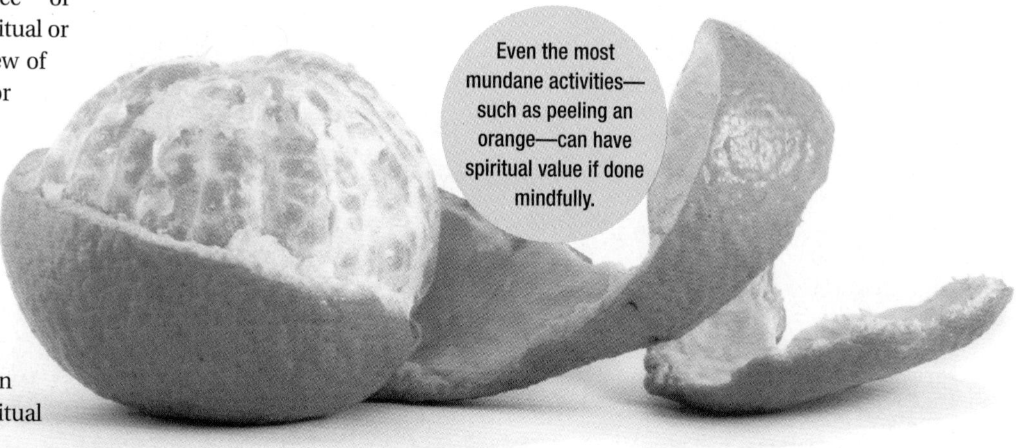

Even the most mundane activities—such as peeling an orange—can have spiritual value if done mindfully.

GREEN GUIDE

Developing Environmental Mindfulness

In her recent book, *Mindfully Green*, environmentalist Stephanie Kaza emphasizes the connection between mindfulness and environmental consciousness. Kaza argues that more people need "to bring their best ethical and spiritual attention to environmental concerns." We need to base our decisions on "compassion, restraint, and acceptance of universal responsibility for the well-being of the earth."

To be mindfully green, Kaza claims, requires us to contemplate a wide variety of troubling questions, to answer them for ourselves, and to commit to taking the right actions that result from our reflection. These questions include, but are not limited to, the following:

✳ How can I investigate the nature of desire?
✳ How can I challenge its allure for me, as a consumer?

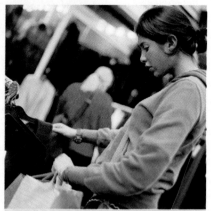

To be mindfully green requires us to ask ourselves some tough questions, such as, what is my fair share? and how much do I really need?

✳ What do I actually need?
✳ What is my fair share?
✳ How do my choices influence the resources available to others?

✳ Can I both practice restraint and cultivate contentment?
✳ Am I willing to witness suffering?
✳ How can I recognize, evaluate, and work to reduce environmental harm?
✳ How can I cultivate kindness toward birds, trees, waters, and lands?
✳ Can I acknowledge my responsibility to inflict no unnecessary harm?
✳ How shall I respond to the harm inflicted by others?
✳ How can I more fully recognize my interdependence with all living organisms and with all elements of the natural world?

In short, Kaza explains that being mindfully green is "about staying present, one action at a time, always asking, What is the kind thing to do now?"

Source: S. Kaza, *Mindfully Green* (Boston: Shambhala, 2008).

---

each day. The **Green Guide** above will help you begin.

Meditation **Meditation** is a practice of emptying the mind, of cultivating stillness. Although the precise details vary with different schools of meditation, the fundamental task is the

39%

of Americans meditate at least once a week.

same: to quiet the mind's noise (variously referred to as the "chatter," "static," or "monkey mind"). As the twentieth-century spiritual teacher J. Krishnamurti explains, "Can the mind—which is chattering, always in movement; which is thought always looking back, remembering, accumulating knowledge, constantly changing—be completely still?"[26]

Why would you want to cultivate the stillness of meditation? For thousands of years, human beings of different cultures and traditions have found that achieving periods of meditative stillness each day enhances their spiritual health. Today, researchers are beginning to discover why. The NCCAM reports that by using brain scanning techniques, researchers have found that experienced meditators show a significantly increased level of *empathy*, the ability to understand and share another person's experience.[27] Similarly, another recent study found that meditation increased the capacity for forgiveness among college students.[28]

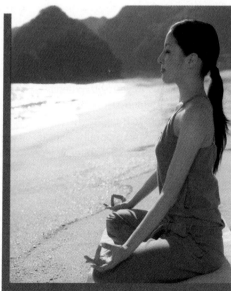

Is meditation boring?

Once you get the hang of it, meditation is anything but boring. As expert Jon Kabat-Zinn notes, "[When] you pay attention to boredom, it gets unbelievably interesting."

And there are other benefits, too. Studies suggest that meditation improves the brain's ability to process information, reduces stress, improves sleep, and relieves chronic pain.[29]

So how do you meditate? Detailed instructions are beyond the scope of this text, but most teachers advise beginning by sitting in a quiet place with low lighting where you can be certain you won't be interrupted. Many advocate assuming a "full lotus" position, with both legs bent fully at the knees, and each ankle over the opposite knee. However, this position can be painful for beginners, people with poor flexibility, and people with joint pain. Thus, you may want to assume a modified lotus position, in which your legs are simply crossed in front of you. Lying down is not recommended because you may fall asleep. Rest your hands palm upward on your knees. This position uncrosses the two bones of the forearm. Your eyes can be open, half-open, or closed, but if you are a beginner, you may find it easier to meditate with your eyes closed.

Once you're in a position conducive to meditation, it's time to start emptying your mind. Different schools of meditation teach different methods to achieve this. For example:

- **Mantra meditation.** Focus on a *mantra*, a single word such as *Om*, *Amen*, *Love*, or *God*. Keep repeating this word silently to yourself. When a distracting thought arises, simply set it aside. It may help to imagine the thought as a leaf, and mentally place it on a gently flowing stream that carries it away. Do not fault yourself for becoming distracted. Simply notice the thought, release it, and return to your mantra.
- **Breath meditation.** Count each breath: Pay attention to each inhalation, the brief pause that follows, and the exhalation. Together, these equal one breath. When you have counted ten breaths, return to one. As with mantra meditation, as distractions

prayer Communication with a transcendent Presence.

arise, release them and return to the breath.
- **Color meditation.** When your eyes are closed, you may perceive a field of color, such as a deep blue "pearl" or "flame." Focus on this color. Treat distractions as for other forms of meditation.
- **Object meditation.** With your eyes open, focus on an object, such as a picture of a religious symbol or figure, or a flower or stone. Allow your eyes to soften as you meditate on this object. Treat distractions as for other forms of meditation.
- **Loving-kindness meditation.** Send yourself loving-kindness. Once you feel enveloped in this embrace, send loving-kindness to family members, friends, and acquaintances, then to strangers, then to those you may ever have perceived as your enemies, and finally to all sentient beings.

After several minutes of meditation, and with practice, you may come to experience a sensation sometimes described as "dropping down," in which you feel yourself release into the meditation. In this state, which can be likened to a wakeful sleep, distracting thoughts are far less likely to arise, and yet you may suddenly receive surprising insights.

When you're just starting out, try meditating for just 10 to 20 minutes a session, once or twice a day. In time, you can increase your sessions to 30 minutes or more. As you meditate for longer periods, you will likely find yourself feeling more rested and less stressed throughout your day, and you may begin to experience the increased

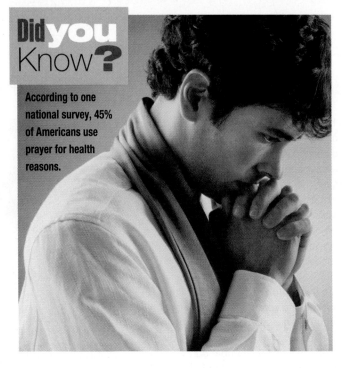

levels of empathy recorded among expert meditators.

Prayer In **prayer,** rather than emptying the mind, an individual focuses the mind in communication with a transcendent Presence. Spiritual traditions throughout the world distinguish several forms that this communion commonly takes, including adoration, petition and intercession, and thanksgiving.

For many, prayer begins with *adoration* (also known as *praise*), which may be explicitly stated or may take the form of simply sitting still and allowing yourself to feel the transcendent Presence beside you or enveloping you. Adoration is often followed by *petition* and *intercession*, that is, sharing your concerns for yourself and others, and promising to be open to guidance. This listening to the Presence, which continues long after the formal prayer is over, can make each moment of daily life a prayer. Note that petition and intercession do not have to include a request for something specific, such as acceptance into a graduate program or healing of a loved one. Rather, these forms of prayer can be offered for the

Finding Your Spiritual Side through Service

Recognizing that we are all part of a greater system and that we have responsibilities to and for others is a key part of spiritual growth and development. Volunteering your time and energy is a great way to connect with others and help make the world a better place while improving your own health. Here are some ways you can go about this:

✳ Help elderly neighbors shape up their yards and homes. Offer to mow the lawn, weed the garden, haul away trash and debris, or add caulking or insulation to make their homes energy efficient for the winter.

✳ Volunteer for Meals on Wheels, a local soup kitchen, a food bank, or another program to help neighbors with low food security.

✳ Organize or participate in an after-school or summertime activity for neighborhood children, such as a book group or a basketball, jump rope, chess, or cooking club.

✳ Participate in a highway, beach, or neighborhood cleanup, restoration of park trails and rivers, or other environmental preservation projects.

✳ Volunteer at the local humane society walking dogs, petting and grooming cats, cleaning, fostering pets in your home, or raising money for spaying and neutering.

✳ Join a Big Brother or Big Sister program and work to instill self-esteem and community values among those who may face significant challenges or have poor role models.

✳ Join a student organization working on a cause such as global warming or hunger, or start one yourself. Think that's impossible? Check out these inspiring examples: Students Against Global Apathy (SAGA) was founded by a University of Alberta student confronting global poverty and injustice; Students for the Environment (S4E) was founded by students at the University of Delaware to focus on local issues affecting the environment, as well as national and global environmental issues. And the National Student Campaign Against Hunger and Homelessness is a project of student-level Public Interest Research Groups.

✳ Spend your vacation volunteering in a neighborhood challenged by poverty, low literacy, or a natural disaster. Or volunteer with an organization such as Habitat for Humanity to build homes or provide other aid to developing communities.

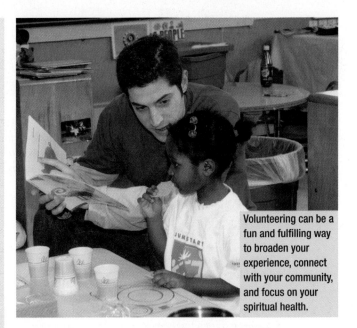

Volunteering can be a fun and fulfilling way to broaden your experience, connect with your community, and focus on your spiritual health.

benefit of all of humanity. Prayer traditionally concludes with *thanksgiving*, that is, an expression of gratitude for the many blessings in your life. Even in times of trial, an acknowledgment of blessings can bring strength.

Reach Out to Others

Altruism, the giving of oneself out of genuine concern for others, is a key aspect of a spiritually healthy lifestyle. Volunteering to help others, choosing to work for a not-for-profit organization, donating money or other resources to a food bank or other

program—even spending an afternoon picking up litter in your neighborhood—all of these are ways to serve others and simultaneously enhance your own spiritual health.

Community service can also take the form of **environmental stewardship,** which the Environmental Protection Agency (EPA) defines as the responsibility for environmental quality shared by all those whose actions affect the environment.[30] Responsibility manifests in action. At home, simple actions such as reducing and recycling packaging, turning off the lights, making sure the heat or air-conditioning maintains an ecofriendly room temperature, replacing old lightbulbs with energy-efficient varieties, and taking shorter showers are all part of environmental stewardship.

For more strategies to enhance your spiritual health by reaching out to others, refer to the **Skills for Behavior Change** box at left.

altruism The giving of oneself out of genuine concern for others.
environmental stewardship A responsibility for environmental quality shared by all those whose actions affect the environment.

Assess yourself

What's Your Spiritual IQ?

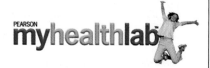

At least a dozen tools are now available for assessing your spiritual intelligence. Although each differs significantly according to its target audience (therapy clients, business executives, church members, and so on), most share certain underlying principles, reflected in the questionnaire below. Answer each question as follows:

0 = not at all true for me
1 = somewhat true for me
2 = very true for me

_____ 1. I frequently feel gratitude for the many blessings of my life.

_____ 2. I am often moved by the beauty of Earth, music, poetry, or other aspects of my daily life.

_____ 3. I readily express forgiveness toward those whose missteps have affected me.

_____ 4. I recognize in others qualities that are more important than their appearance and behaviors.

_____ 5. When I do poorly on an exam, lose an important game, or am rejected in a relationship, I am able to know that the experience does not define who I am.

_____ 6. When fear arises, I am able to know that I am eternally safe and loved.

_____ 7. I meditate or pray daily.

Fill out this assessment online at www.pearsonhighered.com/myhealthlab or www.pearsonhighered.com/donatelle.

_____ 8. I frequently and fearlessly ponder the possibility of an afterlife.

_____ 9. I accept total responsibility for the choices that I have made in building my life.

_____ 10. I feel that I am on Earth for a unique and sacred reason.

Scoring

The higher your score on this quiz, the higher your spiritual intelligence. To improve your score, apply the suggestions for spiritual practices from this chapter.

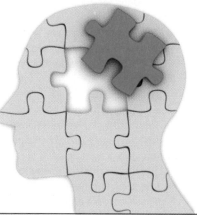

YOUR PLAN FOR CHANGE

The **Assess yourself** activity gave you the chance to evaluate your own spiritual intelligence, and the chapter introduced you to some practices used successfully by millions of people over many generations to enhance their spiritual health. If you are interested in cultivating your own spirituality further, consider taking some of the small but significant steps listed below to start you on your journey.

Today, you can:

◯ Find a quiet spot; turn off your cell phone; close your eyes; and contemplate, meditate, or pray for 10 minutes. Or spend 10 minutes in quiet mindfulness of your surroundings.

◯ In a journal or on your computer, begin compiling a numbered list of things you are grateful for. Today, list at least ten things. Include people, pets, talents and abilities, achievements, favorite places, foods . . . whatever comes to mind!

Within the next 2 weeks, you can:

◯ Explore the options on campus for beginning psychotherapy, joining a spiritual or religious student group, or volunteering with a student organization working for positive change.

◯ Think of a person in your life with whom you have experienced conflict. Spend a few minutes contemplating forgiveness toward

this person, then write him or her an e-mail or letter apologizing for any offense you may have given and offering your forgiveness in return. Wait for a day or two before deciding whether or not you are truly ready to send the message.

By the end of the semester, you can:

◯ Develop a list of several spiritual texts that you would like to read over your break.

◯ Begin exploring options for volunteer work next summer.

References

1. Higher Education Research Institute, *Spirituality in Higher Education: A National Study of College Students' Search for Meaning and Purpose* (Los Angeles: Higher Education Research Institute, University of California Los Angeles, 2007).

2. National Center for Complementary and Alternative Medicine (NCCAM), "Prayer and Spirituality in Health: Ancient Practices, Modern Science," *CAM at the NIH* 12, no. 1 (2005): 1–4.

3. H. G. Koenig, M. McCullough, and D. B. Larson, *Handbook of Religion and Health: A Century of Research Reviewed* (New York: Oxford University Press, 2001).

4. Ibid.

5. Pew Forum on Religion & Public Life, *U.S. Religious Landscape Survey Religious Beliefs and Practices: Diverse and Politically Relevant* (Washington, DC: Pew Research Center, 2008).

6. Ibid.

7. A. Huxley, *The Perennial Philosophy* (New York: Harper Modern Classics, 2004 edition).

8. B. L. Seaward, *Health of the Human Spirit: Spiritual Dimensions for Personal Health.* (Boston: Allyn & Bacon, 2001), 85–90.

9. D. Zohar, *ReWiring the Corporate Brain: Using the New Science to Rethink How We Structure and Lead Organizations* (San Francisco: Berrett Koehler, 1997).

10. R. A. Emmons, *The Psychology of Ultimate Concerns: Motivation and Personality in Spirituality* (New York: Guilford Press, 2003).

11. A. Moreira-Almeida and H. G. Koenig, "Retaining the Meaning of the Words Religiousness and Spirituality," *Social Science and Medicine* 63, no. 4 (2006): 843–45.

12. National Center for Complementary and Alternative Medicine (NCCAM), "Prayer and Spirituality in Health," 2005.

13. A. J. Weaver and H. G. Koenig, "Religion, Spirituality, and Their Relevance to Medicine: An Update," *American Family Physician* 73, no. 8 (2006) 1336–37; R. F. Gillum, D. E. King, T. O. Obisesan, and H. G. Koenig, "Frequency of Attendance at Religious Services and Mortality in a U.S. National Cohort," *Annals of Epidemiology* 18, no. 2 (2008): 124–29.

14. M. E. McCullough and B. L. B. Willoughby, "Religion, Self-Regulation, and Self-Control: Associations, Explana-tions, and Implications," *Psychological Bulletin* 135, no. 1 (2009): 69–93.

15. National Cancer Institute, "Spirituality in Cancer Care," Modified March 6, 2009, www.cancer.gov/cancertopics/pdq/supportivecare/spirituality/patient.

16. F. A. Curlin, S. A. Sellergren, J. D. Lantos, and M. H. Chin, "Physicians' Observa-tions and Interpretations of the Influence of Religion and Spirituality on Health," *Archives of Internal Medicine* 167, no. 7 (2007): 649–54.

17. M. Baetz and R. Boewn, "Chronic Pain and Fatigue: Associations with Religion and Spirituality," *Pain Research & Management* 13, no. 5 (2008): 383–88.

18. G. Ironson, R. Stuetzle, and M. A. Fletcher, "An Increase in Religiousness/Spirituality Occurs after HIV Diagnosis and Predicts Slower Disease Progression over 4 Years in People with HIV," *Journal of General Internal Medicine* 21, no. 5 (2006): S62–S68.

19. A. Moreira-Almeida and H. G. Koenig, "Religiousness and Spirituality in Fibromyalgia and Chronic Pain Patients," *Current Pain and Headache Reports* 12, no. 5 (2008): 327–32; B. R. Doolittle and M. Farrell, "The Association between Spirituality and Depression in an Urban Clinic," *Primary Care Companion to the Journal of Clinical Psychiatry* 6, no. 3 (2004): 114–18; National Cancer Institute, "Spirituality in Cancer Care," 2009.

20. M. Javnbakht, R. Hejazi Kenari, and M. Ghasemi, "Effects of Yoga on Depression and Anxiety of Women," *Complementary Therapies in Clinical Practice* 15, no. 2 (2009): 102–04; A. Wool-ery, H. Myers, B. Sternlieb, and L. Zeltzer, "A Yoga Intervention for Young Adults with Elevated Symptoms of Depression," *Alternative Therapies in Health and Medicine* 10, no. 2 (2004): 60–63.

21. National Center for Complementary and Alternative Medicine (NCCAM), "Prayer and Spirituality in Health," 2005; National Cancer Institute, "Spirituality in Cancer Care," 2009.

22. G. G. Ano and E. B. Vasconcelles, "Reli-gious Coping and Psychological Adjust-ment to Stress: A Meta-Analysis," *Journal of Clinical Psychology* 61, no. 4 (2005): 461–80; U. Winter, D. Hauri, S. Huber, J. Jenewein, U. Schnyder, and B. Kraemer, "The Psychological Outcome of Religious Coping with Stressful Life Events in a Swiss Sample of Church Attendees," *Psychotherapy and Psychosomatics* 78, no. 4 (2009): 240–44.

23. A. Chiesa and A. Serretti, "Mindfulness-Based Stress Reduction for Stress Man-agement in Healthy People: A Review and Meta-Analysis," *Journal of Alternative and Complementary Medicine* 15, no. (2009): 593–600.

24. J. A. Astin, S. L. Shapiro, D. M. Eisenberg, and K. L. Forys, "Mind-Body Medicine: State of the Science, Implications for Practice," *Journal of the American Board of Family Practice* 16, no. 2 (2003): 131–47; J. Bishop et al. "Mindfulness: A Proposed Operational Definition," *Clinical Psychology: Science and Practice* 11 (2004): 230–41.

25. J. Kabat-Zinn, *Coming to Our Senses: Healing Ourselves and the World through Mindfulness* (New York: Hyperion, 2005).

26. J. Krishnamurti, *This Light in Oneself: True Meditation* (Boston: Shambhala, 1999), 5.

27. National Center for Complementary and Alternative Medicine (NCCAM), "Research Spotlight: Meditation May Increase Empathy," Modified April 2009, http://nccam.nih.gov/research/results/spotlight/060608.htm.

28. D. Oman, S. Shapiro, C. Thoreson, T. Plante, and T. Flinders, "Meditation Lowers Stress and Supports Forgiveness among College Students: A Randomized Controlled Trial," *Journal of American College Health* 56, no. 5 (2008): 425–31.

29. National Center for Complementary and Alternative Medicine (NCCAM), "Research Spotlight: Meditation May Make Information Processing in the Brain More Efficient," Modified April 2009, http://nccam.nih.gov/research/results/spotlight/082307.htm; A. Chiesa and A Serretti, "Mindfulness-Based Stress Reduction for Stress Management in Healthy People, 2009; N. Y. Winbush, C. R. Gross, and M. J. Kreitzer, "The Effects of Mindfulness-Based Stress Reduction on Sleep Disturbance: A Systematic Review. *EXPLORE: The Journal of Science and Healing* 3, no. 6 (2007): 585–91; N. E. Morone, C. S. Lynch, C. M. Greco, H. A. Tindle, and D. K. Weiner, "'I Felt Like a New Person.' The Effects of Mindfulness Meditation on Older Adults with Chronic Pain: Qualita-tive Narrative Analysis of Diary Entries," *Journal of Pain* 9, no. 9 (2008): 841–48.

30. Environmental Protection Agency (EPA), "Environmental Stewardship," Updated April 30, 2009, www.epa.gov/stewardship.

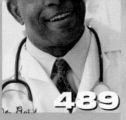
489
What questions should I ask my health care provider about proposed tests, treatments, or medications?

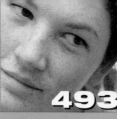
493
Can I count on my school's health care plan to cover my medical needs?

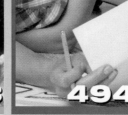
494
What should I consider when choosing health insurance?

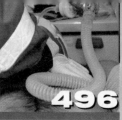
496
What happens if I don't have insurance and I need medical care?

16 Savvy Health Care Consumerism

Objectives

✱ Explain why it is important to be a responsible health care consumer and how to encourage health care consumers to take action.

✱ Understand what factors to consider when making health care decisions.

✱ Describe the U.S. health care system in terms of types of insurance; the changing structure of the system; and issues concerning cost, quality, and access to services.

✱ Understand the role health insurers play in providing health care.

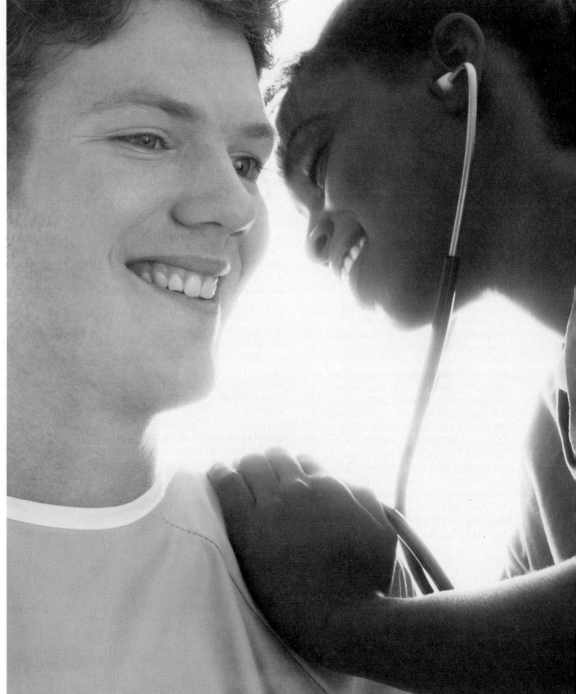

Have there been times when you wondered whether you were sick enough to go to your campus health clinic? Have you left visits with your health care provider feeling like you had more questions than you did when you arrived? Do you engage in risky behaviors, such as skateboarding without a helmet, and don't know where or how you would be treated if you were injured? Are you one of the 20 percent of college students without health insurance? If any of these is true, you will find the information in this chapter valuable in helping you to become a better health care consumer.

There are many reasons for you to learn to make better decisions about your health and health care. Most important, you have only one body—if you don't treat it with care, you will pay a major price in terms of financial costs and health consequences. Doing everything you can to stay healthy and to recover rapidly when you do get sick will enhance every other part of your life. Throughout this book we have emphasized the importance of healthy preventive behaviors. Learning how to navigate the health care system is an important part of taking charge of your health.

Taking Responsibility for Your Health Care

As the health care industry has become more sophisticated in seeking your business, so must you become more sophisticated in purchasing its products and services. Acting responsibly in times of illness can be difficult, but the person best able to act on your behalf is you.

If you are not feeling well, you must first decide whether you really need to seek medical advice. Not seeking treatment, whether because of high costs or limited coverage, or trying to medicate yourself when more rigorous methods of treatment are needed, is potentially dangerous. Being knowledgeable about the benefits and limits of self-care is critical for responsible consumerism.

Self-Help or Self-Care

Individuals can practice behaviors that promote health, prevent disease, and minimize reliance on the formal medical system. We can also treat minor afflictions without seeking professional help. Self-care consists of knowing your body, paying attention to its signals, and taking appropriate action to stop the progression of illness or injury. Common forms of self-care include the following:

● Diagnosing symptoms or conditions that occur frequently but may not require physician visits (e.g., the common cold, minor abrasions)
● Using over-the-counter remedies to treat minor infrequent pains, scrapes, or cold or allergy symptoms.
● Performing monthly breast or testicular self-examinations
● Learning first aid for common, uncomplicated injuries and conditions

● Checking blood pressure, pulse, and temperature
● Using home pregnancy tests and ovulation kits
● Using home HIV test kits
● Doing periodic checks for blood cholesterol
● Learning from reliable self-help books, websites, and DVDs
● Benefiting from meditation and other relaxation techniques and nutrition, rest, and exercise

When to Seek Help

Effective self-care also means understanding when to seek medical attention rather than treating a condition yourself. Deciding which conditions warrant professional advice is not always easy. Generally, you should consult a physician if you experience *any* of the following:

● A serious accident or injury
● Sudden or severe chest pains especially if they cause breathing difficulties
● Trauma to the head or spine accompanied by persistent headache, blurred vision, loss of consciousness, vomiting, convulsions, or paralysis
● Sudden high fever or recurring high temperature (over 102°F for children and 103°F for adults) and/or sweats
● Tingling sensation in the arm accompanied by slurred speech or impaired thought processes
● Adverse reactions to a drug or insect bite (shortness of breath, severe swelling, dizziness)
● Unexplained bleeding or loss of body fluid from any body opening
● Unexplained sudden weight loss
● Persistent or recurrent diarrhea or vomiting
● Blue-colored lips, eyelids, or nail beds
● Any lump, swelling, thickness, or sore that does not subside or that grows for over a month
● Any marked change or pain in bowel or bladder habits
● Yellowing of the skin or the whites of the eyes

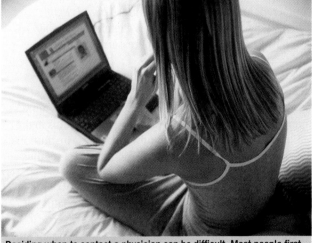

Deciding when to contact a physician can be difficult. Most people first try to diagnose and treat a condition themselves.

35 million

Americans are admitted to the hospital each year.

- Any symptom that is unusual and recurs over time
- Pregnancy

With the vast array of home diagnostic devices available, it seems relatively easy for most people to take care of themselves. But some caution is in order here: Although many of these devices are valuable for making an initial diagnosis, home health tests are no substitute for regular, complete examinations by a trained practitioner. See the **Skills for Behavior Change** box at right for information on taking an active role in your own health care.

Assessing Health Professionals

Suppose you decide that you do need medical help. You must then identify what type of help you need and where to obtain it. Selecting a professional may seem simple, yet many people have no idea how to assess the qualifications of a health care provider.

Numerous studies document the importance of good communication skills: The most satisfied patients are those who feel their health care provider explains diagnosis and treatment options thoroughly and involves them in decisions regarding their own care.[1]

When evaluating a health care provider, be sure to consider the following questions:

- What professional educational training have they had? What license or board certification(s) do they hold? Note that there is a difference between "board certified" and "board eligible" physicians. *Board certified* indicates that the physician has passed the national board examination for his or her specialty (e.g., pediatrics) and has been certified as competent in that specialty. In contrast, *board eligible* merely means that the physician is eligible to take the specialty board's exam, but not necessarily that he or she has passed it.
- Are they affiliated with an accredited medical facility or institution? The Joint Commission is an independent nonprofit organization that evaluates and accredits more than 15,000 health care organizations and programs in the United States. Accreditation requires that these institutions verify all education, licensing, and training claims of their affiliated practitioners.
- Are they open to complementary or alternative strategies? Would they refer you for different treatment modalities if appropriate?
- Do they indicate clearly how long a given treatment may last, what side effects you might expect, and what problems you should watch for?

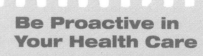

Be Proactive in Your Health Care

The more you know about your body and the factors that can affect your health, the better you will be at communicating with health care providers. The following points can help:

* Know your own and your family's medical history.
* Research your condition—causes, physiological effects, possible treatments, and prognosis. Don't rely on the health care provider for this information.
* Bring a friend or relative along for medical visits to help you review what the doctor says. If you go alone, take notes.
* Ask the practitioner to explain the problem and possible treatments, tests, and drugs in a clear and understandable way. If you don't understand something, ask for clarification.
* If the health care provider prescribes any medications, ask whether you can take generic equivalents that cost less.
* Ask for a written summary of the results of your visit and any lab tests.
* If you have any doubt about the health care provider's recommended treatment, seek a second opinion.
* After seeing a health care professional, write down an accurate account of what happened and what was said. Be sure to include the names of the health care provider and all other people involved in your care, the date, and the place.
* When filling prescriptions, ask the pharmacist to show you the package inserts that list medical considerations. Request detailed information about potential drug and food interactions.

- Are their diagnoses, treatments, and general statements consistent with established scientific theory and practice?
- Who will be responsible for your care when your physician is on vacation or off call?
- Do they listen to you, respect you as an individual, and give you time to ask questions? Do they return your calls, and are they available to answer questions?

Asking the right questions at the right time may save you personal suffering and expense. Many patients find that writing their questions down before an appointment helps them get answers to all their questions. You should not accept a defensive or hostile response; asking questions is your right as a patient.

Active participation in your treatment is the only sensible course in a health care environment that encourages

defensive medicine. A recent study examined over 4,000 routine preventive health checkups. In 43 percent of the checkups, doctors ordered a urinalysis, an electrocardiogram, or an X ray, despite the fact that the patient showed no symptoms that would have caused the physician to ask for such tests.[2] Unnecessary drugs and procedures are not likely to improve health outcomes and in some cases may create new health problems.

In addition to asking the suggested questions above, being proactive in your health care also means that you should be aware of your rights as a patient:[3]

1. The right of informed consent means that before receiving any care, you should be fully informed of what is being planned; the risks and potential benefits; and possible alternative forms of treatment, including the option of no treatment. Your consent must be voluntary and without any form of coercion. It is critical that you read any consent forms carefully and amend them as necessary before signing.

2. You are entitled to know whether the treatment you are receiving is standard or experimental. In experimental conditions, you have the legal and ethical right to know if any drug is being used in the research project for a purpose not approved by the Food and Drug Administration (FDA), and if the study is one in which some people receive treatment while others receive a placebo. (See the **Health Today** box on page 490 for more on placebos and the placebo effect.)

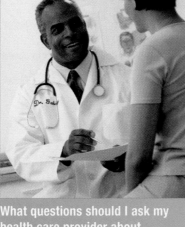

What questions should I ask my health care provider about proposed tests, treatments, or medications?

It's important to understand recommendations that your health care provider makes. Questions to ask include how often the practitioner has performed a procedure, the proportion of successful outcomes for the treatment or procedure, any side effects and whether they can be treated or reduced, whether a hospital stay will be required, and why a test has been ordered.

Choosing Health Products

Recall from Chapter 7 that prescription drugs can be obtained only with a written prescription from a physician, while over-the-counter drugs can be purchased without a prescription. Just as making wise decisions about providers is an important aspect of responsible health care, so is making wise decisions about medications.

Prescription Drugs

In about two-thirds of doctor visits, the physician administers or prescribes at least one medication. In fact, prescription drug use has risen by 25 percent over the past decade. Even though these drugs are administered under medical supervision, the wise consumer still takes precautions. Hazards and complications arising from the use of prescription drugs are common.

Consumers have a variety of resources available to determine the risks of various prescription medicines and can make educated decisions about whether to take a certain drug. One of the best resources is the U.S. FDA Center for Drug Evaluation and Research

defensive medicine Actions taken by a health care provider, such as ordering unnecessary tests, for the sake of avoiding potential malpractice claims rather than for the health of the patient.

91% of U.S. physicians admitted that they sometimes order unnecessary medical tests because they are concerned about being sued for malpractice.

3. You have the right to privacy, which includes the source of payment for treatment and care. It also includes protecting your right to make personal decisions concerning all reproductive matters.

4. You have the right to receive care. You also have the legal right to refuse treatment at any time and to cease treatment at any time.

5. You are entitled to have access to all of your medical records and to have those records remain confidential.

6. You have the right to seek the opinions of other health care professionals regarding your condition.

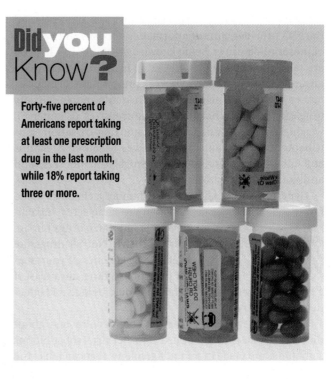

Did you Know?

Forty-five percent of Americans report taking at least one prescription drug in the last month, while 18% report taking three or more.

HEALTH Today

THE PLACEBO EFFECT: MIND OVER MATTER?

The *placebo effect* is an apparent cure or improved state of health brought about by a substance, product, or procedure that has no generally recognized therapeutic value. Patients often report improvements in a condition based on what they expect, desire, or were told would happen after receiving a treatment, even though the treatment was, for example, simple sugar pills instead of powerful drugs.

Researchers are investigating how and why placebos work on some people. One theory is that expecting a positive outcome activates the same natural pathways in the brain as some medications do. One recent study involved patients with Parkinson's disease. The patients who thought that they were receiving the real treatment but actually received a placebo had the same changes in their brains on positron-emission tomography (PET) scans as those who received the medication. Similar chemical changes on brain imaging tests were seen with placebos in studies of pain and depression.

In another recent trial, a sample of alcohol-dependent patients received

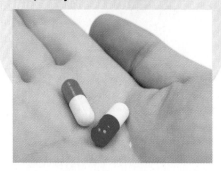

Is it a real medicine or a placebo? In some cases, it may not make a difference.

either the drugs naltrexone or acamprosate, or a placebo for a period of 12 weeks. They were also asked whether they thought they were receiving an active medication or a placebo. Those who believed they had been taking medication consumed fewer alcoholic drinks and reported less alcohol dependence and cravings, regardless of whether they really were receiving the drug.

Placebos are also used in clinical research studies. Patients with a particular condition are given either the treatment that is being tested or a placebo. If the patients receiving the treatment have a more beneficial outcome than the patients receiving the placebo, then the treatment can be considered effective. The patients and the doctors running the study are not told until the study ends who had the real treatment and who had the placebo.

People who mistakenly use placebos when medical treatment is needed increase their risk for health problems. However, what we learn from the ways in which placebos work may someday help us harness the mind's power to treat certain diseases and conditions.

Sources: J. Friedman and R. Dubinsky, "The Placebo Effect," 2008, www.neurology.org/cgi/content/full/71/9/e25#R1-20; R. de la Fuente-Fernandez et al., "Expectation and Dopamine Release: Mechanism of the Placebo Effect in Parkinson's Disease," *Science* 293 (2001): 1164–66; N. Diederich and C. Goetz, "The Placebo Treatments in Neurosciences: New Insights from Clinical and Neuroimaging Studies," *Neurology* 71 (2008): 677–84; *Journal of Psychotherapy and Psychosomatics*, "Learning More about the Placebo Effect," 2009, *ScienceDaily*, www.sciencedaily.com/releases/2009/06/090622064701.htm.

---

website (www.fda.gov/cder). This consumer-specific section of the FDA provides current information on risks and benefits of prescription drugs. Being knowledgeable about what you are taking or thinking about taking is a sound strategy to ensure safety. Common types of prescription drugs discussed in this text include antidepressants and antianxiety drugs (Chapter 2), hormonal contraceptives (Chapter 6), weight-loss aids (Chapter 10), smoking-cessation aids (Chapter 8), stimulants and sedatives (Chapter 7), statins and other cholesterol-lowering drugs (Chapter 12), and antibiotics (Chapter 13).

Generic drugs, medications sold under a chemical name rather than a brand name, contain the same active ingredients as brand-name drugs but are less expensive. Not all drugs are available as generics. If your doctor prescribes a drug, always ask if a generic equivalent exists and if it would be safe and effective for you to try.

Be aware, though, that there is some controversy about the effectiveness of generic drugs, because substitutions sometimes are made in minor ingredients that can affect the

generic drugs Medications marketed by chemical names rather than brand names.

way the drug is absorbed, potentially causing discomfort or even allergic reactions in some patients. Always note any reactions you have to medications and tell your doctor about them.

Over-the-Counter (OTC) Drugs

Over-the-counter (OTC) drugs are nonprescription substances used in the course of self-diagnosis and self-medication. More than one-third of the time, people treat their routine health problems with OTC medications. In fact, American consumers spend billions of dollars yearly on OTC preparations for relief of everything from runny noses to ingrown toenails.

The FDA has categorized 26 types of OTC preparations. Those most commonly used are analgesics; cold, cough, allergy, and asthma relievers; stimulants; sleeping aids and relaxants; and dieting aids (Table 16.1).

Despite a common belief that OTC products are safe and effective, indiscriminate use and abuse can occur with these drugs as with all others. For example, people who frequently drop medication into their eyes to "get the red out" or pop

Type/Name of Drug	Use	Examples	Potential Hazards/Common Side Effects
Acetaminophen	Pain reliever, fever reducer	Tylenol	Bloody urine, painful urination, skin rash, bleeding and bruising, yellowing of the eyes or skin, difficulty in diagnosing overdose because reaction may be delayed up to a week; liver damage from chronic low-level use
Antacids	Relieve "heartburn"	Tums Maalox	Reduced mineral absorption from food; possible concealment of ulcer; reduced effectiveness of anticlotting medications; interference with the function of certain antibiotics (for antacids that contain aluminum); worsened high blood pressure (for antacids that contain sodium); aggravated kidney problems
Anticholinergics	Often added to cold preparations to reduce nasal secretions and tears	atropine scopolamine	None of the preparations tested by the FDA have been found to be Generally Recognized as Effective (GRAE) or Generally Recognized as Safe (GRAS). Some cold compounds contain alcohol in concentrations greater than 40%.
Antihistamines	Central nervous system depressants that dry runny noses, clear postnasal drip and sinus congestion, and reduce tears	Claritin Benadryl Xyzal	Drowsiness, sedation, dizziness, disturbed coordination
Aspirin	Pain reliever; reduces fever and inflammation	Bayer Bufferin	Stomach upset and vomiting; stomach bleeding; worsening of ulcers; enhancement of the action of anticlotting medications; hearing damage from loud noise; severe allergic reaction; association with Reye's syndrome in children and teenagers; prolonged bleeding when combined with alcohol
Decongestants	Reduce nasal stuffiness due to colds	Sudafed DayQuil Allermed	Nervousness, restlessness, excitability, dizziness, drowsiness, headache, nausea, weakness, and sleep problems
Diet pills, caffeine	Aid to weight loss	Dexatrim	Organ damage or death from cerebral hemorrhage; nervousness; irritability; dehydration
Expectorants	Loosen phlegm, which allows the user to cough it up and clear congested respiratory passages.	Mucinex	Safety issues may arise when combined with other medications, particularly in frail or very ill individuals. Effectiveness is sometimes in question.
Ibuprofen	Pain reliever; reduces fever and inflammation	Advil Motrin	Allergic reaction in some people with aspirin allergy; fluid retention or swelling (edema); liver damage similar to that from acetaminophen; enhancement of anticlotting medications; digestive disturbances
Laxatives	Relieve constipation	Ex-lax Citrucel	Reduced absorption of minerals from food; dehydration; dependency
Naproxen sodium	Pain reliever; reduces fever and inflammation	Aleve Naprosyn	Potential bleeding in the digestive tract; possible stomach cramps or ulcers
Sleep aids and relaxants	Help relieve occasional sleeplessness	Nytol Sleep-Eze Sominex	Drowsiness the next day; dizziness; lack of coordination; reduced mental alertness; constipation; dry mouth and throat; dependency

antacids after every meal are likely to become dependent. Many people also experience adverse side effects because they ignore the warnings on the labels or simply do not read them.

The FDA has developed a standard label that appears on most OTC products (see **Figure 16.1** on the next page). It provides directions for use, warnings, and other useful information. Diet supplements, which are regulated as food products, have their own type of label that includes a Supplement Facts panel.

Choices in Medical Care

Most people believe that **allopathic medicine,** or traditional Western medical practice, is based on scientifically validated methods. But be aware that not all allopathic treatments have had the benefit of the extensive clinical trials and long-term studies of outcomes

allopathic medicine Conventional, Western medical practice; in theory, based on scientifically validated methods and procedures.

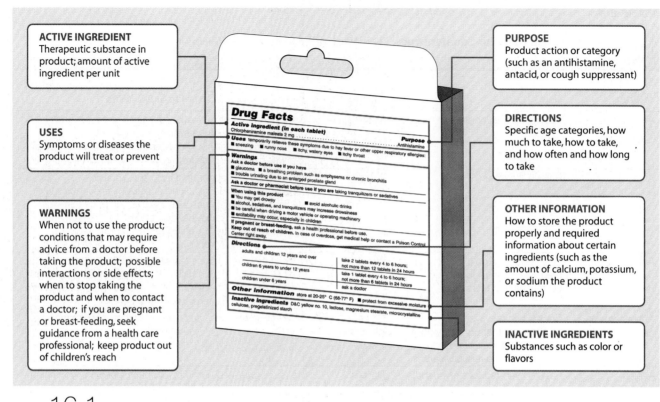

ACTIVE INGREDIENT
Therapeutic substance in product; amount of active ingredient per unit

USES
Symptoms or diseases the product will treat or prevent

WARNINGS
When not to use the product; conditions that may require advice from a doctor before taking the product; possible interactions or side effects; when to stop taking the product and when to contact a doctor; if you are pregnant or breast-feeding, seek guidance from a health care professional; keep product out of children's reach

PURPOSE
Product action or category (such as an antihistamine, antacid, or cough suppressant)

DIRECTIONS
Specific age categories, how much to take, how to take, and how often and how long to take

OTHER INFORMATION
How to store the product properly and required information about certain ingredients (such as the amount of calcium, potassium, or sodium the product contains)

INACTIVE INGREDIENTS
Substances such as color or flavors

FIGURE 16.1 The Over-the-Counter Medicine Label

Source: Adapted from Consumer Healthcare Products Association, "Check the OTC Label," 2009, www.otcsafety.org/publications.

that would be necessary to conclusively prove effectiveness in different populations. Even when studies appear to support the health benefits of a particular treatment or product, other studies with equal or better scientific validity often refute these claims. Also, today's recommended treatment may change dramatically in the future as new technologies and medical advances replace older practices. Like other professionals, medical doctors are only as good as their training, continued acquisition of knowledge, and resources allow them to be.

primary care practitioner (PCP)
A medical practitioner who treats routine ailments, advises on preventive care, gives general medical advice, and makes appropriate referrals when necessary.

osteopath General practitioner who receives training similar to a medical doctor's but with an emphasis on the skeletal and muscular systems; often uses spinal manipulation as part of treatment.

ophthalmologist Physician who specializes in the medical and surgical care of the eyes, including prescriptions for glasses.

optometrist Eye specialist whose practice is limited to prescribing and fitting lenses.

dentist Specialist who diagnoses and treats diseases of the teeth, gums, and oral cavity.

Selecting a **primary care practitioner (PCP)**—a medical practitioner whom you can visit for routine ailments, preventive care, general medical advice, and appropriate referrals—is not an easy task. The PCP for most people is a family practitioner, an internist, a pediatrician, or an obstetrician/gynecologist (OB/Gyn). Many people routinely see nurse practitioners or physician assistants who work for an individual doctor or a medical group, and others use nontraditional providers as their primary source of care. As a college student, you may opt to visit a PCP at your campus health center. The reputation of health care providers on college campuses is

excellent. In national surveys, students have indicated that the health center medical staff is their most trusted source of health information.[4]

Doctors undergo rigorous training before they can begin practicing. After 4 years of undergraduate work, students typically spend 4 years studying for their medical degree (MD). After this general training, some students choose a specialty, such as pediatrics, cardiology, cancer, radiology, or surgery, and spend 1 year in an internship and several years doing a residency. Some specialties also require a fellowship; in all, the time spent in additional training after receiving an MD can be up to 8 years.

Other specialists include **osteopaths,** general practitioners who receive training similar to that of a medical doctor but who place special emphasis on the skeletal and muscular systems. Their treatments may involve manipulation of the muscles and joints. Osteopaths receive the degree of doctor of osteopathy (DO) rather than MD.

Eye care specialists can be either ophthalmologists or optometrists. An **ophthalmologist** holds a medical degree and can perform surgery and prescribe medications. An **optometrist** typically evaluates visual problems and fits glasses but is not a trained physician. If you have an eye infection, glaucoma, or other eye condition needing diagnosis and treatment, you need to see an ophthalmologist.

Dentists are specialists who diagnose and treat diseases of the teeth, gums, and oral cavity. They attend dental school for 4 years and receive the title of doctor of dental surgery (DDS) or doctor of medical dentistry (DMD). They must also pass both state and national board examinations before receiving their licenses to practice. The field of dentistry includes many specialties. For example, *orthodontists* specialize in the alignment of teeth. *Oral surgeons* perform surgical procedures to correct problems of the mouth, face, and jaw.

Nurses are highly trained and strictly regulated health professionals who provide a wide range of services for patients and their families, including patient education, counseling, community health and disease prevention information, and administration of medications. They may choose from several training options. There are over 2.4 million licensed registered nurses (RNs) in the United States who have completed either a 4-year program leading to a bachelor of science in nursing (BSN) degree or a 2-year associate degree program. More than half a million lower-level licensed practical or vocational nurses (LPN or LVN) have completed a 1- to 2-year training program, which may be based in either a community college or a hospital.

Nurse practitioners (NPs) are nurses with advanced training obtained through either a master's degree program or a specialized nurse practitioner program. Nurse practitioners have the training and authority to conduct diagnostic tests and prescribe medications (in some states). They work in a variety of settings, particularly in HMOs (health maintenance organizations), clinics, and student health centers. Nurses and nurse practitioners may also earn the clinical doctor of nursing degree (ND), doctor of nursing science (DNS and DNSc degrees), or a research-based PhD in nursing.

More than 68,000 **physician assistants (PAs)** currently practice in the United States. Physician assistants are licensed to examine and diagnose patients, offer treatment, and write prescriptions under a physician's supervision. An important difference between a PA and an NP is that the PA must practice under a physician's supervision. Like other health care providers, PAs are licensed by state boards of medicine.

Health Insurance

Whether you're visiting your regular doctor, consulting a specialist, or preparing for a hospital stay, chances are that you'll be using some form of health insurance to pay for your care. Insurance typically allows you, the consumer, to pay into a pool of funds and then bill the insurance carrier for health care charges you incur. The fundamental principle of insurance underwriting is that the cost of health care can be predicted for large populations. This is how health care premiums (payments) are determined. Policyholders pay premiums into a pool, which is held in reserve until needed. When you are sick or injured, the insurance company pays out of the pool, regardless of your total amount of contribution. Depending on circumstances, you may never pay for what your medical care costs, or you may pay much more for insurance than your medical bills ever total. The idea is that you pay affordable premiums so that you never have to face catastrophic bills. In today's profit-oriented system, insurers prefer to have healthy people in their plans who pour money into risk pools without taking money out.

Unfortunately, not everyone has health insurance. Over 46 million Americans are uninsured—that is, they have no private health insurance and are not eligible for Medicare, Medicaid, or other government health programs.[5] Lack of health insurance has been associated with delayed health care and increased mortality. *Underinsurance* (i.e., the inability to pay out-of-pocket expenses despite having insurance) also may result in adverse health consequences. Another 25 million Americans between the ages of 19 and 64 are estimated to be underinsured (at risk for spending more than 10% of their income on medical care because their insurance is inadequate).[6]

Contrary to the common belief that the uninsured are unemployed, 75 percent of them are either workers or the dependents of workers. One-quarter of all the uninsured are children under age 16. Among young adults 18 to 24 years of age, 30 percent reported being uninsured at some point in time. This age group is more than twice as likely to be uninsured as are people 45 to 64 years of age. However, for young adults who are college students, the statistics are different. According to a recent survey, approximately 8 percent of college students report not having health insurance, and another 5 percent are unsure whether they have health insurance.[7]

For the uninsured and many of the underinsured, health care from any source may be too expensive to be obtainable. People without health care coverage are less likely than other

nurse Health professional who provides many services for patients and who may work in a variety of settings.

nurse practitioner (NP) Professional nurse with advanced training obtained through either a master's degree program or a specialized nurse practitioner program.

physician assistant (PA) A midlevel practitioner trained to handle most standard cases of care under the supervision of a physician.

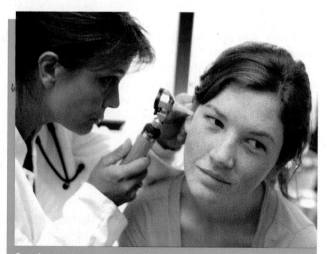

Can I count on my school's health care plan to cover my medical needs?

If you are enrolled in your parents' health insurance plan, coverage will end at age 23 or if you are not enrolled in school full time. Most university insurance plans are short term and noncatastrophic and have low upper limits of benefits, all of which are problematic in the event of an emergency illness or accident. If you are covered only under your school's health care plan, you should consider buying a higher level catastrophic plan in case of costly illness or accident.

Americans to have their children immunized, seek early pre-natal care, obtain annual blood pressure checks, and seek attention for serious symptoms. Experts believe that this ultimately leads to higher system costs, because their conditions deteriorate to a more debilitating and costly stage before they are forced to seek help.

Private Health Insurance

Originally, health insurance consisted solely of coverage for hospital costs (it was called *major medical*), but gradually it was extended to cover routine physicians' treatment and other areas, such as dental services and pharmaceuticals. These payment mechanisms laid the groundwork for today's steadily rising health care costs. Hospitals were reimbursed for the costs of providing care plus an amount for profit. This system provided no incentive to contain costs, limit the number of procedures, or curtail capital investment in redundant equipment and facilities. Physicians were reimbursed on a fee-for-service (indemnity) basis determined by "usual, customary, and reasonable" fees. This system encouraged physicians to charge high fees, raise them often, and perform as many procedures as possible. At the same time, because most insurance did not cover routine or preventive services, consumers were encouraged to use hospitals whenever possible (the coverage was better) and to wait until illness developed to seek care instead of seeking preventive care. Consumers were also free to choose any provider or service they wished, including even inappropriate—and often very expensive—levels of care.

Private insurance companies have increasingly employed several mechanisms to limit potential losses: cost sharing (in the form of deductibles, co-payments, and coinsurance), exclusions, "preexisting condition" clauses, waiting periods, and upper limits on payments. *Deductibles* are front-end payments (commonly $250 to $1,000) that you must make to your provider before your insurance company will start paying for any services you use. *Co-payments* are set amounts that you pay per service received, regardless of the cost of the service (e.g., $20 per doctor visit or per prescription). *Coinsurance* is the percentage of the bill that you must pay throughout the course of treatment (e.g., 20% of the total bill). *Preexisting condition clauses* limit the insurance company's liability for medical conditions that a consumer had before obtaining coverage (i.e., if a woman takes out coverage while she is pregnant, the insurance company may

managed care Cost-control procedures used by health insurers to coordinate treatment.
capitation Prepayment of a fixed monthly amount for each patient without regard to the type or number of services provided.

cover pregnancy complications and infant care but may not cover charges related to "normal pregnancy"). Because many insurance companies use a combination of these mechanisms, keeping track of the costs you are responsible for can become very difficult.

Group plans of large employers (e.g., government agencies, school districts, and corporations) generally do not have pre-existing condition clauses in their plans, but smaller group plans (a group may be as small as two people) often do. Some plans never cover preexisting conditions, whereas others specify a *waiting period* (e.g., 6 months) before they will provide coverage. All insurers set some limits on the types of services they cover (e.g., most exclude cosmetic surgery, private rooms, and experimental procedures). Some insurance plans may also include an *upper* or *lifetime limit*, after which coverage will end. Although $250,000 may seem like an enormous sum, medical bills for a sick child or chronic disease can easily run this high within a few years.

what do you think?

Why is it important that private insurance cover preventive or lower-level care as well as hospitalization and high-technology interventions?
● What kinds of incentives would cause you to seek care early rather than delay care?

Managed Care

Managed care describes a health care delivery system consisting of the following elements:

1. A network of physicians, hospitals, and other providers and facilities linked contractually to deliver comprehensive health benefits within a predetermined budget, sharing economic risk for any budget deficit or surplus
2. A budget based on an estimate of the annual cost of delivering health care for a given population
3. An established set of administrative rules requiring patients to follow the advice of participating health care providers in order to have their health care paid for under the terms of the health plan

Types of managed care plans include health maintenance organizations (HMOs), preferred provider organizations (PPOs), and point of service (POS). Approximately 64 million Americans are enrolled in HMOs, the most common type.[8]

Many managed care plans pay their contracted health care providers through **capitation,** that is, prepayment of a fixed monthly amount for each patient without regard for the type or number of health

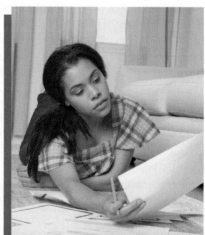

What should I consider when choosing health insurance?

Choosing a health insurance plan can be confusing. Some things to think about include how comprehensive your coverage needs to be, how convenient your care must be, how much you are willing to spend on premiums and co-payments, what the overall cost will be, and whether the services of the plan meet your needs.

services provided. Some plans pay health care providers a salary, and some are still fee-for-service plans. As with other insurance plans, enrollees are members of a risk pool, and it is expected that some persons will use no services, some will use a modest amount, and others will have high-cost usage over a given year. Doctors have the incentive to keep their patient pool healthy and avoid catastrophic ailments that are preventable; usually such incentives come back in terms of increased salaries, bonuses, and other benefits. As such, prevention and health education to reduce risk and intervene early to avoid major problems are often capstone components of such plans.

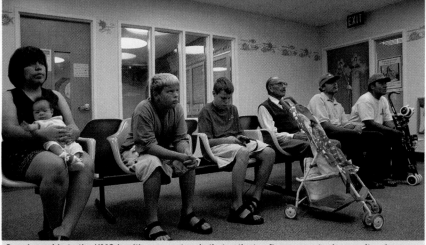

One downside to the HMO health care system is that patients often encounter long waits when they need to see their health care provider.

Managed care plans have grown steadily over the past decade with a proportionate decline of enrollment in traditional indemnity insurance plans. The reason for this shift is that indemnity insurance, which pays providers and hospitals on a fee-for-service basis with no built-in incentives to control costs, has become unaffordable or unavailable for most Americans.

Health Maintenance Organization Health maintenance organizations (HMOs) provide a wide range of covered health benefits (e.g., checkups, surgery, doctor visits, lab tests) for a fixed amount prepaid by the patient, the employer, Medicaid, or Medicare (discussed later). Usually, HMO premiums are the least expensive form of managed care (saving between 10 and 40 percent more than other plans) but also are the most restrictive (offering little or no choice in doctors and certain services). These premiums are 8 to 10 percent lower than for traditional plans, there are low or no deductibles or coinsurance payments, and co-payments are approximately $20 per office visit.

The downside of HMOs is that patients are typically required to use the plan's doctors and hospitals and to get approval from a "gatekeeper" or PCP for treatment and referrals. As more and more people enroll in HMOs, criticisms about them are mounting. Concerns about HMOs include questions about care allocation, profit-motivated medical decision making, and the degree of focus on prevention and intervention.

Preferred Provider Organization Preferred provider organizations (PPOs) are networks of independent doctors and hospitals that contract to provide care at discounted rates. Although they offer greater choices in doctors than HMOs do, they are less likely to coordinate a patient's care. Members do have a choice of seeing doctors who are not on the preferred list, but this choice may come at considerable cost (e.g., having to pay 30% of the charges out of pocket, rather than 10 to 20% for PPO doctors and services).

Point of Service Point of service (POS)—a hybrid of the HMO and PPO types—provides a more acceptable form of managed care for people used to the traditional indemnity plan of insurance, which probably explains why it is among the fastest growing of the managed care plans. Under POS plans, patients can go to providers outside their HMO for care but must pay for the extra cost.

Medicare and Medicaid

Medicare is a federal insurance program that covers a broad range of services except long-term care. Medicare covers 99 percent of individuals over age 65, all totally and permanently disabled people (after a waiting period), and all people with end-stage kidney failure—currently over 45 million people, or one in seven Americans, in all.[9] By 2030, it is estimated that one in five—or 77 million—Americans will be insured by Medicare. As the costs of medical care have continued to increase, Medicare has placed limits on the amount of reimbursement to providers. As a result, some physicians and managed care programs have stopped accepting Medicare patients.

To control hospital costs, in 1983 the federal government set up a prospective payment system based on **diagnosis-related groups (DRGs)** for Medicare. Using a complicated formula, nearly 500 groupings of diagnoses were created to establish how much a hospital would be reimbursed for a particular patient. If a hospital can treat the patient for less than that amount, it can keep the difference. However, if a patient's care costs more than the set amount, the hospital must absorb the difference (with a few exceptions that must be reviewed by a panel). This system gives hospitals the incentive to discharge patients quickly after doing as little as possible for them, to provide more ambulatory care, and to admit only patients with favorable (profitable) DRGs. Many private health insurance companies have followed the federal government in adopting this type of reimbursement. In 1998, the federal Health Care Financing Administration (HCFA) expanded the prospective payment system to include payments for outpatient surgery and skilled nursing care.

diagnosis-related groups (DRGs) Diagnostic categories established by the federal government to determine in advance how much hospitals will be reimbursed for the care of a particular Medicare patient.

In its continuing effort to control rising costs, the HCFA has encouraged the growth of prepaid HMO senior plans for

Medicare-eligible persons. Under this system, commercial managed care insurance plans receive a fixed per capita premium from the HCFA and then offer more preventive services with lower out-of-pocket co-payments. These managed care plans encourage providers and patients to utilize health care resources under administrative rules similar to commercial HMO plans.

In contrast to Medicare, Medicaid, covering approximately 46 million people, is a federal–state matching funds welfare program for people who are defined as poor, including many who are blind, disabled, elderly, or receiving Aid to Families with Dependent Children. Medicaid relies on matching funds provided by federal and state sources.[10] Because each state determines income eligibility and payments to providers, there are vast differences in the way Medicaid operates from state to state.

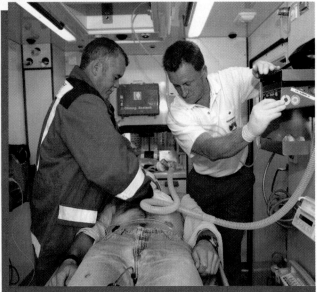

Issues Facing Today's Health Care System

Many Americans believe that our health care system needs fundamental reform. In recent years, the number of individuals who are underinsured has risen dramatically, and, without reform, the rise will likely continue. Individuals with preexisting conditions, and those who are self-employed are just two groups who often find themselves unable to find or afford health care. The significant costs of a major procedure, course of treatment, or hospital stay mean many families are one catastrophic illness or accident away from financial ruin. In addition to cost and access, malpractice, restricted choices in providers and treatments, unnecessary procedures, complicated and cumbersome insurance rules, and dramatic ranges in quality are also issues of concern. See the **Green Guide** on the next page for a discussion of another concern about the

What happens if I don't have insurance and I need medical care?

People without insurance can't gain access to preventive care, so they seek care only in an emergency or crisis. Because emergency care is extraordinarily expensive, they often are unable to pay, and the cost is absorbed by those who can pay—the insured or taxpayers. Using the emergency room for anything other than a real crisis contributes to higher health care costs and diminished access to emergency care for everyone. If you need nonemergency health care, there are often community-based resources, such as free or low-cost clinics, that can provide preventive care.

health care system: the amount of waste it produces and its impact on the environment.

Cost

Both per capita and as a percentage of gross domestic product (GDP), we spend more on health care than any other nation. Yet, unlike the rest of the industrialized world, we do not provide access for our entire population. Already, we spend over $2 trillion annually on health care, over $7,200 for every man, woman, and child (Figure 16.2). This translates into 16.3 percent of our GDP. Does this sound like a lot? Consider that health care expenditures are projected to grow by 6.2 percent each year, reaching over $4 trillion annually by 2018—nearly 20 percent of our projected GDP.[11]

Why do health care costs continue to skyrocket? Many factors are involved: excess administrative costs; duplication of services; an aging population; growing rates of obesity, inactivity, and related health problems; demand for new diagnostic and treatment technologies; an emphasis on crisis-oriented care instead

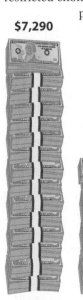

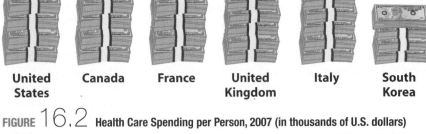

FIGURE 16.2 **Health Care Spending per Person, 2007 (in thousands of U.S. dollars)**

United States	Canada	France	United Kingdom	Italy	South Korea
$7,290	$3,895	$3,601	$2,992	$2,686	$1,688

Source: Data are from Organisation for Economic Co-operation and Development, *OECD Health Data 2009*, 2009, www.oecd.org/health.

GREEN GUIDE

The Perils of Medical Waste

The health care system in the United States is massive, and it affects many aspects of our daily lives, including our environment. Medical and pharmaceutical waste have been shown to have negative environmental impacts on air and water resources, as well as on human and animal health.

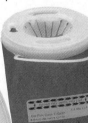

MEDICAL WASTE

The Medical Waste Tracking Act of 1988 defines medical waste as "any solid waste that is generated in the diagnosis, treatment, or immunization of human beings or animals, in research pertaining thereto, or in the production or testing of biologicals." This definition includes, but is not limited to, blood-soaked bandages; culture dishes and other glassware; discarded surgical gloves; discarded surgical instruments; discarded needles used to give shots or draw blood (e.g., medical sharps); cultures, stocks, or swabs used to inoculate cultures; removed body organs (e.g., tonsils, appendices, limbs); and discarded lancets.

Due to concern about the spread of infectious diseases, especially in hospital and clinic settings, there is a vital need for sterility. This leads to excessive one-time-use items such as latex gloves, needles, bandages, and much more. All these items contribute substantially to the amount of medical waste.

Some estimate that the volume of hospital-generated medical waste is as much as 2 million tons each year. Approximately 10 percent of potentially infectious medical waste is combined with medical waste that is not deemed infectious and then disposed of in landfills. As water percolates through solid-waste disposal sites such as landfills, it collects contaminants and forms a substance called

Extra precautions must be taken when disposing of medical waste.

leachate. This can contaminate groundwater and surface water. Pollution in the ocean is also a major problem, as it directly affects all sea life and indirectly affects human health. In 1988, the EPA banned dumping waste into the ocean, but the ban wasn't enforced until January 1992. Most of the waste that was dumped in the 1980s and early 1990s is still there today.

Currently, the vast majority—over 90 percent—of potentially infectious medical waste in the United States and around the world is incinerated, resulting in carbon emissions and other pollution such as particulate matter. Alternatives to incineration of medical waste include thermal treatment, such as microwave technologies; steam sterilization, such as autoclaving; and chemical mechanical systems that break down organic and inorganic wastes without polluting.

PHARMACEUTICAL WASTE

In addition to medical waste, hospitals generate a substantial amount of pharmaceutical waste—both hazardous and nonhazardous—that requires proper disposal. Generally, this waste comprises drugs that have been dispensed but not completely used. There is also a large amount of individual-generated pharmaceutical waste. Studies have shown that nearly 54 percent of consumers put unwanted medications in the trash, and 35 percent flush them down the toilet.

Prescription drug waste can contaminate our water supply through a number of avenues. First, medicines disposed of down the toilet or drain can easily be incorporated into groundwater, lakes, rivers, and streams. This may harm fish and wildlife that live in lakes, rivers, and

the ocean. In addition, these drugs can end up back in our drinking water supply. This leads to elevated levels of chemicals that many water treatment facilities are not equipped to filter. Pharmaceutical drugs have been detected in the drinking water supplies of major metropolitan areas all across the United States. To date, the federal government has not set limits on the amount of pharmaceutical drugs in drinking water and doesn't require any testing for their presence.

Prescription drugs that are thrown away rather than flushed add to our growing landfills and can contribute to the toxicity of leachate. However, many sources still encourage throwing away unused prescription drugs, as it is a better method of disposal than flushing or dumping down the drain. Alternatively, here are some more green ways to manage unused medications:

✱ Send your medicine to those in need. Some organizations collect unused, unexpired medicine to send to other countries where prescription drugs are harder to access. Recently, nine states (Florida, Nebraska, Nevada, New Jersey, Oklahoma, Texas, Wisconsin, Indiana, and South Dakota) have passed legislation for recycling unused medications in nursing homes with nine more considering similar practices. Nonprofits, like the Iowa Prescription Drug Corporation (www .iowapdc.org), have developed and administered statewide drug-donation programs.

✱ Take your drugs back to the pharmacy. Many community pharmacies are starting take-back programs for unused or unneeded prescriptions. The pharmacy then disposes of these drugs safely. In some cases, pharmacies return unused pharmaceuticals to manufacturers for processing; in other cases, unused prescription medications are destroyed safely. It is still recommended to throw away (instead of flush) nonprescription drugs such as aspirin or ibuprofen.

of prevention; and inappropriate use of services by consumers.

Our system has more than 2,000 health insurance companies, each with different coverage structures and administrative requirements. This lack of uniformity prevents our system from achieving the *economies of scale* (bulk purchasing at a reduced cost) and administrative efficiency realized in countries where there is a single-payer delivery system. According to the Health Insurance Association of America, commercial insurance companies commonly experience administrative costs greater than 10 percent of the total health care insurance premium, whereas the administrative cost of the government's Medicare program is less than 4 percent. These administrative expenses contribute to the high cost of health care and force companies to require employees to share more of the costs, cut back on benefits, and drop some benefits altogether. These costs are largely passed on to consumers in the form of higher prices for goods and services. See **Figure 16.3** for a breakdown of how health care dollars are spent.

Access

Over 90 million people in the United States suffer from chronic health conditions that should be at least monitored by medical practitioners.[12] Their access to care is largely determined by whether they have health insurance. Catastrophic or chronic illness among only 10 percent of the population accounts for 75 percent of all health expenditures.[13] Since we cannot perfectly predict who will fall into that 10 percent, every American is potentially vulnerable to the high cost and devastating effects of such illnesses.

Access to health care is determined by numerous factors, including the supply of providers and facilities, proximity to care, ability to maneuver in the system, health status, and insurance coverage. Although there are approximately 700,000 physicians in the United States, many Americans lack adequate access to health services because of insurance barriers or maldistribution of providers. There is an oversupply of higher-paid specialists and a shortage of lower-paid primary care physicians (family practitioners, pediatricians, internists, OB/Gyns, geriatricians). Inner cities and some rural areas face constant shortages of physicians.

Until recently, many employees lost their insurance benefits when they changed jobs; this led the federal government to pass legislation mandating the "portability" of health insurance benefits from one job to the next, thereby guaranteeing

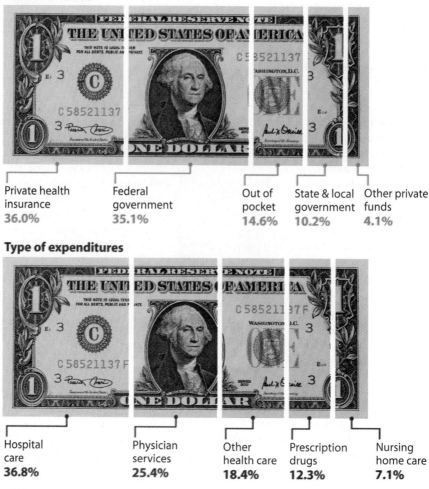

Source of funds

Private health insurance **36.0%**

Federal government **35.1%**

Out of pocket **14.6%**

State & local government **10.2%**

Other private funds **4.1%**

Type of expenditures

Hospital care **36.8%**

Physician services **25.4%**

Other health care **18.4%**

Prescription drugs **12.3%**

Nursing home care **7.1%**

Total expenditures = $1.8 trillion

FIGURE 16.3 **Where Do We Spend Our Health Care Dollars?**

Source: Data are from National Center for Health Statistics, *Health, United States, 2008, with Chartbook on Trends in the Health of Americans* (Hyattsville, MD: National Center for Health Statistics, 2009).

coverage during the transition. Today, individuals who leave their jobs can continue their group health insurance benefits under the Consolidated Omnibus Budget Reconciliation Act (COBRA). COBRA allows former employees, retirees, spouses, and dependents to continue their insurance at group rates. COBRA beneficiaries pay a higher amount than when they were employed, as they're covering both the personal premium and the amount previously covered by the employer. As a result, COBRA benefits are more expensive than benefits through an employer, but less expensive than purchasing individual insurance. COBRA coverage is only temporary, and usually lasts for up to 18 months.

Managed care health plans determine access on the basis of participating providers, health plan benefits, and administrative rules. Often this means that consumers do not have the freedom to choose specialists, facilities, or treatment options beyond those contracted with the health plan and recommended by their PCP. In the United States, consumer demand has led to an expansion of benefits to include nonallopathic therapies such as chiropractic and acupuncture (see

Chapter 17). However, many nonallopathic treatments remain unavailable, even to a limited degree, through current health plans.

Quality and Malpractice

The U.S. health care system has several mechanisms for ensuring quality services: education, licensure, certification/registration, accreditation, peer review, and the legal system of malpractice litigation. Some of these mechanisms are mandatory before a professional or organization may provide care, whereas others are purely voluntary. (Be aware that licensure, although mandated by the state for some practitioners and facilities, is only a minimum guarantee of quality.) Insurance companies and government payers may also require a higher level of quality by linking payment to whether a practitioner is board certified or a facility is accredited by the appropriate agency. In addition, most insurance plans now require prior authorization and/or second opinions, not only to reduce costs but also to improve quality of care.

Consumer, provider, and advocacy groups focus on the great variation in quality as a major problem. A new form of quality measurement uses "outcome" as the primary indicator for measuring health care quality at the individual level. With outcome measurements, we don't look just at what is done to the patient, but at what subsequently happens to the patient's health status. Thus, mortality rates and complication rates (e.g., infections) become important in assessing individual practitioners and facilities.

Medical errors and mistakes do happen. An Institute of Medicine report indicates that as many as 44,000 to 98,000 people die in U.S. hospitals each year as the result of medical errors.[14] Clearly, we must be proactive in our health care.

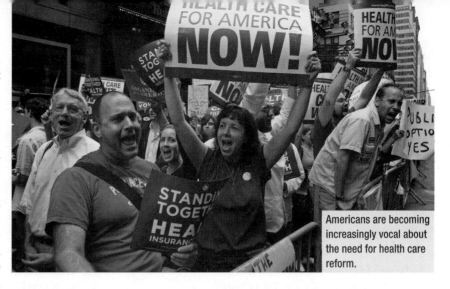

Americans are becoming increasingly vocal about the need for health care reform.

what do you think?

Do you believe prospective patients should have access to information about practitioners' and facilities' malpractice records? ● How about their success and failure rates or outcomes of various procedures?

The Debate over National Health Insurance

The United States has seen four major political movements supporting national health insurance during the past century, but none has succeeded. Most recently, the Obama administration put health care reform at the top of its domestic agenda. Whether universal coverage will—or should—be achieved and through what mechanism remain hotly debated topics.

Proponents of reform argue that health care should be available and affordable for everyone, and often state the view that health care is a right, not a privilege. They point to other Western countries, such as Canada and France, that currently have successful universal coverage. Opponents of health care reform feel that the high cost of changing the system is more than the United States can afford, and often state that the government should not interfere in what has been a largely free-market industry. Both sides of the debate have articulated valid arguments and concerns.

However, analysts believe that health care reform has failed in the past due to a combination of less valid factors that have little to do with the quality of the nation's health. Lobbying efforts by the insurance industry and the medical community, proposed plans that were too complicated, and interest groups that contended that the plans either went "too far" or "not far enough" have all played a role in thwarting reform in the past. Some people also believe that our current system serves people well.

One critical point must be made, though: We are paying for the most expensive system in the world without obtaining full coverage. We pay for people who don't have insurance through increased premiums and taxes, and we spend more than necessary, because prevention and early treatment are not emphasized. We also pay for much duplication of services and technologies, for practitioners who practice defensive medicine, and for the vast bureaucracy made inevitable by the vast number of private health insurance companies.

The Institute of Medicine, a nonpartisan organization that advises the federal government on health issues, recommends a single-payer, tax-financed scheme that severs insurance ties from employment.[15] Similar to the Canadian model, it would cover everyone—regardless of income or other factors such as health status. It would offer many different ways to tailor a plan to the needs of U.S. citizens. A single federal plan or a privately administered plan paid for by general tax funds or earmarked taxes could be created. Thus, all (or most) private insurers would be eliminated or would see their role limited to that of fiscal administrators. While a single-payer system might be the most equitable and efficient health care model, it is not realistically on the table for the United States, due to the size and influence of the current health care industry. The closest viable alternative is the "public option," which would implement a government-run insurer, similar to Medicare, that consumers could choose instead of a traditional provider.

Are You a Smart Health Care Consumer?

PEARSON
myhealthlab

Fill out this assessment online at
www.pearsonhighered.com/myhealthlab
or www.pearsonhighered.com/donatelle.

Answer the following questions to determine what you might do to become a better health care consumer.

	Yes	No
1. Do you have health insurance, and do you understand the coverage available to you under your plan?	○	○
2. Do you know which health care services are available for free or at a reduced cost at your student health center or local clinic? If so, what are they?	○	○
3. When you receive a prescription, do you ask the doctor or pharmacist if a generic brand could be substituted?	○	○
4. When you receive a prescription, do you ask the doctor or pharmacist about potential side effects, including possible food and drug interactions?	○	○
5. Do you report any unusual drug side effects to your health care provider?	○	○
6. Do you take medication as directed?	○	○

	Yes	No
7. When you receive a diagnosis, do you seek more information about the diagnosis and treatment?	○	○
8. If your health care provider recommends surgery or an invasive type of treatment, do you seek a second opinion?	○	○
9. Do you seek health information only from reliable and credible sources? Can you name three examples of such sources?	○	○
10. Do you read labels carefully before buying over-the-counter (OTC) medications?	○	○
11. Do you have a health care provider?	○	○

12. How much of a role do you think advertising plays in your decision to purchase a new product?

None ○ Some ○ A lot ○

YOUR PLAN FOR CHANGE

Once you have considered your responses to the **Assess yourself** questions, you may want to change or improve certain behaviors in order to get the best treatment from your health care provider and the heath care system.

Today, you can:

○ Research the insurance plan under which you're covered. Find out which health care providers and hospitals you can visit, the amounts of any co-payments and premiums you will be responsible for, and the drug coverage of your plan.

○ Clean out your medicine cabinet. Get rid of any expired prescriptions or OTC medications (see the Green Guide on page 497 for information on safe drug disposal) and take stock of what you have. Keep on hand a supply of basic items, such as pain relievers, antiseptic cream, bandages, cough suppressants, and throat lozenges, and replenish the supply if you're running low.

Within the next 2 weeks, you can:

○ Find a regular health care provider if you do not have one and make an appointment for a general checkup and interview.

○ Think about health conditions you would benefit from knowing more about—such as those that run in your family or that you've experienced in the past—and do some research on them. Write down any unanswered questions so you can discuss them with your health care provider.

By the end of the semester, you can:

○ Ask if a generic version is available when filling your next prescription.

○ Become an advocate for health insurance for all. Write to your congressperson or state legislature to express your interest in health care reform.

Summary

* Self-care and individual responsibility are key factors in reducing rising health care costs and improving health status. Advance planning can help you navigate health care treatment in unfamiliar situations or emergencies. Assess health professionals by considering their qualifications, their record of treating problems like yours, and their ability to work with you.
* In theory, allopathic (conventional Western) medicine is based on scientifically validated methods and procedures. Medical doctors, specialists of various kinds, nurses, physician assistants, and other health care professionals practice allopathic medicine.
* Prescription drugs are administered under medical supervision. Generic drugs often can be substituted for more expensive brand name products. Over-the-counter (OTC) drugs include analgesics; cold, cough, allergy, and asthma relievers; stimulants; sleeping aids and relaxants; and dieting aids. Consumers should be aware of the potential side effects and interactions of both prescription and OTC drugs.
* Health insurance is based on the concept of spreading risk. Insurance is provided by private insurance companies (which charge premiums) and the government Medicare and Medicaid programs (which are funded by taxes). Managed care (in the form of HMOs, POS plans, and PPOs) attempts to control costs by streamlining administrative procedures and stressing preventive care, among other initiatives.
* Concerns about the U.S. health care system include cost, access, choice of treatment modality, quality and malpractice, and fraud and abuse.

Pop Quiz

1. Which of the following is not a condition that would indicate a visit to a physician is needed?
   a. recurring high temperature (over 103°F in adults)
   b. persistent or recurrent diarrhea
   c. the common cold
   d. yellowing of the skin or the whites of the eyes

2. Which is a common type of over-the-counter drug?
   a. antibiotics
   b. hormonal contraceptives
   c. antidepressants
   d. antacids

3. What medical practice is based on procedures whose objective is to heal by countering the patient's symptoms?
   a. allopathic medicine
   b. nonallopathic medicine
   c. osteopathic medicine
   d. chiropractic medicine

4. Jack evaluates visual problems and fits glasses but is not a trained physician. Jack is a(n)
   a. osteopath.
   b. ophthalmologist.
   c. optometrist.
   d. physician assistant.

5. What mechanism used by private insurance companies requires that the subscriber pay a certain amount directly to the provider before the insurance company will begin paying for services?
   a. coinsurance
   b. cost sharing
   c. co-payments
   d. deductibles

6. Deborah, 28, is a single parent on welfare. Her medical bills are paid by a federal health insurance program for the poor. This agency is
   a. an HMO.
   b. Social Security.
   c. Medicaid.
   d. Medicare

7. The federal insurance program that covers 99 percent of adults over 65 years of age is
   a. Medicare.
   b. Medicaid.
   c. COBRA.
   d. HMO.

8. The most restrictive type of managed care is
   a. fee-for-service.
   b. health maintenance organizations.
   c. point of service.
   d. preferred provider organizations.

9. Lauren has diabetes, and because of a job change she had to choose a new health insurance provider. The new insurance company refused to cover her diabetic care expenses under a clause in the contract which stated that Lauren has
   a. a coinsurance limit.
   b. a preexisting health condition.
   c. already exceeded the lifetime upper limit.
   d. no major medical coverage on her policy.

10. A specialist who diagnoses and treats diseases of the teeth, gums, and oral cavity is a(n)
    a. dentist.
    b. orthodontist.
    c. oral surgeon.
    d. osteopath.

Answers for these questions can be found on page A-1.

Think about It!

1. List several conditions (resulting from illness or accident) for which you wouldn't need to seek medical help. When would you consider each condition to be bad enough to require medical attention? How would you decide to whom and where to go for treatment?

2. Describe your rights as a patient. Have you ever received treatment that violated these rights? If so, what action, if any, did you take?

3. What are the inherent benefits and risks of managed care organizations?

4. Explain the differences between traditional indemnity insurance and managed health care. Which would you feel more comfortable with? Should insurance companies dictate rates for various medical tests and procedures in an attempt to keep prices down?

5. Discuss how medical and pharmaceutical waste has a negative impact on the environment. What are two ways in which you personally can reduce such waste?

Accessing Your Health on the Internet

The following websites explore further topics and issues related to personal health. For links to the websites below, visit the Companion Website for *Health: The Basics*, Green Edition at www.pearsonhighered.com/donatelle.

1. *Agency for HealthCare Research and Quality (AHRQ)*. A gateway to consumer health information. Provides links to sites that can address health care concerns and provide information on what questions to ask, what to look for, and what you should know when making critical decisions about personal care. www.ahrq.gov

2. *Food and Drug Administration (FDA)*. News on the latest government-approved home health tests and other health-related products. www.fda.gov

3. *HealthGrades*. This company provides quality reports on physicians as well as hospitals, nursing homes, and other health care facilities. www.healthgrades.com

4. *The Leapfrog Group*. A nationwide coalition of more than 150 public and private organizations, the Leapfrog Group focuses on identifying problems in the U.S. hospital system that can lead to medical errors and on devising solutions. www.leapfroggroup.org

5. *National Committee for Quality Assurance (NCQA)*. The NCQA assesses and reports on the quality of managed care plans, including HMOs. www.ncqa.org

6. *National Library of Medicine*. Supports Medline/Pubmed information retrieval systems in addition to providing public health information for consumers. www.nlm.nih.gov

7. *HealthReform.Gov*. Provides up-to-date information regarding health care reform in America. www.healthreform.gov

References

1. American Academy of Orthopaedic Surgeons, "Information Statement: The Importance of Good Communication in the Physician-Patient Relationship," September 2005, www.aaos.org/about/papers/advistmt/1017.asp.

2. D. Merenstein et al., "Use and Costs of Nonrecommended Tests during Routine Preventive Health Exams," *American Journal of Preventive Medicine*, 30 (2006): 521–27.

3. Consumer Health, "Patient Rights: Informed Consent," 2008, www.emedicinehealth.com/informed_consent/article_em.htm.

4. American College Health Association, *American College Health Association-National College Health Assessment (ACHA-NCHA) Reference Group Data Report Fall 2008* (Baltimore: American College Health Association, 2009).

5. C. DeNavas-Walt, B. Proctor, and J. Smith, *Income, Poverty, and Health Insurance Coverage in the United States: 2008*, U.S. Census Bureau, Current Population Reports, P60-236 (Washington, DC: U.S. Government Printing Office, 2009).

6. C. Schoen et al. "How Many Are Underinsured? Trends among U.S. Adults, 2003 and 2007," *Health Affairs* Web Exclusive (June 10, 2008): w298–w309.

7. National Center for Health Statistics, *Health, United States, 2007, with Chartbook on Trends in the Health of Americans* (Hyattsville, MD: National Center for Health Statistics, 2008).

8. Kaiser Family Foundation, "Total HMO Enrollment, June 2008," Statehealthfacts.org, 2009, www.statehealthfacts.org/comparemaptable.jsp?ind=348&cat=7.

9. Centers for Medicare and Medicaid Services, "Medicare Enrollment: National Trends 1966–2008," 2009, www.cms.hhs.gov/MedicareEnRpts/Downloads/HISMI08.pdf.

10. Centers for Medicare and Medicaid Services, "Medicaid Data Sources," 2008, www.cms.hhs.gov/MedicaidDataSourcesGenInfo.

11. National Center for Health Statistics, *Health, United States, 2008 with Chartbook on Trends in the Health of Americans*, 2009; Centers for Medicare and Medicaid Services, "National Health Care Expenditures Projections: 2008–2018," 2008, www.cms.hhs.gov/NationalHealthExpendData/Downloads/proj2008.pdf.

12. Centers for Disease Control and Prevention, "Indicators for Chronic Disease Surveillance," *Morbidity and Mortality Weekly Report, Recommendations and Reports* 53, no. RR11 (2004): 1–6, www.cdc.gov/mmwr/preview/mmwrhtml/rr5311a1.htm.

13. National Center for Chronic Disease Prevention and Health Promotion, "Chronic Disease Overview," 2008, www.cdc.gov/nccdphp/overview.htm.

14. Institute of Medicine, "The Chasm in Quality: Select Indicators from Recent Reports," May 2006, www.iom.edu.

15. Institute of Medicine, "Insuring America's Health: Principles and Recommendations," January 2004, www.iom.edu/CMS/3809/4660/17632.aspx.

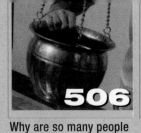
506
Why are so many people using alternative medicine?

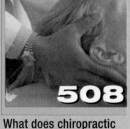
508
What does chiropractic medicine do?

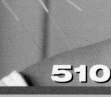
510
How does acupuncture work?

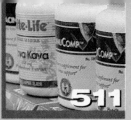
511
Do herbal remedies have any risks or side effects?

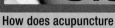
17

Complementary and Alternative Medicine

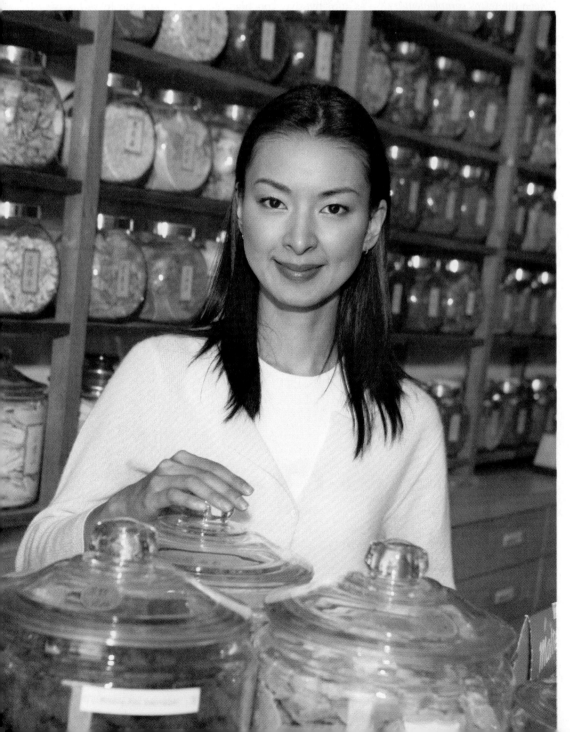

Objectives

* Describe complementary and alternative medicine (CAM), and identify its typical domains.

* Explain major types of complementary and alternative medicine providers and common treatments they offer.

* Discuss the various types of complementary and alternative medicines used today, who is most likely to use them, their patterns of use, and their potential benefits and risks.

* Understand how to evaluate testimonials and claims related to complementary and alternative products, services, and practitioners to ensure that you are getting accurate information and safe treatment.

* Summarize the challenges and opportunities related to complementary and alternative medicine in ensuring our health and wellness.

An increasingly popular trend in self-care and health promotion focuses on **complementary and alternative medicine (CAM).** These therapies are defined as a group of diverse medical and health care systems, practices, and products that are not currently considered part of conventional medicine.[1] Various products and services offer today's consumers a broad range of health choices and an opportunity for greater control over their own health.

Complementary and Alternative Medicine: What Is It and Who Uses It?

Although often used interchangeably when referring to therapies, there is a distinction between the terms *complementary* and *alternative*. **Complementary medicine** is used *together with* conventional medicine, as part of the modern integrative-medicine approach. An example of complementary medicine is to use massage therapy along with prescription medicine to treat anxiety.[2] **Alternative medicine** has traditionally been used *in place of* conventional medicine, such as following a special diet or herbal remedy to treat cancer instead of using radiation, surgery, or other conventional treatments. However, as some alternative medical approaches have gained scientific credibility, they are used along with conventional treatment. A survey conducted by the National Center for Complementary and Alternative Medicine (NCCAM) revealed that 38 percent of adults use some form of CAM.[3] **Figure 17.1** shows more results from this study.

complementary and alternative medicine (CAM) Forms of treatment distinct from traditional allopathic medicine that until recently were neither taught widely in U.S. medical schools nor generally available in U.S. hospitals.
complementary medicine Treatment used in conjunction with conventional medicine.
alternative medicine Treatment used in place of conventional medicine.
holistic Relating to or concerned with the whole body and the interactions of systems, rather than treatment of individual parts.

Conventional medicine is practiced by holders of MD (medical doctor) or DO (doctor of osteopathy) degrees and by allied health professionals, such as physical therapists, psychologists, and registered nurses (see Chapter 16). Other terms for conventional medicine include *allopathy, Western, mainstream, orthodox,* and *biomedicine*. In general, practitioners of allopathic medicine treat disease by using remedies that include pharmaceutical drugs or surgery, have graduated from U.S.-sanctioned schools of medicine or nursing, or are licensed practitioners recognized by the American Medical Association (AMA), American Nurses Association (ANA), or other certification board. Some conventional medical practitioners are also CAM practitioners.

The list of practices that are considered CAM changes continually as therapies become accepted as "mainstream." In general, CAM therapies serve as alternatives to the conventional Western system of medicine, which some people regard as too invasive, too high-tech, and too toxic in terms of laboratory-produced medications. CAM therapies incorporate a **holistic** approach to medicine that focuses on treating both the mind and the whole body, rather than just an isolated part of the body. Often CAM users seek what they perceive as a more natural, gentle approach to healing. Other CAM patients distrust the traditional medical approach and believe that alternative practices will give them greater control over their own health care. CAM therapies can vary based on whether they have been scientifically studied and whether those studies have shown them to be beneficial. Research has shown that many types of CAM, including acupuncture and massage therapy, are beneficial in treating conditions such as chronic back pain and cancer.[4]

As the NCCAM survey indicates, more than one-third of adults in the United States have used CAM. Why do so many people seek alternative therapy? Distinct patterns of CAM use emerge from this survey:[5]

● More women than men
● People with higher educational levels

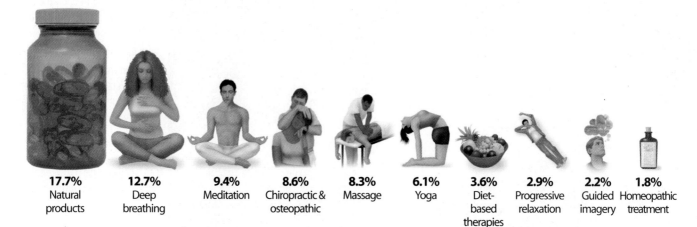

17.7%	12.7%	9.4%	8.6%	8.3%	6.1%	3.6%	2.9%	2.2%	1.8%
Natural products	Deep breathing	Meditation	Chiropractic & osteopathic	Massage	Yoga	Diet-based therapies	Progressive relaxation	Guided imagery	Homeopathic treatment

FIGURE 17.1 The 10 Most Common CAM Therapies among U.S. Adults

Source: Data are from National Center for Complementary and Alternative Medicine, "The Use of Complementary and Alternative Medicine in the United States," NCCAM Publication no. D434, 2008.

36% of 18- to 29-year-olds report having used some form of CAM.

- People who had been hospitalized in the past year
- Former smokers (compared with current smokers or those who have never smoked)
- People with back, neck, head, or joint aches or other painful conditions
- People with gastrointestinal disorders or sleeping problems

Figure 17.2 summarizes the conditions for which respondents to the NCCAM survey used CAM.

As with traditional Western medicine, practitioners of most complementary and alternative therapies spend years learning their practice. Various forms of CAM are increasingly being taught in U.S. medical schools and are available to patients in some clinics and hospitals. Some, such as acupuncture, are even covered under many health insurance policies. However, it is important to note that complementary and alternative therapies vary widely in terms of the nature of treatment, extent of therapy, and types of problems for which they offer help. There is no national training or licensure standard, and states differ in their practices (this is also true for conventional

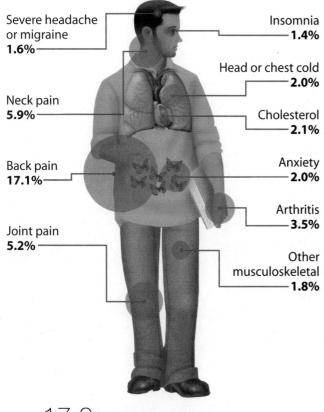

Severe headache or migraine
1.6%

Neck pain
5.9%

Back pain
17.1%

Joint pain
5.2%

Insomnia
1.4%

Head or chest cold
2.0%

Cholesterol
2.1%

Anxiety
2.0%

Arthritis
3.5%

Other musculoskeletal
1.8%

FIGURE 17.2 Diseases and Conditions for Which CAM Is Most Frequently Used among Adults, 2007

Source: Data are from P. M. Barnes, B. Bloom, and R. Nahin, "Complementary and Alternative Medicine Use Among Adults and Children: United States, 2007," *CDC National Health Statistics Report,* no. 12 (December 2008).

medicine). Whereas practitioners of conventional medicine have graduated from U.S.-sanctioned schools of medicine or are licensed medical practitioners recognized by the AMA—the governing body for all physicians—each CAM domain has a different set of training standards, guidelines for practice, and licensure procedures.

Alternative Medical Systems

Alternative (whole) medical systems are built on specific systems of theory and practice. There are many alternative systems of medicine that have been practiced by various cultures throughout the world. Some have evolved from centuries-old practices, such as traditional Chinese medicine and Ayurveda, which are at the root of much of our CAM thinking today. Other alternative medical systems include homeopathy and naturopathy.

Traditional Chinese Medicine

Traditional Chinese medicine (TCM) emphasizes the proper balance or disturbances of *qi* (pronounced "chi"), or vital energy, in health and disease, respectively. Diagnosis is based on personal history, observation of the body (especially the tongue), palpation, and pulse diagnosis, an elaborate procedure requiring considerable skill and experience by the practitioner. Techniques such as acupuncture, herbal medicine, massage, and *qigong* (a form of energy therapy) are among the TCM approaches to health and healing.

TCM practitioners within the United States must complete a graduate program at a college or university approved by the Accreditation Commission for Acupuncture and Oriental Medicine (ACAOM). Graduate programs vary based on the specific area of concentration within TCM but usually involve an extensive 3- or 4-year clinical internship. In addition, an examination by the National Commission for the Certification of Acupuncture and Oriental Medicine, a standard for licensing in the United States, must be completed. Specific practices incorporated in TCM are discussed later in the chapter under the different CAM domains.

alternative (whole) medical systems Complete systems of theory and practice that involve several CAM domains.

traditional Chinese medicine (TCM) Ancient comprehensive system of healing that uses herbs, acupuncture, and massage to bring the body into balance and to remove blockages of vital energy flow that lead to disease.

qi Element of traditional Chinese medicine that refers to the vital energy force that courses through the body; when *qi* is in balance, health is restored.

Ayurveda (Ayurvedic medicine) A comprehensive system of medicine, derived largely from ancient India, that places equal emphasis on the body, mind, and spirit, and strives to restore the body's innate harmony through diet, exercise, meditation, herbs, massage, exposure to sunlight, and controlled breathing.

Ayurveda

Ayurveda (Ayurvedic medicine) relates to the "science of life," an alternative medical system that began and evolved over thousands of years in India. Ayurveda seeks to integrate and balance the body, mind, and spirit and to restore harmony in the individual.[6] Ayurvedic practitioners use various techniques, including questioning, observing, touching patients, and classifying patients into one of three body types, or *doshas,* before establishing a treatment plan. The goals of Ayurvedic treatment are to eliminate impurities in the body and reduce symptoms. Dietary modification and herbal remedies drawn from the vast botanical wealth of the Indian subcontinent are common. Treatments may also include animal and mineral ingredients, powdered gemstones, yoga, stretching, meditation, massage, steam baths, exposure to the sun, and controlled breathing.

Training of Ayurvedic practitioners varies. There is no national standard for certifying or training Ayurvedic practitioners, although professional groups are working toward licensure. Specific practices incorporated in Ayurvedic medicine are discussed later in the chapter under the different CAM domains.

Homeopathy

Homeopathic medicine is an unconventional Western system based on the principle that "like cures like." In other words, the same substance that in large doses produces the symptoms of an illness will in very small doses cure the illness. It was developed in the late 1700s by Samuel Hahnemann, a German physician, as an approach to medicine that was not as harsh as other treatments of the time, such as bloodletting and blistering.[7] Homeopathic physicians use herbal medicine, minerals, and chemicals in extremely diluted forms to kill infectious agents or ward off illnesses that are caused by more potent forms or doses of those substances.

Homeopathic training varies considerably and is offered through diploma programs, certificate programs, short courses, and correspondence courses. Laws that detail requirements to practice vary from state to state.

Naturopathy

Naturopathic medicine views disease as a manifestation of an alteration in the processes by which the body naturally heals itself. Disease results from the body's effort to ward off impurities and harmful substances from the environment. Naturopathic physicians emphasize restoring health rather than curing disease. They employ an array of healing practices, including diet and clinical nutrition; homeopathy; acupuncture; herbal medicine; hydrotherapy (the use of water in a range of temperatures and methods of application); spinal and soft-tissue manipulation; physical therapies involving electric currents, ultrasound, and light therapy; therapeutic counseling; and pharmacology.

Several major naturopathic schools in the United States and Canada provide training, conferring the *naturopathic doctor (ND)* degree on students who have completed a 4-year graduate program that emphasizes humanistically oriented family medicine.

Other Alternative Medical Systems

Native American, Aboriginal, African, Middle Eastern, and South American cultures also have their own unique alternative systems. As the number of alternative therapists grows and systems become intertwined, so do the number of options available to consumers. Before considering any treatments, wise consumers will consult the most reliable resources to thoroughly evaluate risks, the scientific basis of claimed benefits, and any contraindications to using the CAM product or service. Avoid practitioners who promote their treatments as a cure-all for every health problem or who seem to promise remedies for ailments that have thus far defied the best scientific efforts of mainstream medicine. In short, apply the same strategies to researching CAM as you would to choosing allopathic care (see Chapter 16).

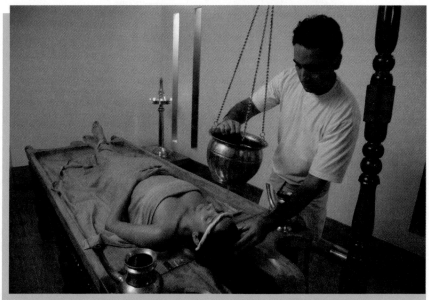

Why are so many people using alternative medicine?

People use alternative medicine for multiple reasons, and many treatments can benefit a variety of physical and mental ailments. For example, *shirodhara*—a traditional Ayurvedic treatment in which warm herbalized oil is poured over the forehead in guided rhythmic patterns—is said to relieve stress and anxiety, treat insomnia and chronic headaches, and improve memory.

Major Domains of Complementary and Alternative Medicine

The U.S. government has created the National Center for Complementary and Alternative Medicine (NCCAM) within the National Institutes of Health (NIH) to provide a mechanism for reliable information about CAM practices. The NCCAM serves as a clearinghouse for CAM information and a focal point for research initiatives, policy development, and general recommendations. It has grouped the many varieties of CAM into four domains of practice (Figure 17.3), recognizing that the domains may overlap and aspects of them may be part of larger alternative medical systems:

- **Manipulative and body-based practices** are based on manipulation or movement of one or more body parts. Examples include chiropractic or osteopathic manipulations and massage.
- **Energy medicine** involves the use of energy fields, such as magnetic fields or biofields (energy fields that some believe surround and penetrate the body). Examples include Reiki and therapeutic touch.
- **Mind–body medicine** uses a variety of techniques to enhance the mind's ability to affect bodily function and symptoms. Some examples include support groups, meditation, and the use of cognitive behavioral theory.
- **Biologically based practices** use substances found in nature, such as herbs, special foods, or vitamins (in doses outside those used in conventional medicine). This includes the use of natural but sometimes unproven therapies, such as dietary supplements and herbal products.

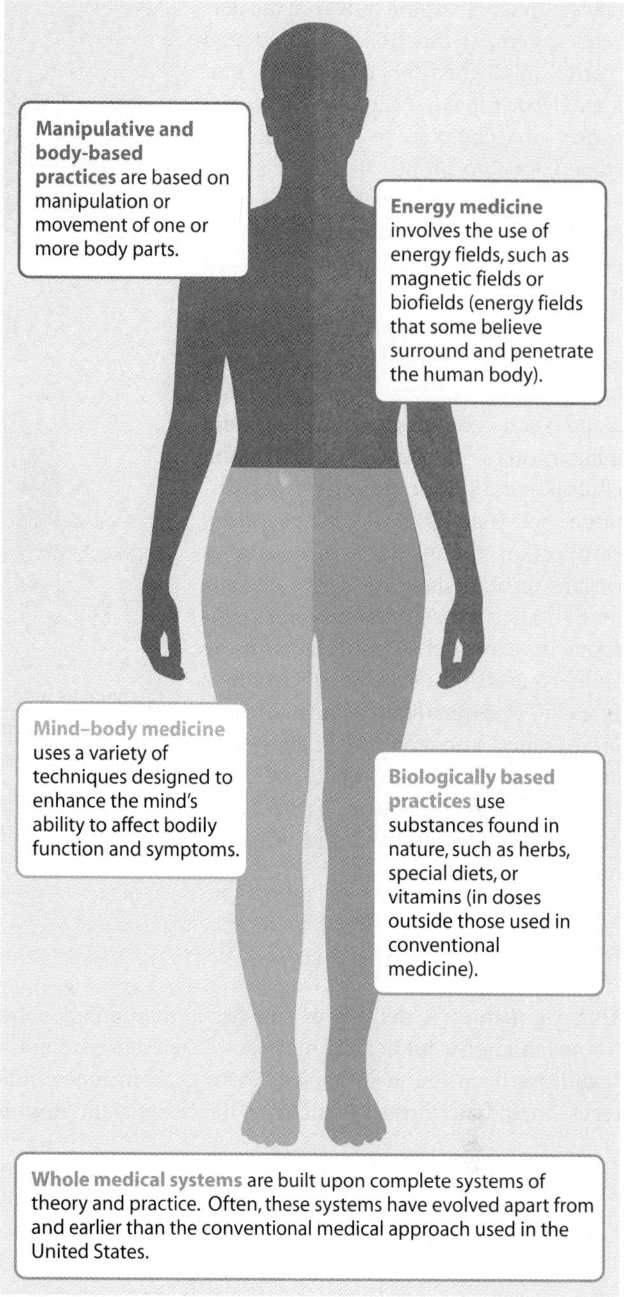

Manipulative and Body-Based Practices

The CAM domain of **manipulative and body-based practices** includes methods that are based on manipulation or movement of the body. For example, chiropractors focus on the relationship between the body's structures (primarily the spine) and function and on how that relationship affects the preservation and restoration of health. Massage therapists use various hand techniques to move muscles and soft tissues to increase the flow of blood and oxygen to these areas or to release muscle tension.

Chiropractic Medicine

Chiropractic medicine has been practiced for more than 100 years and focuses on manipulation as a key therapy.[8] A century ago, allopathic medicine and chiropractic medicine were in direct competition. Today, however, many health care organizations work closely with chiropractors, and many

Manipulative and body-based practices are based on manipulation or movement of one or more body parts.

Energy medicine involves the use of energy fields, such as magnetic fields or biofields (energy fields that some believe surround and penetrate the human body).

Mind–body medicine uses a variety of techniques designed to enhance the mind's ability to affect bodily function and symptoms.

Biologically based practices use substances found in nature, such as herbs, special diets, or vitamins (in doses outside those used in conventional medicine).

Whole medical systems are built upon complete systems of theory and practice. Often, these systems have evolved apart from and earlier than the conventional medical approach used in the United States.

FIGURE 17.3 **The Domains of Complementary and Alternative Medicine**

NCCAM groups CAM practices into four domains, recognizing there can be some overlap. In addition, NCCAM studies CAM whole medical systems, which cut across all domains.

Source: National Center for Complementary and Alternative Medicine, "The Use of Complementary and Alternative Medicine in the United States," NCCAM Publication no. D434, 2009.

insurance companies will pay for chiropractic treatment, particularly if recommended by a medical doctor. More than 20 million Americans now visit chiropractors each year.

Chiropractic medicine is based on the idea that a life-giving energy

manipulative and body-based practices Treatments involving manipulation or movement of one or more body parts.

chiropractic medicine Manipulation of the spine to allow proper energy flow.

flows through the spine by way of the nervous system. If the spine is subluxated (partly misaligned or dislocated), that force is disrupted. Chiropractors use a variety of techniques to manipulate the spine back into proper alignment so the energy can flow unimpeded. It has been established that their treatment can be effective for back pain, neck pain, and headaches.

The average chiropractic training program requires 4 years of intensive courses in biochemistry, anatomy, physiology, diagnostics, pathology, nutrition, and related topics, combined with hands-on clinical training. Many chiropractors continue their training to obtain specialized certification, for instance, in neurology, geriatrics, or pediatrics. There are currently 16 accredited programs and 2 chiropractic educational institutions in the United States. Most state boards require 2 years of undergraduate education, and more states are requiring a bachelor's degree in addition to the doctor of chiropractic degree for licensure. The practice of chiropractic is licensed and regulated in all 50 states.[9]

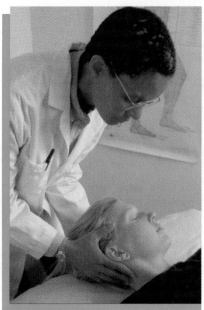

What does chiropractic medicine do?

Chiropractic medicine is often used to treat body pains. Chiropractors manipulate the alignment of the spine, allowing energy to flow freely throughout the body.

Massage Therapy

Massage therapy is defined as soft-tissue manipulation by trained therapists for healing purposes.[10] References to massage have been found in ancient writings from many cultures, including those of ancient Greece, ancient Rome,

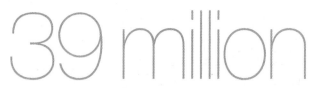

39 million

American adults per year get massages.

Japan, China, Egypt, and the Indian subcontinent.[11] Today, massage therapy is used as a means of treating painful conditions, including low back pain (see the **Health Headlines** box at right); relaxing tired and overworked muscles; reducing stress and anxiety; rehabilitating sports injuries; and promoting general health.[12] This is accomplished by manipulating soft tissues to improve the body's circulation and to remove waste products from the muscles. There are many different types of massage therapy; the following are some of the more popular:

● **Swedish massage** uses long strokes, kneading, and friction on the muscles and moves the joints to aid flexibility.

● **Deep tissue massage** uses patterns of strokes and deep finger pressure on parts of the body where muscles are tight or knotted, focusing on layers of muscle deep under the skin.
● **Trigger point massage** (also called *pressure point massage*) uses a variety of strokes but applies deeper, more focused pressure on myofascial trigger points— "knots" that can form in the muscles, are painful when pressed, and cause symptoms elsewhere in the body as well.
● **Shiatsu massage** uses varying, rhythmic pressure from the fingers on parts of the body that are believed to be important for the flow of vital energy.

Other varieties include massage of specific body parts, such as the feet or fingers, application of hot rocks, water massage, or other techniques. Massage techniques are important aspects of both traditional Chinese medicine and Ayurvedic medicine.

There are about 1,300 massage therapy schools, college programs, and training programs in the United States. The course of study typically covers subjects such as anatomy and physiology; kinesiology; therapeutic evaluation; massage techniques; first aid; business, ethical, and legal issues; and hands-on practice. These educational programs vary in respect to length, quality, and whether they are accredited. Many require 500 hours of training, which is the same number of hours that many states require for certification. Some therapists also pursue specialty or advanced training. Massage therapists work in an array of settings both private and public: private offices, studios, hospitals, nursing homes, fitness centers, and sports medicine facilities, for example.[13]

Bodywork

Bodywork actually consists of several forms of exercise. The *Feldenkrais method* is a system of movements, floor exercises, and bodywork designed to retrain the central nervous system to find new pathways around areas of blockage or damage. It is gentle and effective in rehabilitating trauma victims. *Rolfing*, a more invasive form of bodywork, aims to restructure the musculoskeletal system by working on patterns of tension held in deep tissue. The therapist applies firm—sometimes painful—pressure to different areas of the body. Rolfing can release repressed emotions as well as dissipate muscle tension. *Shiatsu* is a traditional healing art from Japan that applies firm finger pressure to specified points on the body and is intended to increase the circulation of vital energy. *Trager bodywork* employs gentle, shaking motions of the patient's limbs in a rhythmic fashion to induce states of deep, pleasant relaxation.[14]

Health Headlines

THE BENEFITS OF MASSAGE FOR LOW BACK PAIN

With 31 percent of adults who get massages using massage therapy for medical purposes, recent American Massage Therapy Association (AMTA) consumer surveys show that massage therapy is a growing trend. Massage has been credited with alleviating a wide variety of ailments, including migraines, carpal tunnel syndrome, and anxiety. In particular, massage has been looked at as a useful treatment for low back pain (LBP). More than 100 million Americans suffer from LBP, and nearly $25 billion a year is spent in search of relief. In the Centers for Disease Control and Prevention's (CDC's) thirtieth annual report on the nation's health status, *Health, United States, 2006*, LBP was the most commonly reported type of pain, the most common cause of job-related disability, and a leading contributor to missed work and reduced productivity.

Medication may still be the most common way to treat LBP, but increasing evidence suggests it is neither the most effective nor the safest treatment method. The need for more effective solutions to this problem has led many health care organizations to increase research for alternative treatments such as massage therapy. A recent study in the *Annals of Internal Medicine* showed that massage therapy produced better results and reduced the need for painkillers by 36 percent when compared to other therapies, including acupuncture and spinal modification.

As evidence that massage therapy is increasingly on the public's mind, the AMTA reports that 13 percent of Americans discussed massage therapy with their health care provider in 2008. Moreover, 57 percent of doctors recommended massage therapy when their patients inquired about it. Nearly half of all chiropractors (48%) and physical therapists (47%) also recommended massage to their patients. Despite lingering pessimism from some in the conventional medical community, an impressive 25 million more Americans each year are getting massages today than they did in 1997, according to a 2006 AMTA study. Many people are coming to believe massage is not just a luxury but a medical necessity, but Medicare and Medicaid have not yet supported insurance coverage for massage as a remedy for LBP, and many insurance companies offer only limited

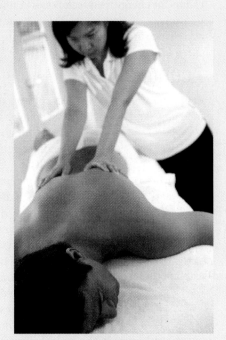

Oh, my aching back? Try massage!

coverage for it. Because massage therapy, as with most CAM care, is paid for by the patients, it is not accessible to all Americans. Only those who can afford the out-of-pocket costs have access to broader choices in their health care.

Sources: Adapted from M. Vivo, "Making a Statement about Massage," *Massage Today*, Vol. 7, no. 2. Copyright © 2007 MPA Media. Used with permission. www.massagetoday.com/mpacms/mt/article.php?id=13538; American Massage Therapy Association, "2009 Massage Therapy Fact Sheet," 2009, www.amtamassage.org/news/MTIndustryFactSheet.html.

Energy Medicine

Energy medicine therapies focus either on energy fields thought to originate within the body (biofields) or on fields from other sources (electromagnetic fields). The existence of these fields has not been experimentally proven. Some forms of energy therapy manipulate biofields by applying pressure and/or manipulating the body by placing the hands in, or through, these fields.[15]

Popular examples of biofield therapy include qigong, Reiki, and therapeutic touch. *Qigong*, a component of traditional Chinese medicine, combines movement, meditation, and regulation of breathing to enhance the flow of vital energy *(qi)*, improve blood circulation, and enhance immune function. *Reiki*, whose name derives from the Japanese word representing "universal life energy," is based on the belief that by channeling spiritual energy through the practitioner, the spirit is healed, and it in turn heals the physical body. *Therapeutic touch* derives from the ancient technique of "laying on" of hands and is based on the premise that the healing force of the therapist brings about the patient's recovery and that healing is promoted when the body's energies are in balance. By passing the hands over the body, the healers identify bodily imbalances.

energy medicine Therapies using energy fields, such as magnetic fields or biofields.

Bioelectromagnetic-based therapies involve the unconventional use of electromagnetic fields—such as pulsed fields, magnetic fields, or alternating current or direct current fields—to treat asthma, cancer, pain, migraines, and other conditions. There is little scientific documentation to support claims for energy field techniques at this point. However, two derivatives of energy medicine have gained much wider acceptance in recent years: acupuncture and acupressure.

Acupuncture

Acupuncture, one of the oldest forms of traditional Chinese medicine (and one of the most popular among Americans), is sought for a wide variety of health conditions, including musculoskeletal dysfunction, mood enhancement, and wellness promotion. It describes a family of procedures that involve stimulating anatomical points of the body with a series of precisely placed needles. The placement and manipulation of acupuncture needles is based on traditional Chinese theories of life-force energy *(qi)* flow through *meridians,* or energy pathways, in the body. Following acupuncture, most respondents and participants in clinical studies report high levels of satisfaction with the treatment, improved quality of life, improvement in or cure of the condition, and reduced

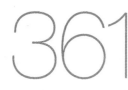

acupuncture Branch of traditional Chinese medicine that uses the insertion of long, thin needles to affect flow of energy *(qi)* along pathways (meridians) within the body.
acupressure Branch of traditional Chinese medicine related to acupuncture. Uses application of pressure to selected body points to balance energy.
mind–body medicine Techniques designed to enhance the mind's ability to affect bodily functions and symptoms.

361 **points along 14 meridians exist on the human body, according to classic acupuncture theory.**

reliance on prescription drugs and surgery. In particular, results have been promising in the treatment of nausea associated with chemotherapy, dental pain, and knee pain.[16]

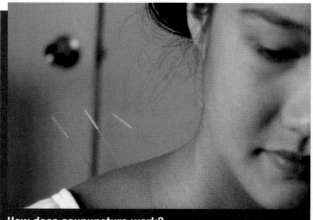

How does acupuncture work?

In acupuncture, long, thin needles are inserted into specific points along the body. This is thought to increase the flow of life-force energy, providing many physical and mental benefits.

Some Western researchers believe that acupuncture may work through stimulating or repressing the autonomic nervous system.[17]

Acupuncturists in the United States are state licensed, and each state has specific requirements regarding training programs. Most acupuncturists either have completed a 2- to 3-year postgraduate program to obtain a master of traditional Oriental medicine (MTOM) degree or have attended a shorter certification program in North America or Asia.

Acupressure

Acupressure is similar to acupuncture but does not use needles. Instead, the practitioner applies pressure to points critical to balancing *yin* and *yang,* the two Chinese principles that interact to influence overall harmony (health) of the body. Practitioners must have the same basic training and understanding of energy pathways as do acupuncturists.

Mind–Body Medicine

Mind–body medicine employs a variety of techniques designed to facilitate the mind's capacity to affect bodily function and symptoms. Many therapies fall under this category, but some areas, such as biofeedback and cognitive-behavioral techniques, have been so well investigated that they are no longer considered alternative. However, meditation, yoga, tai chi, certain uses of hypnosis, dance, music and art therapy, prayer and mental healing, and several others are still categorized as complementary and alternative. (See Chapter 11 for more on yoga and tai chi; see Chapters 2 and 3 and **Focus On: Your Spiritual Health** beginning on page 474 for more on the mind–body connection.)

Psychoneuroimmunology

As discussed in Chapter 3, *psychoneuroimmunology (PNI)* is a relatively new field of study. It is defined as the "interaction of consciousness *(psycho),* the brain and central nervous system *(neuro),* and the body's defense against external infection and internal aberrant cell division *(immunology).*"[18] Many researchers have postulated over the years that excessive stress and maladaptive coping can lead to immune system dysfunction and can increase the risk of disease. Scientists are exploring ways in which relaxation, biofeedback, meditation, yoga, laughter, exercise, and activities that involve either conscious or unconscious mind "quieting" may counteract negative stressors.

A classic study of PNI and mind–body health attempted to assess the effects of relaxation and coping techniques on the immune system by studying nursing home patients. Participants were divided into three groups: those who were taught relaxation techniques, those who were provided with abundant social contact, and those who received no special techniques or contact. After 1 month, immune system function greatly improved in participants who received stress management therapy as compared to the other groups. Several studies have shown promising positive effects of mind–body techniques that encourage relaxation and other stress-reduction strategies for people with cancer or other health problems.[19]

what do you think?

Why do you think more and more people are opting for complementary and alternative treatments? ● What are the potential benefits of these treatments? ● What are the potential risks?

Biologically Based Practices

Biologically based practices are perhaps the most controversial domain of CAM therapies because of the sheer number of options available and the many claims that are made about their effects. Many of these claims have not been thoroughly investigated, and regulation of this aspect of CAM has been slow in coming. Biologically based practices include natural treatments, interventions, and products, many of which overlap with conventional medicine's use of dietary supplements. The FDA defines dietary supplements as "products (other than tobacco) that are intended to supplement or add to the diet; that contain one or more of the following ingredients: vitamins, minerals, amino acids, herbs, or other substances that increase total dietary intake; that are intended for ingestion in the form of a capsule, powder, soft gel, or gelcap; and are not represented as a

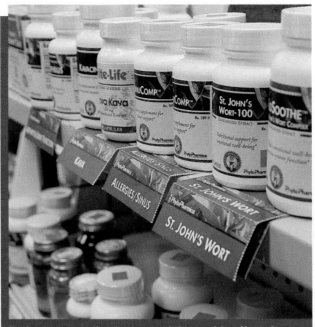

Do herbal remedies have any risks or side effects?

Herbs do have the potential to cause negative side effects. St. John's wort, for example, has potentially dangerous interactions with some prescription antidepressants and should never be taken with them. Other herbs, such as kava, can have negative effects even when taken alone.

conventional food."[20] Included among biologically based practices are herbal remedies, special dietary supplements, individual biological therapies, and functional foods.[21] Typically, people take these supplements and remedies—often without guidance from any CAM practitioner—to improve health, prevent disease, or enhance mood.

Herbal Remedies

People have been using herbal remedies for thousands of years. Herbs were the original sources for compounds found in approximately 25 percent of the pharmaceutical drugs we use today, including aspirin (white willow bark), the heart medication digitalis (foxglove), and the cancer treatment Taxol (Pacific yew tree plant). In addition, scientists continue to make pharmacological advances by studying the herbal

biologically based practices Treatments using substances found in nature, such as herbs, special diets, or vitamin megadoses.

remedies used in cultures throughout the world. With conventional scientists now recognizing the benefits of herbs, it is no wonder that more and more consumers are turning to herbal products.

However, herbal remedies are not to be taken lightly. Just because something is natural does not necessarily mean that it is safe. For example, in recent years, the FDA has warned that certain herbal products containing kava may be associated with severe liver damage.[22] Even rigorously tested products can be risky. Many plants are poisonous, and some can be toxic if ingested in high doses. Others may be dangerous

GREEN GUIDE

Sustainable Supplements

As herbal supplement use becomes increasingly common, environmentally conscious health consumers can take steps toward supporting herbal supplement manufacturers who adhere to sustainable environmental practices. One way to promote sustainability is to purchase fair trade herbal supplement products.

In brief, fair trade advocates that manufacturers pay suppliers a fair price while supporting social and environmental standards. Fair trade–certified sales commonly involve exports of coffee, cocoa, and sugar from developing nations

to developed nations. As a multibillion-dollar industry, fair trade–certified product sales continue to grow each year. Fair trade teas and herbs are a relatively new idea, with many products only becoming available during the last several years. By purchasing fair trade herbal supplements, you can assist with supporting sustainable farming methods and providing a living wage to farmers and workers. Further, fair trade practices seek to enhance communities by providing funding for social and business development.

One U.S. organization, TransFair USA (www.transfairusa.org), is a third-party certifier

of fair trade products, such as herbal teas, and allows consumers to search their website for companies that are devoted to fair trade. The company's parent organization, Fairtrade Labelling Organizations International (FLO; www.fairtrade.net), is a global network of fair trade organizations that offer the Fairtrade Certification Mark. Standards for a product to earn certification include buyers paying at least the fair trade price set by FLO, buyers paying a fair trade premium that is used for community development, and buyers establishing a long-term relationship with the seller.

---

when combined with prescription or over-the-counter drugs, could disrupt the normal action of the drugs, or could cause unusual side effects.[23] Properly trained herbalists and homeopaths have received graduate-level training in special programs such as herbal nutrition or traditional Chinese medicine. These practitioners have been trained in diagnosis; in mixing herbs, titrations, and dosages; and in the follow-up care of patients.

Herbal remedies come in several different forms. **Tinctures** (extracts of fresh or dried plants) usually contain a high percentage of grain alcohol to prevent spoilage and are among the best herbal options. Freeze-dried extracts are very stable and offer good value for your money. Standardized extracts, often available in pill or capsule form, are also among the more reliable forms of herbal preparations. Increasingly, herbal preparations of many forms are being made available through environmentally responsible means and companies (see the **Green Guide** above for more information).

In general, herbal medicines tend to be milder than chemical drugs and produce their effects more slowly; they also are much less likely to cause toxicity because they are diluted rather than concentrated forms of drugs. But diluted or not, and no matter how natural they are, herbs still contain many of the same chemicals as synthetic prescription drugs. Too much of any herb, particularly one from nonstandardized extracts, can cause problems.

tinctures Herbal extracts usually combined with grain alcohol to prevent spoilage.

nutraceuticals Term often used interchangeably with *functional foods;* refers to the combined nutritional and pharmaceutical benefit derived through use of foods or food supplements.

Table 17.1 gives an overview of some of the most common herbal supplements on the market.

Special Supplements

Not all the supplements on the market today are directly derived from plant sources. In recent years, there have been increasing reports in the media on the health benefits of various vitamins, minerals, amino acids, and other specific biological compounds. Table 17.2 on page 514 lists popular nonherbal supplements and their risks and benefits.

The Role of Functional Foods in CAM Therapies

Changes to the diet are often part of CAM therapies, and such changes commonly involve increased intake of certain *functional foods*— foods or supplements designed to improve some specific aspect of physical or mental functioning. Sometimes referred to as **nutraceuticals** for their combined nutritional and pharmaceutical benefit,

> Garlic is often considered a functional food.

Common Herbs and Herbal Supplements: Benefits, Research, and Risks

Herb	Claims of Benefits	Research Findings	Potential Risks
Echinacea (purple coneflower, *Echinacea purpurea*, *E. angustifolia*, *E. pallida*)	Stimulates the immune system and increases the effectiveness of white blood cells that attack bacteria and viruses. Useful in preventing and treating colds or the flu.	Many studies in Europe have provided preliminary evidence of its effectiveness, but a recent controlled study in the United States indicated that it is no more effective than a placebo in preventing or treating a cold.	Allergic reactions, including rashes, increased asthma, gastrointestinal problems, and anaphylaxis (a life-threatening allergic reaction). Pregnant women and those with diabetes, autoimmune disorders, or multiple sclerosis should avoid it.
Ephedra (ma huang, Chinese ephedra, *Ephedra sinica*)	Useful for weight loss and athletic performance.	Comprehensive research has found that ephedra has only limited positive effects on weight loss and athletic performance but has numerous adverse effects.	Heart attack, stroke, heart palpitations, psychiatric problems, upper gastrointestinal effects, tremor, insomnia, and death. The FDA has banned the sale of supplements containing ephedra.
Flaxseed (*Linum usitatissimum*)	Useful as a laxative and for hot flashes and breast pain; the oil is used for arthritis; both flaxseed and flaxseed oil have been used for cholesterol level reduction and cancer prevention.	Study results are mixed on whether flaxseed decreases hot flashes or lowers cholesterol levels.	Delays absorption of medicines, but otherwise has few side effects. Should be taken with plenty of water.
Ginkgo (*Ginkgo biloba*)	Useful for depression, impotence, premenstrual syndrome, dementia and Alzheimer's disease, diseases of the eye, and general vascular disease.	Some promising results have been seen for Alzheimer's disease and dementia, and research continues on its ability to enhance memory and reduce the incidence of cardiovascular disease.	Gastric irritation, headache, nausea, dizziness, difficulty thinking, memory loss, and allergic reactions.
Ginseng (*Panax ginseng*)	Affects the pituitary gland, increasing resistance to stress, affecting metabolism, aiding skin, muscle tone, and sex drive; improves concentration and muscle strength.	Studies have raised questions about appropriate dosages. Because the potency of plants varies considerably, dosage is difficult to control and side effects are fairly common.	Nervousness, insomnia, high blood pressure, headaches, chest pain, depression, and abnormal vaginal bleeding.
Green tea (*Camellia sinensis*)	Useful for lowering cholesterol and risk of some cancers, protecting the skin from sun damage, bolstering mental alertness, and boosting heart health.	Although some studies have shown promising links between green and white tea consumption and cancer prevention, recent research questions the ability of tea to significantly reduce the risk of breast, lung, or prostate cancer.	Insomnia, liver problems, anxiety, irritability, upset stomach, nausea, diarrhea, or frequent urination.
Kava (*Piper methysticum*)	Useful for relaxation; relief of anxiety, insomnia, and menopausal symptoms; sometimes used topically as a numbing agent.	Scientific studies provide some evidence that kava may be beneficial for the management of anxiety.	Increases the effect of alcohol and other drugs; causes drowsiness; the FDA has issued a warning that using kava supplements has been linked to a risk of severe liver damage.
St. John's wort (SJW, Klamath weed, *Hypericum perforatum*)	Useful for depression, anxiety, and sleep disorders.	There is evidence that SJW is useful for treating mild to moderate depression, but two large studies showed that it was no more effective than a placebo in treating major depression of moderate severity.	Gastrointestinal upset, fatigue, dry mouth, anxiety, sexual dysfunction, dizziness, skin rashes, itching, and extreme sensitivity to sunlight.
Valerian (*Valeriana officinalis*)	Useful for relaxation, sleep disorders, anxiety, headaches, depression, irregular heartbeat, and trembling.	Research suggests it may be helpful for insomnia, but there is not enough evidence to determine whether it works for anxiety, depression, or headaches.	Mild side effects, such as headaches, dizziness, upset stomach, and tiredness the morning after use.

Sources: National Center for Complementary and Alternative Medicine, "Herbs at a Glance," 2009, http://nccam.nih.gov/health/herbsataglance.htm; Office of Dietary Supplements, National Institutes of Health, "Dietary Supplement Fact Sheets," 2009, http://ods.od.nih.gov/Health_Information/Information_About_Individual_Dietary _Supplements.aspx; U.S. Food and Drug Administration, "Final Rule Declaring Dietary Supplements Containing Ephedrine Alkaloids Adulterated Because They Present an Unreasonable Risk," 2008, www.fda.gov/Food/GuidanceComplianceRegulatoryInformation/GuidanceDocuments/DietarySupplements/ucm072997.htm; American Cancer Society, "Green Tea," 2008, www.cancer.org/docroot/ETO/content/ETO_5_3x_Green_Tea.asp.

17.2 Common Nonherbal Supplements: Benefits, Research, and Risks

Supplement	Claims of Benefits	Research	Potential Risks
Dehydroepiandrosterone (DHEA) (hormone)	Fights aging, boosts immunity, strengthens bones, and improves brain functioning.	No antiaging benefits proven.	Could increase cancer risk and lead to liver damage, even when taken briefly.
Vitamin E (vitamin)	Reduces risk of heart disease; better chance of survival after heart attack.	Research results on prevention of heart disease are mixed. Some researchers are curious to see if it is most protective for young, healthy people against eventual heart disease.	High doses cause bleeding when taken with blood thinners.
Glucosamine (biological substance that helps the body grow cartilage)	Useful for arthritis and related degenerative joint diseases; relieves swelling and decreases pain.	When it is taken with chondroitin sulfate, preliminary research shows that it helps reduce pain in people with moderate to severe joint pain.	Few side effects noted.
L-Carnitine (amino acid derivative)	Improves athletic performance, increases fat-burning enzymes, used to combat fatigue and aging.	No consistent evidence that it improves performance in healthy athletes. Some evidence that it enhances mental function in older adults with mild cognitive impairment.	Nausea, vomiting, abdominal cramps, diarrhea, "fishy" body odor; more rarely, muscle weakness, seizures in patients with seizure disorders; interacts with some medications.
Melatonin (hormone)	Useful in regulating circadian rhythms and sleep patterns and treating insomnia; claims of antiaging benefits.	Some evidence supports its usefulness in regulating sleep patterns. No scientific support for antiaging claims.	Nausea, headaches, dizziness, blood vessel constriction; possibly a danger for people with high blood pressure or other cardiovascular problems.
SAMe (pronounced "sammy") (biological compound that aids over 40 functions in the body)	Useful in treatment of mild to moderate depression and in treatment of arthritis pain.	Studies have supported its usefulness in treating depression and arthritis pain.	Fewer side effects than prescription antidepressants have. Questions remain over how much a person should take, in what form, and whether there are long-term side effects.
Zinc (mineral)	Supports immune system; used to lessen duration and severity of cold symptoms; aids wound healing.	Research results are mixed, possibly due to the wide variety of cold viruses and differences of formulations and dosages in zinc lozenges.	Excessive intake associated with reduced immune function, reduced levels of high-density lipoproteins ("good" cholesterol).

Source: Office of Dietary Supplements, National Institutes of Health, "Dietary Supplement Fact Sheets," 2009, http://ods.od.nih.gov/Health_Information/Information_About_Individual_Dietary_Supplements.aspx.

several are believed to work in much the same way as pharmaceutical drugs in making a person well or bolstering the immune system.

In recent years, the most commonly advertised functional foods are those containing *antioxidants.* Antioxidants are chemicals that combat free radicals and oxidative damage in cells. They are present in many plant foods (including green tea). Though covered in depth in Chapter 9, it should be noted here that antioxidants are among the most sought-after functional foods on the market. Primary antioxidants include beta-carotene, selenium, vitamin C, and vitamin E.

Other common functional foods and their purported benefits include the following:

- **Plant stanols/sterols.** Can lower "bad" (LDL) cholesterol.

- **Oat fiber.** Can lower LDL cholesterol; serves as a natural soother of nerves; stabilizes blood sugar levels.
- **Sunflower.** Can lower risk of heart disease; may prevent angina.
- **Soy protein.** May lower heart disease risk by reducing LDL cholesterol and triglycerides.
- **Garlic.** Lowers cholesterol and reduces clotting tendency of blood; lowers blood pressure; may serve as form of antibiotic.
- **Ginger.** May prevent motion sickness, stomach pain, and stomach upset; discourages blood clots; may relieve rheumatism.
- **Yogurt.** Yogurt that is labeled "Live Active Culture" contains active, friendly bacteria that can fight off infections.

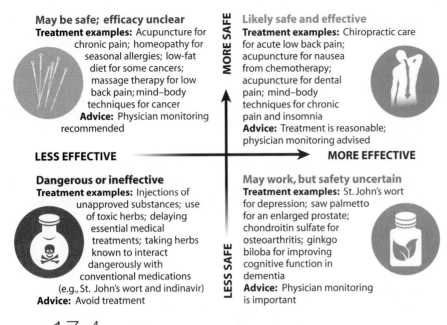

May be safe; efficacy unclear
Treatment examples: Acupuncture for chronic pain; homeopathy for seasonal allergies; low-fat diet for some cancers; massage therapy for low back pain; mind–body techniques for cancer
Advice: Physician monitoring recommended

Likely safe and effective
Treatment examples: Chiropractic care for acute low back pain; acupuncture for nausea from chemotherapy; acupuncture for dental pain; mind–body techniques for chronic pain and insomnia
Advice: Treatment is reasonable; physician monitoring advised

MORE SAFE

LESS EFFECTIVE

MORE EFFECTIVE

LESS SAFE

Dangerous or ineffective
Treatment examples: Injections of unapproved substances; use of toxic herbs; delaying essential medical treatments; taking herbs known to interact dangerously with conventional medications (e.g., St. John's wort and indinavir)
Advice: Avoid treatment

May work, but safety uncertain
Treatment examples: St. John's wort for depression; saw palmetto for an enlarged prostate; chondroitin sulfate for osteoarthritis; ginkgo biloba for improving cognitive function in dementia
Advice: Physician monitoring is important

FIGURE 17.4 **Assessing the Risks and Benefits of CAM Treatments**
Medical experts devised this chart to gauge the potential liability of recommending alternative treatments, but by categorizing treatments according to their relative safety and effectiveness, it can also help patients and consumers make appropriate choices.

Source: M. H. Cohen and D. M. Eisenberg, "Potential Physician Malpractice Liability Associated with Complementary and Integrative Medical Therapies," *Annals of Internal Medicine* 136, no. 8 (2002): 596–603. Copyright © 2002 American College of Physicians. Used with permission.

Protecting Consumers and Regulating Claims

Although many CAM procedures and products appear promising, be aware that most of them are not currently regulated in the United States as strictly as are food, drugs, and Western medical procdures. Supplement regulation in particular is in sharp contrast to nations such as Germany, where the government holds companies to strict standards for ingredients and manufacturing. In the United States, new FDA regulatory controls are just starting to take place. While FDA regulations of supplements are being phased in and until other regulations of CAM are in place, it is important to have as much information as possible to make a smart decision when evaluating CAM options (**Figure 17.4**).

In the United States, supplements are becoming more heavily regulated.

Strategies to Protect Supplement Consumers' Health

The burgeoning popularity of nutraceuticals and functional foods concerns many scientists. Although some alternative therapies, such as acupuncture, have been widely studied, there is little quality research to support the many claims in the area of nutraceuticals and supplements. If you are considering using herbal supplements or functional foods, start your own research at the websites for NCCAM (http://nccam.nih.gov) and the Cochrane Collaboration's review on complementary and alternative medicine (www.cochrane.org).

Herbal supplements and functional foods can currently be sold without FDA approval. This raises issues of consumer safety to new levels. Even when products are dispensed by CAM practitioners, the situation can be risky. Some homeopaths and herbalists who mix their own tonics may not use standardized measures. Lack of standard regulation means that some unskilled and untrained people may be treating patients without fully understanding the potential chemical interactions of their preparations.

Pressure has mounted to establish consistent standards for herbal supplements and functional foods similar to those used in Germany and other countries. Many scientists have advocated a more stringent FDA approval process for supplements sold in the United States. As a result, the FDA has instituted new regulations to oversee the manufacture of dietary supplements, including herbal supplements. These new regulations require manufacturers to evaluate the identity, purity, strength, and composition of the supplements to ensure they contain what the label claims. These regulations are due to phase in by June 2010.[24] The official public standards-setting authority for all medicines, supplements, and other health care products manufactured and sold in the United States is the U.S. Pharmacopeia, which tests select products, including herbal supplements, to ensure that they comply with safety and purity standards. Products that meet these standards display a "USP Dietary Supplement Verified" seal.

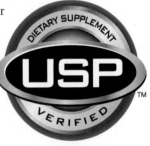

Source: U.S. Pharmocopeia, 2009, www.uspverified.org.

The Future of CAM Therapy

Clearly, CAM appears to serve a very real need for consumers. But while consumers are making the adjustment to CAM in record numbers, members of the health care delivery system seem slow to act. Although progress has been noted, there is still a long way to go before CAM therapies become fully accepted in mainstream medical practice.

Enlisting Support from Insurers and Providers

More and more insurers are covering alternative care, at least to some degree. This is especially true as criticisms of managed care increase and government agencies get involved.

Today, nearly all health insurance providers cover at least one form of CAM, with acupuncture and massage therapy the most common. In spite of this progress, many patients will continue to pay out of pocket for alternative therapies until the scientific evidence supporting these alternative medical care choices is impossible to ignore. What is known is that the numbers are increasing despite a reimbursement system that is biased in favor of traditional treatments.

Support from professional organizations, such as the AMA, is also increasing as more physician training programs require or offer electives in alternative treatment modalities. In many cases, medical schools are educating doctors to be better prepared to advise patients about the pros and cons of alternative treatments and how to follow integrative practices. Although alternative medicine is becoming increasingly integrated into today's health care programs and plans, there is still a long way to go. As we learn more, we will be better able to apply both traditional and alternative care.

See the **Skills for Behavior Change** box at right for specific tips on how to ensure you get the best possible care.

As we enter a new era of medicine, more than ever you are being called on to take responsibility for what goes into your body. This means you must educate yourself. CAM can offer new avenues toward better health, but it is up to you to make sure that you are on the right path.

CAM and Self-Care

Today, we face an exciting array of possible health choices. To help you make the best decisions, consider these pointers:

✳ Take charge of your health by being an informed consumer. Find out what scientific studies have been done on the safety and effectiveness of the CAM treatment in which you are interested. Consult only reliable sources—texts, journals, periodicals, and government resources. Start with the websites listed at the end of this and every chapter.

✳ Remember that decisions about treatment should be made in consultation with your health care provider and based on your own condition and needs. If you use any CAM therapy, inform your primary health care provider. It is particularly important to talk with your provider if you are thinking about replacing your prescribed treatment with one or more supplements, are currently taking a prescription drug, have a chronic medical condition, are planning to have surgery, are pregnant or nursing, or are thinking about giving supplements to children or pets.

✳ If you use a CAM therapy such as acupuncture, choose the practitioner with care. Check with your insurer to see if the services will be covered.

✳ Remember that *natural* and *safe* are not necessarily synonymous. Many people have become seriously ill from seemingly harmless "natural" products. Be cautious about combining herbal medications, just as you should be cautious about combining other drugs. Seek help if you notice any unusual side effects.

✳ Realize that no one is closely monitoring the purity of herbal supplements and that dosage levels in many herbal products are in the process of getting regulated. Look for the word *standardized* or the "USP Dietary Supplement Verified" seal on any herbal product you buy, and look for reputable manufacturers. German manufacturers are legally required to produce identical batches of herbal remedies.

Are You A Savvy CAM Consumer?

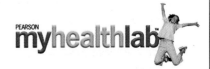

PEARSON
myhealthlab

If you are like millions of Americans, you've already tried one or more CAM therapies (including the use of supplements) or may be considering one. Take this quiz to assess your knowledge of complementary and alternative medicine. For each statement, indicate whether you believe the following items are true or false.

Fill out this assessment online at www.pearsonhighered.com/myhealthlab or www.pearsonhighered.com/donatelle.

1. When considering a CAM technique, it is important to do some research and identify scientific findings of the specific CAM therapy. **T F**

2. Researching the credentials of a CAM practitioner is an important step to take before receiving any type of CAM treatment. **T F**

3. CAM therapies can be used with traditional medical treatments. **T F**

4. I should inform new practitioners of all the treatments I am currently receiving, including all CAM and traditional therapies. **T F**

5. If my friend or family member didn't have success with a CAM therapy, then it probably won't work for me either. **T F**

6. I should ask if the CAM therapy is covered by insurance before receiving the treatment. **T F**

7. Learning about CAM therapies can be a proactive way to maintain good health. **T F**

8. Taking supplements is a good idea, because even if a product isn't helpful, it isn't likely to be harmful. **T F**

9. The word *natural* on a supplement package means that the product is healthful and safe. **T F**

10. When buying supplements, I should choose those with the USP (United States Pharmacopeia) seal on their labels. **T F**

11. Any potentially dangerous supplement product is required to have cautionary information on the label. **T F**

12. A recall of a harmful product guarantees that all such harmful products will be immediately and completely removed from the marketplace. **T F**

13. There is no reason for me to consult a physician before taking a supplement. **T F**

14. Fewer than 10 percent of Americans use dietary supplements. **T F**

Scoring Key

1. *True.* Finding out scientific evidence on a particular CAM therapy can help to identify its effectiveness.

2. *True.* CAM techniques require rigorous training, and it is important to receive treatment from only those practitioners who have received extensive training and are licensed for their particular CAM technique. Inadequate training can result in injury, transmission of disease, and improper balancing of energy.

3. *True.* CAM techniques can be used with traditional medical treatment and can provide additional benefits for a comprehensive treatment plan.

4. *True.* Any new practitioner, whether CAM or traditional, should be aware of all therapies you are receiving to prevent any complications if a new therapy is introduced and to allow all providers to communicate with one another to provide the best overall care.

5. *False.* Individuals respond differently to CAM therapies. You should consult your physician when considering CAM therapies.

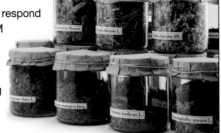

6. *True.* Many CAM therapies are not covered by insurance. If the procedure is covered, you may still have to pay a percentage of the total amount. It is important to find this out before pursuing the treatment.

7. *True.* A recent study showed that those who inquired about CAM therapies were more health conscious than those who did not.

8. *False.* When consumed in high enough amounts, for a long enough time, or in combination with certain other substances, all chemicals can be toxic, including nutrients, plant components, and other biologically active ingredients.

9. *False.* The word *natural* on labels is not well defined and is sometimes used ambiguously to imply unsubstantiated

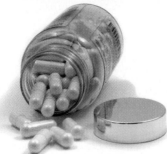

benefits or safety. For example, many weight-loss products claim to be "natural" or "herbal," but this doesn't necessarily make them safe. Their ingredients may interact with drugs or may be dangerous for people with certain medical conditions.

10. *True.* Because FDA regulations are in the process of being implemented, the USP symbol is currently the best way to tell if the supplement has been tested and dissolves properly in the body.

11. *False.* Dietary supplement manufacturers may not necessarily include warnings about potential adverse effects on their product labels. If consumers want to know about the safety of a specific dietary supplement, they should contact the manufacturer of that brand directly.

12. *False.* A product recall of a dietary supplement is voluntary, and although many manufacturers do their best, a recall does not necessarily remove all harmful products from the marketplace.

13. *False.* Supplements can interact with prescription medications, so telling your doctor what you intend to take can help him or her check for such interactions.

14. *False.* National surveys indicate that about half of all Americans use dietary supplements. Research shows that people who take supplements tend to have better diets and generally healthier habits than those who don't. They also tend to have higher levels of both education and income.

Interpreting Your Score

Add up the number of items you got right: The higher your score, the better your knowledge of the potential risks and benefits of supplements and other CAM techniques. Any incorrect responses may indicate areas you need to learn more about in order to be an informed consumer. Ultimately, you are the one most responsible for your health and safety, so think about ways to increase your awareness and understanding of the CAM methods you consume.

Sources: Adapted from NCCAM, "Are You Considering Using CAM?" 2009 http://nccam.nih.gov/health/decisions/consideringcam.htm; Council of Colleges of Acupuncture and Oriental Medicine, 2008, www.ccaom.org/aom .asp; NCCAM, "Selecting a CAM Practitioner," 2009, http://nccam.nih.gov/ health/decisions/practitioner.htm; NCCAM, "CAM Use in America: Up Close," *CAM at the NIH: Focus on Complementary and Alternative Medicine* 15, no. 1 (2008): 8–9, http://nccam.nih.gov/news/newsletter/pdf/2008april.pdf; D. Sinovic, "Choosing and Using Supplements," Meriter Healthy Living, Created for Wellness Library, 2006, http://meriter.staywellsolutionsonline .com/InteractiveTools/Quizzes/40,SupplementsVitaminsMQuiz; Council for Responsible Nutrition, "The Benefits of Nutritional Supplements Test Your Supplement Savvy," 2007, www.crnusa.org/benpdfs/CRN00benefits _quiz.pdf.

YOUR PLAN FOR **CHANGE**

The **Assess**yourself activity gave you the chance to evaluate your understanding of responsible use of CAM treatments. Depending on the results of the assessment, and your own interest in pursuing CAM therapies, you may consider investigating CAM further.

Today, you can:

◯ Take a few moments to close your eyes and think of a calm place or activity you enjoy. Perhaps you are lying on a tropical beach or are curled up in front of a fireplace. Clear your mind of everything else, and use relaxation to improve your health.

◯ Go to a credible website and look up information on a CAM therapy. What are the scientific findings? What are the benefits?

Within the next 2 weeks, you can:

◯ Check with your insurance provider and see what CAM therapies are covered. Ask what expenses you'll be responsible for, and if you are limited to a certain network of practitioners.

◯ Check with your college's health clinic and find out what types of alternative therapies it offers.

By the end of the semester, you can:

◯ Schedule an appointment with your current health care provider to discuss any CAM therapies you are considering.

◯ Make relaxation and mind–body stress-reducing techniques a part of your everyday life. This can simply mean practicing meditation, deep breathing, or even taking long walks in nature. You don't need to visit a CAM practitioner or follow a specific therapeutic practice to benefit from methods of relaxation, meditation, and spiritual awakening. See Chapter 3 and Focus On: Your Spiritual Health for suggestions on ways to reduce stress and enhance your mind–body awareness.

Summary

❋ Throughout the world people are using complementary and alternative medicine (CAM) in increasing numbers. Much of the influence of CAM strategies may be traced to other cultures, particularly those that are part of traditional Chinese medicine, such as acupuncture, or Ayurvedic medicine, such as yoga.

❋ Alternative medical systems include traditional Chinese medicine (TCM), Ayurveda, homeopathy, and naturopathy. TCM emphasizes the proper balance of vital energy, or *qi*. Ayurveda seeks to integrate and balance the body, mind, and spirit. Homeopathic medicine is based on the principle that "like cures like." Naturopathic medicine views disease as an alternation in the processes by which the body heals itself.

❋ Manipulative and body-based practices are based on movement of one or more body parts, and include chiropractic medicine and massage. Energy medicine, such as reiki and therapeutic touch, involves the use of energy fields. Mind–body medicine, including mediation or cognitive behavioral therapy, enhances the mind's ability to affect bodily function and symptoms. Biologically based practices use substances found in nature, such as herbs, special foods, or vitamins, in doses outside those used in conventional medicine.

❋ Herbal remedies include ginkgo biloba, St. John's wort, echinacea, ginseng, and green tea. Nonherbal supplements include glucosamine, SAMe, vitamins, minerals, hormones, and other biological compounds. Functional foods may also serve as healing agents.

❋ Although many positive effects are associated with CAM, there are also many risks. As a consumer, you must be aware of the risks and remember that research into CAM is ongoing.

Pop Quiz

1. CAM therapies focus on treating both the mind and the whole body, which make them part of a
   a. natural approach.
   b. psychological approach.
   c. holistic approach.
   d. gentle approach.

2. What type of medicine addresses imbalances of *qi*?
   a. chiropractic medicine
   b. naturopathic medicine
   c. traditional Chinese medicine
   d. homeopathic medicine

3. The alternative system of medicine based on the principle that "like cures like" is
   a. naturopathic medicine.
   b. homeopathic medicine.
   c. Ayurvedic medicine.
   d. chiropractic medicine.

4. Chiropractic treatment is based on the theory that diseases can be caused by
   a. misalignment of the bones.
   b. poor eating habits.
   c. taking too many drugs.
   d. muscle atrophy.

5. The use of techniques to improve the psychoneuroimmunology of the human body is called
   a. acupressure.
   b. mind–body medicine.
   c. Reiki.
   d. body work.

6. What system places equal emphasis on body, mind, and spirit and strives to restore the innate harmony of the individual?
   a. Ayurvedic medicine
   b. homeopathic medicine
   c. naturopathic medicine
   d. traditional Chinese medicine

7. The domain of CAM that uses substances found in nature, including herbal treatments, dietary supplements, or functional foods, is
   a. manipulative and body-based practices.
   b. energy medicine.
   c. mind–body medicine.
   d. biologically based practices.

8. Plant sterols, oat fiber, sunflower, and soy protein are examples of
   a. antioxidants.
   b. herbal remedies.
   c. nutraceuticals.
   d. phytomedicines.

9. The energy therapy derived from the ancient technique of "laying on" of hands is
   a. Reiki.
   b. qigong.
   c. therapeutic touch.
   d. acupressure.

10. The "USP Dietary Supplement Verified" seal indicates that a supplement is
    a. safe and pure.
    b. effective.
    c. low cost.
    d. child safe.

Answers for these questions can be found on page A-1.

Think about It!

1. What are some of the potential benefits and risks of CAM? Why do you think these practices and products are becoming so popular?

2. What are the major domains of CAM treatments? Have you tried any of them? Would you feel comfortable trying any new ones? Why or why not?

3. What are the major herbal remedies? Special supplements? What are some of the risks and benefits associated with each?

4. What can you do to ensure that you are receiving accurate information regarding CAM treatments or medicines? Which federal agency oversees CAM in the United States?

5. What is being done in the United States to ensure continued growth of CAM?

Accessing Your Health on the Internet

The following websites explore further topics and issues related to personal health. For links to the websites below, visit the Companion Website for *Health: The Basics*, Green Edition at www.pearsonhighered.com/donatelle.

1. *National Center for Complementary and Alternative Medicine (NCCAM).* A division of the National Institutes of Health dedicated to providing the latest information and research on complementary and alternative practices. http://nccam.nih.gov

2. *ClinicalTrials.gov.* Includes the latest information on CAM research and clinical trials. Search for results from NCCAM and complementary and alternative medicine. http://clinicaltrials.gov

3. *Acupuncture.com.* Provides resources for consumers regarding traditional Asian therapies; geared to students and practitioners. www.acupuncture.com

4. *National Institutes of Health, Office of Dietary Supplements.* An excellent resource for information on dietary supplements. Includes access to a database of federally funded research projects pertaining to dietary supplements. http://dietary-supplements.info.nih.gov

References

1. National Center for Complementary and Alternative Medicine, "What Is CAM?" NCCAM Publication no. D347, Updated February 2007, http://nccam.nih.gov/health/whatiscam/overview.htm.
2. Mayo Clinic Staff, "Complementary and Alternative Medicine: What Is It?" Mayo Clinic, 2007, www.mayoclinic.com/health/alternative-medicine/PN00001.
3. National Center for Complementary and Alternative Medicine, "The Use of Complementary and Alternative Medicine in the United States," 2008, http://nccam.nih.gov/news/camstats/2007/camsurvey_fs1.htm.
4. J. Tsao, "Effectiveness of Massage Therapy for Chronic, Non-Malignant Pain: A Review," *Evidence Based Complementary and Alternative Medicine* 4, no. 2 (2007): 165–79; American Medical Student Association, "EDCAM: CAM and Medical Education Report," 2007, www.amsa.org; National Cancer Institute, "Acupuncture: Human/ Clinical Studies," 2008, www.cancer.gov/cancertopics/pdq/cam/acupuncture/HealthProfessional/page6.
5. National Center for Complementary and Alternative Medicine, "The Use of Complementary and Alternative Medicine in the United States," 2008.
6. National Center for Complementary and Alternative Medicine, "Ayurvedic Medicine: An Introduction," NCCAM Publication no. D287, 2009, http://nccam.nih.gov/health/ayurveda.
7. American Institute of Homeopathy, "Homeopathy: Efficacy and Evidence Base," 2007, http://homeopathyusa.org/homeopathy-now.html; Health Alternatives Online, "Homeopathy," 2008, www.healthalternativesonline.com/homeopathy.html.
8. National Center for Complementary and Alternative Medicine, "Chiropractic: An Introduction," NCCAM Publication no. D403, 2009, http://nccam.nih.gov/health/chiropractic.
9. Bureau of Labor Statistics, U.S. Department of Labor, "Chiropractors," *Occupational Outlook Handbook, 2008–09 Edition,* 2007, www.bls.gov/oco/ocos071.htm.
10. J. Tsao, "Effectiveness of Massage Therapy for Chronic, Non-Malignant Pain," 2007.
11. National Center for Complementary and Alternative Medicine, "Massage Therapy: An Introduction," NCCAM Publication no. D327, 2009, http://nccam.nih.gov/health/massage.
12. Mayo Clinic Staff, "Massage: A Relaxing Method to Relieve Stress and Pain" Mayo Clinic, 2008, www.mayoclinic.com/health/massage/SA00082; National Center for Complementary and Alternative Medicine, "Massage Therapy as CAM," 2009.
13. Bureau of Labor Statistics, U.S. Department of Labor, "Massage Therapists," *Occupational Outlook Handbook, 2008–09 Edition,* 2007, www.bls.gov/oco/ocos295.htm.
14. National Center for Complementary and Alternative Medicine, "What Is CAM?" Updated February 2007; U.S. Trager Association, "The Trager Approach," 2008, www.trager-us.org/trager-approach.html.
15. National Center for Complementary and Alternative Medicine, "What Is CAM?" Updated February 2007.
16. American Cancer Society, "Acupuncture," 2008, www.cancer.org/docroot/ETO/content/ETO_5_3X_Acupuncture.asp.
17. National Center for Complementary and Alternative Medicine, "Acupuncture: An Introduction," NCCAM Publication no. D404, 2009, http://nccam.nih.gov/health/acupuncture.
18. B. Seaward, *Managing Stress.* 6th ed. (Sudbury, MA: Jones and Bartlett, 2009); D. Tosevski et al., "Stressful Life Events and Physical Health," *Current Opinions in Psychiatry* 19, no. 2 (2009): 184–89.
19. J. Robins et al., "Research in Psychoneuroimmunology: Tai Chi as a Stress Management Approach for Individuals with HIV Disease," *Applied Nursing Research* 19, no. 1 (2006): 2–9; M. Opp et al., "Sleep and Psychoneuroimmunology," *Neurology Clinician* 24, no. 3 (2006): 493–506; A. Starkweather et al., "Immune Function, Pain, and Psychological Stress in Patients Undergoing Spinal Surgery," *Spine* 31, no. 18 (2006): E641–E647.
20. Office of Dietary Supplements, National Institutes of Health, "Dietary Supplements: Background Information," 2009, http://ods.od.nih.gov/factsheets/dietarysupplements.asp.
21. National Center for Complementary and Alternative Medicine, "What Is CAM?" Updated February 2007.
22. National Center for Complementary and Alternative Medicine, "Kava," 2009, http://nccam.nih.gov/health/kava/ataglance.htm.
23. Mayo Clinic Staff, "Herbal Supplements: What to Know before You Buy," 2009, www.mayoclinic.com/health/herbal-supplements/SA00044.
24. C. Paddock, "FDA Tightens Up Dietary Supplement Manufacturing and Labeling," *Medical News Today,* June 26, 2007, www.medicalnewstoday.com/articles/75250.php.

Answers to Chapter Review Questions

Chapter 1
1. d; 2. b; 3. c; 4. d; 5. a;
6. a; 7. a; 8. a; 9. a; 10. c

Chapter 2
1. a; 2. b; 3. a; 4. b; 5. c;
6. c; 7. b; 8. b; 9. c; 10. b

Chapter 3
1. c; 2. c; 3. d; 4. d; 5. c;
6. d; 7. c; 8. c; 9. c; 10. b

Chapter 4
1. a; 2. a; 3. c; 4. d; 5. d;
6. c; 7. a; 8. c; 9. b; 10. a

Chapter 5
1. b; 2. c; 3. c; 4. c; 5. a;
6. c; 7. d; 8. c; 9. b; 10. c

Chapter 6
1. c; 2. d; 3. a; 4. c; 5. b;
6. a; 7. c; 8. d; 9. c; 10. a

Chapter 7
1. d; 2. a; 3. c; 4. d; 5. c;
6. c; 7. a; 8. a; 9. d; 10. b

Chapter 8
1. c; 2. d; 3. b; 4. d; 5. c;
6. c; 7. b; 8. d; 9. c; 10. a

Chapter 9
1. c; 2. a; 3. a; 4. b; 5. b;
6. a; 7. d; 8. b; 9. d; 10. c

Chapter 10
1. c; 2. b; 3. b; 4. b; 5. c;
6. b; 7. a; 8. a; 9. d; 10. a

Chapter 11
1. d; 2. a; 3. b; 4. a; 5. c;
6. b; 7. a; 8. d; 9. c; 10. c

Chapter 12
1. b; 2. a; 3. a; 4. c; 5. b;
6. b; 7. c; 8. c; 9. b; 10. d

Chapter 13
1. a; 2. d; 3. d; 4. b; 5. c;
6. a; 7. a; 8. c; 9. c; 10. b

Chapter 14
1. b; 2. b; 3. b; 4. a; 5. d;
6. a; 7. a; 8. c; 9. c; 10. d

Chapter 15
1. b; 2. c; 3. d; 4. a; 5. a;
6. d; 7. b; 8. b; 9. d; 10. c

Chapter 16
1. c; 2. d; 3. a; 4. c; 5. d;
6. c; 7. a; 8. b; 9. b; 10. a

Chapter 17
1. c; 2. c; 3. b; 4. a; 5. b;
6. a; 7. d; 8. c; 9. c; 10. a

Photo Credits

Frontmatter p. iv: Jamie Grill/Getty Images; p. v left: Ekaterina Monakhova/iStockphoto; right: Mindbodysoul/Alamy; p. vi left: Purestock/Getty Images; right: Donna Coleman/iStockphoto; p. vii left: Alamy; right: iStockphoto; p. viii top left: Brian Leatart/FoodPix/Jupiter Images; bottom left: K.J. Pargeter Images/iStockphoto; right: Masterfile; p. ix: Andrew Manley/iStockphoto; p. x top: Dan Bosler/Getty Images; bottom: Ariel Skelley/Corbis; p. xi left: SuperStock, Inc.; right: K-King Media Co. Ltd/Getty Images; p. xiii: John Giustina/Getty Images.

Chapter 1 Opener: Laura Doss/Corbis; Small images left to right: AP Photos; AP Photos; Randy Faris/Corbis; Mitchel Gray/SuperStock/Jupiter Images; p. 2: Masterfile; fig. 1.1: Ale Ventura/Jupiter Images; fig. 1.2: IT STOCK FREE/AGE Fotostock; p. 6: AP Photos; p. 8: iStockphoto; p. 9: Suzy Allman/Getty Images; p. 11: AP Photos; p. 13: Liz Van Steenburgh/iStockphoto; p. 15: Randy Faris/Corbis; p. 16: Andrew Manley/iStockphoto; p. 18: Mitchel Gray/Jupiter Images; p. 22: Jacob Wackerhausen/iStockphoto; p. 23: Lisa F. Young/iStockphoto; p. 24 top: iStockphoto; bottom: Boris Yankov/iStockphoto.

Chapter 2 Opener: RubberBall/SuperStock; Small images left to right: Pascal Broze/AGE Fotostock; Randy Faris/Corbis; Comstock/Jupiter Images; Alamy Images; fig. 2.2 left: Thinkstock/Jupiter Images; right: Terry Vine/Blend Images/Getty Images; p. 32: Pascal Broze/AGE Fotostock; p. 34: Ed Bock/Corbis; p. 35: Image Source; p. 36: Randy Faris/Corbis; p. 38: Photolibrary.com; p. 40: Comstock/Jupiter Images; p. 41: Alamy Images; p. 43: David H. Seymour/Shutterstock; p. 44: Losevsky Pavel/Shutterstock; p. 45: John Bell/iStockphoto; p. 46: Monte S. Buchsbaum, MD, Mt. Sinai School of Medicine, New York, NY; p. 47: Alamy Images; p. 49: George Doyle/Getty Images; p. 51: Jon Helgason/iStockphoto; p. 52: iStockphoto.

Chapter 3 Opener: Jupiter Images; Small images left to right: Jupiter Images/Getty Images; Ryan McVay/Photodisc/Getty Images; Chuck Savage/Corbis; Alamy Images; p. 57: Sam Chrysanthou/Photolibrary.com; fig. 3.2: Sam Diephuis/zefa/Corbis; fig. 3.3: Michael Krinke/iStockphoto; p. 62: Alamy Images; p. 63 top: Jupiter Images/Getty Images; bottom: David De Lossy/Blend Images/Getty Images; p. 64: Daniel Garcia/Agence France Presse/Getty Images; p. 65: Ryan McVay/Photodisc/Getty Images; p. 66: Marili Forastieri/Getty Images; p. 67: Bridget Montgomery/AP Wide World Photos; p. 68: Ekaterina Monakhova; p. 70: Chuck Savage/Corbis; p. 72: Jamie Grill/Getty Images; p. 73: DEX IMAGE/Jupiter Images; p. 74: Alamy Images; p. 75: iStockphoto; p. 76: Creatas Images/Jupiter Images; fig. 3.4: Andy Crawford/Dorling Kindersley; fig. 3.5: John Dowland/Photolibrary .com; p. 79: iStockphoto; p. 80: Sharon Dominick/iStockphoto; p. 81 top: Gerville Hall/iStockphoto; bottom: fred goldstein/iStockphoto.

FOCUS ON Your Sleep Opener: Rubberball/Getty Images; Small images left to right: Patrick Keen/iStockphoto; Brooklyn Production/Corbis; GoGo Images/Jupiter Images; Radius Images/Jupiter Images; p. 88 top: Ryan McVay/Getty Images; bottom: Patrick Keen/iStockphoto; p. 90: Rob Melnychuk/Digital Vision/Getty Images; p. 91: Brooklyn Production/CORBIS; p. 93: GoGo Images/Jupiter Images; p. 94: Stockxpert/Jupiter Unlimited; p. 95: Mark Douet/Getty Images; p. 96: Radius Images/Jupiter Images; p. 97 top: stephanie phillips/iStockphoto; bottom: Emrah Turudu/iStockphoto.

Chapter 4 Opener: Chris Rout/Alamy; Small images left to right: D. Hurst/Alamy; Paula Bronstein/Getty Images; Bill Aron/PhotoEdit; William Thomas Cain/Getty Images; fig. 4.1: Jochen Tack/Alamy; p. 103: D. Hurst/Alamy; p. 105: iStockphoto; p. 106: AP/Wide World Photos; p. 107: Paula Bronstein/Getty Images; p. 108: Hill Creek Pictures/Getty Images; p. 111: Bill Aron/PhotoEdit; p. 112: Peter M. Fisher/Corbis; p. 114: Jochen Tack/Alamy; p. 115: William Thomas Cain/Getty Images; p. 116: Justin Sullivan/Getty Images; p. 118: Mindbodysoul/Alamy; p. 119: eddie linssen/Alamy; p. 120: Gerville Hall/iStockphoto; p. 121 top: Daniel Deitschel/iStockphoto; bottom: Eric Ferguson/iStockphoto.

Chapter 5 Opener: JGI/Jamie Grill/Getty Images; Small images left to right: Jose Luis Pelaez/Corbis; David Young-Wolff/PhotoEdit; Kevin Dodge/Masterfile; Orenstein/Photodisc/Getty Images; p. 127: Jose Luis Pelaez/Corbis;

p. 129: Masterfile; p. 130: Dave Nagel/Getty Images; p. 131: Mitja Bezensek/iStockphoto; p. 132: David Young-Wolff/PhotoEdit; p. 133: Purestock/Getty Images; p. 135: Purestock/Jupiter Images; p. 136: Ryan McVay/Photodisc/Getty Images; p. 137: Bruce Ayres/Stone/Getty Images; p. 138: Marina Krasnorutskaya/Shutterstock; p. 139: Rick Gomez/Masterfile; p. 142: Kevin Dodge/Masterfile; p. 143: Scott Wintrow/Getty Images; p. 150: Allison Michael Orenstein/Photodisc/Getty Images; p. 151: Sieto Verver/iStockphoto; p. 153: BananaStock/Jupiter Images; p. 154: Yanik Chauvin/iStockphoto.

Chapter 6 Opener: Gary John Norman/Getty Images; Small images left to right: Adam Hart-Davis/Photo Researchers; Michael Newman/PhotoEdit; AFP PHOTO/Brendan Smialowski/Newscom; Leland Bobbe/Stone/Getty Images; p. 161: Corbis; fig. 6.2: Dorling Kindersley; fig. 6.3: Jules Selmes and Debi Treloar/Dorling Kindersley; fig. 6.4a: Reproduced with permission from FemCap Inc. and Alfred Shihata, MD; fig. 6.4b: Allendale Pharmaceuticals, Inc.; p. 166: Adam Hart-Davis/Photo Researchers; p. 167 top: NuvaRing Inc., Organon USA, Inc.; bottom: www.orthoevra.com; p. 168: Duramed Pharmaceuticals, Inc., a subsidiary of Barr Pharmaceuticals, Inc.; p. 169: Michael Newman/PhotoEdit; p. 174: Newscom; p. 178: Leland Bobbe/Stone/Getty Images; fig. 6.12: Lisa Spindler Photography, Inc./Getty Images; fig. 6.13a: Claude Edelman/Photo Researchers; fig. 6.13b–c: Petit Format/Nestle/Photo Researchers; p. 186: Donna Coleman/iStockphoto; p. 187 left: Christoph Achenbach/iStockphoto; right: Marc Dietrich/iStockphoto.

Chapter 7 Opener: Falko Updarp/Corbis; Small images left to right: Alamy; Arnd Wiegmann/Reuters/Corbis; Luc Beziat/Getty Images; Kristy-Anne Glubish/Jupiter Images; p. 192: Dove Shore/Contributor/Getty Images; p. 193: Alamy; p. 194: Denis Pepin/iStockphoto; p. 195: Antonio Mo/Getty Images; fig. 7.1: Image Source/Getty Images; p. 197: Craig Wactor/Shutterstock; p. 198: Lori Sparkla/Shutterstock; p. 199: Arnd Wiegmann/Reuters/Corbis; p. 200: Brian Chase/Shutterstock; p. 201: Colin Edwards/Photofusion Picture Library/Alamy; fig. 7.2: Image Source/Getty Images; p. 206: Charles Tatlock; p. 207: iStockphoto; p. 208: Jamie Grill/Iconica/Getty Images; p. 209: Gregor Buir/Shutterstock; p. 210: David Hoffman/Alamy Images; p. 212 top: Luc Beziat/Getty Images; bottom: Bob Cheung/Shutterstock; p. 213: Martyn Vickery/Alamy Images; p. 214: Andy Hayt/Getty Images; p. 215: Kristy-Anne Glubish/Jupiter Images; p. 217: iStockphoto.

Chapter 8 Opener: Leland Bobbe/Photonica Amana America/Getty Images; Small images left to right: Getty Images; Goodshoot/Jupiter Images; Rayman/Getty Images; David Young-Wolff/PhotoEdit; p. 222: Getty Images; p. 223: Rafael Laguillo/iStockphoto; p. 224: Alamy Images; p. 227: Goodshoot/Jupiter Images; fig. 8.5: Digital Vision/Getty Images; p. 230: Benjamin Brandt/iStockphoto; fig. 8.6a: CNRI/SPL/Photo Researchers; fig. 8.6b: Martin M. Rotker/Photo Researchers; p. 232: Kenneth C. Zirkel/iStockphoto; p. 236: SuperStock; p. 239: Rayman/Getty Images; p. 240: David Young-Wolff/PhotoEdit; fig. 8.9: TPH/allOver Photography/Alamy Images; p. 242: Image courtesy of Romano & Associates, Inc./Oral Health America; fig. 8.10a: James Steveson/Photo Researchers; fig. 8.10b: James Steveson/Photo Researchers; p. 244: Tony Cenicola/The New York Times/Redux; p. 246: John Howard/Digital Vision/Getty Images; p. 247: Tek Image/SPL/Photo Researchers; p. 249 left: iStockphoto; right: Milos Luzanin/iStockphoto; p. 250: Stanislav Fadyukhin/iStockphoto.

Chapter 9 Opener: Radius Images/Getty Images; Small images left to right: Mohr Images-Stockfood Munich/Stockfood; Peter Nicholson/Stone/Getty Images; Brian Hagiwara/Jupiter Images; Reg Charity/Corbis; p. 255: Ariel Skelley/Corbis; p. 256: HO/Reuters/Corbis; fig. 9.1 top to bottom: Fotocrisis/iStockphoto; Flashon Studio/Shutterstock; Chris Bence/Shutterstock; Westmacott Photography/iStockphoto; JR Trice/Shutterstock; Stargazer/Shutterstock; Morgan Lane Photography/Shutterstock; fig. 9.2: webphotographeer/iStockphoto; p. 259: design56/Shutterstock; fig. 9.3: PLG/Pearson Science; p. 261: Brian Leatart/FoodPix/Jupiter Images; p. 262: Mohr Images-Stockfood Munich/Stockfood; p. 266: Monika Adamczyk/iStockphoto; Table 9.2 top to bottom: Brand Pictures/AGE Fotostock; Brand Pictures/AGE Fotostock; Corbis; Photodisc/Getty Images; Corbis; Corbis; Table 9.3 top to bottom: Brand Pictures/AGE Fotostock; Corbis; Corbis; Brand Pictures/AGE Fotostock; p. 269: pixhook/iStockphoto; Table 9.4 top to bottom: Brand Pictures/AGE Fotostock; Brand Pictures/AGE Fotostock; Corbis; Brand Pictures/AGE Fotostock; Corbis; Table 9.5 top to bottom: Corbis; Corbis; Corbis; Photodisc/Getty Images; p. 272: Peter Nicholson/Stone Allstock/Getty Images; p. 274: Barbara Ayrapetyan/Shutterstock; p. 278: Brian Hagiwara/Jupiter Images; p. 279: Michael Newman/PhotoEdit; p. 280 left: Eric Gevaert/iStockphoto; right: rtyree1/iStockphoto; p. 281: MorePixels/iStockphoto; p. 283: Denise Kappa/iStockphoto; p. 284 top: Алексей Пинчу/iStockphoto; bottom: Jaimie Duplass/iStockphoto.

Chapter 10 Opener: Erik Isakson/age footstock; Small images left to right: Jim Esposito Photography LLC/Getty Images; Alex Mares-Manton/Getty Images; UPI/Brian Kersey/Newscom; Evan Vucci/AP Photo; fig. 10.2: Big Cheese Photo LLC/Alamy; p. 291: Richard B. Levine/Newscom; p. 292: Jim Esposito Photography LLC/Getty Images; fig. 10.4 top to bottom: PhotoEdit; Brown/Custom Medical Stock Photo; Phototake NYC; BSIP/Phototake NYC; Life Measurement, Inc; p. 295: Alex Mares-Manton/Getty Images; p. 296: UPI/Brian Kersey/Newscom; p. 297: Anton J. Geisser/age footstock; p. 298 all: Brand X Pictures/Getty Images; p. 299 top: Jose Luis Pelaez, Inc./Getty Images; bottom: Brand X Pictures/Jupiter Unlimited; p. 300: Polka Dot/Getty Images; p. 302: Evan Vucci/AP Photo; fig. 10.6 left: Girl Ray/Stone/Getty Images; right: Image Source Pink/Getty Images; p. 304: Aleksei Potov/Shutterstock; Table 10.2: Christopher Dodge/Shutterstock; p. 306: Kevin Winter/American Idol 2009/Getty Images for FOX; p. 308 top: Catherine Lane/iStockphoto; bottom: Sharon Dominick/iStockphoto; p. 309: Angelika Schwarz/iStockphoto; p. 310: Kristen Johansen/iStockphoto.

FOCUS ON Your Body Image Opener: Stockbyte/Getty Images; Small images left to right: CBS Photo Archive/Getty Images; Bettmann/Corbis; Travel Ink/Alamy; Simona Ghizzoni/Contrasto/Redux Pictures; Pascal Broze/Getty Images; fig. 1 left: Custom Medical Stock Photo/Alamy; right: Sakala/Shutterstock; p. 317 top (left): CBS Photo Archive/Getty Images; (top right): Bettmann/Corbis; bottom: Travel Ink/Alamy; p. 318: Jupiter Images; fig. 2 left: Brand X Pictures/Jupiter Unlimited; right: gollykim/iStockphoto; fig. 3: Chistopher LaMarca/Redux Pictures; p. 320: Simona Ghizzoni/Contrasto/Redux Pictures; fig. 4: moodboard/Corbis; p. 322: Pascal Broze/Getty Images; p. 323: Lucas Allen White/Shutterstock; fig. 5: Erik Soh/Creatas/Jupiter Images; p. 324: Gustavo Andrade/iStockphoto.

Chapter 11 Opener: Stockbyte/Getty Images; Small images left to right: Blend Images/Getty Images; Goodshoot/Jupiter Images; David Sacks/Getty Images; Dennis Welsh/AGE Fotostock; p. 327: Neo Vision/Getty Images; fig. 11.1 left to right: Teo Lannie/PhotoAlto/Getty Images; Elena Dorfman; Photodisc/Getty Images; SuperStock; JLP/Jose Luis Pelaez/zefa/Corbis; fig. 11.2: Pete Saloutos/zefa/Corbis; p. 330: George Doyle/Stockbyte/Getty Images; p. 331: Blend Images/Getty Images; fig. 11.3 left to right: Dan Dalton/Digital Vision/Getty Images; MIXA/Getty Images; Image Source Pink/Getty Images; Table 11.1 left to right: Elena Dorfman; Elena Dorfman; Creative Digital Visions/HOGGAN Health Industries, Inc., http://www .hogganhealth.com; p. 335: Masterfile; p. 336: Goodshoot/Jupiter Images; p. 337: Najlah Feanny/Corbis; p. 339: David Sacks/Getty Images; p. 340: Getty Images; Table 11.3 top left to right: r Cruz/Dallas Morning News/MCT/Newscom; Craig Veltri/iStockphoto; Paul Maguire/iStockphoto; Tatuasha/Shutterstock; Melvin Levine/Time & Life Pictures/Getty Images; Graca Victoria/Shutterstock; bottom left to right: K.J. Pargeter Images/iStockphoto; enderbirer/iStockphoto; Bob Jacobson/Corbis; Ali Ender Birer/Shutterstock; Dandanian/iStockphoto; p. 344: Masterfile; p. 345: Thomas Northcut/Getty Images; p. 346: Dennis Welsh/AGE Fotostock; p. 347 top: Aleksandr Lobanov/iStockphoto; bottom left: Jac Mat/Jac Mat Communication Marketing; bottom right: Elena Dorfman.

Chapter 12 Opener: Purestock/Getty Images; Small images left to right: John Shearer/WireImage/Getty Images; Thinkstock/Jupiter Images; Philippe Psaila/SPL/Photo Researchers; James Doberman/Getty Images; p. 354: John Shearer/WireImage/Getty Images; p. 361: Ariusz Nawrocki/iStockphoto; p. 362: Petros Tsonis/iStockphoto; p. 363: Thinkstock/Jupiter Images; p. 364: Stefan Ataman/iStockphoto; p. 367 top: Philippe Psaila/SPL/Photo Researchers; bottom: Alamy; p. 369: Gordo25/iStockphoto; p. 372: Garo.Photo Researchers; p. 374: James Doberman/Getty Images; fig. 12.7a: James Stevenson/SPL/Photo Researchers; fig. 12.7b: Dr. P. Marazzi/SPL/Photo Researchers; fig. 12.7c: Dr. P. Marazzi/SPL/Photo Researchers; p. 376: Mikhail Pogosov/Shutterstock; p. 377: Joel Saget/AFP/Corbis; p. 380 top: Mark Stay/iStockphoto; bottom: Max Delson Martins Santos/iStockphoto; p. 381: Wojciech Krusinski/iStockphoto; p. 382: Denise Bush/iStockphoto.

FOCUS ON Your Risk for Diabetes Opener: Radius Images/Alamy; Small images left to right: John Giustina/Getty Images; Terry Vine/Blend Images/Corbis; Stockxpert/Jupiter Unlimited; Jerilee Bennet/Colorado Springs Gazette/Newscom; fig. 2: Richard Schultz/Taxi/Getty Images; p. 389: John Shearer/WireImage/Getty Images; p. 390 top: Elfina Photo Art/iStockphoto; bottom: John Giustina/Getty Images; p. 391: Terry Vine/Blend Images/

Corbis; fig. 3a: Medicimage/Phototake; fig. 3b: ISM/Phototake; p. 393: Stockxpert/Jupiter Unlimited; p. 394: Jerilee Bennet/Colorado Springs Gazette/Newscom; p. 395: Andrew Gentry/Shutterstock.

Chapter 13 Opener: Somos/Veer/Getty Images; Small images left to right: Yellow Dog Productions/Getty Images; Steve Mercer/Image Bank/Getty Images; Gideon Mendel/Corbis; Medical Stock Photo/Alamy; p. 399: John Howard/Getty Images; p. 402: Yellow Dog Productions/Getty Images; fig. 13.4a: Gary Gaugler/Photo Researchers; fig. 13.4b: Dr. Linda Stannard, UCT/Photo Researchers; fig. 13.4c: Steve Gschmeissner/Photo Researchers; fig. 13.4d: Eye of Science/Photo Researchers; fig. 13.4e: Dennis Kunkel/Phototake NYC; p. 406: Michael Krinke/iStockphoto; p. 408: Dai Kurokawa/epa/Corbis; p. 411: Steve Mercer/Image Bank/Getty Images; fig. 13.6: Centers for Disease Control and Prevention; p. 414: Jupiter Images/Getty Images; fig. 13.7: SPL/Photo Researchers; fig. 13.8a: National Archives and Records Administration; fig. 13.8b: ISM/Phototake NYC; fig. 13.9 left: Dr. P. Marazzi/Science Photo Library/Photo Researchers; right: Centers for Disease Control and Prevention (CDC); fig. 13.10: Eye of Science/Photo Researchers; p. 418: John Amis/Associated Press; p. 419: Gideon Mendel/Corbis; p. 422: Stonehill/zefa/Corbis; p. 424: Custom Medical Stock Photo/Alamy; p. 425: Elena Dorfman; p. 427 top: Tomaz Levstek/iStockphoto; bottom: iStockphoto; p. 428 top: Simon Valentine/iStockphoto; bottom: Brandon Brown/iStockphoto.

Chapter 14 Opener: Jim Naughten/Taxi/Getty Images; Small images left to right: Avik Gilboa/WireImage/Getty Images; Thinkstock/Getty Images; DreamPictures/Blend Images/Corbis; Bodenham, LTH NHS Trust/Photo Researchers; p. 433 top: Ronnie Kaufman/Blend Images/Getty Images; bottom: Avik Gilboa/WireImage/Getty Images; p. 435: Markos Dolopikos/Alamy Images; p. 436: Klaus Guldbrandsen/Photo Researchers; fig. 14.2: Moodboard/Corbis; p. 438: Ariel Skelley/Corbis; p. 439: Karen Massler/iStockphoto; p. 440: Dan Bosler/Getty Images; p. 441 top: John Henley/Corbis; bottom: Thinkstock/Getty Images; p. 444: DreamPictures/Blend Images/Corbis; p. 447: Bodenham, LTH NHS Trust/Photo Researchers; p. 448: Apex News and Pictures Agency/Alamy; p. 450: Daniel Cardiff/iStockphoto.

Chapter 15 Opener: Alix Minde/Getty Images; Small images left to right: Lonely Planet Images; William Thomas Cain/Getty Images; Real World People/Alamy; Livio Sinibaldi/Photodisc/Getty Images; p. 455: Lonely Planet Images; p. 458: William Thomas Cain/Getty Images; p. 460: Real World People/Alamy; p. 463: Livio Sinibaldi/Photodisc/Getty Images; p. 464: Ari Joseph/Middlebury College; p. 466: Image Source/Corbis; p. 468: Lawrence Lawry/Getty Images; p. 470: christopher conrad/iStockphoto; p. 471 top: stiv kahlina/iStockphoto; bottom left: iStockphoto; bottom right: Brand X Pictures/Jupiter Images.

FOCUS ON Your Spiritual Health Opener: Stephen Shepherd/Alamy; Small images left to right: Jim West/Alamy; Jochem D Wijnands/Getty Images; K-King Media Co. Ltd/Getty Images; DAJ/Getty Images; p. 475: Jim West/Alamy; p. 476: Jochem D Wijnands/Getty Images; p. 478: K-King Media Co. Ltd./Getty Images; p. 479: Blend Images/Alamy; fig. 2: mvp64/iStockphoto; p. 480: Slobo Mitic/iStockphoto; p. 481 top: PhotoAlto/Alamy; bottom: DAJ/Getty Images; p. 482: Blend Images/Alamy; p. 483: Nancy Sheehan Photography; p. 484 top: Alex Slobodkin/iStockphoto; bottom: Aldo Ottaviani/iStockphoto.

Chapter 16 Opener: Darren Kemper/Corbis; Small images left to right: SuperStock; BURGER/PHANIE/Photo Researchers; Bruce Laurance/Getty Images; Jochen Tack/Alamy Images; p. 487: Peter Scholey/Photographer's Choice/Getty Images; p. 489 top: SuperStock; bottom: Steve Snowden/Shutterstock; p. 490: Tatiana Popova/Shutterstock; p. 493: BURGER/PHANIE/Photo Researchers; p. 494: Bruce Laurance/Getty Images; p. 495: Spencer Grant/PhotoEdit; p. 496: Jochen Tack/Alamy Images; p. 497: Comstock Images/Jupiter Unlimited; p. 499: Viviane Moos/Corbis; p. 500: iStockphoto.

Chapter 17 Opener: Barry Austin/Getty Images; Small images left to right: Luca Tettoni/Corbis; Novastock/Stock Connection; Willie Hill, Jr./The Image Works; Michael Newman/PhotoEdit; p. 506: Luca Tettoni/Corbis; p. 508: Novastock/Stock Connection; p. 509: Bananastock/Jupiter Images; p. 510: Willie Hill, Jr./The Image Works; p. 511 left: Photo Researchers; right: Michael Newman/PhotoEdit; p. 512: Vakhrushev Pavlo/Shutterstock; Table 17.1 top to bottom: Elena Elisseeva/Shutterstock; WILDLIFE GmbH/Alamy; Shapiso/Shutterstock; Joanna Wnuk/Shutterstock; WEKWEK/iStockphoto; eAlisa/Shutterstock; bildagentur-online.com/th foto/Alamy; Richard Griffin/Shutterstock; WILDLIFE GmbH/Alamy; p. 515 left: Paul Kline/iStockphoto; right: U.S. Pharmacopeia; p. 517 left: Paul Merrett/iStockphoto; right: Ivan Ivanov/iStockphoto; p. 518 top: jo unruh/iStockphoto; bottom: Mark Fairey/iStockphoto.

Index

Page references followed by *fig* indicate an illustrated figure; by *t* a table; and by *p* a photograph.

A

ABCD rule for melanomas, 374, 374*fig*
Abortion
  debate over, 173–174, 174*p*
  defined, 173
  emotional aspects of, 174
  medical, 175
  mortality rates for women, 175
  rates by weeks pregnant, 174*fig*
  surgical, 174–175, 175*fig*
  worldwide contraceptive use and abortion, 176
Abortion pill (Mifepristone), 175
Abstinence, method of contraception, 170
Academic performance, impediments to, 3*fig*
Academic pressures, 64
ACAOM. *See* Accreditation Commission for Acupuncture and Oriental Medicine
Acceptance, dying and, 443*fig*, 444
Access, to health care, 498–499
Accident-avoidance techniques, 118
Accountability in relationships, 127
Accreditation Commission for Acupuncture and Oriental Medicine (ACAOM), 505
Acetaldehyde, 227
Acetate, 227
Acid (LSD), 211
Acquaintance/date rape, 110, 111*p*
  drugs and, 153
Acquired immunodeficiency syndrome (AIDS), 418–421
  See also HIV/AIDS
ACSM. *See* American College of Sports Medicine
ACTH. *See* Adrenocorticotropic hormone
Action, 17
Active euthanasia, 447
Activities of daily living (ADLs), 5
Activity reinforcers, 18
Acupressure, 510
Acupuncture, 510, 510*p*
Acute stress response, 59*fig*
Adaptive response, 58
Adaptive thermogenesis, 296
Addiction
  compulsive spending, 194, 194*p*
  defined, 192
  effects on family and friends, 195
  to exercise, 194
  to gambling, 193–194
  signs of, 192
  to technology, 194–195, 195*p*
  to tobacco, 239–240

  See also Alcohol abuse/alcoholism; Drug abuse; Drugs
Addiction treatments, 214–216, 215*p*
  for alcoholism, 235–237, 236*p*
  for cocaine, 203
  for college students, 216
  for heroin, 210
  recovery programs, 215
  relapse, 236–237
  for smoking/tobacco use, 245, 247*p*, 247–248
Adenosine, 93
Adequate Intake, 272
ADHD. *See* Attention deficit/hyperactivity disorder
ADLs. *See* Activities of daily living
Administration, of drugs, 196–197, 197*p*
Adolescents, drug use by, 196
Adoption, 186
Adoration, 482
Adrenal hormones, 61
Adrenaline, 60
Adrenocorticotropic hormone (ACTH), 60
Adult attention deficit/hyperactivity disorder (ADHD), 38
Adult-onset diabetes (type 2), 262, 388*fig*, 389–390
  See also Diabetes mellitus
Advance directives, 446–447, 447*p*
Advertising, tobacco use and, 237
Aerobic capacity, 331
Aerobic exercise, 329–333
  benefits of, 329–331, 329*fig*
  duration, 333, 333*fig*
  frequency, 331, 332*fig*
  intensity, 331–333, 332*fig*, 333*fig*
  See also Cardiorespiratory fitness; Exercise; Physical fitness programs
Affirmation, 126
African Americans
  alcoholism, 235
  asthma, 424
  college drinking, 223
  diabetes, 391
  obesity, 289
  smoking, 237*t*
  stress and, 65
  See also Race/ethnicity differences
Agatson, Arthur, *South Beach Diet, The*, 305*t*
Aggravated rape, 110
Aggression
  primary, 102
  reactive, 102
  See also Anger
Aging
  alcohol and drug use and abuse, 440–441
  cardiovascular disease and, 363
  defined, 433

  developing and maintaining healthy relationships, 441
  diet and nutrition, 442
  ethical and moral considerations, 435
  exercise and, 441–442, 442*t*
  health care costs and, 434
  housing and living arrangements and, 434–435, 435*p*
  infectious diseases and, 398
  mental changes during, 439–440, 440*p*
  osteoporosis, 438, 438*p*
  physical changes during, 435–439, 437*fig*, 438*p*, 439*p*
  sexual changes, 439
  spiritual health, 441
  successful, 433
  theories of, 435
  websites for, 452
  See also Older adults
Agreeableness, 34
AIDS. *See* HIV/AIDS
Air pollution
  air quality index (AQI), 459, 459*fig*
  carbon dioxide, 458
  carbon monoxide, 458
  cleanest and dirtiest U.S. cities, 457*t*
  defined, 456
  ground-level ozone, 458
  hydrocarbons, 458–459
  nitrogen dioxide, 458
  ozone layer depletion, 461
  particulates, 457–458
  reducing, 462–463
  sulfur dioxide, 456–457
  See also Global warming; Indoor air pollution
Air quality index (AQI), 459, 459*fig*
Alarm phase, of general adaptation syndrome, 58–60, 58*fig*
Alcohol
  beverages and alcohol equivalents, 226*fig*
  college students and, 222–225, 222*p*, 224*p*, 224*fig*, 225*fig*
  consumption trends, 225
  diabetes and, 393
  gender differences and, 4, 227–228
  injuries and, 229
  sexual decision-making and, 229–230
  sleep and, 93
  standard drink defined, 226
  women and, 230
Alcohol abuse/alcoholism
  aging and, 440–441
  alcohol abuse defined, 233
  alcoholism (alcohol dependency) defined, 233
  binge drinking, 222–225, 222*p*, 225*fig*

  biological and family factors, 233–234
  costs to society, 234
  cutting down on drinking, 234
  identifying a problem drinker, 233
  pregnancy and, 178
  prescription drug abuse and, 233
  race/ethnicity differences, 235
  rape and, 110–111
  recovery and treatments, 235–237, 236*p*
  relapse, 236–237
  sex and, 153, 229–230
  social and cultural factors, 234
  violence and, 102–103
  websites for, 252
  women and, 234–235
  See also Addiction treatments; Drug abuse; Substance abuse
Alcohol dehydrogenase, 227
Alcohol effects
  absorption and metabolism, 226–227, 227*p*
  blood alcohol concentration (BAC), 227–228, 228*fig*, 232
  on the body and health, 229*fig*
  chemistry and potency of alcohol, 226
  driving and, 232–233, 232*fig*, 232*p*
  immediate and short-term effects, 228–230, 229*fig*
  long-term effects, 229*fig*, 230–231
  pregnancy and, 231–232
  standard drink equivalents, 226*fig*
  women and, 230
Alcohol poisoning, 230
Alcohol-related neurodevelopmental disorder (ARND), 232
Alcoholic hepatitis, 231
Alcoholics Anonymous (AA), 215, 236
Alcoholism. *See* Alcohol abuse/alcoholism
Allergens, 402, 425
Allergies, 402–403
Allergy shots, 403
Allopathic medicine (traditional Western medical practice), 491, 504
Allostatic load, 60
Alternative insemination, 186
Altruism, 483
Alveoli, 423
Alzheimer's disease, 440
  smoking and, 244
AMA. *See* American Medical Association
American Automobile Association (AAA), accident-avoidance techniques, 118

in college students, 40
gender differences and, 4
in men, 41–42
in older adults, 42
pharmacological treatment for, 42, 44, 43t
professional treatment for, 48–49, 50t
psychotherapeutic treatment for, 42
sleep disorders and, 95
stress and, 63p
symptoms of, 39
types of, 39
in women, 40–41
Desensitization, to violence, 103
Desertification, 12
Detoxification, 215, 236
Developed countries, population growth, 454fig
Developing countries, population growth, 454fig
Dextromethorphan (DXM), 198, 204t
Diabetes mellitus
amputations and, 391, 392fig
assessing yourself, 395
blood tests for diagnosis and monitoring, 392, 392fig
complications of, 393, 394fig
defined, 387
diet and, 261
exercise and, 330, 393–394
gestational, 390, 390p
glucose in healthy people, 387–388, 388fig
insulin injections, 394
lifestyle and, 392–394
metabolic syndrome (MetS), 391
percentage of adults with, 387fig
pre-diabetes leading to type 2 diabetes, 390
prevention, 394
stress and, 62
symptoms of, 391
treatment for, 392–394
type 1, 388fig, 388–389, 389p
type 2, 262, 388fig, 389–390
Diabetic ketoacidosis, 391
Diagnosis related groups (DRGs), 495
Diagnostic and Statistical Manual of Mental Disorders (DSM-IV-TR), 37, 45, 46
Diapers, 184
Diaphragmatic breathing, 77, 77fig
Diaphragms, 160t, 163–164, 163fig
Diastolic pressure, 362, 363t
Diet
diabetes and, 393, 393p
older adults and, 442
Diet aids, 306, 491t
Diet books, 305t
Diet pills, abuse of, 199
Dietary fiber, 262
Dietary Reference Intakes (DRIs), 272
Diets
starvation, 304
yo-yo dieting, 296
See also Weight management
Digestive problems, stress and, 61–62
Digestive process, 258fig
Digitalis, 358
Dilation and evacuation (D&E), 175

Dioxins, 465
Dipping, 240
Disabilities, health disparities and, 9
Disaccharides, 261
Discretionary calories, 276
Discrimination, defined, 104
Diseases/disorders
cancer, 365–379
cardiovascular disease (CVD), 353–365
chronic fatigue syndrome, 425–426
chronic lung diseases, 422–424
diabetes, 386–396
emerging and resurgent diseases, 410–411
headaches, 424–425
HIV/AIDS, 418–422
infectious diseases, 398–411
low back pain, 425–426
mental illnesses, 37–50
noninfectious diseases, 422–426
repetitive motion disorders, 426
sexually transmitted infections (STIs), 411–418
See also headings under specific diseases/disorders; Pathogens
Disenfranchised grief, 444–445
Disordered eating, 318
Disparities, in health, 8, 9
See also Health in a Diverse World
Distillation, 226
Distress, 58
Diuretics, 358
Divine, 480
Divorce, 133, 140–141
DMD. *See* Doctor of medical dentistry
DNA. *See* Deoxyribonucleic acid
Doctor of dental surgery (DDS), 492
Doctor of medical dentistry (DMD), 492
Doctor shopping, 199
Domestic terrorism, 106
Domestic violence, 106–109
causes of, 107
child abuse and neglect, 107–108, 108fig
cycle of violence, 107
defined, 106
elder abuse, 109
homicide, 106
intimate partner violence against men, 108
intimate partner violence against women, 107, 107p
recycled cell phones and, 109
statistics, 106
Donner, Alice, *Be Happy without Being Perfect*, 72
Dopamine, 196
Down syndrome, 179
Downshifting, 75
Dr. Atkins' New Diet Revolution (Atkins), 305t
DRGs. *See* Diagnosis related groups
DRIs. *See* Dietary Reference Intakes
Driving, drinking and, 232–233, 232fig, 232p
Drug abuse
abuse defined, 195–196
addressing, 216
aging and, 441

assessing use/abuse, 217
costs of, 196, 216
gender differences and, 4
misuse defined, 195
of over-the-counter (OTC) drugs, 198–199, 198p
prescription, 199–200
treatment and recovery for, 214–216, 215p
types of drugs of abuse and effects, 204t–205t
websites for, 219
women and, 201
See also Addiction; Alcohol abuse/alcoholism; Drugs
Drug-Induced Rape Prevention and Punishment Act (1996), 153
Drugs
administration routes, 196–197
amphetamines, 203–206, 206p
anabolic steroids, 213–214, 214p
antianxiety, 43t, 95t, 490
antidepressants, 42, 44, 43t, 96, 490
antipsychotics, 43t
for attention deficit/hyperactivity disorder (ADHD), 204–205, 205fig
benzodiazepines and barbiturates, 210–211
the brain and, 196, 197fig
caffeine, 206–207, 207fig
for cardiovascular disease, 358
categories of, 196
club drugs, 211–212, 212p
cocaine, 203
depressants, 209–211
drug interactions, 197–198
fertility, 185–186
hallucinogens, 211–213, 212p, 213p
hormonal birth control, 160t, 165–168, 165fig, 166fig, 166p, 167p
illicit, 200–203, 201p, 202t, 202fig
inhalants, 213
injecting and HIV/AIDS, 419
marijuana/cannabinoids, 207–209, 207p, 208p
misuse defined, 195
mood stabilizers, 43t
opioids, 209–210, 209p
performance-enhancing, 336, 337, 337p
polydrug use, 197
sex and, 153
for smoking cessation, 247–248, 247p
stimulants, 43t, 203
teratogenic (birth defect-causing) effects of, 178–179
for treating mental illness, 42, 44, 43t
for tuberculosis, 405
uses and effects, 204t–205t
for weight loss, 306
See also Drug abuse; Herbal remedies; Medications; Nonherbal remedies; Over-the-counter drugs; Prescription drugs
DSM-IV-TR. See Diagnostic and Statistical Manual of Mental Disorders
DTs. *See* Delirium tremens
du Toit, Natalie, 6p

Dual-energy X-ray absorptiometry, 294fig
Dubos, René, 3–4
Durable power of attorney for health care, 446
Duration, of exercise, 332fig, 333, 333fig
DXM. *See* Dextromethorphan
Dying
defined, 443
final arrangements, 447–449
Kübler-Ross stages of, 443–444, 443fig
right to, 446–447, 447p
websites for, 452
Dysfunctional families, 33
Dysmenorrhea (menstrual cramps), 147
Dysphoria, 211
Dyspnea, 423
Dysthymic disorder, 39

E

Eastwood, Clint, 315, 317p
Eat More, Weigh Less (Ornish), 305t
Eating, sleep and, 93
Eating disorders
anorexia nervosa, 320–321, 320fig, 320p
binge-eating, 322
bulimia nervosa, 321, 321fig
continuum of, 319fig
defined, 318
eating disorders not otherwise specified (EDNOS), 322
helping persons with, 322
risk population, 319–320
treating, 322
See also Body image
Eating disorders not otherwise specified (EDNOS), 322
Eating habits, 302–304
ECG. *See* Electrocardiogram
Echinacea, 513t
Eclampsia, 183–184
Ecological footprint, 455
Economic factors, obesity, 299
Ecosystem, 454
Ecstasy, 211–212
Ectopic pregnancy, 184, 414
Edamame, 269, 269p
EDNOS. *See* Eating disorders not otherwise specified
Ejaculation, 148
Elder abuse, 109
Electrocardiogram (ECG), 364
Electrodessication, 374
ELISA (enzyme-linked immunosorbent assay), 420
Embryo, 180fig, 181, 182fig
Emergency contraception, 160t, 169–170, 169p
Emerging and resurgent diseases, 410–411
Emmons, Robert, 477
Emotional abuse, 113
Emotional health, defined, 5, 31
See also Mental illnesses; Psychosocial health
Emotional responses, managing, 70–71
Emotional stability, 34
Emotions, defined, 31
Empathy, 481
Emphysema, 243, 423
EMR. *See* Exercise metabolic rate